Smith's **BLOOD DISEASES OF INFANCY AND CHILDHOOD**

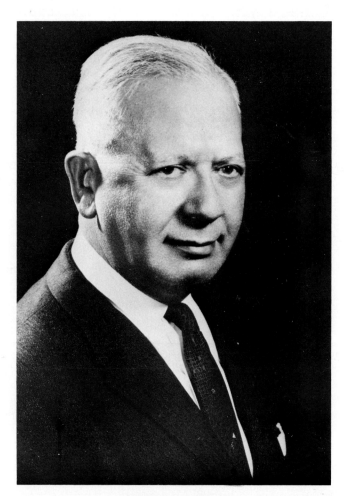

CARL H. SMITH

Smith's
BLOOD DISEASES OF INFANCY AND CHILDHOOD

Editors

DENIS R. MILLER, M.D.

Professor of Pediatrics, Cornell University Medical College;
Chairman, Department of Pediatrics, Memorial Sloan-Kettering Cancer Center;
Attending Pediatrician, New York Hospital–Cornell Medical Center,
New York, New York

HOWARD A. PEARSON, M.D.

Professor and Chairman, Department of Pediatrics,
Yale University School of Medicine; Chief, Pediatric Service, Yale–New Haven Hospital,
New Haven, Connecticut

Associate editors

ROBERT L. BAEHNER, M.D.

Hugh McK. Landon Professor of Pediatrics and Clinical Pathology,
Indiana University School of Medicine; Director, Pediatric
Hematology-Oncology, James Whitcomb Riley Hospital
for Children, Indiana University Medical Center,
Indianapolis, Indiana

CAMPBELL W. McMILLAN, M.D.

Professor of Pediatrics, University of North Carolina at Chapel
Hill School of Medicine; Head, Pediatric Hematology-Oncology Division,
and Attending Pediatrician, North Carolina Memorial Hospital,
Chapel Hill, North Carolina

FOURTH EDITION
with 336 illustrations
including four color plates

The C. V. Mosby Company
Saint Louis   1978

FOURTH EDITION

Copyright © 1978 by The C. V. Mosby Company

All rights reserved. No part of this book may be reproduced in
any manner without written permission of the publisher.

Previous editions copyrighted 1960, 1966, 1972

Printed in the United States of America

The C. V. Mosby Company
11830 Westline Industrial Drive, St. Louis, Missouri 63141

Library of Congress Cataloging in Publication Data

Smith, Carl H.
    Smith's Blood diseases of infancy and child-
hood.

    First-3d ed. published under title: Blood
diseases of infancy and childhood.
    Includes bibliographies and index.
    1. Pediatric hematology.   I.   Miller, Denis R.
II. Pearson, Howard A.   III. Title.   IV. Title:
Blood diseases of infancy and childhood.   [DNLM:
1. Hematologic diseases—In infancy and childhood.
WS300 S644b]
RJ411.S6   1978   618.9′21′5   78-7023
ISBN 0-8016-4691-X

GW/CB/B   9 8 7 6 5 4 3 2 1

Contributors

ROBERT L. BAEHNER, M.D.

Hugh McK. Landon Professor of Pediatrics and Clinical Pathology, Indiana University School of Medicine; Director, Pediatric Hematology-Oncology, James Whitcomb Riley Hospital for Children, Indiana University Medical Center, Indianapolis, Indiana

D. H. BUCHHOLZ, M.D.

Assistant Professor of Laboratory Medicine, Yale University School of Medicine, New Haven, Connecticut

HENRY CHANG, M.D.

Assistant Professor of Pediatrics, Cornell University Medical College; Assistant Attending Pediatrician, Division of Pediatric Hematology-Oncology, New York Hospital–Cornell Medical Center, New York, New York

MARGARET W. HILGARTNER, M.D.

Professor of Pediatrics, Cornell University Medical College; Attending Pediatrician, New York Hospital–Cornell Medical Center; Associate Attending Pediatrician, Hospital for Special Surgery, New York, New York

MARTIN R. KLEMPERER, M.D.

Professor of Pediatrics and of Medicine, University of Rochester School of Medicine; Pediatrician and Physician, Strong Memorial Hospital, Rochester, New York

PHILIP LANZKOWSKY, M.D., F.R.C.P. (Edinburgh), D.C.H. (London)

Professor of Pediatrics, School of Medicine, Health Sciences Center, State University of New York at Stony Brook, New York; Chairman of Pediatrics and Chief of Pediatric Hematology-Oncology, Long Island Jewish–Hillside Medical Center, New Hyde Park, New York

SUE McINTOSH, M.D.

Associate Professor of Pediatrics, Yale University School of Medicine; Attending Pediatrician, Yale–New Haven Hospital, New Haven, Connecticut

CAMPBELL W. McMILLAN, M.D.

Professor of Pediatrics, University of North Carolina at Chapel Hill School of Medicine; Head, Pediatric Hematology-Oncology Division, and Attending Pediatrician, North Carolina Memorial Hospital, Chapel Hill, North Carolina

DENIS R. MILLER, M.D.

Professor of Pediatrics, Cornell University Medical College; Chairman, Department of Pediatrics, Memorial Sloan-Kettering Cancer Center; Attending Pediatrician, New York Hospital–Cornell Medical Center, New York, New York

RICHARD T. O'BRIEN, M.D.

Associate Professor of Pediatrics, University of Utah College of Medicine; Attending Hematologist, Primary Children's Medical Center, Salt Lake City, Utah

RICHARD J. O'REILLY, M.D.

Assistant Professor of Pediatrics, Cornell University Medical College; Director, Bone Marrow Transplantation Program, and Assistant Attending Pediatrician, Memorial Sloan-Kettering Cancer Center, New York, New York

HOWARD A. PEARSON, M.D.

Professor and Chairman, Department of Pediatrics, Yale University School of Medicine; Chief, Pediatric Service, Yale–New Haven Hospital, New Haven, Connecticut

MICHAEL SORELL, M.D.

Assistant Attending Pediatrician, Memorial Sloan-Kettering Cancer Center, New York, New York

RUTH N. WRIGHTSTONE, M.S.

Director, International Hemoglobin Information Center, Medical College of Georgia, Augusta, Georgia

Affectionately dedicated to our
wives and children

Foreword

The French philosopher-scientist of the nineteenth century Auguste Comte said, "To understand a science, it is necessary to know its history." Thus a historical introduction to this textbook of pediatric hematology might offer needed background for the understanding of some of its chapters. However, Ralph Waldo Emerson, another nineteenth century philosopher-essayist, stated, "There is properly no history; only biography." Since I have been involved in the care of children with blood disorders for some 50 years, in this brief biography I may be able to provide some insight into the development and complexities of pediatric hematology. If this personal viewpoint occasionally overlooks some landmarks or slights some contributors, due apologies are offered.

The specialty of pediatric hematology is relatively young. Before the 1920s there were few treatises on this subject or books devoted exclusively to it. In 1924, when the monumental eight-volume multiauthored textbook on pediatrics was published by Abt, it contained six chapters in 217 pages on diseases of the blood by William Palmer Lucas and E. Charles Fleischner and was a fairly complete dissertation on what was then known. Our own discussion of anemias in children was published in 1930 as part of Gorham and Ordway's *Diseases of the Blood,* volume 9, in the series of Oxford Monographs on Diagnosis and Treatment. In the meantime, Barr and Stransky, in 1928, had published their book in German, *Clinical Hematology of Childhood,* and there was no English translation until 1960 when the second edition came out. Therefore its value in this country was minimal.

One of the first hematologic conditions that was recognized as limited to children was a nonspecific disorder known as pseudoleukemic anemia of infancy, or more popularly as von Jaksch's anemia after its describer. It was a popular diagnosis, especially in Europe, and eventually became a large and convenient but useless wastebasket in which was placed any anemia with leukocytosis and splenomegaly in infancy and early childhood.

Most such cases were probably nutritional anemias complicated by the then-prevalent rickets and/or infections, as well as other unrecognized disorders. The eponym was used for many years to imply a nonfatal anemia somewhat resembling leukemia. As more specific diagnostic criteria for specific diseases became identified, e.g., Cooley's erythroblastic anemia or thalassemia, simple iron deficiency with or without rickets, and various hemolytic anemias, the name "von Jaksch's anemia" was abandoned. Even the memory of it has dimmed in the past 50 years.

Before many hematologic disturbances in the young were recognized, the major problem that required resolution was the definition of normal values at various ages for levels of all the blood elements and the fluctuations that required special attention and investigation. While specific blood diseases in infancy and childhood were being detected and reported, hematologic studies of large groups of normal children of all ages were being pursued and standards tabulated for healthy subjects. Only a few of the pioneers in the United States in this necessary groundwork are mentioned here briefly. Lippman in 1924 published a study of the blood cells in the newborn. Lucas and Fleischner gathered what was known regarding normal values for their chapters in Abt's *Pediatrics*. Guest and Brown undertook a horizontal and a 5-year vertical analysis of normal infants' and children's blood values and published the results in 1938. Alfred Washburn followed a group of children in Denver and developed his own set of normal values, which he published in 1934 and 1935; Philip Sturgeon did likewise and combined them with a much-needed review of the normal appearance of the bone marrow in infants and children in 1950 and 1951. Gradually, then, normal values for hematologic measurements and limits of normality were accumulated in infants and children against which abnormalities could be recognized even in their incipiency.

A deficiency that became evident in the 1930s was the absence of data on bone marrow changes in infants and children. In part this was a result of the practice of performing punctures for marrow on the sternum, as was commonly done in adults. With the thin bone and narrow cavity of the sternum in the very young, the danger of pushing into the mediastinum was a hazard that few hematologists were willing to face. In addition, many pathologists insisted that a mere marrow aspirate gave insufficient material for analysis and that a block of marrow tissue was necessary. This required an open biopsy under anesthesia, removal of a block of bone and marrow by a surgeon, and decalcification and staining by several methods, which took several days. Such a major procedure was not undertaken lightly, nor was it justifiable on normal subjects. In fact, this procedure was prohibited at some children's hospitals, as also were marrow aspirations. Not until other safer sites for marrow puncture came into common use were bone marrow aspirates part of the routine work-up of pediatric hematologic problems. A few notable exceptions to this were the early studies and publications of K. Kato (1937) and Peter Vogel (1939).

Throughout the world the anemia resulting from iron deficiency is and probably always has been the most common type in infancy and childhood. Yet its prevalence was unrecognized for many years because it was associated with so many other more striking diseases. First, there were (and unfortunately still are) starvation and malnutrition. Kwashiorkor, marasmus, and growth failure often masked the accompanying anemia. Recurrent acute or chronic infection diverted attention from the underlying or associated iron-deficiency state. And rickets, with its skeletal deformities, at one time so common in heavily populated temperate zones, usually overshadowed the regularly associated anemia from iron deficiency. Part of this may have resulted from the binding of iron in the intestinal tract by large amounts of unabsorbed phosphate. At any rate, rickets with its accompanying iron-deficiency anemia became a great rarity, even in developing countries, when vitamin D concentrates with irradiated ergosterol were introduced and particularly when they were regularly added to milk, infant formulas, and cereals.

The masking factor was also removed by the control of bacterial infection with antibiotics and chemotherapy. Although malnutrition and infection still exist in children throughout the world, even among the economically deprived in the United States, their incidence and combined effects are diminished.

One other development must be recalled in the long-time failure to recognize iron-deficiency anemia. The trial of iron therapy in anemic infants and children was often unsuccessful because the available medications were low in absorbable mineral or were unpalatable and therefore ineffective, often casting doubt on the diagnosis of iron deficiency. Saccharated iron (5% iron), reduced iron (8%), Blaud's mass (10%), and a variety of mixtures were difficult to take in sufficient quantity to be curative even after months of ingestion. In contrast, our present armamentarium of ferrous sulfate (20% iron) and other compounds, even including parenteral medication when necessary, usually effects a cure in a few weeks.

Pathologists and clinical pathologists who have dealt with youngsters also contributed to the accumulation of knowledge in this field. One of the true pioneers in pediatric hematology is Wolf W. Zuelzer. He is credited with a number of "firsts" in describing hematologic entities. He was (and still is, despite "retirement") an outstanding teacher and clinical investigator in this field; with the abundant patient population of the Children's Hospital in Detroit, he trained and stimulated an outstanding group of pediatric hematologists. One of his important contributions was the delineation of megaloblastic anemia in infancy, a common syndrome that responds specifically to folic acid therapy. Although previously there had been rare reports of juvenile pernicious anemia and equally rare instances of macrocytic anemia caused by fish tapeworm infestation and goat milk formula feeding, the typical macrocytes of folic acid deficiency were overlooked. They may have been masked by the predominance of iron-deficiency microcytosis often present in the same patient. In 1946, Zuelzer published his elegant study of twenty-five cases of megaloblastosis in infants in whom "cure" was effected by treatment with folic acid. Thereafter, few such patients were found because many prepared formulas had folic acid added by the manufacturers, and the minute amounts (<1 mg) needed for prevention and cure of this deficiency were given regularly in most cases of suspected nutritional anemia.

In 1925 Thomas Cooley of Detroit had reported a curious anemia he found in five children who had unusual "mongoloid" facies, severe peculiar anemia, enlarged spleens, and striking x-ray changes in the skull and long bones. At first he called it von Jaksch's anemia, since it seemed to fit that descriptive term for a pseudoleukemia, but he soon realized it afflicted older children; was progressively severe, congenital, and familial; and had a very abnormal blood picture, especially in the unusual number of nucleated red cells. The name was changed to erythroblastic anemia, or Cooley's anemia, and still later to thalassemia. Cooley did not realize that he had described an example of what we now classify as a hemoglobinopathy, a qualitative or quantitative abnormality of hemoglobin synthesis caused by a mutation, and of which there now have been recognized several hundred variants.

The wonder is how pediatricians and hematologists could miss such an obvious and unusual condition for so long, one that was especially prevalent in the Mediterranean littoral. One personal experience may help to explain this in part. In 1927, as a house office at the Boston Children's Hospital where I was in charge of three children with Cooley's anemia, I presented them to a visiting pediatrician from southern Europe. He agreed he had seen a number of similar cases but said that they had diagnosed it as chronic malaria and, if we continued to search the blood more diligently we would substantiate their diagnosis! Another visiting foreign dignitary favored the diagnosis of congenital syphilis. Thus, given a locale where either of these conditions was prevalent, it is possible that the less common thalassemia was overlooked. "Atypical familial hemolytic anemia" was the diagnosis an eminent hematologist made when he saw our first patient in 1925. What a missed opportunity! It illustrates an important maxim: An "atypical" form of a typical condition very likely may be a different disease and deserves study and consideration as such. A new entity may thus be discovered.

A striking neonatal condition long unexplained and misunderstood is the now completely resolved disease defined as hemolytic disease of the fetus and newborn. This, too, is an illustration of the fable of the blind men and the elephant. The most severe manifestation in this condition, fetal hydrops, was described in 1892 by Ballantyne, a British physician. In 1910 Rautman, a German pathologist, called attention to the extraordinary red cell proliferation in the fetus and termed the condition erythroblastosis. Severe jaundice of the newborn that increases rapidly in the first week and often occurs in subsequent children in a family was described by the prominent English obstetrician Sir Humphrey Rolliston in 1915 as icterus gravis familiaris. Finally, the late manifestation in surviving infants, who had not had edema or striking jaundice, was profound anemia. These were reported in 1925 simply as congenital anemia of the newborn.

These four manifestations were recognized as parts of a single underlying disease process in our report of 1932. The pathogenesis was missed by us, although B. Darrow in 1938 had hypothesized that it was a hemolytic anemia. It is now clear why we failed to detect and confirm this by the laboratory tests of cross matching the infant's and donor's blood samples, performed routinely prior to transfusion. The standard method for such testing then required suspension of the red cells in normal saline at a dilution of about 2%. The hyperimmune IgG antibodies (anti-Rh and others) did not produce agglutination in the saline medium and thus were missed.

In 1939 a new blood group was revealed through the coincidental occurrence of an inexplicable hemolytic reaction in a woman transfused with her husband's blood shortly after the birth of an infant with erythroblastosis fetalis. Philip Levine, a talented pupil of the great Landsteiner, found that the woman's serum contained a saline-active agglutinin against the donor's red cells. He realized that the maternal antibody, acting on the infant's red cell antigen, inherited from the father, was the cause of erythroblastosis fetalis, the pathogenesis of which was hemolytic disease of the fetus and newborn. Soon this was substantiated all over the country, and a new rapidly expanding field of basic and clinical research came into being. The blood group antigen, erroneously named the Rh factor by Landsteiner and Wiener, was found eventually to have a dozen variants, and other individually inherited red cell factors were soon discovered. In contrast to only three families of blood groups known before 1939 (ABO, MN, and P), eventually at least twelve have been recognized and more than 100 variants are now detectable. The use of these has proved immeasurably valuable in characterizing individuals, in forensic medicine, in anthropology, as well as in clinical problems. Through laboratory tests such as the albumin test, the Coombs test, and others developed for identification of "warm agglutinins," new antibodies and new antigens have been disclosed. Later, when leukocyte and platelet markers were found, immunology received a tremendous stimulus and became the burgeoning and exciting field for research that it is now.

From the viewpoint of the hematologist, the neonatologist, and the pediatrician, erythroblastosis fetalis, which affected between 0.5% and 1.0% of fetuses and newborns in the United States, could be recognized and appropriately treated in the majority of cases after 1946. A mortality of almost 50% for liveborn victims was reduced by exchange transfusion to less than 5%; intrauterine death, with an incidence of 20%, was diminished to less than 10%. In addition exchange transfusion for protection against dangerous hyperbilirubinemia from any cause has made kernicterus a preventable catastrophe. Finally, through the use of anti-Rh γ-globulin, Rh-negative unsensitized pregnant women now can be protected from sensitization by their Rh-positive infants. Erythroblastosis fetalis therefore must soon become a rare disease.

The Rh discovery has also made blood transfusion very much safer, and the Coombs test has become the method for diagnosing autoimmune hemolytic anemia. Other antibody tests developed thereafter play a similarly useful role in the recognition of autoimmune thrombopenia and leukopenia. If the Rh discovery seemed initially to be merely a pebble tossed into the lake of medical research, the waves it produced on distant shores have given it the mass of a huge boulder.

Leukemia was justifiably a much dreaded disease in infancy and childhood in the days before the induction of remission was possible. Most of the easily recognized cases showed high white cell counts with an abundance of immature or "blast" forms in the peripheral blood. The course was rapidly fatal. Only occasionally (in about 10% of one small series) would a spontaneous temporary remission occur. Acute intercurrent pyogenic infection seemed to precede most of these and suggest, in retrospect, an immune mechanism. However, this was not fully appreciated at the time and was not pursued by investigators. The so-called aleukemic leukemia, a confusing and contradictory term, was seen occasionally and was difficult to substantiate unless the peripheral blood showed unmistakable "blasts" or there was a terminal crisis and the development of a typical high white cell count. Biopsy of an enlarged lymph node or bone marrow confirmation of leukemia was not a common practice. By the late 1940s marrow aspiration had become established as a relatively simple and necessary routine for the differential diagnosis of leukemia and other invasive processes, as well as for aplastic anemia, neutropenia, and thrombopenia. In fact, repeated aspirations became necessary with the advent of antileukemic drug therapy. This was an epochal event!

In 1946 and 1947 after noting the acceleration of cell growth in some malignant tumors by large doses of folic acid, the late Sidney Farber, pathologist at Boston Children's Hospital conceived the idea of using a folic acid antagonist to impair such cell proliferation. The brilliant biochemist Y. Subbarow, of the Lederle Company, synthesized a number of antifolates; eventually one of them, aminopterin, was tried in children with leukemia. As reported in 1948 by Farber et al., temporary remissions were induced in ten of sixteen children with acute leukemia. Side effects of this powerful drug were rather severe and a less toxic, equally effective analogue was found in methotrexate. Thus was the antimetabolite therapy of leukemia and other malignancies initiated. It has brought a prolongation of life, greater comfort, even freedom from disease and hope of permanent cure to thousands of victims of leukemias and cancers. There are now at least a dozen different drugs that retard or control malignant cell growth. Their beneficial effects can be exploited to the maximum when used in combination or in sequence.

The contributions of Carl Smith to pediatric hematology have carved a permanent niche for him in the gallery of pioneers in this subspecialty. In addition to publishing in 1960 the first American textbook on blood diseases of infancy and childhood, which went through three editions in a dozen years and was even translated into Spanish, he also contributed more than 100 scientific papers in the 45 years of his active practice. His early studies helped to establish normal standards for leukocyte levels and differential counts in infants and children. He was not a laboratory bench worker nor a researcher on animals but, first and foremost, a clinician who observed and cared for children with hematologic disorders. To him laboratory measurements were only a necessary and important adjunct to the careful history, physical examination, and close scrutiny of the ailing patient. He recorded and reported conditions previously undetected or misdiagnosed, among which was his 1941 description of infectious lymphocytosis, a benign condition that can be confused with leukemia; he also called attention to factor IX deficiency as a cause of hemorrhagic disease of the newborn. Several of his review articles helped guide the practitioner to the correct diagnosis and treatment of the other anemias of infants and young children, especially sufferers from malnutrition. Because his location in the eastern section of New York City brought many children to his clinic with Mediterranean (Cooley's) anemia, he became particularly interested in their welfare, the course of the disease, and its treatment. He established an efficient, economic, and successful outpatient transfusion service for them. He was one of the first to point out the danger of overwhelming infection in splenectomized children and warned against eagerness to resort to this operation.

In addition to pioneering in the subspecialty of pediatric hematology, Carl Smith guided several generations of younger pediatricians to an interest in hematology. He was the patriarch of pediatric hematologists in New York. Yet, with it all, he was a modest person. He liked to consult with his peers and even to refer an occasional "puzzler" to another specialist. His patients idolized him and through their efforts a large fund was established to support research and therapy in hematologic diseases of infants and children at the New York Hospital, a fitting tribute to this dedicated pediatrician and "blood specialist." It is also a great satisfaction that his textbook has been continued and revised under the able editorship of his chosen assistant and successor, Denis Miller.

Louis K. Diamond, M.D.

Adjunct Professor of Pediatrics, University of California, San Francisco; Professor Emeritus of Pediatrics, Harvard Medical School, Boston, Massachusetts

REFERENCES

1. Blackfan, K. D., Baty, J. M., and Diamond, L. K.: In Ordway, T., and Gorham, A. W., eds.: The diagnosis and treatment of diseases of the blood, London, 1930, Oxford University Press.
2. Cooley, T. B., and Lee, P.: Trans. Am. Pediatr. Soc. **37:**29, 1925.
3. Farber, S., Diamond, L. K., Mercer, R. D., Sylvester, R. F., and Wolff, J. A.: N. Engl. J. Med. **238:**787, 1948.
4. Guest, G. M., Brown, E. W., and Wing, M.: Am. J. Dis. Child. **56:**529, 1938.
5. Kato, K.: Am. J. Dis. Child. **54:**209, 1937.
6. Lippman, H. S.: Am. J. Dis. Child. **27:**473, 1924.
7. Sturgeon, P.: Pediatrics **7:**642, 1951.
8. Vogel, P., and Bassen, F. A.: Am. J. Dis. Child. **57:** 245, 1939.
9. Washburn, A. H.: Am. J. Dis. Child. **47:**993, 1934.
10. Zuelzer, W. W., and Ogden, F. N.: Am. J. Dis. Child. **71:**211, 1946.

Preface

In his preface to the first edition of *Blood Diseases of Infancy and Childhood,* written nearly 20 years ago, Carl H. Smith's stated purpose was "to present the essentials of pediatric hematology in concise form" for the student and practitioner "against the background of normal development." The second and third editions introduced advances in pediatric hematology, revised the original text in light of newer concepts, and reviewed current knowledge in the field. The purpose of the fourth edition, separated from the third by a span of 6 years, remains essentially unchanged. Our intent was to meet the informational needs of the medical student, pediatric house staff officer, trainee in pediatric hematology-oncology, pediatrician, family physician, laboratory technologist, pathologist, and internist-hematologist who dabbles in pediatrics. The basic orientation is clinical. We hope that teachers of hematology will find this edition useful as well.

The field of pediatric hematology-oncology has grown tremendously in the two decades since Dr. Smith's first edition was published. A small fraternity 20 years ago, today the subspecialty is vital, vibrant, productive, and at the forefront of major advances in clinical pediatrics and laboratory research. The first subboard examination in pediatric hematology-oncology was given in November, 1974, and today there are over 300 certified pediatric hematologists-oncologists in the United States. Basic knowledge of hematopoiesis and coagulation are as essential to the oncologist as is a thorough understanding of the pharmacologic action of antileukemic myelosuppressive drugs for the hematologist. As in the previous editions, we discuss pediatric blood dyscrasias and hematopoietic malignancies but have excluded malignant solid tumors.

The first three editions are a monument to the vision, breadth, and scope of Carl Smith's vast fund of knowledge. It would be impossible and presumptuous today for a single individual to attempt a text of this kind. The field has grown and expanded exponentially. A single-authored text would require a superhuman effort that is beyond the intellectual and physical capabilities of most mortals. The primary reason for the delay between the publication of the third edition and the completion of the fourth was the stark realization that the day of the single-authored text had reached its zenith and had passed. With this limited multi-authored text we hope to retain the historical perspective and consistent approach of a single author and, at the same time, provide the reader with a critical and useful update of the field.

Although the basic outline of the fourth edition remains unchanged from its antecedent, most chapters have been completely rewritten, and new references, illustrations, and tables have been added. The introductory material in most chapters provides the student with basic background material on normal physiology, biochemistry, function, and metabolism. Obsolete material has been deleted, but the historically important concepts have been recognized and are included. The presentations of disease entities follow a classical format: definition, history, classification, incidence, genetics, pathogenesis, clinical features, laboratory evaluation, differential diagnosis, course and treatment, prognosis, and future perspectives. Rare disorders are given less attention and disorders that are becoming extinct because of advances in therapy (e.g., hemolytic disease of the newborn secondary to Rh incompatibility) are covered more concisely than previously. However, we recognize that some material in previous editions represents classical writing, and it is retained intact. We have not tampered with the section on infectious lymphocytosis, which was first described by Carl Smith in 1941.

Tremendous strides in molecular biology, genetics, biochemistry, and cell metabolism and function have provided the clinician with a much firmer understanding of diverse disorders that heretofore had been lumped under catchall phrases such as "nonspherocytic hemolytic anemia," "lymphoproliferative disorders," "granulocyte dysfunction syndromes," and "thrombopathies." With the use of automated electronic counting equipment, even normal values for red blood cell indices need modification. Blood component therapy and the availability of frozen-thawed red cells, platelet concentrates, granulocytes, and lyophilized clotting factors have improved the outlook for the pancytopenic child with leukemia and the hemophiliac with inhibitors. Iron-deficiency anemia still remains the most common hematologic problem in pediatrics, but we now have a much clearer understanding of iron absorption, metabolism, and excretion and the effects of iron deficiency on cellular metabolism. A number of new disorders involving vitamin B_{12} and folate metabolism have been described recently, adding to the differential diagnosis of megaloblastic anemias.

The recent application of in vitro techniques of bone marrow culture has provided us with exciting new insights relating to normal and abnormal hematopoiesis, the control mechanisms of erythropoiesis and myelopoiesis, and their inhibitors, modulators, and stimulators. Previously poorly understood disorders such as congenital hypoplastic anemia (Diamond-Blackfan syndrome), aplastic anemia, and congenital neutropenia can now be studied in detail using agar or methyl cellulose culture methods.

New inherited disorders involving the three components of the erythrocyte—the membrane, the enzymes, and the hemoglobin molecule—have been described, and the interrelationships between metabolism, structure, function, and premature destruction have been stressed. A remarkable heterogeneity is emerging, even within diseases caused by the same enzyme or protein deficiency. Ruth Wrightstone has provided the reader with a complete listing of every known hemoglobinopathy. The molecular pathology of the thalassemia syndromes is better understood now that we can use cell-free systems to quantify messenger RNA and reverse transcriptase and complimentary DNA to determine whether or not genetic material is deleted. Iron chelation therapy and revised transfusion programs designed to rid the iron-overloaded host of iron and to decrease ineffective erythropoiesis and improve growth and development offer new hope to children with thalassemia

where none existed before. Antenatal detection of hemoglobinopathies and thalassemia is now possible, but effective therapy for sickle cell disease still eludes us.

The interface of immunology and hematology is sharply defined and the collaborative efforts of the two disciplines have increased dramatically and productively during the past 5 years. Dr. Klemperer has reviewed immune mechanisms of hemolysis, and Drs. O'Reilly and Sorell have updated the exciting field of bone marrow transplantation in aplastic anemia, immunodeficiency disorders, and leukemia. This new approach is now advocated as primary treatment for the child with aplastic anemia or severe combined immunodeficiency disease (SCID) who has an HLA- and MLC-compatible donor.

Dr. Baehner has rewritten the entire section on white blood cells. Each step of normal function and metabolism has its counterpart in a granulocyte disorder, often associated with recurrent infection. Abnormalities of production, release, chemotaxis, phagocytosis, and intracellular digestion are described in detail. The chapter covering the hematologic malignancies—leukemia, lymphoma, and Hodgkin's disease—has been rewritten and new concepts relating to diagnosis, etiology, therapy, and supportive care are provided. We now realize that prognosis in childhood acute lymphocytic leukemia varies with certain "frontend" factors, such as the initial white blood cell count and age, and that other factors—lymphoblast markers, cytomorphology, and immunoglobulins—may be equally important. Future therapy will be based on prognostic groups, lessening the toxic risk to patients with a good prognosis and improving the outlook for patients with a high risk of early relapse and death.

Drs. McMillan and Hilgartner have updated the third major section, coagulation. The basic mechanisms and biochemistry of blood clotting, platelet function and metabolism, and modern therapy of plasma clotting deficiencies and platelet disorders are presented.

Controversy regarding etiology, pathogenesis, and therapy for many disorders still exists. Medical knowledge is neither absolute nor immutable. Accordingly we have concluded many sections with an overview of unresolved issues and speculations regarding future research endeavors, questions to be answered in subsequent editions.

Despite the departure from a single-authored text to one with fourteen contributors, our co-

Preface **xvii**

authors have common bonds; we are all first- or second-generation offspring of the Carl H. Smith and Louis K. Diamond era of pediatric hematology. We have been deeply influenced by their teaching, their clinical acumen, their humanity, their insatiable curiosity, and their indefatigable spirit. We owe them both a great debt of appreciation.

This edition demanded the expert editorial assistance of Herta Tishcoff, Patricia Nugent, and Florence Graziano (New York Hospital–Cornell Medical Center), Prakash Kaur and Jessie Ross (Memorial Hospital), Gretchen Umbach and Linda Oliva (Yale), Cathy Devine and Wanda Braxton (North Carolina), Marianne R. Able (Indiana), Christine Collins (Rochester), and Geri Schwartz and Rose Yannaco (Long Island Jewish Medical Center). We are also grateful to our colleagues, fellows, and students for offering many helpful and constructive suggestions, contributions, photographs, and tables. We are especially thankful to the American Society of Hematology for per-mission to use slides from their slide bank in the color plates.

Others deserve special thanks for their support and encouragement: Mrs. Carl H. Smith; Harold Weill, Chairman, and his colleagues of the Children's Blood Foundation; and Wallace W. Mc-Crory, Chairman of the Department of Pediatrics at Cornell, who tolerated two minisabbaticals on Martha's Vineyard so that the fourth edition could become a reality. The zephyrs, sun, surf, clay courts, and bucolic solitude of the Vineyard eased the burden.

Finally, particular gratitude is due those who bore the brunt of the rewriting of this edition—my wife, Johanna, and my children, Karin and Daniel. Without their patience, understanding, and encouragement none of this would have been possible.

With the completion of the fourth edition, plans for a fifth begin immediately. The enduring work of a unique physician and man will be continued by a younger but equally enthusiastic breed.

Denis R. Miller

Contents

COLOR PLATES

PART ONE GENERAL TOPICS

edited by
DENIS R. MILLER
HOWARD A. PEARSON

1 □ Origin and development of blood cells and coagulation factors

Howard A. Pearson

The extraordinarily rapid growth of the human embryo after fertilization imposes an increasing requirement for oxygen transport and delivery. It is therefore not surprising that development of vascular and hematopoietic systems begin early in embryonic life and proceed in parallel. Extant knowledge about embryonic hematopoiesis is principally derived from studies in experimental animals. However, the considerable anatomic and experimental data obtained from these species appear to correlate reasonably well with more limited human material.[3,15,27] Fig. 1-1 depicts the successive anatomic changes and stages that occur during development.[44]

HEMATOPOIESIS
Yolk-stalk (mesoblastic) hematopoiesis

Approximately 2 to 3 weeks after fertilization and implantation of the human ovum, clusters of darkly staining cells appear in the mesenchyma lateral to the primitive streak. These clusters are designated "blood islands" and represent the progenitors of both vascular and hematopoietic systems. The peripheral cells of the blood islands form the primitive endothelium of the developing vascular network. The more central cells arise from the blood vessel wall and become free in the lumen. These are hematocytoblasts. They are deeply basophilic and do not contain hemoglobin.

Primitive erythroblasts appear to arise directly from hematocytoblasts. The red cells of this first generation have a characteristic morphology. They are very large and their nuclei have a coarse, clumped chromatin pattern. This led Ehrlich to compare these embryonic cells with the megaloblasts found in patients with pernicious anemia.[45] Hemoglobin can be demonstrated by benzidine staining in the cytoplasm of these early nucleated cells, and it is likely that the protohemoglobins are the embryonic varieties Hb Gower 1 and 2 and Hb Portland. Infrequent megakaryocytes and granular leukocytes may be seen, even in this earliest stage of yolk stalk hematopoiesis.

By approximately 8 weeks of gestational life the blood islands begin to regress. Intravascular hematopoiesis, accounting for the fact that almost all of the blood cells are nucleated, begins to wane. The large nucleated "megaloblasts," which represent the first generation of erythropoietic cells, disappear from the circulation by 12 to 15 weeks.

Visceral hematopoiesis

At approximately 9 weeks of gestational age hematopoiesis is well established in the liver. Nests of hematopoietic cells appear in the liver sinusoids and rapidly enlarge. Hematopoiesis becomes an extravascular phenomenon. There are distinct morphologic differences between the red

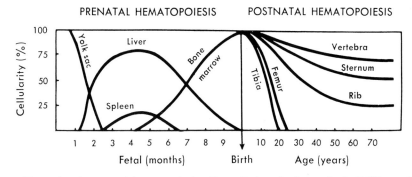

Fig. 1-1. Prenatal and postnatal hematopoiesis. (From Erslev, A. J., et al.: In Williams, W. J., et al., eds.: Hematology, New York, 1972, McGraw-Hill Book Co. Used with permission of McGraw-Hill Book Co.)

cells formed in the liver and the earlier lines of the yolk stalk. They are smaller and have a nuclear structure more closely resembling normoblastic red cell precursors. By 12 to 16 weeks of gestation the red cells are no longer synthesizing the embryonic hemoglobins. Although Hb F overwhelmingly predominates, a small amount of adult hemoglobin is produced. This has permitted midtrimester diagnosis of hemoglobinopathies and thalassemia.[2]

Although circulating granulocytes and platelets are observed, hematopoiesis in the liver is almost exclusively erythropoietic. During this midgestational period some hematopoietic activity is present in the thymus, lymph nodes, and kidneys. Nucleated red cells are also observed in the spleen and probably represent autochthonous production as well as sequestration and destruction. Visceral hematopoiesis reaches its maximum extent at 5 to 6 months of gestational age, then slowly regresses. At term only a few nucleated red cells are normally noted in the viscera. However, in a wide variety of fetal diseases and infections there is a marked increase in extramedullary hematopoiesis.

Medullary hematopoiesis

The final anatomic phase of hematopoiesis is initiated at about 4 months of gestational age. Medullary spaces begin to be formed within the cartilaginous long bone precursors by a process of reabsorption. At first the cellularity within the marrow space is scanty and predominantly leukopoietic. However, rapid proliferation of erythropoietic tissues occurs and by 30 weeks of gestational age the marrow is fully cellular with good representation of all cellular lines, and the marrow becomes the preeminent source of the formed elements of the blood.

From 32 weeks of gestation until birth all of the extant marrow space is filled with hematopoietically active tissue and the marrow is fully cellular. However, the relative marrow volume of the fetus and newborn is considerably smaller than that of the older child and adult. This is because much of the fetal skeleton still is cartilaginous and the long bones of the extremities are proportionately small. In fact it can be shown that the actual volume of the bone marrow is approximately the same as the total volume of hematopoietic cells. Therefore the only way that the fetus and newborn can significantly increase his hematopoietic output and reserve is by reactivated or persistent extramedullary hematopoiesis, especially in the abdominal viscera. The massive visceral hematopoiesis of erythroblastosis fetalis is a clear example of this.

It has been shown that the normal adult or older child can increase his marrow output of red cells six- to eightfold when subjected to a chronic hemolytic stress. This increase is accomplished by converting fatty spaces and yellow marrow to active red marrow. The total marrow potential in early life is not known. However, because the marrow of the fetus and infant is fully active, the marrow output can only be increased by hypertrophy. This probably explains the clinical observation that infants with chronic congenital hemolytic states such as hereditary spherocytosis may initially be very anemic, whereas with passing time they may be able to satisfactorily compensate. It also explains why the phenomenon of extramedullary hematopoiesis is so age related.

ORIGIN AND DIFFERENTIATION OF HEMATOPOIETIC CELLS

For many years controversy has centered on the origin and interrelations of the red cells, granulocytes, and platelets. Proponents of unitarian and trinitarian hypotheses have debated with as much fervor as religious dogmatists. Because of the limitations imposed by purely morphologic techniques, the controversy was unresolvable. Recently certain crucial clinical observations and development of important experimental methods have helped somewhat to resolve the controversy.

In patients with chronic granulocytic leukemia of the adult variety a specific chromosomal abnormality, deletion of the long arms of a G group chromosome, occurs as an acquired defect called the Philadelphia (Ph[1]) chromosome. Study of these patients has demonstrated the Ph[1] chromosome in red cell precursors, young myeloid elements, and megakaryocytes.[12,41]

Even more convincing has been a series of imaginative experiments involving bone marrow transplantation in genetically inbred, lethally irradiated mice. The work of Till and McCulloch[40] confirmed that infusions of bone marrow from isogenic donors prevented hematologic death of lethally irradiated mice. Seven to 10 days following injections of small numbers of marrow cells, nodules consisting of masses of hematopoietic cells were noted in the recipient's spleen. About one half of the spleen colonies were found to consist of "pure" erythropoietic tissues, whereas the remainder were granulocytic and megakaryocytic or mixed. In a second set of experiments cells from the "pure" colonies were retransplanted into another irradiated recipient. Both pure and mixed colonies again occurred in the recipients' spleens. Cytologic studies indicated that the mixed colonies were derived from a single cell and were clonal.[7,46] These studies clearly pointed to the existence of a single, self-perpetuating, multipotential stem cell. In the mouse about 1 of 1,000 marrow cells are believed to be stem cells or colony forming units (CFU). However, differentiation must occur to give rise to the formed elements of the blood. This is believed to be induced or favored by humoral factors such as erythropoietin and the microenvironment into which the stem cells are introduced.

The interrelation between hematopoietic and lymphocytic cell lines is also the subject of intense study and speculation. It may ultimately be proved that there is a common precursor "stem cell" for both of these systems. This is suggested by the recent observation that the abnormal cells seen in the "blast crises" in some cases of chronic myelogenous leukemia have histologic characteristics of lymphoblasts and may contain high levels of the enzyme terminal deoxynucleotidyl transferase, which is specific for lymphoblasts.[29,30]

HEMOGLOBIN VALUES DURING FETAL LIFE

Only a few descriptions of hemoglobin values during early gestation have been published, principally because of the difficulty in obtaining blood from very young normal fetuses. Recently, the increasing numbers of therapeutic abortions performed have provided an opportunity for a more systematic study of fetal hematology. Walker and Turnbull[43] studied the blood of fetuses obtained at therapeutic abortion and were able to define early hematologic development. In the youngest fetuses, of approximately 10 weeks of gestation, the hemoglobin level was approximately 9.0 gm/dl. Subsequently the level steadily increased and by 24 weeks the average hemoglobin level was 14 to 15 gm/dl. At 38 weeks they found the mean cord blood hemoglobin level to be 15.2 gm/dl, a value generally within the lower range for term infants reported by other investigators.

WHITE BLOOD CELL COUNTS
White blood cell counts in the fetus

Leukocytes can be recognized in the fetal circulation early in gestational life. They are formed at first in the hematopoietic center of the yolk stalk and subsequently in liver, spleen, and marrow.

In the smallest fetuses the nucleated counts are high because of the presence of large number of nucleated red cells. Young granulocytes (myelocytes) are seen at 8 weeks of gestation and mature polymorphonuclear leukocytes at 12½ weeks. The number of granulocytes steadily increases until 28 weeks of gestation.[23,39]

Lymphocytes also show a steady increase in absolute numbers until about 15 weeks of gestation, when the counts level off at approximately 2.5×10^9/liter.

A few eosinophils are seen in the early fetuses. The average number of these cells is about 0.2×10^9/liter after 20 weeks. Monocyte counts show considerable scatter and a range somewhat higher than that of eosinophil counts after 20 weeks.

White blood cell counts in the newborn

The total white blood cell count at birth ranges between 9 and 30×10^9/liter but it is in general high. Neutrophilic granulocytes predominate with a mean at birth of 8×10^9/liter and a range of 4.5 to 13.2×10^9/liter.[47] The neutrophils show a tendency to immaturity (shift to left) with an average of 10% band forms as well as occasional younger elements (myelocytes and metamyelocytes).

The lymphocytes also show a characteristic series of changes during the first 2 weeks.[47] Their absolute number at birth averages 3×10^9/liter. This decreases slightly during the first 3 days and then increases to an average value of 6×10^9/liter by 10 days of age. The increase in lymphocytes, combined with the decreasing number of granulocytes, results in the long recognized lymphocytic predominance of infancy, which is established by 2 or 3 weeks of age.

Monocyte numbers are low (mean 1×10^9/liter) and do not vary during the first 2 weeks. Eosinophils average about 2% with a mean absolute eosinophil count of 0.7×10^9/liter during this time.[47] Absolute numbers of basophils are very low during the newborn period.

The total white blood cell counts of premature infants are approximately 30% lower than those of full-term infants. However, the sequential changes, with a tendency to wide variations, are similar to those previously described for term infants.[47]

"PHYSIOLOGIC ANEMIA" OF THE NEWBORN

The normal newborn is relatively plethoric and has an increased red cell volume, hemoglobin level, and hematocrit when compared to older children and adults. Within the first weeks of life the hemoglobin level begins a progressive decline that persists for approximately 6 to 8 weeks, a decrease that has been generally referred to as the "physiologic anemia" of the newborn. This is actually a misnomer, for the minimal hemoglobin concentration of the full-term infant at its nadir is 10 to 11 gm/dl, and the normal infant does not become truly anemic. The decline cannot be altered by administration of hematinics.

Several factors have been shown to be operative in the genesis of physiologic anemia. These include diminished red cell production, an increased rate of red cell destruction, and relative hemodilution as a result of rapid bodily growth.

Red cell production during this period has been evaluated by a number of techniques. Several studies have produced morphologic evidence of erythroid hypoplasia of the bone marrow in the physiologic anemia of full-term infants.[16,36-38] Garby's ferrokinetic studies with radioactive iron demonstrated that a rapid and profound fall in red cell production occurs after the first week of extrauterine life and persists until about 2 months of age.[13] The meticulous reticulocyte studies of Seip[33] also confirmed relative erythroid hypoactivity during this time.

The abrupt cessation of erythropoiesis probably reflects at least three factors, the first of which is a lack of the hormone erythropoietin. As has been previously described, erythropoietin-mediated control of erythropoiesis is operative in the fetus, for in the relatively hypoxic intrauterine environment, erythropoietin levels are high and erythropoiesis is active. It appears likely that erythropoietin is produced by the fetal liver.[31] When the lung replaces the placenta as the source of oxygen and the arterial oxygen saturation rises from 45% toward 95%, erythropoietin activity of the plasma falls to so low a level that it becomes temporarily undetectable in the plasma after the first week of life.[18] It is not until the hemoglobin level falls to 10 to 11 gm/dl at 2 to 3 months of age that erythropoietin activity can once again be detected in the plasma, and concomitantly significant erythropoiesis resumes.

The second factor operative in the genesis of physiologic anemia of the newborn is presumably the short survival of the fetal red cell. The third contributing factor is the sizeable expansion of blood volume that accompanies the rapid gain of weight during the first 3 months of life and creates a situation that has been aptly described as "bleeding into the circulation."

It is clear that the relative bone marrow inactivity is the most important of these three causes of an anemia that should be viewed as physiologic adaptation to extrauterine life. Shortening of red cell survival should not in itself result in anemia, since compensation could be realized by an increase in red cell production of only 1½ to 2 times. The lack of such response is not caused by refractoriness of the bone marrow; infants with cyanotic congenital heart disease and severe postnatal hypoxic stress do not develop physiologic anemia.[28] Hemodilution also is inadequate to explain physiologic anemia without invoking markedly diminished production as well.

The premature infant also develops a physiologic anemia, but with a decline in hemoglobin level that is not only more extreme but also more rapid. Minimal hemoglobin levels of 7 to 9 gm/dl commonly occur by 3 to 7 weeks of age, whereas in very small premature infants, levels as low as 6 to 7 gm/dl may be observed after a faster decrease.[21,34] The same factors operative in the

physiologic anemia of term infants are also present but exaggerated. Although they appear to explain the greater anemia after premature birth, the specific reasons for this quantitative difference between premature and term infants are undetermined. In premature infants significant inverse correlations were noted between hemoglobin levels and oxygen unloading capacity compared to plasma erythropoietin levels.[35] This erythropoietin excretion is appropriate, albeit perhaps less than in later life.[20]

Within this setting of diminished red cell production, shortened red cell survival, and rapidly expanding blood volume, it is easy to see how physiologic anemia, particularly in the premature infant, can be aggravated by any process that further taxes an already precarious erythropoietic equilibrium. Diseases associated with markedly increased hemolysis, such as erythroblastosis fetalis, hereditary spherocytosis, and other congenital hemolytic anemias, are often associated with quite severe anemia in the early weeks of life. In erythroblastosis fetalis an additional contributory factor may be antibody damage to red cell precursors, because the bone marrow is unregenerative, even in the face of extreme anemia, until the transplacentally derived antibody is eliminated.[19]

Dietary factors may also aggravate physiologic anemia. Iron deficiency is frequently invoked as a cause of anemia during infancy. It has been estimated that the full-term infant has a sufficient iron endowment to sustain normal hemoglobin levels until about 5 months of age, whereas the premature infant has enough iron endowment to sustain hemoglobin synthesis for at least 3 months.[5] However, in the absence of significant pre- or perinatal blood loss, iron deficiency should not be invoked as a cause of anemia in the first 2 months of life.

As another important hematinic substance, folic acid requires consideration. Biochemical abnormalities suggestive of folic acid deficiency are frequently found in premature infants.[32] Typical cases of folic acid–responsive megaloblastic anemia have also been described.[17] Diarrhea, starvation, parenteral alimentation, and consumption of a diet unusually low in folic acid (such as goat's milk) are known causes of such anemia in the first 3 months after term birth. The premature infant, however, can develop folic acid–responsive megaloblastic anemia even in the absence of such recognized causes. Human milk contains about 20 μg folic acid/liter; cow's milk and most proprietary infant formulas contain 30 to 100 μg/liter. These amounts are sufficient to prevent deficiency. (See also Chapter 7.)

Vitamin E deficiency has also been implicated

as a cause of a hemolytic anemia in premature infants at 4 to 8 weeks of age.[44] In its full-blown form this deficiency state produces a hemolysis associated with acanthocytic red cells and increased susceptibility of erythrocytes to hydrogen peroxide,[26] as well as thrombocytosis and clinical edema.[26] A relationship between vitamin E, polyunsaturated fatty acids, and iron-supplemented infant formulas in inducing hemolysis has recently been pointed out.[44] This has led to significant changes in the composition of infant formulas. These modifications have prevented the development of hemolysis in premature infants consuming them.

When viewed as a developmental process, physiologic anemia usually requires no therapeutic considerations other than assurance that the diet of the infant contains sufficient amounts of essential nutriments, especially iron, folic acid, and vitamin E, for normal hematopoiesis. If the premature infant is feeding well and growing normally, transfusions are rarely indicated. Occasionally, particularly in very small infants, transfusions are considered necessary because of a very low hemoglobin level or a complicating medical condition. If transfusion is utilized, only small amounts of blood should be given, with the object of increasing the hemoglobin level only to approximately 8 gm/dl. Larger transfusions are not indicated and may in fact delay spontaneous recovery by suppressing normal erythropoiesis.

COAGULATION
Coagulation in the fetus

Circulating levels of most of the coagulation factors are maintained within well-defined but quite wide ranges throughout life. It seems likely that the coagulation factors do not cross the placental barrier to any significant degree. Certainly there is no correlation between maternal and fetal levels of factor VIII.[24] Newborn infants with hemophilia as a result of inherited deficiencies of factor VIII, and probably of factor IX, are born to mothers without such deficiencies, but the diagnostically low levels of these factors in cord blood permit recognition of hemophilia at birth.[10] A similar lack of transplacental transmission of factor I has been demonstrated in a newborn with congenital afibrinogenemia.[25]

A nearly complete placental barrier for factors I, VII, and X was proved by the lack of significant difference in the levels in umbilical venous and arterial samples in the face of a large maternal-fetal difference.[4] All of these studies preclude significant maternal-fetal transmission and support the hypothesis that the clotting factors in the circulation of the newborn have been synthesized as a fetus.

Table 1-1. Levels of coagulation factors in full-term infants*

Factor	Level†
I	240 ± 40 mg/dl
	217 ± 41 mg/dl
II	56% ± 10%
	60% ± 38%
V	92% ± 41%
	172% ± 41%
VII	25%-40%
	5%-50%
VIII	137% ± 40%
	96% ± 33%
IX	28% ± 6%
	43% ± 7%
X	43% ± 7%
	21% ± 54%
XI	36% ± 15%
	13%-85%
XII	54% ± 16%
XIII	100%
Prothrombin time	14.5 ± 1.0 sec.
Thromboplastin time	41 ± 21.0 sec.

*From Pearson, H. A.: In Smith, C. A., and Nelson, N. N., eds: The physiology of the newborn, ed. 4, Springfield, Ill., 1976, Charles C Thomas, Publisher.
†Defined as a percentage of the normal adult level, arbitrarily set at 100%.

Coagulation in the full-term infant

Although the clotting times of full-term newborn infants are the same or even more rapid than those of adults, factor assays show definite and characteristic differences. Moderately low activities are apparent for factors II, VII, IX, and X, yet these decreases do not ordinarily affect the prothrombin time or partial thromboplastin time, which are either normal or only slightly prolonged in full-term infants at birth; levels of factors V, VIII, and XIII are within normal range or even elevated during the newborn period[22] (Table 1-1).

Hemorrhagic disease of the newborn

The levels of coagulation factors (II, VII, IX, X) synthesized in the liver under the influence of vitamin K[8] are, as has been noted in Table 1-1, lower in the cord blood than the adult normal levels. Following birth the levels of these so-called vitamin K–dependent factors decrease rapidly, reaching a nadir at 48 to 72 hours of life. From their low point at 2 or 3 days of life, levels of these factors rise slowly, but they do not approach normal adult levels until 9 months of age or even later.

In most full-term infants these postnatal decreases, although definite, are of no clinical consequence, but in about 10% of infants the drop is so profound that a spontaneous hemorrhagic state may develop. This exaggeration of the physiologic postnatal decrease of the vitamin K–dependent coagulation factors is the basis of the syndrome long known as hemorrhagic disease of the newborn.[42]

The rise in the levels of the vitamin K–dependent factors on the second or third day of life is not spontaneous but indicates a response to diet. Since the vitamin K content of human milk is considerably lower than that of cow's milk,[9] hemorrhagic disease of the newborn is virtually confined to breast-fed infants.[14] Whatever the milk intake, in full-term infants a significant postnatal decline of the vitamin K–dependent factors, and virtually every possibility of hemorrhagic disease, can be prevented by administration of prophylactic vitamin K to the newborn infant. Only 25 μg of vitamin K prevents the postnatal decline of the coagulation factors.[1] The Committee on Nutrition of the American Academy of Pediatrics has recommended administration of 1.0 mg of Vitamin K_1 oxide intramuscularly to all infants shortly after birth.[6] Larger doses are not necessary, for they have no greater therapeutic effect. Synthetic vitamin K (K_3) should not be used; this compound may produce hemolysis when given in large doses.

Coagulation in premature infants

The plasma of premature infants has marked depression of many coagulation factors. The more immature the infant, the more profound are these

Table 1-2. Levels of coagulation factors in premature infants*

Factor	Level†
I	270 ± 150 mg/dl
	180 ± 267 mg/dl
II	46%-70%
	25%
V	49%-65%
	60%-100%
VII	37%
VIII	21%-67%
	64%-100%
	26%
IX	8%-12%
X	12%-46%
	46%
XI	5%-18%
XIII	100%
Prothrombin time	16-35 sec
Thromboplastin time	73-147 sec

*From Pearson, H. A.: In Smith, C. A., and Nelson, N. N., eds.: The physiology of the newborn, ed. 4, Springfield, Ill., 1976, Charles C Thomas, Publisher.
†Defined as a percentage of the normal adult level, arbitrarily set at 100%.

deficiencies. Considerable individual variability is seen, so that levels of some factors in some premature infants may be expected to lie in the same range as in normal term neonates, whereas severe degrees of coagulation impairment may be expected in others. This wide variation of activity reflects differences in hepatic maturity and rates of synthesis (Table 1-2).[22]

The complex deficiency of multiple coagulation factors characteristically seen in small premature infants has been designated "secondary" hemorrhagic disease of the newborn and may be an important factor contributing to hemorrhage in premature infants.[1]

REFERENCES

1. Aballi, A. J., and DeLamerens, S.: Coagulation changes in the neonatal period and in early infancy, Pediatr. Clin. North Am. **9**:785, 1962.
2. Alter, B. P., Modell, C. B., and Fairweather, D.: Prenatal diagnosis of hemoglobinopathies: a review of 15 cases, N. Engl. J. Med. **295**:1443, 1976.
3. Bloom, W., and Barlelmitz, G. W.: Hematopoiesis in young human embryos, Am. J. Anat. **67**:21, 1940.
4. Cade, J. F., Hirsh, J., and Martin, M.: Placental barrier to coagulation factors: its relevance to the coagulation defect at birth and of haemorrhage in the newborn, Brit. Med. J. **2**:281, 1969.
5. Committee on Nutrition, American Academy of Pediatrics: Iron supplementation for infants, Pediatrics **58**:765, 1977.
6. Committee on Nutrition, American Academy of Pediatrics: Vitamin K compounds and the water soluble analogues: use in therapy and prophylaxis in pediatrics, Pediatrics **20**:272, 1957.
7. Curry, J. L., and Trenton, J. J.: Hemopoietic cell colony studies. I. Growth and differentiation, Dev. Biol. **15**:395, 1967.
8. Dam, H., Dyggne, H., Larson, H., and Plum, P.: The relation of vitamin K deficiency to hemorrhagic disease of the newborn, Adv. Pediatr. **5**:129, 1952.
9. Dam, H., Glavend, J., Larson, E., and Plum, P.: Investigations into the cause of the physiological hypopiothrombinemia in newborn children IV. The vitamin K content of woman's milk and cow's milk, Acta. Med. Scand. **112**:210, 1942.
10. Didisheim, P., and Lewis, J. H.: Congenital disorders of the mechanisms for coagulation of blood, Pediatrics **22**:478, 1958.
11. Erslev, A. J.: Production of erythrocytes. In Williams, W. J., Beutler, E., Erslev, A. J., and Rundles, R. W., eds.: Hematology, New York, 1972. McGraw-Hill Book Co., p. 162.
12. Fialkow, P. J., Gartler, S. M., and Yoshida, A.: Clonal origin of chronic myelocytic leukemia in man, Proc. Soc. Nat. Acad. Sci. **58**:1468, 1967.
13. Garby, L., Sjolin, S., and Viulle, J. C.: Studies on erythrokinetics in infancy. III. Disappearance from plasma and red cell uptake of radioactive iron injected intravenously, Acta Paediatr. **52**:537, 1963.
14. Gillis, S. S., and Lyon, R. A.: The influence of the diet of the newborn infant on the prothrombin index, J. Pediatr. **19**:495, 1941.
15. Gilmour, J. R.: Normal haemopoiesis in intra-uterine and neonatal life, J. Pathol. Bacteriol. **52**:25, 1941.
16. Glaser, K., Lamarzi, L. R., and Poncher, H. G.: Cellular composition of the bone marrow in normal infants and children, Pediatrics **6**:789, 1950.

17. Guy, O. P., and Butler, E. B.: Megaloblastic anemia in premature infants, Arch. Dis. Child. **40:**53, 1965.
18. Halvorsin, S.: Plasma erythropoetin levels in cord blood and in blood during the first weeks of life, Acta Paediat. **52:**425, 1963.
19. Hyman, C. B., and Sturgeon, P.: Observations on the convalescent phase of erythroblastosis fetalis, Pediatrics **16:**15, 1955.
20. Nathan, D. G.: Regulation of erythropoiesis, N. Engl. J. Med. **296:**684, 1977.
21. O'Brien, R. T., and Pearson, H.: Physiologic anemia of the newborn infant, J. Pediatr. **79:**132, 1971.
22. Pearson, H. A.: The blood. In Smith, C. A., and Nelson, N. N., eds.: The physiology of the newborn, ed. 4, Springfield, Ill., 1976, Charles C Thomas, Publisher.
23. Playfaw, J. H. L., Wolfendale, M. R., and Kay, H. E. M.: The leucocytes of peripheral blood in the human foetus, Brit. J. Haematol. **9:**336, 1963.
24. Preston, A. E.: The plasma concentration of factor VIII in the normal population. I. Mothers and babies at birth, Bri. J. Haematol. **10:**110, 1964.
25. Prichard, R. W., and Vann, R. I.: Congenital afibrinogenemia: report of a child without fibrinogen and review of literature, Am. J. Dis. Child. **88:**703, 1954.
26. Ritchie, J. H., Mathews, B. F., McMasters, V., and Grossman, M.: Edema and hemolytic anemia in premature infants: a vitamin E deficiency syndrome, N. Engl. J. Med. **279:**1185, 1968.
27. Rosenberg, M.: Fetal hematopoiesis, Blood **33:**66, 1969.
28. Rudolph, A. M., Nadas, A. S., and Borges, W. H.: Hematologic adjustments and cyanotic congenital heart disease, Pediatrics **11:**454, 1953.
29. Sarin, P. S., Anderson, P. M., and Gallo, R. C.: Terminal deoxynucleotidyl transferase activities in human blood leukocytes and lymphoblast cell lines: high levels in lymphoblast cell lines and in blast cells of some patients with chronic myelogenous leukemia in acute phase, Blood **47:**11, 1976.
30. Sarin, P. S., and Gallo, R. C.: Terminal deoxynucleotidyl transferase in chronic myelogenous leukemia, J. Biol. Chem. **249:**8051, 1974.
31. Schooley, J. C., and Mahylamm, L. J.: Extrarenal erythropoietin production by the liver in the weanling rat, Proc. Soc. Exp. Biol. Med. **145:**1081, 1974.
32. Shojania, A. M., and Gross, S.: Folic acid deficiency and prematurity, J. Pediatr. **64:**323, 1964.
33. Siep, M.: The reticulocyte level and the erythrocyte production judged from reticulocyte studies in newborn infants during the first week of life, Acta. Paediatr. **44:**355, 1955.
34. Sisson, T. R. C., Whalen, L. E., and Tilek, A.: Blood volume of infants. II. The premature infant during the first year of life, J. Pediatr. **55:**430, 1959.
35. Stockman, J. A., Gancia, J. F., and Oski, F. A.: The anemia of prematurity: factors governing the erythropoietin response, N. Engl. J. Med. **296:**647, 1977.
36. Sturgeon, P.: Volumetric and microscopic patterns of bone marrow in normal infants and children: volumetric pattern, Pediatrics **7:**577, 1951.
37. Sturgeon, P.: Volumetric and microscopic patterns of bone marrow in normal infants and children: cytologic pattern, Pediatrics **7:**642, 1951.
38. Sturgeon, P.: Volumetric and microscopic patterns of bone marrow in normal infants and children, Pediatrics **7:**774, 1951.
39. Thomas, D. B., and Yaffey, J. M.: Human foetal haemopoiesis. I. The cellular composition of foetal blood, Br. J. Haematol. **8:**290, 1962.
40. Till, J. E., and McCulloch, E. A.: A direct measurement of the radiation sensitivity of normal mouse bone marrow, Radiat. Res. **14:**213, 1961.
41. Townsend, C. W.: The haemorrhagic disease of the newborn, Arch. Pediatr. **11:**559, 1894.
42. Tryjillo, J. M., and Ohno, S.: Chromosomal alteration of erythropoietic cells in chronic myeloid leukemia, Acta Haematol. **29:**311, 1963.
43. Walker, J. L., and Turnbull, E. P. N.: Haemoglobin and red cells in the human fetus and their relation to the oxygen content of the blood in the vessels of the umbilical cord, Lancet **2:**312, 1953.
44. Williams, M. L., Shott, R. J., O'Neal, P. L., and Oski, F. A.: Role of dietary iron and vitamin E deficiency anemia of infancy, N. Engl. J. Med. **292:**887, 1975.
45. Wintrobe, M. M., and Shumacker, H. B., Jr.: Comparison of hematopoiesis in the fetus and during recovery from pernicious anemia, J. Clin. Invest. **14:**837, 1935.
46. Wu, A. M., Till, J. E., Simmovitch, L., and McCulloch, E. A.: A cytological study of the capacity for differentiation of normal hemopoietic colony-forming cells, J. Cell Physiol. **69:**177, 1967.
47. Xanthow, M.: Leukocyte blood picture in healthy full-term and premature babies during neonatal period, Arch. Dis. Child. **45:**242, 1970.

2 □ Normal values and examination of the blood: perinatal period, infancy, childhood, and adolescence

Denis R. Miller

BLOOD CHANGES DURING GROWTH

Knowledge of the normal blood values during the dynamic period of growth is a prerequisite to the interpretation of a particular blood response in infancy and childhood. For this reason the normal developmental changes in hematologic values are included in this discussion. It is recognized that the values cited are subject to wide variations, both in each individual and among members of an age group. These values are presented as yardsticks and are in general agreement with the composite data available in standard texts and articles dealing with this subject.* Not only are there numerical variations during infancy and childhood but there are also important changes in the structure and function of blood cells.

Blood volume and placental transfusion

The blood volume of the full-term infant at birth is approximately 85 ml/kg and that of the premature infant averages 108 ml, the difference mainly being the result of an excess of plasma in the latter.[74] Placental transfusion may significantly increase the blood volume. The placental vessels contain approximately 150 ml of whole blood with a range from 50 to 200 ml.[37] In infants of diabetic mothers the residual blood volume is at least twice as large as that of control groups.[49] A transfusion of placental blood usually takes place within seconds of birth, and approximately 45 ml of this volume may be accommodated in the pulmonary circulation. A contributory cause of the large residual placental blood volume in infants of diabetic mothers is related to the late onset of respiration and shallow breathing.

Using iodinated human albumin to measure serial blood volume in normal full-term infants, Usher et al.[85] found that the blood volume at the moment of birth was 78 ml/kg, with a venous packed cell volume of 48%. A delay in cord clamping increases the blood volume. It is estimated that the placenta contains a reservoir of 125 to 150 ml of blood and that delayed clamping may account for the addition of as much as 100 ml of blood to the circulation of the newborn infant. A 5-minute delay in cord clamping may increase the blood volume by 60% (to 126 ml/kg). The amount of blood received by the infant depends on the time after delivery at which the cord is clamped. One fourth of the placental transfusion occurs in the first 15 seconds of birth, 50% in the first minute after delivery, 80% in 5 minutes, and 90% in 10 minutes. The effect of stripping the umbilical cord on the blood volume is controversial. In one study stripping of the cord during the first 5 minutes after birth did not increase the volume of the transfusion,[16] whereas in another study no significant difference was found in the erythrocyte count in the neonatal period with respect to the time of clamping *unless* the cord was deliberately stripped.[92]

During the first 4 hours a 30% decrease in the blood volume (126 to 89 ml/kg) occurs in infants who received a placental transfusion. This reduction is caused by transudation of one half of the original plasma volume. A rise in the venous hematocrit from 48% to 64% by 4 hours is noted concomitantly. In those infants in whom placental transfusion was prevented by immediate clamping of the cord no changes in blood volume occurred. The differences at 72 hours in blood volume, red cell, mass, plasma volume, and venous hematocrit between infants receiving and not receiving a placental transfusion are shown in Table 2-1.

Table 2-1. Average values 72 hours after placental transfusion

	No transfusion	Placental transfusion
Blood volume (ml/kg)	82	93
Red cell volume (ml/kg)	31	49
Plasma volume (ml/kg)	51	44
Venous hematocrit (%)	44	60

---

*References 4, 34, 53, 55, 64, 95.

Thus during the first 3 days infants who had received a placental transfusion maintained a red cell mass about 60% larger than those who had not. However, at 3 months the mean hemoglobin level in early-clamped infants was exactly the same as in those clamped later.[52] The advantages of late clamping of the umbilical cord may be of importance to the premature infant in whom total iron stores are decreased.

Neonatal polycythemia and twin-to-twin transfusion

The upper limits of normal for venous hemoglobin and hematocrit values during the first week of life are 22 gm/dl and 65%, respectively.[93] Abnormally high values have been reported in a number of disorders, including placental hypertransfusion, placental insufficiency, maternal toxemia, intrauterine growth retardation, asphyxia, certain metabolic and endocrine abnormalities such as maternal diabetes, congenital adrenal hyperplasia and neonatal thyrotoxicosis, rare tumors associated with excessive erythopoietin production, trisomy 21, and the hyperplastic visceromegaly syndrome.

Plethora and polycythemia of unknown etiology have been reported in infants with anorexia, lethargy, cyanosis, and convulsions but without congenital malformations.[27,98] The hematocrits ranged between 73% and 80%, hemoglobin levels between 21 and 25 gm/dl, and red cell counts over 7×10^{12}/liter. Hyperbilirubinemia, hypocalcemia, hypoglycemia, thrombocytopenia, and decreased concentration of fetal hemoglobin for age have been associated laboratory findings. The demonstration of significant numbers of maternal erythrocytes in the infant's blood by differential agglutination implicated a maternal-fetal transfusion as the cause of plethora in some of these infants. Ordinarily a fetus might lose blood into the mother and be born anemic, the pressure gradients within the placenta favoring such a transfer. Conceivably an anatomic abnormality in the placentas of the infants accounted for the reverse situation—maternal-fetal transfusion.[57]

Intrauterine hypoxia and asphyxia result in increased production of erythropoietin,[18] increased erythropoiesis, and higher reticulocyte and nucleated red blood cell counts. Flod and Ackerman[19] found that perinatal asphyxia causes the transfer of blood in utero from placenta to fetus with resultant decreased residual placental blood volume.

A twin-to-twin transfusion may occur in the presence of an arteriovenous shunt between the supposedly separate placental circulations of single-ovum twins, resulting in a parabiotic circulatory system.[7,51] Unequal functioning between the two circulations accounts for polycythemia in one twin and anemia in the other.[43] Hemoglobin values

of 25.2 and 3.7 gm/dl and red cell counts of 7.47 and 1.85×10^{12}/liter, respectively, have been reported.[51]

Usually newborn polycythemic levels drop to normal spontaneously and without ill effect to the infant. The polycythemic twin is subject to the hazards of hemorrhage, venous thrombosis, cardiac failure, pulmonary edema, and hyperbilirubinemia. If cardiopulmonary or central nervous system symptoms threaten the plethoric newborn infant, partial exchange transfusion with fresh plasma should be performed to reduce the venous hematocrit below 65% to 60%. Above this level blood viscosity is markedly increased and blood flow is significantly reduced.[33] The anemic twin should be treated with small packed red cell transfusions.

Postmortem examination of eleven pairs of twins showed that hyaline membrane disease was present in both members of four twin pairs.[59] In the recipient twin myocardial hyperplasia involving all chambers developed with a corresponding increase of muscle about the arteries of both major circulatory beds, suggesting antenatal hypertension. In contrast, small hearts and reduced arterial muscle masses found in the anemic twins suggested a relative hypotension in the circulatory beds. In twins with the syndrome the anemic member was on the arterial side and the polycythemic sibling on the venous side of one or more placental arteriovenous shunts.

In 130 monochorial twin pregnancies studied in one institution, the twin transfusion syndrome was diagnosed nineteen times.[71] In ten instances both twins died in the perinatal period, in five only one twin died, and in four both twins survived. Most of the deaths occurred in utero early in pregnancy. The twin transfusion syndrome accounts for a significant number of fetal and neonatal deaths in twin pregnancies and appears to be the cause of a large part of the higher fatality rate noted in monochorial, in contrast to dichorial, twin gestation. It has been suggested that infants surviving the twin transfusion syndrome have persistent alterations in comparative growth and development.

Life span of newborn cells

During the first week of life the decline in hemoglobin and red cells in the peripheral blood is at a minimum. This initial stationary period is followed by a definite decline. The postnatal adjustment is characterized by a normal or slightly increased rate of blood destruction accompanied by diminished or stationary hematopoietic activity. During this period the drop in red cells occurs within the limits of normal survival—100 to 120 days, or approximately 0.8%/day.

Estimates of the life span of the red cell in premature and full-term infants have not always been in agreement. In one study fetal red blood cells obtained from the umbilical cord and tagged with ^{51}Cr had a shortened half-life of 15 to 23 days, as compared with a range of 24 to 35 days in normal adults.[44] Similarly tagged placental red cells also transfused into adult recipients had a mean half-life of 22.8 days (range 17 to 28 days) and 15.8 days (range 10 to 18 days) for cells of full-term and premature infants, respectively, compared with an autologous survival of 27.5 days for adult cells.[20] Another study demonstrated a normal half-life (25 to 35 days) during the first 5 days of life of full-term infants, whereas in premature infants the half-life was less than 20 days.[46] In the third to ninth week of life the ^{51}Cr-labeled erythrocyte half-life is similar to full-term and premature infants (12 to 34 days).

These findings indicate that survival of erythrocytes in full-term infants' is normally at adult levels during the first 5 days of life, whereas in premature infants it is invariably shortened. On the other hand, when glycine ^{15}N was fed to premature infants in the first 48 hours of life, the rate of elimination of newly formed tagged erythrocytes was identical with that seen in normal adults similarly treated—120 days.[14] The normal results in these observations, as compared with the shorter red cell life span of premature infants reported by others, may be a result of differences between adult-type erythrocytes produced postnatally and red cells of shortened survival produced in utero.

Characteristics of newborn red cells

The metabolic, functional, and structural characteristics of the newborn's erythrocytes differ considerably from their counterparts in older infants, children, and adults and are listed here[64]:

A. Membrane
  1. Phospholipid content
     a. Increased sphingomyelin, decreased lecithin
     b. Increased lipid phosphorus and cholesterol per cell
     c. Decreased linoleic acid*
  2. Transport and permeability
     a. Decreased ouabain-sensitive ATPase*
     b. Decreased potassium influx*
     c. Decreased permeability to glycerol and thiourea*
     d. Greater affinity for glucose*
  3. Deformability and integrity
     a. Decreased deformability*
     b. Altered morphology with storage or incubation*
     c. Decreased membrane sulfhydryl groups

4. Antigenicity
     a. Presence of i antigens*
B. Hemoglobin
  1. Increased oxygen affinity*
  2. Increased methemoglobin content and formation*
  3. Decreased methemoglobin reduction (NADH-dependent methemoglobin reductase)*
  4. Increased susceptibility to oxidative denaturation* (Heinz body formation)
  5. Increased oxygen consumption and H_2O_2 production*
C. Enzymes and metabolism
  1. Carbohydrate metabolism
     a. Increased glucose consumption
     b. Increased galactose utilization, galactokinase, and galactose-1-phosphate uridyltransferase*
     c. Decreased activity of sorbitol pathway*
  2. Embden-Meyerhof (anaerobic) pathway
     a. Increased activity of hexokinase, phosphoglucose isomerase,* aldolase, glyceraldehyde-3-phosphate dehydrogenase,* phosphoglycerate kinase, phosphoglycerate mutase, enolase,* pyruvate kinase, and lactic dehydrogenase
     b. Decreased phosphofructokinase*
     c. Increased ATP
     d. Accelerated decline of 2,3-DPG* and ATP
  3. Pentose phosphate (aerobic) shunt
     a. Increased G-6-PD, 6-phosphogluconic dehydrogenase, and glutathione reductase
     b. Decreased glutathione stability, glutathione peroxidase,* and glutathione synthetase*
  4. Nonglycolytic enzymes
     a. Decreased catalase,* carbonic anhydrase,* and adenylate kinase*
     b. Increased glutamic oxaloacetic transaminase

Generally the red cell membranes of the newborn contain more sphingomyelin; less lecithin (phosphotidylcholine); and more total lipids, phospholipid cholesterol, and polyunsaturated fatty acid than do cells from older individuals.[60] The membranes of red cells of premature and newborn infants are much more susceptible to lipid peroxidation. The decreased quantity of ATPase is associated with decreased potassium influx. Furthermore, the deformability of the newborn erythrocyte is decreased (increased rigidity) and marked morphologic alterations characterized by crenation and fragmentation occur with incubation and storage. Normal and abnormal membrane structure and function are discussed in greater detail in Chapter 11.

In addition to the increased affinity of hemoglobin for oxygen, hemoglobin in newborn erythrocytes is more susceptible to oxidation and oxidative denaturation. The content of methemoglobin in increased, and the quantity of the major

---

*Uniquely characteristic.

enzyme involved in methemoglobin reduction, NADH-dependent methemoglobin reductase, is decreased. Increased oxygen consumption and increased hydrogen peroxide production in red cells of neonates contribute to the oxidative denaturation of hemoglobin.

The red cells of premature and full-term infants consume more glucose than those of adults, but when glycolysis in the cells of neonates is compared with that of older patients with a comparable reduction in the mean age of their erythrocyte population, the glycolytic rate is actually lower in neonates than in older individuals.[65] The newborn cells do not consume as much glucose as would be expected from cells of a similar young mean cell age primarily because of the relative deficiency of a key rate-limiting enzyme of glycolysis, phosphofructokinase. The activities of all of the other enzymes of the Embden-Meyerhof, or anaerobic, pathway are increased and commensurate with the youth of the cell population.[63]

Although the concentration of ATP is higher in the red cells of neonates, the decline of ATP with incubation or storage is accelerated. Decreased ATP content severely impairs membrane cation and lipid transport, decreases cell deformability, and causes increased oxygen affinity and decreased synthesis of glutathione.

The activities of a number of enzymes of the pentose phosphate shunt are increased in the erythrocytes of newborns, and decreased generation of NADP is not responsible for the ease with which neonatal cells develop oxidative denaturation of hemoglobin.[62] However, glutathione is unstable and its concentration decreases when erythrocytes are incubated in the presence of a potent oxidant stress. The activities of glutathione synthetase and glutathione peroxidase are decreased as well; the activity of the latter does not approach normal adult values until the age of 6 months. A fuller discussion of erythrocyte metabolism is presented in Chapter 12.

Carbonic anhydrase, a zinc metalloenzyme, is important in the physiologic transport of carbon dioxide. Normal full-term newborn infants have approximately 25% of the enzymatic activity of adults.[50,66] Premature infants without the respiratory distress syndrome (RDS) averaged 13% of the adult enzyme activity and those with RDS averaged only 5% of adult activity. Two carbonic anhydrase fractions, designated B and C, are detected on starch-gel electrophoresis of human erythrocyte lysates.[90] Levels of both isoenzymes are lower in infancy and reach their adult intensity at the second to third year of life. Carbonic anhydrase activity is markedly elevated in red cells from patients with megaloblastic anemia secondary to vitamin B_{12} deficiency and in folic acid de-

ficiency. Decreased carbonic anhydrase activity with a newborn isoenzyme pattern has been described in a number of hematologic disorders associated with certain but not necessarily all other fetal red cell characteristics, including raised levels of fetal hemoglobin, i antigen, decreased or absent Hb A_2, and a fetal pattern of hexokinase isoenzymes. These conditions include juvenile chronic granulocytic leukemia, paroxysmal nocturnal hemoglobinuria, and the refractory anemias with hyperplastic bone marrow, acute leukemias, aplastic anemia, and certain tumors.[90] A true reversion to fetal erythropoiesis and protein synthesis appears to occur solely in juvenile chronic granulocytic leukemia; it could represent the emergence of undifferentiated cells or reflect a more general phenomenon common to malignant transformation, in which the reappearance of fetal proteins is part of the neoplastic process.

Blood of premature infants

The mean hemoglobin values of small-for-gestational age infants (17.1 ± 2.1 gm/dl) born between 36 and 46 weeks of gestation was significantly higher than for comparable normal infants (16.2 ± 2.3 gm/dl). Sex differences in mean cord hemoglobin values of low birth weight infants born between 28 and 42 weeks of pregnancy have been observed. In males the cord hemoglobin value reaches a maximum at 32 weeks and remains constant with a mean of 16.2 gm/dl until 38 weeks. The hemoglobin values of females are lower than those of males until 38 weeks of gestation. The linear relation between hemoglobin values and duration of pregnancy in the female fetus can be expressed by the following formula:

cord Hb (gm/dl) = 7 + gestational age in lunar months,
$$\text{or}$$
$$= 7.016 + 0.245(\text{gestational age in weeks})$$

Although Burman and Morris[10] could find no significant correlation between cord hemoglobin and birth weight in small-for-date infants, there was a negative correlation with placental weight and placental weight/birth weight ratios.

From the twelfth to the thirty-fourth week of gestation, the hemoglobin level increases from 8.0 to 15.0 gm/dl, the hematocrit from 33% to 47%, and the red cell count from 1.5 to 4.4 × 10^{12}/liter. The mean corpuscular volume decreases from 180 to 118 fl, the mean corpuscular hemoglobin declines from 60 to 38 pg, and the mean corpuscular hemoglobin concentration remains in the normal range of 32% to 34%. The reticulocyte count decreases from 40% to approximately 10%, and the percentage of normoblasts decreases from 8% to 0.1% or 0.2% (10 to 20/100 white blood cells).

Thus the number of immature erythrocytes in the peripheral blood of the premature infant reflects gestational age and any additional in utero hypoxic stress. Polycythemia at birth may be exaggerated in the premature infant because of differences in the proportions of blood volume in the body and the placenta. Whereas the amount of blood in the placenta remains fairly constant during the third trimester of pregnancy, that in the body increases steadily. The effect of the transfer of placental blood in the infant after birth therefore would produce a greater relative effect in the premature infant than in the full-term infant, especially when tying of the cord is delayed and the full complement of blood is obtained from this source.

At the end of the decline in the second and third months the hemoglobin levels of the premature infant are 1 gm/dl or more below the values of 11 gm/dl for full-term infants. Thereafter a gradual recovery sets in, with values approximating normal full-term levels at about 1 year of age.

Platelet counts below 100×10^9/liter in premature infants are extremely unusual and should be considered pathologic. Aballi et al.[1] found that in the first 2 days of life platelet counts of premature infants were somewhat lower than those observed in full-term infants.[2] The differences, although statistically significant, were not marked. A steady rise in platelet count, albeit slower in the premature infant, was generally observed during the first month of life, irrespective of the birth weight. In another study of seventy-three premature infants, Fogel et al.[21] found that the majority had platelet counts corresponding to those of adults, with a range of 156 to 300×10^9/liter and a mean of 212×10^9/liter. The earlier findings[56] of platelet counts in premature infants ranging from 31 to 197×10^9/liter in the first 5 days of life and a decrease below 50×10^9/liter by 10 to 20 days of age in small (less than 1,700 gm) premature infants has been attributed to a pathologic process. It seems apparent that significant thrombocytopenia in premature infants should be considered abnormal, not physiologic, and possible causes should be sought.[68] Thrombocytopenia is discussed in Chapters 3 and 24.

There is evidence that premature infants, as compared with their full-term counterparts, have higher granulocyte, lower lymphocyte, and lower total white blood cell counts.

Bone marrow changes

The bone marrow hematopoietic tissue reaches a maximum intrauterine level at about 30 weeks of gestation and remains at this level for the last 10 weeks of gestation.[45] On the day of birth nucleated red cells are relatively numerous, ranging from 30% to 65%; their numbers fall to 12% to 40% by

Table 2-2. Mean and range of bone marrow differential counts (percentages) in premature infants

	0-24 hours	3 weeks
Myeloblasts	4.2 (1.0-9.0)	5.8 (1.5-12.0)
Promyelocytes	4.3 (1.5-12.0)	5.2 (2.0-8.3)
Myelocytes and metamyelocytes	25.4 (11.0-38.3)	24.5 (13.0-29.5)
Bands	4.5 (1.5-8.0)	4.9 (1.5-8.3)
Segmented neutrophils	15.5 (4.5-37.5)	8.7 (6.0-14.0)
Eosinophils	1.2 (0.5-3.5)	1.2 (0.5-2.3)
Basophils	—	—
Pronormoblasts	1.8 (0.8-3.8)	0.9 (0.5-2.0)
Normoblasts	20.4 (6.0-36.0)	20.2 (14.5-29.8)
Lymphocytes	14.6 (5.3-28.3)	15.2 (10.0-21.5)
Monocytes	3.2 (0.3-7.5)	—
Plasma cells	0.4 (0.0-1.0)	2.6 (0.5-5.5)
M:E ratio	2.48	2.38

the seventh day and 8% to 30% by the fourteenth day, with an average of about 10%. Erythroid cells then increase gradually, reaching the normal childhood level of about 20% at 3 to 4 weeks of age.[28] The total cellularity of the bone marrow averages 136×10^9/liter on the first day, 35×10^9/liter on the ninth day, and 201×10^9/liter at 3 months.[22]

Although bone marrow aspirate preparations from premature infants are usually more cellular than those of full-term infants,[54] there are no differences in the differential counts of marrow elements in full-term and premature infants.[24] Composites of bone marrow differential counts derived from reported studies of premature infants and normal infants and children are presented in Tables 2-2 and 2-3.

Normal blood values (Table 2-4)

Hemoglobin concentration. The mean cord blood hemoglobin value varies between approximately 16.6 and 17.1 gm/dl of blood.[25,34] In our laboratory the hemoglobin values averaged 16.4 gm/dl, with a range of 14 to 19 gm/dl. During

Table 2-3. Mean and range of bone marrow differential counts (percentages) during infancy and childhood*

	0-24 months	1 week	1 month	3 months	6 months	12 months	1-4 years	4-12 years	Adult
Myeloblasts	0.3 (0-1)	1.2 (0.4-1.9)	2.5	0.4	0.7	0.3	0.5 (0-1.2)	0.9 (0.75-1.1)	0.9 (0.3-5.0)
Promyelocytes	1.0 (0.5-1.5)	1.8 (1.0-2.5)	4.5	1.6	2.6	1.1	1.6 (0.6-3.5)	1.9 (1.8-2.1)	3.3 (1-8)
Myelocytes	1.6 (0.6-2.4)	4.3 (2.5-7.2)	5.4	1.5	4.8	2.1	1.6 (0-3.7)	10.5 (2.4-18.7)	12.7 (8-16)
Metamyelocytes	2.0 (0.7-3.0)	5.5 (3.1-9.1)	6.9	2.0	6.2	2.7	2.1 (0-4.8)	13.4 (3.1-23.8)	15.9 (9-25)
Bands	19.0 (13-23)	22.9 (17-32)	33.2 (14-52)	8.3	15.7	11.7	16.3 (4-31)	13.9 (7-20)	12.4 (9-15)
Segmented neutrophils	23.3 (9.6-39)	22.0 (8.7-30.2)	5.8 (4.0-7.6)	8.1 (3.7-11.5)	10.6	29.8 (11.0-48.5)	25 (9.6-66.9)	13.9 (9.7-14.6)	7.4 (3-11)
Eosinophils	1.3 (1-3)	2.9 (1.9-5.3)	6.0	3.9	3.2	1.9	2.9 (0-4.6)	4 (5-7)	3.1 (1-5)
Basophils	<0.1 (0-0.2)	<0.1 (0-0.2)	2.5 (0-5)	0.1	0.2	0	0.2	0.2 (0.2-1.8)	<0.1 (0-0.2)
Pronormoblasts	1.6 (0.4-2.5)	0.8 (0.4-1.1)	1.3	0.3	0.2	0.4	0.7 (0-1.4)	1.0 (0.2-2.5)	0.6 (0.2-1.3)
Normoblasts	37.8 (21-54)	19.1 (12-25)	13.9	18.4 (13-24)	10.4	5.9 (2.4-9.5)	22.2	23.4 (19-29)	25 (18-36)
Lymphocytes	6.1 (3.7-8.0)	14.5 (9.5-19)	12.1 (4-20)	51	37.2	27.6 (24-31)	22.0 (11-29)	24.3 (14-28)	16.2 (11-23)
Monocytes	5.3 (2.0-7.3)	5.2 (3-10)	6.8	5.0	8.0	3.4 (0-7)	6.1	6.3 (2-12)	0.3 (0-0.8)
Plasma cells	—	0.2 (0-0.2)	—	—	0.2	0.2	0.2 (0-0.4)	0.8 (0.6-0.9)	1.3 (0.4-3.9)
M:E ratio	1.24	2.91	3.83	1.40	3.83	3.9	2.5	2.71	1.5-3.3

*Data from references 24, 28, 45, 54, 77, and 82.

Table 2-4. Average normal blood values in infancy and childhood*

Age	Hemoglobin (gm/dl)	RBC (×10¹²/liter)	Hematocrit (%)	MCV (fl)	MCH (pg)	MCHC (%)	Reticulocytes (%)
Cord blood	16.8	5.25	63	120	34	31.7	3.2
1 day	19.0	5.14	61	119	36.9	31.6	3.2
3 days	18.7	5.11	62	116	36.5	31.1	3.8
7 days	17.9	4.86	56	118	36.2	32.0	0.5
2 weeks	17.3	4.80	54	112	36.8	32.1	0.5
3 weeks	15.6	4.20	46	111	37.1	33.9	0.8
4 weeks	14.2	4.00	43	105	35.5	33.5	0.6
2 months	10.7	3.40	31	93	31.5	34.1	1.8
3 months	11.3	3.70	33	88	30.5	34.8	0.7
6 months	12.3	4.60	36	78	27	34	1.4
8 months	12.1	4.6	36	77	26	34	1.1
10 months	11.9	4.6	36	77	26	34	1.0
1 year	11.6	4.6	35	77	25	33	0.9
2 years	11.7	4.7	35	78	25	33	1.0
4 years	12.6	4.7	37	80	27	34	1.0
6 years	12.7	4.7	38	80	27	33	1.0
8 years	12.9	4.7	39	80	27	33	1.0
10-12 years	13.0	4.8	39	80	27	33	1.0
Adult men	16.0	5.4	47	87	29	34	1.0
Adult women	14.0	4.8	42	87	29	34	1.0

*Based on standard sources[35,55] and observations made at The New York Hospital–Cornell Medical Center.

the first day of life an elevation of the hemoglobin level occurs. This is caused by the shift of fluid (plasma) from the vascular to the extravascular compartment. The postnatal rise in hemoglobin level (and packed cell volume) takes place within a few minutes of birth and is complete within 1 to 2 hours, increasing by 17% to 20% of the initial values and reaching a value of 19.1 ± 2.4 gm/dl in 1 to 8 hours. The extent to which placental blood transfer contributes to this rise has been controversial, but early cord clamping is associated with a less marked rise in hemoglobin level.[16]

Blood samples from a heel puncture show a higher concentration of hemoglobin than those from a vein. This may be a result of the stasis of newborn macrocytic cells in the peripheral blood and their decreased deformability. Mollison and Cutbush[58] give the following comparative normal hemoglobin values for newborn infants: cord blood, 13.6 to 19.6 gm/dl; venous blood, 14.5 to 22.5 gm/dl; skin prick, 15.4 to 22.8 gm/dl. These variations are important in the management of erythroblastosis (Chapter 10).

The gradual drop in hemoglobin level reaches a nadir at 2 months of age and is followed by a rise, reaching a maximum at 14 years of 16 gm/dl for males and 14 gm/dl for females, with an average of 15 gm/dl for both sexes (Table 2-4).

The hematologic changes that occur in early infancy are usually orderly and gradual and appear to be directed toward the establishment of hematopoietic equilibrium designed to function at a low-

er level than exists at birth. Although hemolysis accounts for the decrease in hemoglobin level and number of red cells, the continued drop represents a diminished rate of compensatory regeneration. The fall in hemoglobin level represents a gradual adjustment to the increased oxygen saturation of the blood that prevails when the lung replaces the placenta as a source of oxygen. The oxygen saturation at birth is elevated from about 65% in the umbilical vein to 95% a few hours after birth.[22]

Other factors contributing to the decreased hematopoietic drive are the decline in the concentration of fetal hemoglobin and the increase in β-globin and adult hemoglobin synthesis. The oxygen affinity of fetal hemoglobin is much higher than that of adult hemoglobin and is in part related to the decreased reactivity of fetal hemoglobin with 2,3-diphosphoglycerate (2,3-DPG), a glycolytic intermediate that reversibly and allosterically binds with hemoglobin and decreases oxygen affinity. With the normal decline in the concentration of fetal hemoglobin during the first few months of life (Fig. 2-1), a progressive decline in oxygen affinity and a rightward shift in the oxygen dissociation curve occur (Fig. 2-2). The net effect is the maintenance of adequate tissue oxygenation despite a decrease in the concentration of hemoglobin.

Spurious elevations in hemoglobin concentration can be found using the Coulter Model S counter in patients with triglyceridemia, especially if the values exceed 1,000 mg/dl.[61] Triglycerides

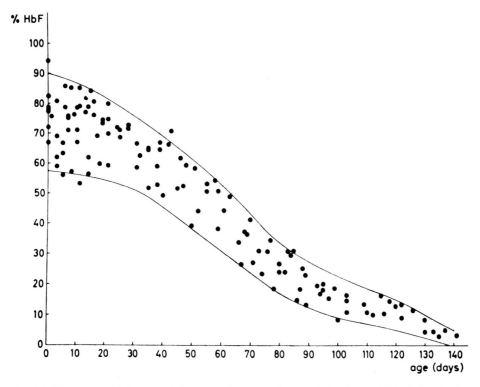

Fig. 2-1. Time course of the normal decline in the concentration of fetal hemoglobin during the first few months of life. (From Garby, L., and Sjolin, S.: Acta Paediatr. Scand. **51:**245, 1962.)

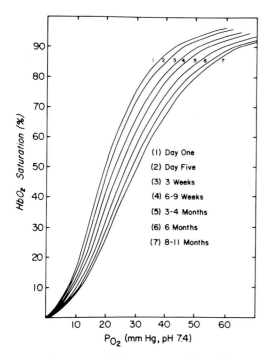

Fig. 2-2. Oxygen equilibrium curve of blood from term infants at different postnatal ages. P_{50} is 19.4 ± 1.8 mm Hg on day 1 and has shifted to 30.3 ± 0.7 at age 11 months. (Normal adult value = 27.0 ± 1.1 mm Hg.) (From Delivoria-Papadopoulos, M., et al.: Pediatr. Res. **5:**235, 1971.)

cause turbidity that interferes with the automated spectrophotometric determination of hemoglobin and accordingly the derived values for mean corpuscular hemoglobin and mean corpuscular hemoglobin concentration are also elevated. In such instances, a manual hemoglobin determination using the patient's turbid plasma as a blank should correct the artifact.

Erythrocyte count. The red cell count is high at birth and averages 5.2×10^{12}/liter with a range from 4.7 to 5.9×10^{12}/liter. The red cells are macrocytic at birth. They range in size from 8 to 9 μ in diameter, decrease to their smallest diameter of about 5 μ after 3 to 6 months, and increase to adult dimensions of 7.2 to 7.5 μ at 8 months.[35]

The red blood cell count averages 4.6×10^{12}/liter at the end of the first year and 4.8×10^{12}/liter at 12 years. At 14 years of age and over, red cell counts in males average 5.4 and in females average 4.8×10^{12}/liter.

Hematocrit (volume of packed red cells). The hematocrit obtained after centrifugation of a given amount of blood averages 55% at birth. The hematocrits together with the hemoglobin values increase sharply during the first few hours of life and then slowly decrease, so that by the end of the first week of life they approximate the initial cord blood values. The hematocrit of the capillary blood in healthy newborn infants is 63% ± 3.2% and decreases to 54% ± 2.5% by the tenth day of life.[26] At 1 week of age the mean capillary hematocrit (57.8% ± 2.4%) is significantly higher than the mean venous hematocrit of 55.8% ± 2.0%.

The hematocrit declines to 30% by the second month, increases to 35% at 1 year of age and 38% at 3 years of age, and achieves normal adult values of about 47% for males and 42% for females in adolescence. These changes simulating polycythemia are transient and benign, revert to normal in the postadolescent period, and require no treatment.

Hematocrits in adolescence. A large-scale survey performed in the United States in 1966-1970 has provided data on hematocrits in youths 12 to 17 years of age.[40] In boys, mean hematocrits increase consistently with age from a low of 40.5% for 12-year-olds to a high of 45.8% for 17-year-olds, an increase in hematocrit of about 1%/year. This increase of hematocrits with age does not occur in girls, the mean hematocrits remaining within the range of 40.3% to 40.7% throughout adolescence (Fig. 2-3). The differences between mean hematocrits of male and female adolescents increases consistently with age. The sex difference in hematocrits is unrelated to geography, race, or socioeconomic factors. However, the mean hematocrits are higher in white youths and those with higher family income and parental education

than in black adolescents and those in lower socioeconomic groups. Among white boys and girls in all age groups a consistent increase in mean hematocrit was found both with increase in family income and with increase in parental education.

Red blood cell indices. Quantification of indices of erythrocytes based on ratios of packed red cell volume, red blood cell count, and hemoglobin concentration provides a useful means of designating anemias. The normal indices are not constant during infancy and childhood.

Mean corpuscular volume. The mean corpuscular volume (MCV) represents the mean or average volume of a single red cell. The result is expressed in femtoliters (fl, or 10^{-15} liter). It is also expressed in cubic microns (μ^3).

$$MCV = \frac{\text{volume packed red cells (liter/liter)} \times 1,000}{\text{red blood cell count } (\times 10^{12}/\text{liter})}$$

For example, if the red blood cell count is 5×10^{12}/liter and the volume of packed red cells (hematocrit) is 0.45 liter/liter (45%):

$$MCV = \frac{0.45 \times 1,000}{5}$$
$$= 90 \text{ fl}$$

The normal range of MCV is 80 to 94 fl. An MCV of more than 94fl indicates macrocytes; 80 to 94 fl, normocytes; and less than 80 fl, microcytes. The MCV is unusually large at birth, with an average cord blood value of 119 fl and a range of 110 to 128 fl.[4,35] According to Guest and Brown,[34] the MCV in the newborn averages 113 ± 0.8 fl, and at 1 week it averages 106 ± 6 fl. At 6 months it drops to 78 ± 0.7 fl; at 1 year it is 73 ± 1.1 fl; and at 14 years it is 81 ± 1.1 fl. The lower limit of normal (80 fl) for children and adults is reached at 4 to 5 years.[35]

Mean corpuscular hemoglobin. Mean corpuscular hemoglobin (MCH) represents the average *quantity (weight)* of hemoglobin per individual red cell. Results are expressed in picograms (pg) or micromicrograms ($\mu\mu$g, or 10^{-12} gm).

$$MCH = \frac{\text{hemoglobin (gm/liter)}}{\text{red blood cell count } (\times 10^{12}/\text{liter})}$$

For example, if the red blood cell count is 5×10^{12}/liter and the hemoglobin level is 15 gm/dl (150 gm/liter):

$$MCH = \frac{150}{5}$$
$$= 30 \text{ pg}$$

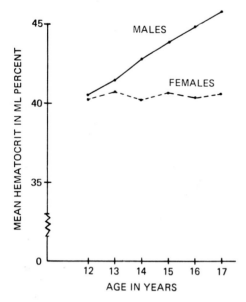

Fig. 2-3. Mean hematocrits for youths aged 12 to 17 years, by age and sex: United States, 1966-1970. (From Heald, F., et al.: Pub. No. 75-1628, Vital and Health Statistics Series 11 No. 146, U.S. Department of Health, Education, and Welfare, 1974.)

The normal range of MCH is 27 to 32 pg. The decline in MCH parallels the MCV fairly closely. An MCH with normal hemoglobin content is called normochromic; above normal, hyperchromic; below normal, hypochromic.

Mean corpuscular hemoglobin concentration. The mean corpuscular hemoglobin concentration (MCHC) represents the average *concentration* of hemoglobin in the individual red cell as calculated from the amount of hemoglobin per 100 ml of cells rather than of whole blood. The result is expressed as a percentage or more accurately in grams of hemoglobin per deciliter of packed red cells (gm/dl, or gm/100 ml).

$$\text{MCHC} = \frac{\text{hemoglobin (gm/dl)}}{\text{volume packed red cells (liter/liter)}}$$

For example if the hemoglobin level is 15 gm/dl and the volume of packed red cells (hematocrit) is 0.45 liter/liter:

$$\text{MCHC} = \frac{15}{0.45}$$
$$= 33 \text{ gm/dl}$$

The MCHC remains constant throughout infancy and childhood. The adult MCHC of 33 gm/dl (33%) is reached at about 6 months of age.

Red cells with an MCHC of less than 33 gm/dl are hypochromic. At approximately 34 gm/dl the normal erythrocyte contains a maximal number of hemoglobin molecules. Hyperchromia in reality describes an increased intensity of staining of red cells.

• • •

Standardization, calibration, and quality control of electronic and automated instruments is critically essential for accurate and reproducible results.

Discrepancies between the given values for red cell indices in the older literature and those in more recent studies are in part related to differences in methodology and instrumentation.[55] The error inherent in performing a red blood cell count by the hemocytometer method is notoriously high compared with the precision of 1% to 2% when red cells are counted electronically. Some automatic cell counters (e.g., Coulter Model S) compute the hematocrit electronically from the measured red cell count and MCV.

Reticulocytes. According to Windle,[93] there are about 90% reticulocytes in the blood of the human fetus at 3 months of gestation and 15% to 30% at 6 months of gestation. Lower values, 40% at 12 weeks of gestation and 5% to 10% at 24 weeks of gestation, have been reported more recently.[64] Reticulocytes number 4% to 6% at birth and reflect active red cell formation in fetal life. The reticulocytosis at birth remains constant for about 3 days.[75] From the fourth day to the sixth day there is a pronounced drop, and from the sixth to the seventh day there is a further and slower decrease to a low level of 0.5%. A slight increase in reticulocytes

is again noted at approximately 2 months of age, followed by a slight decline from 3 months until 2 years, when adult levels are attained.

Normoblasts. Normoblasts are frequently observed in the normal infant on the first day of life but usually disappear during the first week, in most instances by the third to the fifth day. The average number at birth ranges from 3 to 10/100 white blood cells, or 0.3 to 3×10^9/liter. Occasional nucleated red cells are observed in the peripheral blood of an older infant with acute infection associated with anemia or in severe hemolytic anemias. The presence of normoblasts in the blood of older patients with pancytopenia is indicative of bone marrow embarrassment and frequently invasion of the marrow by tumor or replacement by leukemia. With hypoxia and anemia associated with blood loss and hemolysis or in infections such as congenital syphilis or rubella, sepsis, or the occasional case of cytomegalic inclusion disease, increased numbers of normoblasts appear in the peripheral blood at birth and in the neonatal period.

Platelets. Variable numbers of platelets have been given for the neonatal period. Some workers have found fewer platelets during the first 48 hours than in older infants. Figures reported at the time of birth range from 150 to 350×10^9/liter. In a series of 204 platelet counts in 105 normal full-term newborn infants, the normal range in the first 96 hours of life was 100 to 300×10^9/liter.[2] At 2 weeks of age the average platelet count is 300×10^9/liter. The smaller number of platelets at birth has been attributed to birth trauma.

The platelets of the newborn infant also show greater variation in size and shape than those of adults, in whom larger platelets are found in appreciable numbers[84] and are considered to represent younger platelets.[48] Adult values of 250 to 350×10^9/liter are reached at about 6 months of age. The platelet count in premature infants is discussed on p. 14.

White blood cells. The total leukocyte count is high at birth, ranging from 9 to 30×10^9/liter during the first 2 days of life, with an average of 22×10^9/liter at the end of 12 hours.[4] In the first week the white blood cell count drops to an average of 12×10^9/liter with a range of 5 to 21×10^9/liter. At the end of the first year the white blood cell count averages 12×10^9/liter with a gradual decline to values of 8 to 10×10^9/liter by the fourth year. The white blood cell count and absolute granulocyte count are lower genetically in blacks[76] and in Yemenite Jews[17] than in whites.

Neutrophilic leukocytes. Neutrophilic leukocytes average 60% at birth, with a range from 40% to 80%, and may include a small percentage of metamyelocytes and myelocytes. The average drops to 40% by the tenth day and then to 30% in the fourth to the sixth month. It remains at this level until the fourth year, when a rise to 40% occurs. In the sixth year adult values of 55% to 60% are attained.

Eosinophils and basophils. Levels of eosinophils and basophils are maintained at 2% to 3% and 0.5%, respectively, throughout infancy and childhood.

Lymphocytes. Lymphocytes average 30% at birth and rise to 60% in the fourth to sixth month. These values are maintained until they drop to 50% in the fourth year, to 40% at the end of the sixth year, and to 30% by the eighth year.

Monocytes. Monocytes number 6% at birth and, except for a rise to 9% in the second and third weeks, remain at levels of about 5% during infancy and childhood.

Plasma cells. Plasma cells are not found in the embryo but appear after birth in interstitial, lymphoid, and glandular tissue. Increased numbers of plasma cells have been noted in patients with infections in whom hypergammaglobulinemia is found. On the other hand, patients with agammaglobulinemia regularly exhibit a deficiency of plasma cells in hematopoietic centers and in inflammatory exudates.[6,30]

Summary of white blood cell changes. Certain approximate values may be designated for comparative purposes. At birth a leukocytosis is present with mean counts of 18×10^9/liter and 60% neutrophils. At the end of the second month of life leukocytes total 12×10^9/liter with 35% granulocytes and 60% lymphocytes. These values are maintained until the fourth and fifth years, when the total white cell count drops to 8×10^9/liter and the differential percentage is reversed to 60% granulocytes and 35% lymphocytes. From the sixth to the fourteenth year there is a gradual numerical shift to adult values of 7×10^9 white blood cells/liter with 65% neutrophilic granulocytes and 30% lymphocytes. Newborn infants with total leukocyte counts at either extreme should be investigated for existing abnormalities.

EXAMINATION OF BONE MARROW

Aspiration and biopsy of the bone marrow constitute useful laboratory aids in the diagnosis of blood disorders. The accessibility of the marrow, its responses to stimuli producing depression or hyperplasia, its availability for repeated examinations, and the comparative ease of identifying the cellular elements account for the frequency with which aspiration is performed.[80] Disturbances of each of the principal blood elements are frequently reflected earlier or are more conspicuous in the bone marrow than in the peripheral blood. In patients with leukemia, for instance, the bone marrow may be extensively infiltrated with leukoblas-

tic cells, whereas they appear in the peripheral blood in such scant numbers as to be overlooked. In patients with hypoplastic-aplastic anemias and in those with the hemolytic anemias, bone marrow studies permit quantitative estimation of the cell types involved. Improved needles permit the simultaneous performance of bone marrow aspiration and biopsy, the latter of particular importance to determine more accurately marrow cellularity and architecture and to detect the presence of tumor or storage cells.[15] Bone marrow examination serves as a guide to therapy with hematinic and chemotherapeutic agents.

Technique of bone marrow aspiration

The sternal manubrium is rarely the optimal site for bone marrow aspiration in children and should be avoided. Other areas offer the advantages of being less dangerous, less painful, and less emotionally traumatic to the patient. Such sites are the posterior and anterior superior iliac crests, the lower thoracic and lumbar vertebral spinous processes, and, in the first few months of life, the tibial tuberosity. In children older than 18 months to 2 years, the iliac crests are the most popular and safest areas. It is probably wise to reserve use of the tibia for exceptional circumstances, since fractures or lacerations of major blood vessels have resulted from punctures at this site.

For children who are uneasy, frightened, or even hysterical about bone marrow aspiration, the combination of the following drugs may be administered orally or intramuscularly approximately 1 hour before the procedure: meperidine (Demerol), 2 mg/kg; promethazine (Phenergan), 1 mg/kg; and chlorpromazine (Thorazine), 1 mg/kg. The cooperation of the patient for subsequent bone marrow studies is directly proportional to the painlessness and ease of the initial examination. Every effort should be made to ensure that a skilled and experienced individual performs the procedure. Thus sedatives and their attendant side effects may be obviated for future attempts, and an adequate sample should be obtained.

Skin preparation should include the use of povidone-iodine (Betadine) or a similar topical antiseptic. Local anesthesia is obtained by the use of 1% procaine or lidocaine (Xylocaine) solution. This is performed with a 25-gauge needle. Following the intradermal injection of approximately 0.2 ml of the local anesthetic agent, a short time is necessary to allow adequate anesthetic effect to occur. The subcutaneous tissue is next injected with proper care to avoid touching the periosteum. Another short interval will allow further injection of the periosteal layer with minimum discomfort to the patient.

A spring-loaded jet gun injector is commercially available.* Intradermal, subcutaneous, and periosteal infiltration are accomplished in a single quick procedure, obviating needle infiltration. In our experience local anesthesia is much better in thinner children with easily palpated crests or spines than in obese children.

An 18-gauge 1½ - or 2-inch bone marrow needle with an obturator is used in the majority of children, although a smaller gauge and length may be employed for very young infants. Gripping the needle between the thumb and forefinger with the hub firmly against the thenar eminence provides excellent control of direction during the procedure. The needle should be guided at the skin's surface by the fingers of the operator's nondominant hand to prevent it from slipping off the bony prominence while pressure is being exerted. Laceration of the skin with a scalpel blade is unnecessary if the needle tip is sharp and should be avoided. The skin should be entered at an angle. The point of insertion should be in the midpoint of the superior spine of the posterior iliac crest, 1 cm below the lip of the ilium, or the midpoint of the spinous process. The angle of insertion into the periosteum should be perpendicular to the iliac crest or spinous process. A slow, steady, forceful, clockwise, circular motion should be used to advance the needle in bone. Once the tip of the needle has been inserted through the periosteum, the needle is advanced a few millimeters with added pressure until it is firmly fixed within the bone. A sense of "give" is occasionally felt as the needle enters the marrow cavity.

Moisture on the stylet or pain on its removal often indicates the intramedullary location of the needle. A 10 ml plastic syringe is attached to the needle. The actual aspiration of marrow contents is usually painful and it is wise to prewarn the patient that if pain occurs it will signify the end of the aspiration procedure. To minimize admixture with blood, only 0.2 to 0.3 ml of marrow is withdrawn into the syringe. *One should then release the suction in the syringe.* This maneuver is necessary to avoid spreading the aspirate along the walls of the syringe when the needle is being removed from the bone. The needle, still attached to the syringe, is removed from the puncture site and the aspirate is expelled onto a clean, alcohol-washed, dry glass slide. At this time speed is essential to avoid coagulation and loss of cells, especially megakaryocytes. Bone marrow particles (fragments or spicules) will settle on the slide, which may be tipped to permit drainage of blood or aspirated with gentle suction. Smears are made on glass slides. Wright's stain is satisfactory for routine use, but Wright-Giemsa–stained prepara-

tions provide better cellular detail. Enough smears should be made for special histochemical studies, such as for iron, glycogen (periodic acid–Schiff), lipids, peroxidase, esterases, and other intracellular enzymes as indicated. Smears from spicules offer a more accurate estimate of cellular content and arrangement of the bone marrow than smears from the total aspirate. Some centers add a small aliquot of the aspirated whole marrow sample to a solution of EDTA, centrifuge in a Wintrobe sedimentation tube, and measure the bone marrow hematocrit and nucleated cell layer (buffy layer) to estimate marrow cellularity. Smears are then prepared from this concentrated specimen as well as from the direct marrow aspirate. In most laboratories a minimum of 300 nucleated cells are counted.

A total nucleated cell count is made by diluting the fluid marrow as for a peripheral white blood cell count using an automatic cell counter or chamber. Aspirated marrow samples are often cultured for bacteria, fungi, and viruses and provide cells for chromosome analysis or for in vitro bone marrow culture.[70]

Technique of bone marrow biopsy

The posterior iliac crest is the preferred site for bone marrow biopsy, a procedure that has added another dimension to diagnostic morphology.[80] The aspiration smear does not invariably give a correct idea of the relative distribution of the cell types present. Architectural derangements of the marrow and especially the significance of the "dry top" are interpreted more reliably and accurately by biopsy. A generous plug of bone marrow can be obtained consistently and easily without recourse to a surgical procedure. The technique permits both aspiration and biopsy in a single procedure. The Vim-Silverman needle consists of three parts: an outer needle, an obturator, and cutting blades. The biopsy needle is placed into the marrow cavity and the obturator is removed and replaced by the cutting blades. The Jamshidi needle has a tapered cutting edge, a sharp inner stylet that projects beyond the tapered distal portion of the cutting edge, and a probe. The stylet is removed just before the marrow cavity is entered. A further advance of the needle provides a more adequate and usually a less distorted and crushed sample of bone marrow than that obtained with the Vim-Silverman needle. "Touch" preparations on slides are made immediately; the core is then placed in Zenker's solution for standard sections and stains.

Normal values

The figures in Table 2-3 represent the approximate range and average values of the cellular ele-

*Styrijet, Mizzy Co., Clifton Forge, Va.

ments in samples of the bone marrow obtained from normal infants and children. Erythroid hyperplasia is characteristically present at birth, but by the first week the granulocytic series predominates. By 1 to 3 months the lymphocytes increase in number, and they often reach levels of 50% of the nucleated cells in the marrow during the first year. The presence of a lymphocytosis of this magnitude need not give rise to unnecessary concern, provided that the cells are morphologically normal. Immature white blood cell precursors, including lymphoblasts and myeloblasts, may comprise up to 10% of the marrow cells in the first few months of life. Between 4 and 8 years of age, the granulocytic precursors and granulocytes equal the lymphocytes numerically, and eventually they predominate, reaching adult values at about 12 years of age.

Myeloid:erythroid ratio. The myeloid:erythroid (M:E) ratio provides an index of depression or hyperactivity of the granulocytic elements as compared with nucleated red cells. In the newborn infant the M:E ratio rises from 1.2:1 on the first day of life to about 4:1 to 6:1 in the first and second weeks, indicative of a decline of erythrocyte production. Beyond infancy, the M:E ratio is 2.5:1 to 3.5:1.[96]

Characteristics of primitive blood cells

Primitive cells of both the red and white cell series possess similar structural characteristics and in their maturation reveal many points in common. The early blast forms are large, the cytoplasm is deeply basophilic, the nucleus occupies more space and stains less deeply than the cytoplasm (leptochromatic), the chromatin is finely granular, and one or more nucleoli are present. At this stage, classification of primitive cells is facilitated by comparison with more mature cells with which they are associated by noting morphologic similarities. Maturation is accompanied by the following features: in the primitive cell in each series the nucleus becomes progressively smaller, the cytoplasm content decreases, the basophilia (paralleling ribonucleic acid content) of the cytoplasm lessens, the chromatin becomes more condensed, its original purplish color changes to dark blue, and the nucleoli disappear early. In the red cell the basophilia is replaced by hemoglobin. In the mature granulocyte the cytoplasm is faintly pink with specific granulation; in the lymphocyte a hyaline or sky-blue color; and in the monocyte, a gray-blue with fine reddish blue granules.

Stages in maturation of red blood cells

The normal progression of red cell maturation is based on intracellular chemical changes. A knowledge of these changes aids in identification of individual cells.

Nucleic acids and cellular growth. Cellular growth and multiplication of cells are closely identified with the content of the nucleic acids, deoxyribonucleic acid (DNA) and ribonucleic acid (RNA). Although they occur together, the former predominates in the chromatin of the cell nucleus and the latter in the cytoplasm and nucleolus. Rapid growth of all cellular types, especially during mitosis, is accompanied by increased concentrations of the nucleic acids.[31]

DNA, present in the nuclear material of all living cells, is the principal component of the genes. DNA consists of two polynucleotide chains forming an interlocking helix about the central axis. Sugar-phosphate backbones make up the lines of the helix, while purines (adenine and guanine) and pyrimidines (cytosine and thymine) point inward toward the center. The genetic information for protein structure (structural genes) and for the amount of protein synthesized (control genes) is encoded in DNA. The nuclear DNA code is transferred to messenger RNA (mRNA) by *transcription* by an enzyme, DNA-dependent RNA polymerase. The amino acid sequence along the polypeptide chain of a protein is determined by the sequence of three nucleotide bases (codon) transcribed from the DNA template to mRNA. The specific sequence of the three nucleotide bases controls the insertion of one of the twenty amino acids into a polypeptide chain. The actual assembly of amino acids into proteins occurs in cytoplasmic RNA ribosomes and requires mRNA, transfer RNA, amino acids, various enzymes, initiation factors, elongation factors, and chain terminators. A fuller discussion of protein synthesis is found in Chapter 13 and in several excellent reviews.[88,89]

Polychromasia and stippling. Admixtures of basophilic substance and hemoglobin in intermediate stages of red cell maturation produce polychromatophilia of the cytoplasm. Stippling (punctate basophilia) refers to the fine or coarse bluish violet granules (ribosomal RNA) found in red cells stained with Wright's or similar Romanowsky stains. Stippled cells are noted in a variety of clinical conditions such as lead poisoning and hemolytic and nutritional anemias of varying severity.

Basophilia. Deep basophilia of the cytoplasm characterizes the stem cell and red and white cell precursors at the "blast" level of immaturity. The high content of RNA parallels the maximal cytoplasmic basophilia. The basophilic staining is ascribed to the affinity of cytoplasmic RNA for the basic component (methylene blue) of Wright's stain or other polychromatic stains. In all cell types basophilia recedes with increasing maturity, and in the red cell its gradual replacement by hemoglobin results in an increased affinity for acid dyes (eosin).

Normal erythrocyte maturation (Plate 1)

In normal maturation the cytoplasm and nucleus mature simultaneously and synchronously. The stages of normal red cell development and their chief distinguishing morphologic and staining characteristics as determined by light microscopy are as follows.

Pronormoblast (proerythroblast). The diameter of a pronormoblast is 14 to 19 μ. The cytoplasm is narrow rimmed and deeply basophilic except for a small pale area at the periphery of the nucleus. The nucleus is light purplish, vesicular, and granular; there is slight chromatin clumping; and one or more nucleoli are present.

Basophilic normoblast (early normoblast or erythroblast). The basophilic normoblast is smaller than the pronormoblast (12 to 17 μ in diameter). The cytoplasm is basophilic. The nucleus is darker purplish staining; chromatin clumping is more marked; there may be a cartwheel arrangement of chromatin; and nucleoli are absent.

Polychromatophilic normoblast (intermediate normoblast, late erythroblast). The diameter of a polychromatophilic normoblast is 12 to 15 μ. The cytoplasm is less basophilic, with traces of hemoglobin present. The nucleus is shrunken and more mature, and the chromatin is bluish black, coarse, and clumped; a light area resembling hemoglobin is often seen at one pole of the nucleus.

Orthochromic normoblast (late normoblast). The orthochromic normoblast has a diameter of 8 to 12 μ. The cytoplasm is almost completely filled with hemoglobin, late forms staining red, or eosinophilic. In the nucleus the chromatin is a condensed, dark, homogeneous structureless mass referred to as pyknotic.

Reticulocytes. A reticulocyte is slightly larger than a normal erythrocyte, and the nucleus has been extruded. The reticulum or filamentous substance, varying in amounts and arrangements, stains deep blue with supravital stains such as brilliant cresyl blue or new methylene blue; the smallest amounts of staining are seen in those that are nearly mature. Reticulum, a precipitate material composed of ribosomal RNA, corresponds to the basophilia of the cytoplasm and is not related to nuclear remnants, mitochondria, or hemoglobin. Reticulocytes formed during periods of rapid cell production differ from those formed under normal conditions.[41,42,79] They are known as stress or shift reticulocytes; they are delivered prematurely from the marrow pool into the circulating blood and require 1 to 3 days longer than the normal reticulocytes to lose their reticulum (1 to 2 days). These immature or stress reticulocytes are recognizable through their relatively large size and increased basophilia. They are of greater diameter, contain more reticulum and ATP, and are of lower density than the normal reticulocyte; approximately 25%

of stress reticulocytes are destroyed within 10 days, whereas the remainder have a longer life span.

The normal erythrocyte. The erythrocyte is the mature end stage of erythropoiesis. It is a round, flat, biconcave, nonnucleated disc with a diameter of 7 to 8.5 μ. It cannot be mistaken for any other cell. The mean thickness of normal erythrocytes is between 1.64 and 2.14 μ,[94] the mean volume is about 87 fl, and the surface area is about 140 μ^2.[94]

Normal leukocyte maturation

The leukocytes present in the normal blood comprise three main groups: the granulocytic or mycloid series, the lymphocytes, and the monocytes. The individual types of white cells differ from one another in structure and function. For practical purposes, development of leukocytes may be regarded as proceeding in definitive lines: the myeloblast gives rise to myelocytes and granulocytes, the lymphoblast to lymphocytes, and monoblasts to monocytes. A pluripotential stem cell is thought to be the primitive precursor of the specific blast cell. Primitive cells of both red and white cell series possess similar structural and staining characteristics and in their maturation reveal many common features. The immature forms of all white cells (the myeloblast, lymphoblast, and monoblast) are not found in the peripheral blood of the normal person, but their differentiation assumes importance in persons with leukemia in whom they infiltrate both bone marrow and blood.

Myeloid series (Plate 1). Myeloid maturation is characterized by the development of dark bluish primary granules that increase in number and are replaced by specific secondary granules, differing in their staining affinity for Romanowsky dyes. The granules of basophils are stained blue with basic dyes; the granules of eosinophils are stained reddish orange with acidic dyes; and the granules of neutrophils do not stain intensely with either dye. With increasing maturity the nuclei of basophilic, eosinophilic, and neutrophilic precursors become progressively smaller and multilobular.

Myeloblast. Myeloblasts have a diameter of 15 to 20 μ. Their cytoplasm is abundant, with no specific granules, peripheral tags, or buds. The nucleus has a fine chromatin network with finely divided particles; a smooth, thin nuclear membrane; and two or more distinct nucleoli with indefinite nucleolar membranes. Supravital staining shows fine, spherical mitochondria diffusely scattered in cytoplasm. The morphologic differences between the myeloblast, monoblast, and lymphoblast, when stained by Wright's method, are listed in Table 2-5.

Promyelocyte. Promyelocytes are the same size or larger than myeloblasts. The cytoplasm is deep-

Table 2-5. Morphologic differences between myeloblast, monoblast, and lymphoblast

	Myeloblast	Monoblast	Lymphoblast
Diameter	14 to 20 μ	12 to 18 μ	8 to 20 μ
Cytoplasm	Abundant, agranular	Abundant, blunt pseudopodia	Scanty
Nuclear membrane	Smooth and thin	Prominent	Dense
Nucleus	Round or oval	Indented, lobulated	Round or oval
Chromatin	Fine network, finely divided	Sparse, fine, lacy	Coarse, some aggregation
Nucleoli	Prominent, 2 to 5	Prominent, 2 to 4	1 to 2
Nucleolar membrane	Indefinite		Distinct
Mitochondria (supravital staining)	Fine, spheric, scattered diffusely	Fine, numerous	Larger, oval, close to nucleus
Peroxidase reaction	Positive	Negative or weakly positive	Negative
Periodic acid–Schiff reaction (PAS)	Negative	Negative or weakly positive	Positive
Naphthol-AS-acetate esterase reaction	Positive	Positive (inhibited by NaF)	Negative

ly basophilic and may be abundant or confined to a narrow margin around the nucleus. The granules are relatively few (the earliest forms have no more than ten granules), overlie the nucleus, are nonspecific, stain deep red to dark blue, and increase in number as the cell matures. The granules are peroxidase positive. The nuclei are round, the chromatin is coarser, and the nucleoli are not so numerous and so sharply demarcated as those in the myeloblast.

Myelocytes. Myelocytes are about the same size or smaller than promyelocytes. The cytoplasm stains reddish purple and contains numerous dark granules that are scattered throughout and also cover the nucleus. As the myelocytes mature, the granules assume a definitive neutrophilic, eosinophilic, and basophilic character. Each of these cells in turn becomes a progenitor of the respective fully mature granulocyte. The nuclei are round, oval, or flattened on one side, the chromatin is thick and unevenly stained, and the nucleoli are indistinct.

Metamyelocyte. Metamyelocytes are smaller than myelocytes. The cytoplasm is less basophilic than that in the myelocyte, and an eosinophilic cast predominates. Granules are smaller, stain less deeply, and are clearly differentiated as neutrophilic, eosinophilic, or basophilic. Ameboid motion initially observed in the late myelocyte is definitely established and characterizes the more mature cells. The nucleus is oval, slightly indented, or kidney shaped. Chromatin strands are coarse but not so deeply stained as those in more mature cells. The nuclear membrane is sharply defined, and nucleoli are not observed. The cytoplasm and nucleus may not develop evenly (asyn-

chronous maturation), so that precise classification as late myelocyte and metamyelocyte is not always possible.

Band or nonsegmented forms. Band forms are slightly smaller than metamyelocytes. The cytoplasm consists of small, evenly distributed granules staining various shades of pink or blue in the neutrophil series, reddish orange in eosinophils, and deep bluish purple in basophils. The nucleus is horseshoe shaped with deep indentations. There is irregular condensation of the nucleus with a pyknotic area at each end. The nonsegmented polymorphonuclear neutrophils number 4% to 5% of the total number of leukocytes.

Segmented forms

NEUTROPHILS. The polymorphonuclear neutrophil measures 9 to 12 μ, with an average diameter of 10 μ. The cytoplasm is faintly pink, with minute granules that fill the cell and stain pink, or blue-violet. The nucleus is deep purple, with coarsely condensed chromatin strands. The nucleus consists of two to five lobes connected by a thin strand or filament of chromatin.

SEX DIFFERENCE IN NEUTROPHILS. A sex difference in the nuclear structure of the human polymorphonuclear neutrophilic leukocyte has been described.[55] In the female a solitary "drumstick" with a well-defined solid round head, 1.5 μ in diameter, is joined by a single fine chromatin strand to one of the main lobes of the nucleus (Fig. 2-4). These structures are rarely found in the unsegmented forms, nonneutrophils, or precursors. This distinctive nuclear appendage has been found in females of all ages and in blood specimens from the umbilical cord.[83] They are present in males with Klinefelter's syndrome (XXY karyotype) and

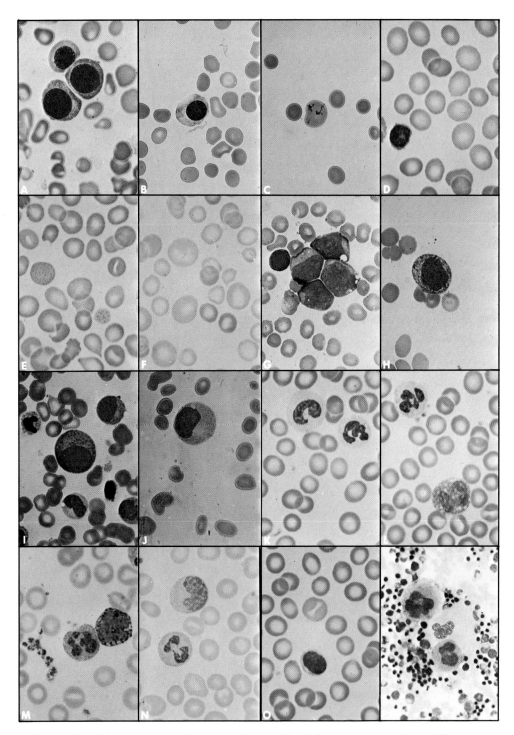

Plate 1. Normal bone marrow and peripheral blood cells. **A,** Pronormoblast and basophilic normoblasts. **B,** Polychromatophilic and orthochromic normoblasts. **C,** Reticulocytes. **D,** Normal red blood cell. **E,** Basophilic stippling. **F,** Stress macrocytes in polychromasia. **G,** Myeloblast. **H,** Promyelocyte. **I,** Myelocyte. **J,** Metamyelocyte. **K,** Band and neutrophil. **L,** Eosinophil. **M,** Basophil. **N,** Monocyte. **O,** Lymphocyte. **P,** Megakaryocyte.

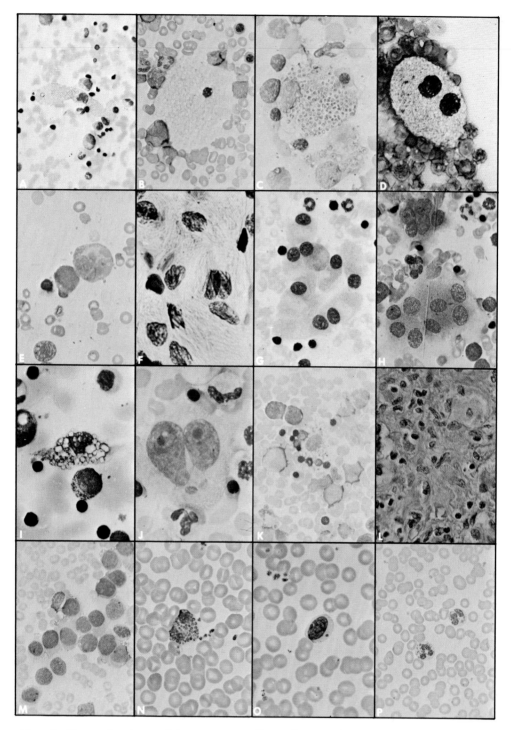

Plate 2. Abnormal and normal bone marrow cells. **A**, Letterer-Siwe disease. **B**, Neurovisceral lipidosis. **C**, Histoplasmosis. **D**, Niemann-Pick disease. **E**, Erythrophagocytosis. **F**, Gaucher's disease. **G**, Osteoblasts. **H**, Osteoclasts. **I**, Cystine storage disease. **J**, Hodgkin's disease (Reed-Sternberg cell). **K**, Rhopheocytosis. **L**, Chronic granulomatous disease. **M**, Metastatic rhabdomyosarcoma. **N**, Eosinophils in Chediak-Higashi disease. **O**, Lymphocytes in Chediak-Higashi disease. **P**, Neutrophils in Chediak-Higashi disease.

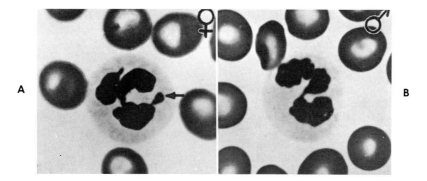

Fig. 2-4. A, Neutrophil in a blood film from a chromosomal female illustrating the accessory nuclear lobule that is present in an average of 2% to 3% of neutrophils in females. **B,** A similar accessory nuclear lobule does not occur in neutrophils of chromosomal males. (×1,800.) (From Grumback, M. M., and Barr, M. L.: In Pincus, G., ed.: Recent progress in hormone research, vol. 14, New York, 1958, Academic Press, Inc.)

absent in females with Turner's syndrome (XO karyotype). These appendages are not to be confused with sessile nodules and related structures that are attached to the nucleus of the polymorphonuclear cell in both the female and male.

A small mass, usually adjacent to the nuclear membrane, which stains deeply with hematoxylin, Feulgen reagent, and thionin, is known as the sex chromatin or Barr body.[5] It is present in 80% to 90% of the somatic cells of the normal female.

EOSINOPHILS. The eosinophil is a polymorphonuclear granulocyte the same size or a little larger than the neutrophil. The cytoplasm has large, coarse, spheric granules with an affinity for the eosin stain. Granules are scattered throughout the cytoplasm and superimposed on the nucleus, which is bilobed or has a band form. Eosinophils are less motile and more fragile than neutrophils and represent 1% to 40% of the total number of leukocytes.

BASOPHILS. Basophils are somewhat smaller than mature neutrophils. The cytoplasm contains large, round, coarse bluish black and azurophilic granules that obscure the nucleus by their number and intensity of staining. The granules are peroxidase negative. The background cytoplasm stains faint pink to lilac. The nucleus is round, kidney shaped, or slightly lobulated. The basophils number 0% to 0.5% in children and adults, are motile, and contain two very important compounds—heparin and histamine. These agents are released when the cell undergoes degranulation to participate in anaphylactic and lipemia-clearing reactions.[78]

Monocyte series (Plate 1)

Monoblasts. Monoblasts are difficult to differentiate from the corresponding myeloblasts and promyelocytes. Their diameter is 12 to 18 μ. The cells possess an irregular outline caused by the presence of blunt pseudopodia and are nonmotile.

The cytoplasm is deeply basophilic with a grayish blue cast, differing in this way from the blasts of other cell series. The cytoplasm contains vacuoles but no granules. The nucleus is large, round, or often kidney shaped, horseshoe shaped, or convoluted like the mature cell. The chromatin is fine and lacy and stains lighter than that in the mature monocyte. Nucleoli may or may not be present. The peroxidase reaction is negative or poorly defined. The naphthol-AS-acetate esterase reaction is positive and is inhibited by sodium fluoride. The presence of monocytes and promonocytes in the same smear facilitates the identification of the primitive monoblasts.

Promonocyte. The promonocyte is similar to the monoblast in terms of cell size and nuclear characteristics. The cytoplasm contains dustlike reddish blue granules and vacuoles. The cell is somewhat larger, and the cytoplasm is perhaps less granular than that in the older cell, the monocyte.

Monocyte. The diameter of a monocyte is 13 to 20 μ, larger than most cells found in the peripheral blood. The cytoplasm is abundant in relation to the nucleus; stains a dull gray, muddy blue color; is filled with large numbers of evenly spread, fine, lilac and reddish blue granules, interspersed among which are a lesser number of unevenly distributed azurophilic granules and occasional vacuoles. The granules are peroxidase positive but they are much fewer and finer than those in the granulocytes. The gray-blue cytoplasm of the monocyte contrasts with the clear light blue of the lymphocyte. The nucleus is somewhat eccentric, possessing a skeinlike or lacy structure that stains lighter than that of the lymphocyte or metamyelocyte. The chromatin is loosely arranged with light spaces and grooves in contrast to the clumped chromatin of the lymphocyte. The nucleus is indented, multilobulated, and convoluted, often presenting a folded appearance. The nuclear folds with the heavier staining at their margins are characteristic.

The monocyte is a motile cell with slow ameboid motion, in contrast to the more active neutrophil. The monocyte phagocytoses other blood cells, cellular fragments, particulate matter, microorganisms, and the incompletely lysed nuclei of other cells, as occurs in the formation of the "tart" cell. Monocytes represent 5% to 10% of the leukocytes.

Lymphoid series (Plate 1)

Lymphoblast. Lymphoblasts have a diameter of 8 to 20 μ. The cytoplasm is scanty, usually clear blue or deeply basophilic, and nongranular. The peroxidase stain is negative. The nucleus is large and round or oval, and it stains reddish purple with fine granular chromatin that is slightly more coarse than that found in the myeloblast. Deep nuclear clefts may be seen. One or two nucleoli are present, and the nuclear membrane is well defined. The PAS stain is positive.

Prolymphocytes (young lymphocytes). The diameter of prolymphocytes is 10 to 14 μ. The cytoplasm is deeply basophilic, homogeneous, and agranular. The nucleus is less compact than that of more mature lymphocytes, with light spaces between chromatin threads and indistinct nucleoli. Prolymphocytes are occasionally found in normal blood and more frequently in the blood of children, especially those with chronic upper respiratory tract infections with associated tonsillar and cervical node enlargement.

Large lymphocytes. Large lymphocytes have a diameter of 10 to 15 μ. The cytoplasm is more abundant than in the small lymphocyte and frequently contains azurophilic granules; the edges are frequently scalloped and stain clear light blue. Vacuoles may be present. A perinuclear clear zone is a differentiating feature. The nucleus is larger than that in the small lymphocyte; it is round, slightly indented, and thickened at the margins. The chromatin is paler and not nearly so markedly condensed as in the smaller lymphocytes.

During the first months of life small numbers of lymphocytes that resemble large lymphocytes

and the atypical lymphocytes found in patients with infectious mononucleosis are occasionally observed in the blood smears from normal infants. These cells, however, bear no relationship to this disease or any other related condition. Scattered vacuoles may be found normally in the rim of deeply staining blue cytoplasm. These cells are to be differentiated from the heavily vacuolated cells, producing a foamy appearance characterizing the lymphocytes of infectious mononucleosis.

Atypical lymphocytes are not specifically diagnostic but occur in a wide variety of diseases of suspected viral etiology, such as infectious mononucleosis, hepatitis, the posttransfusion syndrome, and drug sensitivities.[97]

Megakaryocytes

Megakaryocytes arise from mononuclear precursors.[36] In the earlier forms of megakaryocytes, the megakaryoblast and promegakaryocyte, the cytoplasm stains deep blue, is nongranular, and shows no evidence of platelet formation. In the mature megakaryocyte the cytoplasm is abundant and basophilic and contains numerous azurophilic granules. Masses of mature platelets often adhere to the periphery of the cells. The number of nuclei doubles with each mitosis. In normal bone marrow about 65% of the megakaryocytes contain eight diploid nuclei, 25% have sixteen nuclei, and 10% have four nuclei. The nuclei are large and are joined together in an irregular lobulated ring. According to Harker,[36] the cell accumulates cytoplasm in direct proportion to the number of nuclei formed during nuclear proliferation. In bone marrow smears and biopsies from normal individuals the megakaryocytes constitute 1 to 4/1,000 nucleated cells (0.1% to 0.4%). The morphologic features of the megakaryocytic series are listed in Table 2-6.

Miscellaneous bone marrow cells (Plate 2)

Histiocytes. Histiocytes are occasionally seen in the bone marrow. They are derivatives of the reticuloendothelial or macrophage-monocyte system and are also referred to as macrophages, clasmatocytes, and endothelial phagocytes. They are larg-

Table 2-6. Morphologic features of megakaryocytic series

Cell type	Cytoplasmic granules	Cytoplasmic tags	Platelets	Nuclear number and characteristics
Megakaryoblast	Absent	Present	Absent	Single, fine chromatin structure, nucleoli present
Promegakaryocyte	Few	Present	Absent	Double
Megakaryocyte	Numerous	Usually present	Absent	Two or more nuclei
Mature megakaryocyte	Aggregated	Absent	Present	Four or more nuclei

er than other cells of the peripheral blood (15 to 80 μ in diameter). The nucleus is larger and lighter in color than that of either the monocyte or lymphocyte. The cell outline is irregular because of the pseudopodial formation of the cytoplasm. Many of the histiocytes are actively phagocytic; the cytoplasm is vacuolated and may contain intact erythrocytes, remnants of other blood elements, and often peculiar reddish rodlike structures or granules. The granular form of histiocyte is also termed a Ferrata cell. The nucleus is usually oval or may be indented or elongated. The nuclear chromatin is coarse and one or more bluish nucleoli are readily demonstrable.

The macrophages or histiocytes are increased in number in patients with chronic inflammatory disorders, chronic myelocytic leukemia, agranulocytosis, aplastic anemia, viral diseases; in patients exposed to radioactive materials and chemicals; and in the tissues of patients with histiocytosis. Distinctive abnormal foamy histiocytes are seen in the bone marrow aspirations in patients with various lipid storage diseases.

Plasma cell (plasmacyte). The plasma cell is larger than the lymphocyte and has a round, oval, or elongated shape with abundant intensely basophilic cytoplasm. The cell diameter varies from 15 to 25 μ. They constitute approximately 1% of the nucleated marrow cells in adults and older children but are virtually absent in the newborn's bone marrow and comprise fewer than 0.2% of the marrow cells in infants under 12 months of age.[9] Blue staining is deeper than that of the lymphocyte or the pronormoblast. The nucleus is small and eccentrically placed with chromatin characteristically arranged in coarse clumped masses with a cartwheel distribution. A well-defined clear zone is present in the cytoplasm adjacent to the nucleus. The cytoplasm may contain sparse azure granules or prominent spheric hyaline bodies or globules that take an acidophilic stain. These masses, termed Russell bodies, occur singly or in clusters and consist of mucoprotein. There is also abundant evidence that Russell bodies contain γ-globulin.[29] These structures can be found in the bone marrow of patients with plasmacytosis from any cause and are often noted to be numerous within areas of chronic inflammation. They are not the product of a degenerative process.[91]

Mature plasma cells are derived from lymphocytes (plasmablasts), with intermediate forms constituting young plasma cells. Plasma cells rarely appear normally in the peripheral blood but are present in the bone marrow, lymph nodes, spleen, and other areas. They are found in greatly increased numbers in the peripheral blood in patients with multiple myeloma, plasma cell leukemia, and to a lesser extent measles, rubella, chickenpox,

serum reactions, skin disorders, and other hypersensitivity reactions. The so-called myeloma cell is a derivative of the early plasma cells and shows the main features of the plasmablasts.

Osteoblasts and osteoclasts. Osteoblasts and osteoclasts may be confused with normal constituents of the bone marrow (Fig. 2-5). Osteoblasts superficially resemble plasma cells since both have a basophilic cytoplasm and an eccentric nucleus containing one to three nucleoli. The cells are oval, 25 to 50 μ in diameter. Osteoclasts are giant cells about the size of a megakaryocyte, with which they may be confused. The diameter often exceeds 100 μ. The cells contain several nuclei scattered loosely throughout the cytoplasm. The nuclear chromatin is dense. Osteoblasts and osteoclasts are seen most frequently in fetal and infant marrow.

Tissue mast cells (tissue basophils). The tissue mast cell is a granular basophil that shows little mobility as compared with the active basophils. The separation of the tissue mast cells from the circulating basophils has been a subject of controversy.[67,81] Both have in common metachromasia of the granules. The cytoplasm of the mast cells is filled with granules that stain well with methylene blue, Wright-Giemsa stain, or toluidine blue.

Tissue mast cells can be differentiated from blood basophils and are not interchangeable with them. Tissue mast cells do not possess myeloid precursors as do basophilic leukocytes. Functionally the two cells have much in common in the production of several biologically active substances, especially in the associated content of heparin and histamine in their granules.[72] Serotonin (5-hydroxytryptamine) has also been isolated from the tissue mast cell. There is evidence that serotonin and histamine act in conjunction to cause capillary permeability, hyperemia, and edema, which constitute the vascular response to acute inflammation.[73]

Morphologically tissue mast cells can be differentiated from basophilic leukocytes. The former possess a normal vesicular nucleus, which is rarely indented, but the cytoplasmic contours vary widely, being round, irregularly oval, spindle, or star shaped. The bluish cytoplasm may be hidden because of the densely packed granules, which do not overlie the nucleus as they do in the basophil. By contrast the blood basophils usually have a small cell body with a polymorphic or lobulated nucleus typical of leukocytes. The granules tend to be irregularly distributed.[87] Accumulations of mast cells are observed in both the macular and papular type of urticaria pigmentosa, a dermatologic disorder occurring principally in childhood, and in basophilic leukemia, a disease of adults.

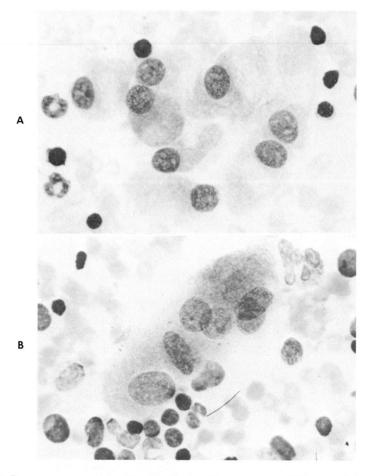

Fig. 2-5. A, Bone marrow aspirate with osteoblasts with eccentric, partially extruded nucleus. **B,** Bone marrow aspirate with multinuclear osteoclasts. (Courtesy Dr. Julius Rutzky, Royal Oak, Mich.)

EXAMINATION OF PERIPHERAL BLOOD

Of all of the laboratory procedures available to the hematologist-oncologist, the most important for its diagnostic value, yet the simplest, is the examination of the peripheral blood smear. Although corroborative evidence from auxiliary sources may be required to establish a final diagnosis, the stained film constitutes a visual representation of the effect on morphology of the factors involved in the pathogenesis of a specific anemia. It also permits an evaluation of platelet and leukocyte morphology and number.

There are relatively few morphologic changes of red cells, leukocytes, or platelets that are indicative of a particular disorder. For example, target cells, elliptocytes, hypochromic macrocytes, basophilic stippling, and hypochromic microcytes appear in varying percentages in certain stages of many anemias and therefore cannot be regarded as distinguishing features of a single disease. They are significant with the support of other pertinent information. The specific abnormalities of size and shape of erythrocytes in various anemias and other diseases are presented in Chapter 5.

Cell stains

Romanowsky stains. Romanowsky stains, of which Wright's stain is a modification, consist of a combination of methylene blue with eosin. Depending on their acidic and basic affinities, the red and blue structures of cells are identified in contrasting colors. For example, the nuclei of white cells stain purplish blue with clear separation of basichromatin and oxychromatin, neutrophilic granules stain light pink or lavender, and the granules of eosinophils and basophils stain red and deeply azurophilic, respectively. For bone marrow preparations a combination of Wright-Giemsa staining often enhances cellular and particularly nuclear detail.

Supravital staining. Supravital staining[12] permits the examination of cytoplasmic structure of blood cells in the living motile state. The reticulocyte stain and stains for erythrocyte inclusion bodies or Heinz bodies are supravital. In nucleated cells mitochondria are stained by Janus green and the specific granules and vacuoles of the cytoplasm by neutral red dye. The nucleus and cytoplasm are left unstained, but the nuclear outlines are readily discerned. Mitochondria are most plentiful in the blast cells and decrease in numbers progressively as the cells mature, being reduced in late myelocytes and frequently absent in the mature polymorphonuclear leukocyte, lymphocyte, and monocyte.

At times the blue-green stain may serve in differentiating the blast cell by the shape and size of the mitochondria and their location. In the myeloblast the mitochondria are numerous and extremely fine and are scattered diffusely or packed in a segment of the cytoplasm. In the lymphoblast they are short, thick, oval, or spheric and may be clustered around the nucleus or scattered diffusely. In the monoblast they exist as fine, slender rods scattered throughout the cell. In the monocyte the supravital stain is particularly diagnostic since the neutral red bodies are characteristically clustered as a rosette in the indention of the nucleus. Supravital staining serves as an adjunct to the fixed smear in the identification of cells and as an aid in visualizing their physiologic activity.

Peroxidase stain. The presence of an oxidative ferment in the cytoplasm of myeloid cells provides an added means of differentiating these from other cells. In the commonly used techniques (such as the Goodpasture method and the copper peroxidase method of Sato and Sekiya), this ferment causes the oxidation and precipitation of benzidine by hydrogen peroxide. Cells of the granulocytic series, including promyelocytes, give a strong peroxidase reaction as contrasted with lymphocytes, plasma cells, and red cells, which are peroxidase negative. Monocytes show fewer and less well-defined peroxidase-positive granules than do granulocytes. The peroxidase reaction in myeloblasts may show faint localized positivity, occasionally accompanied by positively staining Auer rods, but the reaction is less intense than in more mature myeloid cells. When used with the Sudan black B stain, in which myeloblasts stain positively, the peroxidase reaction is of diagnostic use in separating these cells from lymphoblasts. For more extensive discussions and methods of peroxidase and related stains, other references should be consulted.[11,13,38,39]

Miscellaneous stains. Leukocyte alkaline phosphatase is an enzyme capable of hydrolyzing phosphorus from a wide variety of phosphomonoesters.[47] This enzyme is present in the cytoplasm of leukocytes of the granulocyte series and can be assayed chemically or roughly quantitatively by cytochemical staining. With histochemical methods the granules representing alkaline phosphatase activity stain from a pale brown color to deep black. In blood from patients with infection, polycythemia vera, myelofibrosis, and leukemoid reactions, alkaline phosphatase staining is increased, whereas in acute and chronic myeloid luekemia and in paroxysmal nocturnal hemoglobinuria the reaction is decreased. The test is valuable therefore in distinguishing a nonleukemic myeloid (leukemoid) reaction from chronic myelocytic leukemia.

The presence of DNA can be demonstrated by a microchemical reaction.[32] With Feulgen's stain the intensity of the nuclear reaction in leukocytes and nucleated red cells correlates with the concentration of DNA. The clear definition of nucleoli (unstained spaces) is sometimes of help in differentiating lymphoblasts (one to two nucleoli) from myeloblasts (two to four nucleoli).

Methyl green–pyronine also stains, to some degree, the ribonucleic acids of leukocytes.[69]

The periodic acid–Schiff (PAS) reaction is widely used in hematology for demonstrating glycogen and related mucopolysaccharides.[39] Lymphoblasts may stain positively with PAS reagent. Mature polymorphonuclear leukocytes are strongly positive, and monocytes and occasionally lymphocytes have a weakly positive reaction. Normal erythroid precursors and erythrocytes are always PAS negative. Erythroblasts in patients with erythroleukemia and with thalassemia may be PAS positive.

Sudan black B stains for lipids and is useful for identifying myeloblasts and all other myeloid cells. Lymphoblasts, lymphocytes, and erythroblasts are not sudanophilic; monocytes show a weakly positive reaction.

Phase contrast microscopy

Phase contrast microscopy provides a useful means by which the details of living cells can be examined. The papers by Ackerman and Bellios[3] and by Bessis,[8] among others, provide a background for this technique. Phase contrast intensifies relatively minute differences in optical density and permits the detection of intimate details of cells. It allows important structures of living cells to be examined in detail.[8] Granulocytes and monocytes are observed to spread on supporting surfaces. The movements of the pseudopodia of granulocytes can be seen readily. The centrosome appears as a region more transparent than the surrounding cytoplasm and devoid of granules. In its neighborhood, however, the granules are arranged radially.

Red cells examined with phase contrast microscopy reveal a scintillating effect, probably resulting from differences in thickness due to molecular movement. This scintillation disappears at the moment when the sickle cell becomes rigid. Phase contrast gives a very detailed image of the spherocyte, stomatocyte, and erythroblast. Platelets are seen so distinctly with this method that they can be counted directly on a special counting chamber.

Electron microscopy

The introduction of methods for transmission electron microscopy and scanning electron microscopy in hematology has contributed significantly to our knowledge of the ultrastructure, function, and three-dimensional surface characteristics of blood cells. The degree of resolution (1 nm) and magnification (100,000×) are far superior to the limits imposed by light microscopy.

REFERENCES

1. Aballi, A., Puapondh, Y., and Desposito, F.: Platelet counts in thriving premature babies, Pediatrics **42**:685, 1968.
2. Ablin, A. R., Kushner, J. H., Murphy, A., and Zippin, C.: Platelet enumeration in the neonatal period, Pediatrics **28**:822, 1961.
3. Ackerman, G. A., and Bellios, N. C.: A study of the morphology of living cells of blood and bone marrow in vital films with the phase contrast microscope. I. Normal blood and bone marrow, Blood **10**:3, 1955.
4. Albritton, E. C., ed.: Standard values in blood: biological data, AF Technical Report No. 6039, 1951.
5. Ashley, D. J. B.: The technic of nuclear sexing, Am. J. Clin. Pathol. **31**:230, 1959.
6. Barr, D. P.: The function of the plasma cell, Am. J. Med. **9**:277, 1950.
7. Becker, A. H., and Glass, H.: Twin to twin transfusion syndrome, Am. J. Dis. Child. **106**:134, 1963.
8. Bessis, M.: Phase contrast microscopy and electron microscopy applied to the blood cells, Blood **10**:272, 1955.
9. Bridges, R. A., Condie, R. N., Zak, S. J., and Good, R. A.: The morphologic basis of antibody formation development during the neonatal period, J. Lab. Clin. Med. **35**:331, 1959.
10. Burman, D., and Morris, A. F.: Cord haemoglobin in low birthweight infants, Arch. Dis. Child. **49**:382, 1974.
11. Cartwright, G. E.: Diagnostic laboratory hematology, New York, 1968, Grune & Stratton, Inc.
12. Cunningham, R. S., and Tompkins, E. H.: The supravital staining of normal human blood cells, Folia Haematol. **42**:257, 1950.
13. Dacie, J. V., and Lewis, S. M.: Practical haematology, ed. 4, New York, 1968, Grune & Stratton, Inc.
14. Dancis, J., Danoff, S., Zabriski, J., and Balis, M. E.: Hemoglobin metabolism in the premature infant, J. Pediatr. **54**:748, 1959.
15. Delta, B. G., and Pinkel, D.: Bone marrow aspiration in children with malignant tumors, J. Pediatr. **64**:542, 1964.
16. DeMarsh, Q. B., Windle, W. F., and Alt, A. L.: Blood volume of newborn infant in relation to early and late clamping of umbilical cord, Am. J. Dis. Child. **63**:1123, 1942.
17. Djaldetti, M., Joshua, H., and Kalderon, M.: Familial leukopenia-neutropenia in Yemenite Jews, Bull. Res. Council Israel **E9**:24, 1961.
18. Finne, P. H.: Erythropoietin levels in cord blood as an indicator of intrauterine hypoxia, Acta Paediatr. **55**:478, 1966.
19. Flod, N. E., and Ackerman, B. D.: Perinatal asphyxia and residual placental blood volume, Acta Paediatr. Scand. **60**:433, 1971.
20. Foconi, S., and Sjölin, S.: Survival of Cr^{51}-labelled red cells from newborn infants, Acta Paediatr. **48**(suppl. 117):18, 1958.
21. Fogel, B. J., Arias, D., and Kung, F.: Normal platelet counts in premature infants, J. Pediatr. **73**:108, 1968.
22. Gairdner, D., Marks, J., and Roscoe, J. D.: Blood formation in infancy. I. The normal bone marrow, Arch. Dis. Child. **27**:128, 1952.
23. Gairdner, D., Marks, J., and Roscoe, J. D.: Blood formation in infancy. II. Normal erythropoiesis, Arch. Dis. Child. **27**:214, 1952.
24. Gairdner, D., Marks, J., and Roscoe, J. D.: Blood formation in infancy. IV. The early anaemias of prematurity, Arch. Dis. Child. **30**:203, 1955.
25. Gairdner, D., Marks, J., Roscoe, J. D., and Brettell, R. O.: The fluid shift from the vascular compartment immediately after birth, Arch. Dis. Child. **33**:489, 1958.
26. Gatti, R. A.: Hematocrit values of capillary blood in the newborn infant, J. Pediatr. **70**:117, 1967.
27. Gatti, R. A., Muster, A. J., Cole, R. B., and Paul, M. H.: Neonatal polycythemia with transient cyanosis and cardiorespiratory anomalies, J. Pediatr. **69**:1063, 1966.
28. Glaser, K., Limarzi, L. R., and Poncher, H. G.: Cellular composition of the bone marrow in normal infants and children, Pediatrics **6**:789, 1950.
29. Goldberg, A. F., and Deane, H. W.: A comparative study of some staining properties of crystals in a lymphoplasmacytoid cell and of amyloids; with special emphasis on their isoelectric points, Blood **16**:1708, 1960.
30. Good, R. A.: Agammaglobulinemia, Bull. Univ. Minn. Hosp. **26**:1, 1954.
31. Granick, S.: The chemistry and functioning of the mammalian erythrocyte, Blood **4**:404, 1949.
32. Greig, H. B. W.: A substitute for the Feulgen staining technique, J. Clin. Pathol. **12**:93, 1959.
33. Gross, G. P., Hathaway, W. E., et al.: Hyperviscosity in the neonate, J. Pediatr. **82**:1004, 1974.
34. Guest, G. M., and Brown, E. W.: Erythrocytes and hemoglobin of the blood in infancy and childhood; factors in variability, statistical studies, Am. J. Dis. Child. **93**:486, 1957.
35. Guest, G. M., Brown, E. W., and Wing, M.: Erythrocytes and hemoglobin of the blood in infancy and childhood: variability in number, size and hemoglobin content of the erythrocytes during the first five years of life, Am. J. Dis. Child. **56**:529, 1938.
36. Harker, L. A.: Platelet production, N. Engl. J. Med. **282**:492, 1970.
37. Haselhorst, G., and Allmeling, A.: Die Gewichtszunahme von Neugeborenen infolge postnataler Transfusion, Z. Geburtshilfe Gynäkol. **98**:103, 1930.
38. Hayhoe, F. G. J., Quaglino, D., and Doll, R.: The cytology and cytochemistry of acute leukaemias: a study of 140 cases, London, 1964, Her Majesty's Stationery Office.
39. Hayhoe, F. G. J., Quaglino, D., and Flemans, R. J.: Consecutive use of Romanowsky and periodic-acid-Schiff techniques in the study of blood and bone marrow cells, Br. J. Haematol. **6**:231, 1960.
40. Heald, F., Levy, P. S., Hamill, P. V. V., and Rowland, M.: Hematocrit values of youths 12-17 years, Pub. No. 75-1628, Vital and Health Statistics Series 11, No. 146, U.S. Department of Health, Education, and Welfare, 1974.
41. Hillman, R. S.: Characteristics of marrow production and reticulocyte maturation in normal man in response to anemia, J. Clin. Invest. **48**:443, 1969.

42. Hillman, R. S., and Finch, C. A.: The misused reticulocyte, Br. J. Haematol. **17:**313, 1969.

43. Hodapp, R. V.: The case of the red and white Minnesota twins: intrauterine blood transfer between twins, J. Lancet **82:**413, 1962.

44. Hollingsworth, J. W.: Life span of fetal erythrocytes, J. Lab. Clin. Med. **45:**469, 1955.

45. Kalpaktsoglou, P. E., and Emery, J. L.: The effect of birth on the haemopoietic tissue of the human bone marrow: a biological study, Br. J. Haematol. **11:**453, 1965.

46. Kaplan, E., and Hsu, K. S.: Determination of erythrocyte survival in newborn infants by means of Cr^{51}-labelled erythrocytes, Pediatrics **27:**354, 1961.

47. Kaplow, L. S.: A histochemical procedure for localizing and evaluating leukocyte alkaline phosphatase activity in smears of blood and bone marrow, Blood **10:**1023, 1955.

48. Karpatkin, S.: Heterogeneity of human platelets. I. Metabolic and genetic evidence suggestive of young and old platelets, J. Clin. Invest. **48:**1073, 1969.

49. Kjeldsen, J., and Pederson, J.: Relation of residual placental blood-volume to onset of respiration and respiratory-distress syndrome in infants of diabetic and nondiabetic mothers, Lancet **1:**180, 1967.

50. Kleinman, L. I., Petering, H. G., and Suterland, J. M.: Blood carbonic anhydrase activity and zinc concentration in infants with respiratory-distress syndrome, N. Engl. J. Med. **277:**1157, 1967.

51. Klingberg, W. G., Jones, B., Allen, W. M., and Dempsey, E.: Placental parabiotic circulation of single ovum human twins, Am. J. Dis. Child. **90:**519, 1955.

52. Lanzkowsky, P.: Effects of early and late clamping of umbilical cord on infant's haemoglobin level, Br. Med. J. **2:**1777, 1960.

53. Leichsenring, J. M., Norris, L. M., and Halbert, M. L.: Hemoglobin, red cell count, and mean corpuscular hemoglobin of healthy infants, Am. J. Dis. Child. **84:**27, 1952.

54. Lichtenstein, A., and Nordenson, N. G.: Studies on bone marrow in premature children, Folia Haematol. **63:**155, 1939.

55. Matoth, Y., Zaizov, R., et al.: Postnatal changes in some red cell parameters, Acta Paediatr. **60:**317, 1971.

56. Medoff, H. S.: Platelet counts in premature infants, J. Pediatr. **64:**287, 1964.

57. Michael, A. F., Jr., and Mauer, A. M.: Maternal-fetal transfusion as a cause of plethora in the neonatal period, Pediatrics **28:**458, 1961.

58. Mollison, P. L., and Cutbush, M.: Haemolytic disease of the newborn. In Gairdner, D., ed.: Recent advances in pediatrics, New York, 1954, The Blakiston Co.

59. Naeye, R. L.: Human intrauterine parabiotic syndrome and its complications, N. Engl. J. Med. **268:**804, 1963.

60. Neerhout, R. C.: Erythrocyte lipids in the neonate, Pediatr. Res. **2:**172, 1968.

61. Nosanchuk, J. S., Roark, M. F., and Wanser, C.: Anemia masked by triglyceridemia, Am. J. Clin. Pathol. **62:**838, 1974.

62. Oski, F. A.: Red cell metabolism of the premature infant. II. The pentose phosphate pathway, Pediatrics **39:**689, 1967.

63. Oski, F. A., Brigandi, E., and Noble, L.: Red cell metabolism in the newborn infant. V. Glycolytic intermediates and glycolytic enzymes, Pediatrics **44:**84, 1969.

64. Oski, F. A., and Naiman, J. L.: Hematologic problems in the newborn, ed. 2, Philadelphia, 1972, W. B. Saunders Co.

65. Oski, F. A., Smith, C., and Brigandi, E.: Red cell metabolism in the premature infant. III. Apparent inappropriate glucose consumption for cell age, Pediatrics **41:**473, 1968.

66. Pablete, E., Thibeault, D. W., and Auld, P. A. M.: Carbonic anhydrase in the premature, Pediatrics **42:**429, 1968.

67. Padawer, J.: Studies on mammalian mast cells, Trans. N.Y. Acad. Sci. **19:**690, 1957.

68. Pearson, H. A.: Thrombocytopenia in premature infants—physiological or pathological, J. Pediatr. **73:**160, 1968.

69. Perry, S., and Reynolds, J.: Methyl-green-pyronin as a differential nucleic acid stain for peripheral blood smears, Blood **11:**1132, 1956.

70. Pike, B. L.: Human bone marrow colony growth in vitro, J. Cell. Physiol. **76:**77, 1970.

71. Rausen, A. R., Seki, M., and Strauss, L.: Twin transfusion syndrome: a review of 19 cases studied at one institution, J. Pediatr. **66:**613, 1965.

72. Riley, J. F.: Heparin, histamine and mast cells, Blood **9:**1123, 1954.

73. Rowley, D. A., and Benditt, E. P.: 5-Hydroxytryptamine and histamine as mediators of the vascular injury produced by agents which damage mast cells in rats, J. Exp. Med. **103:**399, 1956.

74. Schulman, I., Smith, C. H., and Stern, G. S.: Studies on the anemia of prematurity, Am. J. Dis. Child. **88:**567, 1954.

75. Seip, M.: The reticulocyte level and the erythrocyte production judged from reticulocyte studies in newborn infants during the first week of life, Acta Paediatr. **44:**355, 1955.

76. Shaper, A. G., and Lwen, P.: Genetic neutropenia in people of African origin, Lancet **2:**1023, 1971.

77. Shapiro, L. M., and Bassen, F. A.: Sternal marrow changes during the first week of life: correlation with peripheral blood findings, Am. J. Med. Sci. **202:**341, 1941.

78. Shelley, W. B., and Juhlin, L.: Functional cytology of the human basophil in allergic and physiologic reactions: technic and atlas, Blood **19:**208, 1962.

79. Shojania, A. M., Roland, M., Simovitch, H., et al.: Alterations in red cell structure and metabolism associated with rapid blood production: the stress reticulocyte, J. Pediatr. **65:**1101, 1964.

80. Smith, C. H.: Bone marrow examination in blood disorders of infants and children, Med. Clin. North Am. **31:**527, 1947.

81. Speirs, R. S.: Physiological approaches to an understanding of the function of eosinophils and basophils, Ann. N.Y. Acad. Sci. **59:**706, 1955.

82. Sturgeon, P.: Volumetric and microscopic pattern of bone marrow in normal infants and children. II. Cytologic pattern, Pediatrics **7:**642, 1951.

83. Tenczar, F. J., and Streitmatter, D. E.: Sex difference in neutrophils, Am. J. Clin. Pathol. **26:**384, 1956.

84. Tocantins, L. M.: Mammalian blood platelet in health and disease, Medicine **17:**155, 1938.

85. Usher, R., Shephard, M., and Lind, J.: The blood volume of the newborn infant and placental transfusion, Acta Paediatr. **52:**497, 1963.

86. Washburn, A. H.: Blood cells in healthy young infants: a study of 608 differential leukocyte counts, with a final report on 908 total leukocyte counts, Am. J. Dis. Child. **50:**412, 1935.

87. Waters, W. J., and Lacson, P. S.: Mast cell leukemia presenting as urticaria pigmentosa: report of a case, Pediatrics **19:**1033, 1957.

88. Watson, J. D.: Molecular biology of the gene, ed. 2, Cambridge, Mass., 1970, Harvard University Press.

89. Weatherall, D. J., and Clegg, J. B.: The thalassemia syndromes, ed. 2, Oxford, 1972, Blackwell Scientific Publications.

90. Weatherall, D. J., and McIntyre, P. A.: Developmental and acquired variations in erythrocyte carbonic anhydrase isozymes, Br. J. Haematol. **13:**106, 1967.

91. Welsh, R. A.: Electron microscopic localization of Russell bodies in human plasma cells, Blood **16:**1307, 1960.

92. Whipple, G. A., Sisson, T. R. C., and Lund, C. J.: Delayed ligation of the umbilical cord, Obstet. Gynecol. **10:**603, 1957.

93. Windle, W. F.: Development of the blood and changes in the blood picture at birth, J. Pediatr. **18:**538, 1941.

94. Wintrobe, M. M.: Clinical hematology, ed. 7, Philadelphia, 1974, Lea & Febiger.

95. Wolman, I.: Laboratory applications in clinical pediatrics, New York, 1957, The Blakiston Co.

96. Wolman, I. J., and Dickstein, B.: Clinical applications of bone marrow examination in childhood, Am. J. Med. Sci. **214:**677, 1974.

97. Woo, T. A., and Frenkel, E. P.: The atypical lymphocyte, Am. J. Med. **42:**923, 1967.

98. Wood, J. L.: Plethora in the newborn infant associated with cyanosis and convulsions: a review of postnatal erythropoiesis, J. Pediatr. **54:**143, 1959.

3 □ Maternal-fetal interactions

Sue McIntosh
Howard A. Pearson

The fetus, surrounded by the mother's body and a layer of amniotic fluid, occupies a protected environment. However, the insulation is not complete, for there is direct opposition of the fetal and maternal circulations, separated only by a few layers of cells. Many substances, particularly those proteins and drugs of low molecular weight, diffuse freely across the placental barrier and occasionally may produce significant problems in the fetus. The placental barrier may also permit direct exchange of particulate material, including the cellular elements of the blood.

Most of the placental mass consists of chorionic villi bathed in maternal blood. Fetal and maternal blood are separated from each other by only two layers of cells at the trophoblastic endothelial junction of each villus. The maternal blood constantly circulates between the individual villi and is then drained by the decidual sinuses into placental veins (Fig. 3-1).

Maternal arterial blood enters the intervillous space at a pressure of 60 to 70 mm Hg higher than the existing pressure in this area and is then dissipated by lateral dispersion. The difference between the umbilical arterial blood pressure and that in the intervillous space produces a pressure gradient from fetus to mother. Fetal blood may follow a similar course, and this is the probable mechanism for maternal isoimmunization to red cells, white cells, and platelets in pregnancy.

Cellular elements of both the fetus and mother may pass through the placental trophoblastic lining in either direction during normal gestation. The transplacental passage of maternal sickle cells[68,137] and elliptocytes[88] into the fetal circulation has been demonstrated. White cells and plate-

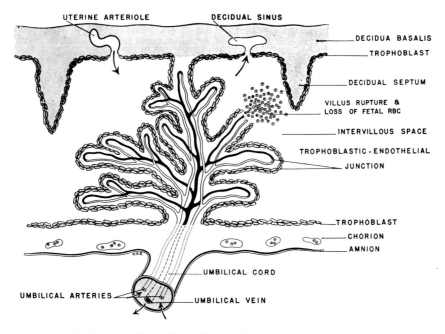

Fig. 3-1. Schematic diagram of the placental circulation showing rupture of a villus at the trophoblastic endothelial junction, permitting the mixing of fetal and maternal blood and the entrance of fetal red blood cells into the maternal circulation. (Modified from Javert, C. T., and Reiss, C.: Surg. Gynecol. Obstet. **94:**257, 1952.)

lets labeled with quinacrine (Atabrine) and injected into the maternal circulation have been subsequently detected in the fetus.[44] Fetal lymphocytes have been identified in the maternal blood stream in some primiparous women,[200,231,248] and maternal leukocytes are frequently found in aborted fetuses.[200] Of more clinical importance is the passage of red blood cells across the placenta.

FETAL HEMORRHAGE INTO MATERNAL CIRCULATION (FETAL-MATERNAL TRANSFUSION)

Wiener[233] was the first to suggest the possibility of fetal bleeding into the maternal circulation. His concept was confirmed by Chown,[31] who reported a case of neonatal anemia in which a high concentration of fetal hemoglobin as well as fetal red cells were found in the maternal blood soon after delivery.

Transplacental bleeding from the fetus can be demonstrated by agglutination procedures demonstrating a population of red cells in the maternal circulation that differ in ABO, Rh, or other blood group antigens from the mother's own red cells but are identical with those of her newborn infant. Postpartum elevation of maternal-fetal hemoglobin concentration that subsequently disappears constitutes further proof of the passage of fetal blood into the maternal circulation.[158] Entrance of fetal red cells into the maternal circulation just before delivery has been adduced from the reported appearance in group O mothers of immune anti-A antibodies (from group A infants) 10 to 20 days after delivery when none had been present at birth.[49]

Fetal-maternal transfusion of erythrocytes occurs primarily during labor and parturition, although small numbers of fetal red cells may gain access to the maternal circulation prior to the third trimester.* In as many as one third of normal births fetal erythrocytes are found in maternal blood immediately postpartum.[174,200] The frequency and magnitude of fetal-maternal hemorrhage is increased by obstetric instrumentation, manual removal of the placenta, preeclampsia, antenatal hemorrhage, and cesarean section.[158,174] Parturitional transfusion of fetal cells can be reduced significantly by allowing the placental end of the cut umbilical cord to bleed freely prior to delivery of the placenta. This maneuver may also decrease the risk of sensitization in Rh-negative mothers.[118,218]

Clinical syndromes associated with transplacental hemorrhage

Clinical manifestations of fetal-maternal transfusion vary with the magnitude of the hemorrhage,

the rapidity of the bleeding, and the time at which it occurs with respect to delivery. Massive fetal hemorrhage may produce stillbirth, hypotensive shock, apnea, or severe anemia at the time of birth.* If the hemorrhage occurs immediately before birth, the infant may be in hypovolemic shock and yet the hemoglobin level may be still relatively normal. If the hemorrhage occurs earlier, hemodilution may result in a severe degree of anemia with relatively few signs of acute cardiovascular stress.

A blood picture suggestive of nonimmune hemolysis in the neonatal period, with anemia and reticulocytosis, may in fact represent antenatal fetal hemorrhage, providing that enough time has elapsed after the hemorrhage for a reticulocyte response to be mounted by the fetus. In these infants the Coombs test is negative and jaundice is usually absent.[173] Chronic fetal-maternal hemorrhage may produce the appearance of congenital iron deficiency anemia.† In these infants the quantity of fetal blood in the maternal circulation may actually exceed the blood volume in the fetus.

Laboratory diagnosis. The most sensitive method for confirming fetal-maternal transfusion is the acid elution method of Kleihauer and Betke applied to the maternal blood.[157,158] Adult hemoglobin in maternal cells is denatured and eluted, leaving red cell membranes, or "ghost cells," whereas fetal red cells, containing resistant fetal hemoglobin, remain intact. (Fig. 3-2). This method is less reliable as an indicator of fetal hemorrhage during the first and second trimesters of pregnancy, when a small population of red cells containing Hb F may appear in the maternal blood, presumably resulting from the effects of high levels of chorionic gonadotrophins.[158] The acid elution test may also be falsely positive if the mother has a hematologic condition characterized by elevated levels of Hb F, such as hereditary persistence of fetal hemoglobin, thalassemia, or sickle cell anemia.

Estimation of the amount of fetal blood lost into maternal circulation can be made using the following formula:

$$2{,}400 \times \text{ratio of fetal:maternal cells} = \text{ml of fetal blood}^{157,158}$$

For example, if 1 in 600 red cells in the mother's circulation is fetal, $2{,}400 \times 1/600 = 4$ ml of fetal blood in the maternal circulation. Observation of 1 fetal red cell/1,000 maternal red cells indicates at least 2 ml of fetal blood loss. The Kleihauer-Betke blood smear must be even and thin, and only strongly positive red cells should be counted as fetal red cells. Using this estimate, only 1% of normal deliveries are accompanied by

---

*References 40, 68, 88, 138, 144.

*References 79, 109, 173, 180, 198, 245.
†References 54, 132, 149, 160, 237.

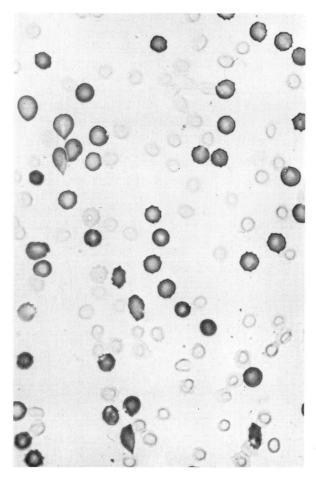

Fig. 3-2. Blood smear prepared from a mixture of adult and cord blood and treated by the acid elution technique (see text). The dark-staining cells contain fetal hemoglobin; the ghostlike cells contain adult hemoglobin. (Courtesy Dr. Alvin Zipursky, Manitoba, Canada.)

more than 3 ml of fetal blood in the maternal circulation and only 0.3% by 10 ml or more.[158]

When ABO incompatibility exists between mother and infant (e.g., the mother is group O and the infant group A or B), fetal red cells are agglutinated and rapidly removed from the maternal circulation. In fact, symptoms suggestive of a maternal transfusion reaction and jaundice have been described.[31,74] In these instances fetal-maternal transfusion may be documented only in the immediate postpartum period.[104] If the red cell blood groups of mother and infant are compatible, fetal red cells may be detected in the maternal blood as long as 100 days after delivery.[180]

Therapy. Therapy for fetal-maternal hemorrhage is dictated by the infant's clinical condition. If the infant is in shock, rapid blood transfusion via an umbilical vein catheter is mandatory. These infants have tachycardia and extreme pallor, and the central venous pressure is low. These findings are in contrast to the infant with shock secondary to intracranial damage (asphyxia pallida), in whom bradycardia and a normal central venous pressure are usual.

Packed cell transfusions are indicated when the infant is anemic but does not show manifestations of hypovolemia. Mildly anemic neonates, because loss of red cells may have depleted their iron endowment, require early supplemental iron therapy.

MATERNAL-FETAL TRANSFUSION

Maternal-fetal transfusion occurs in 10% to 80% of normal deliveries.[200] This can be confirmed by the "reverse Kleihauer-Betke" test, in which increased numbers (>15%) of maternal "ghost" forms are found in the fetal blood. In the blood of fetuses less than 35 weeks of gestational age, all of the red cells are of the fetal type. At 35 weeks of gestation small numbers of cells containing Hb A begin to appear. In the cord blood of term infants, about 5% to 10% of the circulating red cells are of the adult type; the remainder are fetal.[64] When the magnitude of maternal-fetal transfusion is large, the neonate may develop congestive heart failure and other complications. Acute hypervolemia, polycythemia, and hyperviscosity may be relieved by phlebotomy or exchange transfusion. In the symptomatic neonate phlebotomies in increments of 5 ml/kg should be done with simultaneous replacement by fresh plasma or isotonic fluid.

NEONATAL THROMBOCYTOPENIA

Hemostasis in the newborn, as in the older individual, depends on an interaction of the coagulation mechanism and the platelet. When either of these is quantitatively or qualitatively abnormal, hemorrhage may occur. The normal platelet count is $241 \pm 100 \times 10^9$ liter in older children and adults. Albin et al.[4] reported platelet counts ranging from 120 to 300×10^9/liter in 105 healthy term infants; at 4 days of age the mean counts were $224 \pm 100 \times 10^9$/liter. A similar mean and range was described by Aballi et al.[1] in eighty-eight normal full-term infants.

There has been less unanimity about the platelet count of premature infants. Medoff[140] reported that significant thrombocytopenia (less than 100×10^9 platelets/liter) was a common finding during the second and third weeks of life after premature birth. The concept of a "physiologic thrombocytopenia of prematurity" has been disproved by larger series, and it seems likely that platelet numbers, even in small premature infants, do not differ significantly from those in larger newborns.[61] Although the range of normal values is relatively wide, platelet counts of less than 100×10^9/liter in the newborn period are abnormal and require explanation.

Platelet production is usually assessed by inference. If normal numbers of megakaryocytes are found in aspiration or biopsy specimens of bone marrow, platelet production is assumed to be normal, an assumption that is valid in most clinical situations. However, it must be recognized that bone marrow sampling in the newborn, particularly in the premature infant, may be technically difficult because of the very small marrow space. Reports that describe decreased numbers of megakaryocytes in neonatal thrombocytopenic states must be viewed with skepticism unless actual marrow particles or biopsy has been obtained.

The normal platelet life span is about 10 days as determined by radioactive isotopic techniques. Thus in the steady state about 10% of platelets are removed from the circulation and are replaced by new young platelets released from the bone marrow each day. Such recently released platelets have a large volume and can be morphologically identified by their relatively large size on blood smears, and increased platelet production is ac-

companied by increased numbers of these megathrombocytes.[131] Although there have been no systematic studies of platelet kinetics in normal newborns, it is likely that both the rate of production and the life span of the platelets of the neonate are similar to those of later life.

Thrombocytopenia during the newborn period may be caused by a number of specific disease processes. However, in all of these diverse conditions the reduced platelet count is a consequence of the following:

1. Decreased production or release of platelets from the megakaryocytes of the bone marrow
2. An accelerated rate of platelet destruction that exceeds the capacity of the bone marrow to compensate
3. A combination of both of these mechanisms

The important causes of neonatal thrombocytopenia categorized by their pathogenetic mechanisms are listed below:

A. Decreased production of platelets
   1. Congenital megakaryocytic hypoplasia
      a. TAR syndrome
      b. Megakaryocytic hypoplasia without anomalies
      c. Fanconi's anemia
   2. Congenital malignancies
      a. Acute leukemia
      b. Metastatic tumor
      c. Histiocytosis
   3. Inherited thrombocytopenias
      a. Wiskott-Aldrich syndrome
      b. Other X-linked or recessively transmitted thrombocytopenias
B. Increased destruction of platelets
   1. Immune thrombocytopenias
      a. Maternal ITP and lupus erythematosus
      b. Isoimmune neonatal purpura (Pl^{A1} and others)
   2. Maternal drug-induced purpura (quinidine, etc.)
   3. Giant hemangioma syndrome
   4. Disseminated intravascular coagulation
C. Both decreased production and increased destruction
   1. Infections (TORCH syndrome)
   2. Osteopetrosis

Thrombocytopenias resulting primarily from decreased production

Congenital megakaryocytic hypoplasia. Thrombocytopenia is found in a complex syndrome designated TAR (thrombocytopenia–absent radii) syndrome.[81,201] Affected infants are usually small for gestational age and have obvious skeletal deformities. The most striking of these are the absent radii, but other limb abnormalities may also be present, producing phocomelia.[46] Congenital heart disease occurs in about one third of cases. Thrombocytopenia is associated with hemorrhagic manifestations varying from petechial rash to severe gastrointestinal bleeding and fatal intracranial hemorrhage. About two thirds of the infants die in the first year of life. A striking hematologic finding in one half of these infants is a leukemoid blood reaction with total white cell counts exceeding 40×10^9/liter. Bone marrow aspiration reveals a hypercellular marrow resulting from myeloid hyperplasia and a paucity of megakaryocytes.

The TAR syndrome must be distinguished from constitutional aplastic anemia (Fanconi's anemia).[55] Although the skeletal anomalies are similar, constitutional aplastic anemia rarely has hematologic manifestations in infancy. Infants with the TAR syndrome do not have the cytogenetic abnormalities of multiple chromatid breaks and quadriradial configurations found in Fanconi's anemia.[20]

A few infants with isolated thrombocytopenia and megakaryocytic hypoplasia but no congenital anomalies have been reported. In some of these, pancytopenia and frankly aplastic bone marrow have evolved with passing time.[169]

Transfusions of platelet concentrates are efficacious in treating hemorrhage.[13] If fatal hemorrhage can be successfully prevented, hematologic improvement tends to occur with increasing age in infants with TAR syndrome.

Congenital leukemias and histiocytosis. Congenital leukemia, manifested in the first days of life, has been reported in a substantial number of cases.[186] In almost every instance the morphology in these cases has been of the acute myelogenous variety, and hyperleukocytosis (white blood cell count $> 100 \times 10^9$/liter) is usual. Rarely lymphoblastic and monocytic varieties may be seen.[179,229] Extensive leukemic infiltration occurs in liver, spleen, and bone marrow. Thrombocytopenia is a consequence of replacement of the bone marrow by leukemic tissue, and reduced numbers of megakaryocytes are found.

Striking cutaneous manifestations are usually present. These consist of bluish nodules of leukemic infiltration interspersed with petechial hemorrhages. The same kind of lesions are noted on the placenta. Neonatal leukemia responds poorly to therapy, although prolonged remissions (often spontaneous) have been observed.[179]

A leukemia-like disorder has been repeatedly recognized in newborn infants with Down's syndrome.[53] Affected children have profound thrombocytopenia, anemia, and a blood picture resembling acute granulocytic leukemia; nodular skin infiltrations indistinguishable from leukemia have occurred in some cases. Death from infection or hemorrhage has occurred during the first months of life, but spontaneous remissions of extended and indefinite duration have occurred in a number of instances. Whether this syndrome is truly leuke-

mia or rather a leukemoid state unique to infants with Down's syndrome is a moot question. Thrombocytopenic hemorrhage responds to transfusions of platelet concentrates. Cytotoxic antileukemic chemotherapy should be withheld.

A few newborn infants with systemic histiocytosis (congenital Letterer-Siwe disease) have been described. These infants have had profound thrombocytopenia and hepatosplenomegaly and extensive infiltration of the skin and viscera by histiocytes.[90]

Inherited thrombocytopenias. A number of genetically determined syndromes have been described. The most clearly defined of these is the Wiskott-Aldrich syndrome, an X-linked disorder characterized by thrombocytopenia, eczema, elevated IgE level, and a complex immunologic defect predisposing to severe infections.[5,28,113] Thrombocytopenia results from both impaired production and poor survival of small, defective platelets.[78] Megakaryocyte numbers in the bone marrow are normal. Other congenital thrombocytopenias are inherited recessively.[114]

Thrombocytopenia and bleeding may be noted at birth, although eczema and infection may not develop until later. Bleeding responds satisfactorily to transfusion with platelet concentrates, which have a normal survival time.[183]

Therapy. Viable platelets for transfusion are prepared from fresh donor blood collected in citrate-phosphate-dextrose (CPD) anticoagulant in plastic equipment (Chapter 4). Differential centrifugation permits harvesting of most of the platelets in a small, concentrated volume. Following transfusion, platelets have a survival of about 10 days. The incremental increase in count obtained after platelet transfusion depends on the size of the recipient. The platelets concentrated from 500 ml of blood are sufficient to increase the platelet count of a newborn by about 50×10^9/liter. The initial count decreases about 10%/day, returning to baseline levels in about 10 days. If platelet production is constant and low, the sequential change in count following transfusion can be used to estimate platelet life span, for it approximates a survival curve. A drop in platelet count more rapid than the expected 10%/day indicates shortened survival. More accurate definition of platelet survival can be obtained by ^{51}Cr survival studies, but exposure of infants to the radioactive isotope should be justified by the information derived from the study.

Thrombocytopenia associated with increased peripheral destruction

Immune thrombocytopenias. Immune thrombocytopenia is a consequence of a markedly reduced platelet survival. In older individuals the normal bone marrow is able to increase its production of platelets several-fold as a response to increased thrombocytolysis. However, no studies of the capacity of the fetal marrow to increase platelet production have been described.

In contrast to the overt clinical illness of infants with thrombocytopenia complicating infections or neoplasms, newborn infants with immune thrombocytopenia are otherwise normal. Hepatosplenomegaly, hemolytic anemia, intrauterine growth retardation, and other evidence of systemic illness are lacking.

The infant's blood counts are normal except for thrombocytopenia. Bone marrow aspiration reveals large numbers of megakaryocytes. Thrombocytopenia is prolonged and persists for 4 to 8 weeks, regardless of therapy. However, clinical bleeding after the first week of life is unusual. Splenectomy is contraindicated.

Although thrombocytopenia exists in utero and platelet counts in cord blood are severely depressed, petechiae and purpura are not apparent at birth but may appear a few minutes to a few hours after delivery. Because the fetus is subjected to hemostatic stresses during birth that may evoke intracranial hemorrhage, neonatal mortality and serious morbidity are relatively high.[7,120,134]

Thrombocytopenic neonatal purpura secondary to maternal ITP. Idiopathic thrombocytopenic purpura (ITP) in the pregnant woman, particularly in the last trimester of pregnancy, is often associated with profound thrombocytopenia in the newborn infant. Because the circulating antibody in chronic ITP is of the IgG class, it may cross the placenta, causing destruction of fetal platelets.[7,218,219] It has broad reactivity against all platelets. Thirty percent to 70% of infants born to mothers with active ITP have thrombocytopenic purpura at birth.* The fetal risk is much lower when the maternal ITP is in remission. However, persistent circulating maternal antiplatelet antibodies may still affect the infant born of a mother with a remote history of ITP, and the woman herself may have shortened platelet survival in the face of a normal platelet count.[25] We have managed an extreme example of this in the newborn child of a woman who had ITP 30 years previously, when she was only 4 years old. She had a splenectomy at 5 years of age for chronic thrombocytopenia, with an excellent result. During the following 29 years repeated platelet counts were normal, and they were normal at the time of parturition. Her newborn infant had extensive purpura and a platelet count of only 5×10^9/liter and thrombocytopenia persisted for 8 weeks.

The maternal bleeding history may be relatively

unimpressive, and yet the child can be severely affected. The delivery of a thrombocytopenic infant may lead to a diagnosis of ITP in the mother. Affected mothers have a history of chronic but moderate bruising and menorrhagia, and platelet counts of 75 to 100 $\times 10^9$/liter were found in the postpartum period.

TREATMENT. Obstetrical management of the mother with gestational ITP poses significant problems, although pregnancy per se does not necessarily worsen this condition. Splenectomy during pregnancy is technically difficult and is associated with a fetal wastage of 25%.[175,185] Steroid therapy, which may be indicated for control of maternal bleeding, may also benefit the fetus.[92] Dexamethasone crosses the placenta and may afford some protection during delivery. Bleeding does not occur in utero. Before delivery, however, careful consideration of the method of delivery of the infant should be given to assure minimal trauma to the fetal head. Cesarean section is indicated when there is a high probability of the infant being affected,[120,217] as when the mother has active disease. Mortality in affected infants in older series ranged from 15% to 25%, but optimal obstetric and medical management should reduce this high risk.[7]

After birth, corticosteroid therapy (2 mg/kg of prednisone) should be given for several days to a seriously affected infant. Transfusions of platelet concentrates from random donors or the mother are of little value because of their extraordinarily short survival, but they may be used as an emergency measure if potentially serious hemorrhage has occurred. Exchange transfusions with fresh blood preserved in CPD anticoagulant may be transiently effective by simultaneous removal of circulating antiplatelet antibodies and provision of large numbers of viable platelets. Heparin or heparinized blood should not be used because of the added risk of hemorrhage in the thrombocytopenic individual. Fig. 3-3 shows the effectiveness of exchange transfusions in assuring temporary hemostasis in an infant with neonatal thrombocytopenia secondary to maternal ITP. This infant required emergency surgery, which was successfully conducted after the exchange transfusion.

In some cases of systemic lupus erythematosus, antiplatelet antibodies comparable to those in ITP may be present. These may cross the placenta and produce transient neonatal thrombocytopenia.[166] The newborn may also have a transiently positive test for antinuclear and LE factors.[15,26,148] Rarely a lupuslike illness affects the neonate.[227] Management of thrombocytopenic infants should be conducted in a manner similar to that suggested for affected infants born of mothers with ITP.

---

*References 7, 75, 84, 91, 120, 218.

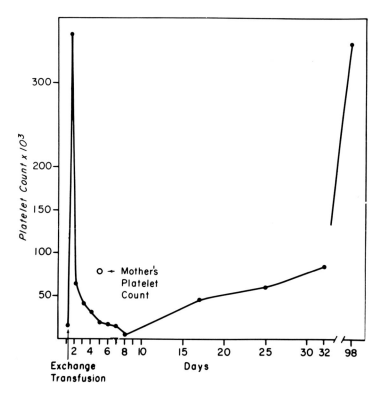

Fig. 3-3. Serial platelet counts of infant with neonatal purpura. Infant was transferred for surgery for imperforate anus. Exchange transfusion with fresh CPD blood produced a dramatic increase in platelet count. Although this was sustained for less than 24 hours, surgery was performed uneventfully. Later it was determined that infant's mother had long history of bruising easily, and her platelet count on the fifth postpartum day was 75×10^9/liter. Diagnosis of chronic ITP was subsequently established. (From Pearson, H. A., and McIntosh, S.: Clin. Haematol. **7:**116, 1978.)

Isoimmune neonatal purpura. When the mother lacks a platelet antigen that is present on the platelets of her fetus, isoimmunization may occur in a manner analogous to isoimmunization against red cell Rh antigens in erythroblastosis fetalis. There are a number of platelet antigens that have been implicated in isoimmune neonatal purpura,[203,204] all of which are inherited as autosomal dominant genes. Some are restricted to platelets; others, such as PlGrLy[B1] and PlGrLy[C1], are shared by leukocytes and may be identical with certain antigens of the HLA system. The platelet antigenic system most commonly associated with isoimmune neonatal purpura has been designated Pl[A1] or Zw[A]. The Pl[A1] antigen occurs only on platelets and is associated with more than 50% of cases of proved isoimmune neonatal purpura.[203] In random populations 98% of individuals are Pl[A1] positive (homozygous or heterozygous). It is the 2% of Pl[A1]-negative women who may have an affected infant. The finding of negativity for the Pl[A1] antigen in the mother of an infant with neonatal thrombocytopenia is strong presumptive evidence of isoimmunization.

Laboratory confirmation of isoimmunization is difficult. Only a few laboratories perform the techniques for determination of the platelet antigen or for detection of complement-fixing and blocking antibodies present in the maternal circulation.[204] Therefore a diagnosis of isoimmune neonatal purpura is often made inferentially. The usual criteria include the following:

1. Congenital thrombocytopenia
2. Normal maternal platelet count and no history of maternal ITP
3. No evidence in the infant of other systemic diseases such as infection or malignancy
4. Recovery of platelet count within 2 to 3 weeks*

Bone marrow aspirations in isoimmune cases have generally revealed many megakaryocytes, but in a few instances a reduced number has been noted. First-born infants are frequently affected, probably because platelets cross into the maternal circulation more easily than red cells during early gestation. Once a mother has been immunized,

---

*References 7, 21, 133, 134, 182, 199.

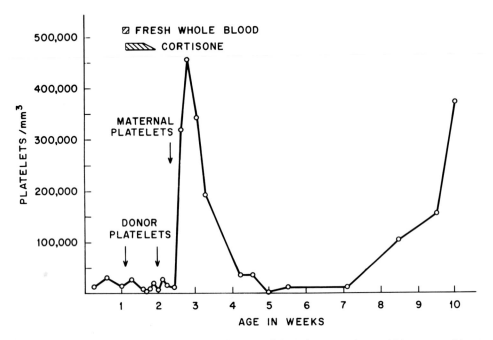

Fig. 3-4. Platelet counts of newborn infant with neonatal thrombocytopenia caused by maternal iso-immunization. Transfusions with random-donor platelets had no effect on two occasions. Transfusion of one unit of maternal platelets produced prompt rise with normal platelet survival. Although these platelets were washed, persistence of thrombocytopenia for several weeks might indicate infusion of maternal antibody with platelets. (From McIntosh, S., O'Brien, R. T., Schwartz, A. D., and Pearson, H. A.: J. Pediatr. **82:**1020, 1973.)

subsequent Pl[A1]-positive infants are affected about 75% of the time.[204]

TREATMENT. Therapy for isoimmune neonatal purpura is somewhat controversial. The disease is self-limited. Even without treatment, thrombocytopenia persists for less than 3 weeks. Because most patients recover without sequellae, some have advocated no active intervention.[7] However, a review of cases reported in the literature suggests that mortality and significant morbidity secondary to intracranial hemorrhage may be as high as 10%, especially in those infants subjected to vaginal delivery.[182] Most of the reported mortality came from a single report.

If the diagnosis is made in the first 12 hours of life or if there is evidence of progressive purpura, bleeding, or neurologic abnormalities, therapy is indicated. Since it is unlikely that platelets from a random donor will be compatible (only 2% of the population is Pl[A1] negative), transfusions of random donor platelet concentrates may be of little immediate value. Exchange transfusion with fresh CPD blood is effective in providing temporary hemostasis.[182]

Because the mother's platelets necessarily lack the antigen responsible for isoimmunization, platelet concentrates prepared from the mother's blood constitute specific and effective therapy.[3,133]

Transfusion of one unit of maternal platelets almost always stops the bleeding and should reduce the risk of serious complications (Fig. 3-4). It is important to remove as much of the maternal plasma as possible from the platelet concentrate because infusion of maternal antibody contained in platelet concentrates may cause a marked prolongation of the period of thrombocytopenia. Washing of maternal platelets with normal plasma to remove antibodies more completely has been advocated.

Repeated transfusions of maternal platelets are usually unnecessary, despite continuing thrombocytopenia in the infant. The infant can be protected from external trauma, and spontaneous and severe hemorrhage is unlikely after the immediate postpartum period. Administration of corticosteroids to the infant to reduce platelet destruction and increase vascular integrity has also been advocated.[3]

It is not possible to anticipate the first case of isoimmune purpura in a given family. However, once an index case has occurred, every effort should be made to obtain determination of the platelet genotypes of the parents. For example, if the father is homozygous Pl[A1] positive and the mother sensitized homozygous Pl[A1] negative, all of their subsequent infants will be heterozygous

Pl^{A1} positive and therefore are likely to be affected.

Obstetric management previously suggested for maternal ITP is also applicable here: immediate prenatal corticosteroid therapy to the mother and elective atraumatic delivery with a strong consideration of cesarean section.[144,206] Washed maternal platelet concentrates should be available for immediate administration to the infant after birth.[134]

Thrombocytopenia associated with maternal drug-induced purpura. A number of pharmacologic agents have the capacity to interact with platelets, making them antigenic and evoking antibody formation. If the sensitized individual subsequently ingests the drug, platelet destruction and thrombocytopenia may occur. All three elements —platelets, antibody, and drug—must be simultaneously present for this to happen.

The drugs most clearly associated with thrombocytopenia are the cardiologic agent quinidine and the related drug quinine.[17,65,224] These drugs are transmitted transplacentally when ingested by the pregnant woman. If a mother has circulating drug-induced antibodies that are IgG globulins, these can also pass into the fetal circulation. The combination of drug, fetal platelet, and maternal antibody may result in neonatal thrombocytopenia.[139] In drug-induced neonatal thrombocytopenia, the mother is also thrombocytopenic.

Other drugs[32,35,95,197] have rarely been implicated in the genesis of neonatal thrombocytopenia. Neonatal thrombocytopenia has been ascribed to maternal administration of thiazide diuretics,[193] but prospective study did not confirm such an association.[146] Exchange transfusion with fresh CPD blood is the preferred therapy if hemorrhage is severe; platelet concentrates from unsensitized donors may also help.

Thrombocytopenia associated with giant hemangioma (Kasabach-Merritt syndrome). Extensive cavernous hemangiomas involving large portions of the body may cause severe and even lethal thrombocytopenic hemorrhage.[202] Large numbers of platelets are sequestered and destroyed in the tortuous vascular channels of these tumors, and consumption of coagulation factors may also occur.[101] Although the giant hemangiomas associated with platelet consumption are usually readily apparent by physical examination, hepatic, splenic, or placental tumors have also sometimes been implicated.[67,219] (See also Chapters 24 and 25.)

Transfusions of platelets and other coagulation factors have only transient effect, but such replacement therapy may hasten involution of the tumor. Although corticosteroid therapy has limited immediate effect, its use may produce tumor involution, especially in very young infants.[63]

Heparinization may result in increases in fibrinogen and other coagulation factors. However, since tumor regression is probably a consequence of vascular thrombosis and infarction, anticoagulation might interfere with this and prolong the problem.

When it is possible, external compression of the hemangioma by firm bandaging may reduce blood flow and platelet trapping. Total surgical excision, when possible, has also corrected thrombocytopenia. Radiation therapy to reduce the size of the hemangioma should be considered when the hemorrhagic manifestations are severe.[34,121]

Disseminated intravascular coagulation. Neonates, particularly premature infants, are susceptible to disseminated intravascular coagulation (DIC) precipitated by a variety of perinatal events. Even in the uncomplicated delivery, placental separation is associated with the transient appearance of fibrin degradation products in the sera of many neonates and some mothers.[51,72,111,213] This "physiologic defibrination" may be incited by the release of thromboplastins during placental separation. Whereas clearance of circulating degradation products is complete within 24 hours in the healthy newborn, their increase in preeclampsia, eclampsia, placental abruption, and intrauterine fetal death and their persistence in some sick infants suggest a pathologic extension of this normal phenomenon.[51,72,111]

Consumption of platelets and coagulation factors occurs frequently in ill neonates.[73,85-87] The classic array of laboratory findings—hemolysis, thrombocytopenia, prolonged prothrombin and partial thromboplastin times, circulating degradation products, and decreased levels of plasminogen and factors V and VIII—occurs infrequently relative to the incidence of "partial" or "incomplete" DIC in which only two or three of these parameters may be abnormal.[85-87] Defibrination may complicate hypoxia, acidosis, infection, respiratory distress, eclampsia, placental abruption, or severe hemolysis or may be produced by giant hemangioma or venous thrombosis.[48,89,135]

Heparin therapy for DIC remains controversial. Purpura fulminans and regional trapping of coagulation factors in hemangiomas or deep vein thrombi are conditions in which heparinization may be beneficial.[2,85-87] Heparin is probably more safely administered by continuous intravenous infusion than intermittently.[196] Heparinization should be accompanied by concomitant infusions of platelet concentrates and fresh frozen plasma to replace consumed elements.[47] Heparinization has not been useful in systemic diseases and should not be applied routinely.[2,85,86] Bleeding infants in whom defibrination is not continuous may be protected by replacement of platelets and coagulation factors. In most cases intravascular coagulation subsides with resolution of the underlying disease.

Thrombocytopenias caused by both decreased production and increased destruction

Infection. Thrombocytopenia is a common finding in severe systemic perinatal infections caused by viral, bacterial, spirochetal, and protozoal organisms. The acronymic designation "TORCH" has been used to encompass the clinical syndromes resulting from neonatal infections: toxoplasmosis, rubella, cytomegalic inclusion disease,[105,141] herpesvirus hominis infection, and others including syphilis,[192,242] malaria,* tuberculosis,[77] and infections with gram-negative bacteria. When infections such as toxoplasmosis, syphilis, herpesvirus, or cytomegalovirus infection are acquired by the pregnant woman, they may be acquired by the fetus by means of hematogenous transplacental spread, cervical or vaginal contamination, or breast milk infection.† Although as many as 5% of all live-born infants may be infected by common organisms, relatively few are clinically ill. Infants with flagrant intrauterine infections are usually small for gestational age and clinically ill, have enlargement of their livers and spleens, and are jaundiced because of hemolysis or hepatitis.

Thrombocytopenia is often present and is manifested clinically as generalized petechiae.‡ The petechial rash may be punctate or a spreading blue-purple macular lesion, an appearance that has been compared to a blueberry muffin.

The mechanism for the thrombocytopenia of severe congenital infections is complex. Hypoplasia of megakaryocytes has been documented in infants with the congenital rubella syndrome, indicating that decreased platelet production is an important cause of thrombocytopenia in some of these cases.[36,86,228,249] Additionally, in many cases increased platelet destruction results from splenomegaly and reticuloendothelial hyperactivity.[249] DIC often complicates these conditions, particularly herpetic infection.[150,164]

When possible, therapy should be directed at the underlying infection. Antibiotics are indicated for bacterial sepsis and syphilis, and treatment of congenital toxoplasmosis with pyrimethamine (Daraprim) and sulfa should also be considered. Newer antiviral agents (iodoxuridine, adenine arabinoside) are being used to treat viral infections,§ especially herpes, but convincing proof of their efficacy is scarce.[243]

Thrombocytopenia does not require specific treatment since life-threatening hemorrhage is unusual. However, replacement therapy with platelet concentrates should be considered if serious bleeding occurs. When thrombocytopenia is predominantly a consequence of decreased platelet production, a sustained increase in platelet count should occur.[36,130,171] Prolonged thrombocytopenia for several months has been observed occasionally in infants with rubella.[249]

Osteopetrosis (marble bone disease). In osteopetrosis the marrow space is progressively obliterated by exuberant osseous growth.[211] Extensive extramedullary hematopoiesis develops in the liver and spleen, but this is quantitatively insufficient to maintain hematologic normalcy. Thrombocytopenia, leukocytosis, and anemia are present, characterized morphologically by teardrop-shaped poikilocytes and nucleated red blood cells (leukoerythroblastic anemia). The spleen also causes an increased rate of destruction of platelets and red cells. The severe form of osteopetrosis with symptoms in the newborn period is inherited as an autosomal recessive trait.[207]

WHITE BLOOD CELL COUNT AND NEUTROPENIA IN THE NEWBORN

The white cells of the blood show considerable variability in numbers and proportions during the neonatal period. Although average values can be listed, they are probably of less significance than are the broad ranges of leukocyte counts observed in normal infants. Wide deviations from an average may therefore be less indicative of clinical abnormalities than at other periods of life.

The total white blood cell count at birth may be anywhere from 9 to 30 × 10^9/liter but is generally high. Neutrophilic granulocytes predominate, with a mean at birth of 8 × 10^9/liter and a range of 4.5 to 13.2 × 10^9/liter.* The neutrophils show a tendency to immaturity (shift to left) with an average of 10% band forms as well as occasional younger elements (myelocytes and metamyelocytes).

Shortly after birth the white blood cell count increases, reaching a high point at 12 hours of age. This increase has often been attributed to hemoconcentration,[234,244] although Xanthou has demonstrated that, as granulocytes increase, the absolute lymphocyte count simultaneously decreases and the numbers of other white blood cells do not change.[247] Therefore hemoconcentration is an unlikely reason for the observed increase in neutrophil count. Mobilization of neutrophils from the so-called marginal pool of granulocytes temporarily sequestered in the lung and other portions of the

---

*References 27, 39, 123, 220, 246.
†References 45, 57, 164, 171, 187, 239, 241.
‡References 36, 52, 56, 58, 108, 151, 171, 240.
§References 9, 20, 30, 82, 107, 190, 212, 237.

---

*References 106, 147, 233, 234, 244.

circulation may be a better explanation.[138] After 12 hours of age the total white blood cell count decreases, and at 2 weeks of age it averages 11.4×10^9/liter with about 35% neutrophils and 5% band forms.

The lymphocytes also show a characteristic series of changes during the first 2 weeks.[247] Their absolute number at birth averages 3×10^9/liter. This decreases slightly during the first 3 days and then increases to an average value of 6×10^9/liter by 10 days of age. The increase in lymphocytes, combined with the decreasing number of granulocytes, results in the long-recognized lymphocytic predominance of infancy, which is established by 2 or 3 weeks of age.

Monocyte numbers are low (mean 1×10^9/liter) and do not vary during the first 2 weeks. Eosinophils average about 2% with a mean absolute eosinophil count of 0.7×10^9/liter during this time.[247] Absolute numbers of basophils are very low in the newborn period.

The total white blood cell counts of premature infants are approximately 30% lower than those of full-term infants. However, the sequential changes with a tendency to wide variations are similar to those previously described for term infants.[247]

Isoimmune neonatal neutropenia

Neonatal neutropenia (absolute neutrophil count $< 1.5 \times 10^9$/liter) may result from fetal or neonatal infection, isoimmunization, or, rarely, congenital immune deficiency.[71] The severely neutropenic infant is susceptible to cutaneous and systemic bacterial infection.

Isoimmune neutropenia may be produced by transplacental passage of IgG antileukocyte antibodies.[23,99,116] Despite the fact that 25% of multiparous women or women who have received transfusions develop leukoagglutins, neonatal neutropenia is uncommon.*

Leukoagglutinins are complex antibodies[222] often directed against lymphocytes,[23] platelets, and placental tissue.[226] Fetal granulocytes, formed at approximately 15 weeks of gestation, and possibly placental antigens[172] evoke chronic stimulation from repeated leakage to the maternal circulation. Desai[44] and Lalezari[117] have suggested that fetal chimerism and the presence of fetal neutrophil antigens might be the basis for development of chronic autoimmune neutropenia in later life. At birth these children appear healthy and neutropenia may only be discovered coincidentally during a routine blood count. The absolute neutrophil count is often lower than 1×10^9/liter. "Maturation arrest" and shift to the left have usually been described in the bone marrow.[23,99]

*References 103, 172, 176-178, 225, 226.

Antibiotic therapy is indicated for actual or probable bacterial infections, but prophylactic antibiotics should not be used. In selected cases granulocyte transfusions may be a beneficial adjunct. Isoimmune neutropenia is a self-limited disease that usually resolves in the early weeks or months of life.

MATERNAL DRUG EXPOSURE

Drugs that are commonly ingested by pregnant women often reach the fetus or nursing neonate by placental transfer or active secretion into breast milk. Medicines taken most commonly during pregnancy include salicylates and other analgesics, antacids, thiazide diuretics, antihistamines, antibiotics, sedatives, and cathartics.[19,94,95] Lipophilic, unionized drugs of low molecular weight are transferred across the placenta and into the breast milk. The transfer is affected by blood flow, pH, and thickness of trophoblastic epithelium.[154,155] In spite of the great number of medicines and toxins that can reach the fetus or nursing infant, relatively few have been clearly implicated as causes

Table 3-1. Drugs associated with blood dyscrasias in the fetus and neonate

Condition	Drug	Reference
Hyperbilirubinemia (nonhemolytic)	Menadione	125, 126, 126
	Oxytocin	11, 42, 205
	Epidural anesthetics	205
	Novobiocin	215
Hemolysis	Naphthalene	8, 43
	Nalidixic acid	14
	Sulfanilamide(?)	70, 125
	Thiazides(?)	83
Thrombocytopenia	Quinine	139
	Tolbutamide(?)	197, 205
	Thiazides(?)	146, 193
	Diethylstilbestrol(?)	33
Neutropenia	Thiouracil	168
	Thiazides(?)	193
Anemia, nonhemolytic	Thiazides(?)	197
Cytoplasmic vacuolization	Alcohol infusion	69, 124, 230
Methemoglobinemia	Prilocaine	32
Bleeding		
Thrombopathy	Aspirin	18, 19, 37
	Promethazine	37
	Alphaprodine	37
Depressed coagulation factors	Phenytoin	93, 96, 112, 160
	Warfarin (Coumadin)	33, 76, 97, 98

of hematologic disease in the fetus and newborn infant[33,95,168] (Table 3-1).

Nonhemolytic hyperbilirubinemia may be caused by large doses of water-soluble vitamin K analogs, even when there is no predisposing enzymatic deficiency such as G-6-PD deficiency.[126,127] Intravenous oxytocin infusion, combined with artificial rupture of membranes,[11,42,205] and epidural anesthesia[205] have also been implicated. White infants with G-6-PD deficiency may develop spontaneous nonhemolytic hyperbilirubinemia as well as severe hemolysis from oxidant drugs.[142,223] Exchange transfusion may be required to prevent kernicterus when severe jaundice occurs.

Two infants with hemolysis and hepatic necrosis whose mothers had received sulfanilamide were reported by Ginzler[70], and Lucey[129] has demonstrated that sulfadiamethoxine, a long-acting sulfa metabolized and excreted by glucuronidation, readily enters the fetal circulation and persists in the neonate for as long as 6 days. Hemolytic jaundice has been associated with maternal ingestion of mothballs,[8] as has nalidixic acid in breast milk.[14]

Methemoglobinemia may accompany hemolysis in infants with G-6-PD deficiency exposed to oxidant drugs and may complicate obstetric epidural anesthesia with prilocaine.[32] Cytoplasmic vacuoles in bone marrow cells may be found in premature infants whose mothers received intravenous infusions of alcohol.[69,124,230]

Drug-induced hemorrhagic tendencies result either from acquired thrombopathy or from the suppression of coagulation factors. Abnormal platelet function has been reported in some healthy neonates with no maternal drug exposure.[161] However, neonatal platelets appear to have a greater sensitivity to drugs that interfere with platelet function than those of adults.[37] Maternal aspirin ingestion within 1 week of delivery produced abnormal aggregation to ADP and collagen and increased the risk of hemorrhage in the neonate, even though maternal platelet function was normal.[18,19,37] Promethazine and alphaprodine, given as adjuncts with narcotics during labor, also depress the aggregation response of neonatal platelets to collagen but are not as potent as aspirin.[37]

Neonates born to mothers taking phenytoin and phenobarbital may bleed during the first 24 hours of life because of low levels of vitamin K–dependent coagulation factors.[96,112,160] Hemorrhage in these infants occurs earlier than that from vitamin K deficiency and tends to be more severe.[160] In cats treated with phenytoin, the bleeding tendency (but not the neurologic effects of the drug) was reversed with vitamin K.[93] Protection of the fetus can be achieved by discontinuation of phenytoin therapy in the mother and administration of aqueous vitamin K to the infant at birth. If fetal hemorrhage is not controlled with vitamin K, replacement of coagulation factors with fresh frozen plasma is recommended.[160]

Complications such as stillbirth and neonatal death from hemorrhage may result from the use of anticoagulants during the last trimester of pregnancy.[24,33,76,97,98] Warfarin (Coumadin) exaggerates the normal postnatal depression of vitamin K–dependent coagulation factors, and its effect can be reversed by administration of vitamin K or fresh frozen plasma. Perinatal risk can be reduced significantly in animals by discontinuing warfarin therapy at least 4 days prior to delivery.[97] If maternal anticoagulation therapy is mandatory during the perinatal period, heparin, a large, charged molecule that does not cross the placenta and is not secreted with breast milk, should be used.

MATERNAL ANEMIA
Hemoglobinopathies

Abnormal hemoglobins, particularly those affecting the β-chains of globin, may produce overt disease in individuals with homozygous or doubly heterozygous genotypes. (See Chapters 13 and 14.) Those in which erythrocyte sickling occurs predispose the pregnant woman, the placenta, and the fetus to adverse effects of infection, infarction, and anemia.

Among pregnancies complicated by maternal sickle cell anemia, sickle cell–β-thalassemia, or sickle cell–Hb C disease, fetal death and perinatal mortality rates are increased to as high as 65%. Live-born infants are often wasted and small for gestational age, and multiple infarcts may be found in the placenta. Risk of maternal obstetric mortality varies from 0% to 25%, and morbidity among pregnant women is significant, even for those with mild sickling disorders.*

Anemia and vaso-occlusive episodes can be prevented by maintaining the pregnant woman on a regimen of regular transfusions, particularly during the third trimester. The hemoglobin level should be kept higher than 10 gm/dl, and the percentage of Hb S should be less than 40% with transfusions of packed red cells, in effect converting the patient's hemoglobinopathy to sickle cell trait. Cautious exchange transfusion has also been recommended to reduce the population of sickled erythrocytes.

In women with nonsickling hemoglobinopathies, such as Hb CC disease, hemolysis and anemia may worsen with advancing gestation. Hypertransfusion is not needed, but supportive transfusions of packed cells should be given as dictated by the severity of anemia.[110]

---

*References 59, 62, 66, 100, 119, 122, 158, 162, 184, 189.

Pregnancy has not been reported in women with transfusion-dependent thalassemia major. Women with heterozygous β-thalassemia and homozygous thalassemia intermedia may become quite anemic during pregnancy and require occasional transfusions.

Neonates born to parents heterozygous for an abnormal hemoglobin or β-thalassemia should be tested for clinically significant major hemoglobinopathies.[181] Abnormalities in the β-chain of hemoglobin are not significant in the neonatal period, since the amount of adult hemoglobin is only 10%-20% of the full-term infant's hemoglobin complement,[64] the remainder being Hb F. At 2 to 3 months of age hemolysis appears and heralds the onset of other symptoms, such as the painful vaso-occlusive episodes of sickle cell anemia.[167]

Nutritional anemias

Maternal iron deficiency, even when severe, has little effect on the fetus. The neonatal blood picture of infants of iron-deficient mothers does not differ from that of normal infants.[129] Folic acid deficiency usually becomes evident only in the last trimester of pregnancy, but infants of folate-deficient mothers have not had significant anemia.

Autoimmune hemolytic anemia

Coombs-positive hemolytic anemia in the mother may necessitate occasional transfusions during pregnancy but usually does not produce deleterious effects on the neonate. A positive Coombs test in cord blood or in the newborn is not unusual and disappears during the early weeks of life. Rarely, particularly when autoimmune hemolysis appears during the third trimester, the neonate may have full-blown hemolytic anemia and hyperbilirubinemia from transplacental passage of the IgG autoantibody.[10] The disease is self-limited but may require exchange transfusion for extreme hyperbilirubinemia and transfusions of packed erythrocytes for severe anemia. A short course of corticosteroids should be considered for severe neonatal hemolysis.

MATERNAL MALIGNANCY

The woman with malignant disease who elects to conceive and wishes to continue the pregnancy presents the physician with the formidable task of providing optimal therapy for her neoplasm while simultaneously reducing risks of malignancy, teratogenicity, drug toxicities, and carcinogenesis in the fetus.

Transmission of active maternal malignancy to the fetus depends on the type of maternal neoplasm, the degree of bloodstream invasion, sequestration or transvillous passage of malignant cells in the placenta, and fetal response.[195] Although the incidence of maternal malignancy during pregnancy approaches 1 in 1,000, fewer than 40 cases of concurrent fetal or placental malignancy have been reported. Rothman[195] reported placental metastasis in 54% of women with disseminated cancer, but fetal malignancy occurred only rarely and only in women with leukemia,[19] lymphoma, and malignant melanoma. Two neonates with disseminated melanoma at birth developed spontaneous resolution of the neoplasm.[29] Two neonates with maternal acquisition of lymphoma and two with acute lymphocytic leukemia died within the first year of life.

Treatment of maternal neoplasms with radiotherapy or chemotherapy predisposes the fetus to damaging effects, particularly in the first trimester. Irradiation of a portal outside the abdomen may be more safely accomplished early in pregnancy than in the third trimester, when the abdominal location of the uterus places the fetus in proximity to scattered radiation. Abdominal or pelvic irradiation in therapeutic doses of several thousand rads usually produces fetal death and in doses of more than 10 rads carries a high probability of carcinogenisis.[12,41,209]

Antineoplastic drugs are potentially toxic, teratogenic, and carcinogenic to the fetus.* Although risks of fetal death and major anomalies appear greater during the first-trimester exposure,[145] the full spectrum of fetal effects is undetermined.

Alternative forms of therapy that can be used in the pregnant woman include surgery, radiotherapy distant from the uterus, interruption of pregnancy for abdominal irradiation or chemotherapy, conventional treatment with acceptance of fetal risks, and no therapy until the child is delivered.

Fetal carcinogenesis from maternal exposure to environmental toxins† and drugs‡ may occur to a greater degree than now realized. As illustrated by the totally unexpected association of diethylstilbestrol therapy during pregnancy with benign and malignant genital lesions in offspring,[16] the teratogenic and neoplastic potential of these agents may not be manifest for years after birth.

THE IMMUNOGLOBULINS

The immunoglobulins comprise a heterogenous group of serum proteins that are crucial for host resistance. These proteins are secreted by differentiated B (bursa-derived) lymphocytes. All of the immunoglobulins have a similar basic structure and contain two pairs of polypeptide chains.[209] Each immunoglobulin molecule has two heavy and two light chains.

---

*References 12, 38, 115, 145, 208, 209, 232.
†References 60, 136, 152, 153.
‡References 16, 38, 94, 115, 145, 168, 232.

The immunoglobulins are classified into five different classes (IgG, IgA, IgM, IgD, and IgE), each of which has a different chain composition.[50,188] Each class of immunoglobulin has a unique type of heavy chain and one of two types of light chain. Molecular formulas for the major immunoglobulin varieties may be represented as follows:

IgG: $\gamma_2\kappa_2, \gamma_2\lambda_2$ IgA: $\alpha_2\kappa_2, \alpha_2\lambda_2$ IgM: $\mu_2\kappa_2, \mu_2\lambda_2$
IgD: $\delta_2\kappa_2, \delta_2\lambda_2$ IgE: $\epsilon_2\kappa_2, \epsilon_2\lambda_2$

The situation is made even more complex by the discovery of four subclasses of γ-heavy chains and two subclasses of α-heavy chains.[166]

IgG is the predominant serum immunoglobulin, constituting 80% of the serum antibody. It has a molecular weight of about 145,000 daltons. Serum antibodies against most viruses and against gram-positive bacteria and polysaccharide antigens are of the IgG type. IgG antibodies can be transmitted transplacentally and therefore constitute the major portion of immunoglobulins in the fetus.

IgM constitutes 10% of serum antibodies. It has a high molecular weight of about 1×10^6 daltons, has a high specificity for endotoxins of gram-negative bacteria as well as cultured virus (Epstein-Barr virus), and fixes complement. Naturally occurring serum isohemagglutinins (anti-A and anti-B) are also of the IgM class.

IgA antibodies predominate in body secretions such as saliva and respiratory mucus and are secreted as dimers by plasma cells located in the epithelial lining.[194]

IgD is a trace immunoglobulin found predominantly in the serum.

IgE antibodies compose the reaginic antibodies of allergic and anaphylactoid reactions.

Developmental aspects of immunoglobulin levels

The immunoglobulin in the cord blood of the newborn infant (600 to 1,200 mg/dl) is derived entirely from the maternal circulation by placental passage (Fig. 3-5). Low immunoglobulin levels are found in fetal blood until the fourth or fifth month of pregnancy, after which they rise gradually to reach maternal concentrations by the eighth to ninth month. At birth the immunoglobulin level in fetal blood is somewhat higher than in maternal blood.[222] The immunoglobulin level is observed to fall steadily in the first month of life, following a simple exponential curve, reaching one third of the birth value at 2 months of age when it is stabilized.[170] No change occurs between 3 and 4 months of age (300 to 600 mg/dl) when the rate of synthesis balances the rate of catabolism. From 4 months of age levels of immunoglobulin rise slowly and progressively; adults levels (900 mg/dl) are reached at 2 years of age.[102] According to these calculations, the half-life of immunoglobulin is approximately 25 days.[215,236]

Although all maternal IgA and virtually all IgM globulins are excluded from the fetus, maternal immunoglobulin is carried across the placental barrier with great efficiency. Consequently the detection of IgA and IgM globulin in umbilical cord blood indicates that the infant was provoked into an antibody response by intrauterine infection. Alford et al.[6] demonstrated that IgM antibodies are the first to appear in the response sequence and,

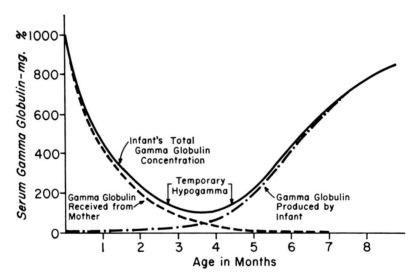

Fig. 3-5. Graph showing levels of γ-globulin in physiologic hypogammaglobulinemia of newborn infants. As level of γ-globulin from mother drops and production by infant begins, there is a temporary drop in γ-globulin concentration. (From Barrett, B., and Volwiler, W.: J.A.M.A. **164**:866, 1957.)

because elevated concentrations of IgM or IgA antibodies in cord serum cannot normally be of maternal origin, their presence in cord serum is indicative of intrauterine infection.

Routine assessment of IgM content of umbilical cord serum can be of particular value in detecting infants with subclinical or unusual types of congenitally acquired infection and is particularly useful in identifying those born after inapparent maternal illnesses.

REFERENCES

1. Aballi, A. J., Puapondh, Y., and Desposito, F.: Platelet counts in thriving premature infants, Pediatrics **42:** 685, 1968.
2. Abildgaard, C. F.: Recognition and treatment of intravascular coagulation, J. Pediatr. **74:**163, 1969.
3. Adner, M. M., Fisch, G. R., Starobin, S. G., and Aster, R. H.: Use of "compatible" platelet transfusion in treatment of congenital isoimmune neonatal purpura, N. Engl. J. Med. **280:**244, 1969.
4. Albin, A. R., Kushner, J. H., Murphy, A., and Zippin, C.: Platelet enumeration in the neonatal period, Pediatrics **28:**822, 1961.
5. Aldrich, R. A., Steinberg,, A. G., and Campbell, D. C.: Pedigree demonstrating a sex-linked recessive condition characterized by draining ears, eczematoid dermatitis, and bloody diarrhea, Pediatrics **13:**133, 1954.
6. Alford, C. A., Schaefer, J., Blankenship, W. J., et al.: A correlative immunologic, microbiologic, and clinical approach to the diagnosis of acute and chronic infections in newborn infants, N. Engl. J. Med. **277:**437, 1967.
7. Anthony, B., and Krivit, W.: Neonatal thrombocytopenic purpura, Pediatrics **30:**776, 1962.
8. Anziulewicz, J. A., Dick, H. J., and Chiarulli, E. E.: Transplacental napthalene poisoning, Am. J. Obstet. Gynecol. **78:**519, 1959.
9. Appleyard, G.: Chemotherapy of viral infections, Br. Med. Bull. **23:**114, 1967.
10. Baumann, R., and Rubin, H.: Autoimmune hemolytic anemia during pregnancy with hemolytic disease in the newborn, Blood **41:**293, 1973.
11. Beasley, J. M., and Alderman, B.: Neonatal hyperbilirubinemia following the use of oxytocin in labour, Br. J. Obstet. Gynecol. **82:**265, 1975.
12. Becker, M. D., and Hyman, G. A.: Management of Hodgkin's disease coexistent with pregnancy, Radiology **85:**725, 1965.
13. Bell, A. D., Mold, J. W., Oliver, R. A. M., and Shaw, S.: Study of transfused platelets in a case of congenital hypoplastic thrombocytopenia, Br. Med. J. **2:**692, 1956.
14. Belton, E. M., and Jones, R. V.: Haemolytic anemia due to nalidixic acid. Lancet **2:**691, 1965.
15. Berlyne, G. M., Short, I. A., and Vickers, C. F. H.: Placental transmission of the L.E. factor, Lancet **1:**15, 1957.
16. Bibbo, M., Gill, W. B., Azizi, F., Blough, R., Fang, V. S., Rosenfield, R. L., Schumacher, G. F. B., Sleeper, K., Sonek, M. G., and Wied, G. L., Follow-up study of male and female offspring of DES-exposed mothers, Obstet. Gynecol. **49:**1, 1977.
17. Bigelow, F. S., and Desforges, J. F.: Platelet agglutination by an abnormal plasma factor in thrombocytopenic purpura associated with quinidine ingestion, Am. J. Med. Sci. **224:**274, 1952.
18. Bleyer, W. A., Au, W. Y. W., Lange, W. A., and Raisz, L. G.: Studies on the detection of adverse drug reactions in the newborn. I. Fetal exposure to maternal medication, J.A.M.A. **213:**2046, 1970.
19. Bleyer, W. A., and Breckenridge, R. T.: Studies on the detection of adverse drug reactions in the newborn. II. The effects of prenatal aspirin on newborn hemostasis, J.A.M.A. **213:**2049, 1970.
20. Bloom, G. E., Warner, S., Gerald, P. S., and Diamond, L. K.: Chromosomal abnormalities in constitutional aplastic anemia, N. Engl. J. Med. **274:**8, 1966.
21. Bluestone, S. S., and Maslow, H. L.: Essential thrombocytopenic purpura in the newborn infant, Pediatrics **4:**620, 1949.
22. Boston Interhospital Virus Study Group and the NIAID-sponsored Cooperative Antiviral Clinical Study: Failure of high dose 5-iodo-2' deoxyuridine in the therapy of herpes simplex virus encephalitis, N. Engl. J. Med. **292:** 599, 1975.
23. Boxer, L. A., Yokoyama, M., and Lalezari, F.: Isoimmune neonatal neutropenia, J. Pediatr. **80:**783, 1972.
24. Brambel, C. E., and Hunter, R. E.: Effect of dicumerol on the nursing infant, Am. J. Obstet. Gynecol. **59:**1153, 1950.
25. Branehog, I.: Platelet kinetics in idiopathic thrombocytopenic purpura (ITP) before and at different times after splenectomy, Br. J. Haematol. **29:**413, 1975.
26. Bridge, R. G., and Foley, F. E.: Placental transmission of the lupus erythematosus factor, Am. J. Med. Sci. **227:**1, 1954.
27. Bruce-Chwatt, L. J.: Acute malaria in newborn infants, Br. Med. J. **3:**283, 1970.
28. Canales, L., and Mauer, A. M.: Sex-linked hereditary thrombocytopenia as a variant of Wiskott-Aldrich syndrome, N. Engl. J. Med. **277:**899, 1967.
29. Cavell, B.: Transplacental metastasis of malignant melanoma, Acta Paediatr. **146**(suppl.):37, 1963.
30. Charnock, E. L., and Cramblett, H. G.: 5-Iodo-2'-deoxyuridine in neonatal herpes virus hominis encephalitis, J. Pediatr. **76:**459, 1970.
31. Chown, B.: Anaemias in the newborn other than haemolytic disease, Pediatr. Clin. North Am. **4:**371, 1957.
32. Climie, C. R., McLean, S., Starmer, G. A., and Thomas, J.: Methaemoglobinaemia in mother and foetus following continuous epidural analgesia with prilocaine, Br. J. Anesth. **39:**155, 1967.
33. Cohlan, S. Q.: Fetal and neonatal hazards from drugs administered during pregnancy, N.Y. State J. Med. **64:** 493, 1964.
34. Colebatch, J. H., Horan, M. B., and Turner, K. K.: Giant hemangioma in newborn. In Gellis, S. S., ed.: Year book of pediatrics, Chicago, 1966-67, Year Book Medical Publishers, Inc. pp. 155-158.
35. Cooper, B. A., and Bigelow, F. S.: Thrombocytopenia associated with the administration of diethylstilbestrol in man, Am. Int. Med. **52:**907, 1960.
36. Cooper, L. Z., Green, R. H., Krugman, S., et al.: Neonatal thrombocytopenic purpura and other manifestations of rubella contracted in utero, Am. J. Dis. Child. **110:** 416, 1965.
37. Corby, D. G., and Schulman, I.: The effects of antenatal drug administration on aggregation of platelets of newborn infants, J. Pediatr. **79:**307, 1971.
38. Cote, C. J., Meuwissen, H. J., and Pickering, R. J.: Effects on the neonate of prednisone and azathioprine administered to the mother during pregnancy, J. Pediatr. **85:**324, 1974.
39. Covell, G.: Congenital malaria, Trop. Dis. Bull. **47:** 1147, 1950.
40. Creger, W. P., and Steele, M. R.: Human fetomaternal passage of erythrocytes, N. Engl. J. Med. **256:**158, 1957.
41. D'Angio, G. J., and Nisce, L. Z.: Problems with the irradiation of children and pregnant patients, J.A.M.A. **223:**171, 1973.

42. Davies, D. P., Gomersall, R., Robertson, R., et al: Neonatal jaundice and maternal oxytocin infusion, Br. Med. J. **1**:476, 1973.

43. Dawson, J. P., Thayer, W. W., and Desforges, J. F.: Acute hemolytic anemia in the newborn infant due to naphthalene poisoning: report of two cases, with investigations into the mechanism of the disease, Blood **13**: 1113, 1958.

44. Desai, R. G., and Creger, W. P.: Maternofetal passage of leukocytes and platelets in man, Blood **21**:665, 1963.

45. Desmonts, G., and Couvreur, J.: Congenital toxoplasmosis, N. Engl. J. Med. **290**:1110, 1974.

46. Dignan, D., Maurer, A. M., and Frantz, C.: Phocomelia with congenital hypoplastic thrombocytopenia and myeloid leukemoid reactions, J. Pediatr. **70**:561, 1967.

47. Donaldson, V. H., and Kisker, C. T.: Blood coagulation and hemostasis. In Nathan, D. G., and Oski, F. A., eds.: Hematology of infancy and childhood, Philadelphia, 1974, W. B. Saunders Co.

48. Dube, B., Bhattacharya, S., and Dube, E. K.: Blood coagulation profile in Indian patients with pre-eclampsia and eclampsia, Br. J. Obstet. Gynaecol. **82**:35, 1975.

49. Dunsford, I.: Proof of fetal antigens entering the maternal circulation. In Official Program of the Sixth International Congress of the International Society of Hematology, Boston, 1956, p. 539.

50. Edelman, G. M.: Antibody structure and molecular immunology, Science **180**:830, 1973.

51. Ekelund, H., Hedner, U., and Nilsson, I. M.: Fibrinolysis in newborns, Acta Paediatr. Scand. **59**:33, 1970.

52. Emanual, I., and Kenny, G. E.: Cytomegalic inclusion disease of infancy, Pediatr. **38**:957, 1966.

53. Engel, R. R., Hammond, D., Eitzman, D. V., et al.: Transient congenital leukemia in seven infants with mongolism, J. Pediatr. **65**:303, 1964.

54. Eshagpour, E., Oski, F. A., Naiman, J. L.: Iron deficiency anemia in a newborn infant, J. Pediatr. **68**:806, 1966.

55. Fanconi, G.: Familial constitutional panmyelopathy: Fanconi's anemia, Semin. Hematol. **4**:233, 1967.

56. Feldman, H. A.: Toxoplasmosis, Pediatrics **22**:559, 1958.

57. Feldman, H. A.: Toxoplasmosis, N. Engl. J. Med. **279**: 1370, 1968.

58. Feldman, H. A.: Toxoplasmosis, N. Engl. J. Med. **279**: 1431, 1968.

59. Fiakpui, E. Z., and Moran, E. M.: Pregnancy in the sickle hemoglobinopathies, J. Reprod. Med. **11**:28, 1973.

60. Finberg, L.: PBB's: the ladies' milk is not for burning, J. Pediatr. **90**:511, 1977.

61. Fogel, B. J., Arias, D., and Jung, F.: Platelet counts in healthy premature infants, J. Pediatr. **73**:108, 1968.

62. Fort, A. T., Morrison, J. C., Berreras, L., et al.: Counselling in the patient with sickle cell disease about reproduction: pregnancy outcome does not justify the maternal risk; Am. J. Obstet. Gynecol. **111**:324, 1971.

63. Fost, N. C., and Esterly, N. B.: Successful treatment of juvenile hemangiomas with prednisone, J. Pediatr. **72**: 351, 1968.

64. Fraser, I. D., and Raper, A. B.: Observations on the change from foetal to adult erythropoiesis, Arch. Dis. Child. **37**:289, 1962.

65. Freedman, A. L., Brody, E. A., and Barr, P. S.: Immunothrombocytopenic purpura due to quinidine, J. Lab. Clin. Med. **48**:205, 1956.

66. Freeman, M. G., and Ruth, G. J.: SS disease, SC disease, and CC disease: obstetric considerations and treatment, Clin. Obstet. Gynecol. **12**:134, 1969.

67. Froehlich, L. A., and Housler, M.: Neonatal thrombocytopenia and chorangioma, J. Pediatr. **78**:516, 1971.

68. Fujikura, T., and Lkionsky, B.: Transplacental passage of maternal erythrocytes with sickling, J. Pediatr. **87**: 781, 1975.

69. Gartner, U., and Ryden, G.: The elimination of alcohol in the premature infant, Acta Paediatr. Scand. **61**:720, 1972.

70. Ginzler, A. M., and Chesner, C.: Toxic manifestations in the newborn infant following placental transmission of sulfanilamide, Am. J. Obstet. Gynecol. **44**:46, 1942.

71. Gitlin, D., Vawter, G., and Craig, J. M.: Thymic alymphoplasia and congenital aleukocytosis, Pediatrics **33**: 184, 1964.

72. Gjønnaess, H., and Fagerhol, M. K.: Studies on coagulation and fibrinolysis in pregnancy, Acta Obstet. Gynecol. Scand. **54**:363, 1975.

73. Glader, B. E., and Buchanan, G. R.: The bleeding neonate. In Smith, C. A., ed.: The critically ill child: diagnosis and management. Philadephia, 1977, W. B. Saunders Co., p. 217.

74. Goodall, H. B., Graham, F. S., Miller, M. D., and Cameron, C.: Transplacental bleeding from the foetus, J. Clin. Pathol. **11**:251, 1958.

75. Goodhue, P. A., and Evans, T. S.: Idiopathic thrombocytopenic purpura in pregnancy, Obstet. Gynecol. Surv. **18**:671, 1963.

76. Gordon, R. R., and Dean, T.: Foetal deaths from antenatal anticoagulant therapy, Br. Med. J. **2**:719, 1955.

77. Gouley, B. A., Blumberg, N., and Grayson, R. J.: Thrombocytopenic purpura associated with tuberculous splenomegaly and tuberculosis of the bone marrow, N. Engl. J. Med. **241**:147, 1949.

78. Grottum, K. A., and Hovig, T.: Wiskott-Aldrich Syndrome: qualitative platelet defects and short platelet survival, Br. J. Haematol. **17**:373, 1969.

79. Gunson, H. H.: Neonatal anemia due to fetal hemorrhage into the maternal circulation, Pediatrics **20**:3, 1957.

80. Haider, S. A.: Polymorphonuclear leukocyte count in diagnosis of infection in the newborn, Arch. Dis. Child **47**:394, 1972.

81. Hall, J. G., Levin, J., Kuhn, J. P., et al.: Thrombocytopenia with absent radius, Medicine **48**:411, 1969.

82. Hanshaw, J. B.: Idoxuridine in herpes virus encephalitis, N. Engl. J. Med. **282**:47, 1970.

83. Harley, J. D., Robin, H., and Robertson, S. E. J.: Thiazide-induced neonatal hemolysis? Br. Med. J. **1**:696, 1964.

84. Harrington, W. J., Sprague, C. C., Minnich, V., et al.: Immunologic mechanisms in idiopathic and neonatal thrombocytopenic purpura, Ann. Intern. Med. **38**:433, 1953.

85. Hathaway, W. E.: Coagulation problems in the newborn infant, Pediatr. Clin. North Am. **17**:929, 1970.

86. Hathaway, W. E.: Disseminated intravascular coagulation. In Snith, C. A., ed.: The critically ill child: diagnosis and management, Philadelphia, 1977, W.B. Saunders, Co.

87. Hathaway, W. E., Mull, M. M., and Pechet, G. S.: Disseminated intravascular coagulation in the newborn, Pediatrics **43**:233, 1969.

88. Hedenstedt, S., and Naeslund, J.: Investigations of the permeability of the placenta with the help of elliptocytes, Acta Med. Scand. **169**(suppl.):126, 1946.

89. Henderson, A. H., Pugsley, D. J., and Thomas, D. P.: Fibrin degradation products in pre-eclamptic toxaemia and eclampsia, Br. Med. J. **3**:545, 1970.

90. Hertz, C. G., and Hambrich, G. W.: Congenital Letterer-Siwe disease, Am. J. Dis. Child. **116**:553, 1968.

91. Heys, R. F.: Child-bearing and idiopathic thrombocytopenic purpura, J. Obstet. Gynaecol. Br. Cwlth. **73**:205, 1966.

92. Heys, R. F.: Steroid therapy for idiopathic thrombocy-

topenic purpura during pregnancy, Obstet. Gynecol. **28:** 532, 1966.

93. Hilgartner, M., Solomon, G. E., and Kutt, H.: Diphenyl-hydantoin-induced coagulation abnormalities, Pediatr. Res. **5:**408, 1971.

94. Hill, R. B.: Prenatal medication—epidemiology and teratology. In Mead Johnson Symposium on Perinatal and Developmental Medicine, No. 5, Evansville, Ind., 1975, Mead Johnson Co.

95. Hill, R. M., and Barton, M. D.: Maternal drugs in the prenatal and intrapartum period and their effect on the neonate, In Mead Johnson Symposium on Perinatal and Developmental Medicine No. 5, Evansville, Ind., 1975, Mead Johnson Co.

96. Hill, R. M., Verniaud, W. M., Horning, M. G., et al.: Infants exposed in utero to anti-epileptic drugs: a prospective study, Am. J. Dis. Child **127:**645, 1974.

97. Hirsh, J., Cade, J. F., and Gallus, A. S.: Fetal effects on coumadin administered during pregnancy, Blood **36:** 623, 1970.

98. Hirsh, J., Cade, J. F., and O'Sullivan, E. F.: Clinical experience with anticoagulant therapy in pregnancy, Br. Med. J. **1:**270, 1970.

99. Hitzig, W. H., and Gitzelmann, R.: Transplacental transfer of leukocyte agglutinins, Vox. Sang. **4:**445, 1959.

100. Horger, E. D. III.: Sickle cell and sickle cell hemoglobin C disease during pregnancy, Obstet. Gynecol. **39:**873, 1972.

101. Inceman, S., and Tangun, Y.: Chronic defibrination syndrome due to a giant hemangioma with microangio-pathic hemolytic anemia, Am. J. Med. **96:**997, 1963.

102. Janeway, C. A., and Gitlin, D.: The gamma globulins. In Levine, S. Z., et al. eds.: Advances in pediatrics, vol. 4, Chicago, 1951, Year Book Medical Publishers, Inc., p. 65.

103. Jensen, K. G.: Leucocyte antibodies in serums of pregnant women, Vox. Sang. **7:**454, 1962.

104. Jones, A. R., and Silver, S.: The detection of minor erythrocyte populations by mixed agglutinates, Blood **13:** 763, 1958.

105. Kalinowski, S. Z., and Walker, J. M.: Thrombocyto-penic purpura in tuberculosis, Br. J. Tuberc. Dis. Chest **50:**239, 1956.

106. Kato, K.: Leukocytes in infancy and childhood. A statistical analysis of 1,081 total and differential counts from birth to fifteen years, J. Pediatr. **7:**7, 1935.

107. Kaufman, H. E.: Chemotherapy of virus disease, Chemotherapy **7:**1, 1963.

108. Kilbrick, S., and Loria, R. M.: Cytomegalovirus infection, Pediatr. Clin. North Am. **21:**518, 1974.

109. Kirkman, H. N., and Riley, H. D.: Posthemorrhagic anemia and shock in the newborn: a review, Pediatrics **24:**197, 1959.

110. Kitay, D. Z., and Perrin, E. V.: Homozygous hemoglobin C disease and pregnancy, Obstet. Gynecol. **32:** 657, 1968.

111. Kleiner, G. J., Merskey, C., Johnson, A. J., and Markus, W. B.: Defibrination in normal and abnormal parturition, Br. J. Haematol. **19:**159, 1970.

112. Kohler, H. G.: Haemorrhage in the newborn of epileptic mothers, Lancet **1:**267, 1966.

113. Krivit, W., and Good, R. A.: Aldrich's syndrome (thrombocytopenia, eczema, and infection in infants), Am. J. Dis. Child. **97:**137, 1959.

114. Kurstjens, R., and Balt, C.: Familial thrombopathic thrombocytopenia, Br. J. Haematol. **15:**305, 1968.

115. Lacher, J. M.: Use of vinblastine sulfate to treat Hodgkin's disease during pregnancy, Ann. Intern. Med. **61:** 113, 1964.

116. Lalezari, P., and Bernard, G. E.: An isologous antigen-antibody reaction with human neutrophiles, related to

117. Lalezari, P., Jiang, A., Yegen, L., and Santorineou, M.: Chronic autoimmune neutropenia due to anti-NA2 antibody, N. Engl. J. Med. **293:**744, 1975.

118. Lapido, O. A.: Management of third stage of labour, with particular reference to reduction of feto-maternal transfusion, Br. Med. J. **1:**721, 1972.

119. Laros, R. K., Jr., and Kalstone, C. E.: Sickle cell-β thalassemia and pregnancy, Obstet. Gynecol. **37:** 67, 1971.

120. Laros, R. K., and Sweet, R. L.: Management of idiopathic thrombocytopenic purpura during pregnancy, Am. J. Obstet. Gynecol. **122:**182, 1975.

121. Lelong, M., Alagille, D., Habib, E. C., and Steiner, A.: Giant hemangioma with thrombopenia in infancy. In Gellis, S. S., ed.: Year book of pediatrics, Chicago, 1965-1966, Year Book Medical Publishers, Inc., pp. 301-304.

122. Levin, J., and Algazy, K. M.: Hematologic disorders. In Burrow, G. N., and Ferris, T. F., eds.: Medical complications during pregnancy, Philadelphia, 1975, W. B. Saunders Co.

123. Logie, D. E., and McGregor, I. A.: Acute malaria in newborn infants, Br. Med. J. **3:**404, 1970.

124. Lopez, R., and Montoya, M. F.: Abnormal bone marrow morphology in the premature infant associated with maternal alcohol infusion, J. Pediatr. **79:**1008, 1971.

125. Lucey, J. F.: Hazards to the newborn infant from drugs administered to the mother, Pediatr. Clin. North Am. **8:** 413, 1961.

126. Lucey, J. F., and Dolan, R. G.: Hyperbilirubinemia in infants, J.A.M.A. **167:**1875, 1958.

127. Lucey, J. F., and Dolan, R. G.: Injections of vitamin-K compound in mothers and hyperbilirubinemia in the newborn, Pediatrics **22:**605, 1958.

128. Lucey, J. F., and Driscoll, T. J.: Hazard to newborn infants of administration of long-acting sulfonamides to pregnant women, Pediatrics **24:**498, 1959.

129. M and R Laboratories: Report of the fifteenth M & R pediatric research conference, 1955, p. 27.

130. McCracken, G. H., Jr., Shinefield, H. R., Cobb, K., et al.: Congenital cytomegalic inclusion disease: a longitudinal study of 20 patients, Am. J. Dis. Child. **117:**522, 1969.

131. McDonald, T. P.: Platelet size in relation to platelet age, Proc. Soc. Exp. Biol. Med. **115:**684, 1964.

132. McGovern, J. J., Driscoll, R., DuToit, C. H., et al.: Iron-deficiency anemia resulting from feto-maternal transfusion, N. Engl. J. Med. **258:**1149, 1958.

133. McIntosh, S.: Neonatal purpura, Contemp. Obstet. Gynecol. **6:**13, 1975.

134. McIntosh, S., O'Brien, R. T., Schwartz, A. D., and Pearson, H. A.: Neonatal isoimmune purpura: Response to platelet infusions, J. Pediatr. **82:**1020, 1973.

135. McKay, D. G.: Hematological evidence of disseminated intravascular coagulation in eclampsia, Obstet. Gynecol. Surg. **27:**399, 1972.

136. McMahon, B., and Levy, M. A.: Prenatal origin of childhood leukemia, N. Engl. J. Med. **270:**1082, 1964.

137. Macris, N. T., Hellman, L. M., and Watson, R. J.: Transmission of transfused sickle-trait cells from mother to fetus, Am. J. Obstet. Gynecol. **76:**1214, 1958.

138. Mauer, A. M., Athens, J. W., Warner, H. R., Ashenbrucker, H., Cartwright, G. E., and Wintrobe, M. M.: An analysis of leukocyte radioactivity curves obtained with radioactive avisopropyl fluorophosphate (DFP³²). In Stohlman, F., ed.: The kinetics of cellular proliferation, New York, 1959, Grune & Stratton, Inc.

139. Mauer, A. M., DeVaux, W., and Lahey, M. E.: Neonatal and maternal thrombocytopenic purpura due to quinine, Pediatrics **19:**84, 1957.

neonatal neutropenia, J. Clin. Invest. **45:**1741, 1966.

140. Medoff, H. S.: Platelet counts in premature infants, J. Pediatr. **64**:287, 1964.

141. Melish, M. E., and Hanshaw, J. B.: Congenital cytomegalovirus infection, Am. J. Dis. Child. **126**:190, 1973.

142. Meloni, T., Costa, S., and Cutillo, S.: Haptoglobin, hemopexin, hemoglobin, and hematocrit in newborns with erythrocyte glucose-6-phosphate dehydrogenase deficiency, Acta Haematol. **54**:284, 1975.

143. Mengert, W. F., Rights, C. S., Bates, C. R., et al.: Placental transmission of erythrocytes, Am. J. Obstet. Gynecol. **69**:678, 1955.

144. Mennuti, M., Schwartz, R. H., and Gill, F.: Obstetric management of isoimmune thrombocytopenia, Am. J. Obstet. Gynecol. **118**:565, 1974.

145. Mennuti, M. T., Shepard, T. H., and Mellman, W. J.: Fetal renal malformation following treatment of Hodgkin's disease during pregnancy, Obstet. Gynecol. **46**:194, 1975.

146. Merenstein, G. B., O'Loughlin, E. P., and Plunket, D. C.: Effects of thiazides on platelet counts of newborn infants, J. Pediatr. **76**:766, 1970.

147. Merritt, K. K., and Davidson, L. T.: The blood during the first year of life, Am. J. Dis. Child. **46**:990, 1933.

148. Mijer, F., and Olsen, R. N.: Transplacental passage of the L.E. factor, J. Pediatr. **52**:690, 1958.

149. Miles, R. M., Maurer, H. M., and Valdes, O. S.: Iron-deficiency anemia at birth: two examples secondary to chronic fetal-maternal hemorrhage, Clin. Pediatr. **10**:223, 1971.

150. Miller, D. R., Hanshaw, J. B., O'Leary, D. S., and Hnilicka, J. V.: Fatal disseminated herpes simplex virus infection and hemorrhage in the neonate, J. Pediatr. **76**:405, 1970.

151. Miller, M. J., Seaman, E., and Remington, J. S.: The clinical spectrum of congenital toxoplasmosis: problems in recognition, J. Pediatr. **70**:714, 1967.

152. Miller, R. W.: Pollutants in breast milk, J. Pediatr. **90**:510, 1977.

153. Miller, R. W.: Relationship between human teratogens and carcinogens, J. Natl. Cancer Inst. **58**:471, 1977.

154. Mirkin, B. L.: Placental transfer and fetal localization of drugs. In The Mead Johnson Symposium on Perinatal and Developmental Medicine, Evansville, Ind., 1974, Mead Johnson Co.

155. Mirkin, B. L.: Perinatal pharmacology: placental transfer, fetal localization and neonatal disposition of drugs, Anesthesiology **43**:156, 1976.

156. Mole, R. H.: Antenatal irradiation and childhood cancer: Causation or coincidence? Br. J. Cancer **30**:199, 1974.

157. Mollison, P. L.: Estimation of the extent of transplacental hemorrhage, Br. Med. J. **3**:31, 1972.

158. Mollison, P. L.: Blood transfusion in clinical medicine, ed. 5, 1972, Blackwell Scientific Publications, Ltd.

159. Morrison, J. C., Roe, P. L., Stahl, R. L., et al.: Heterozygous thalassemia and pregnancy: a twenty-five year experience. J. Reprod. Med. **11**:35, 1973.

160. Mountain, K. R., Hirsh, J., and Gallus, A. S.: Neonatal coagulation defect due to anticonvulsant drug treatment in pregnancy, Lancet **1**:265, 1970.

161. Mull, M. M., and Hathaway, W. E.: Altered platelet function in newborns, Pediatr. Res. **4**:229, 1970.

162. Necheles, T.: Obstetric complications associated with haemoglobinopathies, Clin. Haematol. **2**:497, 1973.

163. Nahmias, A. J.: The TORCH complex, Hosp. Prac., **9**:65, May 1974.

164. Nahmias, A., Alford, C., and Korones, S.: Infection of the newborn with herpes virus hominis, Adv. Pediatr. **17**:185, 1970.

165. Nathan, D. J., and Snapper, I.: Simultaneous placental transfer of factors responsible for L.E. cell formation and thrombocytopenia, Am. J. Med. **25**:647, 1958.

166. Natvig, J. B., and Kunkel, H. G.: Human immunoglobulins: Classes, subclasses, genetic variants, and idiotypes, Adv. Immunol. **16**:1, 1973.

167. O'Brien, R. T., McIntosh, S., Aspnes, G. T., and Pearson, H. A.: Prospective study of sickle cell anemia in infancy, J. Pediatr. **89**:205, 1976.

168. O'Brien, T. E.: Excretion of drugs in human milk, Am. J. Hosp. Pharm. **31**:844, 1974.

169. O'Gorman-Hughes, D. W.: Neonatal thrombodytopenia; Assessment of aetiology and prognosis, Austr. Paediatr. J. **3**:276, 1967.

170. Orlandim, O., Sass-Kortsak, A., and Ebbs, J. H.: Serum gamma globulin levels in normal infants, Pediatrics **16**:575, 1955.

171. Overall, J. C., Jr., and Glasgow, L. A.: Virus infections of the fetus and newborn infant, J. Pediatr. **77**:315, 1970.

172. Overweg, J., and Engelfriet, C. P.: Cytotoxic leucocyte iso-antibodies formed during the first pregnancy, Vox. Sang. **16**:97, 1969.

173. Pai, M. K. R., Bedritis, I., and Zipursky, A.: Massive transplacental hemorrhage: Clinical manifestations in the newborn, Med. Prac. **112**:585, 1975.

174. Papageorgiades, G.: Transplacental passage of fetal red cells into the maternal circulation, Clin. Pediatr. **15**:42, 1976.

175. Paul, J. D., Jr., Pranckun, P. P., and Grosh, J. L.: Splenectomy for thrombocytopenic purpura in pregnancy, Obstet. Gynecol. **28**:236, 1966.

176. Payne, R.: The development and persistence of leukoagglutinins in parous women, Blood **19**:411, 1962.

177. Payne, R.: Neonatal neutropenia and leukoagglutinins, Pediatrics **33**:194, 1964.

178. Payne, R., and Rolfs, M. R.: Fetomaternal leukocyte incompatability, J. Clin. Invest. **37**:1756, 1958.

179. Pearson, H. A., and Diamond, L. K.: Chronic monocytic leukemia in childhood, J. Pediatr. **53**:259, 1958.

180. Pearson, H. A., and Diamond, L. K.: Feto-maternal transfusion, Am. J. Dis. Child. **97**:267, 1959.

181. Pearson, H. A., O'Brien, R. T., McIntosh, S., et al.: Routine screening of umbilical cord blood for sickle cell disease, J. Am. Med. Assoc. **227**:420, 1974.

182. Pearson, H. A., Shulman, N. R., Marder, V. J., and Cone, Jr., T. E.: Isoimmune neonatal thrombocytopenic purpura: clinical and therapeutic considerations, Blood **23**:154, 1964.

183. Pearson, H. A., Shulman, N. R., Oski, F. A., and Eitzman, D. V.: Platelet survival in Wiskott-Aldrich syndrome, J. Pediatr. **68**:754, 1966.

184. Perkins, R. P.: Inherited disorders of hemoglobin synthesis and pregnancy, Am. J. Obstet. Gynecol. **111**: 120, 1971.

185. Peterson, O. H., and Larson, P.: Thrombocytopenic purpura in pregnancy, Obstet. Gynec. **4**:454, 1954.

186. Pierce, M.: Leukemia in the newborn infant, J. Pediatr. **54**:691, 1959.

187. Plotkin, S. A.: Routes of fetal infection and mechanisms of fetal damage, Am. J. Dis. Child. **129**:444, 1975.

188. Porter, R. R.: Structural studies of immunoglobulins, Science **180**:713, 1973.

189. Pritchard, J. A., Scott, D. E., Whalley, P. J., et al.: The effects of maternal sickle cell hemoglobinopathies and sickle cell trait on reproductive performance, Am. J. Obstet. Gynecol. **117**:662, 1973.

190. Prusoff, W. H.: Recent advances in chemotherapy of viral diseases, Pharmacol. Rev. **19**:209, 1967.

191. Rigby, P. G., Hanson, T. A., and Smith, R. J.: Passage of leukemic cells across the placenta, N. Engl. J. Med. **271:**124, 1964.

192. Robinson, R. C. V.: Congenital syphilis, Arch. Dermatol. **99:**599, 1969.

193. Rodriguez, S. U., Leikin, S. L., and Hiller, M. C.: Neonatal thrombocytopenia associated with antepartum administration of thiazide drugs, N. Engl. J. Med. **270:**881, 1964.

194. Rosen, F. S., and Merler, E.: Genetic defects in gamma globulin synthesis. In Stanbury, J. B., and Wyngarden, J. B., eds.: The metabolic basis of inherited disease, ed. 3, New York, 1972, McGraw-Hill Book Co.

195. Rothman, L. A., Cohen, C. J., and Astarloa, J.: Placental and fetal involvement by maternal malignancy: a report of rectal carcinoma and review of the literature, Am. J. Obstet. Gynecol. **116:**1023, 1973.

196. Salzman, E. W., Deykin, D., Shapiro, R. M., and Rosenberg, R.: Management of heparin therapy: controlled prospective trial, N. Engl. J. Med. **292:**1046, 1975.

197. Schiff, D., Aranda, J. V., and Stern, L.: Neonatal thrombocytopenia and congenital malformations associated with administration of tolbutamide to the mother, J. Pediatr. **77:**457, 1970.

198. Schiller, J. G.: Shock in the newborn caused by transplacental hemorrhage from fetus to mother, Pediatrics **20:**7, 1957.

199. Schoen, E. J., King, A. L., and Duane, R. T.: Neonatal thrombocytopenic purpura, Pediatrics **17:**72, 1956.

200. Schröder, J.: Transplacental passage of blood cells, J. Med. Gen. **12:**230, 1975.

201. Seip, M.: Hereditary hypoplastic thrombocytopenia, Acta Paediatr. **52:**370, 1963.

202. Shin, W. K. T.: Hemangiomas of infancy complicated by thrombocytopenia, Am. J. Surg. **116:**896, 1968.

203. Shulman, N. R., Aster, R. H., Pearson, H. A., and Hiller, M. C.: Immunoreactions involving platelets. VI. Reaction of maternal isoantibodies responsible for neonatal purpura. Differentiation of a second platelet antigen system, J. Clin. Invest. **41:**1059, 1962.

204. Shulman, N. R., Marder, V. J., Hiller, M. C., and Collier, E. M.: Platelet and leukocyte isoantigens and their antibodies: serologic, physiologic, and clinical studies, Prog. Hematol. **4:**222, 1964.

205. Sims, D. G., and Neligan, G. A.: Factors affecting the increasing incidence of severe non-haemolytic neonatal jaundice, Br. J. Obstet. Gynecol. **82:**863, 1975.

206. Sitarz, A. L., Driscoll, J. M., and Wolff, J. A.: Management of isoimmune neonatal thrombocytopenia, Am. J. Obstet. Gynecol. **124:**39, 1976.

207. Sjolin, S.: Studies on osteopetrosis. II. Investigations concerning the nature of the anemia, Acta Paediatr. **48:**529, 1959.

208. Smith, R. B. W., Sheehy, T. W., and Rothberg, H.: Hodgkin's disease and pregnancy, Ann. Intern. Med. **102:**777, 1958.

209. Smith, R. T.: Human immunoglobulins: a guide to nomenclature and clinical application, Pediatrics **37:**822, 1966.

210. Sokal, J. E., and Lessmann, E. M.: Effects of cancer chemotherapeutic agents on the human fetus, J.A.M.A. **172:**1765, 1960.

211. Solcia, E., Rondini, G., and Capella, C.: Clinical and pathological observations on a case of newborn osteopetrosis, Helv. Paediatr. Acta **23:**650, 1968.

212. South, M. A., and Rawls, W. E.: Treatment of neonatal herpes virus infection, J. Pediatr. **76:**497, 1970.

213. Stiehm, E. R., and Clatanoff, D. V.: Split products of fibrin in the serum of newborns, Pediatrics **43:**770, 1969.

214. Stiehm, E. R., Vaerman, J. P., and Fudenberg, H. H.: Plasma infusions in immunologic deficiency states: metabolic and therapeutic states, Blood **28:**918, 1966.

215. Sutherland, J. M., and Keller, W. H.: Novobiocin and neonatal hyperbilirubinemia, Am. J. Dis. Child. **101:**447, 1961.

216. Tancer, M. L.: Idiopathic thrombocytopenic purpura and pregnancy, Am. J. Obstet. Gyn. **79:**148, 1960.

217. Territo, M., Finklestein, J., Oh, W., et al.: Management of autoimmune thrombocytopenia in pregnancy and in the neonate, Obstet. Gynecol. **41:**579, 1973.

218. Terry, M. F.: A management of the third stage to reduce feto-maternal transfusion, J. Obstet. Gynaecol. Br. Cwlth. **77:**129, 1970.

219. Thatcher, L. G., Clatanoff, D. V., and Stiehm, E. R.: Splenic hemangioma with thrombocytopenia and afibrinogenemia, J. Pediatr. **73:**345, 1968.

220. Thompson, D., Pegelow, C., Underman, A., and Powars, D.: Congenital malaria: a rare cause of splenomegaly and anemia in an American infant, Pediatrics **60:**209, 1977.

221. Tullis, J. L.: Prevalence, nature, and identification of leukocyte antibodies, N. Engl. J. Med. **258:**569, 1958.

222. Vahlquist, B.: Transfer of antibodies from mother to offspring. In Levine, S. Z., et al., eds.: Advances in pediatrics, vol. 10, Chicago, 1958, Year Book Medical Publishers, Inc.

223. Valaes, T., Karaklis, A., Stravrakakis, D., et al.: Incidence and mechanism of neonatal jaundice related to glucose-6-phosphate dehydrogenase deficiency, Pediatr. Res. **3:**448, 1969.

224. Van der Weerdt, C. M.: Thrombocytopenia due to quinidine or quinine, Vox. Sang. **12:**265, 1967.

225. Van Rood, J. J., Eernisse, J. G., and van Leeuwen, A.: Leukocyte antibodies in sera from pregnant women, Nature **181:**1735, 1958.

226. Van Rood, J. J., van Leeuwen, A., and Eernisse, J. G.: Leucocyte antibodies in sera of pregnant women, Vox. Sang. **4:**427, 1959.

227. Vonderheid, E. C., Koblenzer, P. J., Ming, P. M. L., and Burgoon, C. F.: Neonatal lupus erythematosus: report of four cases with review of the literature, Arch. Dermatol. **112:**698, 1976.

228. Vossaugh, P., Leikin, S., Avery, G., et al.: Neonatal thrombocytopenia in association with rubella, Acta Haematol. **35:**158, 1966.

229. Wagner, H. P., Tonz, O., and Greyerz-Gloor, R. D.: Congenital lymphoid leukemia, Helv. Paediatr. Acta **23:**591, 1968.

230. Wagner, L., and Wagner, G.: Effect of alcohol on premature newborn infants, Am. J. Obstet. Gynecol. **108:**308, 1970.

231. Walknowska, J., Conte, F. A., and Grumbach, M. M.: Practical and theoretical implication of fetal-maternal lymphocyte transfer, Lancet **1:**1119, 1969.

232. Warkany, J., Beaudry, P. H., and Hornstein, S.: Attempted abortion with aminopterin (4-amino-pteroylglutamic acid) malformations of the child, Am. J. Dis. Child. **97:**274, 1959.

233. Washburn, A. H.: Blood cells in healthy young infants: a study of 608 differential leukocyte counts, with a final report on 908 total leukocyte counts, Am. J. Dis. Child. **50:**412, 1935.

234. Wegelius, R.: On changes in peripheral blood picture of newborn infant immediately after birth, Acta Paediatr. **35:**1, 1948.

235. Weiner, A. S.: Diagnosis and treatment of anemia of the newborn caused by occult placental hemorrhage, Am. J. Obstet. Gynecol. **56:**717, 1948.

236. Weiner, A. S.: The half-life of passively acquired anti-

body globulin molecules in infants, J. Exp. Med. **94:** 213, 1951.

237. Weinstein, L., and Chang, T. W.: The chemotherapy of viral infections, N. Engl. J. Med. **289:**725, 1973.

238. Weisert, O., and Marstrander, J.: Severe anemia in a newborn infant caused by protracted feto-maternal transfusion, Acta Paediatr. Scand. **49:**426, 1960.

239. Weller, T. H.: The cytomegaloviruses: ubiquitous agents with protean clinical manifestations. I, N. Engl. J. Med. **285:**203, 1971.

240. Weller, T. H.: The cytomegaloviruses: Ubiquitous agents with protean clinical manifestations. II, N. Engl. J. Med. **285:**267, 1971.

241. Weller, T. H., and Hanshaw, J. B.: Virologic and clinical observations on cytomegalic inclusion disease, N. Engl. J. Med. **266:**1233, 1962.

242. Whitaker, J., Sartain, P., and Sheheedy, M.: Hematologic aspects of congenital syphilis, J. Pediatr. **66:**629, 1965.

243. Whitley, R. J., Soong, S., Dolin, R., Galasso, G. J., Ch'ien, L. T., Alford, C. A., and the Collaborative Study Group: Adenine arabinoside therapy of biopsy-proved herpes simplex encephalitis, N. Engl. J. Med. **277:**289, 1977.

244. Windle, W. F.: Development of the blood and changes in the blood picture at birth, J. Pediatr. **18:**538, 1941.

245. Woodrow, J. C., and Finn, R.: Transplacental hemorrhage, Br. J. Haematol. **12:**297, 1966.

246. Woods, W. G., Mills, E., and Ferrieri, P.: Neonatal malaria due to Plasmodium Vivax, J. Pediatr. **85:**669, 1974.

247. Xanthou, M.: Leukocyte blood picture in healthy full-term and premature babies during the neonatal period, Arch. Dis. Child. **45:**242, 1970.

248. Zilliacus, R., de la Chapelle, A., Schröder, J., et al.: Transplacental passage of foetal blood cells. Scand. J. Haematol. **15:**333, 1975.

249. Zinkham, W. H., Medearis, D. N., and Osborn, J. E.: Blood and bone-marrow findings in congenital rubella, J. Pediatr. **71:**512, 1967.

4 □ Blood groups and blood component transfusion

D. H. Buchholz

Blood groups

Although blood has been administered to humans since the mid-1600s, early transfusions frequently ended in disaster since nothing was known about blood group antigens or antibodies. Hemolytic transfusion reactions were common, especially following infusion of blood obtained from animals.[10,65] It was not until Landsteiner's description of the ABO blood groups in 1900 that the study of blood group serology began to proceed on a scientific basis.

Landsteiner[36] collected blood from several of his associates, separated serum from the red blood cells, and mixed each serum with the red cells of each donor. He noted agglutination in some cell-serum mixtures and concluded that the agglutination was caused by serum antibodies directed against specific substances present on the red cells that defined three different blood groups, later called A, B, and O. The following year the fourth group, AB, was described.

It was not until over a quarter century later that the next blood group systems, MN and P, were identified using antibody produced in rabbits immunized with human red blood cells.[37,38] Another significant advance in blood grouping came about in 1939 when Levine and Stetson found an antibody in the serum of a woman who had delivered a stillborn fetus; the woman had a severe transfusion reaction after she was transfused with her husband's blood. Her serum agglutinated her husband's red cells as well as 80 of 104 samples tested. The antibody was clearly not related to the known ABO, MN, or P blood group systems and appeared to define a new blood group system.[40] At about the same time Landsteiner and Wiener[39] immunized rabbits and guinea pigs with red cells from the monkey *Macacus rhesus* and harvested an antibody that agglutinated about 85% of the human red cells tested. These investigators called the cells that were agglutinated Rh (for *rhesus*) positive and those that were not, Rh negative. The antibody described by Landsteiner and Wiener had a slightly different specificity than the one described by Levine; the latter antibody is now called anti-Rh, whereas the former has been renamed anti-LW in honor of Landsteiner and Wiener.

Since then, many more blood group antigens have been described and the total of known antigens is nearly 400.[33] The ABO and Rh systems are much more important than the others and are the only groups routinely determined when blood is to be transfused.

BLOOD GROUP TERMINOLOGY

Blood group antigen terminology is confusing. In some systems antigens are indicated by a capital letter (A, B, O, M, N) or by a capital letter and a numerical or alphabetical subscript (A_1, A_2, A_x, A_m). While the genes responsible for these antigenic determinants may be alleles, this information is not indicated by the terminology. Other systems use capital and lower case letters to represent antigens produced by genes that are allelic (K and k, S and s, I and i); in others alleles are indicated by a capital and a lower case letter followed by an alphabetical superscript (Jk^a and Jk^b; Fy^a and Fy^b). Some antigens are called by their alphabetical letter (P, M, N, I), whereas the letter(s) represent(s) a specific name in others (K for Kell, k for Cellano, Fy for Duffy, Le for Lewis). Genes are usually written in italics *(Fy^a, Jk^a)* and antibodies are indicated by the term "anti-" plus the blood group antigen designation (anti-Fy^a, anti-Jk^a).

The general terms used to refer to antigens and antibodies have also led to confusion. Since the ABO system was discovered first and the presence of agglutination defined the presence of the antigen, a terminology based on this phenomenon developed: Antibodies were called agglutinins (or isoagglutinins), and the antigens they determined were named agglutinogens. These names were not only awkward and confusing but also were not appropriate after the later discovery of antibodies that bound to the red cell membrane but did not produce agglutination. Those antibodies, usually best detected using antihuman globulin, have also been called incomplete antibodies, in contrast to those that produce agglutination directly and are termed complete.

Basic to the understanding of blood group serology is the concept that antigens are defined by their respective antibodies. Without antibody (produced as a result of transfusion, pregnancy, or deliberate immunization) an antigen cannot be detected. For practical purposes the ABO blood group system is the only one in which antibodies are regularly found in the plasma without prior host exposure to red cell A or B antigens. Antibodies defining most other blood groups result only from immunization, either inadvertant or intentional. Normally only persons who lack a particular antigen on their red cell membrane have the potential to produce antibody specific for that antigen.

An antigen is a substance capable of eliciting an immune response when suitably presented to an immunocompetent host lacking that antigen. In general the terms "antigen" and "immunogen" refer to the entire molecule, whereas the term "antigenic determinant" is reserved for the portion of the molecule that determines specificity in the reaction with antibody. Although exposure to a foreign antigenic determinant can lead to both cellular and humoral immune responses, the humoral or antibody-producing phase is of most importance in blood transfusion.

Since antibodies define antigens, it is apparent that antibodies can be used to detect the presence of specific antigens on red blood cell membranes. Alternatively, however, red cells with a known representation of antigenic determinants can be used to detect the presence and specificity of antibodies as shown in Table 4-1. In this example the red cells of four persons have been tested for the Rh system antigens C, D, and E using specific antisera. The presence or absence of the antigen is represented by a + or 0, respectively. Cells from persons 1 and 2 have the C and D antigenic determinants but not E, the cells of the third person have D but lack C and E, and the fourth person's cells lack C but have D and E. Once the antigen composition of each cell is known, if serum sus-

pected of containing an Rh blood group antibody is tested with each of the four types of cells, the resultant pattern of cell reactivity may allow identification of the antibody. For example, if cells 1 and 2 but not 3 and 4 are agglutinated, the likely specificity would be anti-C, since only cells 1 and 2 possess the C antigen. Similarly, if only cell 4 is agglutinated, the antibody might be anti-E, while if all four cells are agglutinated, anti-D might be suspected.

If only the C, D, and E antigens of the test cells are known and if only four types of cells are used, it is impossible to identify antibodies other than anti-C, anti-D, and anti-E. This problem can be avoided by testing each cell for antigens in addition to C, D, and E and by using more than four types of cells. In practice, eight to ten cells whose antigen composition has been carefully characterized are used to identify antibodies. Comparison of patterns of cell reactivity with the known antigen composition of the test cells usually allows identification of antibody specificity as described above. Occasionally specificity cannot be determined, especially if the antibody is directed against antigens with an extremely high ("public") or low ("private") incidence.

DETECTION OF ANTIGEN-ANTIBODY REACTIONS

Several methods of detection are utilized for recognition of blood group antigens and antibodies, but most ultimately rely on red blood cell agglutination. IgM (19S) antibodies of the ABO, MNSs, P, and Lewis blood group systems usually produce in vitro agglutination of saline-suspended red cells at room temperature although a few, such as those of the I/i blood group system, react preferentially at lower temperatures. IgM antibodies may fix complement and occasionally produce in vitro hemolysis, seen most often in the ABO and Lewis systems.

Most antibodies produced consequent to transfusion are IgG (7S); these antibodies often react with membrane antigenic determinants but cannot produce in vitro agglutination since they are smaller than IgM molecules and cannot bridge the distance between two erythrocytes. Some IgG molecules can agglutinate red cells if bovine albumin or other colloidal material is added to the test mixture or if the cells are treated with proteolytic enzymes such as papain or ficin, but most do not. Because of this, IgG antibodies could not readily be detected until the development of the antiglobulin (Coombs) test popularized by Coombs et al.[17] although originally described by Moreschi.[52] These workers immunized rabbits with human immunoglobulin and were able to produce "anti-antibody" capable of agglutinating human

Table 4-1. Determination of antibody specificity

Cell No.	Antigens			Reactivity of unknown antibody
	C	D	E	
1	+	+	0	Agglutination
2	+	+	0	Agglutination
3	0	+	0	No agglutination
4	0	+	+	No agglutination

red cells coated with nonagglutinating IgG blood group antibodies. This technique allowed detection of otherwise unrecognizable antigen-antibody reactions and resulted in a significant advancement in safe blood transfusion therapy as well as the discovery of a multitude of new blood group antigens.

ANTIGEN TESTING

Although there are hundreds of blood group antigens, only the ABO and Rh groups are routinely determined prior to transfusion. It is necessary to know the ABO group because group A, B, and O persons have anti-A and/or anti-B antibody in their plasma that can destroy transfused red cells with the corresponding antigens; Rh testing is done because the Rh antigen is a potent immunogen and can stimulate antibody production in about 70% of Rh-negative persons.[57] When antibody is produced following exposure to antigens of a member of the same species, the process is termed *alloimmunization*. Although any blood group antigen has the *potential* to induce antibody formation, alloimmunization following transfusion is uncommon since most antigens other than ABO and Rh are relatively poor immunogens. The most frequently encountered antibodies that pose cross matching problems are listed in Table 4-2.

Table 4-2. Frequently encountered blood group antibodies*

Antibody	Blood group system	Relative potency of antigen (%)†	Antigen frequency in unselected donors (%)‡
Anti-D	Rh	70	85
Anti-K	Kell	5.0	9
Anti-Le^a	Lewis	§	22
Anti-Le^b	Lewis	§	72
Anti-E	Rh	1.69	30
Anti-c	Rh	2.05	80
Anti-Fy^a	Duffy	0.23	67
Anti-P₁	P	§	79
Anti-M	MNSs	§	78
Anti-C (or Ce)	Rh	0.11	70
Anti-e	Rh	0.56	98
Anti-Jk^a	Kidd	0.07	77
Anti-S	MNSs	0.04	55
Anti-Jk^b	Kidd	0.03	73
Anti-s	MNSs	0.03	89
Anti-k	Kell	1.50	99.8

*Modified from Giblet, E. R.: Transfusion **1**:233, 1961.
†Percentage of antigen-negative recipients expected to form antibody after exposure to the antigen by transfusion.
‡Percentage of unselected whole blood that would be incompatible.[33,59]
§These antibodies are sometimes "naturally occurring" (i.e., present without known previous exposure to the antigen), and no estimate of antigen potency can be made.

Transfusion of a single unit of blood leads to antibody formation in about 1% of recipients[25]; the incidence becomes greater as the number of transfusions increases.[45] Since alloimmunization occasionally occurs, it might be argued that cells with antigens that the recipient lacks (and that thus could lead to antibody formation) should not be used for transfusion. While this has a theoretical appeal, the impossibility of providing "identical" red blood cells is illustrated in the following example. Suppose a recipient is group B, Rh negative, and lacks the following antigens: K (Kell), Fy^b (Duffy b), Jk^a (Kidd a), and Rh system C and E. Suppose additionally that a pool of 100,000 blood donors exists from which "identical" red cells can be chosen. Since about 9% of persons are group B, 9,000 of the original donor pool will be selected for further consideration. Of these, 15% will be Rh negative, leaving 1,350. Kell is a low-frequency antigen occurring in 9% of whites; this reduces the donor pool to 1,229. Of these, however, only 17% will be Fy^b negative (leaving 209 potential donors), while 23% will be Jk^a negative, reducing the number to 48. Finally, since 30% of persons lack the C antigen and 70% lack E, only 10 of the original 100,000 donors could provide red cells "identical" with those of the recipient. Although only 7 of the nearly 400 red cell antigens have been discussed in this example, it is obvious that it is impossible to provide red cells that lack the potential to induce antibody formation.

GENOTYPES AND PHENOTYPES

Blood group antigens are under the control of genes located on various chromosomes. Assignment of individual genes to specific chromosomes has not yet been firmly established except for the Duffy and Rh blood group systems (chromosome 1),[47,61] the MNSs system (chromosome 2),[24] the ABO system (chromosome 9),[78] and the genes that control histocompatibility (chromosome 6).[75] Each gene occupies a defined space on a chromosome, termed a locus. Although only one gene can occupy a given locus, more than one gene may have the potential to occupy that locus; such genes are called alleles. Genes may be dominant, recessive, or codominant; the gene products that result vary according to the combination of genes inherited. For example, three allelic genes, *A, B,* and *O,* determine the ABO blood group. If a child inherits an *O* gene from each parent, his blood will be group O. If he inherits one *O* gene with an *A* (or *B*) gene, group A (or B) red cells will result since *A* (or *B*) is dominant to *O*. If both *A* and *B* are inherited, the blood group will be AB since *A* and *B* are codominant. The representation of genes at a given locus on two homologous chromosomes is known as the genotype, and the representation of detectable products produced by action of those genes is termed the phenotype. Although in many instances the phenotype indicates the genotype, this is not always the case. (For example, the genotypes *A/A* and *A/O* both result in blood of phenotype A.)

Many blood group systems are composed of antigens produced by pairs of antithetical allelic genes; i.e., inheritance of the *same* gene from each parent results in the presence of one antigen on the cell membrane and the regular absence of a corresponding antigen. Jk^a and Jk^b behave as antithetical genes; if a person inherits Jk^a from both parents (genotype Jk^a/Jk^a), his red cells react with anti-Jk^a and not with anti-Jk^b. If only anti-Jk^b is used to test the cells, the presence of the Jk^a antigen can reasonably be assumed if the cells do not react with the anti-Jk^b antiserum.

Based upon the presence (+) or absence (−) of reactivity with specific antisera, a person's phenotype can be represented by an antigen symbol and the appropriate + or −; the gene pair of Jk^a and Jk^b could thus produce three phenotypes: Jk(a+b−) (genotype Jk^a/Jk^a), Jk(a−b+) (genotype Jk^b/Jk^b), and Jk(a+b+) (genotype Jk^a/Jk^b). If there were only two codominant genes acting at a given locus, the genotype could always be implied from the phenotype if antisera were used that recognized the specificity of the two antigens produced by the genes. Although this appears to be the case in many blood group systems, the inference of genotype cannot be made from the phenotype with certainty.

For example, suppose a rare third allele, Jk^c, acts at the Kidd locus; six genotypes rather than three will be possible (Jk^a/Jk^a, Jk^a/Jk^b, Jk^a/Jk^c, Jk^b/Jk^b, Jk^b/Jk^c, and Jk^c/Jk^c). If cells are tested only with anti-Jk^a and anti-Jk^b, the presence or absence of the Jk^c antigen cannot be determined, and the incorrect genotype will be inferred for those persons who inherit the Jk^c gene; i.e., the phenotypes of persons who have the Jk^c antigen (*true* genotypes Jk^a/Jk^c, Jk^b/Jk^c, and Jk^c/Jk^c) will appear to be Jk(a+b−), Jk(a−b+), and Jk(a−b−), respectively. If the genotype is inferred from the phenotype in this instance, it will be incorrect.

DIRECT AND INDIRECT ANTIGLOBULIN TESTS

The antiglobulin (Coombs) test is termed direct or indirect depending on whether red cells are tested to detect antibody that has been attached to the cell in vivo (direct) or artificially in vitro (indirect). The principles of the indirect antiglobulin test are illustrated in Fig. 4-1. Red cells are incubated with serum suspected of containing a blood group antibody, the cells are washed, and antihuman globulin is added. If antibody is present in the serum and binds to the antigenic determinant on the red cell membrane, it will not be removed by washing and the cells will be agglutinated when

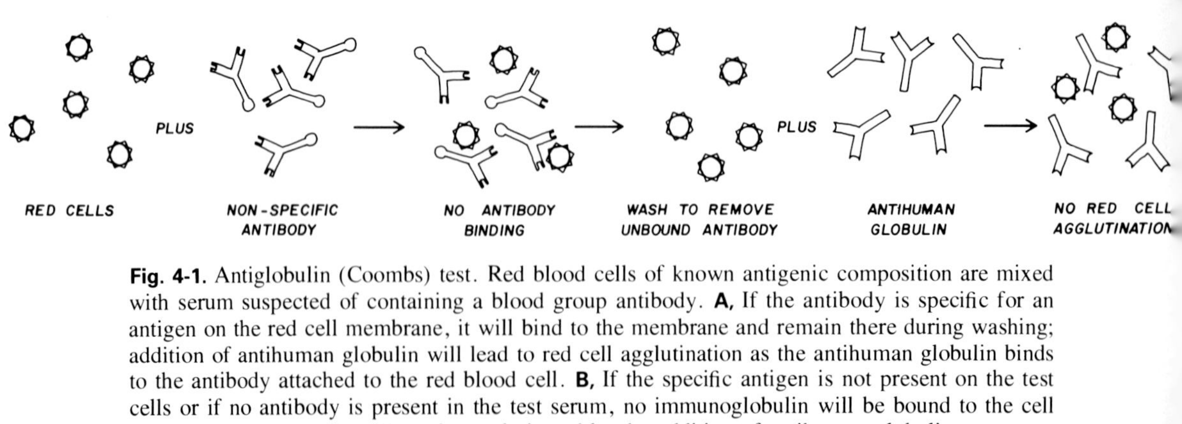

Fig. 4-1. Antiglobulin (Coombs) test. Red blood cells of known antigenic composition are mixed with serum suspected of containing a blood group antibody. **A,** If the antibody is specific for an antigen on the red cell membrane, it will bind to the membrane and remain there during washing; addition of antihuman globulin will lead to red cell agglutination as the antihuman globulin binds to the antibody attached to the red blood cell. **B,** If the specific antigen is not present on the test cells or if no antibody is present in the test serum, no immunoglobulin will be bound to the cell membrane and the cells will not be agglutinated by the addition of antihuman globulin.

the antihuman serum is added; agglutination thus indicates the presence, but not the specificity, of antibody in the serum. Depending on the size and character of the agglutinates, positive reactions are graded from +1 to +4 and roughly quantify the amount of antibody on the cell membrane. Lack of agglutination is presumptive evidence that no antibody is attached to the cell membrane.

Compatibility testing (cross matching) is performed to detect antigen-antibody reactions between the cells and serum of recipient and donor. The antiglobulin test is routinely used as part of the cross matching procedure. In addition, most blood banks also test recipient serum for the presence of unexpected blood group antibodies using cells that carry the clinically important red cell antigens. In this way, antibody that might be undetected by the cross matching can be recognized and the blood bank alerted to potential cross matching difficulties that might occur if additional blood is needed.

Occasionally, some blood group antibodies display "dosage"; i.e., cells homozygous for an antigen (for example, cells of genotype Fy^a/Fy^a) may react with a weak antibody, but heterozygous cells (genotype Fy^a/Fy^b) may not. In this instance, if the antibody has been detected by other tests, it is important to identify the antibody and test red cells that appear compatible with a potent specific antiserum to prevent the infusion of cells that could be rapidly destroyed following transfusion.

The *direct* antiglobulin test allows recognition of red cells that have been coated with antibody in vivo, for example, the cells of persons with autoimmune hemolytic anemia. Red cells are washed to remove any globulin not immunologically bound to the cell, and then antihuman globulin is added. As with the indirect antiglobulin test, cell agglutination indicates the presence of antibody. In reality the test is identical with the indirect antiglobulin test except that the "antibody incubation" portion occurs in a patient rather than in a test tube. Persons with a positive direct antiglobulin test may also have antibody in their serum, although if present, it may be too weak to allow determination of specificity. In this case the antibody sometimes can be eluted from the red cell membrane by heat, ether, or acid and the eluate tested with cells of known antigenic specificity analogous to what is done to identify serum antibodies. The direct antiglobulin test may also be positive following treatment with certain drugs such as cephalothin, penicillin, stibophen, and α-methyldopa.[54] The development of hemolytic anemia following use of these drugs is rare.

ABO, LEWIS, AND SECRETOR SYSTEMS

The ABO blood group system differs from most others in that antibody with A or B specificity or both is regularly present in the plasma of persons who have never been exposed to red cell A or B antigens. The plasma of group A persons contains anti-B; anti-A is found in group B plasma. Most group AB persons have no anti-A or anti-B, whereas group O persons have both antibodies. Inhalation or ingestion of materials such as bacteria with A- or B-like specificity may stimulate production of these antibodies.[69] Newborns usually have only passively transferred maternal anti-A or anti-B, although by age 3 to 6 months infants actively produce antibody.

Anti-A and anti-B are either IgM (sometimes called "naturally occurring") or IgG ("immune") antibodies. Both forms fix complement and can rapidly destroy cells containing the corresponding antigen. Most group A and B persons have predominately IgM anti-B or anti-A, whereas both IgM and IgG antibodies are found in group O persons; this probably explains the greater incidence of ABO hemolytic disease of the newborn in infants of group O mothers, since only IgG antibodies can cross the placenta.

The approximate frequency of the six ABO blood groups is shown in Table 4-3. Because persons whose red cells lack the A or B antigens usually have the corresponding antibody present in the plasma (except neonates), group-specific transfusions are usually given to avoid destruction of transfused cells by recipient antibody or destruction of recipient red cells by transfused antibody. Thus the concept of group O blood as a "universal donor" and a group AB person as a "universal recipient" is of limited usefulness since anti-A or anti-B in transfused plasma will destroy *recipient* red blood cells if the antibody is potent. In an

Table 4-3. ABO blood group system

Geno-type	Pheno-type	Approximate frequency*	Red cell antigens	Plasma antibodies
O/O	O	43.5%	(H)	anti-A, anti-B
A_1/A_1 A_1/A_2 A_1/O	A_1 A_1 A_1	34.8%	A_1	anti-B
A_2/A_2 A_2/O	A_2 A_2	9.9%	A_2	anti-B, rarely anti-A_1 (2%)
B/B B/O	B B	8.6%	B	anti-A
A_1/B	A_1B	2.6%	A_1 and B	None
A_2/B	A_2B	0.6%	A_2 and B	anti-A_1 (25%)

*As reported by Ikin et al.[29]

Table 4-4. ABO, H/h, Lewis, and secretor gene interaction

H/h genes	ABO genes	Le/le genes	RBC phenotype	Se/se genes	RBC phenotype	Antigens in secretions[†]
H/H or *H/h* → H substance	*A/O* or *A/A* — Group A *B/O* or *B/B* — Group B *A/B* — Group AB *O/O* — Group O	*Le/Le* or *Le/le*	A, Le(a+b−) B, Le(a+b−) AB, Le(a+b−) O, Le(a+b−)	*Se/Se* or *Se/se*	A, Le(a−b+)* B, Le(a−b+)* AB, Le(a−b+)* O, Le(a−b+)*	A, H, Le^a, and Le^b B, H, Le^a, and Le^b A, B, H, Le^a, and Le^b H, Le^a, and Le^b
				se/se	A, Le(a+b−) B, Le(a+b−) AB, Le(a+b−) O, Le(a+b−)	Le^a Le^a Le^a Le^a
		le/le	A, Le(a−b−) B, Le(a−b−) AB, Le(a−b−) O, Le(a−b−)	*Se/Se* or *Se/se*	A, Le(a−b−) B, Le(a−b−) AB, Le(a−b−) O, Le(a−b−)	A and H B and H A, B, and H H
				se/se	A, Le(a−b−) B, Le(a−b−) AB, Le(a−b−) O, Le(a−b−)	None None None None
h/h → Precursor substance unchanged	*A/O* or *A/A* — Bombay O$_h^A$ *B/O* or *B/B* — Bombay O$_h^B$ *A/B* — Bombay O$_h^{AB}$ *O/O* — Bombay O$_h^O$					

*Some Le^a may be present.
†Plasma, saliva, etc.

emergency, group O Rh-negative *packed cells* and group AB plasma may be used for transfusion to recipients of *any* blood type (if the recipient is Rh-positive, however, O-positive red cells should be used).

An A_1, A_2, B, or O gene is inherited from each parent, and ten different genotypes and six phenotypes are possible (Table 4-3). The A_1, A_2, and B genes are codominant, and all are dominant to O. The product of the A gene is a transferase that adds the sugar N-acetyl-galactosamine to a precursor known as H substance; this provides group A specificity. Similarly the B gene directs the addition of galactose to H substance and confers B specificity.[77] If both sugars are added, group AB red cells result. The O gene acts as an amorph; i.e., it does nothing. If an O gene is inherited from both parents, no sugars are added to the H substance and the cells are said to be group O, although if an A or B gene is inherited with an O gene, A or B antigens will be present since both the A and B genes are dominant to the O gene.

Short of performing family studies, there is no easy way to determine the genotype of group A or B persons since the red cells of heterozygous (A/O or B/O) persons react as strongly with anti-A or anti-B as the cells of homozygotes (A/A or B/B). Eighty percent of group A adults have an antigen, termed A_1, that reacts with group B serum previously adsorbed with A_2 cells, as well as with a lectin derived from the seeds of the plant *Dolichos biflorus*. The A_1 antigen is not well developed on the cell membranes of newborns and cannot be reliably detected until a later age. Nearly all of the remaining group A persons have a "weak" form of A, called A_2, which does not react with anti-A_1. Anti-A_1 is present in the plasma of 1% to 2% of A_2 persons and about 25% of A_2B persons who have never received transfusions[73]; the reason for this is not known. Even weaker (A_3, A_4, A_x, A_m) antigens are found on the cells of a small number of persons.[59]

Inheritance of ABO antigens is closely related to three other gene systems: H/h, Se/se (secretor), and Le/le (Lewis). The H, Se, and Le genes are dominant to the h, se, and le genes, respectively. The H gene is thought to code for the addition of a molecule of the sugar fucose to an oligosaccharide chain on the red cell membrane with the resultant formation of H substance; this then serves as a precursor substance for the product of the A and B genes.[77] Nearly all people are H/H; the rare recessive gene, h, does not produce H substance. If an h gene is inherited from each parent, A and B antigens cannot be produced even though the A or B gene or both are present, since the required H precursor substance is not available (Table 4-4). Such persons have a blood type termed Bombay.[9]

Their red cells react as group O when tested with anti-A and anti-B, irrespective of the true ABO genotype. Since there is nothing wrong with their ABO genes, they can transmit them normally to their children; as long as the child receives an H gene from the other parent, the ABO genes inherited from both the normal and the Bombay parent will be expressed.

The Le (Lewis) gene produces a plasma antigen, Le^a, which is adsorbed onto the red cell and is therefore not a true membrane antigen although it confers specificity when cells are tested with anti-Le^a.[68] About 22% of whites have Le^a on their red cells. Le^a substance is also found in saliva, semen, urine, breast milk, and gastrointestinal tract secretions. If the Le gene is not inherited (i.e., the genotype is le/le), Le^a is not present on red cells or in plasma secretions.

Another Lewis antigen, Le^b, is formed by interaction of the Le gene and the Se (secretor) gene. The Se gene is present in about 80% of persons and is responsible for production of soluble forms of A, B, or H substance if the A, B, or H gene, respectively, is present. The recessive gene, se, if inherited from both parents, produces no A, B, or H substance in body fluids although it does not interfere with the expression of the ABH antigens on the red cell membrane. The dominant Se gene also influences the Lewis system and acts in conjunction with the Le gene to convert Lewis a substance to Lewis b substance.[13,28] About 72% of persons have Le^b adsorbed to their red cell membranes. The complex interaction of the H/h, ABO, Lewis, and Secretor genes is represented schematically in Table 4-4.

Anti-Le^a and anti-Le^b antibodies may occur in the small number of le/le persons lacking both Le^a and Le^b; anti-Le^b may be present in persons with the Lewis (Le) gene who lack the secretor (Se) gene (and who are thus Le[a+b−]), but anti-Le^a is not seen in Le(a−b+) persons because the Le^a antigen is genetically represented but its expression modified by the presence of the Se gene. Lewis antibodies are usually IgM and may fix complement, but they rarely cause hemolytic transfusion reactions. A few Lewis antibodies develop after transfusion, although most appear to occur spontaneously.[51] Lewis system antibodies do not cause hemolytic disease of the newborn because IgM antibodies cannot cross the placenta; in addition, the Lewis antigens are not present in the plasma in large amounts at the time of birth and thus do not adsorb on fetal red cells.[4]

Rh BLOOD GROUP SYSTEM

Rh terminology is especially confusing owing to numerous antigens that comprise the system and to the use of three systems of nomenclature. Fisher[23] and Race[58] proposed that the Rh antigens are controlled by three closely linked allelic gene pairs, which produce the antigenic determinants C or c, D or d, and E or e, respectively. A gene from each allelic pair is inherited from each parent; thus a person can inherit two *C* genes, two *c* genes, or one *C* and one *c* gene. Similar combinations of the other genes are thought to result in expression of other membrane antigens. Antibodies defining the C, D, E, c, and e antigenic determinants have been described, although no antibody with d specificity has been found. In spite of this, when red blood cells are tested with anti-C, -D, -E, -c, and -e antisera, a phenotype can be represented, such as CcDee, ccddee, and CcDEe (the presence of dd is assumed if the cells do not react with anti-D). Based on the frequencies of various gene combinations determined through family studies, the likely genotype of a person can be *suggested* from the phenotype; i.e., a white with the phenotype CcDee is more likely to be genotype *CDe/cde* than *Cde/cDe* because the gene frequencies of *CDe* and *cde* are greater than those of *Cde* and *cDe*.[59]

Since the d antigen postulated by the Fisher-Race theory has never been found and since the theory also fails to account for certain variant antigenic forms, many workers utilize a second terminology described by Wiener[80,81] (or more often, *both* terminologies). Wiener suggested that one rather than three genes determines the expression of Rh system antigens. Each gene produces what Wiener called an agglutinogen (antigen), which is comprised of several blood factors (similar to antigenic determinants). Thus the gene R^1 produces the agglutinogen Rh_1 which is comprised of several factors including Rh_0, rh', and hr'' (which correspond with D, C, and e, respectively, in the Fisher-Race terminology). Other allelic genes produce agglutinogens composed of different combinations of blood factors; for instance, the gene R^2 produces the factors Rh_0, hr', and rh'' (D, c and E), while the R^0 gene produces Rh_0, hr', and hr'' (D, c and e), etc.[82]

Although Wiener's theory is thought to be correct, use of this nomenclature is difficult since the blood factors are not easily deduced from the symbol for the agglutinogen or gene, whereas this is readily apparent when the Fisher-Race terminology is used. For example, it is obvious that the gene combination of *CDe* but not *cDE* will result in the presence of e (hr'') on the red cell membrane although this is not easily seen when the gene symbols R^1 and R^2 are compared. Therefore, for ease of understanding, the Fisher-Race terminology will be used throughout this chapter. Table 4-5 lists the common Rh system antigenic determinants using both systems of nomenclature and indicates their frequency in the white population.

Table 4-5. Frequency of common Rh system antigens*

Fisher-Race nomenclature	Wiener nomenclature	Frequency
C	rh'	70%
D	Rh_0	85%
E	rh''	30%
c	hr'	80%
(d)	—	—
e	hr''	98%

*From Issitt, P. D., and Issitt, C. H.: Applied blood group serology, Oxnard, Calif., 1975, Becton, Dickinson & Co.

At least 35 Rh system antigens have been described[59]; a third system of nomenclature, in which antigens are represented by numbers,[60] has also been proposed and has the advantage of being devoid of genetic implication, but it is not in wide use.

The designation "Rh positive" is given to red blood cells that possess the D antigen; cells that lack it are called Rh negative. Although other Rh system antigens can stimulate antibody formation following transfusion or pregnancy, they are much weaker immunogens than D (Table 4-2). The D antigen occurs on the cells of about 85% of whites; if D-positive blood is given to an Rh-negative recipient, there is a 70% chance that the recipient will form anti-D.[57] This usually does not cause problems in an Rh-negative recipient given Rh-positive blood for the *first* time, since in a primary immune response relatively little antibody is produced and red cells are not rapidly removed by the reticuloendothelial system. If, however, the same person is reexposed to Rh-positive cells at a later time, it is likely that the cells will be rapidly destroyed by the much larger amount of antibody produced in an anamnestic or secondary immune response. Rh-negative persons should be given only Rh-negative red cells unless the administration of Rh-positive blood may be lifesaving; if a recipient has made anti-D antibody, he must receive *only* Rh-negative red cells.

D^u

A weakened form of the *D* gene, termed D^u, which produces an antigen that reacts with some but not all anti-D antisera, was described in 1946.[70] The antigen is best detected by performing the antiglobulin test on cells after incubation with anti-D. Since D^u can alloimmunize Rh-negative persons, donor blood that appears to be Rh negative is routinely tested for D^u. A D^u-positive person can receive Rh-positive blood although, as described below, rarely he may produce a form of anti-D. Ordinarily, if a *D* gene is inherited from either parent, the red cells will react as Rh positive when tested with anti-D; under certain circumstances, however, they may appear to be D^u. Persons with the phenotype CcDdee have red cells that react as D^u if their genotype is *Cde/cDe* but not if it is *CDe/cde*.[15] The D antigen is expressed normally if the *D* gene is on the same chromosome as the *C* gene but not if *C* and *D* are on opposite chromosomes.

D^u also results when a portion of the Rh mosaic is missing. The D antigen of most persons is composed of four subunits, Rh^A, Rh^B, Rh^C, and Rh^D.[33] Most Rh antibody recognizes all four subunits. Occasionally one or more of these may be missing, with the result that the red cells can react as D^u. In this circumstance transfusion with Rh-positive blood (Rh^A, Rh^B, Rh^C, and Rh^D) may induce antibody directed against a missing subunit; i.e., anti-Rh^B might be formed in a person with Rh^A, Rh^C, and Rh^D. This could result in the paradoxical situation of an ''Rh-positive'' (as determined by testing with a potent anti-Rh^{ABCD}) person who has no evidence of autoantibody (negative direct antiglobulin test) but who has anti-D in his circulation (really anti-Rh^B, but since nearly all Rh-positive cells contain Rh^B, the antibody appears to define anti-D). While this occurs rarely, it may cause considerable confusion.

Rh_{null}

The complete absence of Rh system antigens was described in an Australian aborigine in 1961 and the condition termed Rh_{null}.[76] Since that time several additional examples have been noted and, although the condition is rare, it appears to arise via two different mechanisms. In one type a gene that converts a precursor substance to the substrate on which the Rh gene complex appears is inhibited or absent[44] (similar to the absence of the *H* gene in the ABO system, which results in the Bombay phenotype). Persons with this deficiency can transmit an Rh gene to their children if the gene controlling conversion of the precursor substance is inherited from the other parent. Rh_{null} cells also occur in persons homozygous for an allelic gene that acts as an amorph (i.e., does nothing) at the Rh locus.[31] In this instance, children of affected persons will appear to be homozygous for the C or c, D or (d), and E or e antigens inherited from the nonaffected parent, since the affected parent cannot transmit a gene complex that can produce Rh antigens. For example, children of an amorphic Rh_{null} person (genotype $---/---$) and a person of genotype *CDe/cde* will have the phenotype CDe/CDe or cde/cde (but never any other combination) since their genotype will be either *CDe/$---$ or cde/$---$*.

The Rh system antigens appear to be important

constituents of the red cell membrane since persons with the Rh_{null} phenotype have a mild to moderate hemolytic anemia with stomatocytosis.[66,72] Rh-specific antibody has been seen in these persons without known antigenic stimulus, and antibody frequently is produced following transfusion or pregnancy. Partial deletions of other Rh system antigens have also been reported and are discussed in detail by Race and Sanger.[59]

Rh antibodies are usually IgG, although IgM forms are occasionally seen. Anti-D is a common cause of hemolytic disease of the newborn, although anti-C, anti-c, anti-E, and anti-e can also destroy fetal red blood cells. Rh system antibodies virtually never fix complement, and Rh system–mediated red cell destruction occurs only in the reticuloendothelial system. For reasons that are unclear, some persons with autoimmune hemolytic anemia have antibody with apparent anti-c or anti-e specificity. In other persons even those antibodies thought to be ''nonspecific'' can often be shown to have Rh system specificity in that they fail to react with cells with partial or complete (Rh_{null}) deletions of Rh antigens.[32]

KELL BLOOD GROUP SYSTEM

The Kell system is composed of at least sixteen antigenic determinants, and several are important in transfusion practice. The Kell (K) antibody, for which the system is named, was found in 1946[18]; an antibody that defined an apparent allelic antigen k (Cellano) was found three years later.[41] Cellano is present on the red cells of 99.8% of the population, whereas Kell occurs on the cells of about 9% of whites and 3% of blacks. Kell is a relatively potent immunogen and frequently leads to the production of anti-K if Kell-negative persons are exposed to Kell-positive red cells.

In addition to K and k, two other antigen pairs produced by antithetical genes are part of the Kell system: Kp^a and Kp^b (Penney and Rautenberg, respectively[1]) and Js^a and Js^b (Sutter and Matthews, respectively[71]). Many antibodies and antigens in the Kell system, as well as in other blood group systems, were named after the person in whom the antibody was first discovered; symbols were later assigned when it became apparent that certain antibodies defined antigens produced by allelic genes, although it was not appreciated that Sutter and Matthews belonged to the Kell system when the symbols Js^a and Js^b were given. There are also other antigens in the Kell system, which are sometimes represented by a letter and numerical designation, i.e., K12, K13, etc.[59] One antigen, termed K_x, is on the erythrocytes, granulocytes, and monocytes of normal persons but is regularly absent from the cells of persons with chronic granulomatous disease.[48]

Table 4-6. Antigen frequency in Kell blood group system*

Antigen symbol	Antigen name	Frequency	
		Whites	Blacks
K (K1)	Kell	9.0	3.5
k (K2)	Cellano	99.8	>99.9
Kpᵃ (K3)	Penney	2.0	<0.1
Kpᵇ (K4)	Rautenberg	>99.9	>99.9
Jsᵃ (K6)	Sutter	<0.1	19.5
Jsᵇ (K7)	Matthews	>99.9	98.5

*From Issitt, P. D., and Issitt, C. H.: Applied blood group serology, Oxnard, Calif. 1975, Becton, Dickinson & Co.

For practical purposes the cells of nearly everyone contain the k, Kpᵇ, and Jsᵇ antigens. The corresponding antibodies are rare. This is fortunate, since if any one of the antibodies is present, compatible red cells are difficult to obtain owing to the high frequency of the antigens in the donor population. On the other hand, although the K, Kpᵃ, and Jsᵃ antigens are relatively uncommon (Table 4-6), the respective antibodies are seen more frequently than anti-k, anti-Kpᵇ, or anti-Jsᵇ, since many persons lack the antigens and are capable of producing antibody following exposure to the antigen. Anti-Kell is the most important of the Kell system antibodies and is seen much more frequently than any of the others.

Most Kell system antibodies are IgG and are best detected using the antiglobulin test. In general they do not bind complement and do not cause intravascular hemolysis in vivo. Anti-K, anti-k, anti-Kpᵃ, anti-Kpᵇ, anti-Jsᵃ, and anti-Jsᵇ all have caused transfusion reactions and all but anti-Kpᵃ have been responsible for hemolytic disease of the newborn.

DUFFY BLOOD GROUP SYSTEM

The Duffy system was discovered in 1950 when an antibody was found in a person named Duffy that defined an antigen present on the red blood cells of about two thirds of the population.[21] The next year anti-Fyᵇ was found and appeared to detect the product of a gene antithetical to *Fyᵃ*.[30] Using anti-Fyᵃ and anti-Fyᵇ the three expected phenotypes, Fy(a+b−), Fy(a−b+), and Fy(a+b+) were detected, and it was initially thought that two genes, *Fyᵃ* and *Fyᵇ*, controlled this blood group system and that the three observed phenotypes were expressions of the three genotypes *Fyᵃ/Fyᵃ*, *Fyᵇ/Fyᵇ*, and *Fyᵃ/Fyᵇ*, respectively. The finding that 68% of blacks lacked both the Fyᵃ and Fyᵇ antigens, however, led to the postulation of a third allelic gene, termed *Fy*.[63] Although initially the *Fy* gene was thought to be an amorph

and produce nothing (similar to the *O* gene in the ABO system), recent evidence has suggested that the *Fy* gene does produce a specific antigen, which has been termed Fy4,[8] although only one example of anti-Fy4 (which reacts with Fy[a+b−], Fy[a−b+], and Fy[a−b−] but not Fy[a+b+] cells) has been described. It is of interest that the Fyᵃ and Fyᵇ antigens appear to be important as red cell membrane receptor sites for invading merozoites of *Plasmodium knowlesi* in vitro and *Plasmodium vivax* in vivo. Red cells lacking both antigens (i.e., Fy[a−b−]) are resistant to malarial parasites, whereas cells with either or both antigens can be infected.[49]

Whites lacking the Fyᵃ or Fyᵇ antigens can produce anti-Fyᵃ or anti-Fyᵇ following transfusion, and anti-Fyᵃ can cause hemolytic disease of the newborn.[27] Anti-Fyᵃ is seen more often than anti-Fyᵇ, although both of the corresponding antigens are comparatively weak immunogens. Duffy antibodies are usually IgG and can best be detected using antihuman globulin; some have the ability to fix complement and can cause hemolytic transfusion reactions. In contrast to many other blood group antigens, the Fyᵃ and Fyᵇ antigens are destroyed by treatment of red cells with enzymes. Although it might be expected that Duffy antibodies would occur much more often in blacks, since 68% are Fy(a−b−) and would thus be expected to make antibody following transfusion of Fyᵃ- or Fyᵇ-positive cells, anti-Fyᵃ or anti-Fyᵇ occurs only rarely, possibly because the presence of a Duffy precursor substance on the red cells prevents host recognition of Fyᵃ or Fyᵇ as foreign.[33] The frequency of the four common phenotypes is shown in Table 4-7.

LUTHERAN BLOOD GROUP SYSTEM

An antibody that defined Luᵃ (Lutheran a) specificity was discovered in 1945,[12] and the antibody detecting Luᵇ was found 11 years later.[20] Luᵃ occurs on the red cells of about 7.7% of whites, whereas Luᵇ is present on the red cells of nearly everyone (99.85%).[59] Two genes, *Luᵃ* and *Luᵇ*, account for the three phenotypes Lu(a+b−), Lu(a+b+), and Lu(a−b+). In addition, there appears to be a third gene, *Lu*, that, like the *O* gene, acts as a silent allele; the inheritance of *Lu/Lu* results in the phenotype (Lu[a−b−]).[22] This phenotype also arises when a rare dominant inhibitor gene, independent of the Lutheran gene locus, is inherited.[19] In recent years several additional antigenic specificities have been added to the Lutheran system; most of these have been indicated by the Lu abbreviation and a numerical designation, i.e., Lu4, Lu5, etc.[59]

The strength of the Luᵃ and Luᵇ antigens on the red cell varies considerably from person to person,

Table 4-7. Duffy blood group system*

	Whites			Blacks		
		Antigen frequency			Antigen frequency	
Phenotype	Phenotype frequency	Fy^a	Fy^b	Phenotype frequency	Fy^a	Fy^b
Fy(a+b−)	17%	66%		9%	10%	
Fy(a+b+)	49%		83%	1%		23%
Fy(a−b+)	34%			22%		
Fy(a−b−)	<0.1%			68%		

*From Issitt, P. D., and Issitt, C. H.: Applied blood group serology, Oxnard, Calif., 1975, Becton, Dickinson & Co.

and Lutheran antibodies usually display dosage. Anti-Lu^b is a most uncommon blood group antibody, and nearly all examples that have been found react only with the antiglobulin method. Anti-Lu^a, although also rare, is usually an agglutinating antibody and can be detected without the use of antihuman globulin. Both antibodies have caused transfusion reactions, although they have rarely caused hemolytic disease of the newborn, both because the antibodies are so unusual and because the Lu antigens are not well developed on neonatal red cells.[59]

KIDD BLOOD GROUP SYSTEM

The Kidd blood group system is similar to the Duffy and Lutheran systems in that there are two common antithetical genes, *Jk^a* and *Jk^b*,[56] which produce two common antigens, and a third rare recessive gene, *Jk,* which produces neither the Jk^a nor Jk^b antigens.[55] Jk^a occurs on the cells of about 77% of whites, 93% of American blacks and 50% of Chinese.[59] Jk^b is present on the erythrocytes of about 73% of whites. Only a few persons, most of whom are of Polynesian origin, appear to be Jk(a−b−) and thus presumably of genotype *Jk/Jk.*

Kidd antibodies are usually IgG and most bind complement; they react best with red cells that have been treated with enzymes such as papain. Both antibodies have caused transfusion reactions and hemolytic disease of the newborn. In contrast to many other antibodies, anti-Jk^a and anti-Jk^b usually cannot be detected for more than a few months after alloimmunization has occurred. Although the antibodies have a short half-life, they reappear very rapidly following a second exposure to the antigen. Previously alloimmunized persons are often inadvertently transfused with red cells that appear compatible but that cause the rapid reappearance of antibody a few days later. The antibody is often sufficiently potent to cause the intravascular destruction of transfused cells with concurrent hemoglobinemia and hemoglobinuria. A profound hemolytic anemia may be seen in persons who have received many units of blood before the antibody has reappeared, since either antibody will react with the cells of about three of four donors.

MNSs BLOOD GROUP SYSTEM

The MN blood group system was described in 1927 after anti-M and anti-N were produced in rabbits immunized with human erythrocytes.[37] Although *M* and *N* appear to behave as antithetical genes, it has been suggested that *N* may control production of a precursor substance N, on which two codominant allelic *M* and *m* genes act. Presence of the *M* gene in a single *(M/m)* or double dose *(M/M)* would then confer MN and MM specificity, respectively, while presence of *m/m* would leave the N precursor unchanged.[33] Regardless of the mechanism, three phenotypes result: M/M, M/N, and N/N. The *MN* genes are closely linked[62] to a second set of genes, *S* and *s,* which account for three phenotypes, S/S, S/s, and s/s. The frequency of each of the six phenotypes is shown in Table 4-8. For practical purposes, the M and N antigens are present on the red cells of about 75% of donors; s is quite common (89%), and S occurs on the cells of slightly more than one half of donors.

Anti-M is the most frequently encountered antibody in the MNSs system, although anti-N, anti-S, and anti-s have all been implicated in hemolytic transfusion reactions and in hemolytic disease of the newborn.[59,74] Occasionally anti-M, anti-N, or anti-S appears in the plasma of persons not exposed to the antigens by transfusion or pregnancy; these antibodies are generally IgM, react best in vitro at low temperatures, and do not cause significant transfusion problems. Indeed, some persons have apparent M- or N-specific autoantibodies that do not affect autologous red cells, possibly because the N and M antigens may be a mosaic similar to Rh^ABCD.[33] Occasionally IgG antibodies are produced after transfusion or pregnancy; these antibodies react in vitro at body temperature and have caused hemolytic transfusion

Table 4-8. MNSs antigen frequency*

Pheno-type	Phenotype frequency	Antigen frequency			
		M	**N**	**S**	**s**
M/M	28%	78%			
M/N	50%				
N/N	22%		72%		
S/S	11%			55%	
S/s	44%				
s/s	45%				89%

*From Issitt, P. D., and Issitt, C. H.: Applied blood group serology, Oxnard, Calif., 1975, Becton, Dickinson & Co.

reactions, although most do not fix complement. Anti-M, anti-N, and anti-S frequently display dosage. Antibodies defining several other related antigens have also been described and are reviewed by Issitt and Issitt.[33]

I/i BLOOD GROUP SYSTEM

The I/i blood group system is unique in that the erythrocytes of most persons possess the I antigen although a naturally occurring anti-I antibody is regularly present in the plasma. The expression of the I antigen on the erythrocyte membrane is inversely related to the expression of another antigen termed i: Cells of newborns are rich in i and poor in I; by age 18 months the I-rich/i-poor pattern of the adult is attained.[46] Although the strength of the I antigen varies from person to person, the red cells of nearly all adults react in vitro with anti-I at cold (4° C) temperatures, hence the name "cold agglutinin" for this antibody. Changes in the I/i antigen strength with a reversion to the neonatal i-rich/I-poor form are regularly seen in certain diseases, such as thalassemia, sideroblastic anemia, and leukemia,[26] although the reason for this is unclear.

Anti-I is present in the plasma of many persons. The antibody is usually IgM and reacts best at low temperatures, but occasionally it reacts at higher temperatures and can produce apparent incompatibility in the cross match. In spite of this in vitro reactivity, transfused red cells survive normally, because the antibody is usually weak and because most anti-I is nonreactive at body temperature. Anti-I is regularly seen in association with *Mycoplasma* pneumonia,[67] while another "cold agglutinin," anti-i, is sometimes seen in patients with myeloid leukemia or infectious mononucleosis.[34] The anti-I that produces cold hemagglutinin disease is usually of very high titer[83] and the range of thermal activity is such that antigen-antibody reactions occur in the cooler parts of the body, such as the extremities, with resultant erythrocyte destruction.

P BLOOD GROUP SYSTEM

The P blood group system was identified in 1927 using an antibody produced in rabbits immunized with human erythrocytes.[38] Four antigens comprise the system: P_1, P_2, P^k, and p. The red cells of about 80% of whites and 90% to 95% of blacks carry the P_1 antigen[33]; these persons do not usually have antibody to other antigens of the P system. The strength of the P_1 antigen varies from person to person; the cells of some individuals react much more strongly with anti-P_1 than do the cells of others. A second antigen, P_2, is present on the red cells of the remaining 20% of persons, and about 90% of these have anti-P_1 in their plasma. This antibody is usually IgM and agglutinates red cells at low temperature, although a few react at body temperature and cause hemolytic transfusion reactions.[53]

The P_1 and P_2 antigens are absent from the cells of a small percentage of persons; these persons have either P^k or p on their erythrocyte membranes. P^k persons regularly have antibody that reacts with P_1 and P_2 cells but not with p cells, while persons with the p phenotype have antibody that reacts with P^k cells as well as P_1 and P_2 cells. The latter antibody has caused severe hemolytic transfusion reactions[42] and hemolytic disease of the newborn.[33] This antibody was formerly known as anti-Tj[a] before its place in the P blood group system was appreciated, and it was once thought to be the Donath-Landsteiner antibody seen in persons with paroxysmal cold hemoglobinuria; however, recent studies have shown that the D-L antibody is specific for only the P_1 and P_2 antigens.[43]

HISTOCOMPATIBILITY ANTIGENS (HLA)

Just as erythrocytes possess many antigens, other antigenic determinants are found on leukocytes, platelets, and tissue cells. Some of these appear specific for the platelet (Table 4-9)[84] or the granulocyte,[35] whereas others that appear important in transplantation are shared by lymphocytes, granulocytes, platelets, and tissue cells.

Five closely linked genes on chromosome 6 control transplantation antigens, graft rejection, and the immune response. Three of the gene loci that produce the histocompatibility antigens were formerly called LA, FOUR, and AJ but have recently been renamed HLA-A, HLA-B, and HLA-C, respectively, by a joint committee of the World Health Organization and the International Union of Immunological Societies.[79] Each locus may be occupied by one of several allelic genes, and a gene is inherited from each parent at each of the three loci, resulting in two HLA-A genes, two HLA-B genes, and probably two HLA-C genes as well. The combination of related genes on a single chromosome is called the *haplotype*.

Transplantation antigens can be studied using leukocyte agglutination, complement fixation, or lymphocytotoxicity[11,16]; the last technique is most widely utilized. In it, serum that contains antibody to one or more of the transplantation antigens is incubated with a suspension of fresh human lymphocytes and a source of complement. If the serum contains an antibody that reacts with an antigen on the test cells, complement is fixed and causes cell death. A dye such as trypan blue or eosin is often used to detect killed cells: Viable cells exclude the dye, whereas dead cells cannot. The appearance of many dead cells that have taken up the dye thus indicates that the cells possess the antigen recognized by the antibody. Antibodies to histocompatibility antigens are often found in the serum of multiparous women, in transplant recipients, and in persons who have received blood transfusions. Indeed, the development of HLA antibodies following transfusion often interferes with subsequent platelet transfusion, as will be discussed later.

Leukocyte antibodies have been studied in many laboratories with the result that the same antigens and antibodies were often known by many different names. Since this posed problems in communication, a series of international workshops was held with the purpose of adopting a uniform histocompatibility antigen terminology. As a result, allelic genes have been given an alphabetical designation based on the locus to which they belong plus a numerical designation to indicate the gene (*HLA-A1, HLA-B8,* etc.) when international agreement has been reached as to specificity. Those genes with only provisional specificity are indicated by the letter w before the numeric designation (*HLA-Aw33*). HLA-A and HLA-B have been much more extensively studied than HLA-C. Antigenic specificities 1, 2, 3, 9, 10, 11, 28, and 29 have been assigned to the HLA-A locus, and the specificities 5, 7, 8, 12, 13, 14, 18, and 27 are

Table 4-9. Frequency of platelet-specific antigens*

Antigen	Frequency
Pl^{A1} (Zw^a)	97%
Pl^{A2} (Zw^b)	26%
Pl^{E1}	99%
Pl^{E2}	5%
Ko^a	14%
Ko^b	99%

*From Yankee, R. A.: In Baldini, M. G., and Ebbe, S., eds.: Platelets: production, function, transfusion and storage, New York, 1974, Grune & Stratton, Inc. Used by permission.

Table 4-10. Recognized HLA specificities*

HLA-A locus†		HLA-B locus‡		HLA-C locus§		HLA-D locus‖	
New	**Old**	**New**	**Old**	**New**	**Old**	**New**	**Old**
HLA-A1	HL-A1	HLA-B5	HL-A5	HLA-Cw1	T1	HLA-Dw1	LD 101
HLA-A2	HL-A2	HLA-B7	HL-A7	HLA-Cw2	T2	HLA-Dw2	LD 102
HLA-A3	HL-A3	HLA-B8	HL-A8	HLA-Cw3	T3	HLA-Dw3	LD 103
HLA-A9	HL-A9	HLA-B12	HL-A12	HLA-Cw4	T4	HLA-Dw4	LD 104
HLA-A10	HL-A10	HLA-B13	HL-A13	HLA-Cw5	T5	HLA-Dw5	LD 105
HLA-A11	HL-A11	HLA-B14	W14			HLA-Dw6	LD 106
HLA-A28	W28	HLA-B18	W18				
HLA-A29	W29	HLA-B27	W27				
HLA-Aw19	Li	HLA-Bw15	W15				
HLA-Aw23	W23	HLA-Bw16	W16				
HLA-Aw24	W24	HLA-Bw17	W17				
HLA-Aw25	W25	HLA-Bw21	W21				
HLA-Aw26	W26	HLA-Bw22	W22				
HLA-Aw30	W30	HLA-Bw35	W5				
HLA-Aw31	W31	HLA-Bw37	TY				
HLA-Aw32	W32	HLA-Bw38	W16.1				
HLA-Aw33	W19.6	HLA-Bw39	W16.2				
HLA-AW34	Malay 2	HLA-Bw40	W10				
HLA-Aw36	Mo	HLA-Bw41	Sabell				
HLA-Aw43	BK	HLA-Bw42	MWA				

*From WHO-IUIS Terminology Committee: Transplant. Proc. **8:**109, 1976. Used by permission.
†Formerly LA.
‡Formerly FOUR.
§Formerly AJ.
‖Formerly MLC (MLR).

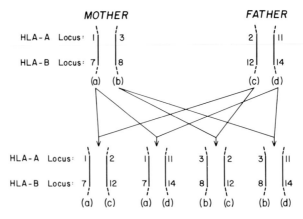

Fig. 4-2. Schematic representation of HLA inheritance. (See text for discussion.)

controlled by HLA-B. Symbols for genes are conventionally written in italics and symbols for antigens are not. At least ninety different antigenic specificities are known at the present time.[3] The association of some HLA antigens with certain disease states (such as HLA-B27 and disease of the spine and sacroiliac joints) has not yet been explained.[64] Table 4-10 lists agreed and provisionally agreed on specificities using both the new and old terminology.

In addition to the three loci that control expression of the transplantation antigens, a fourth locus appears to control the ability of lymphocytes to react to foreign histocompatibility antigens by undergoing blast transformation in tissue culture and by causing the graft versus host response in vivo.[6,7,50] This locus, previously termed MLC (for *m*ixed *l*eukocyte [or *l*ymphocyte] *c*ulture) or MLR (for *m*ixed *l*eukocyte [*l*ymphocyte] *r*esponse), is now called HLA-D.[79] A gene that in some way is involved in immunoregulation is also closely linked to the HLA loci and is called the *Ir* (immune response) gene.[5]

HLA-A, HLA-B, HLA-C, and *HLA-D* are closely linked, and the genes corresponding to each locus are usually transmitted as a unit.[3,14] The lymphocytes of most HLA-identical siblings do not stimulate one another in mixed lymphocyte culture; the occasional stimulation seen in some identical siblings suggests that antigenic determinants other than HLA-A, HLA-B, and HLA-C may be recognized by the HLA-D locus. The inheritance of the histocompatibility complex is shown schematically in Fig. 4-2; for simplicity only the HLA-A and HLA-B loci are shown. In this example *HLA-A1* and *HLA-B7* are carried on one maternal chromosome *(a)*, while *HLA-A3* and *HLA-B8* are found on the other *(b)*. In a similar manner the genes for *HLA-A2* and *HLA-B12* are located on one paternal chromosome *(c)*, while *HLA-A11* and *HLA-B14* are carried on the remaining one *(d)*. Since the

chromosomes segregate independently, maternal chromosome *a* can combine with either paternal chromosome *c* or *d, or* chromosome *b* can pair with either *c* or *d*. As a result children will inherit one of the four possible chromosome combinations *(a/c, a/d, b/c, b/d)*; since the association is random, the chance that any given chromosome pair will be inherited is one in four, and siblings thus have a 25% chance of being "HLA identical" with one another. As in the red cell blood group systems, most persons have the potential to form antibody against antigens that they lack if exposed by pregnancy, transplantation, or transfusion. The clinical relevance of HLA will be discussed in more detail in the section on platelet transfusion and in Chapter 17.

Blood component transfusion

Blood may be used to restore oxygen-carrying capability, to replenish intravascular volume, to correct bleeding tendencies, and to prevent or treat infection. It is rare that all or even most of these indications are present, and as a result the use of specific blood components or fractions to correct specific deficiencies has been increasingly emphasized. Ten to 12 million units of blood are drawn in the United States each year.[125] If all of these were used as whole blood, it would be impossible to provide adequate therapy for patients with thrombocytopenia, leukopenia, and congenital or acquired coagulation defects; indeed, the plasma from nearly 3 million units of blood is required annually just to treat patients with hemophilia.[125] The intelligent use of blood components allows a maximal number of persons to receive optimal transfusion therapy. The following list gives the many components, fractions, and derivatives that can be prepared from whole blood.

1. Packed red cells
2. Leukocyte-poor red cells
3. Frozen thawed red cells
4. Fresh frozen plasma
5. Single-donor plasma
6. Plasma protein fraction
7. Albumin
8. Cryoprecipitate
9. Factor VIII concentrate
10. Factor II-VII-IX-X concentrate
11. Fibrinogen
12. γ-Globulin
13. Specific hyperimmune globulins
14. Platelet-rich plasma
15. Platelet concentrate

Red cell, platelet, and granulocyte transfusion will be discussed in the remainder of this chapter; plasma replacement therapy will be dealt with in Chapter 24.

RED BLOOD CELL TRANSFUSION

Packed red blood cells are the treatment of choice to restore oxygen-carrying capacity unless there is concurrent marked hypovolemia induced by trauma, surgery, or severe hemorrhage. Even in these instances, packed red blood cells may be used with isotonic saline, Ringer's lactate, hydroxyethyl starch,[110] fresh frozen plasma, plasma protein fraction, or albumin to restore volume. The use of protein solutions generally provides a more lasting effect than crystalloid solutions, but both are effective in the acute treatment of hypovolemia. Coagulation factors such as factor V and factor VIII deteriorate rapidly in stored bank blood (approximately 35% of factor V and about 75% of factor VIII are lost after 7 days of storage).[133] Administration of fresh frozen plasma, which contains all of the coagulation factors, may be necessary if there has been massive transfusion with bank blood.

Anticoagulants

Until a few years ago most blood in the United States was collected in acid-citrate-dextrose (ACD) solution; at present a different anticoagulant, citrate-phosphate-dextrose (CPD), is used since it results in better red cell preservation and function. Because both ACD and CPD act as anticoagulants by chelating ionic calcium, transient hypocalcemia may occur in recipients who receive massive transfusion or in those with severe liver dysfunction who are unable to metabolize citrate at a normal rate. Hypocalcemia is usually heralded by circumoral paresthesias and may progress to tetany or cardiac arrest unless the rate of transfusion is slowed or intravenous calcium (0.5 to 1.0 ml of 10% calcium gluconate/100 ml of blood infused) is administered. Calcium should not be added to the blood bag or given through the same intra-

venous line as the blood, since clotting will result.

Other anticoagulants are only rarely used. Blood is occasionally collected in heparin solution for use in special circumstances such as exchange transfusion or open heart surgery. Unlike ACD and CPD, heparin anticoagulant does not contain dextrose (glucose) to maintain erythrocyte metabolism, and red cells collected with this anticoagulant can be stored only 48 hours. Salts of ethylenediaminetetraacetic acid (EDTA) were once used in the preparation of platelet concentrates, but this practice has been abandoned since it was learned that platelet ultrastructure was damaged by the anticoagulant.

Red cell storage

The energy needs of the erythrocyte are provided by the glycolytic and the hexose-monophosphate metabolic pathways.[115] (See Chapter 12.) The end product of glucose metabolism is lactate; this compound progressively accumulates during blood storage since red cells, which lack mitochondria and thus the citric acid metabolic cycle, cannot metabolize it further. The increasing concentration of lactate causes a fall in pH, which in turn leads to inhibition of further cell glucose metabolism and a decrease in the energy-rich compound adenosine triphosphate (ATP). ATP is necessary to preserve erythrocyte viability. As the intracellular ATP level drops, there is a loss of membrane lipid, the membrane becomes rigid, and the cell changes shape from a disc to a sphere[107]; after transfusion, cells that have undergone such changes are rapidly removed from the circulation by the reticuloendothelial system. In spite of this, at least 70% of the red cells survive normally after transfusion even if blood has been stored for up to 21 days.

Even though erythrocytes may *survive* normally after transfusion, they may transiently *function* poorly in delivery of oxygen to the tissues depending on the length of time they have been stored.[89] Valtis and Kennedy[129] first noted that red cells progressively increase their affinity for oxygen during storage as reflected by a leftward shift of the oxygen dissociation curve. The net effect of this shift is that at any given partial pressure, oxygen is bound more tightly to hemoglobin and thus is less available to the tissues. This change in affinity is caused by a decrease in the intracellular concentration of 2,3-diphosphoglycerate (2,3-DPG).[98] Although CPD anticoagulant preserves erythrocyte 2,3-DPG better than ACD, the concentration of the compound begins to decline after 7 to 10 days of red cell storage.[101,121] Even though 2,3-DPG is rapidly restored following transfusion,[90,118] there has been concern that administration of 2,3-DPG-depleted erythrocytes might transiently compromise tissue oxygen delivery. Current evidence suggests that the body compensates for increased hemoglobin oxygen affinity by increasing the cardiac output or by increasing the capillary-tissue oxygen gradient or both.[92,109] As a result the concentration of 2,3-DPG may be clinically important only in persons receiving massive transfusion; even then blood stored for less than 7 to 10 days is probably satisfactory since the concentration of 2,3-DPG does not change significantly during this period.[101,121]

Several compounds such as inosine,[86] adenine,[124] ascorbic acid,[135] and dipyridamole[103] have been added to blood to promote cell viability and maintain function during storage. Although adenine causes 2,3-DPG to disappear more rapidly, it allows maintenance of red cell ATP for up to 35 days of storage with good posttransfusion cell survival.[97] Blood collected in CPD-adenine solution is in use in some countries; however, the Food and Drug Administration has not yet licensed its use in the United States. At present blood may be stored a maximum of 21 days, although there is evidence that blood collected in CPD can be stored for as long as 28 days and still provide 70% posttransfusion red cell survival.

Valeri and Zaroulis[128] have restored ATP and 2,3-DPG concentrations of outdated erythrocytes to nearly normal by incubating the cells in a solution of glucose, inosine, pyruvate, and phosphate; the cells can be frozen and stored with good survival after thawing and transfusion. Although it is experimental, use of this technique could salvage much of the blood that is now discarded because of the 21-day limit on storage. It has been estimated that 12.9% of all blood collected for transfusion is discarded because of outdating.[125]

Red cell cryopreservation

Mollison and Sloviter[114] were the first to transfuse red cells that had been stored and frozen; since that time many workers have contributed to the techniques that allow effective use of frozen-thawed red cells. Two procedures are used at the present time. In one method red cells are quick-frozen in liquid nitrogen using 14% glycerol as a cryoprotective agent and stored at very low ($-196°$ C) temperatures.[120] Alternatively red cells may be frozen more slowly and stored at higher ($-85°$ C) temperatures if a higher concentration of glycerol is used.[111] With either technique the glycerol must be gradually removed from the cells after they have been thawed to prevent hemolysis; several instruments are available to remove glycerol from cells. Posttransfusion cell survival is good and it is possible to store cells in the frozen state for long periods of time.

Although the cost of preparation of frozen-thawed red cells is considerable, the cells have several advantages over conventionally stored erythrocytes including a decreased risk of transmitting hepatitis,[96] the feasibility of long-term storage of "rare" red cells, the stockpiling of autologous red cells for use in elective surgery, the maintenance of normal concentrations of ATP and 2,3-DPG if cells are frozen fresh or after rejuvenation,[128] and a significant reduction in the number of leukocytes and platelets present with the red cells.[99] Both platelets and leukocytes contain histocompatibility antigens that may elicit production of HLA antibodies, which in turn may compromise the outcome of organ transplantation. It is probably reasonable to use frozen-thawed erythrocytes exclusively in persons who are organ transplant candidates or recipients.

Frozen-thawed red cells can be used in the treatment of persons with thalassemia or aplastic anemia who require long-term transfusion support to delay the onset of leukocyte alloimmunization and its transfusion-associated reactions of chills and fever. Since frozen red cells are expensive, it may be prudent to use cells rendered relatively leukocyte poor by differential centrifugation techniques[113]; although 15% to 20% of the red cells are lost, more than 70% of leukocytes and about 90% of platelets are also removed. In spite of the small numbers of leukocytes remaining in blood made leukocyte poor in this manner, recipient chill and fever reactions are uncommon, even in persons who regularly react to standard red cell preparations. Miller et al.[112] have shown that HLA immunization occurred in only 15% of uremic patients transfused with leukocyte-poor red cells, compared with more than 50% of patients who received conventional therapy, even though those treated with leukocyte-poor cells were given an average of twice as many transfusions as the control group.

Calculation of volume of blood for simple transfusion

Mollison[51] suggested a simplified method of calculating the amount of blood required for transfusion. The basic principle is that a hemoglobin concentration of 15 gm/dl corresponds to a red cell volume of 30 ml/kg body weight. This constitutes a convenient proportion for the sake of calculation. It implies that a transfusion of 2 ml of red cells/kg body weight will raise the hemoglobin concentration by 1 gm/dl. Anticoagulated blood as supplied by most transfusion services contains approximately one-third its volume of red cells. Thus 6 ml (3 × 2 ml) of ACD or CPD blood per kg of body weight is required to raise the hemoglobin concentration 1 gm/dl.

The expected change in hemoglobin following transfusion can be calculated as follows:

1. Multiply blood volume (70 ml/kg) by hemoglobin level (gm/dl) to get the initial body hemoglobin content in grams.
2. Determine the desired posttransfusion hemoglobin level (e.g., 10 gm/dl); multiply by blood volume to obtain the posttransfusion body hemoglobin content.
3. Calculate the deficit in body hemoglobin by subtracting the initial body hemoglobin level in grams from the desired body hemoglobin level in grams.
4. Assuming that 1 ml of packed red cells has a hematocrit of about 70% and therefore contains 0.23 gm hemoglobin, divide 0.23 gm into the total body hemoglobin deficit. This equals the volume of packed red blood cells to be transfused to raise the hemoglobin to the value determined in No. 2.

The volume of blood to be given depends on the condition of the patient. Generally if there is no underlying or accompanying disease that could predispose to heart failure, 10 to 15 ml/kg may be administered over 2 hours. A more rapid rate of transfusion in a compensated chronically ill and anemic patient with severe renal disease or collagen vascular disease could precipitate congestive heart failure. Obviously a hypovolemic patient suffering from acute blood loss will tolerate a similar quantity of blood given more rapidly.

The precise hemoglobin level at which a child requires transfusion depends on a number of factors. A child who has iron deficiency anemia or anemia of prematurity but is otherwise healthy can tolerate hemoglobin levels as low as 5 to 6 gm/dl. Since fairly rapid elevation can be expected within a matter of weeks, transfusion of such patients is generally not recommended. Patients with sickle cell disease likewise tolerate lower levels of hemoglobin, and unless there is evidence of respiratory infection, septicemia, or aplastic crisis, transfusion is usually not required. Exceptions may be the presence of progressive nephritis or central nervous system infarct. Patients with thalassemia major apparently do best if their hemoglobin level is maintained at 10 gm/dl or above.

Exchange transfusion

Although the incidence of Rh-induced hemolytic disease of the newborn is decreasing and should continue to decrease with use of Rh immunoglobulin preparations to prevent immunization of Rh-negative mothers delivering Rh-positive infants,[102] exchange transfusion is still occasionally required to treat children with blood group incompatibility, hepatic encephalopathy,[127] sickle cell anemia crisis,[93] neonatal isoimmune thrombocy-

topenic purpura,[116] disseminated intravascular coagulation,[106] respiratory distress syndrome,[105] or hemolysis in the newborn resulting from deficiencies of erythrocyte enzymes.[104] Many causes of neonatal hyperbilirubinemia can be effectively managed with phototherapy,[122,126] although occasionally exchange transfusion is required to prevent kernicterus or correct severe anemia.

Blood for exchange transfusion is often cross matched with maternal serum if the exchange is being performed because of erythroblastosis fetalis; however, if the antibody specificity is known or if the exchange is being performed for reasons other than blood group incompatibility, it is probably best to use blood of the same ABO type as the infant (unless the exchange is for ABO incompatibility) since infusion of other types of blood that contain anti-A or anti-B may result in the destruction of the infant's cells that remain after the exchange. If the immunizing antibody is directed against a high-incidence antigen and a compatible donor cannot be found, maternal cells will not have the offending antigen and may be used for exchange transfusion if maternal antibody is removed and the cells are resuspended in group AB plasma.

Exchange transfusion with freshly drawn heparinized blood is probably preferable for treatment of severely afflicted erythroblastotic infants who are also acidotic, since it is slightly alkaline, in contrast to CPD blood, which is acidic. Since it takes from 1 to 2 hours to draw and process heparinized blood, it may be necessary to use CPD blood even in severely ill infants. Blood for exchange transfusion should be no older than 3 or 4 days since potassium and other substances gradually leach from the red cells and reach high concentrations in the plasma during storage.[88] In addition, use of relatively fresh red cells ensures that the concentration of 2,3-DPG is adequate.

A single unit (500 ml) of blood will usually allow a "two-volume" exchange, with removal of 70% to 85% of the infant's blood. The percentage of blood exchanged may be estimated by the following formula:

$$\%R = \left(\frac{V - S}{V}\right)^n$$

R equals the percentage of blood *remaining* in the infant, V is the infant's estimated blood volume (based on 70 to 80 ml/kg), S is the "syringe size" or aliquot volume sequentially removed and infused during exchange, and n is the number of infusion-removal cycles performed.[87] Fig. 4-3 may be used as a guide to exchange efficiency. If bilirubin removal is the primary goal, it is better to perform an exchange with a single unit of blood on two separate occasions than to use two units of

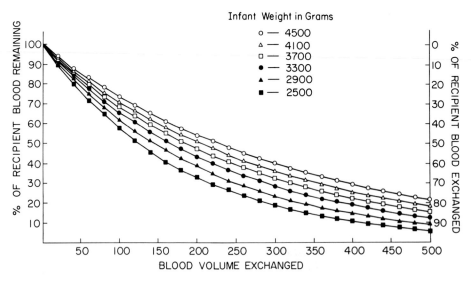

Fig. 4-3. Predicted percent of blood exchanged based on infant weight. Infant blood volume of 75 ml/kg body weight has been assumed. Percent of exchange is based on the formula $\%R = \left(\dfrac{V-S}{V}\right)^n$. (From Buchholz, D. H.: J. Pediatr. **84:**1, 1974.)

blood during a single exchange; the interval between exchanges allows additional bilirubin to diffuse from the tissues and into the bloodstream.

Since exchange transfusion represents a massive transfusion for the neonate, hypocalcemia may occur as a result of the amount of citrate infused in the blood, and it may be necessary to administer supplemental calcium. This problem does not occur when heparinized blood is used for exchange since heparin does not anticoagulate by chelation of calcium; it should be neutralized with protamine sulfate after the exchange. Heparinized blood usually contains 4.5 IU of heparin/ml; the amount of heparin remaining in the infant at the completion of exchange may be approximated by multiplying the product of the estimated infant blood volume and the percentage of blood exchanged by 4.5; from 0.5 to 0.75 mg of protamine should be given for each 100 units of heparin present in the neonatal circulation.[108] For example, an infant with a blood volume of 280 ml who receives an 88% exchange will have 280 × 0.88 × 4.5, or about 1,110 units, of heparin in the circulation; from 5 to 8 mg of protamine is required to neutralize the drug.

Transfusion reactions

One percent to 3% of patients receiving transfusions of blood or components have reactions such as chills, fever, pruritus, urticaria, flushing, headache, dyspnea, and nausea or vomiting[85,123]; rarely hemoglobinemia and hemoglobinuria occur. *Hemolytic transfusion reactions are most often caused by administration of blood to the wrong recipient; great care must be taken to assure the correct identification of specimens sent to the blood bank for cross matching and the identity of the unit of blood and the intended recipient.* Recipients should be observed frequently during transfusion and the infusion discontinued if there is evidence of reaction. Most reactions are caused by leukocyte or platelet antibodies rather than by destruction of transfused red cells. Since symptoms associated with hemolytic reactions are not unique, all reactions should be evaluated to allow detection of those that are potentially serious.

Transfusion reactions can be classed as febrile, allergic, bacterial, or hemolytic. Febrile reactions constitute the bulk of the reactions reported to the blood bank. These usually occur during or shortly after transfusion and are characterized by shaking chills and a 2° to 3° increase in temperature that returns to baseline in a few hours. These reactions occur most often in persons who have received multiple transfusions and in multiparous women; they are thought to be caused by antibodies in either donor or recipient plasma directed against antigens present on leukocytes and platelets. Febrile reactions are usually mild and principally cause patient anxiety and discomfort; acetaminophen is helpful in controlling fever, although this type of reaction can be avoided with the use of red cells made leukocyte poor. Rarely a severe reaction that mimics pulmonary edema is seen. It is characterized by cough, dyspnea, rales, decreased arterial Po_2, and the radiologic appearance of fluffy bilateral perihilar infiltrates without evidence of cardiac enlargement or pulmonary vascular engorgement.[132] Although these reactions usually resolve over 1 to 2 days, one has caused the death of a child with thalassemia who had multiple transfusions.[134] Chill and fever reactions are often seen during leukocyte transfusions and will be discussed later.

Severe reactions characterized by flushing, nausea and vomiting, diarrhea, changes in blood pressure, and frank anaphylaxis have been reported in persons with deficient or absent IgA who have IgG antibodies directed against IgA.[117] Vyas et al.[131] have shown that about 1 in 900 otherwise normal blood donors has no IgA and of these about 20% have antibody to IgA in their circulation. It might be expected that IgA–anti-IgA reactions would be common if a similar percentage of the recipient population possessed anti-IgA; however, this type of reaction is rather rare. Patients known to have anti-IgA should be transfused only with blood or plasma obtained from IgA-deficient donors or with extensively washed red cells. A registry of donors without IgA is maintained by the Irwin Memorial Blood Bank in San Francisco and by the American National Red Cross.

The administration of blood or components contaminated with bacteria may produce a severe reaction characterized by chills, high fever, marked hypotension, disorientation, disseminated intravascular coagulation, and occasionally death. Contamination of blood or components prepared in closed-bag collection systems is unusual, although microorganisms have been recovered from platelet products stored at room temperature,[94,100] and at least three deaths have resulted.[91,95] Examination of a gram-stained smear of bag contents may reveal bacteria, but this cause of reaction should not be ruled out if none are seen. Cultures should be taken of the blood bag as well as the recipient if contamination is suspected, and the patient should be treated with broad-spectrum antibiotics.

Hemolytic reactions occur infrequently but can cause hemoglobinemia, hemoglobinuria, and sometimes hypotension, disseminated intravascular coagulation, acute renal failure, or even death. Symptoms usually consist of flushing, a feeling of apprehension, chest or back pain, chills, fever, and nausea or vomiting; the development of diffuse bleeding may be the only evidence of hemolysis in anesthetized patients at surgery. Cell destruction may be predominantly intravascular, as seen with ABO incompatibilities, or primarily extravascular, as in Rh incompatibility. Intravascular hemolysis is more harmful than the slow extravascular removal of erythrocytes by the reticuloendothelial system.

If hemolysis is suspected, a sample of recipient blood should be centrifuged and the plasma should be examined for hemoglobin. Plasma with a hemoglobin concentration of 20 to 25 mg/dl has a slight pink tinge; when the concentration of hemoglobin is 100 mg/dl or more, it appears red.[130] A direct antiglobulin test may reveal the presence of antibody-coated erythrocytes unless all of the transfused cells have been destroyed intravascularly.

Since the symptoms of the recipient do not provide a clear-cut indication of the type of reaction, it is prudent to terminate all transfusions that produce reactions in the recipient since the consequences of a hemolytic reaction can be catastrophic. If red cell lysis has occurred or is suspected, 10% mannitol and other fluids should be used to promote osmotic diuresis; if good urine output does not result, it may indicate that the patient is in shock or that renal damage has already occurred. Since disseminated intravascular coagulation may accompany hemolytic reactions, the coagulation status of the recipient should also be evaluated. The development of a severe bleeding diathesis may warrant administration of heparin and appropriate components such as fresh frozen plasma and platelets.

PLATELET TRANSFUSION

Thrombocytopenia may result from increased platelet destruction, decreased platelet production, or massive transfusion with bank blood. Bleeding secondary to thrombocytopenia seldom occurs unless the platelet count drops below 50×10^9/liter and serious bleeding episodes are uncommon at counts above 20×10^9/liter. Bleeding can also result from intrinsic or extrinsic platelet dysfunction as in Glanzmann's thrombasthenia,[155] storage pool disease,[181] dysproteinemia,[141] uremia,[176] and the use of certain drugs, especially aspirin.[163]

Preparation of platelets

Although platelet replacement therapy was described in the 1950s, it was not widely used until plastic blood collection systems that permitted easy component preparation became available.[159] Platelets separated from red blood cells by low-gravity centrifugation can be used as platelet-rich plasma or may be concentrated to prepare platelet concentrate. At one time platelets were prepared from whole blood collected in EDTA anticoagulant; EDTA, however, alters platelet morphology and results in poor posttransfusion platelet survival.[139] Anticoagulants containing citrate provide better platelet recovery and survival, and CPD anticoagulant is currently in routine use.[179] Platelets clump when chilled, and concentrates are usually prepared from donor blood before it is refrigerated. Platelets cannot be prepared from blood anticoagulated with heparin since irreversible platelet clumping occurs. An average bag of platelet concentrate contains approximately 0.7×10^{11} platelets, about one-half the number present in a unit of whole blood.

Platelets may also be obtained directly from donors by plateletpheresis, a technique in which the platelets are separated from whole blood and the red cells and most of the plasma are returned to the donor. This allows collection of more than one unit of platelets per donation and permits more frequent collection of platelets than is possible by whole blood donation, in which red cell regeneration time limits donation frequency. Following plateletpheresis the donor platelet count is transiently lowered, but it usually returns to predonation levels within 24 to 48 hours. Although most donors are not plateletpheresed intensively, it is possible to utilize a donor repeatedly as a source of histocompatible platelets for a patient refractory to platelets obtained from random donors.[171]

Platelets can also be harvested using continuous- or semicontinuous-flow centrifugation devices such as the IBM or Aminco Blood Cell Separator[151] or the Haemonetics Model 30 Blood Processor.*[178] These devices separate cells by differential centrifugation and allow platelets from the equivalent of several units of donor blood to be harvested with only modest losses of donor red blood cells. About 4.5×10^{11} platelets, equal to six bags of regular platelet concentrate, can be harvested from a single person in as little as 2 hours.[178]

Platelet administration

Platelets have a life span of about 9 to 10 days but are probably hemostatically effective for only the first 4 or 5.[138] Following production in the bone marrow the cells spend the first 2 days in a nonexchangeable splenic pool[147]; thereafter they enter the circulation, but about one third are retained in the spleen in a pool fully exchangeable with the circulation. Thus in a recipient with a normal spleen only about two thirds of the infused platelets can be accounted for in the circulation after transfusion.

Platelets maintain the hemostatic integrity of small vessels. As the platelet count drops below 100×10^9/liter, the template bleeding time becomes prolonged in proportion to the degree of thrombocytopenia.[156] Most patients do not bleed significantly if the platelet count is 50×10^9/liter or greater, although petechiae, ecchymoses, and the risk of serious bleeding increase dramatically as the platelet count falls below 20×10^9/liter.

Since platelet transfusion can cause alloimmunization and transmit diseases such as hepatitis,

platelets should not be administered unnecessarily. The expected posttransfusion platelet increment can be approximated by the formula:

$$\text{Exp.} = \frac{2}{3}\left(\frac{0.7 \times 10^{11} \times N}{BV}\right)$$

Exp. represents the expected increment, N equals the number of units of platelet concentrate, BV is the recipient's estimated blood volume expressed in microliters, and ⅔ corrects for normal splenic sequestration. The blood volume may be approximated from body weight (70 ml of blood/kg weight). Thus a 25 kg child has an approximate blood volume of 1.75 liters (or $1.75 \times 10^6\ \mu$l). If three units of platelet concentrate are administered, a posttransfusion increment of 80×10^9/liter should occur. Platelet counts of 80×10^9/liter to 100×10^9/liter are adequate for hemostasis, and increasing counts above this increases the risk of alloimmunization without a concomitant increase in hemostasis.

Patients with thrombocytopenia secondary to increased platelet destruction, such as occurs in idiopathic thrombocytopenic purpura, do not respond to platelet infusions and should receive transfusions only if serious hemorrhage occurs. Patients with decreased platelet production, or those who are thrombocytopenic following massive transfusion with bank blood, usually have a good response to transfused platelets unless they are febrile,[149] have organomegaly,[138] have septicemia,[149] or have become alloimmunized to leukocyte or platelet antigens by previous transfusion.[152]

Although it is desirable to provide ABO- and Rh-identical platelets, it is frequently difficult to do so. Consequently many platelet transfusions are given without regard for donor and recipient ABO and Rh group. Potential problems associated with this practice include infusion of plasma containing anti-A or anti-B, which may lead to recipient red cell destruction, impaired posttransfusion survival of ABO-incompatible platelets, and the possibility of Rh alloimmunization if platelets from an Rh-positive donor are given to an Rh-negative recipient.

Each unit of platelet concentrate contains from 30 to 50 ml of plasma (platelets stored at 22° C usually have more plasma than those stored at 4° C); if all donors are group O and the recipient is group A, AB, or B, there may be enough anti-A or anti-B to destroy some recipient red blood cells.[158] Of more concern is the possibility of impaired recovery and survival of group A, B, or AB platelets given to recipients with the corresponding blood group antibody. Aster[137] has reported decreased posttransfusion platelet recoveries in group O normal volunteers transfused

---

*IBM Corp., Princeton, N.J.; American Instrument Co., Silver Spring, Md.; Haemonetics Corp., Natick, Mass.

with group A or AB platelets and has suggested that group A platelets should be given only to group A and AB recipients while group O platelets should be given to group B and group O persons. Lohrmann et al.,[162] however, in a more recent study of refractory thrombocytopenic recipients, showed that ABO incompatibility did not influence posttransfusion platelet recovery when cells from histocompatible donors were utilized.

Finally Rh antigens are not present on the platelet, and their survival is normal in patients with anti-Rh antibody. Sufficient red cells are present in most platelet concentrates to induce alloimmunization to Rh, although Goldfinger showed that only a small percentage of Rh-negative recipients transfused with Rh-positive platelets became immunized to Rh.[150] The recipients described in that study were immunocompromised by either their disease or the therapy for it and may not typify the response seen in recipients with normal immunologic responsiveness. In general, if an Rh-negative recipient will require only short-term *limited* platelet transfusion support, platelets from Rh-negative donors should be given if possible, especially to females. If Rh-positive platelets must be used, one of the Rh immune globin preparations may be given to prevent Rh alloimmunization. It usually is not possible to provide long-term platelet support with cells from Rh-negative donors; use of Rh immune globulin is not indicated in this situation.

Alloimmunization to homologous leukocyte and platelet antigens regularly develops in recipients of multiple transfusions[175,182] and leads to a refractory state in which transfused platelets are rapidly destroyed. In these circumstances platelets from histocompatible related[152] or unrelated[162,183] donors show greatly improved posttransfusion recovery and survival. Even with the use of HLA-compatible cells, however, antibodies directed against leukocyte antigens may develop and cause poor platelet recovery, probably owing to destruction of platelets as "innocent bystanders" when the leukocyte antibody reacts with the white cells in the platelet concentrate. A low-gravity centrifugation, which removes 95% of the leukocytes and less than 20% of the platelets, can restore good posttransfusion platelet recovery in recipients receiving HLA-compatible platelets.[157] Antibody produced to platelet-specific antigens may also cause poor posttransfusion platelet survival.[182]

Unfortunately HLA-compatible platelets are not widely available and as a result most transfusions consist of cells obtained from several donors. Since the likelihood that an unselected donor will be histocompatible with the recipient is remote, patients are exposed to a variety of platelet and leukocyte antigens with each transfusion. Several transfusion services are administering platelets harvested from a single donor using the blood cell separator or the blood cell processor. Since recipients are exposed to the antigens of one rather than several donors, it has been postulated that alloimmunization will be delayed, although this has not yet been established in actual transfusion practice. Every effort should be made to curtail the number of random donor platelet transfusions given to bone marrow transplant candidates or recipients.

Platelet storage

For several years platelets were stored at 4° C although it was recognized that exposure to refrigerator temperature caused poorer posttransfusion recovery and a shorter half-life than when platelets were infused without storage.[161] In 1969 Murphy and Gardner[164] demonstrated that platelets maintained at 22° C showed nearly normal recovery and survival when transfused to normal volunteers. As a consequence most blood banks began to store platelets at room temperature for up to 72 hours. In recent years, however, there has been controversy as to whether storage at 22° or 4° C best preserves platelet function.

During 22° C storage platelet glycogen is markedly decreased, the ability to undergo in vitro aggregation is reduced, lactate accumulates in the plasma, and the pH drops.* If the pH falls below 6.0, platelet viability is lost.[140] Changes in pH are related to both platelet concentration and storage duration; the pH routinely falls below 6.0 after 72 hours if the platelet count is above $2.5 \times 10^6/\mu l$.[160] This can be prevented by storing the platelets in a larger volume of plasma or (experimentally) by use of plastic bags that allow increased diffusion of oxygen and carbon dioxide.[166]

The immediate hemostatic activity of platelets stored at 22° C appears impaired when these cells are given to volunteers who have been treated with aspirin to prolong their bleeding time[153]; transfusion of cells stored 24 hours at that temperature does not correct the bleeding time, although fresh platelets return the bleeding time to normal within 2 hours and restore in vitro platelet aggregation. Platelets stored at ambient temperature appear to require at least 24 hours in the recipient circulation before they correct bleeding time and aggregation responses.[153]

In contrast, platelets kept at 4° C, although morphologically altered, maintain ATP, ADP, pH, structure, and aggregability better than those stored at 22° C.[140,148,173] More important, platelets stored at the lower temperature appear to be more effective in both normal volunteers given aspirin[180] and in thrombocytopenic recipients. Becker

---

*References 140, 165, 166, 173.

et al.[140] studied sixty-eight patients who had low platelet counts and prolonged bleeding times and showed that the bleeding time was decreased in 63% of those given platelets stored at 4° C for 48 to 72 hours, compared with 26% of patients given cells stored at 22° C. Clinical evaluation suggested that platelets stored at 4° C were twice as effective in stopping bleeding as those stored at 22° C.

At the current time the controversy regarding storage temperature has not been resolved. The administration of fresh platelets is ideal but frequently impossible; cells must be stored for use in emergencies and at night and on weekends. Since the defects of platelets stored at 22° C appear to be corrected 24 hours following infusion, it has been suggested that these cells should be given to patients requiring *prophylactic* platelet transfusion with the idea that improved posttransfusion recovery and platelet survival outweigh transient impairment of cell function. Alternatively, since platelets stored at 4° C appear to be hemostatically more effective, these cells should probably be used to treat patients who are *actively bleeding*. Although recovery and survival are not as good as seen with platelets stored at 22° C given to normal volunteers, the differences in posttransfusion recovery and survival tend to disappear in recipients of multiple transfusions, in whom even fresh platelets have short half-lifes.[140]

Platelet cryopreservation

One possible solution to the storage problem is long-term preservation of platelets in the frozen state. Several cryoprotective agents, including glycerol, dimethylsulfoxide, dimethylacetamide, sodium glycerol phosphate, and hydroxyethyl starch have been used to protect platelets during freezing. Although Cohen and Gardner[143] reported good posttransfusion recovery of animal platelets frozen with 12% glycerol, poor posttransfusion recoveries were seen when human platelets were frozen with the same technique. Subsequently several workers have shown that human platelets can be frozen and stored using 5% to 6% dimethylsulfoxide; cell survival after transfusion is moderately good although a significant loss of cells occurs during the freeze-thaw-wash procedure.* Unfortunately dimethylsulfoxide is toxic and produces nausea, vomiting, foul-smelling breath, and phlebitis[146]; it must be removed before transfusion. Dayian and Rowe[145] have used a 5% glycerol–4% glucose mixture for platelet cryopreservation; the thawed platelets can be transfused without washing to remove the cryoprotective agent.

HLA-compatible frozen platelets can also be stockpiled and used in the management of patients with diseases expected to produce further episodes of thrombocytopenia. It is also possible to obtain platelets from patients with leukemia in remission and store them frozen for later use at times of disease relapse,[142,172] although there are questions as to the in vivo effectiveness of platelets obtained in this manner.[144]

Platelet-drug interaction

Platelet function is markedly altered following exposure to certain drugs such as aspirin, antihistamine, sulfinpyrazone, phenylbutazone, and dipyridamole.[174] Administration of as few as two aspirin tablets significantly prolongs the bleeding time of normal persons,[163] apparently by interfering with the platelet ''release'' reaction.[177] Although these cells do not release endogenous ADP and promote aggregation after contact with damaged endothelium, they do aggregate in response to the ADP released from platelets not exposed to aspirin. The hemostatic effectiveness of the entire platelet pool appears to be maintained if as few as 10% of the circulating platelets have not been exposed to the drug.[168] Thus a person who has ingested aspirin need not be rejected as a donor of platelets for an adult since his platelets will likely represent less than 10% of the total platelet pool in the recipient. If the recipient is a child, in which case the platelets of one donor may represent a much higher proportion of the final circulating platelet numbers, donors who have taken aspirin (and therefore have abnormally functioning platelets) should be avoided.

Neonatal thrombocytopenia

Although uncommon, thrombocytopenia is sometimes seen in newborns whose mothers have ingested thiazide diuretics during pregnancy[170] and in infants with congenital rubella, toxoplasmosis, cytomegalic inclusion disease, and herpesvirus infections. Neonatal isoimmune thrombocytopenic purpura is estimated to occur in about 1 in 5,000 births[169] and usually is caused by a maternal antibody produced in response to the Pl^{A1} antigen on fetal cells. The antibody crosses the placenta and destroys platelets in much the same manner that maternal anti-Rh destroys Rh-positive red cells in erythroblastosis fetalis. Usually antibody specificity cannot be rapidly determined. Even if it is known, compatible platelets will be difficult to find since the Pl^{A1} antigen occurs on the cells of about 98% of the population. Maternal antibody in the neonatal circulation will result in destruction of platelets for several days to several weeks; therefore as much antibody as possible should be removed by exchange transfusion[169] using blood without regard to platelet compatibility. After the bulk of antibody has been removed, the infant may be transfused with maternal platelets that have been washed to remove the antibody, since these

---

*References 154, 167, 172, 180.

cells will not contain the offending platelet antigen.[136] Although platelets share many of the HLA antigens with leukocytes, they also possess unique antigens in addition to Pl^A1; the frequency of these antigens is shown in Table 4-9.

GRANULOCYTE TRANSFUSION

Marrow hypoplasia with severe leukopenia and thrombocytopenia frequently follows the aggressive chemotherapeutic treatment of malignancy. Since the advent of platelet transfusion, deaths from hemorrhage have been significantly reduced and at present infection, especially that caused by gram-negative organisms, is the leading cause of death in many patients.[198] The risk of development of infection rises dramatically as the absolute granulocyte count drops below 1×10^9/liter.[189] Newer antibiotics and the use of protected environments such as the life island or the laminar air flow room may help to reduce or delay the onset of infection; however, the severely neutropenic patient remains at risk until marrow function returns.

Granulocyte collection

Although platelet transfusions have become routine in the management of patients with thrombocytopenia, until very recently granulocyte transfusion therapy has been considered experimental and limited to a few large centers. In contrast to platelets, which can be easily separated from whole blood by centrifugation, granulocytes have cell densities similar to those of the least dense red blood cells and are difficult to separate and purify in appreciable numbers by standard centrifugation techniques.

In the mid-1960s it was shown that administration of granulocytes obtained from donors with chronic myelogenous leukemia appeared to be helpful in the treatment of infected neutropenic patients with acute leukemia and aplastic anemia. Although only a small percentage of transfused cells appeared in the circulation following transfusion, many patients responded to transfusion with a reduction in fever and a clearance of bacteria from the bloodstream. Although occasional short-term engraftment of cells occurred, seven of thirteen patients with *Pseudomonas* septicemia survived.[194]

This work stimulated efforts to develop methods whereby granulocytes could be collected from normal donors rather than persons with chronic leukemia. Although the "buffy coat" formed after routine centrifugation procedures has been removed and used as a source of granulocytes, cells from 30 to 40 units of blood are needed to provide enough leukocytes for a single transfusion. This exposure to numerous donors greatly increases the risk of alloimmunization and disease transmission and makes this approach undesirable.

In the past few years several instruments have been devised to semiselectively harvest granulocytes from normal donors. The continuous-flow blood cell separator, developed jointly by the IBM Corporation and the National Cancer Institute, utilizes continuous-flow differential centrifugation to separate granulocytes, lymphocytes, and platelets from the blood of normal donors.[197] Blood is removed from the donor and passed into a small centrifuge bowl in which platelets, leukocytes, and erythrocytes are separated on the basis of cell density. Semipure leukocytes are removed and collected for later transfusion use, and red blood cells, platelets, and plasma are returned to the donor. A typical donation takes 3 to 4 hours; in that time from 8 to 14 liters of donor blood may be processed. Unfortunately granulocyte collection using this technique is inefficient unless the donor is treated with steroids to increase the circulating granulocyte count[197,203,211] and/or given rouleaux-inducing agents[207,211] to improve red cell sedimentation characteristics. Even then, appreciable numbers of lymphocytes contaminate the collected granulocytes. The Aminco Celltrifuge and the Haemonetics Model 30 Blood Processor are also in use and are based on the same principle of cell harvest by differential centrifugation.[205]

A second technique for obtaining granulocytes involves the use of nylon fiber filters as described by Djerassi et al.[191] and modified by other workers.[187,201] When heparinized blood is passed through filters containing nylon fibers, granulocytes and monocytes selectively adhere to the fibers, whereas lymphocytes, red blood cells, plasma, and most platelets do not and return to the donor. Large numbers of nearly pure granulocytes can be harvested by eluting the trapped cells from the fibers after several liters of blood have been processed. This technique routinely produces greater granulocyte yields than techniques using differential centrifugation, although some of the collected cells appear morphologically damaged[213] and show diminished chemotactic, phagocytic, and bactericidal activity when compared with normal cells, depending on the method of elution.* With either method of cell collection it is possible to use the same donor repeatedly, even for several days.[186] Although large numbers of donor granulocytes are removed, donors do not become severely leukopenic and are not at increased risk of developing infection consequent to donation.

Granulocyte administration

Just as with red cell and platelet transfusion, granulocyte transfusion exposes the recipient to granulocyte and lymphocyte antigens that may result in alloimmunization. Granulocytes probably

---

*References 200, 201, 213, 216.

share some HLA antigens but also possess cell-specific antigens.[206] The use of family member donors is at least theoretically desirable if HLA-matched siblings are available, especially if the recipient has preformed leukoagglutinins or lymphocytotoxic or granulocytotoxic antibodies directed against the cells of most random donors. Transfusion of leukocytes to persons with such antibodies may lead to a serious recipient transfusion reaction; in addition there is evidence that cell phagocytic ability and bactericidal capacity may be significantly reduced in the presence of cell-specific antibody.[196]

Granulocytes should be ABO compatible with the recipient since with either technique of cell collection from 25 to 50 ml of red blood cells are present with collected leukocytes.[186] If necessary, red cells can be removed by dextran or hydroxyethyl starch sedimentation, although some leukocytes will also be removed. This loss makes the use of ABO-compatible donors desirable whenever possible. Granulocytes are usually administered slowly over 3 to 6 hours and frequently produce chills and fever, especially if cells collected by filtration leukapheresis are used.[202] The occurrence of chills or mild elevation in temperature is not necessarily an indication to discontinue the transfusion if *granulocytes* are being administered. Premedication with antihistamine, acetaminophen, and steroids may help control recipient reactions, as will slowing or even temporarily stopping the transfusion. More serious reactions have occurred, with fevers to 105° or 106° F, disorientation, dyspnea, bronchospasm, cyanosis, or changes in blood pressure; there has also been a recipient death immediately following leukocyte infusion.[202] If reactions of a severe nature are noted, the transfusion should be stopped and appropriate therapy begun.

Therapeutic granulocyte transfusion

At the present time granulocyte transfusions have progressed beyond the investigational stage but are not yet as common as platelet transfusions. Several studies have suggested that granulocyte transfusion is helpful in the management of infected neutropenic patients. In 1972 Graw et al.[198] showed that 46% of patients with documented septicemia treated with antibiotics and granulocytes survived, compared with only 30% of those treated with antibiotics alone. Several uncontrolled studies have also suggested leukocyte transfusion therapy is helpful.*

In a prospectively randomized controlled study of patients with documented infection, Higby et al.[204] demonstrated that by day 20 only five of

nineteen (26%) patients treated with antibiotics alone were alive, compared with fifteen of seventeen (88%) in the group treated with antibiotics and granulocytes collected by filtration leukapheresis. Graw et al.[199] have also shown in a similar study that five of fourteen (36%) persons with gram-negative septicemia treated only with antibiotics survived, compared with thirteen of sixteen (81%) in the group additionally treated with leukocytes. No differences were seen between cells collected by centrifugation and filtration, and recipient survival was not related to posttransfusion leukocyte increments or to HLA compatibility.[199] Granulocytes also appear to be beneficial in the management of patients with severe burns[215] and in bone marrow transplant recipients.[188]

Several factors make evaluation of granulocyte transfusion difficult. Among these are variation in the criteria required for initiation of transfusion, the occurrence of suspected versus documented infection, the method of cell collection, the dose of cells given, the duration of therapy, and the return of recipient marrow function. A significant number of patients with malignancy develop fever without documented evidence of bacterial infection. Alavi et al.[185] have shown that about half of hospitalized patients with malignancy who develop fever above 101° F for 24 hours do not have infection and usually survive the febrile episode regardless of whether granulocytes are given. In contrast, those with infection appear to benefit from the administration of leukocytes.

The role of transfusion is also difficult to evaluate in patients who have return of marrow function during the course of transfusion therapy; however, granulocytes appear to be of significant benefit to those who are infected but who continue to have marrow hypoplasia.[185,199,204] The optimal dose of cells is not known, although low doses of cells are probably not helpful.[184,193] Similarly the ideal duration of therapy is not known; however, recipient response appears to be better with repeated transfusions.[198,210] The function of cells collected by filtration leukapheresis has been shown to be slightly impaired in vitro compared with control cells, but no differences in clinical efficacy have been demonstrated between cells collected in this manner and those harvested by differential centrifugation.

Because of the many variables involved, only general guidelines can be given with respect to granulocyte transfusion. Most workers select as candidates those with an absolute granulocyte count of less than 0.5×10^9/liter who have concurrent documented infection. ABO-compatible donors are preferred to avoid recipient destruction of transfused donor erythrocytes; the role of HLA compatibility in granulocyte transfusion does not

---

*References 195, 208, 210, 212, 214.

appear to be as important as it is in platelet transfusion. The recipient should not have leukocyte antibodies directed against donor cells. In general, once transfusions are initiated, as many cells as can be collected per donation should be given and the transfusions should be continued until there is clear-cut improvement, return of marrow function, or death. Occasionally transfusion may have to be discontinued as a consequence of severe reactions resulting from recipient alloimmunization.

Prophylactic granulocyte transfusion

The possible role of prophylactic leukocyte transfusion to prevent the development of infection in leukopenic patients is currently being evaluated. Ford studied the effect of alternate-day administration of an average of 14×10^9 granulocytes to a group of previously untreated adults with acute nonlymphocytic leukemia; no benefit of prophylaxis was noted and one transfused recipient died of graft versus host disease.[192] Clift et al.[190] have evaluated the effect of prophylactic transfusion given *daily* to recipients of bone marrow grafts. Three of sixteen transfused patients developed infection, compared with six of fifteen who did not receive granulocytes. Since granulocytes normally remain in the circulation for only short periods of time, daily administration may be important and account for the apparent ineffectiveness seen when given on alternate days.

Mannoni et al.[209] have also administered cells on a daily basis (except weekends) and have shown that none of ten patients with acute myelocytic leukemia developed severe infection or died, whereas nine of seventeen of the control group developed severe infection and six (35%) died, even though the control group received transfusion after infection was documented. These results, although preliminary, suggest that prophylactic cell administration may someday play a role in the management of transiently neutropenic patients.

LIMITATIONS AND HAZARDS OF TRANSFUSIONS

Increased experience and investigation of untoward reactions have provided a greater measure of safety in the administration of transfusions. Of the limitations and hazards included in the following list the most common are reactions to nonerythroid cellular blood elements and perhaps plasma proteins, hepatitis, and circulatory overload.

A. Hemolytic transfusion reactions
  1. Incompatible blood
  2. Interdonor incompatibility in multiple transfusion
B. Nonhemolytic transfusion reactions
  1. Leukocyte or platelet antibodies

  2. Plasma protein antibodies (anti-IgA, anti-Gm, etc.)
C. Transmission of infection
  1. Bacterial contamination
  2. Hepatitis A and B
  3. Malaria
  4. Syphilis
  5. Epstein-Barr virus (posttransfusion pseudomononucleosis)
  6. Cytomegalovirus infection
  7. Toxoplasmosis
  8. Rocky Mountain spotted fever
  9. Colorado tick fever
D. Circulatory overload
E. Suppression of erythropoiesis
F. Excessive iron deposition
  1. Hemosiderosis
  2. Exogenous hemochromatosis
G. Antibody formation
H. Allergic reactions
I. Massive transfusion and extracorporeal circulation
J. Air embolism
K. Electrolyte disturbances
  1. Hyperkalemia
  2. "Citrate intoxication"
L. Graft versus host disease

Hemolytic and nonhemolytic transfusion reactions have been discussed on pp. 70 and 71.

Transmission of infection

No discussion of blood components is complete without mention of diseases transmitted by transfusion. Cytomegalovirus infection, toxoplasmosis, infectious mononucleosis, syphilis, Rocky Mountain spotted fever, malaria, Colorado tick fever, and brucellosis have all been documented following blood transfusion.[235]

Significant bacterial contamination of a unit of blood is a rare event, inasmuch as these instances often result in a fatality. The transmission of malaria is common in areas where it is endemic, and Americans and Europeans returning from these areas are usually proscribed from donating blood except for fractionation.

The spirochete that causes syphilis rarely survives refrigeration, and syphilis transmitted by transfusion is rare. Since spirochetemia often occurs before a positive serologic test for syphilis develops, preparation of fresh components may result in transmission of this disease.

Finally, there has been observed in a significant number of patients who underwent surgical procedures, particularly associated with extracorporeal circulation, an infectious mononucleosis–like syndrome, transmitted with cytomegalovirus or the Epstein-Barr (EB) virus.

Hepatitis. Hepatitis represents the major cause of transfusion-induced morbidity and mortality. In the United States each year 1,500 to 3,000 deaths are estimated to occur following the administration of blood containing hepatitis virus; an additional 20,000 to 30,000 persons require hospitalization for the disease,[224] and many more persons develop subclinical illness.

Both hepatitis A ("infectious" hepatitis, short-incubation hepatitis, MS-1, epidemic hepatitis) and hepatitis B ("serum" hepatitis, long-incubation hepatitis, MS-2, "syringe" hepatitis, "posttransfusion" hepatitis) can be transmitted by blood transfusion; however, the incidence of transfusion-induced hepatitis A is low.[217,248]

Until recently there was no way to detect blood capable of transmitting hepatitis, although it was appreciated that blood products prepared from large pools of donor plasma (such as fibrinogen, fibrinogen-rich factor VIII, pooled plasma, factor VIII concentrate, and factor II-VII-IX-X concentrate) had a much greater hepatitis risk than single units of blood or components. In 1965 Blumberg et al.[221] described the presence of an antigen in the serum of an Australian aborigine that has subsequently been shown to be present in the blood of persons with type B viral hepatitis. The antigen (which has been referred to variously as Australia antigen, Au antigen, Hepatitis Associated Antigen, HAA, and—more correctly—hepatitis B surface antigen, or HB_sAg) has been shown by electron microscopy to be comprised of spherical and tubular particles 16 to 25 nm in diameter.[236] These particles are synthesized in the cytoplasm of infected hepatic cells and serve as an outer coat for the virus, which is replicated in the cell nucleus. Much more surface antigen is produced by the infected cells than is needed as coat material by the replicated virus, and large amounts of the material are released into the circulation. Although the presence of the surface antigen in blood correlates well with infectivity, the surface antigen itself is probably not infective.

Routine tests to detect hepatitis B are based on the detection of the surface antigen; for several years relatively crude techniques (immunodiffusion in agar gel, counterimmunoelectrophoresis, or complement fixation) were used to detect the antigen, although a much more sensitive radioimmunoassay has been in use since 1973. Even so, not all units of blood that can transmit hepatitis B can be detected, and the disease continues to occur following transfusion. Blood obtained from commercial sources (i.e., paid donors) has consistently been associated with a much greater incidence of hepatitis than blood obtained from volunteer sources, even though all units are tested for HB_sAg.[217,233] Goldfield et al.[233] have shown a risk of HB_sAg-associated hepatitis of 0.9/1,000 units of volunteer blood transfused, compared with 4.3/1,000 when commercially acquired blood was used. When *all* cases of posttransfusion icteric hepatitis are considered, the use of commercial blood may be associated with a twentyfold greater risk.[233] As a consequence, vigorous efforts are being made to abolish commercial blood centers and to rely exclusively on blood obtained from volunteer donors.

In addition to the surface antigen particles, small numbers of double-layered particles about 42 nm in diameter, composed of an inner core and outer lipoprotein coat containing the surface antigen, have been described by Dane et al.[225] and may represent the actual hepatitis B virus. Both the core (HB_cAg) and the surface lipoprotein (HB_sAg) appear antigenically distinct and both usually lead to the production of specific antibodies in the infected host. Following an incubation period of 6 weeks to 6 months, HB_sAg can be detected in the circulation for several days prior to the onset of clinical symptoms associated with hepatitis. The core antigen and a DNA polymerase produced by the virus as it replicates may also be detected prior to the disease onset.[239]

After the development of clinical symptoms, HB_sAg usually disappears (unless the person is destined to develop persistent hepatitis or chronic active hepatitis) concurrent with the development of circulating antibody to HB_sAg. Antibody to HB_cAg is also often present and is frequently seen before antibody to the surface antigen appears. Both antibodies are present for months to years following an infection, although antibody to the surface antigen usually persists longer than antibody to HB_cAg.[251] The presence of either antibody is presumptive evidence of prior exposure to hepatitis B virus, although blood is *not* routinely tested for either antibody. Transfusion of blood negative for HB_sAg but containing anti-HB_s antibody does not appear to be either protective or harmful.[233] Blood containing anti-HB_c, however, may be infective.[238,251]

At the present time only a single antigenic specificity has been noted for the core antigen, although several antigenic subtypes have been described for the surface antigen. It appears that all subtypes of the surface antigen contain an antigen termed *a;* in addition, they also contain one or the other of two pairs of antigens (*d* or *y* and *w* or *r*). The four different subtypes of surface antigen (HB_sAg/adw, HB_sAg/adr, HB_sAg/ayw, and HB_sAg/ayr) *may* define different but related forms of the hepatitis B virus.[237,247] Antibody produced either in humans or in animals can be used to determine the subtype of the surface antigen and is useful for epidemiologic purposes; infection induced by a virus with a particular antigenic subtype regularly results in production of surface antigen of the same subtype in the infected host.[237] In addition to these well-defined specificities, there appear to be additional determinants *(x, n, t, q)* that may prove to be of importance.[237] Even more intriguing is another antigen, designated *e,* found in the serum of HB$_s$Ag-positive individuals. There is some evidence to suggest that its presence may correlate with infectivity, whereas its absence or the presence of anti-e may indicate lack of infectivity.[218,243,244]

In addition to techniques for detection of hepatitis B virus, it has recently become possible to detect both hepatitis A antigen (HA Ag) and antibody (anti-HA). The hepatitis A antigen is associated with 27 nm viruslike particles and has been isolated from the stool and liver of animals experimentally infected with hepatitis A virus as well as from the stool of infected humans.[231] HA Ag and anti-HA were first detected in 1973; before that time posttransfusion hepatitis A was thought to be common inasmuch as patients who developed hepatitis but did not have detectable hepatitis B antigen or antibody were considered to have contracted hepatitis A, even though many of the cases clinically resembled hepatitis B. The recent ability to detect HA Ag and anti-HA has lead to the postulation of an unidentified agent ("non A–non B" hepatitis, hepatitis "C") that may account for a significant number of cases of transfusion-induced disease.[232]

Purcell et al.[248] examined serum from patients who by clinical and epidemiologic grounds were thought to have hepatitis A and found anti-HA in 100%; no anti-HA was found in patients with documented hepatitis B infections, and it was found in only two of seventy-three persons who had drug abuse or posttransfusion hepatitis clinically similar to hepatitis B but who lacked the corresponding antigen or antibody. It is this large last group, which failed to make antibody to either HA Ag or HB$_s$Ag, that may be representative of hepatitis C infection.

Several studies are currently under way to evaluate the role of active and passive immunization in the prevention of hepatitis B infection. Although administration of γ-globulin is generally thought to prevent or modify disease caused by hepatitis A virus, several studies of the value of γ-globulin in the prevention of hepatitis B have provided conflicting results, due in part to differences in the amount of specific HB$_s$ antibody contained in different lots of γ-globulin and to the inability until recently to distinguish hepatitis B from disease induced by Epstein-Barr virus, cytomegalovirus, or the so-called hepatitis C virus. Several recent studies have suggested that high-titered specific hepatitis B immune globulin may protect persons with accidental needle puncture,[234] spouses of patients with hepatitis B,[249] and persons un-

dergoing hemodialysis[246] but will probably not be effective in preventing disease caused by blood transfusion.[240] Active immunization using heat-inactivated preparations of serum known to cause hepatitis B has been shown to be feasible,[241,242] and preliminary studies in chimpanzees have suggested that immunization with purified hepatitis B surface antigen may protect against transfusion-induced hepatitis B.[222,247] Whether the latter approach will prove successful in humans remains as yet unknown.

Circulatory overload

The administration of excessively large quantities of blood, or even smaller amounts if given rapidly, may precipitate cardiac failure from circulatory overload. In the course of a transfusion or shortly thereafter, precordial pain, dyspnea, cyanosis, and a dry cough are indicative of a rising venous pressure and pulmonary edema. In patients with severe anemia and evidence of congestive heart failure, preliminary digitalization may occasionally be required. Packed red cell suspensions are useful whenever it is essential to provide blood with the least possible disturbance to the patient's blood volume. Another expedient to prevent overloading the circulatory system is to give half the calculated amount of blood on successive days.

In erythroblastosis death may result from cardiac failure caused by administering more blood than has been removed. Preliminary withdrawal of 30 to 50 ml of blood from the severely anemic infant may be necessary,[51] or a deficit of even larger amounts (40 to 80 ml) should be established within a short time after the exchange is begun when venous pressures are excessively high.[87]

Suppression of erythropoiesis

One of the limitations of transfusion that deserves comment and that has received scant attention is its potential depressant effect on erythropoiesis. That transfusions possess this inhibitory effect was recognized in the treatment of pernicious anemia before the advent of specific therapy and has been confirmed in several studies.* Although retardation of erythropoiesis in a minor degree may accompany a single transfusion, it is overshadowed by the major corrective effects.

Two sets of observations document the thesis that transfusions administered at frequent intervals retard erythropoiesis.[252,253] These data are based on an intensive study of a small group of children with thalassemia major in whom transfusions could be interrupted following splenectomy. By the methods designed to permit quantitative differentiation between donor and recipient blood

---

*References 219, 226, 230, 245.

and by serial examinations of the total red cell mass and circulating hemoglobin levels, it was possible to demonstrate that erythropoietic suppression was most marked from the first to the third week following transfusion. Not until donor blood had been entirely eliminated from the circulation were pretransfusion hemoglobin levels restored in the patient. The depressant effect of transfusion was further substantiated by another means. The presence of large amounts of fetal hemoglobin provides a biologic tag of endogenous hemoglobin synthesis. Transfusions resulted in a depression of the component, which increased sharply as donor cells left the circulation. The diminution in fetal hemoglobin persisted in one patient for the first 7 weeks after transfusion, and in two others the decrease amounted to 50%. Paralleling these observations is a report that, in patients with sickle cell anemia who received multiple transfusions, a period of maximum depression of erythropoiesis occurred from the twelfth to the twenty-fifth day, with the percentage of sickle cells decreasing from 100% to 5%.[227] Suppression of synthesis of sickle cell hemoglobin by transfusion therapy may be beneficial to patients with prolonged painful crises.

In other situations it may be advisable to withhold treatment. Occasionally it may be advisable to determine innate marrow function in patients with chronic anemia. In critical periods of growth, such as in the anemia of prematurity, it may be undesirable to interfere with bone marrow function by transfusions. It has been suggested that in erythroblastosis a similar retardation can result from a persistent effort to maintain normal hemoglobin levels.[223] These studies suggest the need for a less empirical and more individualized orientation, not only in patients with refractory anemias but also in those with other diseases requiring frequent transfusions. The spacing and size of transfusions and levels of hemoglobin to be attained require constant reexamination and appraisal. The effect of anemia on oxygen affinity and any shift in the oxygen dissociation curve must receive as much attention as the hemoglobin level itself.

Hemosiderosis

Studies in iron metabolism have extended into an investigation of "iron overload" or hemosiderosis resulting from repeated transfusions. It should be remembered that 1 gm of hemoglobin contains 3.4 mg of iron and that 100 ml of transfused packed cells provides 70 mg of iron to the recipient. The total amount of iron in a normal adult is approximately 4 to 5 gm, of which 15% to 20% represents the iron reserve, stored principally in the liver as ferritin and hemosiderin. In children storage iron normally represents 8.5 to 10.5 mg/kg body weight. In states of iron deficiency in infancy caused by inadequate diet and periods of rapid growth, storage depots are taxed and may be depleted. Iron otherwise accumulates and, except for the normal excretion of approximately 1 mg daily, cannot leave the body except through blood loss.

Excessive amounts of iron from destroyed transfused red cells become available for storage in patients receiving multiple transfusions. Under such conditions hemosiderin deposits in normal storage depots increase greatly, and, in addition, accessory sites assume the function of iron storage. Hemosiderosis refers to increased iron stores without tissue damage and hemochromatosis to the development of tissue damage in persons with prolonged iron excess (Chapter 6). The amount of iron present in organs such as the liver may exceed the amount given by repeated transfusions, indicating excessive absorption of iron from the gastrointestinal tract.[229]

Whether iron from transfused blood actually may produce hemochromatosis is still controversial, but there is evidence that excessive iron storage is potentially injurious.[228] Studies in thalassemia major have shown, however, that hemosiderosis and fibrosis frequently coexist, although there was no uniformity about the progression.[229] The development of true hepatic cirrhosis and fibrosis of the pancreas that characterizes hemochromatosis associated with transfusion hemosiderosis may depend on the intervention of accessory factors such as continued hypoxia in addition to large iron deposits, which are a prerequisite for this pathologic process. Free radical generation and lipid peroxidation may also be involved.

From these considerations it would seem that the iron derived from an occasional transfusion is harmless. A contrary situation may prevail, however, in the patient receiving multiple transfusions over prolonged periods. In view of the risk involved, the most prudent course is to restrict the number of transfusions to the minimum compatible with comfort and moderate activity. Effective chelation therapy should permit a more liberal use of transfusions.

Antibody formation in the course of multiple transfusions

Patients who receive large numbers of transfusions may develop precipitins. These precipitins may react in agar gel double diffusion experiments with specific human serum lipoproteins found in other individuals. Antilipoprotein isoprecipitins were found in approximately 30% of forty-seven patients with thalassemia who had received transfusions.[220] This parallels the frequency of antileukocyte (37%) and antiplatelet (32%)

antibodies but is considerably greater than that of antierythrocyte antibodies (12.8%).

Allergic reactions

About 1% to 5% of blood transfusions are followed by allergic reactions, principally urticaria and less often angioneurotic edema and asthma. These reactions are especially common in children with refractory anemias requiring multiple transfusions. Although not well studied, allergic reactions are usually attributed to interaction of antigen with reagenic antibody derived from either donor or recipient, and they are common in persons with a history of atopy. Such affected children benefit from oral premedication with an antihistamine and aspirin given 30 minutes before transfusion. Prednisone has been useful in children in whom other medications have proved ineffective in preventing severe allergic and febrile reactions.

Recommended dosages of aspirin, antihistamine, and prednisone for allergic reactions are listed in Table 4-11.

Massive transfusion

The administration of large quantities of blood that has been stored for more than a week may result in a decrease in platelet levels and a decrease of the labile coagulation factors. Although this is not a common problem, it is well to evaluate the circulating level of these factors in any patient receiving massive transfusion of bank blood. Following extracorporeal circulation using large amounts of nonautologous blood, unexpected decreases in blood volume have been observed. The etiology of this "homologous blood syndrome" is poorly understood.

Table 4-11. Recommended dosages of aspirin, antihistamine, and prednisone for allergic reactions to multiple transfusions*

Aspirin	
Up to 5 years	60 mg/year
5 years and over	600 mg
Tripelennamine (Pyribenzamine)†	
Up to 5 years	25 mg
5 years and over	25 to 50 mg
Prednisone	5 to 10 mg given ½ to 1 hr before transfusion, if previous experience demonstrated difficulties with other drugs

*From Baker, R. J., Moinichen, S. L., and Nyhus, L. M.: Ann. Surg. **169**:684, 1969.
†Other antihistamines (e.g., diphenhydramine [Benadryl]) may be substituted.

Air embolism

The use of plastic blood containers has almost totally eliminated the possibility of air embolism. Whenever blood or other fluid is being administered under pressure, it is important to normalize the pressure before the bag is completely empty.

Electrolyte disturbances

In blood stored under refrigeration the potassium content of red cells decreases and that of plasma increases, both factors being intensified during prolonged storage. Marked electrocardiographic changes do not occur until the potassium level reaches approximately 8 mEq/liter.[51] Hyperkalemia induced in patients during exchange transfusion is transient, but the potential risk of toxic effects should be kept in mind. The latter can be minimized by the use of relatively fresh blood, the removal of part of the plasma, the use of packed cells, and the judicious use of calcium during replacement transfusions with citrated whole blood.[245] Patients with heart disease, especially those receiving digitalis, patients with kidney disease who are already hyperkalemic, and newborn infants, are particularly susceptible to the harmful effects of excess potassium.

Graft versus host disease

Graft versus host disease is a potentially fatal complication that has occurred in patients receiving high-dose immunosuppressive therapy or chemotherapy. Irradiated (2,000 R) blood products should be used for prevention.

REFERENCES
Blood groups
1. Allen, F. H., and Lewis, S. J.: Kpª (Penney), a new antigen in the Kell blood group system, Vox Sang. **2**:81, 1957.
2. Allen, F. H., Diamond, L. K., and Niedziela, B.: A new blood group antigen, Nature **167**:482, 1951.
3. Amos, D. B.: Genetics of the human histocompatibility system HL-1, Transplant. Proc. **6**:27, 1974.
4. Andresen, P. H.: Blood group with characteristic phenotypical aspects, Acta Pathol. Microbiol. Scand. **24**:616, 1947.
5. Bach, F. H., and Van Rood, J. J.: The major histocompatibility complex: genetics and biology, N. Engl. J. Med. **295**:806, 1976.
6. Bach, F. H., and Van Rood, J. J.: The major histocompatibility complex: genetics and biology, N. Engl. J. Med. **295**:872, 1976.
7. Bach, F. H., and Van Rood, J. J.: The major histocompatibility complex: genetics and biology, N. Engl. J. Med. **295**:927, 1976.
8. Behzad, O., et al.: A new anti-erythrocyte antibody in the Duffy system: anti-Fy4, Vox Sang. **24**:337, 1973.
9. Bhende, Y. M., Despande, L. K., Bhata, H. M., et al.: A "new" blood-group character related to the ABO system, Lancet **1**:566, 1952.
10. Bird. G. W. G.: The history of blood transfusion, Injury **3**:40, 1971.
11. Bruning, J. W.: Serologic recognition of the histocom-

patibility antigens using agglutination and cytotoxicity techniques, Semin. Hematol. **11:**263, 1974.

12. Callender, S., et al.: Hypersensitivity to transfused blood, Br. Med. J. **2:**83, 1945.

13. Ceppellini, R.: On the genetics of secretor and Lewis characters: a family study, Proc. 5th Cong. Int. Soc. Blood Transf., Paris, 1955.

14. Ceppellini, R., and Van Rood, J. J.: The HL-A system. I. Genetics and molecular biology, Semin. Hematol. **11:**233, 1974.

15. Ceppellini, R., et al.: An interaction between alleles at the Rh locus in man which weakens the reactivity of the Rh_0 factor (D^u), Proc. Nat. Acad. Sci. **41:**283, 1955.

16. Colombani, J., and Colombani, M.: Serologic recognition of histocompatibility antigens using complement fixation, Semin. Hematol. **11:**273, 1974.

17. Coombs, R. R. A., et al.: A new test for the detection of weak and "incomplete" Rh agglutinins, Br. J. Exp. Pathol. **26:**255, 1945.

18. Coombs, R. R. A., et al.: In-vivo isosensitization of red cells in babies with haemolytic disease, Lancet **1:**264, 1946.

19. Crawford, M. M., et al.: The phenotype Lu(a−b−) together with unconventional Kidd groups in one family, Transfusion **1:**228, 1961.

20. Cutbush, M., and Chanarin, I.: The expected blood-group antibody anti-Lu^b, Nature **178:**855, 1956.

21. Cutbush, M., Mollison, P. L., et al.: A new human blood group, Nature **165:**188, 1950.

22. Darnborough, J., et al.: A "new" antibody anti-Lu^aLu^b and two further examples of the genotype Lu(a−b−), Nature **198:**796, 1963.

23. Fisher, R. A., cited by Race, R. R.: An "incomplete" antibody in human serum, Nature **153:**771, 1944.

24. German, J. L., et al.: MN blood-group locus: data concerning the possible chromosomal location, Science **162:**1014, 1968.

25. Giblett, E. R.: A critique of the theoretical hazard of inter- vs. intra-racial transfusion, Transfusion **1:**233, 1961.

26. Giblett, E. R., and Crookston, M. C.: Agglutinability of red cells by anti-i in patients with thalassemia major and other hematological disorders, Nature **201:**1138, 1964.

27. Greenwalt, T. J., et al.: Further examples of hemolytic disease of the newborn due to anti-Duffy (anti-Fy^a), Vox Sang. **4:**138, 1959.

28. Grubb, R.: Observations on the human group system Lewis, Acta Pathol. Microbiol. Scand. **28:**61, 1951.

29. Ikin, E. W., et al.: The distribution of the A_1 A_2 B O blood groups in England, Ann. Eugen. Lond. **9:**409, 1939.

30. Ikin, E. W., et al.: Discovery of the expected haemagglutinin, anti-Fy^b, Nature **168:**1077, 1951.

31. Ishimori, T., and Hasekura, H.: A Japanese with no detectable Rh blood group antigens due to silent Rh alleles or deleted chromosomes, Transfusion **7:**84, 1967.

32. Issitt, P. D.: Auto-immune hemolytic anemia, Am. J. Med. Tech. **40:**479, 1974.

33. Issitt, P. D., and Issitt, C. H.: Applied blood group serology, Oxnard, Calif., 1975, Becton, Dickinson & Co.

34. Jenkins, W. J., et al.: Infectious mononucleosis: an unsuspected source of anti-i, Br. J. Haematol. **11:**480, 1965.

35. Lalezari, P., and Radel, E.: Neutrophil-specific antigens: immunology and clinical significance, Semin. Hematol. **11:**281, 1974.

36. Landsteiner, K.: On agglutination of normal human blood, (A. L. Kappus, trans.), Transfusion **1:**5, 1961.

37. Landsteiner, K., and Levine, P.: A new agglutinable factor differentiating individual human bloods, Proc. Soc. Exp. Biol. N.Y. **24:**600, 1927.

38. Landsteiner, K., and Levine, P.: Further observations on individual differences of human blood, Proc. Soc. Exp. Biol. N.Y. **24:**941, 1927.

39. Landsteiner, K., and Wiener, A. S.: An agglutinable factor in human blood recognized by immune sera for rhesus blood, Proc. Soc. Exp. Biol. N.Y. **43:**223, 1940.

40. Levine, P., and Stetson, R. E.: An unusual case of intra-group agglutination, J.A.M.A. **113:**126, 1939.

41. Levine, P., et al.: A new human hereditary blood property (Cellano) present in 99.8% of all bloods, Science **109:**464, 1949.

42. Levine, P., et al.: Isoimmunization by a new blood factor in tumor cells, Proc. Soc. Exp. Biol. **77:**403, 1951.

43. Levine, P., et al.: The specificity of the antibody in paroxysmal cold hemoglobinuria (PCH), Transfusion **3:**278, 1963.

44. Levine, P., et al.: A second example of − − −/− − − blood or Rh_{null}, Nature **204:**892, 1964.

45. Lostumbo, M. M., et al.: Isoimmunization after multiple transfusions, N. Engl. J. Med. **275:**141, 1966.

46. Marsh, W. L.: Anti-i: a cold antibody defining the iI relationship in human red cells, Br. J. Haematol. **7:**200, 1961.

47. Marsh, W. L., et al.: Mapping human autosomes: evidence supporting assignment of Rhesus to the short arm of chromosome No. 1, Science **183:**966, 1974.

48. Marsh, W. L., et al.: Antigens of the Kell blood group system on neutrophils and monocytes: their relationship to chronic granulomatous disease, J. Pediatr. **87:**1117, 1975.

49. Miller, L. H., et al.: The resistance factor to *Plasmodium vivax* in blacks: the Duffy blood group genotype, *FyFy*, N. Engl. J. Med. **295:**302, 1976.

50. Moller, E.: The MLC reaction, Tissue Antigens **3:**235, 1973.

51. Mollison, P. L.: Blood transfusion in clinical medicine, Oxford, 1972, Blackwell Scientific Publications, Ltd.

52. Moreschi, C.: Neue tatsachen über die blutkörperchen agglutinationen, Zentralbl. Bakteriol. **46:**49, 1908.

53. Moureau, P.: Les réactions post-transfusionnelles, Rev. Belge Sci. Med. **16:**258, 1945.

54. Petz, L. D., and Fudenberg, H. H.: Immunologic mechanisms in drug-induced cytopenias. In Brown, E. B., ed.: Progress in hematology, New York: 1975, Grune & Stratton, Inc.

55. Pinkerton, F. J., et al.: The phenotype Jk(a−b−) in the Kidd blood group system, Vox Sang. **4:**155, 1959.

56. Plaut, G., Skin, E. W., et al.: A new blood group antibody, anti-Jk^b, Nature **171:**431, 1953.

57. Pollack, W., et al.: Studies on Rh prophylaxis. I. Relationship between doses of anti-Rh and size of antigenic stimulus, Transfusion **11:**333, 1971.

58. Race, R. R.: The Rh genotypes and Fisher's theory, Blood **3**(suppl. 2):27, 1948.

59. Race, R. R., and Sanger, R.: Blood groups in man, Oxford, 1975, Blackwell Scientific Publications, Ltd.

60. Rosenfield, R. E., et al.: A review of Rh serology and presentation of a new terminology, Transfusion **2:**287, 1962.

61. Ruddle, F., et al.: Somatic cell genetic assignment of peptidase C and the Rh linkage group to chromosome a-1 in man, Science **176:**1429, 1972.

62. Sanger, R., et al.: An antibody which subdivides the human MN blood groups, Heredity **2:**131, 1948.

63. Sanger, R., et al.: The Duffy blood groups of New York Negroes: the phenotype Fy(a−b−), Br. J. Haematol. **1:**370, 1955.

64. Schaller, J. G., and Omenn, G. S.: The histocompatibility system and human disease, J. Pediatr. **88:**913, 1976.

65. Schmidt, P. J.: Transfusion in America in the eighteenth

and nineteenth centuries, N. Engl. J. Med. **279:**1319, 1968.

66. Schmidt, P. J., and Vos, G. H.: Multiple phenotypic abnormalities associated with Rh$_{null}$ ($---/---$), Vox Sang. **13:**18, 1967.

67. Schmidt, P. J., et al.: *Mycoplasma* (pleuropneumonia like organism) and blood group I: associations with neoplastic disease, Nature **205:**371, 1965.

68. Sneath, J. S., and Sneath, P. H. A.: Transformation of the Lewis groups of human red cells, Nature **176:**172, 1955.

69. Springer, G. F., et al.: Origin of anti-human blood group B agglutinins in "germfree" chicks, Ann. N.Y. Acad. Sci. **78:**272, 1959.

70. Stratton, F.: A new Rh allelomorph, Nature **158:**25, 1946.

71. Stroup, M., MacIlroy, M., Walker, R., and Aydelotte, J. V.: Evidence that Sutter belongs to the Kell blood group system, Transfusion **5:**309, 1965.

72. Sturgeon, P.: Hematological observations on the anemia associated with blood type Rh$_{null}$, Blood **36:**310, 1970.

73. Taylor, G. L., et al.: Frequency of the iso-agglutinin α_1 in the serum of the subgroups A_2 and A_2B, J. Pathol. Bacteriol. **54:**514, 1942.

74. Telischi, M., et al.: Hemolytic disease of the newborn due to anti-N, Vox Sang. **31:**109, 1976.

75. Van Someran, H., et al.: Human antigen and enzyme markers in man—Chinese hamster somatic cell hybrids: evidence for synteny between the HL-A, PGM_3, ME_1, and IPO-B loci, Proc. Nat. Acad. Sci. **71:**962, 1974.

76. Vos, G. H., Vos, D., Kirk, R. L., and Sanger, R.: A sample of blood with no detectable Rh antigens, Lancet **1:**14, 1961.

77. Watkins, W. M.: Blood group substances, Science **152:** 172, 1966.

78. Westerveld, A., et al.: Assignment of the AK_1:Np:ABO linkage group to human chromosone 9, Proc. Nat. Acad. Sci. **73:**895, 1976.

79. WHO-IUIS Terminology Committee: Nomenclature for factors of the HL-A system, Transplant. Proc. **8:**109, 1976.

80. Wiener, A. S.: Fundamentals of immunogenetics, with special reference to the human blood groups, Am. J. Hum. Genet. **17:**457, 1965.

81. Wiener, A. S.: The Rh-Hr blood types: serology, genetics and nomenclature, Trans. N.Y. Acad. Sci. **13:**198, 1951.

82. Wiener, A. S., and Wexler, I. B.: An Rh-Hr syllabus, New York, 1963, Grune & Stratton, Inc., p. 46.

83. Wiener, A. S., Unger, L. J., Cohen, I., and Feldman, J.: Type-specific cold auto-antibodies as a cause of acquired hemolytic anemia and hemolytic transfusion reactions: biologic test with bovine red cells, Ann. Intern. Med. **44:**221, 1956.

84. Yankee, R. A.: HL-A antigens and platelet therapy. In Baldini, M. G., and Ebbe, S., eds.: Platelets: production, function, transfusion and storage, New York, 1974, Grune & Stratton, Inc.

Red blood cell transfusion

85. Ahrons, S., and Kissmeyer-Nielsen, F.: Serological investigation of 1358 transfusion reactions in 74,000 transfusions, Dan. Med. Bull. **15:**257, 1968.

86. Akerblom, O., et al.: Restoration of defective oxygen-transport function of stored red blood cells by addition of inosine, Scand. J Clin. Lab. Invest. **21:**245, 1968.

87. Allen, F. H., Jr., and Diamond, L. K.: Erythroblastosis fetalis, Boston, 1957, Little, Brown & Co.

88. Bailey, D. N., and Bove, J. R.: Chemical and hematological changes in stored CPD blood, Transfusion **15:** 244, 1975.

89. Beutler, E.: The maintenance of red cell function during liquid storage. In Schmidt, P. J., ed.: Progress in transfusion and transplantation, Chicago, 1972, American Association of Blood Banks.

90. Beutler, E., and Wood, L.: The in vivo regeneration of red cell 2,3-diphosphoglyceric acid (DPG) after transfusion of stored blood, J. Lab. Clin. Med. **74:**300, 1969.

91. Blajchman, M. A., et al.: Vacuum tubes as the source of platelet concentrate contamination producing *Serratia marcescens* sepsis. Paper presented at the 29th annual meeting of the American Association of Blood Banks, San Francisco, Nov. 4, 1976.

92. Bowen, J. C., and Fleming, W. H.: Increased oxyhemoglobin affinity after transfusion of stored blood: evidence for circulatory compensation, Ann. Surg. **180:**760, 1974.

93. Brody, J. I., et al.: Symptomatic crises of sickle cell anemia treated by limited exchange transfusion, Ann. Intern. Med. **72:**327, 1970.

94. Buchholz, D. H., et al.: Bacterial proliferation in platelet products stored at room temperature: transfusion-induced *Enterobacter* sepsis, N. Engl. J. Med. **285:**429, 1971.

95. Buchholz, D. H., et al.: Detection and quantitation of bacteria in platelet products stored at ambient temperature, Transfusion **13:**278, 1973.

96. Carr, J. B., et al.: Decreased incidence of transfusion hepatitis after exclusive transfusion with reconstituted frozen erythrocytes, Ann. Intern. Med. **78:**693, 1973.

97. Chanutin, A.: The effect of the addition of adenine and nucleosides at the beginning of storage on the concentrations of phosphates of human erythrocytes during storage in acid-citrate-dextrose and citrate-phosphate-dextrose, Transfusion **7:**120, 1967.

98. Chanutin, A., and Curnish, R. R.: Effect of organic and inorganic phosphates on the oxygen equilibrium of human erythrocytes, Arch. Biochem. Biophys. **121:**96, 1967.

99. Crowley, J. P., and Valeri, C. R.: The purification of red cells for transfusion by freeze preservation and washing. II. The residual leukocytes, platelets, and plasma in washed freeze-preserved red cells, Transfusion **14:**196, 1974.

100. Cunningham, M., and Cash, J. D.: Bacterial contamination of platelet concentrates stored at 20 C, J. Clin. Pathol. **26:**401, 1973.

101. Dawson, R. B., Jr., et al.: Hemoglobin function and 2,3-DPG levels of blood stored at 4 C in ACD and CPD, Transfusion **10:**299, 1970.

102. Freda, V. J., et al.: Prevention of Rh hemolytic disease: ten years' clinical experience with Rh immune globulin, N. Engl. J. Med. **292:**1014, 1975.

103. Gibson, J. G., and Lionetti, F. J.: The effect of dipyridamole on the adenosine triphosphate level of stored human blood, Transfusion **6:**427, 1966.

104. Gilman, P. A.: Hemolysis in the newborn infant resulting from deficiencies of red blood cell enzymes: diagnosis and management, J. Pediatr. **84:**625, 1974.

105. Gottuso, M. A., et al.: The role of exchange transfusions in the management of low-birth-weight infants with and without severe respiratory distress syndrome, J. Pediatr. **89:**279, 1976.

106. Gross, S., and Melhorn, D. K.: Exchange transfusion with citrated whole blood for disseminated intravascular coagulation, J. Pediatr. **78:**415, 1971.

107. Haradin, A. R., et al.: Changes in physical properties of stored erythrocytes: relationship to survival in vivo, Transfusion **9:**229, 1969.

108. Heustis, D. W., et al.: Practical blood transfusion, Boston, 1976, Little, Brown & Co.

109. Jesch, F., et al.: Oxygen dissociation after transfusion of blood stored in ACD or CPD solution, J. Thorac. Cardiovasc. Surg. **70:**35, 1975.

110. Maurer, P. H., and Berardinelli, B.: Immunologic studies with hydroxyethyl starch (HES)—a proposed plasma expander, Transfusion **8:**265, 1968.

111. Meryman, H. T., and Hornblower, M.: A method for freezing and washing red blood cells using a high glycerol concentration, Transfusion **12:**145, 1972.

112. Miller, W. V., et al.: Simple methods for production of HL-A antigen poor red blood cells, Transfusion **13:**189, 1973.

113. Miller, W. V., et al.: Effect on cytotoxicity antibodies in potential transplant recipients of leucocyte-poor blood transfusions, Lancet **1:**893, 1975.

114. Mollison, P. L., and Sloviter, H. A.: Successful transfusion of previously frozen human red cells, Lancet **2:** 862, 1951.

115. Oski, F. A., and Delivoria-Papadopoulos, M.: The red cell, 2,3-diphosphoglycerate, and tissue oxygen release, J. Pediatr. **77:**941, 1970.

116. Pearson, H. A., et al.: Isoimmune neonatal thrombocytopenic purpura-clinical and therapeutic considerations, Blood **23:**154, 1964.

117. Pineda, A. A., and Taswell, H. F.: Transfusion reactions associated with anti-IgA antibodies: report of four cases and review of the literature, Transfusion **15:**10, 1975.

118. Procter, H. J., et al.: Alternations in erythrocyte 2,3-diphosphoglycerate in postoperative patients, Ann. Surg. **173:**357, 1971.

119. Rapaport, S. I.: Defibrination syndromes. In Williams, W. J., Beutler, E., Erslev, A. J., and Rundles, R. W., eds.: Hematology, New York, 1972, McGraw-Hill Book Co.

120. Rowe, A., et al.: A low glycerol-rapid freeze procedure, Cryobiology **5:**119, 1968.

121. Shafer, A. W., et al.: 2,3-Diphosphoglycerate in red cells stored in acid-citrate-dextrose and citrate-phosphate-dextrose: implications regarding delivery of oxygen, J. Lab. Clin. Med. **77:**430, 1971.

122. Sisson, T. R., et al.: Phototherapy of jaundice in newborn infants. I. ABO blood group incompatibility, J. Pediatr. **79:**904, 1971.

123. Stephen, C. R., et al.: Antihistaminic drugs in treatment of nonhemolytic transfusion reactions, J.A.M.A. **158:** 525, 1955.

124. Strumia, M. M., et al.: The preservation of blood for transfusion. VII. Effect of adenine and inosine on the adenosine triphosphate and viability of red cells when added to blood stored from zero to seventy days at 1° C., J. Lab. Clin. Med. **75:**244, 1970.

125. Summary report: NHLI's blood resource studies, Publication No. (NIH)73-416, Department of Health, Education, and Welfare, June 30, 1972.

126. Tan, K. L.: Comparison of the effectiveness of phototherapy and exchange transfusion in the management of nonhemolytic neonatal hyperbilirubinemia, J. Pediatr. **87:**609, 1975.

127. Trey, C., et al.: Treatment of hepatic coma by exchange blood transfusion, N. Engl. J. Med. **274:**473, 1966.

128. Valeri, C. R., and Zaroulis, C. G.: Rejuvenation and freezing of outdated stored human red cells, N. Engl. J. Med. **287:**1307, 1972.

129. Valtis, D. J., and Kennedy, A. C.: Defective gas-transport function of stored red blood cells, Lancet **1:**119, 1954.

130. Verschoyle, M. J.: Laboratory diagnosis: biochemical. In A seminar on hemolytic transfusion reactions, New York, 1967, American Association of Blood Banks.

131. Vyas, G. N., et al.: Healthy blood donors with selective absence of immunoglobulin A: prevention of anaphylactic transfusion reactions caused by antibodies to IgA, J. Lab. Clin. Med. **85:**838, 1975.

132. Ward, H. N.: Pulmonary infiltrates associated with leuko- agglutinin transfusion reactions, Ann. Intern. Med. **73:** 689, 1970.

133. Weisert, O., and Jeremic, M.: Preservation of coagulation factors V and VIII during collection and subsequent storage of bank blood in ACD-A and CPD solutions, Vox Sang. **24:**126, 1973.

134. Wolf, C. F. W., and Canale, V.: Fatal pulmonary hypersensitivity reaction to HL-A incompatible blood transfusion: report of a case and review of the literature, Transfusion **16:**135, 1976.

135. Wood, L., and Beutler, E.: The effect of ascorbic acid on the 2,3-DPG level of stored blood, Clin. Res. **20:** 186, 1972.

Platelet transfusion

136. Adner, M. M., et al.: Use of "compatible" platelet transfusions in treatment of congenital isoimmune neonatal thrombocytopenic purpura, N. Engl. J. Med. **280:**244, 1969.

137. Aster, R. H.: Effect of anticoagulant and ABO incompatibility on recovery of transfused human platelets, Blood **26:**732, 1965.

138. Aster, R. H.: Pooling of platelets in the spleen: role in the pathogenesis of "hypersplenic" thrombocytopenia, J. Clin. Invest. **45:**645, 1966.

139. Aster, R. H., and Jandl, J. H.: Platelet sequestration in man, J. Clin. Invest. **43:**843, 1964.

140. Becker, G. A., et al.: Studies of platelet concentrates stored at 22° C and 4° C, Transfusion **13:**61, 1973.

141. Borchgrevink, C. F.: Platelet adhesion in vivo in patients with bleeding disorders, Acta Med. Scand. **170:**245, 1965.

142. Buchholz, D. H.: Blood transfusion: merits of component therapy. I. The clinical use of red cells, platelets and granulocytes, J. Pediatr. **84:**1, 1974.

143. Cohen, P., and Gardner, F. H.: Platelet preservation. IV. Preservation of human platelet concentrates by controlled slow freezing in a glycerol medium, N. Engl. J. Med. **274:**1400, 1966.

144. Cowan, D. H., and Haut, M. J.: Platelet function in acute leukemia, J. Lab. Clin. Med. **79:**893, 1972.

145. Dayian, G., and Rowe, A. W.: Cryopreservation of human platelets for transfusion, Cryobiology **13:**1, 1976.

146. Djerassi, I., et al.: Preparation and in vivo circulation of human platelets preserved with combined dimethylsulfoxide and dextrose, Transfusion **6:**572, 1966.

147. Ebbe, S.: Origin, production and life span of blood platelets. In Johnson, S., ed.: The circulating platelet, New York, 1971, Academic Press, Inc.

148. Filip, D. J., et al.: The effect of platelet concentrate storage temperature on adenine nucleotide metabolism, Blood **45:**749, 1975.

149. Freireich, E. J., et al.: Response to repeated platelet transfusion from the same donor, Ann. Int. Med. **59:** 277, 1963.

150. Goldfinger, D., and McGuinniss, M. H.: Rh-incompatible platelet transfusions: risks and consequences of sensitizing immunosuppressed patients, N. Engl. J. Med. **284:**942, 1971.

151. Graw, R. G., Jr., et al.: Leucocyte and platelet collection from normal donors with the continuous flow blood cell separator, Transfusion **11:**94, 1971.

152. Grumet, F. C., and Yankee, R. A.: Long term platelet support of patients with aplastic anemia: effect of splenectomy and steroid therapy, Ann. Int. Med. **73:**1, 1970.

153. Handin, R. I., and Valeri, C. R.: Hemostatic effectiveness of platelets stored at 22° C, N. Engl. J. Med. **258:** 538, 1971.

154. Handin, R. I., and Valeri, C. R.: Improved viability of previously frozen platelets, Blood **40:**509, 1972.

155. Hardisty, R. M.: Haemorrhagic disorders due to func-

tional abnormalities of platelets, J. R. Coll. Physicians **3:**182, 1969.

156. Harker, L. A., and Slichter, S. J.: The bleeding time as a screening test for evaluation of platelet function, N. Engl. J. Med. **287:**155, 1972.

157. Herzig, R. H., et al.: Correction of poor platelet transfusion responses with leukocyte poor HL-A matched platelet concentrates, Blood **46:**743, 1975.

158. Heustis, D. W., et al.: Practical blood transfusion, Boston, 1976, Little, Brown & Co.

159. Klein, E., et al.: A practical method for the aseptic separation of human platelet concentrates without loss of other blood elements, N. Engl. J. Med. **254:**1132, 1956.

160. Kunicki, T. J., et al.: A study of variables affecting the quality of platelets stored at "room temperature," Transfusion **15:**414, 1975.

161. Levin, R. H., and Freireich, E. J.: Effect of storage up to 48 hours on response to transfusions of platelet rich plasma, Transfusion **4:**251, 1964.

162. Lohrmann, H.-P., et al.: Platelet transfusions from HL-A compatible unrelated donors to alloimmunized patients, Ann. Int. Med. **80:**9, 1974.

163. Mielke, C. H., et al.: The standardized normal Ivy bleeding time and its prolongation by aspirin, Blood **34:**204, 1969.

164. Murphy, S., and Gardner, F. H.: Platelet preservation. Effect of storage temperature on maintenance of platelet viability: deleterious effect of refrigerated storage. N. Engl. J. Med. **280:**1094, 1969.

165. Murphy, S., and Gardner, F. H.: Platelet storage at 22° C: metabolic, morphologic, and functional studies, J. Clin. Invest. **50:**370, 1971.

166. Murphy, S., and Gardner, F. H.: Platelet storage at 22° C: role of gas transport across plastic containers in maintenance of viability, Blood **46:**209, 1975.

167. Murphy, S., et al.: Platelet preservation by freezing: use of dimethylsulfoxide as cryoprotective agent, Transfusion **14:**139, 1974.

168. O'Brien, J. R.: Effect of salicylates on human platelets, Lancet **1:**779, 1968.

169. Pearson, H. A., et al.: Isoimmune neonatal thrombocytopenic purpura: clinical and therapeutic considerations, Blood **23:**154, 1964.

170. Rodriguez, S. U., et al.: Neonatal thrombocytopenia associated with antepartum administration of thiazide drugs, N. Engl. J. Med. **270:**881, 1964.

171. Schiffer, C. A., and Buchholz, D. H.: Intensive multiunit platelet-pheresis of normal donors, Transfusion **14:**388, 1974.

172. Schiffer, C. A., and Buchholz, D. H.: Frozen autologous platelets in the supportive care of patients with leukemia, Transfusion **16:**321, 1976.

173. Schively, J. A., et al.: The effect of storage on adhesion and aggregation of platelets, Vox Sang. **18:**204, 1970.

174. Schwartz, A. D., and Pearson, H. A.: Aspirin, platelets and bleeding, J. Pediatr. **78:**558, 1971.

175. Shulman, N. R.: Immunological considerations attending platelet transfusion, Transfusion **6:**39, 1966.

176. Stewart, J. H., and Castaldi, P. A.: Uraemic bleeding: a reversible platelet defect corrected by dialysis, Q. J. Med. **36:**409, 1967.

177. Stuart, M. J., et al.: Platelet function in recipients of platelets from donors ingesting aspirin, N. Engl. J. Med. **287:**1105, 1972.

178. Szymanski, I. O., et al.: Efficacy of the Latham blood processor to perform plateletpheresis, Transfusion **13:**405, 1973.

179. Tranum, B. L., and Haut, A.: In vivo survival of platelets prepared in CPD anticoagulant, Transfusion **12:**168, 1972.

180. Valeri, C. R.: Hemostatic effectiveness of liquid-pre-served and previously frozen human platelets, N. Engl. J. Med. **290:**353, 1974.

181. Weiss, H. J.: Abnormalities in platelet function due to defects in the release reaction, Ann. N.Y. Acad. Sci. **201:**161, 1972.

182. Yankee, R. A.: HL-A antigens and platelet therapy. In Baldini, M. G., and Ebbe, S., eds.: Platelets: production, function, transfusion and storage, New York, 1974, Grune & Stratton, Inc.

183. Yankee, R. A., et al.: Selection of unrelated compatible platelet donors by lymphocyte HL-A matching. N. Engl. J. Med. **288:**760, 1973.

Granulocyte transfusion

184. Aisner, J., et al.: Evaluation of factors influencing the results of granulocyte transfusions. Paper presented at the Second International Symposium on Leucocyte Separation and Transfusion, London, October 11-13, 1976.

185. Alavi, J. B., et al.: Filtration leukapheresis transfusions in leukema. Paper presented at the Second International Symposium on Leucocyte Separation and Transfusion, London, October 11-13, 1976.

186. Buchholz, D. H., et al.: Granulocyte harvest for transfusion: donor response to repeated leukapheresis, Transfusion **15:**96, 1975.

187. Buchholz, D. H., et al.: Granulocyte transfusion: a low cost method for filtration leukapheresis. In Goldman, J. R., and Lowenthal, R. M., eds.: Leucocytes: separation, collection and transfusion, London, 1975, Academic Press, Inc., Ltd.

188. Buckner, C. D., et al.: Granulocyte transfusions in marrow transplantation. Paper presented at the Second International Symposium on Leucocyte Separation and Transfusion, London, October 11-13, 1976.

189. Bodey, G. P., et al.: Quantitative relationships between circulating leukocytes and infection in patients with acute leukemia, Ann. Int. Med. **64:**328, 1966.

190. Clift, R. A., et al.: A study of the value of prophylactic granulocyte transfusions. Paper presented at the Second International Symposium on Leucocyte Separation and Transfusion, London, October 11-13, 1976.

191. Djerassi, I., et al.: Continuous flow filtration leukapheresis, Transfusion **12:**75, 1972.

192. Ford, J. M., et al.: Alternate day prophylactic granulocyte transfusions: results of a randomized prospective controlled trial in adults with acute leukemia. Paper presented at the Second International Symposium on Leucocyte Separation and Transfusion, London, October 11-13, 1976.

193. Fortuny, I. E., et al.: Granulocyte transfusion: a controlled study in patients with acute nonlymphocytic leukemia, Transfusion **15:**548, 1975.

194. Freireich, E. J., et al.: The function and fate of transferred leukocytes from donors with chronic myelocytic leukemia in leukopenic recipients, Ann. N.Y. Acad. Sci. **113:**1081, 1964.

195. Goldman, J. R., and Lowenthal, R. M., eds.: Leucocytes: separation, collection and transfusion, London, 1975, Academic Press, Inc., Ltd.

196. Goldstein, I. M., et al.: Leukocyte transfusions: role of leukocyte alloantibodies in determining transfusion response, Transfusion **11:**19, 1971.

197. Graw, R. G., Jr., et al.: Leukocyte and platelet collection from normal donors with the continuous flow blood cell separator, Transfusion **11:**94, 1971.

198. Graw, R. G., Jr., et al.: Normal granulocyte transfusion therapy. Treatment of septicemia due to gram-negative bacteria, N. Engl. J. Med. **287:**367, 1972.

199. Graw, R. G., Jr., et al.: Treatment of gram negative septicemia with normal human granulocyte transfusions and antibiotics: results of a prospective randomized con-

trolled trial. Paper presented at the Second International Symposium on Leukocyte Separation and Transfusion, London, October 11-13, 1976.

200. Harris, M. B., et al.: Polymorphonuclear leukocytes prepared by continuous flow filtration leukapheresis: viability and function, Blood **44:**707, 1974.

201. Herzig, G. P., et al.: Granulocyte collection by continuous flow filtration leukapheresis, Blood **39:**554, 1972.

202. Herzig, G. P., et al.: Impaired transfusion response to granulocytes collected by filtration leukapheresis. In Goldman, J. M., and Lowenthal, R. M., eds.: Granulocytes: separation, collection and transfusion, New York, 1975, Academic Press, Inc.

203. Higby, D. J., et al.: The effect of a single or double dose of dexamethasone on granulocyte collection with the continuous flow centrifuge, Vox Sang. **28:**243, 1975.

204. Higby, D. J., et al.: Filtration leukapheresis for granulocyte transfusion therapy, N. Engl. J. Med. **292:**761, 1975.

205. Huestis, D. W., et al.: Use of hydroxyethyl starch to improve granulocyte collection in the Latham blood processor, Transfusion **15:**559, 1975.

206. Lalezari, P., and Radel, E.: Neutrophil-specific antigens: immunology and clinical significance, Semin. Hematol. **11:**281, 1974.

207. Lowenthal, R. M., and Park, D. S.: The use of dextran as an adjunct to granulocyte collection with the continuous-flow blood cell separator, Transfusion **15:**23, 1975.

208. Lowenthal, R. M., et al.: Granulocyte transfusions in treatment of infections in patients with acute leukaemia and aplastic anaemia, Lancet **1:**353, 1975.

209. Mannoni, P., et al.: Effectiveness of normal granulocyte transfusions in the management of post-chemotherapy aplasia. Paper presented at the Second International Symposium on Leukocyte Separation and Transfusion, London, October 11-13, 1976.

210. McCredie, K. B., and Hester, J. P.: Leukocyte collection and transfusion. In Cohen, E., and Dawson, R. B., eds.: Leukapheresis and granulocyte transfusions, Washington, D.C., 1975, American Association of Blood Banks.

211. McCredie, K. B., et al.: Increased granulocyte collection with the blood cell separator and the addition of etiocholanolone and hydroxyethyl starch, Transfusion **14:** 357, 1974.

212. Schiffer, C. A., and Buchholz, D. H.: Clinical experience with transfusion of granulocytes obtained by continuous flow filtration leukapheresis, Am. J. Med. **58:**373, 1975.

213. Ts'ao, C., and Ruder, E. A.: Ultrastructural damage of leukocytes procured by the leukopak: vulnerability of leukocytes to mechanical injury, Transfusion **16:**336, 1976.

214. Vallejos, C. S., et al.: White blood cell transfusions for control of infections in neutropenic patients, Transfusion **15:**28, 1975.

215. Workman, R. D., et al.: Granulocyte transfusions in patients with severe thermal burns. Paper presented at the twenty-ninth annual meeting of the American Association of Blood Banks, San Francisco, November 5, 1976.

216. Wright, D. G., et al.: Functional abnormalities of human neutrophils collected by continuous flow filtration leukapheresis, Blood **46:**901, 1975.

Limitations and hazards of transfusions

217. Alter, H. J., et al.: The emerging pattern of posttransfusion hepatitis, Am. J. Med. Sci. **270:**329, 1975.

218. Alter, H. J., et al.: Type B hepatitis: the infectivity of blood positive for e antigen and DNA polymerase after accidental needlestick exposure, N. Engl. J. Med. **295:** 909, 1976.

219. Birkhill, F. R., Maloney, M. A., and Lewenson, S. M.: Effect of transfusion polycythemia upon bone marrow activity and erythrocyte survival in man, Blood **6:**1021, 1951.

220. Blumberg, B. S., et al.: Multiple antigenic specificities of serum apoproteins detected with sera of transfused patients, Vox Sang. **9:**128, 1964.

221. Blumberg, B. S., et al.: A "new" antigen in leukemic sera, J.A.M.A. **191:**541, 1965.

222. Buynak, E. B.: Vaccine against human hepatitis B, J.A.M.A. **235:**2832, 1976.

223. Cathie, I. A. B.: The treatment of erythroblastosis fetalis, Arch. Dis. Child. **21:**229, 1946.

224. Chalmers, T. C.: Viral hepatitis on the threshold of control, Am. J. Med. Sci. **270:**3, 1975.

225. Dane, D. S., et al.: Virus-like particles in serum of patients with Australia-antigen-associated hepatitis, Lancet **1:**695, 1970.

226. Dacie, J. V.: Transfusion of saline-washed red cells in nocturnal haemoglobinuria (Marchiafava-Micheli disease), Clin. Sci. **7:**65, 1948.

227. Donegan, C. C., Jr., et al.: Hematologic studies on patients with sickle cell anemia following multiple transfusions, Am. J. Med. **17:**29, 1954.

228. Dubin, I. N.: Idiopathic hemochromatosis and transfusion siderosis: a review, Am. J. Clin. Pathol. **25:**514, 1955.

229. Ellis, J. T., Schulman, I., and Smith, C. H.: Generalized siderosis with fibrosis of liver and pancreas in Cooley's (Mediterranean) anemia, with observations on the pathogenesis of the siderosis and fibrosis, Am. J. Pathol. **30:** 287, 1954.

230. Elmlinger, P. J., Huff, R. L., and Oda, J. M.: Depression of red cell iron turnover by transfusion, Proc. Soc. Exp. Biol. Med. **79:**16, 1952.

231. Feinstone, S. M., et al.: Hepatitis A: detection by immune electron microscopy of a virus-like antigen associated with acute illness, Science **182:**1026, 1973.

232. Feinstone, S. M., et al.: Transfusion-associated hepatitis not due to viral hepatitis type A or B, N. Engl. J. Med. **292:**767, 1975.

233. Goldfield, M., et al.: The consequences of administering blood pretested for HB$_s$ Ag by third generation techniques: a progress report, Am. J. Med. Sci. **270:**335, 1975.

234. Grady, G. F., and Lee, V. A.: Prevention of hepatitis from accidental exposure among medical workers, N. Engl. J. Med. **293:**1067, 1975.

235. Greenwalt, T. J., and Jameson, G. A., eds: Transmissible disease and blood transfusion, New York, 1974, Grune & Stratton, Inc.

236. Hall, W. T.: Ultrastructural features of Australia antigen. In Vyas, G. N., Perkins, H. A., and Schmid, R., eds.: Hepatitis and blood transfusion, New York, 1972, Grune & Stratton, Inc.

237. Holland, P. V.: Hepatitis B antigen subtypes: history, significance and immunogenicity, Am. J. Med. Sci. **270:**161, 1975.

238. Hoofnagle, J. H., et al.: Antibody to hepatitis B core antigen: a sensitive indicator of hepatitis B virus replication, N. Engl. J. Med. **290:**1336, 1974.

239. Kaplan, P. M., et al.: DNA polymerase associated with human hepatitis B antigen, J. Virol. **12:**995, 1973.

240. Krugman, S.: Hepatitis: current status of etiology and prevention, Hosp. Pract. Nov. 1975, pp. 39-46.

241. Krugman, S.: Viral hepatitis: recent developments and prospects for prevention, J. Pediatr. **87:**1067, 1975.

242. Krugman, S., and Giles, G. P.: Viral hepatitis, type B (MS-2 strain): further observations on natural history and prevention, N. Engl. J. Med. **288:**755, 1973.

243. Magnius, L. O., et al.: A new antigen-antibody system: clinical significance in long-term carriers of hepatitis B surface antigen, J.A.M.A. **231:**356, 1975.

244. McAuliffe, V. J., et al.: e: a third hepatitis B antigen? N. Engl. J. Med. **294:**779, 1976.

245. Miller, G., et al.: Studies of serum electrolyte changes during exchange transfusion, Pediatrics **13:**412, 1954.

246. Prince, A. M., et al.: Efficacy of prophylactic HBIG against dialysis-associated hepatitis, N. Engl. J. Med. **293:**1063, 1975.

247. Purcell, R. H., and Gerin, J. L.: Hepatitis B subunit vaccine: a preliminary report of safety and efficacy tests in chimpanzees, Am. J. Med. Sci. **270:**395, 1975.

248. Purcell, R. H., et al.: Relationship of hepatitis A antigen to viral hepatitis, Am. J. Med. Sci. **270:**61, 1975.

249. Redeker, A. G., et al.: Prophylactic hepatitis B immune globulin for spouses exposed to hepatitis B, N. Engl. J. Med. **293:**1055, 1975.

250. Robertson, D. H.: The effects of experimental plethora on blood production, J. Exp. Med. **26:**221, 1917.

251. Robinson, W. S., and Lutwick, L. I.: The virus of hepatitis, type B, N. Engl. J. Med. **295:**1232, 1976.

252. Smith, C. H., Schulman, I., et al.: Studies in Mediterranean (Cooley's) anemia. I. Clinical and hematological aspects of splenectomy with special reference to fetal hemoglobin synthesis, Blood **10:**582, 1955.

253. Smith, C. H., Schulman, I., et al.: Studies in Mediterranean (Cooley's) anemia. II. The suppression of hematopoiesis by transfusions, Blood **10:**707, 1955.

PART TWO **RED BLOOD CELLS**

edited by
DENIS R. MILLER
HOWARD A. PEARSON

5 □ Anemias: general considerations

Denis R. Miller

Anemia may be defined as a condition in which the concentration of hemoglobin or the number of red blood cells, either singly or in combination, is reduced below normal. The volume of packed red blood cells per 100 ml of blood measured by the hematocrit undergoes a simultaneous but not always parallel reduction. The physiologic defect caused by the anemia is a decrease in the oxygen-carrying capacity of the blood and a reduction in the oxygen available to the tissues.

A humoral regulatory mechanism that appears to be responsive to the changes in the relation between oxygen supply and tissue requirements exists as a homeostatic control over erythropoiesis.[43] An intracellular metabolic mechanism exists that is capable of altering oxygen delivery as well.

CLASSIFICATION
Physiologic classification

On an etiologic basis anemia results from an increased loss or destruction of red blood cells or a decreased rate of production. Blood loss is caused by acute or chronic hemorrhage or excessive hemolysis from intracorpuscular defects or extracorpuscular factors. Impaired hemoglobin and red cell formation result from a deficiency of genetic, humoral, or nutritional substances required for their synthesis. Defects of the red cells may be congenital or acquired, but in either case the shortened life span frequently results in anemia when red cell production fails to keep pace with red cell destruction. Erythropoiesis also may be depressed by toxic, chemical, or physical agents; by space-occupying or infiltrative lesions of the bone marrow; or by unrecognized causes. It will be noted that the classifications may overlap. For example, in β-thalassemia major anemia may result from a combination of excessive destruction of erythrocytes and inadequate or ineffective compensatory erythropoiesis. In the hemolytic anemia associated with a deficiency of the enzyme glucose-6-phosphate dehydrogenase (G-6-PD), an interaction of an intracellular abnormality and an extracellular factor (exposure to oxidant drugs) is required. (For general considerations of hypoplastic anemias, see Chapter 8; hemolytic anemias, see Chapter 9; and immune hemolysis, see Chapter 10.)

The following is a physiologic classification of the anemias based on etiology.

A. Blood loss: acute and chronic hemorrhage
  1. Internal
  2. External
B. Excessive blood destruction
  1. Intracorpuscular or intrinsic defects, usually hereditary
    a. Defects of membrane: hereditary spherocytosis, elliptocytosis (ovalocytosis), stomatocytosis, increased phosphatidylcholine
    b. Defects of hemoglobin
      (1) Structural anomalies: sickle cell anemia, Hb C disease, unstable hemoglobinopathies, other anomalies
      (2) Synthetic anomalies: thalassemia syndromes, combinations with other hemoglobinopathies
    c. Defects of enzymes
  2. Extracorpuscular factors
    a. Immune mechanisms
      (1) Naturally occurring isoagglutinins (anti-A, anti-B transfusion reactions)
      (2) Acquired antibodies: Rh factor, autoimmune hemolytic anemia (idiopathic or secondary), paroxysmal cold hemoglobinuria
    b. Nonimmune mechanisms
      (1) Infectious agents; parasitism, bacterial toxins, or hemolysins
      (2) Chemical agents: heavy metals, oxidants
      (3) Physical trauma, microangiopathy, thermal injury, exertional (march) hemoglobinuria, hemolytic-uremic syndrome, Waring blender syndrome
      (4) Secondary hemolytic anemia: associated with acute and chronic infections and renal disease, chronic inflammatory disorders, malignancy
      (5) Miscellaneous causes: hypersplenism and splenomegaly
  3. Interaction of intra- and extracorpuscular factors
    a. Associated with membrane defect: paroxysmal nocturnal hemoglobinuria (complement lysis)
    b. Associated with enzyme defect: favism, G-6-PD deficiency
    c. Lead poisoning
    d. Nutritional deficiencies: iron, vitamin B_{12}, folic acid

C. Decreased or impaired production
  1. Deficiency of substances required for hemoglobin and red cell formation: iron, vitamin B_{12}, folic acid, ascorbic acid, pyridoxine, copper, riboflavin, protein
  2. Depression or inhibition of bone marrow
    a. Infection, chemicals, physical agents, metabolic products, immune mechanisms
    b. Idiopathic depression, failure, and aplasia with or without congenital anomalies
  3. Mechanical interference and replacement by abnormal cells
    a. Osteopetrosis, myelofibrosis
    b. Malignancies: leukemia, Hodgkin's disease, neuroblastoma
  4. Secondary relative marrow failure associated with infection, chronic inflammatory disease, renal disease, liver disease, malignancy, and endocrine disorders
  5. Dyserythropoiesis (ineffective erythropoiesis)
    a. Primary dyserythropoietic anemias: types I, II (HEMPAS),[17] III, IV
    b. Secondary dyserythropoiesis
      (1) Nutritional deficiencies: vitamin B_{12}, folic acid
      (2) Defects of heme or globin synthesis: iron deficiency, sideroblastic anemias, thalassemia syndromes
      (3) Bone marrow failure: aplastic anemia, myelosclerosis, paroxysmal nocturnal hemoglobinuria
      (4) Malignancies: erythroleukemia, myeloblastic leukemia
      (5) Miscellaneous: hereditary orotic aciduria, infections, other refractory anemias

Morphologic classification

In addition to a physiologic classification, the anemias may also be classified morphologically, a system based on the values of mean corpuscular volume (MCV) and mean corpuscular hemoglobin concentration (MCHC). In this classification anemias fall into one of four general categories: normochromic normocytic anemia (MCV, 80 to 100 fl; MCHC, 32 to 36 gm/dl), microcytic normochromic anemia (MCV, 60 to 80 fl; MCHC, 32 to 36 gm/dl), microcytic hypochromic anemia (MCV, 60 to 80 fl; MCHC, 20 to 30 gm/dl), and macrocytic normochromic anemia (MCV 101 to 160 fl; MCHC 32 to 36 gm/dl). These results for MCV are based on red blood cell counts enumerated by electronic particle counters and are about 8% higher than results previously obtained by manual procedures.

The following is a condensed classification of the anemias based on morphology.

A. Normocytic normochromic anemia
  1. Acute blood loss
  2. Hemolytic anemias: intracorpuscular, extracorpuscular, interacting types

3. Hemoglobin–erythrocyte mass deficit: chronic disease, toxic agents, malignancy, splenomegaly, bone marrow failure, endocrine disorders
B. Microcytic normochromic anemia
  1. Hemoglobin–erythrocyte mass deficit: chronic disease, toxic agents, malignancy, splenomegaly, endocrine disorders
C. Microcytic hypochromic anemia
  1. Iron deficiency anemia
  2. Chronic lead poisoning
  3. Thalassemia syndromes: thalassemia trait, intermedia, major
  4. Miscellaneous rare disorders: vitamin B_6 (pyridoxine) abnormality, sideroblastic anemia, familial hypochromic-microcytic anemia
D. Macrocytic normochromic anemia
  1. Pernicious anemia: congenital, associated with endocrinopathy, specific vitamin B_{12} malabsorption
  2. Megaloblastic anemias of infancy, pregnancy, and puerperium
  3. Gastrointestinal abnormalities: malabsorption syndromes, anomalies, surgical resections, inflammatory disease, acute and chronic liver disease
  4. Dietary deficiency of vitamin B_{12}, folic acid, vitamin C
  5. *Diphyllobothrium latum* infestation
  6. Ingestion of anticonvulsant drugs and antifolic acid antimetabolites
  7. Bone marrow failure or hypoplasia: aplastic anemia, Diamond-Blackfan syndrome, uremia
  8. Associated with reticulocytosis of marrow response to hemolysis or hemorrhage
  9. Associated with bone marrow infiltration: myeloid metaplasia, myelophthisis, miliary tuberculosis

ORIENTATION

The anemias constitute the major category of blood disorders of infancy and childhood. Anemia is a syndrome of multiple etiology in which the origins are sometimes difficult to discern for reasons inherent in the developmental processes of the pediatric period. Many of the anemias undoubtedly are conditioned by factors operative in fetal life dating from the critical first months of gestation when hematopoiesis is established. Others are influenced by the postnatal anatomic and physiologic changes that originate within and outside the hematopoietic system. Still others represent inherited disorders of metabolism. The conditioning factors influencing the blood picture in the neonatal period and early infancy are given in the following list.[72] Each of these items is discussed elsewhere in the text. (See Chapters 1 and 3.)
  1. Results of maternal isoimmunization by fetal blood factors
  2. Hemolytic anemia from maternal transmission of ingested drugs or chemical compounds

3. Fetal hemorrhage into maternal circulation
4. Bleeding from the placental surface: abruptio placentae, placenta previa, and other complications of delivery
5. Fluctuations in blood volume as related to early or late clamping of the cord
6. Anemia from congenital bleeding disorders: overt or obscure hemorrhage
7. Possibility that a blood dyscrasia may represent a developmental or congenital defect
8. Effects of prematurity
9. Aregenerative phase of erythropoiesis
10. Substitution of adult for fetal hemoglobin
11. Physiologic variations in the metabolism, structure, and survival of neonatal erythrocytes
12. Tendency for hematopoietic system to react excessively to a stimulus; reactivation of extramedullary foci of hematopoiesis
13. Effects of rapid body growth
14. Inadequate fetal stores of iron from prematurity or from severe maternal deficiency

DIAGNOSIS

The problems of diagnosis in the infant and young child are complicated by the fact that the anemias tend to develop insidiously so that the complete hematologic picture with its specific criteria may be slow in emerging. Despite these apparent difficulties, it is possible with minimal laboratory equipment to make an appropriate diagnosis by the judicious appraisal of data derived from the following sources.

A. History and physical examination
B. Reference to age periods of most frequent occurrence
C. Basic blood studies: complete blood count, red blood cell indices, reticulocyte count, platelet count, interpretation of blood smear, morphologic classification
D. Comparison with normal range of blood values for each age period
E. Bone marrow examination: aspiration, biopsy, culture, special stains
F. Radiologic examination
G. Study of hereditary factors
H. Specialized laboratory procedures
  1. Essential tests
    a. Stool guaiac test
    b. Serum bilirubin determination
    c. Blood urea nitrogen determination
    d. Coombs test
    e. Red cell osmotic fragility
    f. Hemoglobin electrophoresis
    g. Urinalysis including microscopic examination
  2. Helpful tests
    a. Tests of serum iron, total iron binding capacity, and iron saturation
    b. Bone marrow iron determination
    c. Tests of serum vitamin B_{12} and folate levels
    d. Assays of red blood cell enzymes and metabolites
    e. Quantitation of and histochemical stain for fetal hemoglobin
    f. Liver function tests
    g. Diagnostic use of radioisotopes
      (1) Radioactive chromium (^{51}Cr) determination of red cell mass, plasma volume, red cell life span, blood loss, and organ sequestration (liver, spleen, lungs, bone marrow, heart)
      (2) Radioiron (^{59}Fe) determination of plasma clearance rate, plasma iron transport rate, appearance rate in erythrocytes,[24] and amounts appearing in body sites such as bone marrow, liver, and spleen; ^{52}Fe for sites of active erythropoiesis[79]
      (3) Radioactive B_{12} (^{60}Co–vitamin B_{12}) urinary excretion test for B_{12} absorption (Schilling test) in diagnosis of pernicious anemia

The large number of items included illustrates the wide scope of available information and the simpler technical procedures on which the diagnosis is based. A number of simple screening tests are available for enzyme deficiency disorders, hemoglobinopathies, and acquired hemolytic anemias (e.g., methemoglobin reduction test for G-6-PD deficiency, heat stability or isopropanol test for unstable hemoglobins, and the "sugar water" test for paroxysmal nocturnal hemoglobinuria). More elaborate or technically demanding investigations may be required in obscure cases of anemia. However, an insight into the nature of anemia actually requires that relatively few of these topics be probed. Under ordinary circumstances a thorough history, physical examination, and basic blood studies, in conjunction with a simple classification based on etiology, are usually sufficient to arrive at a correct diagnosis. The "shotgun approach" accomplishes little except excessive expense.

History and physical examination

Interrogation along broad lines of causation should include the following: any change of behavior pattern (such as irritability), anorexia, inactivity, fatigability, onset of pallor or jaundice, exertional dyspnea, palpitations, orthopnea, ankle edema, headache, vertigo, faintness, tinnitus, cold sensitivity, decreased mental concentration, menstrual irregularities, urinary frequency, and low-grade fever. All of these are symptoms of decreased oxygen delivery with associated organ dysfunction.

Inquiry should extend into a history of prematurity; exacerbations of pallor and jaundice; purpura; hemetemesis; loss of blood from the bowel; infection with animal parasites; allergy; ingestion of drugs or household products known to depress hematopoiesis or cause hemolysis; exposure to radiation; frequency of respiratory infections and other infections; preexisting cardiac, gastrointestinal, endocrine, or renal diseases; skeletal pain; and joint swelling. A complete dietary history with documentation of food fadism and of the quantity of milk, meats, and solid foods, vitamins, and minerals ingested should be obtained.

Valuable aspects of the family and social history include ethnic and geographic origins, socioeconomic background, presence of consanguinity, and any family history of anemia, gallbladder disease, or splenectomy. Foreign or unusual travel should be documented.

Physical examination should include scrutiny of such diverse features as pallor; jaundice; skin pigmentation; pinkness of palmar creases, nailbeds, conjunctivae, lips, and mucous membranes of the mouth; enlargement of spleen, liver, and lymph nodes; petechiae; and purpura. In iron-deficiency anemia, leukemia, and profound loss of blood the skin has a waxy whiteness. The sallow complexion of iron deficiency is often interpreted as "yellow" by parents. In homozygous forms of thalassemia as well as in other conditions requiring multiple transfusions, such as aplastic anemia and congenital hypoplastic anemia, pallor is replaced by dark pigmentation and bronzing of the skin. In patients in whom hemosiderosis is present, retardation of secondary sexual maturation is noted with absence of facial, axillary, and pubic hair; underdeveloped breasts and genitalia; and lack of deepening of the voice. Malleolar ulcers can occur in sickle cell anemia and thalassemia but are rarely seen nowadays.

Increasing jaundice from the first day of life differentiates hemolytic disease of the newborn from its slower development in physiologic jaundice of the newborn.

In patients with advanced and chronic hemolytic anemia there may be obvious frontal bossing, prominent malar eminences, and maxillary dental malocclusion. The facies of β-thalassemia major are characteristic.

Eye ground changes in anemia include profound pallor of the retina, tortuous vessels with microaneurysms in sickle cell anemia, and retinal hemorrhages in severe anemia.

Tachycardia, increased arterial and capillary pulsation, bruits, and increased rate and depth of respiration may be present, depending on the severity and duration of anemia. Systolic pressure is usually normal in the absence of shock, but the diastolic pressure is decreased. Cardiac enlargement and signs of cardiac failure may be present. Gallop rhythms of the S_3 and S_4 type may be present as well as atrial or ventricular arrhythmias. A loud systolic murmur heard best at the apex and less commonly over the pulmonic area is frequently regarded as being of organic origin before the severe underlying anemia is discovered. These murmurs are of hemic origin and reflect increased pulse rate, cardiac output, and stroke volume; decreased viscosity of the blood; and decreased peripheral resistance. The murmurs usually disappear following transfusions.

Splenomegaly is most noticeable in infants and children with disorders attended by blood destruction such as erythroblastosis fetalis, hereditary and acquired hemolytic anemias, and malignancies. The spleen is occasionally enlarged in patients with iron-deficiency anemia and those with megaloblastic anemia of infancy. It is not palpable in infants and children with aplastic or hypoplastic anemias. It should be remembered that a spleen palpable about 1 to 3 cm below the costal margin is present in a substantial number of normal pediatric patients. The soft edge of the spleen in these children is in contrast with the hard edge found in patients with pathologic conditions. Enlargement of the liver is occasionally found in patients with congestive heart failure and in those with sudden severe anemia from any cause. It is often enlarged in patients with hemolytic anemia, especially in those receiving frequent transfusions who have developed secondary hemochromatosis.

Except for the anemia associated with infection or with leukemia, lymphadenopathy is not a conspicuous feature of anemia. Enlarged cervical nodes, frequently associated with a palpable spleen, occur in the child with anemia as a result of recurrent infections in the upper respiratory tract. The peripheral lymph nodes may be slightly enlarged in patients with thalassemia major and sickle cell anemia but not usually in those with the other intrinsic anemias. Generalized lymphadenopathy in the presence of a refractory anemia and leukopenia should arouse suspicion of leukemia.

Neurologic abnormalities may include residual defects related to earlier vaso-occlusive crises of the central nervous system occurring in sickle cell anemia or long tract defects of combined degeneration of the spinal cord.

Age incidence in relation to diagnosis

When infection, which is responsible for the major number of anemias in the pediatric age group, is excluded, the remaining hematologic disorders can be grouped for orientation according to the age of their most common occurrence: newborn period, infancy, childhood, and adolescence.

In the newborn infant the anemia is usually

caused by blood loss or hemolysis. Acute fetal blood loss during labor and delivery, frequently resulting in posthemorrhagic shock, may be a result of fetal bleeding from the placenta, occult transplacental loss of fetal blood into the maternal circulation, or rupture of a normal or shortened umbilical cord.[38] In the neonate the reticulocyte count provides important information because it becomes elevated with a hemolytic process or hemorrhage. If the reticulocyte count is decreased, aregenerative anemia or some infiltrative disease should be considered, and bone marrow examination is required to establish the diagnosis. When reticulocytosis is present and obstetric hemorrhage has been eliminated, a positive direct Coombs test will identify those infants who have been immunized with Rh, A, B, or minor blood group factors. If the Coombs test is negative, other types of hemolytic disease as well as occult bleeding should be considered.

Anemia of the newborn associated with hypochromic microcytes may stem from fetal-maternal hemorrhage or twin-to-twin transfusion. A search for fetal red cells in the mother's circulation will reveal transplacental loss of fetal blood. Spherocytes, elliptocytes, stomatocytes, and pyknocytes found in the peripheral smear of the newborn provide important diagnostic information. Enzymatic defects such as G-6-PD deficiency or pyruvate kinase deficiency may be present. Hemolytic anemia in the newborn period may be caused by a number of infections such as cytomegalic inclusion disease, toxoplasmosis, congenital rubella, herpes simplex, and congenital syphilis and are usually accompanied by jaundice, prominent hepatosplenomegaly, and thrombocytopenic purpura. Other infections may also be responsible for anemia and jaundice; for these infections blood and urine cultures may reveal the cause of an obscure hemolytic anemia during the first weeks of life.

Anemia caused by iron deficiency occurs most commonly between 6 months and 2 years of age, especially in the premature infant, in the rapidly growing infant, and in any infant whose dietary iron is restricted. Iron-deficiency anemia also occurs during infancy as a result of chronic gastrointestinal bleeding from embryonic structural defects such as diverticula. Megaloblastic anemia of infancy occurs chiefly between the ages of 2 and 18 months. Congenital hypoplastic anemia (Diamond-Blackfan syndrome) is usually apparent at the age of 2 or 3 months or later in the first year. When the infant is approximately 6 months to 2 years old, the clinical and hematologic features of β-thalassemia major, sickle cell anemia, and hereditary spherocytosis are sufficiently conspicuous to be diagnosed. They can be distinguished even earlier in cases suspected because of a familial

background. The laboratory diagnosis of intrinsic abnormalities of red cells during the first 3 months of life may be clouded by the unique structural and metabolic characteristics of fetal erythrocytes. Thus extensive investigations of the membrane, hemoglobin, or enzymes are best postponed until after fetal erythrocytes have left the circulation.

Fanconi's aplastic anemia usually manifests its hematologic features after 3 or 4 years of age. At about this time, too, Banti's syndrome and other disorders are encountered that are associated with splenomegaly and varying degrees of a hypersplenic blood picture, such as that seen in Gaucher's disease.

During adolescence the major cause of anemia is iron deficiency.[21] In fact, more than 10% of American high school students have iron-deficiency anemia related to this period of accelerated body growth and notoriously inadequate diets. Vitamin B_{12} and folate deficiency with megaloblastic anemias are less common in adolescence. An extremely rare form of vitamin B_{12} deficiency and pernicious anemia in adolescents is associated with endocrinopathies (thyroid, parathyroid, and adrenal diseases), low IgA levels, and candidiasis. Aplastic anemia (idiopathic, Fanconi's, or drug-induced) may be manifested during adolescence. During the adolescent period children with hereditary hemolytic anemias begin to develop the complications of their disorders—cholelithiasis, hypoplastic crises, hypersplenism, cardiac enlargement and failure, skeletal changes, and failure of secondary sexual maturation. Autoimmune hemolytic anemias associated with systemic lupus erythematosis and non-Hodgkin's lymphoma are also more common during adolescence. Finally pregnant adolescents are particularly at risk of becoming anemic because of nutritional deficiencies of iron and folic acid and the hydremia of pregnancy.

Basic blood studies

Volume of packed red cells (hematocrit). In all anemias the measurement of the volume of packed red blood cells by the hematocrit constitutes an essential guide for diagnosis and therapy. This determination reflects the total mass of cells in a unit volume of blood and has proved to be of fundamental value in the study of all anemias in which considerable alterations occur in size, shape, and thickness of red blood cells. It has the advantage of being reliable and least subject to error in quantitative interpretation. In patients with iron-deficiency anemia, for instance, the extremely low hematocrit reflects the state of anemia more accurately than does the moderate reduction or even normal value for the number of red blood cells. Also, in the thalassemia trait the volume of packed red cells frequently remains at the same level in spite of wide fluctuations in the number of red cells.

Because of the variations noted in available studies, it is difficult to state the optimum packed cell volume for different age groups. As a working base, a hematocrit of 34% may be regarded as the lower limit of normal in infants after the first month of life, 36% from 2 to 12 years of age, and 40% in older children.

Reticulocyte count. The reticulocyte count reflects the state of erythroid activity of the bone marrow, assuming that erythropoiesis is effective; hence this determination is useful in the determination of both deficiency and hemolytic anemias and in gauging the response to treatment. Normally from 0.5% to 1.5% of the red blood cells are reticulocytes; levels lower than 0.5% represent inactive or depressed erythropoiesis. A persistent depression in the percentage of reticulocytes usually occurs in patients with aplastic or hypoplastic anemia. In those with anemia caused by a deficiency a reticulocyte response from previously low levels follows appropriate treatment. In patients with hemolytic anemias the values for reticulocytes are constantly elevated unless a hypoplastic crisis supervenes. The high levels that are maintained represent intensified bone marrow regeneration.

Diagnostic features of the blood smear—morphologic abnormalities. Of all laboratory procedures the most important, yet the simplest, is the examination of the peripheral blood smear. Although corroborative evidence from auxiliary sources may be required to establish a final diagnosis, the stained blood film constitutes a visual representation of the effect on morphology of the factors involved in the pathogenesis of a specific anemia. There are few specific red cells that are indicative of a particular disorder. Target cells, oval cells, hypochromic macrocytes, spherocytes, basophilic stippling, and hypochromic microcytes appear in varying percentages in certain stages of many anemias and therefore cannot be regarded as distinguishing features of a single disease. They are significant with the support of other pertinent information. Similar morphologic abnormalities in diverse anemias reflect common pathways of red cell destruction, altered function and structure, or abnormal production and metabolism. Thus spherocytosis, indicating membrane fragmentation and a decreased surface area: volume ratio, may be observed in hereditary spherocytosis, in autoimmune hemolytic anemia, in ABO incompatibility, and after thermal injury. The morphologic changes of the red cells in the most common anemias of infancy and childhood are summarized in Tables 5-1 and 5-2.

Table 5-1. Diagnostic features of blood smear in anemias of early infancy

Type of anemia	Diagnostic features
Hemolytic disease of newborn	Hyperchromic polychromatophilic nucleated red blood cells
ABO incompatibility	Above plus spherocytes
Hemorrhagic anemia	
Acute blood loss	Normocytic normochromic red cells
Chronic blood loss	Hypochromic microcytes
Anemia of prematurity	
Early	Normocytic normochromic red blood cells
Later	Hypochromic microcytes
Megaloblastic anemia of infancy	Large macrocytes, microcytes, occasional nucleated red blood cells, hypersegmented neutrophils
Iron-deficiency anemia	Hypochromic microcytes, poikilocytes, target cells, elliptocytes, basophilic stippling, fragments

Each of these disorders is discussed elsewhere in this book. Although overlapping occurs and differentiation from the normal is often subtle, the following represent the most conspicuous alterations in size, shape, and structural changes and staining peculiarities of the erythrocytes.

Abnormalities in size. The following abnormalities of size may be noted in erythrocytes.

ANISOCYTOSIS. Excessive variation in size of the red cells (average diameter 7.5 mμ) is termed anisocytosis.

POIKILOCYTE. Marked irregularity in the shape of the red cell is termed poikilocytosis. The red cells are called poikilocytes.

MICROCYTES. Microcytes are cells with diameters of less than 6.5 mμ and usually characterize the blood smear of a patient with iron-deficiency anemia or thalassemia trait.

MACROCYTES. Macrocytes are large cells with a diameter of 8.5 mμ or more, are thicker than the normocyte, are well filled with hemoglobin, and have a larger volume than normal. They are found in patients with aplastic anemias and megaloblastic anemias (pernicious anemia and folic acid deficiency). Polychromatophilic macrocytes are seen in patients with hemolytic anemia.

HYPOCHROMIC MACROCYTES. Hypochromic macrocytes are found in large numbers in the blood of patients with thalassemia of varying grades of severity; they are of special value in the diagnosis of thalassemia minor. Patients with many of the

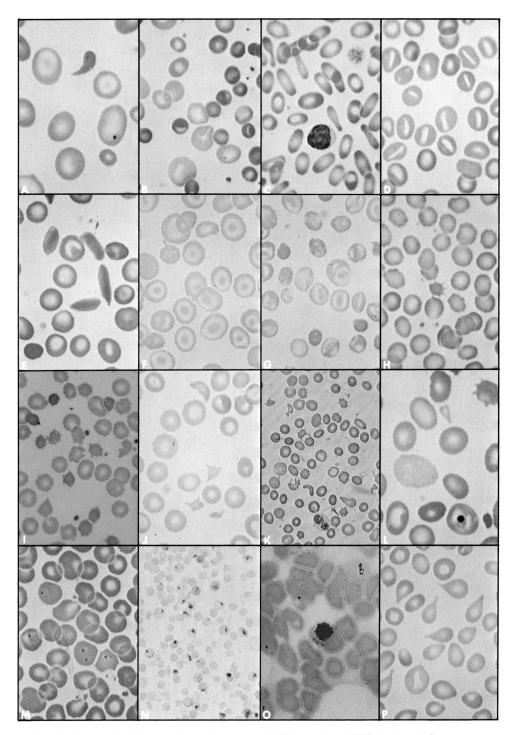

Plate 3. Abnormal red blood cells. **A,** Macrocytes. **B,** Spherocytes. **C,** Elliptocytes. **D,** Stomatocytes. **E,** Sickle cells. **F,** Target cells. **G,** Leptocytes. **H,** Echinocytes. **I,** Acanthocytes. **J,** Schistocytes. **K,** Pyknocytes. **L,** Howell-Jolly bodies. **M,** Malaria. **N,** Heinz bodies. **O,** Sideroblasts and sidero-cytes. **P,** Dacryocytes (teardrops).

Table 5-2. Diagnostic features of blood smear in anemias of later infancy and childhood

Type of anemia	Diagnostic features
Aplastic, hypoplastic, and aregenerative anemia	Normochromic macrocytic red blood cells
Anemia of infection	Normocytic normochromic, occasionally microcytic, hypochromic red blood cells; with iron deficiency, hypochromic microcytes predominate
Acquired hemolytic anemia	Moderate spherocytosis, marked polychromasia, reticulocytosis
Hereditary spherocytosis	Spherocytes, polychromasia, reticulocytosis
Hereditary enzymopathies	Normocytic normochromic red blood cells, occasionally macrocytosis, polychromasia, anisocytosis, poikilocytosis, spherocytes, reticulocytosis
Sickle cell anemia	Sickle cells, target cells, microcytes, occasional nucleated red blood cells, reticulocytosis
Thalassemia major	Leptocytes (large, thin, hypochromic macrocytes), microcytes, nucleated red blood cells, marked poikilocytosis, anisocytosis, reticulocytosis
Thalassemia minor (trait)	Hypochromic macrocytes, microcytes, basophilic stippling, target and oval cells

chronic anemias may have small numbers of these cells.

Abnormalities in shape. Another morphologic abnormality of erythrocytes is irregularity of shape.

SPHEROCYTES (MICROSPHEROCYTES). Spherocytes are globular, thick red cells of lessened diameter with a normal volume enclosed within a greatly diminished surface area; hence they are readily hemolyzed in hypotonic solutions of sodium chloride. The small, deeply stained spherocytes are observed in hereditary spherocytosis, acquired hemolytic anemia (immune and nonimmune types), erythroblastosis fetalis as a result of sensitization by the AB antibodies, and less frequently other hereditary hemolytic anemias, leukemia, conditions of stasis within the spleen, and stored blood.

ELLIPTOCYTES (OVALOCYTES). Oval or elliptical cells occur typically as a dominant hereditary

anomaly in which they constitute from 25% to 90% of all erythrocytes.[47] The cells vary in shape from the rod or elongated forms to oval shape, all being abundantly filled with hemoglobin. Nucleated red cell precursors show no abnormalities of shape. Elliptical cells occur in smaller numbers in the blood of patients with sickle cell anemia[60,80]; unlike sickle cells, however, elliptocytes cannot be made to sickle in an environment of lowered oxygen tension.

Oval and elliptical cells are often noted in association with marked anisocytosis and poikilocytosis.[44] It is necessary therefore to differentiate symptomatic from hereditary elliptocytosis,[53] since oval-shaped cells appear in variable numbers in the blood of newborn infants[82] and of patients with thalassemia, severe iron-deficiency anemia, pernicious anemia, anemia of infection, leukemia, and familial hypochromic microcytic anemia with splenomegaly affecting male members.[61] A more extensive discussion of hereditary elliptocytosis appears in Chapter 11.

STOMATOCYTES. Stomatocytes are erythrocytes that in stained films have a linear, slit, or mouth-like unstained area across the center instead of the normal circular area of pallor.[45] In wet preparations and with an electron microscope, the erythrocytes appear as uniconcave, bowl-shaped, or cup-shaped spheres rather than biconcave discs. Others may resemble pinch-bottles or *knizocytes.*[49] Stomatocytosis may occur as a hereditary hemolytic anemia but these oddities of cell shape may be seen in thalassemia trait, in lead poisoning, in liver disease, and in vitro after incubation with phenothiazines.[40,65,76] The hereditary syndromes are usually associated with aberrations of intracellular cation content and transport and exhibit abnormalities of osmotic fragility.

SICKLE CELLS (DREPANOCYTES). The characteristic sickle cells are elongated and narrow with rounded, pointed, or filamentous ends. Although they appear in the stained smear of the homozygous patient with sickle cell anemia, they are greatly increased in number in sealed wet films with reduced oxygen tension. Reversion to the normal form occurs in cells not irreversibly transformed with reexposure to oxygen or carbon monoxide. Frequently the cells assume a holly leaf appearance, exhibiting numerous superficial spines. The mature orthochromic normoblast can be made to sickle slowly, although stained bone marrow smears show no morphologic changes in the nucleated red cells. The sickling phenomenon requires a minimum of 20% Hb S to elicit the sickling phenomenon.[69]

Elliptocytosis has been observed in association with the sickle cell trait with both varieties of cells in the peripheral blood.[22] The sickle cell trait has been reported coexistent with thalassemia, other hemoglobinopathies, and hereditary hemolytic anemias.

TARGET CELLS. In target cells hemoglobin is concentrated in the periphery and in the center, producing concentric light and dark zones after staining. The deeply stained central area gives the impression of a bull's-eye in a target. Target cells are a variety of leptocytes, or thin cells, in which the cell membrane or surface area is too large and out of proportion to its meager contents. This accounts for the decreased osmotic fragility in hypotonic salt solutions. Thus target cells are the morphologic expression of an increased surface area: volume ratio. Cooper and Jandl[16] have shown that the red cell membrane accumulates cholesterol in obstructive jaundice as a consequence of the elevated levels of bile salts. In so doing the red cells assume the features of target cells on stained smear and in fresh wet preparations.

Target cells are nonspecific and are found in increased numbers in patients with many anemias, with hepatitis, with extrahepatic biliary tract obstruction and hypochromic anemia, following splenectomy, and especially with abnormal hemoglobins. Target cells are present in patients with thalassemia syndromes and thalassemia trait (usually up to 10%), are further increased in those with sickle cell anemia, and appear in large numbers in patients with microdrepanocytic or thalassemia–sickle cell disease. These cells are prominent also in the blood of patients with other pathologic hemoglobins. In those with sickle cell–Hb C disease, for instance, target cells comprise 40% to 85% of all red blood cells.[34] It has been suggested that large numbers of target cells in the blood smear indicate the presence of Hb C. Whereas numbers of target cells are also increased in patients with Hb E disease, perhaps less than in those with Hb C, few or no target cells have been noted in reported cases of sickle cell–Hb D disease.[75]

LEPTOCYTES. Leptocytes are abnormally thin erythrocytes. Some are bowl shaped and assume the appearance of target cells following drying and preparation of the smear. A preponderance of leptocytes occurs in patients with hypochromic microcytic anemia and homozygous thalassemia. Other cells found in thalassemia are not target cells but are extremely thin, leaflike, and transparent.

CRENATION (CRENATED DISCOCYTES AND ECHINO-CYTES). In blood smears that dry slowly the red cell envelope becomes exposed to a hypertonic medium, which causes wrinkling of the surface with the appearance of a moderate number of knoblike (scalloped) or prickly, spiny projections. In suspension, metabolically deprived red cells also undergo reversible changes in shape. The process,

known as crenation, occurs normally and is part of the physiologic transformation of a smooth, biconcave discocyte to a crenated disc, thence to a crenated sphere (echinocyte),[7] and finally to a smooth spherocyte. The echinocyte resembles the egg of a sea urchin. Unfortunately semantic confusion has resulted from the proliferation of descriptive terms that bear little if any relationship to pathophysiologic mechanisms. Accordingly "spur" cells, "spiculated" or "spicule" cells, "burr" cells, acanthocytes, acanthrocytes, pyknocytes, and "helmet" cells are all representative of erythrocytes that have undergone some degree of transformation or fragmentation of the membrane. To distinguish crenation produced by drying artifacts from truly crenated erythrocytes, fresh wet preparations and phase-contrast microscopy are particularly useful.

The appearance of echinocytes after splenectomy[73] has been attributed to the absence of the "culling" or phagocytic function of the spleen. The "culling" function[18] describes the unique ability of this organ to scrutinize circulating red cells and remove those that do not meet the requirements for survival. The normal spleen is a particularly effective filter that clears abnormal cells from the circulation.

ACANTHOCYTES. In the stained film acanthocytes (thorny red cells, from the Greek *akantha,* thorn) look like spherocytes with spiny pseudopodia. The projections are large, coarse, and irregularly spaced. These malformed cells were first observed in a patient with atypical retinitis pigmentosa[70] and they are pathognomonic of acanthocytosis or a-β-lipoproteinemia[39] (Chapter 11). Differentiation between acanthocytes and burr cells may be difficult. Erythrocytes with minimal spiny projections or spurs resembling acanthocytes have been observed in patients with hepatic cirrhosis and hemolytic anemia.[15,27,68,74]

SCHISTOCYTES (FRAGMENTED CELLS). The striking feature of schistocytosis, or presence of fragmented red blood cells, is the presence of bizarre poikilocytes in the peripheral blood, characterized by triangular, crescentic, and half-moon–shaped cells. Spheroidal fragments, or spheroschizocytes, may be seen also. Schistocytes can be produced in vitro by a clothesline effect as red cells are fractured transversely by fibrin strands. These cells are seen especially in syndromes of microangiopathic hemolytic anemia (renal failure,[2] hemolytic-uremic syndrome, thrombotic thrombocytopenic purpura, and cardiac valvular prostheses) and have also been observed in aplastic anemia,[42] after mechanical injury to the red cells,[9] in cirrhosis of the liver,[68] in metastatic carcinoma,[63] and in disseminated intravascular coagulation.[10]

KERATOCYTE ("HORNED" CELL, "BURR" CELL). A schistocyte possessing one to several spiny projections along its periphery is a keratoschistocyte. The horny projections are larger and more irregularly spaced and appear more pointed than those in the crenated red cell, which are short, blunt, and more regularly spaced. The sequence of events ending in a keratocyte appears to be the formation of a vacuole at the periphery of the red cell that subsequently ruptures through the membrane, leaving a crater and a deformed erythrocyte in the shape of a half-moon or spindle.[5]

PYKNOCYTES. In the first few months of life distorted, hyperchromic, contracted erythrocytes, or *pyknocytes* (Greek *pykno,* dense), appear in small numbers in normal full-term and premature infants. The percentages range from 0.3% to 1.9% in full-term infants and from 1.3% to 5.6% in premature infants, increasing with age to at least 2 to 3 months.[36,77] This cell most closely resembles a crenated spherocyte. The cells may be associated with an acute severe hemolytic anemia early in life, in which case they may increase up to 50%, a condition referred to as infantile pyknocytosis.[1,77] Pyknocytosis has been described in association with deficiencies of red cell G-6-PD[83] and pyruvate kinase[55] and of vitamin E.[57]

Abnormalities in staining characteristics: intracellular inclusions and debris. Abnormalities of staining characteristics of erythrocytes are considered in the following discussions. Certain features require special staining techniques; others are detected in Romanowsky-prepared smears.

HYPOCHROMIA AND HYPERCHROMIA. Hypochromia is observed in cells with a lack of hemoglobin and is represented by an increase in central pallor. Deeply and homogeneously stained red cells lacking central pallor because of complete hemoglobinization are termed hyperchromic. A macrocyte with a normal concentration of hemoglobin contains more of this substance than a normocyte only because of its size. Since oversaturation with hemoglobin (MCHC > 36 gm/dl) does not occur, the cell cannot be truly hyperchromic. Nevertheless, according to common usage, hyperchromic anemias identify conditions in which macrocytes prevail. Spherocytes and acanthocytes (pp. 97 and 98) are also hyperchromic cells.

POLYCHROMATOPHILIC ERYTHROCYTES. Polychromatophilic erythrocytes in the peripheral smear represent young reticulocytes with a mean diameter nearly 30% greater than that of mature cells. Polychromatophilic erythrocytes normally constitute 5% or less of the circulating reticulocytes. With moderate anemia or hypoxia an increase to between 10% and 20% occurs; in severe anemia greater than 20% are seen. However, in anemias unaccompanied by elevated erythropoietin levels (e.g., renal failure) no such response is observed.

In disorders of the marrow stroma (myelophthisis, myelofibrosis, metastatic tumor) the increase in polychromatophilic erythrocytes appears disproportionate to the degree of anemia present. Polychromatophilic erythrocytes in the peripheral blood provide a simple means of identifying increased erythropoietin stimulation of the bone marrow.

BASOPHILIC STIPPLING. Basophilic stippling or punctate basophilia describes the presence of round, fine, or coarse bluish violet or dark blue granules scattered in the cytoplasm or polychromatophilic red blood cells. The stippling represents precipitated ribosomal RNA and reflects active erythropoiesis, regeneration, or immaturity of the cell. Basophilic stippling is sometimes best observed in slightly thicker and moderately overstained blood smears and is associated with all chronic anemias, leukemia, iron-deficiency anemia, thalassemia trait, pyrimidine 5-nucleotidase deficiency,[78] and lead poisoning, in which the granules are particularly dense. Punctate basophilia is to be differentiated from the network found in reticulocytes in cresyl blue preparations.

HOWELL-JOLLY BODIES. Howell-Jolly bodies are small, rounded, densely staining nuclear remnants occurring singly, doubly, or rarely more frequently; they are eccentrically placed. They stain a reddish blue or dark violet with Wright's stain and are prominent after splenectomy, with splenic agenesis, and in many anemias, such as severe iron-deficiency anemia, pernicious anemia, hereditary spherocytosis, dyserythropoietic anemias, and leukemia. The origin of these bodies has been ascribed to abnormal mitosis in the late pronormoblast stage when single chromosomes or groups of chromosomes become detached, fail to be included in the formation of the interphase nucleus, and remain free in the cytoplasm as DNA remnants.[32]

CABOT RINGS. Cabot rings are basophilic rings, circular or twisted into a figure-of-eight, which occur occasionally in red blood cells of patients with hemolytic anemias, untreated pernicious anemia, leukemia, and lead poisoning. They stain reddish purple with Wright's stain. They are thought to represent remnants of nuclear membranes or the mitotic spindle apparatus, but their exact origin remains unknown.[62]

HEINZ BODIES (HEINZ-EHRLICH BODIES). Heinz bodies are moderately sized, round, or irregularly shaped protein containing granules lying at or close to the periphery of the red blood cell. Single or multiple, these inclusion bodies are observed only after supravital staining (e.g., brilliant cresyl blue and methyl violet). The Romanowsky dyes such as Wright's stain obscure their presence. They are easily detected as refractile bodies in unstained wet preparations or under phase or Nomarsky optics.

These intracellular inclusions are agglomerations of denatured or precipitated globin,[29] the result of (1) an imbalance in the synthesis of globin chains (thalassemia syndromes), (2) structurally unstable hemoglobins, (3) intrinsic defects of enzymes of the pentose phosphate shunt (G-6-PD deficiency, glutathione deficiency), or (4) drug- or toxin-induced oxidant injury to the red cells. Sulfonamides, primaquine, phenylhydrazine,[8] naphthalene, phenacetin, and the fava bean are prominent among compounds that cause the denaturation of hemoglobin and formation of Heinz bodies.[23] They appear in increased numbers in patients with hemolytic anemias and leukemia, following splenectomy,[66] and in patients with agenesis of the spleen.[26]

The presence of target cells, normoblasts, Howell-Jolly bodies, Heinz bodies and siderocytes in varying combinations in the peripheral blood of a young infant prompts consideration of agenesis of the spleen, especially when associated with levocardia, congenital anomalies of the heart, and situs inversus of the abdominal viscera.[12] The diagnosis of asplenia can be made with confidence in infants with cyanotic congenital heart disease who are polycythemic and whose peripheral blood contains numerous Howell-Jolly and Heinz bodies.[46] A liver-spleen scan will confirm the clinical impression based on the physical examination and careful evaluation of the peripheral blood.

SIDEROCYTES AND SIDEROBLASTS.[19] Siderocytes are red blood cells containing nonhemoglobin iron particles that are visible when stained by the Prussian blue technique and counterstained with safranin.[14] Sideroblasts are normoblasts containing similar iron inclusions. Both types of cells appear in moderate numbers in the peripheral blood and bone marrow, respectively, of normal persons. Their numbers are increased in chronic infection and aplastic and hemolytic anemias and are markedly decreased in iron-deficiency anemias.[33] Siderocytes increase significantly in number after splenectomy. Sideroblasts may be seen in states of excessive hemolysis, with dyserythropoiesis, and in sideroblastic anemias associated with "ring" sideroblasts.

Siderocytes are to be differentiated from basophilic stippling. Siderotic granules fail to stain with basophilic dyes, and the RNA-containing granules of basophilic stippling are not stained by Prussian blue. Basophilic and siderotic granules occasionally coexist in the same cell.

PAPPENHEIMER BODIES. Pappenheimer bodies are present in red blood cells as single or double granules or dots and appear in largest numbers in the peripheral blood in certain cases of hemolytic anemia following splenectomy.[59] They stain a darker shade of blue than does the filamentous material of reticulocytes. They represent aggregates of mitochondrial ferric iron within autophagic vacuoles or phagosomes of reticulocytes[37] that contain other cellular remnants including mitochondria and ribosomes. They stain with Prussian blue and basophilic dyes. These granules closely resemble the iron-staining granules of the siderocyte which stain with Prussian blue but fail to stain with basophilic dyes.[6]

POCKED ERYTHROCYTES. A study of red cell surface morphology using interference or contrast microscopy revealed striking differences in premature and term infants, in infants of various ages, and in normal adults.[31] In normal adults 2.6% of erythrocytes had small (0.2 to 0.5 mμ) pits or craters on their surface. By contrast, premature and term infants had a mean of 47.2% and 24.3% cells, respectively; adult values were reached at 2 months of age in term infants and somewhat later in premature infants. An inverse correlation was observed between birth weight and the number of pitted cells.

The finding of increased numbers of pitted cells in the neonate may reflect reticuloendothelial or splenic hypofunction since this type of cell has been observed with such frequency only in patients without a spleen. Holroyde and Gardner[30] demonstrated that the indentations seen with interference-contrast microscopy are largely optical illusions that reflect the presence of erythrocyte inclusions and autophagic vacuoles beneath the cell membrane. The evidence further suggested that mature normal erythrocytes may continuously form vacuoles and that the majority are removed by the normal spleen.

In summary, the types of concretions within the red blood cell are numerous.[54] The red cell is derived from a nucleated precursor filled with the equipment for ferritin and hemoglobin synthesis with bits of nuclei (Howell-Jolly bodies), nuclear membranes (Cabot rings), remnants of ribosomes and RNA (basophilic stippling), ferrugonous granules (Pappenheimer bodies), traces of endoplasmic reticulum (reticulocytes), and inclusions of precipitated hemoglobin (Heinz bodies). These solid wastes are found in developing as well as in newly formed or more mature erythrocytes.

Bone marrow examination

Aspiration and biopsy of the bone marrow constitute a useful laboratory aid in the diagnosis of anemias.[11,71] The accessibility of the tissue, its responses to stimuli producing depression or hyperplasia, its availability for repeated examinations, and the comparative ease of identifying the cellular elements account for the frequency of performing these procedures. Disturbances of each of the principal blood elements are frequently reflected earlier or are more conspicuous in the bone marrow than in the peripheral blood. The technique and normal values in infancy and childhood are presented in Chapter 2.

Diagnostic features. Although the proliferation and differentiation of one cell type in the bone marrow progresses independently of the others, total hematopoietic stimulation is often observed in patients with hemolytic anemias and most regularly in those with acute hemolytic anemia. In the latter, regeneration of the red blood cells is associated with an increase in the number of granulocytes and platelets. The reverse occurs in patients with aplastic anemia in whom values for the three types of blood cells are depressed simultaneously. In persons with congenital or acquired hypoplastic anemia the production of red blood cells is inhibited without equal depression of myelopoiesis and platelet production. In persons with iron-deficiency anemia and in those with chronic loss of blood an increase in early erythroid precursors and megakaryocytes is often seen.

In patients with the hemolytic anemias the bone marrow is hyperplastic and there is an increased proliferation of normoblasts and, to a lesser extent, of pronormoblasts. Granulopoiesis may be active, especially in persons with acquired hemolytic anemia. In patients with these disorders the increase of nucleated red cells to more than 50% of all nucleated elements in the marrow constitutes an important diagnostic feature (Table 5-3).

Aplastic anemia is associated with profound anemia, leukopenia, neutropenia, and thrombocytopenia. The bone marrow shows a progressive decrease in cellularity, and there is a sharp reduction in the myeloid elements, nucleated red cells, and megakaryocytes with a relative increase in normal lymphocytes. Occasionally, acute lymphoblastic leukemia in the leukopenic stage may simulate aplastic anemia, and the diagnosis is difficult without histologic examination of the bone marrow.

Invasion of bone marrow by foreign cells. Abnormal elements characterizing a specific pathologic condition occasionally appear in the bone marrow and are associated with anemia. In younger patients these consist most commonly of metastatic neoplastic cells such as are found in patients with neuroblastoma and lymphosarcoma and less often the abnormal histiocytes of Letterer-Siwe disease or the lipid storage cells of Gaucher's disease, Niemann-Pick disease, or the generalized gangliosidoses.

Bone marrow smears obtained by aspiration from seventy-nine children with a variety of neoplasms were examined.[20] Tumor cells were found in marrow of twenty-one of thirty patients with metastatic neuroblastoma, three of eighteen with embryonal rhabdomyosarcoma, one of two with retinoblastoma, two of six with osteogenic sarcoma, and one of eight with Ewing's sarcoma. All children with recognizable bone marrow invasion died within 6 months. Although no cases of Wilms' tumor with bone marrow metastases were reported in this series, infrequently tumor cells can be demonstrated by routine aspiration.[56]

Characteristic tumor cells are found so commonly in patients with metastatic neuroblastoma that bone marrow examination is essential when this disease is expected. The presence of tumor cells in the bone narrow is not dependent on the existence of radiovisible bone lesions.[25] Ball-like masses or clusters of large immature cells form syncytial clumps or pseudorosettes with a mosaic pattern.[35] The individual cells are large, with nuclei possessing a finely dispersed chromatin pattern that stains deep blue. The cytoplasm is scant, faintly basophilic, and without granules.[25] Neuroblastoma may occasionally be confused with leukemia on bone marrow aspiration. The presence of discrete syncytia and scattered cells resembling lymphoblasts with indistinct or absent nucleoli are more likely to be diagnostic of neuroblastoma. The presence of immunologically active young lymphocytes, so-called immunoblasts, occurring singly in

Table 5-3. Diagnostic features of bone marrow in common anemias of infancy and childhood

Type of anemia	Diagnostic features
Hemolytic anemias	Hyperplastic marrow with increase of nucleated red cells, chiefly normoblasts; granulopoiesis may also be active; occasionally during crises, marrow aplastic instead of hyperplastic
Iron-deficiency anemia	Hyperplastic marrow with increase in basophilic normoblasts; granulopoiesis is unchanged; megakaryocytes sometimes increased
Hemorrhagic anemia	Hyperplastic marrow with increase in nucleated red cells, chiefly late normoblasts; granulopoiesis active in acute hemorrhage and unchanged in chronic loss of blood
Aplastic anemia	Usually decreased cellularity to acellular; sharp reduction in myeloid, erythroid, and megakaryocytic elements; increase in lymphocytes, and reticulum cells
Congenital hypoplastic anemia	Normal marrow except for absence of nucleated red cells

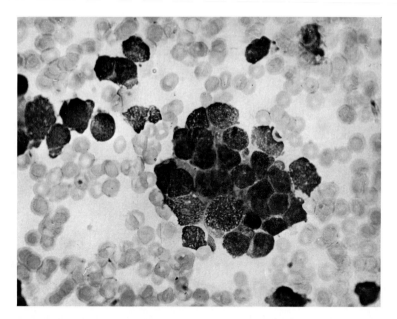

Fig. 5-1. Bone marrow smear in a case of neuroblastoma with splenomegaly and pancytopenia. Note tumor cells in ball-like clusters with scattering of cells resembling stem cells of leukemia in proximity. Diagnostic pseudorosettes are present in other portions of the smear. (×720.)

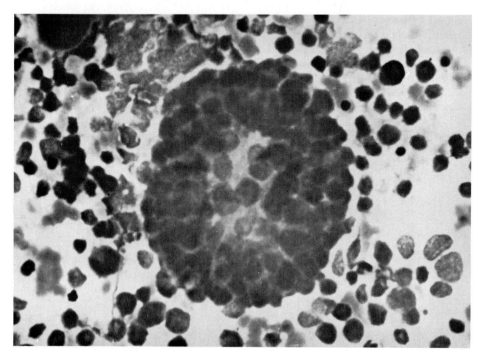

Fig. 5-2. Bone marrow smear in neuroblastoma in a 7-year-old child. Note the striking circular appearance of the rosette and the diffuse infiltration of neuroblastoma cells in the bone marrow. (Courtesy Dr. Philip Lanzkowsky, New York, N.Y.)

the marrows of patients with localized neuroblastoma should not be confused with metastatic neuroblastoma cells (Figs. 5-1 to 5-3).

Roentgenographic examination

The greater value of the roentgenogram in the diagnosis of anemia and other blood dyscrasias in infancy than in later childhood and adult life can be related to the developmental features of the bone marrow. The fact that all the bones are filled with red marrow is advantageous to the anemic infant and young child in whom the demand for erythropoiesis is so great. Fat appears in substantial amounts in the long bones at about 7 years of age. Only with the appearance of nonfunctioning yellow marrow in the older child and its extension in the young adult is a potential reservoir available for the emergency formation of blood. In the absence of yellow marrow, the infant or young child requiring increased blood formation reactivates extramedullary fetal sites of hematopoiesis. In addition, the marrow hypertrophies and expands by absorption and atrophy of the bony trabeculae and the cortex. These changes are observed in the roentgenograms and are of value in diagnosis. More detailed discussions of the radiologic changes are described in connection with the specific blood disorders in this book and in the books by Moseley[51,52] and by Caffey.[13]

The skeletal changes in the anemias of infancy and childhood are listed in Table 5-4.

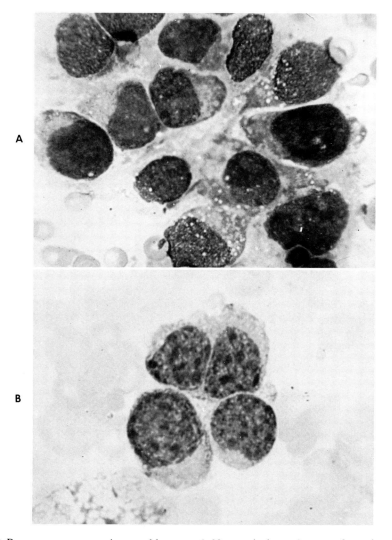

Fig. 5-3. Bone marrow smears in neuroblastoma. **A,** Note typical pseudorosette formation around a fibrillar network. **B,** Same formation as **A,** showing finer detail of individual cells in circular grouping. (×1,200.) (**A** courtesy Dr. Ralph L. Engle, Jr., New York, N.Y.)

Table 5-4. Skeletal changes in anemias of infancy and childhood

Diagnosis	Radiologic skeletal changes
Iron deficiency anemia	Skull: widened diploetic space, thin outer table, radial striation of trabeculae (''hair-on-end'')
	Long bones: widened marrow spaces, thinned cortices, coarsened trabeculae
Congenital hypoplastic anemia (Diamond-Blackfan syndrome)	Retarded bone maturation, triphalangeal thumb,[60] extra thumb, hypoplasia of middle phalanges of fifth fingers
Fanconi's aplastic anemia	Upper extremities: hypoplasia or aplasia of radial elements (thumb, first metacarpal, radial carpals, radius), hypoplasia of middle phalanx, fifth finger with clinodactyly
	Other: congenital dislocation of hip, flatfeet, clubfoot, extra terminal phalanges, Klippel-Feil deformity
Hereditary hemolytic anemias	
Hereditary spherocytosis	General roentgenographic evidence of marrow hyperplasia, improvement following splenectomy
Enzymopathies	Skeletal changes of marrow hyperplasia
Sickle cell anemia	Marrow hyperplasia, ''hand-foot'' syndrome
	Long bones: osteomyelitis, infarction, bone within bone, aseptic necrosis
	Vertebral column: osteoporosis, ''step deformity'' or depression of end-plate
Mixed hemoglobinopathies (S-C, S-thalassemia, S-D)	Osteoporosis of dorsolumbar spine, step deformity of end-plates, aseptic necrosis
Thalassemia major and intermedia	Severe manifestations of marrow hyperplasia, localized radiolucencies, skeletal dwarfism, premature fusion of epiphysis (humerus, femur, tibia, fibula)
	Skull and face: severe hair-on-end, inhibition of pneumatization of maxillary sinuses, maxillary overbite, ocular hypertelorism, malocculsion
	Thorax: ''rib-within-rib,'' notching of margins, bulbous expansion of posterior rib ends
	Vertebrae: demineralization
Thalassemia trait[67]	Widening of diploetic space, radial spiculation, osteoporosis
Osteopetrosis	Individual bones and skull opaque, heavy, lacking in fine structure; fractures, slipping of epiphyses
Leukemia	Destruction of spongiosa, erosion of cortex, periosteal elevation, osteoporosis, moth-eaten appearance, cystic rarefaction, transverse zones of diminished density in metaphyses

Hereditary factors in diagnosis

The genetic aspects of disease are manifested in a variety of anemias, notably erythroblastosis fetalis, the hemoglobinopathies, G-6-PD deficiency, hereditary spherocytosis, and elliptocytosis and the coagulation defects. Specific genetic implications are discussed in connection with each entity elsewhere in this book. The discovery of hereditary factors depends on the application of a painstaking family history and selected laboratory tests of the affected patient and asymptomatic relatives. Tests in common use include examination of the blood smear for morphologic abnormalities, fragility tests, serologic studies (complete blood grouping and HLA typing) for linkage and paternity, hemoglobin electrophoresis and quantification of minor hemoglobins, haptoglobin typing, isoenzyme characterization, and coagulation studies. An analysis of the data obtained from complete family studies usually provides insight into the genetic control of these disorders.

Thalassemia, sickle cell anemia, and hereditary spherocytosis may be cited as examples of familial diseases in which the hereditary trait may be recognized by suitable blood studies. Their hereditary nature is reflected in the relatively high incidence in members of the same family. The diagnosis of these diseases in a child with an obscure anemia of moderate severity often can be made earlier in its course and useless therapy avoided by detection of the trait in parents and siblings. In the patient with thalassemia, for instance, the most important element in the diagnosis of the milder form with the simpler means immediately available to the practitioner is the discovery of qualitatively similar alterations in the blood of other family members. These persons are asymptomatic and have either mild anemia or no anemia. Regardless of the hemoglobin level, their blood usually shows hypochromic macrocytes, stippled erythrocytes, polycythemia, low MCV, increased resistance of the red cells to hemolysis in hypotonic solutions of

Table 5-5. Therapy of common anemias of infancy and childhood

Therapeutic agent	Type of anemia
Iron	Iron-deficiency anemia, anemia of prematurity, chronic blood loss, pregnancy
Folic acid, vitamin B_{12}	Megaloblastic anemias
Corticosteroids	Autoimmune hemolytic anemia, congenital hypoplastic anemia, aplastic anemia
Androgenic steroids	Aplastic anemia
Transfusion	Exchange transfusion in erythroblastosis fetalis, acute and chronic blood loss, aplastic and hypoplastic anemias, hereditary and acquired hemolytic anemias, leukemia and other malignancies, coagulation defects
Splenectomy	Hereditary spherocytosis, selected red cell enzyme deficiency diseases (pyruvate kinase), thalassemia major and intermedia, hypersplenism, autoimmune hemolytic anemia
Bone marrow transplantation	Aplastic anemia

sodium chloride, and less frequently target or oval cells. The evidence is conclusive that, in every family with a child having thalassemia major requiring periodic transfusions, both parents reveal evidence of the trait, assuming that nonpaternity is excluded. In rare cases of the silent carrier state, more demanding determinations of the synthetic ratio of α-and non-α-globin chains must be performed. When this bilateral inheritance of the gene for thalassemia is nonexistent, a search should be made for the presence of another abnormal hemoglobin in the seemingly unaffected parent.

PRINCIPLES OF TREATMENT

The information gathered thus far has provided a sufficiently firm foundation with respect to etiology to warrant a consideration of therapy. In Table 5-5 are listed some of the available agents in current use designed to correct an underlying deficiency or to ameliorate the disorder by accessory means when direct remedies are not available. The constant emphasis on the use of specific rather than indiscriminate mixtures of antianemia substances[81] applies with particular force to children. Iron salts given orally in the ferrous form without the aid of supplementary minerals or vitamins still constitute the most effective treatment of iron-deficiency anemia. Treatment with iron salts in patients with other conditions may be not only futile but also potentially harmful. The anemias for which transfusions are indicated consist of two groups: those in which this measure constitutes a temporary expedient until spontaneous recovery occurs and those in which, in the absence of specific therapy, the need for restoration of optimum levels of hemoglobin is continuous or urgent. Transfusion therapy is discussed in detail in Chapter 4. The indications for splenectomy in the anemias are discussed under specific disease entities.

REFERENCES

1. Ackerman, B. D.: Infantile pyknocytosis in Mexican-American infants, Am. J. Dis. Child. **117:**417, 1969.
2. Aherne, W. A.: The "burr" red cell and azotaemia, J. Clin. Pathol. **10:**252, 1957.
3. Barrett, A. M.: Special forms of erythrocytes possessing increased resistance to hypotonic saline, J. Pathol. Bacteriol. **46:**603, 1938.
4. Bassen, F. A., and Kornzweig, A. L.: Malformation of the erythrocytes in a case of atypical retinitis pigmentosa, Blood **5:**381, 1950.
5. Bell, R. E.: The origin of "burr" erythrocytes, Br. J. Haematol. **9:**552, 1963.
6. Beritic, T.: Siderotic granules and granules of punctate basophilia, Br. J. Haematol. **9:**185, 1963.
7. Bessis, M., and Bricka, M.: Aspect dynamique des cellules du sang. Son étude par la microcinématographic en contrast de phase, Rev. Hématol. **7:**407, 1952.
8. Bevan, G. H., and White, J. C.: Oxidation of phenylhydrazines in the presence of oxyhemoglobin and the origin of Heinz bodies in erythrocytes, Nature **173:**389, 1954.
9. Brain, M. C., Dacie, J. V., and Hourihane, D. D. B.: Microangiopathic haemolytic anaemia, the possible role of vascular lesions in pathogenesis, Br. J. Haematol. **8:**358, 1962.
10. Bull, B. S., Rutenberg, M. L., Dacie, J. V., and Brain, M. C.: Microangiopathic haemolytic anaemia: mechanisms of red cell fragmentation, in vitro studies, Br. J. Haematol. **14:**643, 1968.
11. Burney S. W.: Bone marrow examination: technique and diagnostic value of a bone marrow biopsy using a Silverman needle, J.A.M.A. **195:**171, 1966.
12. Bush, J. A., and Ainger, L. E.: Congenital absence of the spleen with congenital heart disease, Pediatrics **15:**93, 1955.
13. Caffey, J.: Pediatric x-ray diagnosis, Chicago, 1956, Year Book Medical Publishers, Inc.
14. Cartwright, G. E., and Deiss, A.: Sideroblasts, siderocytes, and sideroblastic anemia, N. Engl. J. Med. **292:**185, 1975.
15. Cooper, R. A.: Anemia with spur cells. A red cell defect acquired in serum and modified in the circulation, J. Clin. Invest. **48:**1820, 1969.
16. Cooper, R. A., and Jandl, J. H.: Bile salts and cholesterol in the pathogenesis of target cells in obstructive jaundice, J. Clin. Invest. **47:**809, 1968.
17. Crookston, J. H., Crookston, M. C., Burnie, K. L., et al.: Hereditary erythroblastic multinuclearity associated with a positive acidified-serum test: a type of congenital dyserythropoietic anemia, Br. J. Haematol. **17:**11, 1969.
18. Crosby, W. H.: Normal functions of the spleen relative to the red cells: a review, Blood **14:**399, 1959.
19. Dacie, J. V., and Mollin, D. L.: Siderocytes, sidero-

blasts, and sideroblastic anemia, Acta Med. Scand. **445**(suppl.): 237, 1966.

20. Delta, B. G., and Pinkel, D.: Bone marrow aspiration in children with malignant tumors, J. Pediatr. **64:**542, 1964.
21. Duffy, T. P.: Anemia in adolescence, Med. Clin. North Am. **59:**1481, 1975.
22. Fadem, R. S.: Ovalocytosis associated with sickle cell trait, Blood **4:**505, 1949.
23. Fertman, M. H., and Fertman, M. A.: Toxic anemia and Heinz bodies, Medicine **34:**131, 1955.
24. Finch, C. A., and Noyes, W. D.: Erythrokinetics in diagnosis of anemia, J.A.M.A. **175:**1163, 1961.
25. Gaffney, P. C., Hausman, C. F., and Fetterman, G. H.: Experience with smears of aspirates from bone marrow in the diagnosis of neuroblastoma, Am. J. Clin. Pathol. **31:**213, 1959.
26. Gasser, C., and Wili, H.: Spontane Innenkörpubildung bei milzagenesia, Helvet. Paediatr. Acta **7:**369, 1952.
27. Grahn, E. P., Dietz, A. A., Stefani, S. S. and Donnelly, W. J.: Burr cells, hemolytic anemia and cirrhosis, Am. J. Med. **45:**78, 1968.
28. Guest, G. M., and Brown, E. W.: Erythrocytes and hemoglobin of the blood in infancy and childhood. III. Factors in variability; statistical studies, Am. J. Dis. Child. **93:**486, 1957.
29. Harley, J. D., and Mauer, A. M.: Studies on the formation of Heinz bodies. II. The nature and significance of Heinz bodies, Blood **17:**418, 1961.
30. Holroyde, C. P., and Gardner, F. H.: Acquisition of autophagic vacuoles by human erythrocytes; physiologic role of the spleen, Blood **36:**566, 1970.
31. Holroyde, C. P., Oski, F. A., and Gardner, F. J.: The "pocked" erythrocyte: red-cell surface alterations in reticuloendothelial immaturity of the neonate, N. Engl. J. Med. **281:**516, 1969.
32. Hutchinson, H. E., and Ferguson-Smith, M. A.: The significance of Howell-Jolly bodies in red cell precursors, J. Clin. Pathol. **12:**451, 1959.
33. Kaplan, E., Zuelzer, W. W., and Mouriguand, C.: Sideroblasts: a study of stainable nonhemoglobin iron in marrow normoblasts, Blood **9:**203, 1954.
34. Kaplan, E., Zuelzer, W. W., and Neil, J. F.: Further studies on hemoglobin C: the hematologic effects of hemoglobin C alone and in combination with sickle cell hemoglobin. Blood **8:**735, 1953.
35. Kato, K., and Wachter, H. E.: Adrenal sympathicoblastoma in children: with special reference to the biopsy of sternal marrow and of metastatic nodule in the skull, J. Pediatr. **12:**449, 1938.
36. Keimowitz, R., and Desforges, J. F.: Infantile pyknocytosis, N. Engl. J. Med. **273:**1152, 1965.
37. Kent, G., and Minick, O. T.: Autophagic vacuoles in human red cells, Am. J. Pathol. **48:**831, 1966.
38. Kirkman, H. N., and Riley, H. D.: Posthemorrhagic anemia and shock in the newborn: a review, Pediatrics **24:**97, 1959.
39. Kornzweig, A. L., and Bassen, F. A.: Retinitis pigmentosa, acanthocytosis, and heredodegenerative neuromuscular disease, Arch. Ophthalmal. **58:**183, 1957.
40. Kwant, W. D., and van Steveninck, J.: The influence of chlorpromazine on human erythrocytes, Biochem. Pharmacol. **17:**2215, 1968.
41. Lamy, F., Frezal, J., Polonovski, J., et al.: Congenital absence of beta lipoproteins, Pediatrics **31:**277, 1963.
42. Lewis, S. M.: Red-cell abnormalities and haemolysis in aplastic anaemia, Br. J. Haematol. **8:**322, 1962.
43. Linman, J. W.: Physiologic and pathophysiologic effects of anemia, N. Engl. J. Med. **279:**812, 1968.
44. Lipton, E. L.: Elliptocytosis with hemolytic anemia; the effects of splenectomy, Pediatrics **15:**67, 1955.
45. Lock, S. P., Smith, R. S., and Hardisty, R. M.: Stomato-

cytosis; a hereditary red cell anomaly associated with haemolytic anaemia, Br. J. Haematol. **7:**303, 1961.
46. Lyons, W. S., Hanlon, D. G., Helmholz, J. F., Jr., and Edwards, J. E.: Congenital cardiac disease and asplenia; report of seven cases, Proc. Staff Meet. Mayo Clin. **32:**277, 1957.
47. McBryde, R. R., Hewlett, J. S., and Weisman, R., Jr.: Elliptocytosis: a study of erythrocyte survival using radioactive chromium (Cr^{51}), Am. J. Med. Sci. **232:**258, 1956.
48. Meadow, S. R.: Stomatocytosis, Proc. R. Soc. Med. **60:**13, 1967.
49. Miller, D. R., Rickles, F. R., Weed, R. I., et al.: A new variant of hereditary hemolytic anemia with stomatocytosis and erythrocyte cation abnormality, Blood **38:**184, 1971.
50. Miller, G., Townes, P. L., and MacWhinney, J. B.: A new congenital hemolytic anemia with deformed erythrocytes (?"stomatocytes") and remarkable susceptibility of erythrocytes to cold hemolysis in vitro. I. Clinical and hematologic studies, Pediatrics **35:**906, 1965.
51. Moseley, J. E.: Bone changes in hematologic disorders (roentgen aspects), New York, 1963, Grune & Stratton, Inc.
52. Moseley, J. E.: Skeletal changes in the anemias, Semin. Roentgenol. **9:**169, 1974.
53. Motulsky, A. G., Singer, K., Crosby, W. H., and Smith, V.: The life span of the elliptocyte: hereditary elliptocytosis and its relationship to other familial hemolytic diseases, Blood **9:**57, 1954.
54. Nathan, D. G.: Rubbish in the red cell, N. Engl. J. Med. **281:**558, 1969.
55. Nathan, D. G., Oski, F. A., Sidel, V. W., et al.: Studies of erythrocyte spicule formation in haemolytic anaemias, Br. J. Haematol. **12:**385, 1966.
56. O'Neill, P., and Pinkel, D.: Wilms' tumor in bone marrow aspirate, J. Pediatr. **72:**396, 1968.
57. Oski, F. A., and Barness, L. A.: Vitamin E deficiency in recognized cause of hemolytic anemia in the premature infant, J. Pediatr. **70:**211, 1963.
58. Oski, F. A., Nathan, D. G., Sidel, V. W., and Diamond, L. K.: Extreme hemolysis and red cell distortion in erythrocyte kinase deficiency. I. Morphology, erythrokinetics, and family enzyme studies, N. Engl. J. Med. **270:**1023, 1964.
59. Pappenheimer, A. M., Thompson, K. P., Parker, D. D., and Smith, K. E.: Anaemia associated with unidentified erythrocytic inclusions after splenectomy, Q. J. Med. **14:**75, 1945.
60. Qazi, Q. H., and Smithwick, E. M.: Triphalangy of thumbs and great toes, Am. J. Dis. Child. **120:**255, 1960.
61. Rundles, R. W., and Falls, H. F.: Hereditary (?sex-linked) anemia, Am. J. Med. Sci. **211:**641, 1946.
62. Schleicher, E. M.: Origin and nature of the Cabot ring bodies of erythrocytes, J. Lab. Clin. Med. **27:**983, 1942.
63. Schwartz, S. O., and Motto, S. A.: The diagnostic significance of "burr" red blood cells, Am. J. Med. Sci. **218:**563, 1949.
64. Scott, R. B., Crawford, R. P., and Jenkins, M.: Incidence of sicklemia in the newborn Negro infant, Am. J. Dis. Child. **75:**842, 1948.
65. Seeman, P., and Kwant, W. D.: Membrane expansion of the erythrocyte by both the neutral and ionized forms of chlorpromazine, Biochem. Biophys. Acta **183:**512, 1969.
66. Selwyn, J. G.: Heinz bodies in red cells after splenectomy and after phenacitin administration, Br. J. Haematol. **1:**173, 1955.
67. Sfikakis, P., and Stamatoyannopoulos, G.: Bone changes in thalassemia trait, Acta Haematol. **29:**193, 1963.
68. Silber, R., Amorosi, E., Lhowe, J., and Kayden, J. H.: Spur-shaped erythrocytes in Laennec's cirrhosis, N. Engl. J. Med. **275:**639, 1966.

69. Singer, K., and Fisher, B.: Studies on abnormal hemoglobins, Blood **8:**270, 1953.

70. Singer, K., Fisher, B., and Perlstein, M. A.: Acanthrocytosis: a genetic erythrocytic malformation, Blood **7:**577, 1952.

71. Smith, C. H.: Bone marrow examination in blood disorders of infants and children, Med. Clin. N. Am. **31:**527, 1947.

72. Smith, C. H.: Anemias in infancy and childhood: diagnosis and therapeutic considerations, Bull. N.Y. Acad. Med. **30:**155, 1954.

73. Smith, C. H., and Khakoo, Y.: Burr cells: classification and effect of splenectomy, J. Pediatr. **76:**99, 1970.

74. Smith, J. A., Lonergan, E. T., and Sterling, K.: Spur-cell anemia: hemolytic anemia with red cells resembling acantocytes in alcoholic cirrhosis, N. Engl. J. Med. **271:**369, 1964.

75. Sturgeon, P., Itans, H. A., and Bergren, W. R.: Clinical manifestations of inherited abnormal hemoglobins; the interaction of hemoglobin-S with hemoglobin-D, Blood **10:**389, 1955.

76. Steveninck, J. V., Gjosund, W. K., and Booij, H. L.: The influence of chlorpromazine on the osmotic fragility of erythrocytes, Biochem. Pharmacol. **16:**837, 1967.

77. Tuffy, P., Brown, A. K., and Zuelzer, W. N.: Infantile pyknocytosis, a common erythrocyte abnormality of the first trimester, Am. J. Dis. Child. **98:**227, 1967.

78. Valentine, W. N., Fink, K., Paglia, D. E., et al.: Hereditary hemolytic anemia with human erythrocyte pyrimidine 5'-nucleotidase deficiency, J. Clin. Invest. **54:**866, 1974.

79. Van Dyke, D. C., Shkurkin, C., et al.: Differences in distribution of erythropoietic and reticuloendothelial marrow in hematologic disease, Blood **30:**364, 1967.

80. Watson, J., Stahman, A. W., and Bilello, F. P.: The significance of the paucity of sickle cells in newborn Negro infants, Am. J. Med. Sci. **215:**419, 1948.

81. Wintrobe, M. M.: Shotgun antianemic therapy (editorial), Am. J. Med. **15:**142, 1953.

82. Wyandt, H., Bancroft, I. M., and Winship, T. D.: Elliptic erythrocytes in man, Arch. Intern. Med. **68:**1043, 1941.

83. Zannos-Mariolea, L., Kattamis, C., and Paidoucis, M.: Infantile pyknocytosis and glucose-6-phosphate dehydrogenase deficiency, Br. J. Haematol. **8:**258, 1962.

6 □ Iron metabolism and iron-deficiency anemia

Philip Lanzkowsky

Iron-deficiency anemia is the most common nutritional deficiency in children and is widespread in pediatric populations throughout the world. It is especially prevalent in infancy. The trace amounts of iron in many diets, the limited ability of the human body to absorb dietary iron, the need of iron for growth, as well as the high incidence of parasitism and gastrointestinal blood loss in some populations make infants and children especially vulnerable to develop negative iron balance and iron-deficiency anemia. Iron is critical for certain metabolic and enzymatic processes; it is essential for growth; it plays a vital role in the structure of the hemoglobin molecule; and it is present in the body in larger amounts than any other trace metals.

BIOCHEMISTRY OF IRON

Iron, abundant in the earth's crust, has unique and subtle chemical properties and carries out a variety of biologic functions. It is responsible for the transport of oxygen (hemoglobin and myoglobin), the activation of both molecular nitrogen and oxygen (nitrogenases, oxygenases, and oxidases), and electron transport (cytochromes). In addition, because of the propensity of iron to hydrolyze in aqueous solution, special molecules have been designed for its transport (transferrin) and storage (ferritin).

Iron compounds can be classified into the following functional categories:

1. Hemoglobin and myoglobin: heme-containing proteins that combine reversibly with oxygen
2. Cytochromes *a, b,* and *c:* heme-containing proteins involved with electron transport
3. Peroxidases: heme-containing proteins that activate hydrogen peroxide to accept two electrons from various substrates
4. Catalase: heme-containing protein that converts hydrogen peroxide to water and oxygen
5. Succinic dehydrogenase, lactic dehydrogenase, and xanthine oxidase: flavoproteins that are linked to iron and function as electron acceptors
6. Transferrin, ferritin, and hemosiderin: proteins that act as transport or storage iron

The average adult has about 3 to 5 gm of iron in the body, of which 2 to 3 gm is found in the hemoglobin, 1 to 1.5 gm in the body stores as ferritin and hemosiderin, and the rest in myoglobin, respiratory enzymes, and the plasma.

Iron-containing compounds can thus be grouped into two main categories: those serving a metabolic or enzymatic function and those associated with iron storage and transport.

Metabolic or enzymatic function

This category of iron compounds consists almost entirely of heme protein, i.e., proteins with an iron-porphyrin prosthetic group. The compounds that fall into this group consist of: hemoglobin; myoglobin; cytochromes *a, b,* and *c;* peroxidase; and catalase.

The function of all heme protein is related to oxidative metabolism. The heme compounds (hemoglobin and myoglobin) bind oxygen in a reversible way. Heme enzymes (cytochromes, peroxidase, and catalase) make oxygen available for intracellular oxidation.

Hemoglobin is the most abundant of this group and accounts for more than 65% of body iron. Its function is to transport oxygen via the bloodstream. Hemoglobin is a tetramer made up of four globin chains, each associated with a heme group that contains one iron atom. Its molecular weight is 64,450 daltons and it accounts for more than 99% of the protein in the red cell.

Myoglobin is the red pigment of muscle that stores oxygen for utilization during muscle contraction. It accounts for about 3% of the total body iron. Myoglobin has a molecular weight of 17,000 daltons. Its structure is closely related to the monomeric units of hemoglobin, e.g., it is made of one globin chain attached to a heme group with a single iron atom. The myoglobin concentration in human muscle is 1 to 3 mg/gm of tissue.

Cytochromes are the electron transport enzymes located in the mitochondria as well as in other cellular membranes. They are essential for the transfer of electrons from substrates to molecular oxygen with the simultaneous generation of ATP. In the process of electron transfer the iron atoms in the cytochromes are alternately oxidized and reduced. Cytochrome *c,* the best characterized of the cytochromes, is made up of one globin chain and one heme group containing an atom of iron. It has a molecular weight of 13,000 daltons. The concentration of cytochrome *c* is between 5 and 100 μg/gm tissue. The highest concentrations are in tissues that have a high rate of oxygen utilization such as heart muscle.

Catalase and peroxidase are widely distributed in the body and function in the reduction of endogenously generated hydrogen peroxide. Catalase is a large molecule having a molecular weight of about 240,000 daltons; it contains four heme groups, each with one iron atom. The composition of various peroxidases is not well defined. The myeloperoxidase of the granulocyte is known to contain iron, but the presence of iron in glutathione peroxidase in the red cell has not been established.

In addition there is a group of iron proteins that have an enzymatic function but in which the iron is not in the form of heme. A portion of the iron in these nonheme compounds is present in a group of compounds designated as the metalloflavoproteins. These compounds, which include NADH dehydrogenase and succinate dehydrogenase, are all involved in oxidative metabolism and contain iron and flavin prosthetic groups.

Storage and transport function

The iron-containing compounds concerned with iron storage and transport include ferritin, hemosiderin, and transferrin.

Ferritin and hemosiderin are present primarily in the liver, the erythroid precursors of the bone marrow, and the reticuloendothelial cells. Approximately one third of storage iron is in the liver, one third in the bone marrow, and the remaining one third in the spleen and other tissues. The total amount of storage iron in the body is subject to marked variations. Storage iron exists primarily in ferric salt–protein complexes. The protein portion of ferritin, apoferritin, is homogeneous and is believed to consist of twenty-four identical subunits. The subunits form a spherical cluster around hydrated ferric phosphate in a central colloidal core to make up ferritin. Ferritin contains up to 25% iron and has a molecular weight as high as 900,000 daltons.

Hemosiderin is an ill-defined, chemically heterogeneous group of large iron-salt-protein aggregates. This term is usually applied to iron that, after staining with potassium ferrocyanide, can be seen as blue granules in sections of liver or bone marrow. Under the electron microscope it can be seen that such granules may contain anything from closely packed and well-ordered ferritin molecules

to amorphous deposits of iron.[175] The preparations contain more iron than ferritin (about 30% dry weight) with less nitrogen and a higher proportion of phosphorus.[154] The origin of hemosiderin, its function as an iron store, and its relationship with ferritin are not clearly understood.[175]

Transferrin accounts for a small fraction of 1% of the total body iron. Transferrin is a β_1-globulin with a molecular weight of about 74,000 daltons, that is capable of binding two atoms of ferric iron at specific sites on the protein. Its major role is to transport iron released from hemoglobin catabolism or absorbed from the intestinal lumen to the bone marrow for synthesis of hemoglobin. Transferrin can bind many metals, but iron will displace other metals from the complex so that, except for iron, the physiologic significance of the metal binding is uncertain.

There are at least twenty-one variants of transferrin in humans that have been separated by electrophoresis in starch or polyacrylamide gels.[305] Turnbull and Giblett[381] found no evidence for differences in the plasma clearance or utilization of radioiron bound to four different transferrins or in the iron binding in vitro. Transferrin synthesis occurs mainly in the liver in adult animals although synthesis has been demonstrated in a wide variety of tissues.[271] The protein is synthesized on ribosomes of the rough endoplasmic reticulum with attachment of carbohydrate during passage through the smooth endoplasmic reticulum and Golgi vesicles before eventual secretion into the plasma. No single tissue appears to predominate in transferrin breakdown.

Lactoferrin is a transferrin-like protein found in milk and other secretions[245] and in neutrophils.[246] Both lactoferrin and transferrin have the same molecular weight and iron-binding properties although the binding constant for one iron per molecule is greater for lactoferrin than transferrin.[3] There are differences in amino acid sequences[261] and there is little or no immunologic cross-reaction between the two proteins.[94] The function of lactoferrin is still uncertain although it may have a bacteriostatic activity related to its powerful iron-binding activity.[245] Table 6-1 lists the distribution and function of iron compounds.

METABOLISM OF IRON
Absorption

Iron can probably be absorbed from any part of the gastrointestinal tract, although absorption is greatest in the duodenum and diminishes progressively in the more distal portion of the bowel.

This localization is partly related to such intraluminal factors as pH and the redox potential, but a decreasing capacity to absorb iron in the more distal segments of the bowel has been demon-

Table 6-1. Distribution and function of iron compounds

Protein	Mol. wt.	Distribution	Function
Heme-containing			
Hemoglobin	65,000	Red blood cells	Oxygen carrier
Myoglobin	17,000	Muscle	Oxygen carrier
Cytochrome aa_3	180,000	Mitochondria	Terminal oxidase
b	18,000-30,000	Mitochondria	Electron transport
c_1	37,000	Mitochondria	Electron transport
c	12,000	Mitochondria	Electron transport
Catalase	240,000	Red blood cells	Peroxide breakdown
Lactoperoxidase	93,000	Milk	Peroxide breakdown
Nonheme			
Succinate dehydrogenase Fe-S protein	27,000	Mitochondria	Electron transport
Succinate dehydrogenase flavoprotein	70,000	Mitochondria	Electron transport
NADH dehydrogenase		Mitochondria	Electron transport
Xanthine oxidase	275,000	Milk, tissue	Hypoxanthine → uric acid
Transferrin	77,000	Plasma	Iron transport
Lactoferrin	77,000	Milk, secretions	Iron transport
Ferritin	450,000-900,000	All tissues	Iron storage
Hemosiderin		Liver, spleen, bone marrow	Iron storage

strated independent of intraluminal factors. The absorption of food iron, however, occurs mainly if not exclusively in the duodenum.

There appear to be at least two distinct pathways for iron absorption: one for iron attached to heme[38,380,396] and another for iron in the form of ferrous iron (or possibly soluble ferrous chelates).[268] Dietary iron must be converted to one of these two forms to be absorbed. Heme iron is derived from the hemoglobin, myoglobin, and other heme proteins in foods of animal origin and is an important dietary source of iron. In the absorption of hemoglobin iron and presumably iron in all heme compounds, heme is split from its apoprotein by the acid and proteases of gastric juice. The heme moiety enters absorptive cells where iron is split from the porphyrin ring by a process with features of an enzymatic mechanism, possibly involving a xanthine oxidase–dependent peroxidation[91] that effects the release of iron and permits its passage from the mucosal cell into the plasma in the same manner as ionic iron.[396] Since control of iron absorption principally seems to involve regulation of the mechanism that moves iron from mucosa to plasma, a single regulatory system may control iron absorption regardless of the dietary source.

Role of mucosal cell. The mucosal cell has two important roles in iron absorption: (1) mucosal uptake and (2) transfer of iron from the brush border to the lamina propria, where it enters the plasma.[328,399] Both steps represent energy-dependent, active transport processes.

Iron may be present within the cell in two forms —as a labile form rapidly transported across the cell or as ferritin, a more stable form that remains within the cell. Mucosal uptake occurs rapidly at the brush border of the mucosal cell.[14,128] Within a few hours the newly acquired iron is found to be associated with the rough endoplasmic reticulum and with free ribosomes.[14] Some of it may be present in cytoplasm as unbound iron salts or complexes of low molecular weight.[348] A proportion of the iron taken into the cell is delivered into the plasma within a few hours[292]—the labile form. The remainder is incorporated into mucosal ferritin,[52,348] an intracellular iron—a stable form. Much of the mucosal ferritin iron is sloughed into the intestine with the cell after the mucosal cell has completed its 3- to 4-day life span.[70] This represents a modified "mucosal block" theory. In addition to the labile form and the stable form, a "delayed phase" of iron absorption occurs between 3 and 24 hours and may represent mobilization from ferritin or other intracellular binding sites.[292]

The division of iron metabolism into two major pathways within the cell probably exerts a regulatory reaction. If iron metabolism is shunted toward the labile rapid transport route, iron absorption is increased. This occurs when the storage iron is depleted or when red cell production is increased. If iron is shunted toward the more stable ferritin route, the iron stays mostly within the cell and is lost back into the lumen when the cell is sloughed from the villous crypts. Iron absorption would

NORMAL

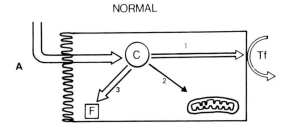

A

IRON DEFICIENT

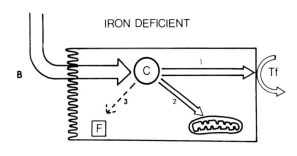

B

IRON LOADED

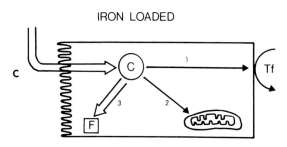

C

Fig. 6-1. Iron uptake and metabolic pathways within the small intestinal epithelial cell. Pathway *1* represents iron transfer from carrier pool *(C)* to plasma; pathway *2*, iron transfer to mitochondria for heme synthesis; and pathway *3*, iron incorporation in ferritin *(F)*. **A,** Normal iron status. **B,** Iron deficiency: increased mucosal uptake because of mitochondrial requirements with increased transfer along pathways *1* and *2* and no transfer along pathway *3*. **C,** Iron overload: normal iron uptake with decreased transfer along pathway *1* and increased ferritin formation via pathway *3*. *Tf,* Transferrin. (From Jacobs, A.: Clin. Haematol. **2:**323, 1973.)

thus be decreased; this occurs when iron storage is excessive or when red cell production rate is decreased. A feedback control mechanism linking erythroid activity and iron stores to the intestinal mucosa seems to be present.

Experiments in rats showed that endogenous iron is incorporated into mucosal cells as they are formed in the crypts of Lieberkühn.[62,70,403] The subsequent absorptive behavior of the mucosal cell is regulated by the amount of iron incorporated into the cell when it is formed in the crypts of Lie-

berkühn. The amount of iron incorporated is thought to be dependent on plasma iron clearance, reflecting mainly iron requirements for hemoglobin synthesis. When iron stores are excessive or erythropoiesis depressed, increased iron is incorporated into newly forming mucosal cells and iron absorption is decreased. On the other hand, when an increase in erythropoiesis occurs, increased amounts of plasma iron would be diverted to the bone marrow and consequently less iron would be incorporated into newly forming mucosal cells. Therefore a decrease occurs either in total iron content of the cell or in the amount of iron incorporated into a specific compound in mucosal cells. This would result in less inhibition of the absorptive mechanism, and an increase in the absorptive capacity occurs.

Depending on the amount of iron incorporated into newly formed mucosal cells, iron taken up from the gut can either proceed into the plasma or be incorporated into ferritin to be sloughed at the end of the life span of the mucosal cell. Mucosal iron has been found to be reduced in a supernatant fraction of mucosal homogenate from both iron-deficient and hemolyzing animals.[348] It is possible that the messenger iron enters a critical subcellular location such as the mitochondria[423] or that it partially saturates a "carrier" essential to absorption.[292,295,375] It is clear therefore that the mucosal cell has a mechanism for transporting iron across the cell into the plasma and a mechanism for trapping iron in the mucosal cell for excretion when the cell sloughs. Wheby has proposed a model, shown in Fig. 6-1, that provides a useful concept of the functioning of the mucosal cell with reference to iron absorption.[398]

This explanation of iron absorption has replaced the "mucosal block" theory of Hahn et al.[139] that considered iron absorption dependent on the degree of "physiologic saturation" of the mucosal receptor, which they speculated to be ferritin or its precursor, apoferritin. This theory was based on observations in dogs that oral administration of iron partially blocked the absorption of a second dose given several hours later and the observations of Granick[127] that, in guinea pigs, oral iron stimulated the mucosal cells to produce a protein, apoferritin, which combines with iron to form ferritin. According to this concept, ferritin acted as a blocking agent. When the ferrous iron in the lumen of the intestine was in equilibrium with the ferric iron in the mucosal cells, no ferrous iron would be absorbed. After the ferric iron content of the cells was diminished by passage of iron from the mucosal ferritin into the bloodstream, iron would pass from the lumen into the mucosa. It was recognized in normal persons or in patients with certain diseases (particularly hemochromatosis) that any blocking mechanism that might exist was not completely effective. Evidence against the existence of mucosal block as a physiologic mechanism was reported by Brown and Justus[34] and Heilmeyer.[156a]

• • •

In addition to the factors already mentioned, the quantity of iron absorbed after digestion is influenced by a number of intraluminal and extraluminal factors.

A. Intraluminal factors
    1. Amount of iron
    2. Type of iron
    3. Relationship to food
       a. Presence or absence of food
       b. Nature of food
       c. Enhancing substances
       d. Inhibiting substances
    4. Role of gastrointestinal tract
       a. Gastric factors
       b. Pancreatic factors
       c. Bile
B. Extraluminal factors
    1. Body iron stores
    2. Erythropoietic activity
    3. Growth

Intraluminal factors

Amount of iron. Increasing the amount of iron ingested increases the amount absorbed, even though the percentage of absorption is smaller with larger amounts of iron.[26,414]

Type of iron. Ferrous iron is absorbed better than ferric iron. Heme iron, which accounts for 80% of the soluble iron compounds in meat, is absorbed in a highly efficient manner and has a high nutritive value in meeting the body's needs for iron. The absorption of heme iron occurs by a mechanism different from that involved in the absorption of nonheme iron present in food or inorganic iron[227] and is not altered by the status of iron stores and iron demand or the presence of ascorbic acid, phytates, or chelating agents.

Relationship to food

PRESENCE OR ABSENCE OF FOOD. Absorption of iron is reduced approximately 50% merely by mixing ferrous salts in food.

NATURE OF FOOD. Food iron ultimately must be converted to the ferrous form to be absorbed.[268] Since the ease with which this conversion is accomplished differs according to the nature of the iron compound, the "availability" of food iron is quite variable.[263] The range of iron absorption from biosynthetically labeled food is 1% to 22%. Meat and animal products are at the upper end and food of vegetable origin at the lower end of this range. Fish muscle and animal muscle have an enhancing effect on the absorption of iron from vegetable foods, whereas milk, butter, and eggs are animal protein foods that do not enhance the absorption of vegetable iron. This has significance to the pediatrician. Iron present in vegetable or plant sources is absorbed less well than iron in animal tissues (a large portion of which is heme iron). If animal and plant sources of food iron are fed in combination, the absorption of iron from the vegetable sources is increased significantly.

The reason for this might be that several of the amino acids, particularly cystine, lysine, and histidine, have been found to be effective in increasing the absorption of ferric iron. Layrisse et al.[227] added nine amino acids to a vegetable diet and demonstrated an increase in the absorption of vegetable iron when the amino acids were present in a proportion similar to that in fish muscle. In foods derived from grains, iron often forms a stable complex of phytates (phosphorus-containing salts of phytic acid) and only small amounts of such iron can be converted to the absorbable form.[347] Similarly the iron in egg yolk is not readily absorbed, probably because it is complexed with phosphates or phosphoproteins.[263] The exact nature of iron in many other foods is not known. However, it appears to be mainly in the ferric state, much of it as ferric hydroxide or loosely bound to organic molecules such as sugars, citrates, lactate, and the amino acids.

ENHANCING SUBSTANCES. Enhancing substances include ascorbic acid and other reducing substances, the presence of amino acids, and the presence of simple sugars such as lactose and fructose to a greater degree than sucrose or glucose. Chelation with these substances greatly enhances subsequent absorption since the chelation in the acid medium of the stomach may maintain inorganic iron in a more soluble and readily absorbable form within the small bowel lumen.

INHIBITING SUBSTANCES. Compounds forming insoluble complexes with iron such as phosphate, phytates, and oxalates decrease absorption.

Role of gastrointestinal tract

GASTRIC FACTORS. The acid gastric juice is a medium in which solubilization and reduction of iron are favored; consequently absorption of ferric iron is impaired in patients with gastrectomy or achlorhydria.*

The gastric juice of healthy persons contains a high molecular weight iron-binding protein that has been designated as gastroferrin.[90] The characteristics of gastroferrin are as follows:

A. Molecular weight 260,000
B. Glycoprotein
    1. Carbohydrate—85%
       a. Glucosamine
       b. Galactosamine

---

*References 66, 177, 258, 274.

c. Galactose
d. Fucose
e. Sialic acid
2. Protein—15%
C. Resistant to pepsin and trypsin digestion
D. Stable pH 1.0 to 8.5

Normally there is sufficient gastric juice to bind the 15 mg of iron present in a typical day's diet. This binding substance is not firm, and iron is rapidly removed from the gastric factor by EDTA and transferrin. The iron-binding protein provides a mechanism, along with other natural ligands, for the chelation of soluble iron in the acid milieu of the stomach, maintaining solubility in the alkaline medium of the duodenum (the site of iron absorption). Levels of this substance are low in patients with hemochromatosis and iron-deficiency anemia resulting from blood loss.[232]

Although some results support the concept that gastroferrin production is concerned with the regulation of iron absorption in health, these observations have been seriously contested. Smith[359] found no differences in the iron-binding content of gastric juice between patients with hemochromatosis and those in the control group; other researchers[324] have found higher levels in iron-deficient patients than in the control group.

PANCREATIC FACTORS. Pancreatic secretions have been implicated in iron absorption. Pancreatic enzymes may split iron-protein complexes and make iron available for absorption. On the other hand, bicarbonate secreted by the pancreas raises the pH and induces formation of poorly absorbed iron complexes. Well-controlled studies of pancreatic insufficiency, however, have failed to show either iron excess or increased absorption of iron. Additionally, more recent studies indicate that the effect of pancreatic extract in iron absorption is nonspecific.[199]

ROLE OF BILE. Bile facilitates iron absorption.[407] Exclusion of bile from the intestine decreases absorption of food iron and iron salts. Bile contains ascorbic acid that forms soluble chelates with iron, thus possibly enhancing iron absorption.[65]

Extraluminal factors

Iron stores. The presence of iron deficiency, even when depleted iron stores are not accompanied by changes in serum iron content, hemoglobin levels, or iron turnover rates, increases iron absorption, e.g., the highest levels of absorption of dietary iron occur during periods of most rapid growth. Increased iron stores are associated with decreased iron absorption. Normal persons absorb 5% to 10% of dietary iron, compared with about 20% in iron-deficient patients.

Erythropoietic activity. An increase in erythropoietic activity in the marrow even if iron stores are already adequate (e.g., as occurs in hemor-rhage, hemolysis, and ascent to a high altitude) increases iron absorption, and diminished erythropoiesis decreases iron absorption.

Growth. Investigators have observed high rates of iron absorption in early infancy, which decrease rapidly with age to the level observed in adults. By means of isotope studies, Garby and Sjölin[115] obtained a mean gastrointestinal absorption rate in three infants of 73% (range 56% to 91%) within the first month of infancy, 56% (range 23% to 96%) in five infants during the second month, and 30% (range 15% to 38%) in three infants at 3 months of age. Schulz and Smith[338] found the mean absorption of radioactive iron in normal infants and children aged 4 to 52 months to be 10% (range 2% to 17%) and demonstrated a significant correlation between decreased iron absorption and increasing age.

Josephs[187] has emphasized that growth is associated with increased demand for iron regardless of hemoglobin level. The percentage of iron absorption, independent of age, is related in a linear way to weight gain.

Gorten et al.[124] found an absorption of ^{59}Fe ranging from 6.8% to 74% (mean 31.5%) in healthy premature infants from 1 to 10 weeks old. There was a highly significant correlation between tagged iron absorption and rate of growth; absorption was unaffected by previous gastrointestinal exposure to iron. The course of absorbed isotopic iron, traced by surface counting of internal organs and blood sampling, revealed a concentration of activity over the sacrum, spleen, and liver at 48 to 72 hours. Incorporation of iron into hemoglobin, calculated from ^{59}Fe activity in red blood cells, displayed a wide range with a mean of 15.3% of the quantity of iron in the test dose. The amount of iron utilized for hemoglobin formation correlated significantly with rate of growth (r = 0.70). The severity of anemia and degree of erythropoietic activity appear to affect positively the immediate utilization of absorbed exogenous iron.

Transport

The plasma iron-binding protein, transferrin, is a glycoprotein with the electrophoretic mobility of a β_1-globulin and a molecular weight of 88,000 to 95,000 daltons. It is a specific transport protein for iron and is essential for the movement of iron from one site to another. It is normally present in a concentration of about 200 mg/dl in plasma. With gel electrophoresis twenty-one different genetic variants have been identified, differing from one another in their electrophoretic mobility resulting from substitution of a single amino acid. They are inherited in an autosomal codominant fashion, and all share the same important chemical and physiologic functions. Transferrin C, which has a mobility between that of the faster B transferrins and slower D transferrins, is the most common in population studies. If no transferrin is present or if iron enters plasma in excess of the transferrin binding capacity, the unbound iron causes flushing, nausea, vomiting, shock, and even death. Each molecule of transferrin binds two atoms in the ferric state at spatially separated sites on the protein.[196] The biologic half-life has been reported to be 12 days in a normal child and from 6.7 to 8.4 days in adults.[120,196]

Transferrin is synthesized chiefly in the liver by the parenchymal cells,[377] but additional synthesis may occur in macrophages of lymphoid tissue. Transferrin acts as a homogenous compartment for transport, and the protein is equally distributed in intravascular and extravascular spaces; exchange takes place between the two compartments at the rate of 5%/hour. The concentration of transferrin in the plasma is about 2.5 gm/liter. More commonly transferrin is quantified in terms of the amount of iron it will bind, the "total iron-binding capacity" (TIBC). In normal persons the plasma iron concentration is about 100 μg/dl and the TIBC is 300 μg/dl. Thus only about one third of the available transferrin binding sites are occupied. There is a diurnal variation in plasma iron concentration with highest value in the morning and lowest in the evening. There is no diurnal variation in TIBC.

In physiologic circumstances the affinity of transferrin for iron is very great. The intrinsic binding constant is of the order 10^{36}, a value much higher than for other known iron chelating agents. The affinity of transferrin for iron can be decreased by lowering the pH or by reducing the iron to the divalent (ferrous) iron. Other metals such as copper, chromium, manganese, and cobalt can be bound by transferrin but with less affinity than iron.

Transferrin functions not only for the transport of iron in the plasma but also in the transfer of iron from the plasma to the developing erythrocytes. Transferrin plays an important role in iron utilization by developing normoblasts and reticulocytes, involves the attachment of the transferrin molecule to the cell membrane.[182,196,197] The iron, which is tightly bound to the transferrin molecule, is transferred into the cell from the transferrin attached to the cell membrane in about 1 minute. The mechanism is energy dependent. The rate of entry of transferrin-bound iron into erythroid cells is affected by several factors:

1. Age of the cells: Younger cells have a larger number of binding sites for transferrin molecules than older cells.
2. Concentration of transferrin-bound iron in the surrounding medium: Uptake increases as the absolute concentration of transferrin iron complex increases and is more important than its relative saturation.
3. The amount of heme in the reticulocytes: This regulates the entrance of iron into the cells by a feedback mechanism. It is decreased in reticulocytes incubated with heme and in sideroblastic anemias; when heme synthesis is inhibited, excessive amounts of nonhemoglobin iron are found in the normoblasts and in the erythrocytes.

The second method of iron accumulation by the erythroid precursors is called rhopheocytosis. Electron microscopy has shown that early erythroid cells contain ferritin. Bessis and Breton-Gorius[20] have demonstrated by electron microscopy that some ferritin is transferred directly from reticulum "nurse" cells to surrounding normoblasts. They termed the process rhopheocytosis to indicate that the nutrient material is transferred by aspiration rather than by micropinocytosis.[20] However, studies by Jandl and Katz[183] and the demonstration that immature red cells assimilate iron from transferrin in vitro much more readily than reticulum cells do[208,209] favor the concept that the direct transfer of iron from the plasma to the young red cell is the normal mechanism. It has also been suggested that ferritin is being transferred from the normoblasts to the reticulum cells rather than the reverse.

Storage

Storage iron is found in numerous sites, but the principal organs are liver, bone marrow, spleen, and skeletal muscles. In the liver iron is stored predominantly in parenchymal cells with relatively small amounts in the reticuloendothelial cells. In the spleen and bone marrow iron is stored chiefly in reticuloendothelial cells. Erythroblasts may contain stainable, nonheme iron and such cells are called sideroblasts.

The extrapyramidal system of the adult human brain contains concentrations of nonheme iron up to 21 mg/100 gm fresh weight, which are equivalent to those found in the liver, a major storage site for iron. The remainder of the brain contains 2 to 5 mg iron/100 gm of tissue (with concentrations proportionate to the phylogenetic age of the brain part), an amount greater than that which can be accounted for by the levels of various known iron-containing enzymes and cofactors.[146] Some of this iron is apparently present in the form of ferritin. Brain iron concentration increases gradually with age, being about 10% of adult values at birth and 50% at age 10 years; and maximal levels are achieved in most parts of the brain between the ages of 20 and 50 years. This gentle rise parallels neither the developmental pattern of brain cytochromes, which increase to adult levels concurrent with myelinization, nor the fluctuations of total body iron stores.[79]

Within the cells iron is stored in two forms: ferritin and hemosiderin. Ferritin is a water-soluble molecule; the protein component, apoferritin, has a molecular weight of about 480,000 daltons. About 25% of ferritin is made up of apoferritin, and the remainder is iron-containing ferritin. Hemosiderin is the other storage form of iron. In contrast to ferritin, it is a complex and heterogeneous product that is insoluble in water and contains variable amounts of proteins, copper hydrates, lipids, nucleotides, and porphyrins. Hemosiderin contains more iron and less protein than ferritin.

Functionally as well as structurally, hemosiderin and ferritin are closely related. The sequence in which iron is incorporated into these compounds varies according to the rate of cellular accumulation of iron. In the usual situation of gradual accumulation, iron appears first in ferritin. Subsequently a portion of iron accumulated in ferritin is transferred to hemosiderin. Iron more recently incorporated into ferritin appears to be preferentially transferred. This preferential handling of newly incorporated iron occurs at increased levels of tissue iron as well as at normal levels. The process of transferring iron from ferritin to hemosiderin probably does not involve release of iron but more likely a direct transformation of ferritin into hemosiderin.

At physiologic levels of tissue iron slightly more ferritin iron is present than hemosiderin iron. Hemosiderin predominates when excess iron develops. At high levels of tissue iron additional stores accumulate as hemosiderin. When iron is mobilized from the stores, ferritin and hemosiderin decrease about equally.[10] Iron stores, however, are not homogeneous. Recently deposited iron is more actively mobilized than older stores, and iron derived from erythrocyte destruction is preferentially used for the production of new red cells.

The iron in both ferritin and hemosiderin can be used for hemoglobin formation. The incorporation of the plasma iron into ferritin in the storage areas is an energy-dependent reaction involving ATP and ascorbic acid. The release of iron from ferritin is controlled by xanthine oxidase. The xanthine oxidase, an enzyme capable of oxidizing hypoxanthine and xanthine, may cause the release of ferritin iron by reducing it to a ferrous form that is readily released. The physiologic significance of this reaction, however, remains to be established. The accelerated release of iron from ferritin stores induced by hypoxia may be mediated by the effects of increasing xanthine oxidase activity.

Iron stores may be measured by a variety of techniques. One of these is repeated phlebotomy at regular intervals until iron-deficiency anemia develops.[25] This method is readily quantitated, removes iron from all sites, and is not subject to sampling error. It is, however, most inconvenient.

Other methods include biopsy of bone marrow or liver and histologic or chemical measurement of iron within the tissue specimen. Another method for evaluating iron stores is measurement of the serum iron concentration and the level of total iron-binding capacity. The value of these measurements is diminished because of the alterations produced by many other factors, including infection, malignancy, and hemolysis.[25]

The recently described plasma ferritin measurement reflects the level of body iron in stores and is quantitative, reproducible, and sensitive and it requires only a small blood sample. This is the most practicable and preferred method today for the estimation of iron stores.

Iron excretion

The body normally conserves iron in a tenacious fashion. Iron in the body is principally located intracellularly, either chelated firmly in the porphyrin ring of hemoglobin, myoglobin, and various intracellular enzymes or bound as the iron-protein complexes ferritin and hemosiderin. Plasma iron is tightly bound to transferrin and is not normally lost into the urine or into the intestinal lumen. Only a very small amount is lost daily as a result of desquamation of cells of the skin and gastrointestinal tract, through the migration of leukocytes into the gastrointestinal tract, by the shedding of hair, and in the excretion of minute amounts of iron in the bile, urine, and sweat. Moore and Dubach[269] found the fecal excretion of normal persons to be 0.3 to 0.5 mg daily, and in iron deficiency the amount may be only one tenth as much. Table 6-2 shows the average body losses of iron.

The conservation of iron is generally advantageous, but the inability of the physiologic mechanism to rid the body of more than a small amount each day allows for the accumulation of iron when excessive amounts gain access to the body as a result of blood transfusion, parenteral injection of iron, or abnormal absorption from the intestine.

Table 6-2. Average body losses of iron

Route	mg/day
Fecal	0.2-0.5
Urine	0.1
Sweating (heavy)	0.5
Menstrual	3.0-4.0 (total 20)

Table 6-3. Basic ferrokinetic measurements*

Measurement†	Calculation†	Average normal value
t½	Graphically, from semilogarithmic plot of plasma radioactivity disappearance	86 minutes
PIT	$\dfrac{0.693}{t\frac{1}{2}} \times$ plasma Fe (mg/ml) $\times$ plasma vol (ml) $\times$ 1,440 min/day *or* $\dfrac{\text{plasma Fe } (\mu g/dl) \times 100 - VPRC}{t\frac{1}{2} \times 100}$	26 mg/day or 0.7 mg/day/dl blood
RCU	$\dfrac{\text{14-day radioactivity/ml blood} \times 100}{\text{0 time radioactivity/ml blood}}$ *or* $\dfrac{\text{14-day radioactivity/ml RBC} \times \text{red cell mass (ml)} \times 100}{\text{total injected radioactivity}}$	80%
EIT	PIT $\times$ RCU	21 mg/day or 0.56 mg/day/dl blood
MTT	Graphically, from a semilogarithmic plot, the time at which 100 − RCU = 50%	3.5 days

*From Wintrobe, M. M.: Clinical hematology, ed. 7, Philadelphia, 1974, Lea & Febiger, p. 165.
†Abbreviations: t½, plasma Fe half-disappearance time; PIT, plasma iron transport rate; RCU, red blood cell utilization; EIT, erythrocyte iron turnover rate; MTT, marrow transport time; VPRC, volume of packed red cells.

Ferrokinetics*

Concentration of iron in plasma represents the balance between (1) iron delivered to the circulating blood from the gastrointestinal tract, hemoglobin breakdown, iron stores, and extracellular fluid, and (2) that removed by heme synthesis, cell metabolism, and deposition into stores and extracellular fluid. Radioisotopes of iron (^{59}Fe) have permitted measurements of the kinetic aspects of iron metabolism. Disappearance of radioactive iron from plasma, its incorporation into erythrocytes, and its appearance at various sites of the body can be measured by counting radioactivity in serial samples of plasma and whole blood and by external counting over appropriate anatomic areas such as sacrum, liver, and spleen.

The close association of iron to hemoglobin synthesis makes it possible with the use of ^{59}Fe tracer to assess the rates and sites of erythropoiesis and to evaluate ineffective and effective erythropoiesis (Chapter 8).

Radioiron is injected directly as ferrous citrate or is first bound to transferrin by incubation with fresh plasma. Serial samples of blood are taken at frequent intervals during the first several hours and daily thereafter. These are analyzed for plasma and red cell radioactivity, plasma iron concentration, and packed red cell volume. The basic measure-

ments calculated from these data are given in Table 6-3.

Radioactive iron injection is followed by a rapid exponential decrease in plasma radioactivity during the first 3 to 5 hours with a clearance of 50% of radioactivity from the circulating plasma in approximately 90 minutes. This 50% clearance or half-life is referred to as the t½ for plasma iron disappearance.

The plasma iron transport rate (PIT) is a measure of the rate at which iron leaves the plasma. It is expressed either as a total daily rate (mg of iron/day) or as a rate per volume (dl) of blood. The latter obviates a determination of plasma volume and assumes that the blood volume is normal. This should not be used if there are clinical reasons to doubt that the plasma volume is normal (e.g., acute hemorrhage, burns, or salt depletion). PIT is a good index of total erythropoiesis—both effective and ineffective.[412]

The erythrocyte iron turnover rate (EIT) is a measure of the rate at which iron moves from marrow to circulating red cells. Like the PIT, it may be expressed as a total daily rate or as a rate per deciliter of blood. It is an index of effective erythropoiesis and correlates well with a corrected reticulocyte index.[412]

The red cell iron utilization (RCU) is less than 100% (usually approximately 80%), because a proportion of the iron leaving plasma does not

*References 24, 107, 168, 298, 412.

Table 6-4. Ferrokinetic data in representative clinical situations*†

	t½ (min)	PIT (mg/day/dl)	RCU (%)	EIT (mg/day/dl)
Normal	86	0.7	80	0.56
Hypoplastic anemia	267	0.45	23	0.10
Hemolytic anemia (hereditary spherocytosis)	24	3.42	57	1.87
Ineffective erythropoiesis (thalassemia major)	21	6.87	18	1.24

*From Wintrobe, M. M.: Clinical hematology, ed. 7, Philadelphia, 1974, Lea & Febiger, p. 167; modified from Bohannon R. A., Hutchison, J. L., and Townsend, S. R.: Ann. Intern. Med. **55:**975, 1961; and Finch, C. A., et al.: Medicine **49:**17, 1970.
† Values are means.

make its appearance in circulating red cells. The reasons are that some iron may be lost with hemoglobin when normoblast denucleation occurs, some may be lost with intramedullary destruction of defective red cells (ineffective erythropoiesis), and some may enter one of several reflux pathways. Because of this there is a discrepancy between the PIT and EIT.[412]

The marrow transit time (MTT) may be used to evaluate the erythropoietin response. This value decreases in proportion to the degree of erythropoietic stimulation.[412]

In addition to these blood determinations it is possible to monitor iron movement within the body by surface counting of the liver, spleen, and sacrum (marrow). This is particularly useful in detecting extra medullary hematopoiesis.

These counts frequently are plotted as ratios of the surface counting rate. Radioactive iron normally accumulates in the bone marrow as plasma radioactivity decreases. Little or no radioactivity accumulates in the liver and spleen. This slight accumulation in organs containing numerous reticuloendothelial cells emphasizes that transferrin-bound iron is not taken up by reticulum cells directly. Diminished incorporation of iron into erythrocytes indicates dilution of radioactivity in increased iron stores, hemolysis, blood loss, or ineffective erythropoiesis rather than a decrease in erythrocyte production. By serial determinations of radioactivity over the organs in which iron uptake may occur, the meaning of changes in ferrokinetics can be clarified.

Variation of ferrokinetic measurements occurs in various hematologic diseases. In hypoplastic anemias, in which erythropoiesis is reduced, the PIT may be normal or slightly reduced but the RCU and EIT greatly reduced. Iron appears early in the liver and is retained there.

In hemolytic anemia, in which erythropoiesis is accelerated, both the PIT and EIT are increased and radioactivity accumulates at the site of destruction, that is the spleen or liver.

In thalassemia major, in which ineffective erythropoiesis occurs, the PIT is greatly increased,

the RCU is reduced, and the EIT is relatively normal. There may be early iron uptake over organs in which the defective cells are destroyed. The ferrokinetic measurements are only approximations of the parameters that they purport to measure. The calculations are based on the incorrect assumption that iron leaves plasma at a single exponential rate. The early part of the plasma disappearance curve approximates a straight line on semilogarithmatic paper. After several hours there is a change in the slope of the line and another exponential disappearance rate is established. This phenomenon is explained by the fact that not all iron leaving the plasma goes to the bone marrow; about 35% of the iron that leaves the plasma refluxes back into it, and some is taken up by liver and other storage cells. It is possible to correct the various ferrokinetic measures for reflux and improve their accuracy. Such correction factors have not yet been employed routinely and the improved accuracy may not be necessary for most clinical purposes. Table 6-4 shows ferrokinetic data in representative clinical situations. (See Fig. 8-10.)

IRON CONTENT OF FETUS AND NEWBORN INFANT

A linear relationship exists between the iron content and body weight of the fetus and newborn infant.[409] Table 6-5 shows the relationship of body weight to iron stores at birth. Although iron transfer to the fetus is negligible during the first two trimesters of pregnancy, it rises to 4 mg daily in the third trimester so that the total amount accu-

Table 6-5. Relationship of body weight to iron stores at birth

Infant weight (kg)	Body stores of iron (mg)
1.5	120
2.0	160
2.5	200
3.0	240
3.5	280

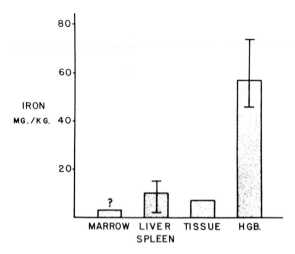

Fig. 6-2. Distribution of body iron at birth. (From Shumway, C. N.: Pediatr. Clin. North Am. **19:**855, 1972; modified from Schulman, I.: J.A.M.A. **175:**118, 1961.)

mulated by the fetus at term approximates 300 mg.[302] This increase in body iron content parallels the rapid increase in fetal weight during this period. In premature infants the deficit in iron at birth is directly proportional to the deficit in total body weight. Since the iron content and the weight of the fetus increase proportionately with age, the fetus maintains a constant iron content of about 75 mg/kg throughout gestation.[112,288,409]

Seventy-five percent of the infant's iron endowment is in the red cell mass and approximately 25% is in the storage sites, predominantly the liver. The liver and spleen have been estimated by Widdowson and Spray[409] to contain 34 mg iron, and Josephs[188] estimated the liver to contain 30 to 35 mg. The amount of the nonhemoglobin iron fraction (myoglobin, cytochromes, and other respiratory enzymes) at birth has been variously estimated at 4 mg/kg,[367] 6 mg/kg,[355] and 7.5 mg/kg[188] (Fig. 6-2).

The amount of iron in the body at the time of birth depends on the total red cell volume and the hemoglobin concentration. The red cell volume is dependent in turn on the blood volume, which is determined by birth weight, the time and method of clamping of the umbilical cord (whether or not a placental transfusion occurs), and the volume of maternal-fetal blood exchange. The *blood volume* is directly related to body weight. In the full-term infant shortly after birth the blood volume may range from 70 to 100 ml/kg of body weight with a mean of 85 ml/kg.* In the premature infant the blood volume ranges from 89 to 105 ml/kg in the first few days of life.[352,382] This increased blood

volume per kilogram in the premature infant is essentially the result of an increased plasma volume, with the red cell volume per kilogram of body weight being similar to that of the term infant. Cassady[45] has observed that in true premature infants the plasma volume decreases with increasing gestational age. Infants with intrauterine growth retardation have greater plasma volumes just after birth than would be expected for infants of comparable weight. The total blood volume of the infant rapidly adjusts after birth, plasma volume decreases and red cell volume remains essentially unchanged.[383]

This results in an increase in red cell count, hematocrit, and hemoglobin concentration shortly after birth. The total hemoglobin mass may be computed by multiplying the blood volume of 85 ml/kg (range 80 to 90 ml/kg) by the hemoglobin concentration per 100 ml of blood. Since each gram of hemoglobin contains 3.4 mg of iron, the total hemoglobin value is multiplied by this figure to convert it to total body iron. With these values Sturgeon[367] calculated that 232 mg of iron is present in circulating hemoglobin, 51 mg in the liver and spleen, and 16 mg as myoglobin and other parenchymal iron in a hypothetical infant weighing 4 kg. In an infant weighing 3 kg at birth the figures accordingly would be 106 mg in circulating hemoglobin, 11 mg in stores, and 12 mg in nonhemoglobin iron.

In both premature and term infants change of the blood volume to normal adult levels occurs during the first months of life. Mean blood volumes of 73 to 70 ml/kg are recorded for infants after the first month of life,[31,323] whereas the normal adult is found to have a blood volume of approximately 77 ml/kg.[119]

The *time of clamping of the umbilical cord* and the volume of the placental transfusion have a profound effect on blood volume (Chapter 2). It has been estimated that the placental vessels contain 75 to 125 ml of blood at birth—or one fourth to one third of the fetal blood volume.[58,93]

The *method of cord clamping* also alters the blood volume. Infants held below the level of the placenta will continue to gain blood; infants held above the placenta may bleed into it.[136] Yao et al.[425] demonstrated that hydrostatic pressure produced by placing the infant 40 cm below the mother's introitus hastened placental transfusion to virtual completion in 30 seconds. When the infant was held above the introitus, the placental transfusion was either markedly reduced or completely prevented.

Work by many investigators indicates that infants with delayed cord clamping usually have higher hemoglobin values during the first week of life.[58,93,220] Lanzkowsky[220] showed a statistically

---

*References 184, 231, 260, 383.

Table 6-6. Effects of immediate and delayed cord clamping on hemoglobin level in 131 infants*

	Number of infants	Hemoglobin level (gm/dl) at age in hours		
		0-12	13-24	72-96
Immediate cord clamping	63	19.8 ± 2.2	18.2 ± 2.0	18.1 ± 1.9
Delayed cord clamping	68	20.1 ± 2.0	19.9 ± 1.9	19.7 ± 1.8
Significance		P > 0.25	P < 0.001	P < 0.001

*From Lanzkowsky, P.: Clin. Endocrinol. Metab. **5:**149, 1976.

significant lower hemoglobin level at 13 to 24 hours and 72 to 96 hours of life in sixty-three infants whose cords were clamped immediately after birth as compared to a group of sixty-eight infants whose cords were clamped after placental separation had occurred and after the cord had been stripped. No significant difference was demonstrated between these groups from birth to 12 hours. There was no statistically significant difference in the hemoglobin level, hematocrit, and mean corpuscular hemoglobin concentration in the mothers of those two groups of infants. Table 6-6 shows these results, indicating that the alteration in blood volume, which occurs as a result of the time and mode of cord clamping, significantly affects the red cell volume and consequently the hemoglobin level and iron endowment of infants after the first 12 hours of life.

Manual stripping of the cord can add as much as 75 ml of whole blood or 40 mg of iron to the storage depots.[367] It has been emphasized that the technique of delayed ligation of the cord does not result in a significant increase in red cell volume unless the cord is initially stripped or milked.[408]

The *volume of maternal-fetal blood exchanged* can have a great effect on the newborn blood volume. It is now recognized that in as many as 50% of pregnancies some fetal cells pass into the maternal circulation at some time during gestation or during the birth process. In 8% of pregnancies these transplacental losses range from 0.5 to 40.0 ml of blood and in about 1% the losses are even greater and may approximate 100 ml.[55]

In contradistinction to this high incidence of fetal-maternal transfusion resulting in a decrease in the newborn's blood volume and lowering of hemoglobin, an infant may occasionally receive a transfusion from the mother, resulting in an increase in blood volume and polycythemia.

These changes in blood volume determine the amount of iron in the body of the infant at the time of birth. The total body iron in newborn infants has a range from 50 to 100 mg/kg with a mean of 78 mg/kg in infants whose birth weights are more than 2 kg. Of this, storage iron is approximately 15 mg/kg. Differences in extremes in

blood volume may cause differences in absolute amounts of body iron of as much as 50 mg.

The only practical indicators of the newborn's iron endowment are body weight and initial hemoglobin level. Measurements of hemoglobin level or hematocrit should be performed in all infants in the neonatal period if such an assessment is sought.

The fetal level of serum iron up to the fifth to sixth month of pregnancy is lower than maternal. After this serum iron in the fetus gradually increases and in the last 2 months the serum iron level is higher in the fetus than in the mother—a relationship that cannot be explained by simple diffusion. Similarly plasma ferritin concentrations, reflecting body iron stores, are markedly higher in cord blood than in maternal blood. Newborn serum iron levels are considerably higher than maternal levels and the transferrin is more nearly saturated. During the first day of life a rapid fall in serum iron occurs.[354,368,383] Serum iron then gradually increases so that by the end of the second week of life it ranges from 125 to 141 mg/dl.[368,383]

Relationship of maternal and fetal iron nutrition

A controversy exists as to the relationship between maternal iron nutrition and iron endowment of the fetus. The hemoglobin concentration in the cord blood of infants born to anemic iron-deficient mothers does not differ from that of infants born to iron-sufficient mothers.[216,351,417] Sisson and Lund,[351] on the other hand, found that the red cell volume and total hemoglobin mass were significantly reduced. Cord serum iron has been found to be dependent to some extent on the maternal value; on average it is twice as high.[426] Sisson and Lund[351] observed that women with low serum iron values tended to have infants with lower than normal serum iron values. However, others* have observed no tendency of the offspring born to anemic mothers to develop iron-deficiency anemia in infancy.

The mean hemoglobin levels in the first 24 hours

*References 74, 113, 216, 417.

Table 6-7. Effect of anemia of mother on hematologic values of newborn*

	Mean maternal values			Mean newborn values		
No. of cases	Hb (gm/dl)	MCHC (%)	Serum iron (μg/dl)	Hb (gm/dl)	MCHC (%)	Serum iron (μg/dl)
15	13.3	34.1	94.5	16.3	31.0	147.6
7	10.0	32.6	61.6	16.1	31.3	144.4
15	7.6	30.4	51.4	17.0	32.1	151.1
8	4.9	27.0	41.4	16.1	31.1	154.3

*Modified from Dabke et al. Indian J. Pediatr. **39:**348, 1972.

of life and at 3 months of age showed no significant statistical difference in two groups of infants: one group born to iron-deficient mothers with a low MCHC (mean 26.0%) and the other born to mothers with a higher MCHC (mean 32.5%). Dabke et al.[74] showed that serum iron levels, iron-binding capacity, and the hematologic status of newborns were not affected by maternal anemia, even profound maternal anemia (Table 6-7). Sturgeon[368] could find no difference in the state of iron nutrition in infants at 6, 12, and 18 months of age, irrespective of whether their mothers had received iron supplements during pregnancy.

Lanzkowsky[217,226b] showed no difference in hemoglobin values during the first 96 hours and at 3 months of age in infants born to mothers who had been given 400 to 1,600 mg of iron-dextran complex by injection at 6 to 7 months' gestation as compared to infants born to mothers not given supplemental iron. Similarly, DeLeeuw et al.[92] could not demonstrate an effect of iron supplementation during pregnancy on the serum iron concentrations of cord blood or on the infant's hemoglobin level during the first year of life.

Recently Rios et al.[314] used plasma ferritin concentrations determined by a two-site immunoradiometric assay to evaluate iron stores at the end of pregnancy in twenty-six women and follow up their healthy full-term infants; they showed that the iron storage status of the mother does not affect the iron status of the infant.

In summary it is clear that maternal iron deficiency itself does not result in iron-deficiency anemia in the newborn period or later in infancy. Factors such as birth weight, rate of growth, subsequent iron nutrition, and blood loss seem to be far more important than the maternal iron status in determining late appearance of iron-deficiency anemia. In the fetus the accumulation of hemoglobin and storage iron is remarkably independent of the mother's iron status.

The preferential maintenance of fetal iron saturation is probably a result of two major factors:

First, fetal transferrin is more saturated with iron than maternal transferrin. The maintenance of this gradient, regardless of maternal iron nutrition, probably ensures that the fetal iron saturation rarely drops below approximately 15%, the level at which iron lack is likely to limit hemoglobin production.

Second, the accumulation of fetal iron stores may be favored by the lack of xanthine oxidase activity in the fetal liver. This iron-containing enzyme is thought to be essential for mobilization of liver iron stores. Its lack presumably makes iron deposition in the liver irreversible until the enzyme increases in activity shortly after birth. These two factors promote positive fetal iron balance.

Maternal-fetal iron transport

Maternal-fetal transport of iron is depicted in Fig. 6-3. The fetus receives its iron from maternal plasma iron, which is transported to the placental villi bound to transferrin. Maternal transferrin does not cross the placenta, but the iron is taken up in the chorionic epithelium of the placenta and stored temporarily in the placenta in three forms: heme, iron bound to transferrin, and nonheme—ferritin and hemosiderin. The intermediate placental uptake is known to occur even in the absence of the fetus, and the placenta can remove iron from the maternal circulation independently of any subsequent transport to the fetus. From the placental depot the iron becomes bound to fetal transferrin and is then transported to fetal tissue; initially most of it can be found in the liver.[113] The accumulation factor for ^{59}Fe is about 200 times larger for the liver and about 50 times larger for the spleen than for other fetal organs following administration of intravenous ^{59}Fe to mothers.[98] The fetus synthesizes its own transferrin for this iron transport, as demonstrated from genetic evidence by Rausen et al.[310]

The amount of iron passing through the maternal plasma depends on the needs of two main acceptor tissues—maternal marrow and fetal tissues that compete for the available iron in the maternal plasma. Murray and Stein[276] showed that in the normal rat an average of 72% of fetal iron originates from maternal iron stores, implying that

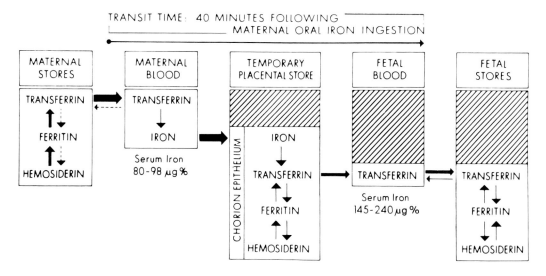

Fig. 6-3. Maternal-fetal transport of iron. (From Lanzkowsky, P.: Clin. Endocrinol. Metab. **5:**149, 1976.)

28% arises from maternal absorption. In maternal iron deficiency fetal iron content is preserved, the fetus obtaining more iron from maternal absorption; conversely in maternal iron overload fetal iron is not increased, the fetus obtaining less iron from maternal absorption.[273] To provide for increased needs incident to the rapid growth of the fetus in the last trimester of pregnancy, iron absorption in the mother is accelerated.[142,300]

The total iron content and total nonheme iron in placentas of women who received a daily supplement of 200 mg of iron were significantly higher than those in placentas of women who had not received iron supplements.[8] The increased amount of nonheme iron as a result of iron supplementation may be considered evidence that an antenatal supplement of iron promotes deposition of greater amounts of ferritin iron in the placenta for subsequent transfer to the fetus and ensures adequate transfer of iron from maternal to fetal tissues. An observed increase in fetal uptake on administration of supplemental iron suggests that the iron uptake by the fetus is to some extent influenced by the "available" iron in the maternal circulation.

Iron transport across the placenta is a unidirectional active process that can occur against a steep concentration gradient in favor of the fetus. Retrograde transfer of iron from the fetus to the mother does not occur. When radioactive iron is injected into the fetal circulation, none passes back into the maternal circulation,[27,302] but within 6 hours of injection of radioactive iron into the maternal plasma 75% or more of the iron extracted by the placenta has been deposited in fetal tissues.[302]

Pommerenke et al.[300] showed that following oral iron administration to pregnant women, iron appears in the fetal circulation within 40 minutes. This observation was confirmed in guinea pigs by Vosburgh and Flexner.[390] Hence iron delivered from maternal plasma is rapidly transported across the placental site, and the absence of any significant holdup suggests that iron entering the placenta does not become mixed with a biologic pool of any important size.[198]

The cells of the placental villi are involved in iron transfer and although the deeper villus tips are more heavily laden with iron, all living cells of the membrane participate. The villi obviously provide an effective cellular barrier between maternal and fetal circulation since the fetal plasma iron concentration is almost twice that in the mother. The difference is particularly remarkable since the iron-binding capacity of the newborn infant is only about one-half that of the mother. This suggests either a higher order of binding on the fetal side or a unidirectional pumping system in the placenta.

Maternal-fetal transport of iron is virtually independent of maternal iron nutrition and of the maternal serum iron level[113,249,303] and may even induce iron deficiency in the mother.[151,198]

It has been shown in the rat that there is diminished uptake of ^{59}Fe by the maternal liver and spleen during rapid accumulation of iron by the fetus. There is a diminished maternal "need" for iron, which makes available to the fetus a greater proportion of circulating maternal iron.[86]

The transfer of iron from the placenta to the fetus depends on an active fetal circulation. There is a close parallel between increasing fetal size and an increasing amount of iron transferred, which implies fine regulation of maternal-fetal iron trans-

port by the fetus.[249] Bothwell et al.[27] demonstrated that in pregnant rabbits the amount of iron
transported from the maternal plasma to the fetus
increased progressively with age and weight of the
fetus. By the end of pregnancy 90% of the plasma
iron turnover was directed to the fetus. This does
not occur through greater "pull" from fetal transferrin, since it is saturated with iron at the time
when fetal uptake is greatest. It also seems unlikely that the uterine blood flow or placental size
accomplishes this adjustment, since changes in
these do not coincide with fetal needs.

POSTNATAL CHANGES IN IRON STATUS
AND MECHANISM OF PHYSIOLOGIC ANEMIA

Erythropoietin-mediated control of erythropoiesis is operative in both the fetus and the neonate.[109,148] In the relatively hypoxic environment
of intrauterine life, erythropoietin levels are high
and erythropoiesis is active.

At birth 75% of the body iron is in the circulating hemoglobin mass. The arterial oxygen saturation rises to 95% from the 45% of the intrauterine life, and after the first week erythropoietin
activity is barely detectable. A significant decrease
in both the hemoglobin concentration and the total
hemoglobin mass begins to occur soon after birth,
reaching a minimum at approximately 7 weeks of
age in the premature infant and at 2 to 3 months in
the full-term infant. This phase, designated as
physiologic anemia of the newborn infant, is highly important in the iron economy of the infant because during the first 6 weeks of life there is marrow depression caused by increased oxygenation
of the blood.[114]

The iron released from red cell breakdown is
stored in the liver, spleen, and bone marrow for
later utilization. At 6 weeks of age only about 40%
of the body iron is present in hemoglobin. The
hemoglobin concentration reaches its lowest level
at approximately 8 weeks of age, with a decrease in the proportion of total body iron within
the circulating hemoglobin mass. During this period the red cell count falls proportionately to hemoglobin so that a normochromic normocytic anemia
develops. It should be emphasized that the anemia
at this stage is caused by a depression of erythropoiesis and hemoglobin synthesis, during which
red cells are destroyed at normal or, at best, slightly increased rates.[165]

At this point significant erythropoietin activity
returns, accompanied by resumption of active
erythropoiesis. With this resumption of active
erythropoiesis the circulating mass expands. In
both full-term and premature infants the amount
of hemoglobin synthesized is limited by the iron
that has accumulated in the stores during the postnatal drop in hemoglobin. This in turn depends

principally on hemoglobin concentration and hemoglobin mass available at birth, a variable component of preexisting iron in the liver and spleen
and the amount of exogenous dietary iron ingested. At about 4 months of age the amount of
iron in the hemoglobin compartment is equal to
that present at the time of birth. Continuing rapid
growth—the trebling of body weight during the
first year of life of a normal infant or the more
rapid weight gain of a low birth weight infant—results in an approximate doubling of the amount of
hemoglobin iron during the first year of life.

The supply of iron becomes strained with rapid
growth so that the infant is exposed to an anemia
caused by the exhaustion of storage iron. Following the period of reutilization of iron for hemoglobin synthesis with an increase in total hemoglobin mass, the supply of iron becomes depleted
unless it is replenished from an adequate diet.
These demands are met in the average full-term infant. The failure to add foods containing significant quantities of iron leads to iron-deficiency anemia, especially if the demands are excessive. Accordingly, iron-deficiency anemia is observed in
clinical practice in infants who are growing rapidly and are fed almost exclusively on diets of milk
and cereals with low iron content.

Plasma ferritin reflects the level of storage iron
and is increased or decreased in proportion to the
body iron stores. In cord blood samples the mean
plasma ferritin level is 113 ng/ml, which is markedly higher than in maternal blood at the time of
delivery. From the second day of life the plasma
ferritin level increases rapidly to a mean of 215
ng/ml,[358] and at 1 month of age the median serum
ferritin concentration is 356 ng/ml.[350] These levels
are maintained until 2 to 3 months of age, when
iron stores are mobilized to meet the demands of
an expanding hemoglobin mass, and beginning
about 6 months of age the level of plasma ferritin
declines to a median level of about 30 ng/ml.[350]
Infants not receiving dietary iron are found to have
no measurable ferritin by 6 months of age, a total
depletion of iron stores. These postnatal changes in
iron status are reflected in the iron content of the
liver, which increases from about 30 mg at birth[409]
to 100 mg at 3 months of age.[357] After 3 months of
age the iron content of liver decreases[357] as
amounts needed for erythropoiesis exceed the
quantity absorbed.

The amount of iron endowment at birth provides sufficient iron to satisfy iron requirements
until 4 to 5 months of age in a full-term infant; dietary iron is needed after 6 months of age to prevent iron-deficiency anemia.

In low birth weight infants this problem is exaggerated because of low iron stores at birth and the
accelerated rate of growth. In these infants the

amount of iron present at birth is sufficient to satisfy requirements until almost 3 months of age; if untreated they develop a more severe iron deficiency at 4 to 5 months of age.

PREVALENCE OF IRON DEFICIENCY

Surveys of preschool children in many countries in the last half century have revealed widespread iron-deficiency anemia. The incidence of the disorder has varied from population to population; it depends on a number of factors such as the age group of the population selected, ethnic composition, dietetic habits, socioeconomic factors, incidence of intestinal parasites, and methods used for the detection of iron deficiency.

The criteria for iron-deficiency anemia vary from one study to another. The World Health Organization (WHO) has proposed that in children of both sexes from 6 months to 6 years of age a hemoglobin concentration of 11 gm/dl or a hematocrit of 33% must be considered the lower limit of normal[421,422] and that a transferrin saturation of less than 16% is diagnostic of biochemical iron deficiency. The serum ferritin level, a most sensitive index of the amount of iron stored in the body, should give an accurate reflection of the true incidence of iron deficiency in any population group. Recent studies by Marner[241] and Moe[257] indicate that the use of the WHO definition results in an underestimation of the incidence of iron deficiency in children.

A number of surveys carried out in various urban areas of the United States during the last 20 years have revealed that the incidence of iron-deficiency anemia in children between 6 and 36 months of age varies from 17% to 44%. The criterion for iron-deficiency anemia in these surveys has been a hemoglobin concentration of less than 10 gm/dl.[106] Andelman and Sered[7] reported from Chicago that by 18 months of age 76% of children had hemoglobin levels below 10 gm/dl, and Gutelius[138] showed a peak incidence of anemia of 65% in children 12 to 17 months of age in Washington, D.C. Guest and Brown[134] reported in 1957 that the prevalence of iron-deficiency anemia in

children younger than 3 years of age in Cincinnati was the same or higher than it was 20 years earlier.

Lanzkowsky et al.[226] carried out a survey of 417 children from 6 to 36 months of age at forty New York City Department of Health well-baby clinics in various boroughs; 21% of black children, 11% of Hispanic children, and 2% of white children had hemoglobin levels of 10.0 gm/dl or less (Table 6-8). The children in this survey with hemoglobin levels below 10 gm/dl also had low MCHC and serum iron levels and high levels of total iron binding capacity. In this survey the peak incidence of iron-deficiency anemia is 10 to 15 months of age, when it reaches 30%. The incidence decreased with increasing age and dropped to less than 5% at 36 months of age. This relatively lower incidence of iron-deficiency anemia in preschool children was also shown by Pearson et al.[290] in a survey of nearly 7,000 preschool children (4 to 6 years of age) of low socioeconomic levels in five cities of the United States. They found that the mean hematocrit was 36.32% ± 2.8%. Severe anemia was unusual and the incidence of significant anemia (hematocrit 31%) showed considerable variation from city to city, ranging from 0.6% to 7.7%. The same investigators reported the effects of a 5-week period of dietary and medicinal iron supplementation on the hematocrit levels of 532 preschool children 4½ to 6½ years of age of low socioeconomic levels.[31] The initial mean hematocrit of the entire group was 35.73% ± 2.5%. A hematocrit of less than 31% was found in only 1.5% of the children. Diet alone and diet plus 30 mg of elemental iron/day were associated with significant increases in the mean hematocrit. A strikingly greater increase in mean hematocrit was seen in the group receiving iron supplements.

Numerous other studies have substantiated the high incidence of iron-deficiency anemia in children younger than 36 months both in American and non-American populations. Even cross-sectional studies involving middle class white populations indicate an incidence of anemia of between 1.4% and 6.3% (Table 6-9). Available figures indicate that incidence has not been substantially altered in several decades.

Although the incidence of iron-deficiency anemia is high in infancy, it also exists to a lesser extent in schoolchildren and during preadolescence. Karp et al.[193] reported that 5.5% of inner city schoolchildren ranging in age from 5 to 8 years had iron-deficiency anemia. They also observed that when iron deficiency is identified in a school-age child, it is likely that other family members are affected. When the school-age child is normal, the similarly aged siblings and mothers are more likely to be normal. Pearson et al.[291] showed an incidence of 2.6% in preadolescent children and

Table 6-8. Children aged 6 to 36 months attending well baby clinics*†

	Black	Hispanic	White
Number	177	158	82
Mean hemoglobin level (gm/dl)	10.9	11.4	12.1
Percentage < 10.0 gm/dl	21	11	2

*From Lanzkowsky, P.: Iron deficiency: a public health problem, Evansville, Ind., 1975, Mead Johnson.
†Significant difference (p < 0.001) among ethnic groups.

Table 6-9. Incidence of iron-deficiency anemia in cross-sectional and middle-class populations*

Reference	Number of patients	Age	Population	Percent anemic <10 gm/dl†
Fuerth, 1971[112a]	526	1 year	Caucasian, middle class, Kaiser plan	6.3%
	367	2 years	Kaiser plan	1.4%
	315	9 months	Caucasian, middle class, Kaiser plan	3.2%
Owen et al., 1970[288a]	5,000	1 to 2 years	Cross-sectional, 40 states	6%

*From Lanzkowsky, P.: Iron deficiency: a public health problem, Evansville, Ind., 1975, Mead Johnson.
†Percentage iron saturation below 15%.

nearly 25% in pregnant teenage girls. Brown et al.[35] showed an incidence among preadolescent and adolescent (12 to 15 years of age) urban black American children varied with age from 5.3% to 18.8% in boys and 11.4% to 27.3% girls.

The accuracy of detecting iron deficiency in population surveys can be substantially improved by employing a battery of laboratory measurements of the iron status and not relying exclusively on one parameter such as hemoglobin level. Because of marked overlap of hemoglobin levels in anemic and normal populations, the definition of anemia based on hemoglobin levels alone results in a large number of false positive and false negative findings. For greater accuracy transferrin saturation, red cell protoporphyrin, and serum ferritin levels should be used.

It has been observed by many investigators* that there is a higher prevalence of iron-deficiency anemia in black than white children. (See Table 6-8.) Although no socioeconomic group is spared, the incidence of iron-deficiency anemia in large population groups is inversely proportional to economic status.[226] Both of the apparent ethnic and socioeconomic factors in the incidence of iron-deficiency anemia are probably related to dietary habits, insofar as high iron content foods or iron-fortified baby foods are probably less available to those groups.

Since anemia is the end result of impaired iron nutrition, it may be viewed as the tip of the iceberg of widespread iron malnutrition. In some of the lowest income urban areas the prevalence of iron deficiency during the first 18 months of life as defined by biochemical assessment is almost 100%.

ETIOLOGIC FACTORS IN IRON-DEFICIENCY ANEMIA

The most common factors that contribute to the development of iron deficiency in children are in-

sufficient dietary intake of iron, rapid growth, and blood loss. Many cases result from a combination of all three factors.

A. Deficient intake: dietary (milk 0.75 mg iron/liter)
B. Increased demand
  1. Low birth weight
  2. Prematurity
  3. Low birth weight twins or multiple births
  4. Adolescence
  5. Cyanotic congenital heart disease
C. Blood loss
  1. Perinatal
    a. Placental
      (1) Transplacental bleeding into maternal circulation
      (2) Retroplacental; e.g., premature placental separation
      (3) Intraplacental
      (4) Fetal blood loss at or before birth; e.g., placenta previa
      (5) Fetofetal bleeding
    b. Umbilicus
      (1) Rupture umbilical cord; e.g., vasa previa
      (2) Inadequate cord tying
      (3) Postexchange transfusion
  2. Postnatal
    a. Gut
      (1) Primary iron-deficiency anemia resulting in gut alteration with blood loss aggravating existing iron deficiency
      (2) Hypersensitivity to whole cow's milk ingestion caused by heat labile protein resulting in blood loss and exudative enteropathy
      (3) Anatomic gut lesions; e.g., varices, hiatus hernia, ulcer, leiomyomata, ileitis, Meckel's diverticulum, duplication of gut, hereditary telangiectasia, polyps, colitis, hemorrhoids, exudative enteropathy as a result of underlying bowel disease, e.g., allergic gastroenteropathy, intestinal lymphangiectasia
      (4) Gastritis due to aspirin ingestion, adrenocortical steroids, indomethacin, phenylbutazone

*References 85, 89, 162, 215, 226a, 272, 283, 287.

Table 6-10. Normal daily iron requirements

	Normal loss	Menses	Pregnancy	Growth	Total requirements
Infants aged 1 year	0.25 mg	—	—	0.8 mg	1.05 mg
Children aged 7 years	0.5 mg	—	—	0.3 mg	0.8 mg
Pubertal females	1.0 mg	0.6 mg	—	0.5 mg	2.1 mg
Menstruating females	1.0 mg	0.6 mg	—	—	1.6 mg
Pregnant females	1.0 mg	—	1.5 mg	—	2.5 mg
Men and postmenopausal women	1.0 mg	—	—	—	1.0 mg

     (5) Intestinal parasites, e.g., hookworm *(Necator americanus)*
     (6) Henoch-Schonlein purpura
  b. Gall bladder: hemocholecyst
  c. Lung: pulmonary hemosiderosis, Goodpasture's syndrome, defective iron mobilization with IgA deficiency
  d. Nose: recurrent epistaxis
  e. Uterus: menstrual loss
  f. Heart: intracardiac myxomas, valvular prostheses or patches
  g. Kidney: traumatic hemolytic anemia; hematuria, Nephrotic syndrome (urinary loss of transferrin), hemosiderinurias (chronic intravascular hemolysis, e.g., paroxysmal nocturnal hemoglobinuria, paroxysmal cold hemoglobinuria, march hemoglobinuria)
  h. Extracorporeal: hemodialysis, trauma
D. Impaired absorption: Malabsorption syndrome, severe prolonged diarrhea, gastrectomy, inflammatory bowel disease

Dietary factors

One of the major factors in the pathogenesis of iron-deficiency anemia is inadequate iron intake.

Iron requirements. The iron stores present at birth in a mature infant are sufficient to supply the infant's iron needs during the first 4 months of life. From 4 months of age until 1 year of age 200 mg of iron is needed, requiring a daily absorption of 0.8 mg. Thus the daily diet of the normal term infant must contain 8 mg of iron by 6 months of age, based on an absorption efficiency of 10%. A term infant with a low initial iron endowment requires this amount by 3 to 4 months of age and the low birth weight infant by two months of age.[336] Sturgeon[366] demonstrated that highest hemoglobin levels were found in infants who consistently had a daily iron intake of about 1.0 mg/kg.

With a 10% rate of absorption an intake of 1.0 mg/kg/day to a maximum of 15 mg/day will provide sufficient iron to maintain normal hemoglobin values in most infants, if begun at an appropriate time with respect to initial iron endowment. This allows a margin for individual variability in absorption and iron endowment. A greater allowance (2.0 mg/kg/day) begun by age 2 months, to a maximum of 15 mg, was recommended by the Committee on Nutrition of the American Academy of Pediatrics[61] for low birth weight infants, infants with low initial hemoglobin values, and those who have experienced significant blood loss. This amount is not ordinarily provided by the diet, even when iron-supplemented cereals are included. Attainment of these larger amounts requires the use of medicinal iron or iron-supplemented milk formula. The Committee recommended that iron-fortified milk or medicinal iron should be prescribed to assure an iron intake of at least 2 mg/day for infants with reduced iron endowment. The marked differences between the iron needs of normal term infants and those in the foregoing special categories require that separate recommendations be stated for the latter.

Table 6-10 shows normal daily iron requirements calculated according to age and condition of various groups of individuals.

In adolescence, because of the growth spurt and menstrual loss, there is an increase in iron requirements. A menstruating adolescent requires 1.2 to 1.6 mg of iron each day as replacement or 12% to 16% absorption of dietary iron. Nonmenstruating females require only 0.5 to 1.0 mg/day as replacement (5% to 10% absorption). Iron required for growth (about 0.5 mg/day, mainly for new hemoglobin) must be added to these figures. In some teenage boys and in many menstruating girls a negative iron balance with loss of iron stores develops despite average nutrition. Iron balance in adolescence is shown in Table 6-11.

In teenage pregnancies additional iron (about 400 to 1,000 mg) is required to satisfy fetal demand, for increased maternal red blood cell volume, and to compensate for blood loss at delivery. Lactation adds 0.5 to 1.0 mg/day to iron losses. Since iron stores are less than 350 mg in at least two-thirds of young women, significant maternal anemia may develop if supplemental iron is not provided during this period.

Iron content of food. A newborn infant is fed predominantly on milk. Breast milk and cow's milk contains less than 1.5 mg iron/1,000 calories (0.5 to 1.5 mg/liter). The iron content of a pre-

Table 6-11. Average iron balance in adolescence

	Male	Female
Iron intake (mg/day)		
Food iron	10-12	10-12
Absorption	10% or less	10% or less
Iron absorbed	1.0-1.2	1.0-1.2
Iron requirements (mg/day)		
Iron losses		
Exfoliation, body fluids	0.75	0.75
Menstrual loss	—	0.60
Total iron losses	0.75	1.35
Growth needs	0.50	0.50
Total iron requirements	1.25	1.85

Table 6-12. Iron content of infant foods

Food	Iron (mg)
Milk	0.5-1.5/liter
Eggs	1.2 each
Cereal—fortified	3.0-5.0/ounce
Vegetables (strained)	
Yellow	0.1-0.3/ounce
Green	0.3-0.4/ounce
Meats (strained)	
Beef, lamb, beef liver	0.4-2.0/ounce
Pork, liver, bacon	6.6/ounce
Fruits (strained)	0.2-0.4/ounce

dominantly unfortified milk diet is always inadequate, and the availability and popularity of milk as an infant food have fostered an abnormally prolonged period of feeding an iron-poor diet. Even the early introduction of solid foods, including iron-fortified cereals, rarely compensates for the low iron content of milk. Since cow's milk often dominates the infant's diet during the first 2 years of life, iron intake may be less than 5% of the recommended amount. Nonfortified cow's milk therefore is totally inadequate in providing the minimum daily requirements of iron for infants. The iron content of typical infant foods is shown in Table 6-12. Thus diet is the major factor in the widespread iron-deficiency anemia that has been demonstrated. The impact of nutritional counseling on altering this dietary pattern has been disappointing. Since bottle feeding can be carried out unattended and is readily accepted by infants, it becomes the path of least resistance, particularly when the triad of low socioeconomic status, working mother, and a large number of young children exists in the household.

However, Saarinen et al.[325] have shown that although cow's milk and breast milk are equally poor in iron, breast-fed infants absorb an average of 49% of a trace dose of extrinsic iron administered during a breast feeding in contrast to about 10% absorbed from cow's milk under similar conditions. As a result of the high bioavailability of breast milk iron, infants fed breast milk during the first 6 to 7 months of life attain greater iron stores than those fed a cow's milk formula.

Growth factors

Growth is particularly rapid during infancy and again during the pubertal growth spurt, and this is reflected in an increased incidence of iron-deficiency anemia at these ages. During the first year of life the weight of the infant trebles, and the weight gain in a low birth weight infant is even greater. Although the proportion of body iron related to body weight at birth is higher than in adults, with the low intake of iron during the first few months it soon drops to adult levels. The blood volume and the total body iron are directly related to body weight throughout life, and so each kilogram gain in weight involves an increase of 35 to 45 mg of body iron. During the first year almost 200 mg of iron is needed to maintain the storage iron in the average infant. Rapid growth, with its concomitant expansion of vascular volume, leads to dilution of hemoglobin mass. For these physiologic reasons infants born with low birth weight (from prematurity or multiple births) and consequently a low hemoglobin mass at birth invariably become iron deficient.

From the age of 2 years to the onset of puberty the growth rate is steady at about 2.5 kg/year, leading to an iron requirement of 100 mg/year or 0.3 mg/day. It is not surprising that, once the deficit of iron frequently found in the first couple of years of life has been corrected, iron deficiency as a clinical problem becomes much less common.

At puberty the weight doubles over a period of 7 years, with a gain of about 30 kg in weight for boys and a little less for girls. This rate requires 1,200 mg iron, or 170 mg/year, or 0.5 mg/day. This estimate is for growth alone; in girls an additional 0.6 mg/day is needed for menstrual loss.

It is clear therefore that precarious iron balance exists in the first 2 years of life as well as during the pubertal growth spurt—during times of major growth rates.

Blood loss

Prenatal, intranatal, or postnatal blood loss can be a factor in iron-deficiency anemia.

Prenatal blood loss. Prenatal blood loss may be transplacental, twin-to-twin, intraplacental, or retroplacental.

Transplacental hemorrhage. In about 50% of all pregnancies some fetal cells can be demonstrated in the maternal circulation.[55,428]

Cohen et al.[55] estimated that in 8% of pregnancies 0.5 to 40.0 ml of fetal blood may enter the maternal circulation, and in 1% of pregnancies the blood loss exceeds 40 ml. Since the transplacental passage of cells may occur as early as the fourth to eighth week of gestation,[428] blood loss may be chronic as well as acute. Bleeding across the placenta may be spontaneous or secondary to certain procedures such as diagnostic amniocentesis or external cephalic version. The incidence of fetal-maternal hemorrhage following diagnostic amniocentesis has been observed to be 10.8% and fatal hemorrhage has been observed following the loss of more than 100 ml of fetal blood as a result of a traumatic amniocentesis.[256]

The diagnosis of fetal-maternal hemorrhage can be made by demonstrating the presence of fetal red cells in the maternal circulation. This can be done by one of several techniques, which include direct differential agglutination,[186] mixed agglutination,[186] fluorescent antibody techniques,[54] and the acid elution method of staining for cells containing fetal hemoglobin.[203]

The Kleihauer technique[349] of acid elution is the simplest method and the one most commonly used for the detection of fetal cells. A diagnosis of fetal-maternal hemorrhage may be missed when there is ABO incompatibility between the mother and the infant, because of rapid clearance of fetal cells from the maternal blood by anti-A or anti-B antibodies.

Twin-to-twin transfusion. Approximately 70% of monozygous twins have monochorial placentas, and twin-to-twin anastomosis occurs in almost every instance, whereas vascular anastomosis is uncommon in dichorionic placentas.[16] Significant twin-to-twin transfusion occurs in at least 15% of all monochorial twins.[309] The anastomosis of the fetal blood vessels in the placenta may be artery-to-artery, vein-to-vein, or artery-to-vein; bleeding from one twin to the other occurs where there is an artery-to-vein communication.

The donor twin is usually smaller than the recipient and may be strikingly pale at birth with evidence of listlessness or shock. Because of blood loss, the donor twin is a candidate for iron-deficiency anemia in the first few days and weeks of life. The recipient twin is usually larger than the donor twin and is plethoric and polycythemic.

A diagnosis of twin-to-twin transfusion should be suspected when a venous hemoglobin difference greater than 5 gm/dl exists between identical twins. In the donor twin the hemoglobin level may range from 3.7 to 18 gm/dl, and an elevated reticulocyte count and increased numbers of nucleated red blood cells may be present as evidence of recent hemorrhage. In the recipient twin the hemoglobin values range from 20 to 30 gm/dl. The plethoric infants have increased bilirubin production, and hyperbilirubinemia and kernicterus may occur. Such transfusion may explain the relatively frequent occurrence of hypochromic anemia in only one twin regardless of similar growth rates and diets.[416] (See Chapter 2 for more discussion of twin-to-twin transfusion.)

Intraplacental and retroplacental hemorrhage. Occasionally blood from the infant does not enter the maternal circulation (transplacental) but may accumulate in the substance of the placenta (intraplacental)[53] or bleeding may occur retroplacentally,[200] and the infant may be born anemic. For this reason careful examination of the placenta is essential for any infant born anemic or who becomes anemic in the first 24 hours of life.

Intranatal blood loss. Hemorrhage may occur during the process of birth as a result of a number of obstetric accidents and malformations of the placenta or the cord.

Rupture of normal umbilical cord. A normal umbilical cord may rupture, generally in the fetal third, from sudden tension during an unattended precipitous delivery.[280] Bleeding is profuse but usually stops spontaneously.

Rupture of varix or aneurysm of cord.[202] Hemorrhage caused by rupture of a varix or aneurysm of the cord has been described, and the site of bleeding may be difficult to find. Occasionally bleeding from this source occurs into the substance of the placenta and external hemorrhage may be absent.

Hematomas of cord.[308] Hematomas of the cord occasionally occur and may contain large volumes of blood.

Rupture of anomalous vessels of cord. Rupture of anomalous vessels of the cord can occur if certain anomalies such as aberrant vessels, velamentous insertion of the cord, or a multilobed placenta are present in the absence of obvious trauma. Occasionally the cord gives rise to one or more aberrant vessels before reaching its point of insertion in the placenta. These vessels are thin and lack protection by Wharton's jelly and therefore may rupture. In a velamentous insertion of the umbilical cord, the umbilical cord enters the amnion and chorion at a point some distance from the placenta. From the point of attachment at some distance from the placenta the vessels divide into fragile branches that pass unprotected between the amnion and chorion and eventually insert into the edge of the placenta. One percent of all pregnancies involve such velamentous insertions of the cord and about 1% to 2% of these bleed.[284]

Multilobular placenta. In a multilobular placenta each lobe sends out fragile communicating veins to the main placenta, and these too are liable to rupture. If any of these vessels overlie the internal os of the cervix, they are termed vasa previa; they may be compressed as well as lacerated during labor.

Obstetric accidents. Severe fetal hemorrhage may result from placenta previa, abruptio placentae, or accidental incision of the placenta or umbilical cord during a cesarean section. About 10% of all infants born following placenta previa are anemic,[285] about 4% of surviving infants born following abruptio placentae are anemic,[122] and in 28 of 879 cesarean sections the placenta was cut with resultant fetal bleeding.[285] Following a cesarean section the placenta and membranes should always be examined from the fetal side for evidence of damage. If there is any question of injury, the hemoglobin level of the infant should be determined at birth and again in 12 to 24 hours because in many cases the initial hemoglobin level may be normal. Such determinations should be performed also on all newborns in cases' of placenta previa, abruptio placentae, or unusual vaginal bleeding.

In women with third trimester bleeding the vaginal blood should be examined for the presence of fetal erythrocytes by employing the acid elution technique.[203]

Postnatal blood loss. Postnatal blood loss from any cause except enclosed or internal hemorrhage (e.g., cephalhematoma or subcapsular hematoma of the liver) may cause iron-deficiency anemia within the first week of life or shortly thereafter. Closed hemorrhage does not cause iron-deficiency anemia, as the blood is absorbed and the iron is reutilized for hemoglobin synthesis.

Postnatal hemorrhage may occur from a number of sites. The common sites are the umbilicus and gut.

Bleeding from umbilicus. Bleeding may occur from the umbilicus because of a slipped ligature around the umbilicus. Exchange transfusion (for hyperbilirubinemia, erythroblastosis fetalis, etc.) may result in anemia and consequently a reduction in the total iron endowment at birth because of the replacement of high-hemoglobin blood by low-hemoglobin bank blood.

Repeated diagnostic venipuncture or the presence of an umbilical arterial line permitting easy blood sampling can result in considerable iatrogenic blood loss, particularly in the ill newborn or in the premature infant with respiratory distress requiring numerous diagnostic tests. This iatrogenic blood loss is common, particularly in

neonatal intensive care units. If this blood loss is not replaced by the administration of blood and iron, it may be a potent cause of iron-deficiency anemia in the neonatal period.

Bleeding from bowel. Bleeding from stress ulcers in ill newborns, duplication of the gut, Meckel's diverticulum, and other anatomic abnormalities of the gut may result in blood loss and in the development of iron-deficiency anemia.

Postnatal hemorrhage may result from a number of mechanisms. These include congenital and acquired plasma factor deficiencies and thrombocytopenia.

Congenital plasma factor deficiency (e.g., factor VIII or IX deficiency) can result in postnatal bleeding and the development of iron deficiency anemia.

Transient hemorrhagic disease of the newborn caused by vitamin K deficiency is a result of decreased levels of factors II, VII, IX, and X. This type of bleeding is responsive to vitamin K therapy, and for this reason the routine use of vitamin K has been advised to prevent its occurrence.

Hepatic immaturity in small premature infants may not respond satisfactorily to vitamin K because of the inability of the liver of small premature infants to synthesize coagulation factors.

Disseminated intravascular coagulopathy is not uncommon in premature infants, and it is thought to be caused by such factors as shock, infection, the presence of thromboplastin-like substances, and hemolysis. The diagnosis of this condition depends on the finding of low levels of factors I, II, V, and VIII; decreased numbers of platelets; normal euglobulin lysis time; and the presence of fragmented red cells in the blood smear and fibrin degradation products in the plasma.

Thrombocytopenia in the newborn, irrespective of its cause, may also cause postnatal hemorrhage. Infants who have congenital and acquired plasma factor deficiencies or thrombocytopenia may manifest bleeding from many sites, such as the umbilicus, venous puncture sites, the bowel, and the brain. If bleeding has occurred externally, these infants are candidates for iron deficiency during the neonatal period.

Blood loss in infancy and childhood. Bleeding can be either occult or apparent. It has been shown by many investigators that occult blood loss occurs in iron-deficiency anemia.[163,307] More than 50% of iron-deficient infants in the United States have guaiac-positive stools, compared to about 7% of normal infants. It is uncertain to what extent this is cause or effect. There is no roentgenographic evidence of gastrointestinal lesions and this blood loss has been considered to be caused by the effects of iron-deficiency anemia on the mucosal lining, e.g., deficiency of iron-containing enzymes in this tissue, that lead to mucosal blood loss. This, of course, sets up a vicious cycle whereby iron-deficiency anemia caused by dietary factors results in mucosal changes that lead to blood loss and further aggravate the anemia. What distinguishes this bleeding from that associated with gross anatomic lesions is that it ceases shortly after iron treatment.

Blood loss from the gut may also occur as a result of an exudative enteropathy caused by a hypersensitivity resulting from ingestion of whole cow's milk or an intestinal intolerance to large amounts of cow's milk.[410] A heat-labile component of milk is the responsible agent that acts as an intestinal irritant or allergen, and heat denaturation of the protein eliminates this effect. Wilson et al.[411] demonstrated that bleeding induced by whole cow's milk did not diminish despite iron therapy as long as whole cow's milk was ingested, but the bleeding was stopped by substituting soya or proprietary milk formulas for the cow's milk. Elegant studies by Woodruff and Clark[418] using iodinated ^{131}I serum albumin showed rapid turnover in seven of twelve patients with iron deficiency indicating significant exudative enteropathy. Treatment with iron dextran had no effect on the albumin turnover. Feeding evaporated milk instead of fresh cow's milk was followed by lengthening of the albumin turnover

half-times, and replacement by a soybean substitute was always followed by a return to normal values.

These observations suggest that cow's milk can result in an exudative enteropathy associated with chronic gastrointestinal blood loss, which is not caused by iron deficiency but results in iron deficiency. Whole cow's milk should be considered the cause of the iron-deficiency anemia in the following clinical circumstances[411]:

1. One quart of whole cow's milk or more consumed per day
2. Iron deficiency accompanied by hypoproteinemia (with or without edema) and hypocupremia (It should be noted that iron-deficiency anemia unassociated with exudative enteropathy is associated with an elevated serum copper level.)
3. Iron-deficiency anemia unexplained by low birth weight, poor iron intake, or excessively rapid growth
4. Iron-deficiency anemia recurring after a satisfactory hematologic response
5. Rapidly developing or severe iron-deficiency anemia
6. Suboptimal response to oral iron
7. Presence of consistently positive stool guaiac tests in the absence of gross bleeding and other evidence of organic surgical lesions

Table 6-13. Classification of iron-deficiency anemia (IDA) in relationship to gut involvement*

Pathogenesis	Gut changes	Result	Treatment
Primary iron deficiency (dietary, rapid growth)			
Mild or severe	No gut involvement or blood loss	IDA	Oral iron
Severe	Leaky gut syndrome		
	1. Loss of red cells only[163,307]	IDA, guiac positive	Oral iron
	2. Loss of red cells, plasma protein, albumin, immunoglobulin, copper, calcium[212,226a]	IDA, exudative enteropathy	Oral iron
	Malabsorption syndrome		
	1. Iron only (?)[201]	IDA refractory to oral iron	IM iron-dextran complex
	2. Xylose, fat, vitamin A, "duodenitis," red cell loss[135,147,278]	IDA, transient enteropathy	IM iron-dextran complex
Secondary iron deficiency			
Cow's milk induced, (?) heat-labile protein	Leaky gut syndrome†: loss of red cells, plasma protein albumin, immunoglobulin, copper, calcium	Recurrent IDA, exudative enteropathy	Discontinue whole cow's milk; soya or milk formula; oral iron
Anatomic lesion, e.g., Meckel's diverticulum, polyp, intestinal duplication, peptic ulcer	Blood loss	Recurrent IDA	Surgery Specific medical management Oral or I.M. iron-dextran complex

*Modified from Lanzkowsky, P.: Iron deficiency: a public health problem, Evansville, Ind., 1975, Mead Johnson.
†References 410, 411, 418, 420.

8. Return of gastrointestinal function and prompt correction of anemia on cessation of cow's milk and substitution by formula

Woodruff et al.[420] compared the effect of fresh cow's milk and a prepared formula on iron nutrition in infants during the first 12 months of life. Fresh cows's milk was associated with a significant degree of microcytosis, ferropenia, and minimal anemia as compared to prepared formula containing the same amount of iron. This study suggested that factors in the diet other than the amount of iron are important in the etiology of iron deficiency. The most likely explanation for these findings might be blood loss or decrease in iron absorption in the fresh cow's milk–fed group. It is probable that an increase in iron intake would prevent the deficiency found in the infants fed fresh cow's milk. The addition of iron to infant formulas may be an appropriate means of preventing iron deficiency in large populations at the present time.

In addition, anatomic gut lesions, e.g., polyps, Meckel's diverticulum, intestinal duplication, hemorrhagic telangiectasia, and other gastrointestinal anomalies, can cause blood loss. It should be suspected when intestinal blood loss or anemia persists or recurs after iron therapy or when severe anemia is detected after the period of peak incidence in infancy. Intestinal parasites, especially hookworm infestation, are a major cause of iron-deficiency anemias in geographic areas where hookworm is prevalent.

Iron-deficiency anemia can cause blood loss from the bowel, and blood loss from the bowel, irrespective of its etiology, can result in iron-deficiency anemia. Iron-deficiency anemia can therefore be classified into various types (Table 6-13), depending on whether blood loss causes iron-deficiency anemia (secondary iron-deficiency anemia) or whether preexisting iron deficiency results in gastrointestinal abnormalities causing blood loss or impaired iron absorption (primary iron-deficiency anemia).

Other sites of blood loss include the nose, uterus, heart (valvular prosthesis), and rarely the gall bladder (hemocholecyst).

In the kidney, blood loss (hematuria), iron loss (hemosiderinuria), and loss of transferrin

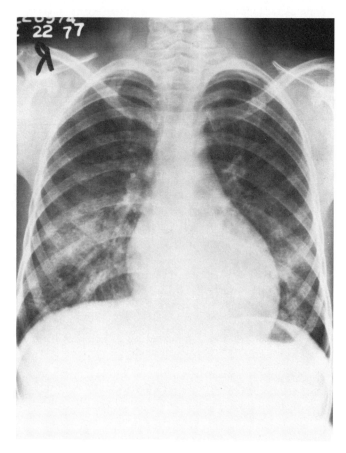

Fig. 6-4. Roentgenogram of chest demonstrating patchy mottling in a patient with idiopathic pulmonary hemosiderosis.

(e.g., nephrotic syndrome)[150] may result in iron-deficiency anemia.

Impaired absorption of iron resulting from a generalized malabsorption syndrome, severe diarrhea, and inflammatory bowel disease are uncommon causes of iron-deficiency anemia and usually occur in older children.

Idiopathic pulmonary hemosiderosis. When chronic pulmonary disease and hypochromic anemia coexist, another cause of iron loss, idiopathic pulmonary hemosiderosis, should be considered. In this case, though, the chronic loss of blood is into the lung parenchyma rather than lost from the body, the iron is unavailable for reutilization and is sequestered in the lungs. The etiology is unknown.

The clinical course is a relapsing one. There are episodes of dyspnea, fever, and cough, usually associated with pallor and at times icterus. During the acute episodes the roentgenograms of the chest demonstrate diffuse or patchy mottling that clears (Fig. 6-4). Initially the hemoglobin concentration may decrease suddenly; subsequently a reticulocytosis develops. After several episodes and progressive iron sequestration in the lungs, a microcytic hypochromic anemia with all the features of iron deficiency secondary to chronic blood loss develops. The appearance of iron-laden macrophages in the lungs and gastric fluid can be demonstrated by gastric washings. In addition to idiopathic pulmonary hemosiderosis, the following conditions are associated with hemosiderin-laden macrophages:

1. Mitral stenosis or chronic venous hypertension
2. Periarteritis nodosa
3. Systemic lupus erythematosis
4. Wegener's granulomatosis
5. Goodpasture's syndrome or antiglomerular basement membrane antibody mediated disease

The course of idiopathic pulmonary hemosiderosis can be quite variable. Progressive pulmonary fibrosis may lead to pulmonary insufficiency and cor pulmonale. Hemoptysis, if severe, may cause death. The disease has been associated with rheumatoid arthritis and myocarditis.[41]

Goodpasture's syndrome. Goodpasture's syndrome has the features of idiopathic pulmonary hemosiderosis in association with glomerulonephritis. Usually the evidence of nephritis is present from the time of clinical manifestations of the disease, but sometimes the onset of urinary findings can be delayed for a few weeks and rarely for a few years.

Etiology of this disease is unknown; the disease is uncommon in children and most frequently appears in young men. Death is most often the consequence of renal failure.

Goodpasture's syndrome should be suspected when the symptoms and findings of pulmonary hemosiderosis are found in association with proteinuria, hematuria, and evidence of progressive renal disability. The hematologic findings are those of iron-deficiency anemia. Confirmation can be obtained by finding iron-laden macrophages in gastric contents and the typical pathologic findings on lung and kidney biopsy.

Defective iron mobilization associated with IgA deficiency. The features of this condition are those of hypochromic hypoferremic anemia responsive to iron therapy. The clinical course of this condition resembles idiopathic pulmonary hemosiderosis with IgA deficiency. It is discussed in more detail on p. 162.

CLINICAL MANIFESTATIONS

It is well established that iron deficiency is a systemic disorder involving multiple systems rather than a purely hematologic condition associated with anemia. It occurs most frequently between the ages of 6 and 24 months and reflects an inadequate supply or excessive demand for iron or blood loss. These factors are interdependent and overlap.

The early phases of iron-deficiency anemia are not associated with clearly recognizable signs or symptoms, and its development is slow and insidious. Pallor, irritability, anorexia, and listlessness usually direct attention to this disorder. These symptoms are noticed only when there has been a significant fall in the hemoglobin level. The precipitating event that brings the child to the physician is frequently an intercurrent infection; the anemia is discovered secondarily. The slow development of anemia allows physiologic adjustment by the infant, and very low hemoglobin levels may go unnoticed by the parents.

Except for pallor of the skin and mucous membranes and occasionally a slightly enlarged spleen, the patient presents no significant physical abnormalities. In patients with severe anemias a soft blowing apical systolic murmur is frequently heard. Koilonychia (concave nails) has been observed in severe long-standing iron-deficiency anemia.

Iron deficiency affects many organ systems in the body.

Hematopoietic system

Effects on the hematopoietic system are discussed on p. 144.

Gastrointestinal tract

Anorexia is a common and early symptom of iron-deficiency anemia, and correction of iron deficiency results in improved appetite. Judisch et al.[190] have demonstrated a marked prepon-

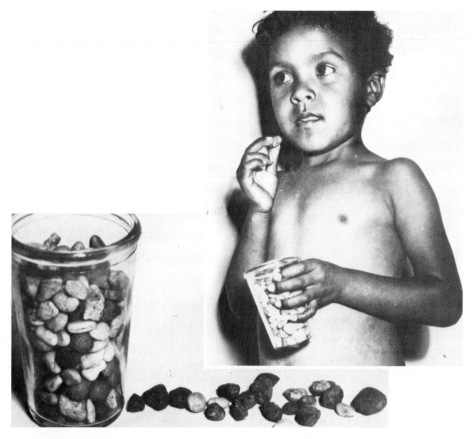

Fig. 6-5. Daily diet of pebbles taken for 3 years by a boy 7½ years of age with pica and iron-deficiency anemia. (From Lanzkowsky, P.: Arch. Dis. Child. **34:**140, 1959.)

derance of underweight children among children with iron-deficiency anemia. When iron is given to these children, there is an accelerated weight gain that produces a normal distribution curve. Anorexia might have important bearing on the maternal-child relationship in the first few years of life and may result in behavioral stresses within the family that might interfere with proper nutrition in general.

Pica, derived from the Latin word meaning magpie, is a perversion of appetite with persistent and purposeful ingestion of apparently unsuitable substances, seemingly of no nutrient value (Figs. 6-5 and 6-6). Pica has been considered to be a symptom of iron-deficiency anemia, even though a number of etiologic factors—nutritional, psychologic, socioeconomic, cultural, and organic—have been implicated in pica. The exact etiology and the relative importance of various etiologic factors remain to be established. Anemia is part of the picture of pica,* and cures after iron therapy have been recorded.[125,221,222]

---

*References 69, 97, 129, 341.

The association of iron-deficiency anemia and pica has been considered to be the result of an intuitive urge of children with iron-deficiency anemia to seek the element they lack. This has many analogies in clinical medicine and in the animal kingdom. It is well known that persons with Addison's disease intuitively eat large amounts of salt, and children with rickets selectively eat cod liver oil rather than other foods.[88] Parathyroidectomized rats selectively choose calcium lactate, and adrenalectomized animals selectively choose sodium chloride.

In the light of these analogies, the iron content of the soil, sand, and clay selectively chosen by these children with pica was determined, and the content of iron as Fe_2O_3 in these samples ranged from 0.38% to 1.04%.[223]

Carlander[44] recorded that 100 patients with pica all had sideropenia and that when treated with iron in adequate doses all patients lost their pica. Similar experience has been reported by Ber and Valero[19] and Catzel.[46] Mohan et al.[259] conducted a study of fifty-eight Indian children with pica comparing the efficacy of iron therapy to that of

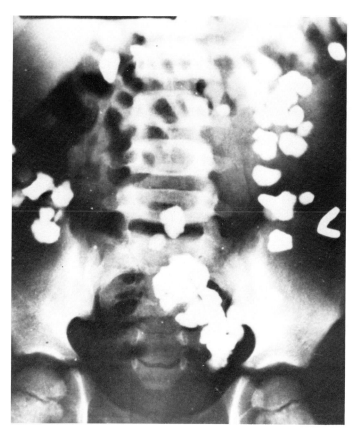

Fig. 6-6. Radiograph of abdomen of boy shown in Fig. 6-5. (From Lanzkowsky, P.: Arch. Dis. Child. **34:**140, 1959.)

a multivitamin tablet without iron. The iron treated group showed a marked decrease in pica compared to the multivitamin treated group. Gutelius et al.[137] showed that children with pica have a significantly lower hemoglobin level than control patients matched for age, but they were unable to prove that iron administration cured pica.

McDonald and Marshall[247] conducted a double-blind trial of the value of iron in the treatment of pica. They used random intramuscular injection of normal saline and concluded that pica can be cured by iron in nearly all cases but that a permanent cure is dependent on the maintenance of an adequate hemoglobin level.

In one series it was found that the overall prevalence of pica was 22.8% in black children, as compared with 14.8% in the white groups, with an overall prevalence of 18.5% for the two groups.[12] In another group of children ranging in age from 1 to 6 years, Millican et al.[255] found that 32.3% of black children had pica, compared with 10% of white children. The prevalence of pica decreases with increasing age over this age range.

Many of these cases were associated with iron deficiency.

Geophagia, the eating of earth or clay, has been observed frequently in children and adults in the Southern and Western United States. Also in New York City a group of nonpregnant patients who had ingested quantities of laundry starch were found to have iron deficiency.[320] Starch ingestion (amylophagia) and clay ingestion varied from 250 to 1,300 gm/day and the average hemoglobin was 6.2 gm/dl. Three patients who were followed received iron but continued to ingest clay or starch despite correction of anemia. It would seem that in adults iron deficiency was not the cause of the pica but that the latter contributed to the anemia. In children, however, there is a loss of pica with correction of the iron deficiency.[247]

Prasad et al.[301] described nine Iranian males with a syndrome characterized by severe iron deficiency (hemoglobin levels ranging from 2.8 to 7.7 gm/dl) hypogonadism, dwarfism, hepatosplenomegaly, and geophagia. The age range was 14 to 21 years. Liver function tests were normal except for elevated serum alkaline phosphatase levels. Patients with this syndrome were also found to be zinc deficient. Further studies of this syndrome by Aksoy et al.[5] suggested that the hepatosplenomegaly in the course of iron-deficiency anemia in this syndrome was a consequence of portal hypertension, possibly caused by liver cirrhosis resulting from nutritional deficiency. Their diet consisted mostly of wheat and rice, with a little milk and rarely meat, vegetables, and fruit. When these patients were properly treated with oral iron, the hemoglobin levels returned to normal and the livers and spleens diminished in size.

Iron lack has been associated with another perversion of appetite characterized by the ingestion of extraordinary amounts of ice—designated as pagophagia. Reynolds et al.[313] found that twenty-three of a group of thirty-eight iron-deficient patients admitted to excessive ice consumption. With iron therapy twenty-two completely lost their ice craving and one was much improved. Reynolds et al. found that this habit best correlated with serum iron levels—the craving disappeared as the serum iron rose above 70 μg/dl. Coltman[60] reported a group of adult women with pagophagia who were iron deficient and consumed at least one ordinary tray of ice daily for a period of more than 2 months. Iron administration in doses insufficient to correct the anemia or to replenish body stores promptly eliminated all craving for ice. The mechanism is related to iron lack but not specifically to iron-lack anemia. Brown and Dyment[36] showed a similar relationship between pagophagia and iron deficiency in adolescent girls.

In addition to pica, food cravings of olives,[50] watercress (an aquatic plant of the mustard family, rich in minerals),[211] carrots,[59] and lettuce[240] in association with iron deficiency have been observed.

Deficiencies of metals other than iron might also be associated with pica. Karayalcin and Lanzkowsky[192] described a child with pica for a zinc-containing scouring material (Comet). The patient's plasma zinc level was low, and this unusual form of pica was corrected by oral zinc replacement. Hambridge and Silverman[149] have also demonstrated rapid improvement in pica after dietary zinc supplementation.

Pica has as its complications lead poisoning[181] and ingestion of the ova of worms. Because available evidence indicates that pica is associated with iron-deficiency anemia and it is cured by iron administration, it seems possible that the widespread eradication of iron deficiency might eventually lead to a reduction in the incidence of pica and consequently lead poisoning.[213]

Atrophic glossitis, dysphagia, esophageal webs (usually at the cricopharyngeal level—Paterson-Kelly syndrome), and atrophic gastritis known to occur in iron-deficiency anemia in adults do not occur in infants and are only rarely observed in children. Although this syndrome is commonly associated with iron deficiency, iron deficiency has not been indicated as the prime factor. It occurs occasionally without evidence of sideropenia, and iron therapy does not necessarily improve the condition.

Reduced gastric acidity, both under basal conditions and following histamine stimulation, has been demonstrated in iron-deficient children.[117]

Iron-deficiency anemia per se may result in loss of blood from the gut.[163,307] These infants have iron-deficiency anemia associated with *guaiac-positive stools.* Correction of the iron-deficiency anemia with iron reverses this process, and bleeding from the gut ceases. This bleeding from the gut is not diet related and is caused by iron-deficiency anemia and corrected by iron administration (p. 128).

Iron-deficiency anemia may result in an *exudative enteropathy* ''leaky gut'' syndrome with a loss of red cells, plasma proteins, albumin, immunoglobulins, copper, and calcium. This exudative enteropathy is caused by iron-deficiency anemia, aggravates existing iron deficiency, and can be completely corrected by iron therapy without any dietary change.[201] Table 6-14 indicates the hematologic and biochemical changes in an infant with iron-deficiency anemia and exudative enteropathy, and the effect of iron treatment on

Table 6-14. Hematologic and biochemical investigations before and after iron therapy*

Investigations	Before iron therapy	8 days after iron therapy	21 days after iron therapy	Normal value
Hemoglobin (gm/dl)	7.5	8.2	12.0	11.0-12.0
MCHC (%)	30	26	34	32-38
Reticulocyte count (%)	2.8	12.7	5.6	0.8-1.6
Copper (μg%)	25	—	135	80-235
Total protein (gm/dl)	3.6	6.0	5.5	6.0-8.0
Albumin (gm/dl)	1.7	2.7	3.4	3.5-5.0
Globulin (gm/dl)	1.9	3.5	2.1	2.5-3.0
IgG (mg/dl)	130	—	560	550-970
IgA (mg/dl)	52	—	76	25-75
IgM (mg/dl)	64	—	120	35-80
Calcium (mg/dl)	7.0	9.6	9.4	8.5-10.5

*From Lanzkowsky, P.: Iron deficiency: a public health problem, Evansville, Ind., 1975, Mead Johnson.

the biochemical parameters. Since these biochemical values returned to the normal range on iron treatment without dietary change, their alteration was intimately related to the presence of iron-deficiency anemia. A similar exudative enteropathy secondary to whole cow's milk ingestion may result in iron deficiency (p. 129).

As iron-deficiency anemia develops, the proportion of iron absorbed from the diet normally increases in a compensatory fashion. When iron deficiency becomes severe this useful adaptation may ultimately fail. Recent work has shown a malabsorption of iron secondary to iron deficiency.[201] Absorption of ^{59}Fe-labeled hemoglobin was shown to be impaired in children with severe dietary iron deficiency and returned to normal after iron repletion. In newly weaned dogs on an iron-deficient diet, absorption of iron was initially increased over the control animals, reaching a maximum value at 5 months of age. Thereafter, despite the increasing severity of iron deficiency, there was a fall in absorption. Decreased levels of cytochrome oxidase and lactase were noted in the mucosa of the iron-deficient dogs. A decrease in iron-containing or iron-dependent enzymes in the mucosa of iron-deficient subjects may be responsible for a secondary malabsorption phenomenon.

Using an iron absorption test, Gross et al.[133] have recently described malabsorption of iron in some children with moderate iron deficiency. However, work done by Lanzkowsky et al.[224] was unable to confirm the finding of selective malabsorption of iron in children with moderately severe iron deficiency. The latter researchers indicate that the iron absorption test is unreliable for a number of reasons, including the fact that variation in iron absorption occurs in the same persons at different times, that healthy individuals have been shown to have flat absorption curves, that the oral iron absorption curve is test dose related (Fig. 6-7), and that the standard recommended test dose of iron of 1 mg/kg is an unreliable indicator of iron absorption. Moreover, the absorption curve following a test dose of oral iron is not only an indication of iron absorption but also a composite of the rate and amount of iron absorption, rate of mucosal iron turnover, and rate and degree of plasma iron clearance. If an oral iron absorption curve is obtained in the investigation of therapeutic failures in the treatment of iron deficiency, a test dose of iron in a conventional therapeutic amount, such as 3 mg/kg, is more likely to yield reliable results.

Many researchers have shown a more generalized *malabsorption syndrome* in iron-deficiency

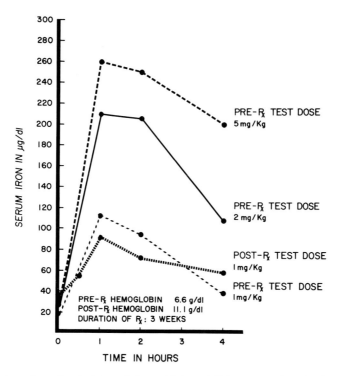

Fig. 6-7. Oral iron absorption test in an infant with iron-deficiency anemia using iron test doses of 1, 2, and 5 mg/kg before iron treatment and 1 mg/kg after iron treatment. (From Lanzkowsky, P., Karayalein, G., Betkerur, U., and Shende, A.: J. Pediatr. **90:**494, 1977.)

anemia.[135,147,278] This has consisted of impaired absorption of xylose, fat, and vitamin A. This enteropathy has been associated with varying degrees of chronic duodenitis, mucosal atrophy on duodenal biopsy, and blood loss from the gut, which aggravates the existing iron deficiency. Following treatment with iron most of these abnormalities revert to normal, indicating a diffuse and reversible enteropathy in children as a result of iron-deficiency anemia.[278]

Guha et al.[135] studied a group of twenty-six 4- to 6-year-old children with iron deficiency. More than two thirds of the children showed evidence of altered gastrointestinal function and structure. Before treatment there was a varying degree of duodenal-jejunal mucosal atrophy and significant shortening of the villi, which were blunted and fused over wide areas. In a high proportion of cases there was occult blood in the stool and impaired absorption of fat and *d*-xylose. Following iron therapy the biochemical and biologic changes in the small bowel disappeared. The severity of the intestinal changes was not directly correlated to the levels of hemoglobin or serum iron. These findings are comparable to the enteropathy caused by iron deficiency in children younger than 3 years that was reported by Naiman et al.[278] In contrast, other workers have found no abnormality in the intestinal mucosa of adults with iron-deficiency anemia[311,326] or minimal changes.[233] The reason for these diverse findings is not clear. Metabolism of intestinal epithelial cells depends on cellular enzymes that require iron, and iron deficiency may affect these enzymes, resulting in alteration in cellular metabolism. Possibly the requirements of iron-containing enzymes for regenerative processes are higher in the growing period. Therefore in iron deficiency the small bowel mucosa is more likely to be affected in children than in adults. It is also possible that with age the mucosa becomes less vulnerable to iron deficiency.

Table 6-13 summarizes the effects of iron deficiency on the gastrointestinal tract (primary iron deficiency) and abnormalities of the gastrointestinal system leading to iron-deficiency anemia (secondary iron deficiency).

Betanin, the red pigment found in beets, appears to be more efficiently absorbed in iron-deficient persons than in normal persons.[379] It is not clear whether this is related to increased passive transport across an abnormal or atrophic intestinal epithelium or to the betanin sharing an active transport mechanism with iron, which accelerates absorption of either substance in iron-deficient patients. The occurrence of red urine, beeturia, in iron-deficient subjects given beet puree is too inconsistent to be a practical diagnostic test, and its exact significance has not been fully determined.

Dallman et al.[84] have found decreased *cytochrome oxidase* activity in the gut epithelium of iron-deficient infants and animals; the rate of renewal after iron therapy depended on the rate of cell renewal. In rats cytochrome *c* activity is decreased to about 30% below control concentrations in intestinal mucosa and skeletal muscle early in the development of iron deficiency.[80] Other organs such as brain and heart muscle show little or no decrease even with severe chronic iron deficiency. The effect on kidney and liver is intermediate.

Central nervous system

The behavioral correlates of sideropenia in animals and man have recently been reviewed by Pollitt and Leibel.[296]

Clinical reports of patients with iron-deficiency anemia indicate that the subjects complain of fatigue, weakness, and lack of ability to concentrate. Some studies suggest that iron-deficient anemic children are irritable and anorexic.[80,153,399] However, Harris and Kellermeyer[153] point out that the subjective response to iron therapy in anemic iron-deficient patients often considerably precedes the rise in hemoglobin values. Thus 3 to 5 days after the institution of iron therapy the patient may note a return of strength, appetite, and a feeling of well-being that could not have been caused by an alteration of red cell mass.[218]

Studies on intellectual function in iron-deficient children have purported to demonstrate varying adverse effects of anemia on one or more cognitive process.[167,369,395]

In one study Sulzer et al.[369] studied more than 230 black 4- to 5-year-olds of both sexes enrolled in a Head Start program in New Orleans. Two batteries of psychologic tests were used. The first included a global, allegedly culture-free IQ test, a vocabulary test, and measures of moral development and grouping behavior. The other battery comprised reaction time, attentive recall, and ranking tasks. The performance of anemic children (hemoglobin levels < 10 gm/dl) was significantly poorer than controls on the vocabulary tests and showed similar but not significant trends on all other measures. The score differentials between groups became more statistically evident when the cutoff point in hemoglobin values was 10.5 gm/dl, which increased the sample of anemic children. Compared with the control group, the anemic children had significantly lower scores on the IQ measure, the vocabulary test, and the latency and associative reaction measures.

This study had a series of methodologic flaws (e.g., the testing environment was far from ideal and there was not time to establish rapport with the children); therefore the investigators considered the results inconclusive.

Howell[167] has reported markedly decreased attentiveness, narrow attention span, and perceptual restriction among 3- to 5-year-old iron-deficient children (hemoglobin levels < 10 gm/dl). Unfortunately, Howell's report is too incomplete to establish the validity of the data.

Iron-deficiency anemia and scholastic achievement in young adolescents were investigated in Philadelphia by Webb and Oski.[393] Subjects were 12- to 14-year-old male and female junior high school students in an economically deprived community. Ninety-two iron-deficient students were compared with a control group of 101 nonanemic students.

The scores of the anemic students in the scholastic performance tests were significantly lower (P < 0.025) than those of nonanemic students. In a subsequent study[395] the subjects' reports on the visualization of an afterimage showed that the iron-deficient anemic children had a longer latency period than the nonanemic subjects.

A third study by Webb and Oski[393] of seventy-four of these ninety-two anemic children and thirty-six control subjects employed a behavior problem checklist and showed a differential trend in behavior between the two groups. The anemic students tended to have more conduct disturbances than the nonanemic students, and the scholastic performance of the anemic children was compromised by disturbances in attention and perception.

It is unclear from these data whether the poor performance, perceptual disturbances, and conduct problems observed in the anemic students were consequences of anemia per se, of iron deficiency alone, or of a general nutritional inadequacy of which iron deficiency was only a readily identifiable component.

The reported investigations in New Orleans and Philadelphia suffer from weak study designs that raise critical questions about their internal validity. They were ex post facto limited to a static-group comparison,[40,251] and neither provided a way to certify that the groups would have been equivalent had it not been for the iron deficiency. It is probably premature for the conclusions of Howell and Webb and Oski to be accepted as evidence that iron deficiency has a detrimental effect on attentional processes, behavioral stability, and scholastic performance.

Some of the behavioral characteristics of iron-deficient children may have been caused by social and economic factors covarying with nutritional deficiency. Unless the environmental conditions in which the children were raised are taken into account, it seems doubtful that the exact nature of the apparent relationship between behavior and nutrition can be clarified.[296]

Given the striking prevalence of iron deficiency in children in the United States—particularly those of less advantaged socioeconomic status—and given the possible contribution of this state to the development of common behavioral and intellectual problems in children, it seems imperative that the nature of the relationship (if any) between these two rather ubiquitous conditions be determined in properly designed studies.

Holowach and Thurston[166] have shown an increased incidence of breath-holding spells in children with iron-deficiency anemia.

Papilledema, although rare, has been observed in infants and children. Because of this observation, iron-deficiency anemia should be considered in the differential diagnosis of pseudotumor cerebri (benign intracranial hypertension).[427]

Cardiovascular system

A reduction in hemoglobin concentration with resultant decrease in the oxygen-carrying capacity of the blood is associated with a compensatory increase in heart rate and cardiac output. Such changes are rarely detectable until the hemoglobin concentration has fallen to 7 gm/dl or less. With increasing severity of anemia, cardiac enlargement and murmurs may develop and decompensation can occur. These features, however, are common to all severe anemias and not specific for iron deficiency.

It is, in fact, notable that iron-deficient children can tolerate extremely low hemoglobin values (< 4 gm/dl) without apparent distress. The development of an intercurrent respiratory infection, however, may precipitate rapid cardiac decompensation.

Oxygen intake and ventilation rate in response to exercise are similar in persons with iron-deficiency anemia and controls but exercise cardiac output is elevated in the anemic group. The increased cardiac output results from an increased heart rate, but the stroke volume is similar in the anemic and control subjects.[82] The severely anemic group has a raised plasma volume and marked decrement in maximum aerobic power. These results suggest that anemia impairs performance during moderate and near-maximum exercise.

Gardner et al.[116] showed higher exercise and recovery heart rates during exercise tests of persons with iron deficiency (146 beats/minute, compared with 120 beats/minute in the iron treatment group) and higher minute ventilation values (42.5 liters/minute, compared to 33.3 liters/minute). This supports the concept that enhanced cardiorespiratory function during exercise is necessary to absorb a given amount of oxygen when hemoglobin levels are reduced.

Tolerance to digitalis in iron-deficient animals is increased. This observation may have some implications concerning the treatment of cardiac failure in anemic patients.[118]

Musculoskeletal system

Glover and Jacobs[121] monitored total and large body movements in Wistar rats using an activity meter and demonstrated considerable reduction in body movement in iron-depleted rats. After 2 and 4 days of iron-repletion therapy an increase in activity was observed, and there was a decline in activity after iron was again withheld.

A well-controlled study of rats by Edgerton et al.[100] showed that iron-deficiency anemia caused a decrement in forced-exercise performance and the decrement was quickly ameliorated by iron therapy. Performance as gauged by a forced exhaustive run and by voluntary activity was more closely related to hemoglobin level and packed cell volume than to levels of iron-containing compounds such as myoglobin or cytochrome in skeletal or heart muscle.

These experiments support the time-honored concept of a correlation between anemia and physical capacity and strongly suggest that the defect is primarily one of reduced oxygen-carrying capacity of the blood because of its decreased content of hemoglobin.

Despite a failure to demonstrate a correlation between physical performance, myoglobin and cytochrome content of the muscles, Edgerton et al.[100] suggested that the apparent salutary effect of iron repletion might not be solely the result of an increment in hemoglobin mass. The reconstitution of tissue iron stores might be a more important factor in the behavioral response to iron therapy.

Available information shows with few exceptions that physical endurance, activity, and manual labor productivity are significantly curtailed in adults with hemoglobin values lower than 11 gm/dl.[13,57,116,388] Basta[13] has shown that there is a significant increment in productivity after iron repletion therapy.

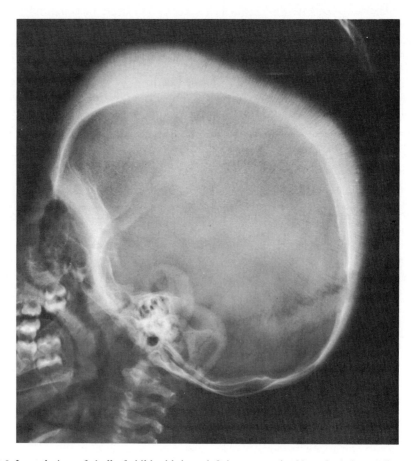

Fig. 6-8. Lateral view of skull of child with iron-deficiency anemia. Note the hair-standing-on-end appearance. (From Lanzkowsky, P.: Am. J. Dis. Child. **116:**16, 1968.)

Lanzkowsky[214] has shown roentgenographic changes in skull and metacarpal bones of fifteen infants and children with iron-deficiency anemia. These radiologic features varied from moderate but definite widening of the diploic space of the skull to widening of the diploic space with prominent vertical striations. The changes of the skull are identical with the ''hair-standing-on-end'' appearance observed on the roentgenogram of patients with the chronic hemolytic anemias.

These radiologic changes are more common in infants with low birth weight as a result of either prematurity or multiple births.* Associated protein deficiency may be a contributing factor in some cases of iron-deficiency anemia with roentgenographic changes.[214] Marrow hyperplasia as a result of an exaggerated erythroid response invoked by the anemia causes the expansion of bone and the radiographic changes. In contrast to the changes observed in thalassemia, these changes are usually but not always confined to the skull (Fig. 6-8).

Rothman et al.[319] have shown that chronic iron-deficiency anemia has an adverse effect on fracture healing as determined by tensile strength and histologic evaluation.

Immunologic system

There is a prevailing opinion that infants and children who have moderate to severe iron-deficiency anemia tend to have more infections than those who do not. This opinion is supported to some extent by morbidity and mortality data in published reports. In 1928 MacKay[239] showed that the morbidity for total attacks of acute illness during a 1-year period was reduced by half in iron-deficient children treated with iron. In a group of infants from a low socioeconomic population in Chicago, Andelman and Sered[7] showed an increased frequency of respiratory infections in the infants with iron deficiency and reduced incidence of such infections in children receiving iron supplements.

These findings have not been confirmed in more recent studies,[37,105] and there is conflicting clinical, laboratory, and theoretical evidence as to the relationship of iron deficiency and infections. Children and adults with severe iron-deficiency anemia or with dimorphic anemia had a lower frequency of bacterial infections compared to patients with other types of severe anemia.[243] Moreover there is considerable experimental evidence to support an argument for increased resistance to bacterial infection in iron-deficient states. It has long been known that several iron-binding proteins, including transferrin, inhibit bacterial growth in vitro by binding iron so avidly that no free iron is avail-

*References 4, 33, 101, 214, 345.

able for growth of the organisms.[331,332] If iron is added to plasma, growth of bacteria remains inhibited until the transferrin becomes saturated with iron.[110] Finally, growth of ordinarily nonpathogenic bacteria has been enhanced in laboratory animals by injections of iron.[174] Thus, although there is widespread belief that iron deficiency predisposes to infection, there is some clinical and a good deal of experimental evidence to the contrary, at least with respect to bacterial infections.

Serum immunoglobulin levels, serum concentration of C3, and serum antibody responses to tetanus toxoid and *Salmonella typhi* are all normal in iron deficiency.[51,237]

With reference to host defenses in iron-deficiency anemia there is a preponderance of evidence suggesting that the iron-deficient host may be compromised in terms of defense against microorganisms.

Joynson et al.[189] and Macdougall et al.[237] reported, respectively, that in vitro lymphocyte responses to the soluble antigens, *Candida,* and purified protein derivative (PPD) and to the mitogen phytohemagglutinin were impaired in patients with iron deficiency. Moreover these two groups of workers found an apparent depression of cell-mediated immunity in vivo in infants with latent and overt iron deficiency and in older iron-deficient persons. A defect in DNA synthesis has been found in iron-deficient lymphocytes, and this may be related to decreased activity of the iron-containing enzyme ribonucleotide reductase.[164] Morphologic abnormalities suggesting metabolic changes have also been demonstrated in the mitochondria of iron-deficient lymphocytes.

Chandra[49] reported that the bactericidal capacity of polymorphonuclear leukocytes of iron-deficient malnourished children was subnormal and suggested that iron deficiency might impair the activity of iron-dependent enzymes important in bacterial killing; a similar decrease in bactericidal function was also found in iron deficiency in the studies reported by Macdougall et al.[237] and Strikantia et al.[362]

Boggs and Miller[22] showed that rats infected orally with *S. typhimurium* were unable to produce and deliver cells containing myeloperoxidase to the gut in sufficient quantity quickly enough to withstand the stress of enteric infection. As the level of myeloperoxidase in the gut increases, the number of *S. typhimurium* organisms decreases. Iron-deficient animals were less able to produce myeloperoxidase-containing cells. Decrease in myeloperoxidase activity has also been demonstrated in iron-deficiency anemia.[160] Kulapongs et al.,[207] however, could not confirm either of these abnormalities, since in vitro studies of lymphocyte responsiveness to phytohemagglutinin and of phagocytosis and killing by polymorphonuclear cells in eight young children with severe iron-deficiency anemia were entirely normal.

The discrepancies between the results of these various studies could be attributed to subject variability or to variability in the laboratory methods used. Subject variability among the iron-deficient patient populations may be related to (1) their state of nutrition and (2) whether they had had recent or intercurrent infections. Except in cases in which the deficiency is clearly a result of blood loss, it is extremely difficult to rule out concomitant deficiencies such as protein malnutrition in iron-deficient infants and children. Some element of general malnutrition may have been present in many of the subjects studied, and variations in the state of nutrition of the patients could account for some of the observed differences in the results of the immunologic tests. More important, however, is that in all such studies it has not been possible to exclude the possibility that intercurrent infection may have been a major factor contributing to the various immunologic abnormalities observed. Decreased delayed skin reactivity and depression of mitogenic lymphocyte transformation in vitro are known to occur in patients infected with or recovering from various infections.

This conflicting evidence is summarized in the following outline:

Effect of iron deficiency on infection

A. Evidence of increased propensity for infection
  1. Clinical evidence
    a. Acute illness in iron-deficient children reduced by iron treatment and rate of recovery better[239]
    b. Increased frequency of respiratory infection in iron deficiency[7]
  2. Laboratory evidence
    a. Impaired lymphocyte transformation[189,237]
    b. Impaired granulocyte killing[49,237] and NBT (nitroblue tetrazolium[51])
    c. Decreased myeloperoxidase in leukocytes[160] and small intestine[22]
    d. Decreased cutaneous hypersensitivity[189,237]
    e. Increased susceptibility to infection in iron-deficient animals[22]
B. Evidence of decreased propensity for infection
  1. Clinical evidence
    a. Decreased frequency of bacterial infection[243]
    b. Increased frequency of infection in iron overload
  2. Laboratory evidence
    a. Inhibition of bacterial growth by transferrin,[331,332] which binds iron so that no free iron is available for growth of microorganisms
    b. Growth of nonpathogenic bacteria enhanced by iron[174]

Cellular metabolism

Red cells. In iron deficiency there is destruction of newly made red cells and red cell precursors within the bone marrow (ineffective erythropoiesis).[297,316] The rate of release of hypochromic microcytic red blood cells to the circulation is decreased. Furthermore as iron deficiency becomes severe, there is progressively diminishing survival of cells to half of normal or less.[238]

Decreased red cell survival appears to be related to the severity of the anemia and the presence of a functioning spleen. Iron-deficient cells survive normally when transfused into a splenectomized recipient, suggesting an intracorpuscular defect. A progressive increase in red cell hexokinase activity (without reticulocytosis) was noted in association with increasing severity of the anemia and decreasing red cell life span. Red cell ATP concentration was normal or slightly decreased and showed marked instability on incubation. Iron-deficient cells that have increased metabolic requirements are more vulnerable to the adverse effects of the splenic environment, a situation that is exaggerated in the most severely anemic patients with the greatest increase in hexokinase activity. Moderate splenic enlargement was present in thirteen (34%) of the iron-deficient children studied by Macdougall et al.,[238] twelve of whom had decreased red cell survival. Iron-deficient cells were found to be more susceptible than normal cells to lysis during 24-hour incubation in glucose-free balanced salt solution (increased autohemolysis). The severely iron-deficient erythrocyte also demonstrated an increased susceptibility to sulfhydryl inhibitors in vitro. Iron-deficient erythrocytes, despite their smaller volume, were found to have an impaired ability to filter through $5~\mu$ Millipore filters.[43]

These studies suggest that the abnormal plasticity or less deformability (rigidity) may lead to excessive trapping of these cells within the narrow vascular channels of the spleen. These metabolically abnormal cells are exposed to hostile conditions of stasis and glucose deprivation, which may then enhance their lysis and account for hemolytic anemia in severe iron deficiency. This sequence of events would explain the improvement noted in survival of the iron-deficient red cells when transfused into asplenic individuals. The increased sequestration of iron-deficient red cells within the spleen may also be responsible for the clinical findings of splenomegaly in patients with severe iron deficiency.

In iron deficiency there is marked decrease in globin synthesis as well as selective decrease in α-chain synthesis relative to β-chain synthesis. Monomers of α-globin, possibly with some $\alpha\beta$ dimers, appear to precipitate on or attach to the cell membrane. Similar findings have been reported in other states of heme deficiency such as sideroblastic anemia and lead poisoning. Utilization of iron and glycine for heme production and glycine for protein synthesis is also decreased.

Macdougall[234] showed a mean decrease in glutathione peroxidase and catalase activity in iron-deficient cells to 60% and 64% of normal, respectively. The reduction in glutathione peroxidase activity has been confirmed by other workers.[318] It is apparent therefore that the enzymatic mechanisms for detoxifying H_2O_2 are inefficient in iron-deficient red cells. This accounts for the fact that Melhorn et al.[254] have demonstrated that iron-deficient red cells are more susceptible to hemolysis by hydrogen peroxide. These observations suggest that a metabolic defect in the iron-deficient red cell may allow oxidative damage of the membrane to occur. Alteration in the membrane may in turn result in increased cellular rigidity, increased sequestration in the spleen and other organs, and ultimately premature cell destruction. It has been proposed that the red cell enzyme glutathione peroxidase may play an important role in protecting the red cell from oxidative changes. The reported increase in glycolysis and amounts of G-6-PD, 6-phosphogluconate dehydrogenase, and glutathione in iron-deficient red cells[236,238] indicates that the glutathione-generating mechanisms of the hexose-monophosphate pathway are intact. The high glutathione concentration presumably confers some protection on the iron-deficient cell and may allow for nonenzymatic oxidation of glutathione should the glutathione peroxidase mechanism prove rate limiting in the presence of peroxide or peroxide-generating drugs, as has been demonstrated in hereditary glutathione peroxidase deficiency.[250,364]

The NADH and methemoglobin reductase activity of human erythrocytes is significantly increased in iron-deficiency anemia. A high methemoglobin reductase activity is important in anemia when the level of hemoglobin is reduced and the need to maintain it in the functional form is greater.[306]

Measurements of 2,3-DPG, ATP, and glutamic oxaloacetic transaminase (GOT) in erythrocytes were performed on normal and iron-deficient patients. The results showed a significant elevation in the level of 2,3-DPG per red blood cell and per gram of hemoglobin and an elevation of GOT in the iron-deficient patients. There was no correlation between rises in the levels of 2,3-DPG and GOT. Neither 2,3-DPG nor GOT correlated with the level of hemoglobin or with the MCHC. The ATP level was not elevated in the iron-deficient patients. Thus elevation of the 2,3-DPG level in iron deficiency cannot be explained only by a decrease in hemoglobin concentration. Other factors such as cell age and intraerythrocytic pH may influence the level of 2,3-DPG in this and possibly other anemia states.[353]

Impairment in DNA and RNA synthesis has been observed in bone marrow cells from iron-deficient patients.[159]

It is evident therefore that iron deficiency not only results in a decrease in hemoglobin synthesis but also has a profound effect on the overall metabolism of hematopoietic tissue.

Other tissues. Beutler[21] has demonstrated deficiencies in heme-containing enzymes (cytochrome *c* and cytochrome oxidase) and iron-dependent enzymes (succinic dehydrogenase and aconitase) in the tissues of animals with latent iron deficiency (sideropenia without significant anemia). Swarup et al.[370] reported a deficiency in aconitase activity of whole blood in nineteen of thirty-nine iron-deficient patients that appeared most severe in the buffy coat and could be attributed to the white cells. Many of the Krebs (tricarboxylic acid) cycle enzymes and cofactors contain iron, and in vitro studies have demonstrated increased oxygen consumption in the leukocytes of iron-deficient patients.[178] A study by Dagg et al.[76] showed tissue (buccal mucosa) cytochrome oxidase deficiency in sideropenic patients but failed to establish a correlation between the enzymopathy and the presence and/or severity of buccal mucosa atrophy. Dallman and Schwartz[82] showed that in rats a mild iron deficiency reduced tissue levels of cytochrome *c* by as much as 30% in intestinal mucosa and skeletal muscle but that little or no decrease in this cytochrome occurred in the brain and cardiac muscle of severely iron-deficient animals.

Another enzyme apparently sensitive to the state of body iron stores is mitochrondrial monoamine oxidase (MAO). Symes et al.[372] have shown that chronic iron deficiency in rats results in decreased MAO activity and that an adequate supply of dietary iron is necessary to maintain normal MAO activity. Voorhess et al.[389] have reported that urinary excretion of norepinephrine is increased in children with untreated iron-deficiency anemia and that the excretion of norepinephrine returns toward normal after 3 or 4 days of parenteral iron therapy.

Given the putative function of various monoamines in brain neurotransmission[67] and the affective and behavioral changes associated with the administration of MAO-blocking agents,[361] it seems possible that at least a portion of the behavioral aberrations commonly attributed to iron deficiency may be caused by impaired MAO function and associated excesses of central nervous system catechols. Voorhess et al.[389] provided evidence of such a conjunction and showed that children with iron-deficiency anemia had elevated urinary nor-epinephrine excretion rates prior to therapy with intramuscular iron. Urinary norepinephrine excretion did not vary directly with the degree of anemia, serum iron level, or percentage of saturation, but patients with anemias unrelated to iron deficiency failed to show any significant alterations in norepinephrine excretion before or after transfusion. The clinical observations regarding the rapidity of symptomatic relief, as opposed to the longer time needed to raise the hemoglobin level in iron-repletion therapy, is particularly interesting in view of the fact that urinary norepinephrine excretion rates were normalized in these patients within 1 week of parenteral iron treatment—before the hemoglobin levels had increased substantially.[389] Tyrosine hydroxylase, the enzyme that converts tyrosine to dihydroxyphenylalanine, requires iron as a cofactor and is inhibited by iron chelators.[361] The iron-deficient state might be expected to suppress the activity of this rate-limiting enzyme in norepinephrine synthesis to partially compensate for the effect of diminished MAO activity.

The effect of iron-deficiency anemia on cellular growth and protein accretion in rats was studied using the parameters of organ weight and protein, DNA, and RNA content. Rats fed an iron-deficient diet from 40 to 143 days of age showed hypoplasia (decreased total DNA) and hypertrophy (increased protein:DNA ratio) of liver cells, hypertrophy of renal cells, and increased total DNA and reduced protein:DNA ratio in spleen.[42] Lanzkowsky et al.[225] have shown that cellular changes in various organs of rats resulting from an iron-deficient diet fed from 21 to 49 days are corrected by iron administration by 147 days of age and are not evidence of permanent cellular damage.

Hyperplasia of cardiac muscles (increase in cardiac DNA) and nonmuscle cells causing cardiomegaly occurs when iron deficiency is induced during early postweaning life in rats whereas iron deficiency occurring during adult life in rats gives rise to hypertrophy of cardiac muscle cells and hyperplasia of cardiac nonmuscle cells.[281]

Dallman et al.[83] showed that a brief period of severe iron deficiency in young rats resulted in a deficit of brain iron that persisted in the adult animals despite an adequate intake of iron and despite the correction of the hematocrit, liver nonheme iron, and liver ferritin levels, which promptly returned to normal after iron treatment. The significance of these observations with reference to iron-deficiency anemia in humans is not clearly understood at present.

Plasma zinc levels have been found to be low in persons with iron deficiency in India.[210] This may be related to the eating of meager amounts of animal protein leading to both iron and zinc deficiency.

The following outline summarizes the tissue effects of iron-deficiency anemia.

A. Gastrointestinal tract
  1. Anorexia
    a. Increased proportion of low-weight percentiles
    b. Depression of growth
  2. Pica
  3. Atrophic glossitis
  4. Dysphagia
  5. Esophageal webs (Paterson-Kelly syndrome)
  6. Reduced gastric acidity
  7. "Leaky gut" syndrome
    a. Guaiac-positive stools
    b. Exudative enteropathy (protein, albumin, immunoglobulins, copper, calcium)
  8. Malabsorption syndrome
    a. Iron only
    b. Generalized malabsorption (xylose, fat, vitamin A, duodenojejunal mucosal atrophy)
  9. Beeturia
  10. Decreased cytochrome oxidase activity, succinic dehydrogenase, and lactose
B. Central nervous system
  1. Irritability
  2. Lower IQ scores (?)
  3. Decreased attentiveness, narrow attention span (?)
  4. Significantly lower scholastic performance (?)
  5. Breath-holding spells
  6. Papilledema
C. Cardiovascular system
  1. Increase in exercise and recovery heart rate and cardiac output
  2. Cardiac hypertrophy
  3. Increase in plasma volume
  4. Increased minute ventilation values
  5. Increased tolerance to digitalis
D. Musculoskeletal system
  1. Deficiency of myoglobin and cytochrome *c*
  2. Decreased physical performance
  3. Roentgenologic changes in bone
  4. Adverse affect on fracture healing
E. Immunologic system: see p. 139
F. Cellular changes
  1. Red cells
    a. Ineffective erythropoiesis
    b. Decreased red cell survival (normal when injected into asplenic individuals)
    c. Increased autohemolysis
    d. Increased red cell rigidity
    e. Increased susceptibility to sulfhydryl inhibitors
    f. Decreased heme production
    g. Decreased globin and α-chain synthesis
    h. Precipitation of α-globin monomers to cell membrane (?)
    i. Decreased glutathione peroxidase and catalase activity
     (1) Inefficient H_2O_2 detoxification
     (2) Greater susceptibility to H_2O_2 hemolysis

(3) Oxidative damage to cell membrane

(4) Increased cellular rigidity

j. Increase in rate of glycolysis—G-6-PD, 6-phosphogluconate dehydrogenase, 2,3-DPG, and glutathione

k. Increase in NADH-methemoglobin reductase

l. Increase in erythrocyte glutamic oxaloacetic transaminase (EGOT)

m. Increase in free erythrocyte protoporphyrin

n. Impairment in DNA and RNA synthesis in bone marrow cells

2. Other tissues

a. Reduction in heme-containing enzymes (cytochrome *c*, cytochrome oxidase)

b. Reduction in iron-dependent enzymes (succinic dehydrogenase, aconitase)

c. Reduction in monoamine oxidase (MAO)

d. Increased excretion of urinary norepinephrine

e. Reduction in tyrosine hydroxylase (enzyme converting tyrosine to dihydroxyphenylalanine) (?)

f. Alterations in cellular growth—DNA, RNA, and protein

g. Persistent deficiency of brain iron following short-term deprivation

h. Reduction in plasma zinc

Permanent sequelae. The reversibility of iron-deficiency anemia following treatment may lead to a false sense of security because all of the easily measured clinical laboratory studies have been corrected. The possibility of long-term and as yet undetermined sequelae deserves more attention. Severe protein-calorie malnutrition in early life results in permanent deficit in growth and intellectual function. Long-term sequelae of iron deficiency, particularly during early development, must be considered within the realm of possibility. The various tissue effects of iron deficiency alert us to the fact that iron deficiency is a systemic disease rather than an abnormality of the blood alone. The readily reversible anemia is not an early finding. Several months must elapse after iron stores are exhausted before a population of red cells substantially deficient in hemoglobin replaces normal cells at a rate of about 1% per day. In the meantime other manifestations of iron deficiency may develop, some of which may not be as readily reversed as anemia. Therefore systemic manifestations of iron deficiency are gradually receiving the increased attention they require.

LABORATORY DATA
Blood

The anemia of iron deficiency is characteristically hypochromic and microcytic (Fig. 6-9). The morphologic changes of hypochromia and microcytosis do not appear until the hemoglobin level has fallen below 10 gm/dl. Because iron deficiency primarily affects hemoglobin synthesis and affects red cell formation to a lesser degree, the red cell count may be normal, near normal, or moderately reduced. Hematocrit levels are lower than normal. The MCHC is less than 32% and is an important index of hypochromic anemia. The MCV (mean cell volume) is usually less than 80 fl, and the MCH (mean corpuscular hemoglobin) less than 29 pg. Associated with the hypochromia is increased resistance to osmotic lysis. Table 6-15 lists typical red cell indices.

Recently red cell volume distribution curves,

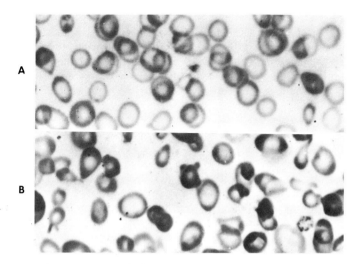

Fig. 6-9. Comparison of blood smears of iron-deficiency anemia and thalassemia major. **A,** Iron-deficiency anemia—note predominance of hypochromic microcytes of fairly uniform size and shape and central pallor. **B,** Thalassemia major before splenectomy—note microcytes, hypochromic macrocytes, marked anisocytosis and poikilocytosis, normoblasts, and teardrop cells.

Table 6-15. Red cell indices

Anemia	MCV (fl)*	MCH (pg)	MCHC (%)
Normocytic	80-96	26-34	32-36
Microcytic hypochromic	50-79	12-29	24-31
Microcytic	70-80	22-26	32-36
Hypochromic	80-96	23-31	28-31

*Older children and adults. In infancy and early childhood levels considerably below 80 fl are normal; e.g., at 1 year the mean MCV is 77 fl, with a range of 72 to 85 fl.[205a]

which are more sensitive than conventional red cell indices, have shown three stages of iron deficiency as it interferes with hematopoietic function[102]:

1. Anisocytosis and an increased percentage of microcytic cells occur at a stage when the hemoglobin is normal and the transferrin saturation is less than 32%.
2. The MCV and MCH decline, the hemoglobin is generally subnormal, and transferrin is usually below 16%.
3. The MCHC declines, the hemoglobin concentration is below 9 gm/dl, and the transferrin saturation is less than 16%.

Analysis of the red cell volume distribution curves is the most sensitive method for detecting persons with low transferrin saturation. In fact the measurements are so sensitive that abnormalities are detectable in persons whose iron deficiency otherwise was either prelatent or latent.

The blood smear shows microcytes, poikilocytes, elliptical and elongated pencil forms, and target cells. Many of the red cells are small. Basophilic stippling and occasional normoblasts may occur as a direct consequence of iron deficiency. In addition to iron-deficiency anemia, basophilic stippling may occur in other causes of hypochromic anemia such as thalassemia, sideroblastic anemia, and lead poisoning. Unless morphologic changes are pronounced, the diagnosis of iron-deficiency anemia from examination of the blood film is difficult and unreliable. Failure to identify patients with iron-deficiency anemia occurs in 10% to 20% of cases when the diagnosis is based on blood smear only, and smears of normal individuals are frequently interpreted as consistent with iron-deficiency anemia when reviewed without knowledge of other clinical or laboratory data. The reticulocyte count is usually normal but in severe iron-deficiency anemia, especially if associated with bleeding, a reticulocyte count of 3% to 4% is occasionally encountered. The absolute reticulocyte count, however, is low.

The platelet count varies from thrombocytopenia to thrombocytosis. Gross et al.[131] showed that thrombocytopenia occurred in 28.3% of iron-deficient infants. Thrombocytopenia is more common in severe iron-deficiency anemia,[155] and thrombocytosis is present when there is associated bleeding from the gut. In one series the mean hemoglobin level of the thrombocytopenic group (platelet counts of 170×10^9/liter) was 4 gm/dl, and for those with increased platelet counts (mean platelet count of 420×10^9/liter) it was 6 gm/dl. Platelet counts rose with iron therapy—much more rapidly with parenteral iron administration. Thrombocytopenia may reflect a depletion of iron, platelets being known to contain iron enzymes, or it may be caused by an associated folate deficiency or a transient thrombopoietin defect.

Iron is necessary for platelet production and when given it increases the number of platelets, but only in the presence of iron deficiency. Administration of parenteral iron to non-iron-deficient control animals has no effect on platelet count or megathrombocyte number.

Karpatkin et al.,[194] as a result of their own and other experiments, suggested that serum iron levels can inhibit, either directly or indirectly, any increase of the platelet count above a steady state level. Conversely low serum iron levels permit an increase above this level, e.g., in the presence of infection or after splenectomy. In both of these situations the serum iron level is usually low.

Other explanations for the thrombocytosis of iron deficiency must, however, be considered. It has been suggested that erythropoietin may increase platelet levels as well as the red cell count in the peripheral blood.[334] Iron deficiency is associated with increased erythropoietin levels, and plasma from rats made anemic by phenylhydrazine induces thrombocytosis when infused into normal animals.[230]

Whatever the mechanism, the increased platelet levels of iron deficiency appear to result from an increased turnover, i.e., increased numbers of megakaryocytes producing increased numbers of platelets that have a normal lifespan.[152]

The leukocyte count is usually normal or slightly reduced. Neutropenia occurs in not more than 10% of patients with iron deficiency.

Bone marrow

The bone marrow shows erythroid hyperplasia with a predominance of polychromatophilic normoblasts, often smaller than normal. The cytoplasm of the normoblasts may be diminished and occasionally ragged, sometimes with vacuolation and delayed cytoplasmic maturation indicative of decreased cellular hemoglobin. Ferrokinetic measurements show ineffective erythropoiesis and hemolysis.

It has been shown in profoundly iron-depleted persons (in whom folic acid and vitamin B_{12} deficiency and diseases associated with dyserythropoiesis have been excluded) that nuclear changes such as karyorrhexis, nuclear budding, multinuclearity, fragmentation, and internuclear bridging occur in the red cell precursors as well as giant granulocytes.[161] The dyserythropoiesis has been attributed to a direct effect of iron deficiency or to a suggested relationship between iron deficiency and defective folate metabolism[47,48,73,387] although the essential connection between them is not known. Although the exact pathogenesis of the abnormalities in iron deficiency is not fully known, it is quite probable that iron has an important role in erythroblast DNA synthesis and conceivably RNA synthesis and that it is necessary for the orderly nuclear maturation in erythropoiesis.

Dallman and Goodman[81] have described enlarged and vacuolated mitochrondria in the erythroblasts of iron-deficient children, underscoring the fact that cellular organization is dependent on an adequate intake of iron.

Neutrophil hypersegmentation has also been observed in pure iron-deficiency anemia.[391] Iron may be required in some way for optimal incorporation of vitamin B_{12} into neutrophils sufficiently to cause neutrophil hypersegmentation.[96]

Megakaryocytes are normal in number and in appearance. They may be increased in patients with high platelet counts. Occasionally when platelets are decreased there are diminished numbers of megakaryocytes associated with evidences of megaloblastic marrow.[131]

Measurement of tissue iron

The amount of iron in the storage cells is a reliable index of the body stores of iron. In iron-deficiency anemia there is a decrease of iron granules in the normoblasts (sideroblasts)[56,187] and almost complete absence of stainable iron or hemosiderin in the marrow sections stained by Prussian blue reaction. Fong et al.[111] showed significantly different amounts of stainable iron in needle biopsy sections compared to aspirated smears in 15% of 251 patients. Usually there is significantly less stainable iron in needle biopsy sections than in aspirated smears. Of clinical importance was the finding of absence of stainable iron in 8% of the needle biopsy sections in contrast to definite deposits observed in the corresponding aspirated smear.

A biopsy specimen of the liver can also be stained for iron or used for the chemical determination of nonheme iron. This provides a good indication of body iron stores, but the procedure is rarely warranted for diagnostic use.

Serum iron and iron-binding capacity

The level of serum iron reflects the balance between the iron absorbed, the iron utilized for

Table 6-16. Normal values of serum iron and iron-binding capacity*

Age	Serum iron (μg/dl)	Latent iron-binding capacity (μg/dl)	Total iron-binding capacity (μg/dl)	Saturation (%)
Birth	168	73	241	69.7
1-2 years	93	319	412	22.0
2-6 years	116	279	395	28.0
6-12 years	127	213	340	38.0

*Modified from Smith, C. H.: Bull. N.Y. Acad. Med. **30:**155, 1954.

Table 6-17. Mean serum iron and iron saturation percentage

Age (years)	Serum iron (μg/dl)	Saturation (%)
0.5-2	68 ± 3.6 (16-120)	22 ± 1.1 (6-38)
2-6	72 ± 3.4 (20-124)	25 ± 1.2 (7-43)
6-12	73 ± 3.4 (23-123)	25 ± 1.2 (7-43)
18 and older	92 ± 3.8 (48-136)	30 ± 1.1 (18-46)

hemoglobin synthesis, the iron released by red cell destruction, and the size of the storage depots. At a particular time the serum iron concentration represents a precise equilibrium between the iron entering and leaving the circulation.

The percentage of transferrin saturation is a more sensitive index of iron status than the serum iron level alone, since total transferrin usually increases in iron deficiency, whereas serum iron decreases. Furthermore the percentage of saturation most accurately reflects the availability of iron for hematopoiesis. When transferrin drops lower than 15% or 16%, iron lack limits hemoglobin production. The values for serum iron and iron-binding capacity in newborn, normal infants, and children at various ages are given in Table 6-16.

Recently Koerper and Dallman[205] have determined normal values for serum iron and iron saturation in children; they excluded children who had any evidence of iron deficiency or hemoglobinopathy (serum ferritin < 12 ng/ml, free erythrocyte protoporphyrin > 3.0 μg/gm hemoglobin, low MCV, low hemoglobin value, or abnormal hemoglobin electrophoresis). The results obtained were much lower than values hitherto accepted as within the normal range. The means ± SEM and 95% confidence limits at various ages are shown in Table 6-17.

If the usual criterion for normal adults, namely 16% iron saturation, were employed, 17% of presumptively normal children would have been designated subnormal.

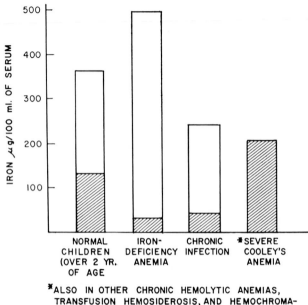

Fig. 6-10. Schematic representation of specific anemias. Shaded areas represent serum iron level and clear areas latent iron-binding capacity. The total iron-binding capacity is the sum of these two fractions. The high serum iron level and absent latent iron-binding capacity in patients with the hemolytic anemias are contrasted with the low serum iron level and greatly expanded latent iron-binding capacity in those with iron-deficiency anemia.

It is of interest that the concentration of serum iron is higher in the morning and lower in the evening. This diurnal variation has been ascribed to the adrenal cortex and to variations in the autonomic nervous system[28]; therefore, blood for serum iron should be drawn in the morning. At 8:00 A.M. serum iron levels normally average 140 μg/dl, yielding a saturation of 47%. This falls throughout the day to a low of 40 μg/dl by 10:00 P.M., or a saturation of 13%.[78] A high degree of variability exists in adolescents with respect to serum iron and iron-binding levels. Boys tend to have higher serum iron levels, slightly lower unsaturated iron-binding capacities, greater saturation of the circulating transferrins, and higher mean hemoglobin levels, hematocrit values, and MCHC.[343]

The average coefficient of variation in serum iron estimations is between 10% and 15%. Therefore 95% of results obtained from a given sample fall within the range of 75% to 125% of the true result.[99]

There is a wide variation of serum iron and saturation according to age, sex, diurnal variation, dietary factors, laboratory methodology, and other factors, resulting in a large normal range. For better accuracy of diagnosis determinations of serum iron and saturation should be used in conjunction with at least one other test of iron status, and the developmental norms for serum iron and saturation must be applied.

In persons with iron-deficiency anemia the depleted stores are represented by a greatly reduced serum iron level, a markedly expanded iron-binding capacity, and a very low percentage of saturation.

In iron deficiency the serum iron level is reduced (varying from 10 to 16 μg/dl), the latent iron-binding capacity of the serum is increased to approximately 450 μg/dl and above, and the saturation of serum iron (serum iron divided by serum iron plus the latent iron-binding capacity) is reduced. Failure of iron supply to the normoblast occurs when the saturation of transferrin falls below 16%, and figures of less than this are invariably associated with iron-deficient erythropoiesis.

The development of iron-deficiency anemia occurs in the following sequence:

1. Depletion of iron stores (usually evident in the bone marrow or by decreased plasma ferritin levels)
2. Elevation of the iron binding capacity of the serum
3. Fall in serum iron level

Table 6-18. Serum and iron-binding capacity in various clinical conditions

	Decreased	Increased
Serum iron	Iron deficiency Infection (acute and chronic) Pregnancy Debilitating diseases (uremia, cancer, and others)	Decreased erythropoiesis Aplastic anemia Acute leukemia Hemolytic anemia Ineffective erythropoiesis Iron overload—hemochromatosis, transfusional hemosiderosis Pernicious anemia (untreated) Cirrhosis Acute hepatitis
Latent iron-binding capacity	Infection Hemolytic disease Debilitating diseases Cirrhosis Hepatitis Pernicious anemia (untreated) Hemochromatosis absent Transfusion hemosiderosis	Iron deficiency Pregnancy

4. Development of normochromic or slightly hypochromic anemia
5. Development of hypochromic microcytic anemia

A reversal of the sequence occurs when the deficiency is treated with oral iron. Serum iron and iron-binding determinations may be employed as useful guides in gauging the adequacy and completeness of therapy in patients with iron-deficiency anemia.

In patients with acute and chronic infection the impairment of hemoglobin synthesis is accompanied by a disturbance in erythropoiesis and a diversion of iron to tissue stores.[317,413] Both the serum iron and the latent iron-binding capacity are significantly reduced, but the percentage of saturation is not decreased to the extent noted in patients with iron-deficiency anemia. In patients with disorders in which hemoglobin synthesis and marrow function are depressed (as in those with untreated pernicious anemia, hypoplastic anemia, and aplastic anemia) the serum iron level is greatly elevated, and the latent iron-binding capacity is reduced or often absent when multiple transfusions have been given. In persons with conditions of iron excess (such as the hemolytic anemias, transfusion hemosiderosis, and hemochromatosis) the body iron is

markedly increased as a result of the preponderance of red cell destruction over formation and in part as a result of increased iron absorption. When the serum iron level is markedly elevated, the latent iron-binding capacity is absent, so that the saturation is 100%. As shown in Fig. 6-10 and Table 6-18, examination of the individual patterns occasionally helps in the differentiation of the various anemias and provides an insight into the separate phases of iron metabolism.

In iron deficiency the copper levels (normal mean, 114; normal limits, 81 to 147 mg/dl) generally are increased except in the small group of infants who have exudative enteropathy caused by iron deficiency or induced by ingestion of whole cow's milk.

The practical assessment of total body iron stores has always been tedious and nonreproducible. The most direct method for measuring storage iron is by quantitative phlebotomy,[176] and the results obtained by this technique provide a standard for comparison with other methods. The alternative methods involve the injection of chelating agents such as desferrioxamine followed by the measurement of urinary iron excretion or the estimation of iron in biopsy samples, either visually or chemically. All these procedures involve some inconvenience for the patient. In addition, chelatable iron is not always directly related to storage iron.

Plasma ferritin

Recently it has become possible to quantify plasma ferritin concentrations. Ferritin is found mainly in the cytoplasm of reticuloendothelial cells and liver cells. It is normally thought to be an intracellular storage compound from which iron is mobilized into the transferrin-bound plasma pool. Before the development of a sensitive immunoradiometric assay method, it was not thought to appear in the plasma or extracellular fluid under normal conditions. It has been shown by these studies that plasma ferritin is increased or decreased in proportion to the levels of storage iron and provides a clinically useful quantitative method of assessing the level of storage iron. The level of serum ferritin reflects the level of body iron stores and is quantitative, reproducible, and sensitive and requires only a small blood sample. It provides a noninvasive method for measuring a segment of the body ferritin pool. The data of Walters et al.[392] suggested that in normal subjects 1 μg of ferritin/liter of serum represents about 8 mg of storage iron.

The mean cord blood concentration of plasma ferritin is 113 ng/ml. Beginning on the second day of life, there is a sharp increase in plasma ferritin to a mean level of 356 ng/ml at 1 month of age. High levels are maintained until 2 to 3 months of

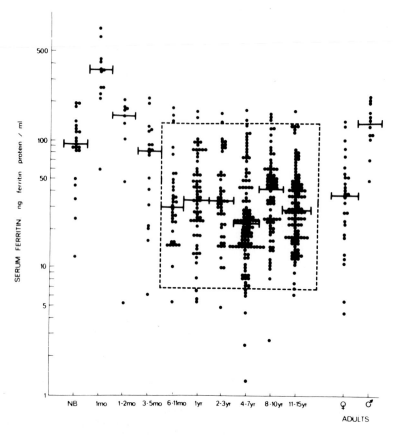

Fig. 6-11. Serum ferritin concentrations during development. Serum ferritin concentrations in healthy nonanemic newborns, infants, and children of various age groups are shown with adult male and female values. The median value in each age group is indicated by a horizontal line. The dashed line encloses a square that includes the 95% confidence limits of the values between the ages of 6 months and 15 years. (From Siimes, M. A., et al.: Blood **43**:581, 1974. Used by permission.)

age when iron stores are mobilized to meet the erythropoietic demands of an expanding hemoglobin mass and the level of plasma ferritin declines. Infants not receiving an available source of dietary iron are found to have no measurable ferritin level by 6 months of age, reflecting complete body iron store depletion. The mean value of plasma ferritin from 6 months through 15 years of age is 30 ng/ml (95% confidence limits of 7 to 142 ng/ml). This value is similar to concentration in iron-depleted adult subjects. The low level of plasma ferritin found in healthy children indicates that there is essentially no accumulation of storage iron during the period of childhood growth. Median concentrations of ferritin in adults are 39 ng/ml in women and 140 ng/ml in men[350] (Fig. 6-11). The mean concentration is higher in men (123 ng/ml) than in women (56 ng/ml) with a range between 12 and 300 ng/ml.[180]

In patients with iron-deficiency anemia concentrations are less than 12 ng/ml and in patients with iron overload the concentration may be as much as 10,000 ng/ml.[180] There is a good correlation between serum ferritin concentration and iron stores mobilized by quantitative phlebotomy,[392] a good correlation between serum ferritin concentration and the concentration of iron in liver biopsy tissue,[228] and a crude relationship between stainable iron in the bone marrow and serum ferritin concentration.[18,173]

The serum ferritin concentration can be used both to evaluate iron stores in patients with suspected iron deficiency and to determine the level of stores after the completion of iron therapy.[17] It is particularly useful for measuring iron stores in patients with chronic disease such as rheumatoid arthritis who may also have a hypochromic microcytic anemia,[18] and in these cases it is the most effective way to determine the need for iron therapy. It has also been used in monitoring the iron status of patients with chronic renal failure on a regular dialysis regime,[173] and in these patients, too, iron therapy can be controlled in a rational manner. Iron overload can be monitored by serial estimations of serum ferritin concentration and in patients with idiopathic hemochromatosis who are undergoing venisection, the assay shows when body iron stores have been fully mobilized. In patients with thalassemia who have been on a regular transfusion regime the effect of chelation therapy can be assessed.[228]

The serum ferritin concentration usually reflects reticuloendothelial storage iron. Changes in reticuloendothelial iron are followed rapidly by changes in the serum concentration of ferritin. In normal persons undergoing venisection the serum ferritin concentration falls rapidly as storage iron is mobilized for hemoglobin synthesis.[179] In the anemia of chronic disease, in which a low serum iron concentration is associated with increased stainable iron in marrow reticuloendothelial cells, the serum iron concentration is no longer a valid index of iron deficiency. The shift of iron from the transferrin and red cell compartments into the storage pool is reflected by a rise in the serum ferritin concentration. This phenomenon has been seen in both rheumatoid arthritis[18] and Hodgkin's disease.[185]

In iron deficiency the serum ferritin assay seems to have an important advantage over determinations of serum iron and iron-binding capacity in that low values are almost invariably diagnostic. Iron-deficiency anemia has sometimes been difficult to distinguish from the anemia of infection, since the serum iron and percent iron saturation can be low in both conditions.[9] The fact that infection is associated with a normal or elevated serum ferritin concentration should add to its diagnostic value. It is uncertain whether a low serum ferritin concentration anticipates a depression in the saturation of serum iron in nutritional iron deficiency as it seems to in blood loss.[179]

Although the serum ferritin concentration seems to reflect the size of iron stores under most conditions, there may be certain exceptions, e.g., acute leukemia. Increased serum ferritin concentrations have been reported in adults with acute myeloblastic leukemia, chronic leukemia, and Hodgkin's disease[185] and in children with acute lymphoblastic leukemia, whether in complete remission or in relapse. Another example of possible failure of serum ferritin to reflect iron stores is found during the course of iron therapy in iron-deficient patients. The serum ferritin concentration rises abruptly during the first week and then stabilizes or falls, a pattern that is unlikely to correspond to iron stores.

There are conditions such as acute hepatocellular disease in which high concentrations of circulating ferritin reflect not high intracellular concentrations of ferritin but abnormal release of the protein from damaged cells. Further investigation

Table 6-19. Serum ferritin concentration in iron deficiency and iron overload in children aged 6 months to 15 years*

	Number	Median (ng/ml)	Range (ng/ml)
Iron-deficiency anemia	13	3.4	1.5-9
Latent iron deficiency†	6	10.6	4.5-41
Thalassemia major	7	850	590-1830
Sickle cell anemia (SS)	14	163	49-180
Chronic hemolytic anemias‡	19	242	96-920
Normal	486	30	7-142§

*From Siimes, M. A., et al.: Blood **43:**581, 1974. Used by permission.
†No anemia, but serum iron saturation less than 16%.
‡Hb SC, Hb H, G6PD deficiency and Coombs-positive hemolytic anemia.
§95% confidence limits.

into the origin of circulating ferritin, its release from the tissues of origin, its biochemical nature, and its clearance from the circulation will make it possible to evaluate the assay in a wider range of clinical conditions.

From the evidence at hand, the serum ferritin assay promises to be a useful tool in the evaluation of iron stores. The sample size required is sufficiently small to be obtainable by finger or heel stick, and thus avoids the need for a venipuncture. This is a particularly important consideration in the age group between 6 months and 3 years, when the incidence of iron deficiency is at its peak. Table 6-19 lists serum ferritin concentrations in iron deficiency and iron overload.

Free erythrocyte protoporphyrin

Protoporphyrin represents the penultimate stage in the biosynthetic pathway of heme immediately prior to the incorporation of iron; failure of iron supply results in an accumulation of unused protoporphyrin in the normoblast and the release of erythrocytes in the circulation with high free protoporphyrin (FEP) levels. Values obtained in one study of erythrocyte protoporphyrin (μg/dl erythrocytes) were as follows: hematologically normal persons, 15.5 ± 8.3; persons with latent iron deficiency, 93 ± 59.8; and patients with iron deficiency, 159.2 ± 96.5. The upper limit of normality is 40 μg/dl erythrocytes.[75]

The FEP/hemoglobin ratio is a useful index of iron deficiency. It increases exponentially in iron deficiency with a decrease in both transferrin saturation and hemoglobin level. The FEP/hemoglobin ratio increases when the iron reserves are exhausted before anemia becomes apparent. In small children an elevation in the FEP/hemoglobin ratio is a better indicator of iron-deficiency anemia than low transferrin saturation.[293] The ratio is normal in thalassemia trait and renal anemia, but it may be elevated in sickle cell anemia and chronic inflammatory processes. An elevation of the FEP/hemoglobin ratio in blood reflects persistent iron deficiency in the marrow. Thus the FEP/hemoglobin ratio remains elevated during iron therapy and returns to normal only after the majority of the cells containing excess FEP formed during iron deficiency are replaced. Protoporphyrin is firmly bound to the hemoglobin in iron deficiency, as in lead intoxication, and persists throughout the life span of the erythrocyte. Accordingly the FEP/hemoglobin ratio is not subject to daily fluctuations and sudden changes as is the transferrin saturation. Measurement of FEP and hemoglobin on filter paper provides a useful tool for the diagnosis of iron deficiency and, in populations at risk, of lead intoxication. FEP is carried out by a simple micromethod from finger puncture samples.[294]

The greatest elevation of FEP levels is observed in lead intoxication, in which values up to 11 times normal may be observed. A level of FEP greater than 160 μg/dl of erythrocytes (equivalent to an FEP/hemoglobin ratio of 5.5 μg/gm of hemoglobin) has been suggested as a convenient cutoff point for the detection of lead intoxication. In iron deficiency anemia the FEP/hemoglobin ratio is only moderately elevated and never exceeds 17.5 μg/gm of hemoglobin (equivalent to 500 μg/dl of erythrocytes). An FEP/hemoglobin ratio in the range of 5.5 to 17.5 μg/gm of hemoglobin may be attributed either to iron-deficiency anemia or to lead intoxication. The latter must be considered and ruled out by direct measurement of blood lead when exposure to lead is possible. When the FEP/hemoglobin ratio is greater than 17.5 μg/gm of hemoglobin, it indicates lead intoxication with or without associated iron deficiency and requires immediate medical attention. The only other syndrome associated with such high values is the rare genetic disorder erythropoietic protoporphyria, in which severe cutaneous photosensitivity is present.

The FEP/hemoglobin ratio is not elevated in individuals with thalassemia trait,[365] and measurements of FEP levels discriminate between the microcytosis of β-thalassemia trait and iron-deficiency anemia. Koenig and Lightsey[204] have made similar observations in α-thalassemia trait.

Free erythrocyte protoporphyrin is thus useful in distinguishing between the principle causes of microcytosis—iron deficiency, α- or β-thalassemia minor, and lead poisoning. In both iron deficiency and lead poisoning the level is elevated, although it remains normal in thalassemia minor. It is much higher in lead poisoning than in iron deficiency.

Cobalt excretion

Cobalt is an element in the same group as iron in the periodic table, and it shares some properties with iron. In iron deficiency both iron and cobalt are absorbed from the gastrointestinal tract at a greater than normal rate.* It is quite possible that this is caused by failure of receptors in the intestinal mucosa to distinguish between cobalt and iron. Simultaneous administration of iron and cobalt results in diminished iron absorption, suggesting competition for the binding sites.

Absorbed cobalt does not appear to be incorporated into storage forms, in contrast to the incorporation of iron into ferritin. Absorbed cobalt is promptly excreted in the urine. This permits a simple and apparently sensitive method for detection of iron deficiency, based on urinary excretion of an orally administered dose of ^{57}Co.[360] In this test cobalt (20 μmoles and 0.5 μCi in 100 ml of 0.01N HCl) is given by mouth, and the urinary excretion of the isotope is measured. In persons 15 to 30 years old a mean of 10% (range 5% to 14%) is excreted into the urine in a 6-hour period. In iron deficiency a mean of 19% is excreted (range 15% to 27%). Thus the test clearly distinguishes iron-deficient persons from normal persons.[386] The results become abnormal as soon as iron stores are depleted, and the test may provide one of the earliest and most sensitive laboratory means for detecting iron deficiency. Although the cobalt excretion test is normal in various anemias not caused by iron deficiency, the excretion is increased in idiopathic hemochromatosis and in other situations in which iron absorption may be increased in the absence of iron deficiency, such as acute blood loss and hemolytic anemia. Since iron absorption may be increased in thalassemia major, it is likely that cobalt excretion will be increased as well.

Falsely low values occur in intrinsic renal disease with renal failure and in patients with nephrectomy. Vomiting or failure to fast completely overnight may lead to low cobalt absorption. Malabsorption caused by intramural disease of the duodenum, such as gluten-sensitive enteropathy, may produce falsely low urinary values in relation to the size of body iron stores, but inflammatory disease of the ileum or ileal resection does not appear to affect cobalt absorption unless associated with moderate to marked steatorrhea.

The amount of ^{57}Co required for such a test is small, and the radiation dosage to the whole body, intestinal mucosa, or hematopoietic tissue is negligible. It is clearly premature to attempt to judge the potential role of this procedure in the diagnosis of iron deficiency. It does not supplant simpler diag-

---

*References 33, 360, 376, 385.

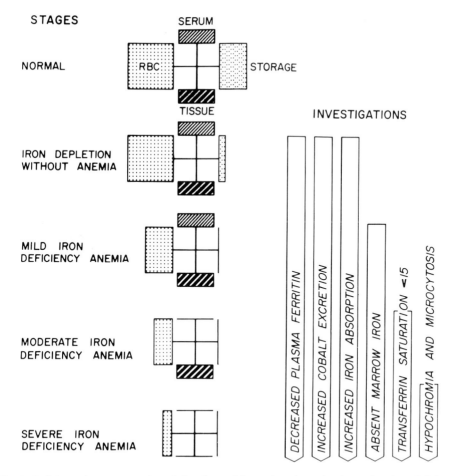

Fig. 6-12. Schematic representation of the place of the various investigations when iron deficiency develops by gradual iron depletion. (Modified from Bothwell, T. H.: N.Z. Med. J. **65**[suppl.]: 880, 1966.)

nostic techniques, but it does provide the clinician with a practical alternative to bone marrow aspiration in the differential diagnosis of hypochromic anemia. In one study 75% of the patients with mild iron-deficiency anemia would not have been recognized by the appearance of the red blood cells on the blood smear, the red cell indices, or transferrin saturation.[386] Thus the test is particularly helpful in differentiating mild iron-deficiency anemia and in differentiating iron-deficiency anemia from anemia from other causes.

Fig. 6-12 is a schematic representation of the place of the various investigations of iron deficiency developing by gradual iron depletion.

Iron absorption

Diminished iron stores generally result in increased intestinal absorption of iron. The investigation of iron absorption as a method for assessing iron balance in a patient is bedeviled by both theoretical and practical problems. The percentage of iron absorbed from a test dose depends on the amount given, the nature of the test dose, the amount of storage iron in the body, and the rate of erythropoiesis, and it is influenced by any pathologic changes affecting the function of the stomach and small intestine. In addition, in patients with sideroblastic anemia or pyruvate kinase deficiency and in children with homozygous β-thalassemia increased iron absorption is found even in the presence of normal or increased iron stores.

Although the measurement of iron absorption may usually indicate whether reduced amounts of storage iron are present, the procedure is inconvenient for the patient and is frought with the inaccuracies mentioned. For these reasons it is not of much clinical value.

The test is done by measuring serial serum iron concentrations or plasma radioactivity following a test dose of an inorganic iron compound or a test dose of radioactive iron (^{59}Fe). Iron absorption may be more accurately determined by the use of the whole body counter.

Desferrioxamine chelation

A technique measuring iron stores utilizing the injection of an iron-chelating agent, desferrioxamine,[10,145] has been described. The quantity of iron excreted in urine after intramuscular injection of this compound correlates well with the size of the iron stores. Although correlation with iron stores is close, other factors such as hemolysis appear to influence the quantity of iron excreted and may impair the usefulness of this test.

Therapeutic trial

In the final analysis, the response to iron therapy is the proof of correctness of the diagnosis of iron deficiency. The physician may not have access to all diagnostic techniques, or on clinical grounds the probability of iron deficiency-anemia may be so high that the patient's response to therapy becomes of primary diagnostic importance. Iron administration in such a therapeutic trial should be by the oral route only, and response should be followed very carefully. A reticulocytosis with a peak occurring between the seventh and tenth days should occur, and a significant rise in hemoglobin should follow. The absence of these changes must be taken as evidence that iron deficiency is not the cause of the anemia. Iron therapy should be discontinued and further diagnostic studies implemented.

The following outline summarizes the diagnostic tests available in the investigation of iron-deficiency anemia.

A. Blood smear: hypochromic microcytic red cells
  1. MCV < 80 fl
  2. MCH < 27.0 pg
  3. MCHC < 30%
B. Bone marrow
  1. Delayed cytoplasmic maturation
  2. Decreased or absent stainable iron
C. Serum iron
  1. Decreased serum iron
  2. Increased iron-binding capacity
D. Plasma ferritin: decreased
E. Free erythrocyte protoporphyrin/hemoglobin ratio: elevated
F. Cobalt excretion test: increased excretion of [57]Co orally administered
G. Iron absorption test: increased
H. Deferoxamine chelation test: iron excretion following injection correlates with iron stores
I. Therapeutic response to oral iron

DIAGNOSIS

The presence of anemia in a child in the absence of other hematologic abnormalities is most likely a result of iron deficiency. The presence of microcytosis (MCV as determined on the Coulter model S of less than 70 fl) and hypochromia (a MCHC of less than 30%) is consistent with the diagnosis.

The easiest and most reliable diagnostic criterion is the response of the anemia to iron. If iron is administered and the hemoglobin has not increased in 3 weeks, the diagnosis of iron-deficiency anemia is probably erroneous unless bleeding has occurred. The characteristic diagnostic features are as follows.

A. Demonstrable cause of iron deficiency, e.g., poor diet or low birth weight
B. Hypochromic microcytic erythrocytes
C. Transferrin saturation of 16% or less
D. Absence of bone marrow iron
E. Low serum ferritin
F. Beneficial response to iron therapy
  1. Reticulocytosis with "peak" 7 to 10 days after institution of therapy
  2. Reappearance of normochromic erythrocytes (dimorphic red blood cell population)
  3. Correction of anemia within 4 weeks

Although hypochromic anemia in children is usually attributed to iron-deficiency anemia, it is not necessarily due to this cause. The causes of hypochromia are given in the following outline.

A. Iron deficiency
B. Hemoglobinopathies
  1. Thalassemia
  2. Hemoglobin Köln
  3. Hemoglobin Lepore
  4. Hemoglobin H
  5. Hemoglobin E
C. Disorders of heme synthesis caused by chemicals
  1. Lead
  2. Pyrazinamide
  3. Isoniazid
D. Sideroachrestic anemias
  1. Hereditary
    a. X-Linked
      (1) Pyridoxine responsive
      (2) Pyridoxine refractory
    b. Autosomal: pyridoxine responsive
  2. Acquired
    a. Idiopathic
      (1) Pyridoxine responsive
      (2) Pyridoxine refractory
    b. Secondary
      (1) Drugs
        (a) Antituberculous drugs (isoniazid, cycloserine)
        (b) Chloramphenicol
        (c) Lead
        (d) Alcohol
        (e) Cytotoxic drugs (nitrogen mustard, azathioprine)
  3. Diseases
    a. Hematologic
      (1) Leukemia
      (2) Polycythemia vera
      (3) Hemolytic anemia
      (4) Megaloblastic anemia
    b. Neoplastic
      (1) Hodgkin's disease

(2) Non-Hodgkin's lymphoma
(3) Carcinoma
c. Inflammatory
(1) Rheumatoid arthritis
(2) Polyarteritis nodosa
(3) Infection
d. Miscellaneous
(1) Myxedema
(2) Thyrotoxicosis
(3) Uremia
(4) Erythropoietic porphyria
(5) Porphyria cutanea tarda
E. Chronic infections or other inflammatory conditions
F. Malignancy
G. Hereditary orotic aciduria
H. Hypo- or atransferrinemia
1. Congenital

2. Acquired, e.g., hepatic disorders, malignancy, protein malnutrition (decreased transferrin synthesis), nephrotic syndrome (urinary transferrin loss)
I. Copper deficiency[191,340]
J. Inborn errors of iron metabolism
1. Congenital defect of iron transport to red cells with parenchymal hepatic accumulation of iron[346]
2. Defective iron mobilization associated with IgA deficiency[206]
3. Idiopathic pulmonary hemosiderosis
4. Goodpasture's syndrome

In some of these cases there is an inability to synthesize hemoglobin normally in spite of a plentiful supply of iron. It is necessary to do additonal investigations such as determinations of serum

Table 6-20. Investigations in differential diagnosis of major causes of hypochromic anemia

	MCV	Serum iron	Total iron-binding capacity	Iron stores	Serum ferritin	Other features
Normal	84-100 fl	80-100 μg/dl	250-400 μg/dl	Normal	Normal*	—
Iron deficiency	Low	Low	High	Absent	Low	—
Anemia of chronic infection	Normal or low	Low	Low	Normal or increased	Normal or increased	Symptoms of primary disorder
Thalassemia (failure of globin synthesis)	Low	High	Normal	Increased or normal	Increased	Increased Hb A$_2$ or Hb F
Sideroachrestic anemia (failure of heme synthesis)	Low or high	High	Normal	Increased	Increased	Ring sideroblasts in marrow

*See Fig. 6-11 for normal serum ferritin values at different ages.

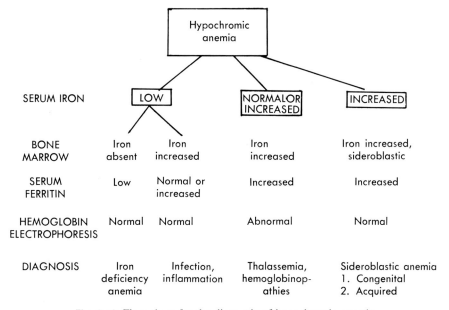

Fig. 6-13. Flow sheet for the diagnosis of hypochromic anemia.

iron and total iron-binding capacity, examination of the bone marrow for stained iron, tests of serum ferritin, and hemoglobin electrophoresis to establish the cause of the hypochromia. Table 6-20 lists the investigations employed in the differential diagnosis of hypochromia, and Fig. 6-13 depicts a flowsheet for the diagnosis of hypochromic anemia.

Iron-deficiency anemia and thalassemia minor are often indistinguishable. The red cells in both conditions may show stippling and target and oval forms, but the larger number of hypochromic macrocytes in the blood smear and the familial hereditary pattern are important diagnostic features of thalassemia minor. The blood smear of patients with thalassemia minor and those with iron deficiency may both show, however, a more or less uniform hypochromic microcytic picture, and other diagnostic aids are necessary.

Confusion with homozygous thalassemia major may occur only in the infant during the first year of life. The large, pale, extremely thin erythrocytes with irregularly distributed hemoglobin and scattered normoblasts interspersed among microcytes in the blood smear are in contrast with the more uniform microcytes of iron-deficiency anemia (Fig. 6-9). The significant splenomegaly and the presence of the trait in both parents and siblings further differentiates thalassemia major from iron-deficiency anemia.

In addition to making a diagnosis of iron-deficiency anemia, it is incumbent on the physician to demonstrate its cause. The history should take into account all factors related to the development of iron deficiency. These should include conditions resulting in low iron stores at birth, careful dietary history, and consideration of all factors leading to blood loss. The commonest site of bleeding is the bowel, and the most important investigation is examination of the stools for occult blood. If found, its cause should be established by examination of the stools for ova, rectal examination, sigmoidoscopy, barium enema, upper GI series, and ^{99}Tc (technetium pertechnetate) scan for Meckel's diverticulum. Occasionally gastroscopy and colonoscopy are required. Results of guaiac tests may be negative, particularly if bleeding is intermittent, and for this reason occult bleeding should be tested for on at least five occasions when gastrointestinal bleeding is suspected. The guaiac test is only sensitive enough to pick up more than 5 ml of occult blood. In menstruating females excessive uterine bleeding, epistaxis, renal blood loss (hematuria), and on rare occasions bleeding into the lung (idiopathic pulmonary hemosiderosis and Goodpasture's syndrome) may all be causes of iron-deficiency anemia. Bleeding into these areas require specific investigations designed to identify the bleeding and determine its cause.

TREATMENT

The treatment of iron-deficiency anemia can be considered in two aspects—treatment of the individual patient and treatment of iron-deficiency anemia as a major public health problem.

Treatment of individual patients

Successful management requires a thorough investigation of the cause of the negative iron balance such as faulty diet, increased iron requirements caused by rapid growth, or blood loss from a structural gastrointestinal defect such as polyps or Meckel's diverticulum.

Nutritional counseling. Most commonly the history reveals a dependence on foods notably poor in iron content such as milk, unfortified cereals, and other carbohydrate foods. Often this situation will have developed unwittingly from a failure of parents to understand the need for a well-balanced diet, particularly in the rapidly growing infant. Restriction of milk to 1 pint a day; the introduction of meat, vegetables, and fruit; and supplementation by an iron preparation will usually suffice to correct the anemia.

Iron-rich foods include the following: commercially prepared, dry, ready-to-serve infants' cereals (0.92 mg of iron/tablespoon), green and yellow vegetables (0.05 mg/tablespoon in spinach, 0.28 mg/tablespoon in green beans), and liver (0.56 mg/tablespoon).

Josephs[187] gives the iron content of milk as it comes from the cow as 0.4 to 0.5 mg of iron/liter. Commercial pasteurization increases the iron to 0.7 to 1 mg/liter. Processed milk, whether powdered or condensed, may contain 1 to 2 mg/liter. Normal children absorb an average of about 10% of the naturally occurring iron in milk, eggs, chicken liver, and iron supplements added to commerically prepared infants' cereals.[338] Iron-deficient children absorb two to three times as much food iron as do normal children.[338]

If iron-deficiency anemia results from a hypersensitivity to whole cow's milk, evaporated milk should be used. If the patient continues to have gastrointestinal dysfunction on evaporated milk, a trial of soybean milk or goat's milk is indicated.

To achieve maximum improvement in hemoglobin concentration, Sturgeon[366] has suggested that the recommended daily allowance (based on data from the Food and Nutrition Board of the National Research Council) of 6 mg of food iron through the first year and 10 mg from 1 to 3 years of age be increased to 6 to 9 mg daily at 3 months of age, 8 to 12 mg by 6 months, and 10 to 15 mg at 12 months. One egg yolk supplies approximately 1 mg of iron, and peaches, the best source of iron among the fruits, provide 0.32 mg/tablespoon.[312]

The average full-term infant requires a total of 8 mg of iron daily from about 6 months of age and with optimal intake may derive this amount from dietary sources alone. The term infant with deficient body iron at birth may require this amount of iron as early as 3 months, and the premature infant at 2 months. In premature infants a total daily intake of about 2 mg/kg should be assured by the third month, gradually decreasing to about 1 mg/kg by the end of the first year.[336] Iron supplementation is indicated for all premature infants; early supplementation produces negligible differences at 3 months but a progressive advantage from the fourth month.[336] Examination of hemoglobin levels during the early periods reveals no substantial elevation of hemoglobin levels.

Oral therapy. Treatment with a soluble iron salt, preferably ferrous iron, corrects the deficiency promptly. Any form of ferrous iron, e.g., ferrous gluconate, ferrous ascorbate, ferrous lactate, ferrous succinate, ferrous fumarate, and ferrous glycine sulfate, is effective. Of the wide variety of ferrous salts available only ferrous succinate is significantly better absorbed than ferrous sulfate without an increase in side effects.[143] Since ferrous sulfate is absorbed so effectively, the 30% improvement in absorption found with ferrous succinate is not a critical therapeutic factor. Ferric irons and heavily chelated iron should not be used, as they are poorly and inefficiently absorbed. Vitamin supplementation or the addition of other heavy metals is unnecessary. Side effects following iron medication include epigastric pain, nausea, diarrhea, and constipation. The side effects are related to the amount of elemental iron and not to the type of preparation. Many preparations reputed to have a lower incidence of side effects also have a lower iron content or are chelated iron, which has a lower therapeutic index.

Dosage and mode of administration. Since the percentage of metallic iron content is a fraction of the entire compound, iron should be prescribed with this in mind. Preparations available are suitably designated according to iron content.

For infants ferrous sulfate is available in concentrated solutions that can be given in a drop dosage in which each drop contains a measured amount of elemental iron. The recommended oral dose is 1.5 to 2 mg/kg of elemental iron given three times daily (4.5 to 6 mg/kg/day).[415] Larger dosages increase the frequency and severity of side effects without significantly speeding the hematologic response.[158] Such side effects are, in fact, a function of dosage, and as a general rule it can be stated that if a compound gives fewer side effects, it is because it contains less iron or the iron is not in an absorbable form. The total daily dose of elemental iron recommended for an infant during the period of iron deficiency (6 to 24 months) ranges from 60 to 90 mg. Ideal treatment consists of the administration of such a soluble iron preparation in divided dosage, preferably between meals.

Theoretically milk has been regarded as being an unfavorable vehicle for iron, either because it combines with phosphates to form insoluble salts or because it shares with other foods of increased phosphorus content a basic difficulty in absorbing iron.[156] Despite these findings, iron salts in therapeutic doses added to milk have produced satisfactory hemoglobin responses in my experience and in that of others.[282]

Oral administration of iron usually results in the stool becoming a deep black color as a result of the increased content of iron sulfides. The absence of this change may serve as a clue to irregular administration of the iron.[356] Ingestion of liquid iron preparations may produce a black staining of the teeth. Brushing the teeth after each administration is of value in reducing this untoward effect, although the staining is only temporary.

For older children tablets of ferrous sulfate or ferrous gluconate are preferable to the concentrated liquid preparations used with infants. Gastric irritation, nausea, vomiting, and abdominal pain are less likely to occur if the tablets are taken with meals. Iron tablets are best taken three times daily at mealtimes. Tablets of ferrous sulfate (0.2 gm) or ferrous gluconate (0.3 gm) given three times daily provide a daily total of 100 to 200 mg of elemental iron.

In the infant, as in the older child, full therapeutic doses of iron should be given for at least 6 to 8 weeks after the hemoglobin level has been restored to normal levels. If oral therapy is withdrawn too soon, the iron stores will remain unreplenished[354] and anemia will eventually recur. The serum ferritin level, reflecting iron stores, rises significantly when oral treatment is continued for two months after the attainment of a normal hemoglobin concentration.[17]

A simple test for the detection of iron in stools was described by Afifi et al.[1] and applied by Macdougall[235] to children with iron deficiency who failed to attain acceptable hemoglobin levels after 3 months of prescribed oral iron therapy. Macdougall[235] found uniformly positive stool tests within 48 hours of initiation of iron therapy. The test depends on the contact of one drop of 0.25% potassium ferricyanide with liquified stool specimen. In positive tests there is an immediate development of a blue crescent (ferrous cyanide) at the junction of this mixture. This test provides a rapid and effective means of determining the reliability of those responsible for administering iron medication.

Adjuvants to oral iron therapy. Adjuvants to iron are unnecessary in the treatment of iron-deficiency anemia. It is unnecessary to add copper, molybdenum, cobalt, vitamin B_{12}, or folic acid in treatment of iron-deficiency anemia. Since iron is absorbed in the ferrous form, the reduction of ferric salts to the bivalent form depends on reducing mechanisms present in the small intestine. Moore et al.[262] demonstrated that the ingestion of vitamin C with ferric salts resulted in an increase in serum iron level, probably by its reducing action. On the other hand, in a study of children of school age Schulze and Morgan[339] used soluble ferric pyrophosphate and small supplements of copper and found that the addition of ascorbic acid was unnecessary for the synthesis of hemoglobin.

Notwithstanding the diverse opinions with regard to ascorbic acid, Brise and Hallberg[32] found that ascorbic acid given in sufficient amounts increased the absorption of ferrous iron and that the absorption-promoting effect increased with increasing amounts of ascorbic acid. The absorption-promoting effect of ascorbic acid is mainly attributed to its reducing action with the gastro-intestinal tract, preventing or delaying formation of insoluble or less dissociated ferric compounds.

In addition to ascorbic acid, sorbitol, mannitol, and *d*-xylose enhance iron absorption but also raise the incidence of side effects.[144] The response to oral iron therapy without additives is so effective with a return of the hemoglobin to normal values in iron-deficiency anemia that for clinical purposes there is no need for adjuvants in the treatment of iron deficiency.

Response to oral iron therapy. Satisfactory response to iron may be heralded by an increase in appetite and improvement in disposition. A peak reticulocyte response is reached on the fifth to the tenth day after institution of iron therapy. The reticulocyte increase is inversely proportional to the severity of the anemia. Following this the hemoglobin rises at an average of 0.25 to 0.4 gm/dl/day, or a 1%/day rise in hematocrit (Fig. 6-14). The magnitude of the response is related to the degree of anemia.

A substantial hemoglobin rise should be ob-

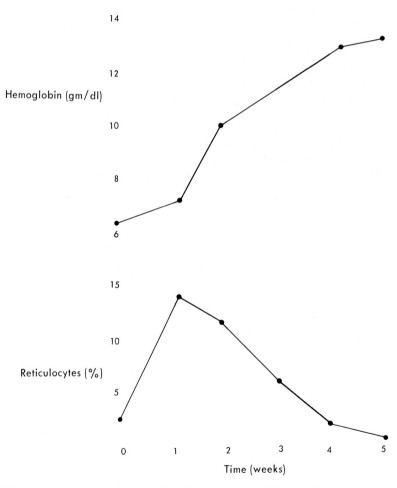

Fig. 6-14. Response to oral iron therapy with reference to hemoglobin level and reticulocyte count. Patient 12 months old and weighing 10 kg received 20 mg elemental iron (as $FeSO_4$) three times daily.

served approximately 3 weeks after beginning iron therapy. The failure to achieve a level of at least 11 gm/dl in this period with adequate iron therapy indicates that the diagnosis of anemia on a purely nutritional basis is to be questioned and suggests continuous blood loss or the continuation of an infectious process, an underlying renal abnormality, or an incorrect diagnosis.

Short-lived macrocytes appear early in iron therapy.[270] Under intense erythroid stimulation with iron therapy there is a shortening of the maturation interval with skipping of cell divisions. As recovery from the anemia progresses, the intensity of the erythroid stimulation decreases and more nearly normal cells are provided. The mechanism of the macrocytic response may be mediated by erythropoietin. Leventhal and Stohlman[229] have demonstrated that in iron-deficiency anemia the red cell size is related to the rate of maturation, which in turn is governed by the level of erythropoietin and the availability of precursors for hemoglobin such as iron. When high doses of iron were given, macrocytes were produced; low doses produced an increased hemoglobin level but with increased production of microcytes; and intermediate doses resulted in the production of normocytes. In the presence of normal or excess iron stores the level of erythropoietin governs the rate of maturation and hence the red cell size. Macrocytes are found with high erythropoietin output together with adequate precursors (iron-deficient group treated with high doses of iron).

Changes in mental status and appetite following iron therapy may occur within 48 to 72 hours (before a hematologic response occurs),[218] suggesting that restoration of enzyme function is a more rapid process than the correction of anemia.

Failure of response to oral iron therapy. When a patient fails to respond to oral iron the following reasons should be sought and examined:

1. Failure of oral iron administration (This can be verified by a change in stool color to gray-black or by testing the stool for iron.)
2. Inadequate iron dose
3. Ineffective iron preparation
4. Persistent or unrecognized blood loss by which the patient loses iron as fast as it is replaced
5. Incorrect diagnosis
6. Coexistent disease that interferes with absorption or utilization of iron, e.g., infection, malignancy, hepatic or renal disease, or concomitant deficiencies (vitamin B_{12}, folic acid, thyroid)
7. Impaired gastrointestinal absorption, e.g., concurrent administration of large amounts of antacids (which will bind iron) as in treatment of peptic ulcer

Parenteral iron therapy. Intramuscular iron should only be administered in the following conditions:

1. Failure to administer or take iron (This occurs when parents fail to administer prescribed iron to their infants or children refuse to take iron. This situation is usually appreciated by the pediatrician when infants with established iron-deficiency anemia fail to respond to prescribed oral iron.)
2. Severe bowel disease (e.g., inflammatory bowel disease) associated with iron-deficiency anemia, in which the use of oral iron might aggravate the underlying disease of the gut
3. Genuine intolerance to oral iron
4. Chronic hemorrhage, e.g., hereditary telangiectasia, menorrhagia
5. Acute diarrheal disorder in underprivileged populations with iron-deficiency anemia

The most commonly used intramuscular iron is iron-dextran complex (Imferon). Iron-dextran is a high molecular weight complex of ferric hydroxide and dextran. Most iron absorption following intramuscular injection occurs in 72 hours; however, at the end of 28 days 10% to 50% of the dose may still remain at the site.

Iron-dextran complex for intramuscular use has proved a valuable adjunct to therapy. It is safe, effective, and well tolerated even in infants with a variety of acute illnesses, including acute diarrheal disorders.[218] The total amount of iron needed to raise the hemoglobin level to normal and replenish stores is calculated as follows:

$$\frac{\text{normal hemoglobin} - \text{initial hemoglobin}}{100} \times$$
$$\text{blood volume (ml)} \times 3.4 \times 1.5$$

1. Normal hemoglobin is 11 to 12 gm in infants, 12.5 to 13.5 gm in children, and 14 to 15 gm at puberty.
2. Blood volume is 80 ml/kg
3. The factor 3.4 converts grams of hemoglobin to milligrams of iron
4. The factor 1.5 provides extra iron to replace depleted tissue stores

EXAMPLE: Infant weighing 10 kg with 5 gm of hemoglobin/dl

Blood volume = 80 ml/kg $\times$ 10 kg = 800 ml
Hemoglobin deficit = 12 (approximately normal for age) − 5 = 7 gm/dl
Total hemoglobin deficit = 7 gm/dl $\times$ 800 ml ÷ 100 = 56 gm
Iron to restore hemoglobin to normal = 56 gm $\times$ 3.4 mg/gm = 190 mg
Addition of iron to replenish stores = 190 mg $\times$ 1.5 = 285 mg
Total dose of iron to be injected = 285 mg

Iron-dextran complex provides 50 mg of elemental iron/ml. Once calculated, the total amount can be given in divided doses but should not be exceeded or repeated.

Injections into the upper outer quadrant of the gluteus muscle are given through skin, which is displaced laterally prior to the injection to prevent superficial staining. Untoward reactions are rare. Occasionally fever lasting 24 to 48 hours occurs. Less commonly staining of the skin occurs when the iron was not given deep enough into the muscle or because of "streaking" along the path of withdrawal of the needle.[218] In rare cases local or generalized reactions, angioneurotic edema, and recurrent arthralgia occur.[344] The carcinogenic risks of iron-dextran complex in laboratory animals appear to have no relevance in clinical medicine.[219]

Newly formed red cells well filled with hemoglobin are recognizable in blood smears within 48 hours after therapy. An increase in the reticulocyte count, probably initiated after 24 hours of therapy, reaches a maximum value about the fifth day of treatment. In patients with severe anemia the hemoglobin level reaches 11 gm/dl after 3 weeks and is higher in patients with moderate anemia. The magnitude of the hemoglobin response varies therefore with the degree of anemia.

A normoblastic response to iron-deficiency anemia may occasionally become excessive. Also a leukoerythroblastosis has been reported[327] when parenteral iron-dextran complex (Imferon) is administered in severe iron deficiency. It has been suggested[29] that in a marrow avid for iron, the rapid delivery of this substance from the iron-dextran combination produces a transient stimulus to granulocytopoiesis as well as erythropoiesis. Such a response should not be confused with leukemia, neoplasia, or a myeloproliferative process. These changes can occur as early as the third day after treatment with iron-dextran complex and can persist for about 10 days.

If hemoglobin values do not rise at least 2 gm in 3 weeks, other possible causes of anemia should be considered and more iron should not be administered. Failure to respond requires further hematologic investigation. The use of iron-dextran intravenously is dangerous and should be avoided because anaphylactic reactions can occur with its use.

A new iron preparation for intramuscular use has been recently introduced.* This is a sterile aqueous solution of iron-polysaccharide (sorbitol-gluconic acid) complex (Ferastral). This preparation appears to be a safe, effective iron preparation. After intramuscular injection it is absorbed exclusively via the lymphatic route. After 48 hours

---

*References 95, 103, 104, 286, 371.

75% of the dose is absorbed, and after 10 days 82% is absorbed.

As with other intramuscular iron preparations, staining at the sight of injection may occur with this product especially in cases in which the solution is accidentally administered into the superficial tissues. Staining is transient, disappearing after a couple of weeks or months. The local inflammatory reaction is slight. Side effects of a general type have occurred in rare cases. In occasional cases there have been complaints of nausea and dizziness.

The dose used is calculated in the same way as for iron-dextran complex. The iron solution contains 50 mg of elemental iron/ml. In adults a single dose of 500 mg has been given. This product has not been demonstrated to be superior to iron-dextran complex.

Blood transfusion. A packed red cell transfusion should be administered because of severe anemia requiring correction more rapidly than is possible with oral iron or parenteral iron or in the presence of certain complicating factors. This should be reserved for debilitated children with infection, especially when signs of cardiac dysfunction are present and hemoglobin is 4 gm/dl or less.

Partial exchange transfusion. Partial exchange transfusion has been recommended in the management of a severely anemic child under two circumstances.[304] One is in the case of a surgical emergency when a final hemoglobin of 9 to 10 gm/dl should be attained to permit safe anesthesia. The other is when anemia is associated with congestive heart failure, in which case it is sufficient to raise the hemoglobin to 4 to 5 gm/dl to correct the immediate anoxia.

Treatment of public health problem

Iron deficiency is the only known vitamin or mineral deficiency disorder still prevalent in an era in which such diseases as scurvy, rickets, and pellagra have become rarities.

Full-term, normal newborn infants with a normal endowment of iron at birth probably do not require supplemental iron if a judicious mixed diet consisting of meat and vegetables contributes to the source of protein and calories for the infant's growth.

It is interesting that breast-fed infants appear to utilize dietary iron more efficiently than a comparable group of infants fed a prepared formula not fortified with iron.[419]

A number of studies have clearly shown that normal full-term infants receiving iron-fortified proprietary formulas are less likely to develop iron-deficiency anemia during infancy than a control group of infants receiving nonfortified milks.[7,172,335] Furthermore if anemia does develop, it tends to be less severe than in the control group.

Low birth weight infants and infants with reduced iron endowment need relatively larger amounts of iron. This can only be provided by iron-fortified staples or medicinal iron supplements.

There are many skeptics who have a laissez-faire attitude to iron-deficiency anemia. It is true that children usually outgrow iron-deficiency anemia. However, both research and clinical observation lead us to the conclusion that a high incidence of iron-deficiency anemia might not be in the best interest of the health and welfare of children. Furthermore it is surprising that the numerous reports made during the past five decades concerning the high incidence of iron-deficiency anemia in underprivileged infants and its effect on various tissues, organs, and health of these children have been accepted with such inertia by members of the profession. This inertia has not been caused by failure to appreciate the problem. In 1969 the Committee on Nutrition of the American Academy of Pediatrics[61] recognized the factors leading to a high incidence of iron-deficiency anemia, the iron needs of normal infants and infants of low birth weight, and the importance of treating iron-deficiency anemia.

The Committee recommended a daily consumption of iron-enriched baby cereal, ¼ ounce dry weight beginning by 6 weeks of age and increasing to ½ ounce dry weight by 6 months of age. This assures an adequate iron intake for all infants except those with low initial endowment. Commercial infant cereals contain 8.6 to 22 mg of iron/ dry ounce of cereal. However, Rios et al.[315] have shown recently that iron as sodium iron pyrophosphate and ferric orthophosphate is poorly absorbed from infant cereal (mean < 1.0%), and these are therefore not dependable sources of iron to meet the nutritional needs of infants. They showed that reduced iron of very small particle size and ferrous sulfate added to cereal are absorbed to a greater extent (mean 4.0% and 2.7%, respectively). For technical reasons these two forms of iron have not been added to commercial cereal products because of discoloration, distribution problems of the iron in the product, and shortened shelf life. Therefore at the present time iron supplementation of infant cereals with sodium iron pyrophosphate, ferric orthophosphate, and reduced iron of large particle size does not provide a predictable and available source of iron to meet the needs of infants. In addition, iron-fortified baby cereals are not used by the segments of the population that have the greatest need for them.

The most effective way to prevent iron deficiency on a large scale is to provide an iron-fortified dietary staple that can be started by 6 weeks of age

for infant consumption. Iron-enriched milk formulas are the most readily available sources of adequate iron intake for infants, and milk fortified with 12 mg of iron as ferrous sulfate per reconstituted quart is effectively utilized.

Several studies have indicated that iron-deficiency anemia can be prevented by the use of cow's milk formula to which iron has been added.[7,242] Recent studies by Rios et al.[315] have shown that supplemental iron as ferrous sulfate in milk- and soy-based formulas gives a mean absorption of 3.4% to 5.4% and can meet the needs for dietary iron and healthy infants.

The availability of iron-supplemented infant formulas containing absorbable iron has been shown to significantly reduce the prevalence of iron deficiency in early life. Studies by Marsh et al.[242] have demonstrated that iron-supplemented infant formula reduces the prevalence of deficiency in the first year of life to well below 10%.

At a Ross conference[321] on iron nutrition in infancy, the following recommendations were made:

1. All infants who are given artificial feeding should receive heat-processed, iron-fortified formula containing 10 to 15 mg of elemental iron/reconstituted quart.
2. Such formula feedings should be continued for the first year of life.
3. All milk formulas and milk-substitute formulas designed for infant feeding should contain adequate iron.
4. The use of iron-fortified cereals should be encouraged during infancy. Implicit in the public health approach to the problem is that steps must be taken to assure that all infants have access to such formulas and that education of the public and medical profession to the need for such an approach be instituted.

The Food and Nutrition Board of the National Academy of Sciences has proposed to increase iron supplementation in flour from the present level of 13 to 16.5 mg/pound to 40 to 60 mg/pound.[68,108] This should assure an adequate iron supply for preschool children and postpubertal girls and women. The most appropriate food selected for iron enrichment may vary in different parts of the world and in different ethnic and social groups. At present such supplemented food staples are not in general use, and efforts to identify and develop suitable vehicles for enrichment are essential if optimal iron nutrition is to be assured.

Because the highest incidence of iron-deficiency anemia is in children younger than 36 months of age, and because the staple food of children of this age is milk, it would appear logical that it should be enriched with iron. Iron-fortified whole milk or evaporated milk should be marketed for infant feeding. This would prevent widespread iron-deficiency anemia. Experience with nutritional deficiencies of sufficient magnitude to constitute public health problems has demonstrated that they can be managed through public health measures.

Federal law requires the enrichment of both canned and powdered milk with vitamin D and although state laws, which control the standards for whole milk, do not require vitamin D enrichment, most companies have elected to add the vitamin to milk. This addition of vitamin D has virtually prevented the development of nutritional rickets in children in the United States and has eliminated rickets as a public health problem. Judicious enrichment programs involving vitamin C have also eliminated scurvy as a public health problem. Likewise judicious enrichment programs with iron will eliminate iron-deficiency anemia in the childhood population.

The addition of iron to milk has a number of advantages compared to medicinal iron therapy. Medicinal iron therapy is more expensive, is potentially dangerous because of the possibility of overdosage, and is not available on such a widespread basis as iron-fortified whole milk.

SPECIAL CONSIDERATIONS IN TREATMENT OF PRETERM INFANTS WITH IRON AND ITS INTERRELATIONSHIP WITH VITAMIN E DEFICIENCY

Unless the diet is supplemented with iron, small preterm infants fed proprietary formulas usually develop iron-deficiency anemia sometime after 6 months of age.* There is evidence to suggest that breast-fed infants are less prone to iron deficiency,[247] but this requires confirmation in premature infants. Although the need for additional iron is universally recognized, there is some disagreement concerning the timing of supplementation and the vehicles that should be used.

Dallman[77] has suggested that iron deficiency may be prevented by either of the following two regimens, which employ the same dose of iron but differ in timing:

1. Administration of iron shortly after birth in the form of ferrous sulfate–supplemented formula (12 mg elemental iron/quart, about 2 mg/100 kcal, or 2.5 mg/kg) (The same dose can be given to breast-fed infants in the form of ferrous sulfate drops.)
2. Administration of iron-supplemented formula, or the same dose of medicinal iron, only when iron stores are first depleted (2 or 3 months of age)

Starting iron administration shortly after birth is the most expedient of these alternatives and is in

*References 61, 123, 289, 337, 342.

accordance with the recommendation of the Committee on Nutrition of the Academy of Pediatrics.[61] It has the advantage of augmenting iron stores during hospitalization to carry the infant through a period at home when dietary insufficiency of iron is more likely to develop because of an early shift from formula to regular cow's milk or erratic administration of drops.

When iron supplementation is delayed until 3 months of age, the dose of 2 to 3 mg iron/kg is still adequate. Gorten and Cross[123] have shown that this dose in the form of iron-supplemented formula is even adequate to treat the established iron-deficiency anemia that had developed after 6 months of age in previously untreated premature infants.

The iron may be given in formula or in medicinal form. The addition of iron and other trace nutrients to formula is the more reliable and convenient of the two methods, but medicinal iron is also effective.

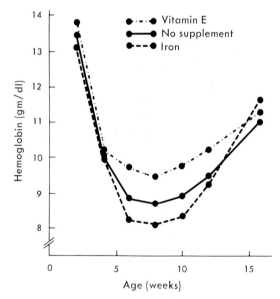

Fig. 6-15. Concentration of hemoglobin in premature infants with birth weights of 1,000 to 1,500 gm. All infants were fed a proprietary formula without added iron and a multiple vitamin preparation containing vitamins A, C, and D. The infants were assigned to one of four groups as follows: no additional supplement; ferrous sulfate, 8 mg elemental iron/kg/day for 2 to 6 weeks of age, then 8 mg/liter of formula; 25 IU/day of α-tocopherol acetate between 2 and 6 weeks of age; or both ferrous sulfate and α-tocopherol acetate. For the sake of clarity, only the first three groups are shown. The highest hemoglobin concentrations were in the vitamin E–supplemented group. Differences between the vitamin E–supplemented and iron-supplemented groups were significant at 6, 8, and 10 weeks of age ($p < 0.01$). (Redrawn from Melhorn, D. K., et al.: J. Pediatr. **79:**569, 1971.)

There are reasons for delaying iron supplementation for a few months. Preterm infants younger than 3 months may develop hemolytic anemia in association with a supplement of 8 mg iron/kg. The risk is greater in those infants not given adequate vitamin E.[253] Whether smaller doses of iron produce a similar effect remains to be determined. Iron supplements may be safe over a broader dosage if vitamin E deficiency can be prevented by α-tocopherol polyethylene glycol 1,000 succinate, as current studies suggest.[132]

The interaction between iron and vitamin E is particularly important during the first few months. Melhorn et al.[253] placed preterm infants on one of four supplementation regimens, in addition to feedings of proprietary formula; iron and vitamin E, iron only, vitamin E only, and no additional supplement. The infants who received solely 8 mg/kg of iron as ferrous sulfate were significantly more anemic (Fig. 6-15) and had higher reticulocyte counts than infants in any of the other groups, suggesting the possibility of hemolysis. Since iron is a cofactor that catalyzes the oxidative breakdown of red cell lipids in vitro through the generation of free radicals, it is postulated that large doses of iron could have the same effect in vivo. The oxidative damage would be most pronounced if vitamin E were not exerting its antioxidant effect. In addition, there is evidence that concurrent administration of 8 mg/kg of iron and 25 mg/day of α-tocopherol results in slightly impaired absorption of α-tocopherol.[252] These observations raise the question of whether iron supplementation may predispose to vitamin E deficiency in the first 2 or 3 months of life. Since iron stores are rarely depleted this early, it may be better to withhold iron supplementation in the preterm infant until 3 months of age.

This might only apply to very small preterm infants weighing between 1,000 and 1,500 gm in whom vitamin E deficiency is more likely to be present. It might not necessarily apply to larger preterm infants, since Gorton and Cross[123] showed accelerated recovery from early low hemoglobin concentrations in a group of premature infants in whom the diet was supplemented in the early weeks with a formula containing 12 mg of elemental iron/quart. These values were significantly higher than for infants not so fed. These studies demonstrate the ability of the infant to absorb and to utilize iron from fortified milk for hemoglobin synthesis. Early routine administration of elemental iron to all premature infants, without depending on the ingestion of a specified quantity of milk, achieves the same results. It should be remembered that, in any case, iron therapy does not alter the initial physiologic drop in hemoglobin but hastens recovery from early low values when

iron contained in the initial circulating hemoglobin mass reaches exhaustion.

In most premature infants iron administration should be continued for several months after the hemoglobin concentration has returned to normal to ensure adequate stores. Periodic hemoglobin determinations are required to assure the maintenance of normal blood values. Prophylaxis by means of parenteral iron (iron-dextran) may be advisable before discharge from the hospital, when it is anticipated that oral administration will be unreliable. The dosage in this case is 100 mg of parenteral iron.

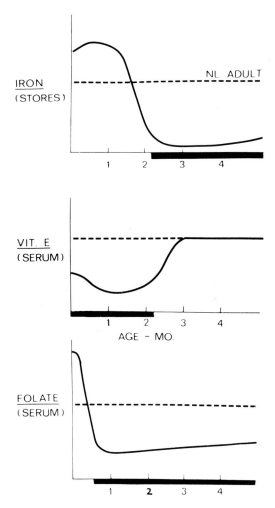

Fig. 6-16. Selected values of iron, vitamin E, and folate nutrition in premature infants. Curves represent estimated changes in concentration of storage iron, serum α-tocopherol, and serum folate levels in premature infants during the first 5 months after birth. Normal values for the adult are indicated by the horizontal dashed line. The horizontal black bars represent the periods during which deficiency is likely to occur. (From Dallman, P. R.: J. Pediatr. **85:**742, 1974.)

In instances in which the hemoglobin level drops to 7 gm/dl or less between 3 and 6 weeks of age, transfusions are required, especially when the infant is listless, sucks poorly, and is not gaining weight. It should be mentioned, however, that in addition to the known complications of transfusions it is possible that repeated administration of blood may suppress inherent hematopoiesis at a time when the bone marrow may have become responsive. Repeated small packed red cell transfusions may be required, especially in small, ill preterm infants from whom multiple blood samples are drawn for blood gases and biochemical tests.

In summary iron deficiency is most likely to occur when mobilizable iron stores have been depleted some time after 2 or 3 months of age. This can be prevented by administration of iron as recommended for premature infants by the Committee on Nutrition: 2 mg/kg of iron during the first year of life in a readily assimilated form such as ferrous sulfate, either in formula or in a medicinal form. Whether it is better to start supplemental iron at 2 or 3 months of age or within a few weeks after birth is unresolved. Doses of iron higher than 3 mg/kg should be avoided, especially in the first 3 months of life when there is likelihood of concurrent vitamin E deficiency.

In addition to iron, preterm infants also require supplementation with vitamin E and folic acid. Vitamin E deficiency is a self-limited problem that requires treatment only during the first 3 months of life. Folate deficiency is likely to develop from 2 weeks to 2 to 4 months after birth, before folate-rich solid foods are introduced in the diet. Regimens for nutritional supplementation of preterm infants should take into account the different periods of risk for each deficiency, as shown in Fig. 6-16.

IRON-DEFICIENCY ANEMIA IN PATIENTS WITH CYANOTIC CONGENITAL HEART DISEASE

In most infants and children with cyanotic congenital heart disease the bone marrow response to the persistent anoxic stimulus is polycythemia, in which the hemoglobin increase approaches the rise in the erythrocyte count. Occasionally the rise in hemoglobin does not keep pace with the erythrocytosis. Hemoglobin levels of 10 to 13 gm/dl, erythrocyte counts of 6 to 8 $\times 10^{12}$/liter, and hematocrit levels of 40%, accompanied by complaints of irritability, anorexia, and poor weight gain, have been observed in young patients.[277] Even hemoglobin levels of 16 to 18 gm/dl may represent relative anemia in the presence of polycythemic blood levels. The administration of iron results in marked improvement in the clinical and hematologic status.[322] Iron therapy is stopped or decreased when the hematocrit level reaches 75%. Experience has shown that patients with appreciable arterial unsaturation function best with a hematocrit of 55% to 75%. Patients with values lower than these require iron medication.[277]

ABNORMALITIES OF IRON METABOLISM
Congenital atransferrinemia

Congenital atransferrinemia is a rare condition characterized by severe hypochromic microcytic anemia present at birth with almost complete absence of serum transferrin. The anemia is severe, requiring multiple transfusions. Iron is absorbed from the intestinal tract and transported to the tissues with the development of hemosiderosis in the myocardium, liver, and spleen. Bone marrow reveals abundant erythroid precursors but no sideroblasts or iron storage cells. The disease is resistant to therapy with hematinics but responds favorably to intravenous iron-free human serum transferrin. It may be inherited in an autosomal recessive manner with both parents having lower than normal amounts of transferrin.[126,157]

Congenital defect of iron transport from transferrin to red cells

A congenital defect of iron transport from transferrin to red cells has been described in two siblings; it was characterized by a hypochromic microcytic anemia, with hemoglobin levels varying from 5.8 to 8.4 gm/dl, associated with an error in iron metabolism.[346] The serum iron values were increased and there was no quantitative or qualitative defect in transferrin or qualitative abnormality in heme synthesis. There was marked discrepancy in iron storage sites. The liver parenchymatous cells were loaded with iron but none was found in the Kupfer cells, the macrophages, or the erythroid cells of the marrow. The presumed defect involved transfer of iron from transferrin to the erythroid cells and macrophages. The anemia was unresponsive to therapy, including purified iron-saturated transferrin.

Two sisters with a similar defect have been described by Stavem et al.[363] These two sisters had a congenital hypochromic anemia (hemoglobin levels varying from 5.2 to 11.0 gm/dl) associated with hyperferremia and a fully saturated serum transferrin. In spite of heavy iron stores in the liver the bone marrow iron was reduced. It was postulated that the disease was caused by a defect in the one-way transport mechanism for iron from transferrin into the red cells.

Defective iron mobilization associated with IgA deficiency

The characteristic features of defective iron mobilization with IgA deficiency are similar to idiopathic pulmonary hemosiderosis with episodic periods of hypochromic anemia, reticulocytosis, progressive lung disease marked by acute exacerbations associated with decreasing hemoglobin values and iron trapping in the lung, and hepatosplenomegaly. Serum iron levels were decreased and the anemia responded to therapy with iron. Iron kinetic data showed that iron was lost into sites from which it could not be reutilized for hematopoiesis, probably because of a generalized dysfunction of the macrophage system. It is suggested that a dysfunction of the pulmonary macrophages could explain the pulmonary "iron trapping" in this disease. The shedding of alveolar-lining cells and the accumulation of hemosiderin-laden macrophages in alveoli may represent the histologic manifestation of such a dysfunction. IgA deficiency occurred in this condition associated with generalized involvement of pathologic iron storage in the macrophages.[206]

The clinical course of this condition resembles idiopathic pulmonary hemosiderosis with IgA deficiency.

Idiopathic pulmonary hemosiderosis and Goodpasture's syndrome

Idiopathic pulmonary hemosiderosis and Goodpasture's syndrome are discussed on p. 130.

REFERENCES

1. Afifi, A. M., Banwell, G. S., Bennison, R. J., Boothby, K., et al.: Simple test for ingested iron in hospital and domiciliary practice, Br. Med. J. **1:**1021, 1966.
2. Agarwal, K. N., and Sharma, M. L.: Red cell survival in iron-deficiency anaemia, J. Indian Med. Assoc. **58:**456, 1972.
3. Aisen, P., and Leibonan, A.: Lactoferrin and transferrin: a comparative study, Biochem. Biophys. Acta **257:**314, 1972.
4. Aksoy, M., Camli, N., and Erdem, S.: Roentgenographic bone changes in chronic iron deficiency: a study of twelve patients, Blood **27:**677, 1966.
5. Aksoy, M., Erdem, S., Dincol, K., Pars, B., and Dincol, G.: On the pathogenesis of the hepatosplenomegaly in chronic iron-deficiency anemia: a study in eleven patients, Paper presented at twelfth congress of the International Society of Hematology, New York, 1968.
6. Al-Rashid, R. A., and Spangler, J.: Neonatal copper deficiency, N. Engl. J. Med. **285:**841, 1971.
7. Andelman, M. B., and Sered, B. R.: Utilization of dietary iron by term infants: a study of 1,048 infants from a low socioeconomic population, Am. J. Dis. Child. **111:**45, 1966.
8. Apte, S. V., Iyengar, L., and Nagarajan, V.: Effect of antenatal iron supplementation on placental iron, Am. J. Obstet. Gynecol. **110:**350, 1972.
9. Bainton, D. F., and Finch, C. A.: The diagnosis of iron-deficiency anemia, Am. J. Med. **37:**62, 1964.
10. Balcerzak, S. P., et al.: Measurement of iron stores using deferoxamine, Ann. Intern. Med. **68:**518, 1968.
11. Balcerzak, S. P., et al.: Idiopathic hemochromatosis: a study of three families, Am. J. Med. **40:**857, 1966.
12. Barltrop, D.: The prevalence of pica, Am. J. Dis. Child. **112:**116, 1966.
13. Basta, S. S.: Nutrition (with particular reference to iron-

14. Bedard, Y. C., et al.: Radioautographic observations on iron absorption by the normal mouse duodenum, Blood **38:**232, 1971.
15. Ben-Basset, I., Mozel, M., and Ramot, B.: Globin synthesis in iron-deficiency anemia, Blood **44:**551, 1974.
16. Benirschke, K.: Accurate recording of twin placenta, Obstet. Gynecol. **18:**334, 1961.
17. Bentley, D. P., and Jacobs, A.: Accumulation of storage iron in patients treated for iron-deficiency anaemia, Br. Med. J. **2:**64, 1975.
18. Bentley, D. P., and Williams, P.: Serum ferritin concentration as an index of storage iron in rheumatoid arthritis, J. Clin. Pathol. **27:**786, 1974.
19. Ber, R., and Valero, A.: Pica and hypochromic anemia: a survey of 14 cases seen in Israel: preliminary communication, J.M.A. Israel **61:**35, 1961.
20. Bessis, M. C., and Breton-Gorius, J.: Iron metabolism in the bone marrow as seen by electron microscopy: a critical review, Blood **19:**635, 1962.
21. Beutler, E.: Iron enzymes in iron deficiency, Blut **6:**160, 1960.
22. Boggs, R. B., and Miller, S. A.: Defects in resistance to salmonella typhimurium in iron-deficient rate, J. Infect. Dis. **130:**409, 1974.
23. Bohannon, R. A., et al.: The use of radioiron in the study of anemia, Ann. Intern. Med. **55:**975, 1961.
24. Bothwell, T. H., and Finch, C. A.: Iron metabolism, J. Clin. Invest. **40:**1, 1967.
25. Bothwell, T. H., and Finch, C. A.: Iron metabolism, Boston, 1962, Little, Brown & Co.
26. Bothwell, T. H., Pirzio-Biroli, G., and Finch, C. A.: Iron absorption. I. Factors influencing absorption, J. Lab. Clin. Med. **51:**24, 1958.
27. Bothwell, T. H., Pribilla, W. F., Mebust, W., and Finch, C. A.: Iron metabolism in the pregnant rabbit: iron transport across the placenta, Am. J. Physiol. **196:**615, 1958.
28. Bowie, J. W., Tauxe, W. N., Sjoberg, W. E., Jr., and Yamaguchi, M. Y.: Daily variation in the concentration of iron in serum, Am. J. Clin. Pathol. **40:**491, 1963.
29. Bowman, H. S.: Hematopoietic responses to iron-dextran (studies on iron-deficiency anemia of infancy), Am. J. Dis. Child. **99:**408, 1960.
30. Brigety, R. E., and Pearson, H. A.: Effect of dietary and iron supplementation on hematocrit levels of preschool children, J. Pediatr., **76:**757, 1970.
31. Brines, J. K., Gibson, J. G., Jr., and Kunkel, P.: Blood volume in normal infants and children, J. Pediatr. **18:**447, 1941.
32. Brise, H., and Hallberg, L.: Effect of ascorbic acid on iron absorption, Acta Med. Scand. **171**(suppl. 376):51, 1962.
33. Britton, H. A., Canby, J. P., and Kohler, C. M.: Iron-deficiency anemia producing evidence of marrow hyperplasia in the calvarium, Pediatrics **25:**621, 1960.
34. Brown, E. B., Jr., and Justus, B. W.: In vivo absorption of radioiron by everted pouches of rat intestine, Am. J. Physiol. **194:**319, 1958.
35. Brown, K., Lubin, B., Smith, R., and Oski, F. A.: Prevalence of anemia among preadolescent and young adolescent urban black Americans, J. Pediatr. **81:**714, 1972.
36. Brown, W. D., and Dyment, P. G.: Pagophagia and iron-deficiency anemia in adolescent girls, Pediatrics **49:**766, 1972.
37. Burman, D.: Haemoglobin levels in normal infants aged 3 to 24 months and the effect of iron, Arch. Dis. Child. **47:**261, 1972.
38. Callender, S. T., et al.: Absorption of haemoglobin iron, Br. J. Haematol. **3:**186, 1957.

deficiency anemia), endurance and productivity, Ph.D. dissertation, Massachusetts Institute of Technology, Cambridge, Mass., 1974.

39. Callender, S. T., et al.: Absorption of haemoglobin iron, International symposium on iron metabolism, Berlin, 1964, Springer Verlag.
40. Campbell, D. T., and Stanley, J. C.: Experimental and quasiexperimental designs for research, Skokie, Ill., 1963, Rand McNally & Co.
41. Campbell, S., and Macafee, C. A. J.: A case of idiopathic pulmonary haemosiderosis with myocarditis, Arch. Dis. Child. **34:**218, 1959.
42. Canale, V., and Lanzkowsky, P.: Cellular growth in specific nutritional deficiency states in rats. I. Iron-deficiency anemia in postweaning rats, Br. J. Haematol. **19:**579, 1970.
43. Card, R. T., and Weintraub, L. R.: Metabolic abnormalities of erythrocytes in severe iron deficiency, Blood **37:**725, 1971.
44. Carlander, O.: Etiology of pica, Lancet **2:**569, 1959.
45. Cassady, G.: Plasma volume studies in low birth weight infants, Pediatrics **38:**1020, 1966.
46. Catzel, P.: Iron deficiency anemia, geophagia and breath holding: excessive milk drinking as a cause, Med. Proc. **10:**439, 1964.
47. Chanarin, I., Bennett, M. C., and Berry, V.: Urinary excretion of histidine derivatives in megaloblastic anaemia and other conditions and a comparison with the folic acid clearance test, J. Clin. Pathol. **15:**269, 1962.
48. Chanarin, L., Rothman, D., and Berry, V.: Iron deficiency and its relation to folic-acid status in pregnancy: results of a clinical trial, Br. Med. J. **1:**480, 1965.
49. Chandra, R. K.: Reduced bactericidal capacity of polymorphs in iron-deficiency anemia, Arch. Dis. Child. **48:**864, 1973.
50. Chandra, P., and Rosner, F.: Olives-craving in iron deficiency anemia, Ann. Intern. Med. **78:**973, 1973.
51. Chandra, R. K., and Saraya, A. K.: Impaired immunocompetence associated with iron deficiency, J. Pediatr. **86:**899, 1975.
52. Charlton, R. W., et al.: The role of the intestinal mucosa in iron absorption, J. Clin. Invest. **44:**543, 1965.
53. Chown, B.: The fetus can bleed, Am. J. Obstet. Gynecol. **70:**1298, 1955.
54. Cohen, F., Zuelzer, W. W., and Evans, M. M.: Identification of blood group antigens and minor cell populations by the fluorescent antibody method, Blood **15:**884, 1960.
55. Cohen, F., Zuelzer, W. W., Gustafson, D. C., and Evans, M. M.: Mechanisms of isoimmunization. I. The transplacental passage of fetal erythrocytes in homospecific pregnancies, Blood **23:**621, 1964.
56. Coleman, D. H., Stevens, A. R., Jr., and Finch, C. A.: The treatment of iron-deficiency anemia, Blood **10:**567, 1955.
57. Collumbine, H.: Hemoglobin and fitness, J. Appl. Physiol. **2:**274, 1949.
58. Colozzi, A. E.: Clamping of the umbilical cord: its effect on the placental transfusion, N. Engl. J. Med. **250:**628, 1954.
59. Coltman, C. A.: Pagophagia, Arch. Int. Med. **128:**472, 1971.
60. Coltman, C. A.: Pagophagia and iron lack, J.A.M.A. **207:**513, 1969.
61. Committee on Nutrition: Iron balance and requirements in infancy, Pediatrics **43:**134, 1969.
62. Conrad, M. E., et al.: The role of the intestine in iron kinetics, J. Clin. Invest. **43:**963, 1964.
63. Conrad, M. E., et al.: Regulation of the intestinal absorption of iron by the rate of erythropoiesis, Br. J. Haematol. **11:**432, 1965.
64. Conrad, M. E., et al.: Intestinal mucosal mechanisms controlling iron absorption, Blood **22:**406, 1963.
65. Conrad, M. E., and Schade, S. G.: Ascorbic acid chelates in iron absorption: a role for HCl and bile, Gastroenterology **55:**35, 1968.
66. Cook, J. D., et al.: The effect of achylia gastrica on iron absorption, J. Clin. Invest. **43:**1185, 1964.
67. Cooper, J. R., Bloom, F. E., and Roth, R. H.: The Biochemical basis of neuropharmacology, Oxford, 1974, Oxford University Press.
68. Council on Foods and Nutrition: Iron in enriched wheat, flour, farina, bread, and rolls, J.A.M.A. **220:**855, 1972.
69. Cragin, F. W.: Observations on cachexia africana or dirt eating, Am. J. Med. Sci. **17:**356, 1835.
70. Crosby, W. H.: The control of iron balance by the intestinal mucosa, Blood **22:**241, 1963.
71. Crosby, W. H.: The control of iron balance by the intestinal mucosa, Am. J. Clin. Nutr. **21:**1189, 1968.
72. Crosby, W. H.: The control of iron balance by the intestinal mucosa, J.A.M.A. **208:**347, 1969.
73. Cusack, R. P., and Brown, W. D.: Achromotricia in iron-deficient rats, Nature **204:**582, 1964.
74. Dabke, A. T., et al.: Serum iron and iron binding capacity in the newborn in relation to maternal anaemia, Indian J. Pediatr. **39:**348, 1972.
75. Dagg, J. H., Goldberg, A., and Lockhead, A.: Value of erythrocyte protoporphyrin in the diagnosis of latent iron deficiency, Br. J. Haematol. **12:**326, 1966.
76. Dagg, J. H., Jackson, G. H., Curry, B., et al.: Cytochrome oxidase in latent iron deficiency (sideropenia), Br. J. Haematol. **12:**331, 1966.
77. Dallman, P. R.: Iron, vitamin E, and folate in the preterm infant, J. Pediatr. **85:**742-752, 1974.
78. Dallman, P. R.: The nutritional anemias. In Nathan, D. G., and Oski, F. A., editors: Hematology of infancy and childhood, Philadelphia, 1974, W. B. Saunders Co.
79. Dallman, P. R.: Tissue Effects of Iron Deficiency. In Jacobs, A., and Wormwood, M., eds.: Iron biochemistry and medicine, New York, 1974, Academic Press, Inc.
80. Dallman, P. R.: Iron restriction in the nursing rat: early effects upon tissue heme proteins, hemoglobin, and liver iron, J. Nutr. **97:**475, 1969.
81. Dallman, P. R., and Goodman, J. R.: Enlargement of mitochondrial compartment in iron and copper deficiency, Blood **35:**496, 1970.
82. Dallman, P. R., and Schwartz, H. C.: Distribution of cytochrome C and myoglobin in rats with dietary iron deficiency, Pediatrics **35:**677, 1965.
83. Dallman, P. R., Siimes, M. A., and Manies, E. C.: Brain iron: persistent deficient following short-term iron deprivation in the young rat, Br. J. Haematol. **31:**209, 1975.
84. Dallman, P. R., Sunshine, P., and Leonard, P.: Intestinal cytochrome response with repair of iron deficiency, Pediatrics **39:**863, 1967.
85. Dannecker, D.: Anemia in selected Allegheny County child health conference populations, Allegheny County Health Department.
86. Davies, J., Brown, E. B., Stewart, D., Terry, C. W., and Sisson, J.: Transfer of radioactive iron via the placenta and accessory fetal membranes in the rabbit, Am. J. Physiol. **197:**87, 1959.
87. Davies, C. T. M., Chukweumeka, A. C., and Van Haaren, J. P. M.: Iron-deficiency anaemia: its effect on maximum aerobic power and responses to exercise in African males aged 17-40 years, Clin. Sci. **44:**555, 1973.
88. Davis, C. M.: Self-selection of diet by newly weaned infants: experimental study, Am. J. Dis. Child. **36:**651, 1928.
89. Davis, L. R., Maren, R. H., and Sarkany, I.: Iron deficiency anemia in European and West Indian infants in London, Br. Med. J. **2:**1426, 1960.

90. Davis, P. S., Luke, C. G., and Deller, D. J.: Reduction of iron-binding protein in haemochromatosis: a previously unrecognized metabolic defect, Lancet **2:**1431, 1966.

91. Dawson, R. B., Jr., Rafal, S., and Weintraub, L. R.: Absorption of hemoglobin iron: the release of iron from heme by intestinal xanthine oxidase. In twelfth congress of the International Society of Haematology, New York, 1968. (Abstract.)

92. DeLeeuw, N. K. M., Lowenstein, L., and Hsieh, Y.-S.: Iron deficiency and hydremia in normal pregnancy, Medicine **45:**291, 1966.

93. DeMarsh, Q. B., Windle, W. F., and Alt. H. L.: Blood volume of newborn infant in relation to early and late clamping of umbilical cord, Am. J. Dis. Child. **63:**1123, 1942.

94. Derechin, S. S., and Johnson, P.: Red proteins from bovine milk, Nature **194:**473, 1962.

95. Domeij, K., Hellström, V., Hogberg, K. G., Lindvall, S., Rydell, G., Wichman, U., and Ortengren, B.: Studies on an iron-poly (sorbitol-gluconic acid) complex for parenteral treatment treatment of iron-deficiency anaemia, Scand. J. Haematol. Suppl. **32:**21, 1977.

96. Doscherholmen, A., Mahmud, K., and Ripley, D.: Hypersegmentation in iron-deficiency anemia, J.A.M.A. **229:**1721, 1974.

97. Duprey, A. J. B.: The anemia of dyspepsia consequent on dirt eating, Lancet **2:**1192, 1900.

98. Dyer, N. C., Brill, A. B., Glasser, S. R., and Goss, D. A.: Maternal-fetal transport and distribution of ^{59}Fe and ^{131}I in humans, Am. J. Obstet. Gynecol. **103:**290, 1969.

99. Eastham, R. D.: Is your iron and iron-binding capacity really necessary? Lancet **1:**1090, 1975.

100. Edgerton, V. R., Bryant, S. L., Gillespie, C. A., and Gardner, G. W.: Iron-deficiency anemia and physical performance and activity of rats, J. Nutr. **102:**381, 1972.

101. Eng, L. L.: Chronic iron-deficiency anaemia with bone changes resembling Cooley's anaemia, Acta Haematol. **19:**263, 1958.

102. England, J. M., Ward, S. M., and Down, M. C.: Microcytosis, anisocytosis, and the red cell indices in iron deficiency, Br. J. Haematol. **34:**589-597, 1976.

103. Evers, J. E. M.: Iron-poly (sorbitol-gluconic acid) complex and iron dextran in the treatment of severe iron-deficiency anaemia, Scand. J. Haematol. Suppl. **32:**377, 1977.

104. Ezem, B. U., Fleming, A. F., and Werblinska, B.: Treatment of severe iron-deficiency anaemia of hookworm infestation with Ferastral, a new intramuscular iron preparation, Scand. J. Haematol. Suppl. **32:**279, 1977.

105. Farquar, J. D.: Iron supplementation during first year of life, Am. J. Dis. Child. **106:**201, 1963.

106. Filer, L. F.: The USA today—is it free of public health nutrition problems? Anemia, Am. J. Pub. Health **59:**327, 1969.

107. Finch, C. A., et al.: Ferrokinetics in man, Medicine **49:**17, 1970.

108. Finch, C. A., and Monsen, E. R.: Iron nutrition and the fortification of food with iron, J.A.M.A. **219:**1462, 1972.

109. Finne, P. H.: Erythropoietin levels in cord blood as an indicator of intrauterine hypoxia, Acta Pediatr. Scand. **55:**478, 1966.

110. Fletcher, J.: The effect of iron and transferrin on the killing of *Escherichia coli* in fresh serum, Immunology **20:**493, 1971.

111. Fong, T. P., Okafor, L. A., Thomas, W., Jr., and Westerman, M. P.: Stainable iron in aspirated and needle-biopsy specimens of marrow: a source of error, Am. J. Hematol. **2:**47, 1977.

112. Friedenthal, H.: Über Säuglingsernährung nach physiologischen Grundsätzen mit Friedenthal schwer Kindermilch und Gemusepülvern, Ber. Klin. Wochenschr. **1:** 727, 1914.

112a. Fuerth, J. H.: Incidence of anemia in full-term infants seen in private practice, J. Pediatr. **79:**562, 1971.

113. Fullerton, H. W.: The iron-deficiency anemia of late infancy, Arch. Dis. Child. **12:**91, 1937.

114. Gairdner, D., Marks, J., and Roscoe, J. D.: Blood formation in infancy. II. Normal erythropoiesis, Arch. Dis. Child. **27:**214, 1952.

115. Garby, L., and Sjölin, J.: Absorption of labelled iron in infants less than three months old, Acta. Pediatr. Scand. **48**(supple. 117):24, 1959.

116. Gardner, G. W., Edgerton, V. R., Bernard, R. J., and Bernauer, E. M.: Cardiorespiratory, hematological, and physical performance responses of anemic subjects to iron treatment, Am. J. Clin. Nutr. **28:**982, 1975.

117. Ghosh, S., Daga, S., Kasthuri, D., Misra, R. C., and Chuttani, H. K.: Gastrointestinal function in iron deficiency states in children, Am. J. Dis. Child. **123:**14, 1972.

118. Giardina, A. C., Gilladoga, A. C., Canale, V., Lanzkowsky, P., and Levin, A. R.: The effect of anemia on digitalis tolerance in rabbits, Atlantic City, N.J., 1971, Society for Pediatric Research.

119. Gibson, J. G., Jr., and Evans, W. A.: Clinical studies of the blood volume. I. Clinical application of a method employing the blue-azo-dye "Evans blue" and the spectrophotometer, J. Clin. Invest. **16:**301, 1937.

120. Gitlin, D., Janeway, C. A., and Farr, L. E.: Studies on the metabolism of plasma proteins in the nephrotic syndrome. I. Albumin, gamma globulin and iron-binding globulin, J. Clin. Invest. **35:**44, 1956.

121. Glover, J., and Jacobs, A.: Activity pattern of iron-deficient rats, Br. Med. J. **2:**627, 1972.

122. Golditch, I. M., and Boyce, N. E.: Management of abruptio placentae, J.A.M.A. **212:**288, 1970.

123. Gorten, M. K., and Cross, E. R.: Iron metabolism in premature infants. II. Prevention of iron deficiency, J. Pediatr. **64:**509, 1964.

124. Gorten, M. K., Hepner, R., and Workman, J. B.: Iron metabolism in premature infants. I. Absorption and utilization of iron as measured by isotope studies, J. Pediatr. **63:**1063, 1963.

125. Gould, A. M.: A case of pica, Boston Med. Surg. J. **94:** 417, 1875.

126. Goya, N., Miyazaki, S., Kodate, S., and Ushio, B.: A family of congenital atransferrinemia, Blood **40:**239, 1972.

127. Granick, S.: Iron metabolism, Bull. N.Y. Acad. Med. **30:**81, 1954.

128. Greenberger, N. J., et al.: Iron uptake by isolated intestinal brush borders, J. Lab. Clin. Med. **73:**711, 1969.

129. Gros, H., Les perversions de l'appetit chez les enfants muslmans de premier age en Algerie, LaCaducee **3:**248, 1903.

130. Gross, S., Keefer, V., and Lieberman, J.: The platelets in cyanotic congenital heart disease, Pediatrics **42:**652, 1968.

131. Gross, S., Keefer, V., and Newman, A. J.: The platelets in iron-deficiency anemia. I. The response to oral and parenteral iron, Pediatrics **34:**315, 1964.

132. Gross, S., and Melhorn, D. K.: Vitamin E-dependent anemia in the premature infant. III. Comparative hemoglobin, vitamin E, and erythrocyte phospholipid responses following absorption of either water-soluble or fat-soluble d-alpha tocopheryl, J. Pediatr. **85:**753, 1974.

133. Gross, S. J., Stuart, M. J. S., Wender, P. T., and Oski, F. A.: Malabsorption of iron in children with iron deficiency, J. Pediatr. **88:**795, 1976.

134. Guest, G. M., and Brown, E. W.: Erythrocyte and hemoglobin of the blood. III. Factors in variability, statistical study, Am. J. Dis. Child. **93**:486, 1957.

135. Guha, D. K., Walia, B. N. S., Tandon, B. N., Deo, M. G., and Ghai, O. P.: Small bowel changes in iron-deficiency anaemia in childhood, Arch. Dis. Child. **43**: 239-244, 1968.

136. Gunther, M.: The transfer of blood between baby and placenta in the minutes after birth, Lancet **1**:1277, 1957.

137. Gutelius, M. F., Milican, F. K., Layman, E. M., Cohen, G. J., and Dublin, C. C.: Nutritional studies of children with pica. I. Controlled study evaluating nutritional status, Pediatrics **29**:1018, 1962.

138. Gutelius, M. F.: The problem of iron-deficiency anemia in preschool Negro children, Am. J. Pub. Health **59**:290, 1969.

139. Hahn, P. F., et al.: Radioactive iron and its metabolism in anemia, J. Exp. Med. **69**:739, 1939.

140. Hahn, P. F., et al.: Radioactive iron and its metabolism in anemia, J. Exp. Med. **70**:443, 1939.

141. Hahn, P. F., et al.: Radioactive iron and its metabolism in anemia, J. Exp. Med. **74**:197, 1941.

142. Hahn, P. F., Carothers, E. L., Darby, W. J., Martin, M., Sheppard, C. W., Cannon, R. O., Beam, A. S., Densen, P. M., Peterson, J. C., and McClellan, G. S.: Iron metabolism in human pregnancy as studied with the radioactive isotope, Fe[59], Am. J. Obstet. Gynecol. **61**: 477, 1951.

143. Hallberg, L., and Sovell, L.: Succinic acid as absorption promoter in iron tablets: Absorption and side effect studies, Acta Med. Scand. **459**(suppl.):23, 1966.

144. Hallberg, L., Sovell, L., and Brise, H.: Search for substances promoting the absorption of iron: studies on absorption and side effects, Acta Med. Scand. **459**(suppl.): 11, 1966.

145. Hallberg, L., Hedenberg, I., and Weinfield, A.: Liver iron and desferrioxamine-induced urinary iron excretion, Scand. J. Haematol. **3**:85, 1966.

146. Hallgren, B., and Sourander, P.: The effect of age on the nonhaemin iron in the human brain, J. Neurochem. **3**:41, 1958.

147. Halstead, J. A., Prasad, A. S., and Nadimi, M.: Gastrointestinal function in iron-deficiency anemia. Arch. Inter. Med. **116**:253, 1965.

148. Halvorsen, S., and Finne, P. H.: Erythropoietin production in the human fetus and newborn, Ann. N.Y. Acad. Sci. **149**:576, 1968.

149. Hambridge, K. M., and Silverman, A.: Pica with rapid improvement after dietary ainz supplementation, Arch. Dis. Child. **48**:567, 1973.

150. Hancock, D. E., Onstad, J. W., and Wolf, P. L.: Transferrin loss into the urine with hypochromic-microcytic anemia, Am. J. Clin. Pathol. **65**:73, 1976.

151. Hancock, K. W., Walker, P. A., and Harper, T. A.: Mobilisation of iron in pregnancy, Lancet **2**:1055, 1968.

152. Harker, L. A., and Finch, C. A.: Thrombokinetics in man, J. Clin. Invest. **48**:963, 1969.

153. Harris, J. W., and Kellermeyer, R. W.: The red cell, Cambridge, Mass., 1970, Harvard University Press.

154. Harrison, P. M., Hoare, R. J., Hoy, T. G., et al.: Ferritin and haemosiderin: structure and function. In Jacobs, A., Worwood, M., eds.: Iron in biochemistry and medicine, New York, 1974, Academic Press, Inc.

155. Heath, C. W., and Patek, A. J.: The anemia of iron deficiency, Medicine (Baltimore) **16**:267, 1937.

156. Hegsted, D. M., Finch, C. A., and Kinney, T. D.: The influence of diet on iron absorption: the interrelation of iron and phosphorus, J. Exp. Med. **90**:147, 1949.

156a. Heilmeyer, L.: In Wallerstern, R. O., and Mettier, S. R., eds.: Iron in clinical medicine, Berkeley, Calif., 1958, University of California Press.

157. Heilmeyer, L., Keller, W., Vivell, O., Betke, F., Wöhler, F., and Keiderling, K.: Die kongenitale Atransferrinämie, Schweiz. Med. Wochenschr. **91**:1203, 1961.

158. Herbert, V.: Oral iron therapy. In Crosby, W. H., ed.: Iron, New York, 1972, prepared for Lakeside Laboratories by Medcom, Inc.

159. Hershko, C., Karsai, A., Eylon, L., and Izak, G.: The effect of chronic iron deficiency on some biochemical functions of the human hemopoietic tissue, Blood **36**:321, 1970.

160. Higashi, O., Sato, Y., Takamatsu, H., and Dyama, M.: Mean cellular peroxidase (MCP) of leukocytes in iron-deficiency anemia, Tohoku J. Exp. Med. **93**:105, 1967.

161. Hill, R. S., Pettit, J. E., Tattersal, M. H. N., Kiley, N., and Lewis, S. M.: Iron deficiency and dyserythropoiesis, J. Haematol. **23**:507, 1972.

162. Hillman, R. W.: Relationship of race and sex to the frequency of local tissue changes suggestive of malnutrition: the five year experience of a district health center nutrition clinic in New York City, Am. J. Clin. Nutritr. **10**: 410, 1962.

163. Hoag, M. S., Wallerstein, R. O., and Pollycove, M.: Occult blood loss in iron-deficiency anemia of infancy, Pediatrics **27**:199, 1961.

164. Hoffbrand, A. V., Ganeshaguru, K., Tattersall, M. H. N., and Tripp, E.: Effect of iron deficiency on DNA synthesis, Clin. Sci. **46**:12p, 1974.

165. Hollingsworth, J. W.: Life span of fetal erythrocytes, J. Lab. Clin. Med. **45**:469, 1955.

166. Holowach, J., and Thurston, D. L.: Breath-holding spells and anemia, N. Engl. J. Med. **268**:21, 1963.

167. Howell, D.: Significance of iron deficiencies: consequences of milk deficiency in children, Extent and meaning of iron deficiency in the United States, Summary Proceedings of Workshop of the Food and Nutrition Board, Washington, D.C., 1971, National Academy of Sciences.

168. Huff, R. L., et al.: Plasma and red cell iron turnover in normal subjects and in patients having various hematopoietic disorders, J. Clin. Invest. **29**:1041, 1950.

169. Huff, R. L., et al.: Ferrokinetics in normal persons and in patients having various hematopoietic disorders, J. Clin. Invest. **30**:1512, 1951.

170. Huff, R. L., et al.: A test for red cell production, Acta Haematol. **7**:129, 1952.

171. Huff, R. L., et al.: Iron turnover abnormalities in patients having anemia: serial blood and in vivo tissue studies with Fe[59], Acta Haematol. **9**:73, 1953.

172. Hunter, R. E.: Frequency of iron deficiency. In Iron nutrition in infancy, Report of the sixty-second Ross Conference on Pediatric Research, Columbus, Ohio, 1970, Ross Laboratories.

173. Hussein, S., Prieto, J., O'Shea, M., Hoffbrand, A. V., et al.: Serum ferritin assay and iron status in chronic renal failure and haemodialysis, Br. Med. J. **1**:546, 1975.

174. Jackson, S., and Burrow, T. N.: The virulence-enhancing effect of iron on nonpigmented mutants of virulent strains of Pasteurella pestis, Br. J. Exp. Pathol. **37**:577, 1956.

175. Jacobs, A.: Iron overload—clinical and pathologic aspects, Semin. Hematol. **14**:89-114, 1976.

176. Jacobs, A.: Erythropoiesis and iron-deficiency anaemia. In Jacobs, A., and Worwood, M., eds.: Iron in biochemistry and medicine, London, 1974, Academic Press, Ltd.

177. Jacobs, A., et al.: Gastric acidity and iron absorption, Br. J. Haematol. **12**:728, 1966.

178. Jacobs, A.: Leukocyte oxygen consumption in iron-deficiency anemia, Br. J. Exp. Pathol. **46:**545, 1965.

179. Jacobs, A., Miller, F., Worwood, M., Beamish, M. R., and Wardrop, C. A.: Ferritin in the serum of normal subjects and patients with iron deficiency and iron overload, Br. Med. J. **4:**206, 1972.

180. Jacobs, A., and Worwood, M.: Ferritin in serum. Clinical and biochemical implications, N. Engl. J. Med. **292:**951, 1975.

181. Jacobziner, H., and Raybin, N. W.: The epidemilogy of lead poisoning in children, Arch. Pediatr. **79:**72, 1962.

182. Jandl, J. H., Inman, J. K., Simmons, R. L., and Allen, D. W.: Transfer of iron from the serum iron-binding protein to human reticulocytes, J. Clin. Invest. **38:**161, 1959.

183. Jandl, J. H., and Katz, J. H.: Plasma-to-cell cycle of transferrin, J. Clin. Invest. **42:**314, 1963.

184. Jegier, W., MacLaurin, J., Blankenship, W., and Lind, J.: Comparative study of blood volume estimation in the newborn infant using I 131-labeled human serum albumen (IHSA) and T-1824, Scand. J. Clin. Lab. Invest. **16:**125, 1964.

185. Jones, P. A. E., Miller, F. M., Worwood, M. R., and Jacobs, A.: Ferritinaemia in leukaemia and Hodgkin's disease, Br. J. Cancer **27:**212, 1973.

186. Jones, R. A., and Silver, S.: The detection of minor erythrocyte population by mixed agglutinates, Blood **13:**763, 1958.

187. Josephs, H. W.: Absorption of iron as a problem in human physiology, Blood **13:**1, 1958.

188. Josephs, H. W.: Iron metabolism and the hypochromic anemia of infancy, Medicine **32:**125, 1953.

189. Joynson, D. H. M., Jacobs, A., Walker, D. M. and Dolby, A. E.: Defect of cell-mediated immunity in patients with iron-deficiency anemia, Lancet **2:**1058, 1972.

190. Judisch, J. M., Naiman, J. L., and Oski, F. A.: The fallacy of the fat iron-deficient child, Pediatrics **37:**987, 1966.

191. Kapel, J. T., and Peden, V. H.: Copper deficiency in long-term parenteral nutrition, J. Pediatr. **80:**32, 1972.

192. Karayalcin, G., and Lanzkowsky, P.: Pica with zinc deficiency, Lancet **2:**687, 1976.

193. Karp, R. J., Haaz, W. S., Starko, K., and Gorman, J. M.: Iron deficiency in families of iron-deficient inner-city school children, Am. J. Dis. Child. **128:**18, 1974.

194. Karpatkin, S., Garg, S. K., and Freedman, M. L.: Role of iron as a regulator of thrombopoiesis, Am. J. Med. **57:**521, 1974.

195. Katz, J. H.: Transferrin and its functions in the regulation of iron metabolism. In Gordon, A. S., ed.: Regulation of hematopoiesis, New York, 1970, Appleton-Century-Crofts.

196. Katz, J. H.: Iron and protein kinetics studies by means of doubly labelled human crystalline transferrin, J. Clin. Invest. **40:**2143, 1961.

197. Katz, J. H., and Jandl, J. H.: The role of transferrin in the transport of iron into the developing red cell. In Gross, F., ed.: Iron metabolism, Berlin, 1964, Springer Verlag.

198. Kaufman, N., and Wyllie, J. C.: Maternofoetal iron transfer in the rat, Br. J. Haematol. **19:**515, 1970.

199. Kavin, H., et al.: Effect of the exocrine pancreatic secretions on iron absorption, Gut **8:**556, 1967.

200. Kevy, S.: Clinical pathological conference, J. Pediatr. **60:**304, 1962.

201. Kimber, C., and Weintraub, L. R.: Malabsorption of iron secondary to iron deficiency, N. Engl. J. Med. **279:**453, 1968.

202. Kirkman, H. N., and Riley, H. D., Jr.: Posthemorrhagic anemia and shock in the newborn: a review, Pediatrics **24:**97, 1959.

203. Kleihauer, E., Braun, H., and Betke, K.: Demonstration von fetalem Hämoglobin in den erythrocyten eines blutausstrichs, Klin. Wochenschr. **35:**637, 1957.

204. Koenig, H. M., and Lightsey, A. L.: The micromeasurement of free erythrocyte porphyrin (FEP) as a means of differentiating alpha-thalassemia trait from iron-deficiency anemia, Pediatr. Res. **8:**404, 1974.

205. Koerper, M. A., and Dallman, P. R.: Serum iron concentration (SI) and transferrin saturation (sat) are lower in normal children than in adults, Pediatr. Res. **11:**473, 1977.

205a. Koerper, M. A., and Dallman, P. R.: J. Pediatri. **91:**870, 1977.

206. Krieger, I., and Brough, J. A.: Gamma-A deficiency and hypochromic anemia due to defective iron mobilization, N. Engl. J. Med. **276:**886, 1967.

207. Kulapongs, P., Vithayasai, V., Suskind, R., and Olson, R. E.: Cell-mediated immunity and phagocytosis and killing function in children with severe iron-deficiency anemia, Lancet **2:**689, 1974.

208. Lajtha, L. G.: In Stohlman, F. R., Jr., Ed: Kinetics of cellular proliferation, New York, 1959, Grune & Stratton, Inc.

209. Lajtha, L. G., and Suit, H. I.: Uptake of radioactive iron (Fe) by nucleated red cells in vitro, Br. J. Haematol. **1:**55, 1955.

210. Lal, A. K., and Saran, A.: Plasma zinc in normal subjects and in cases of cirrhosis and iron-deficiency anaemia, Indian J. Med. Res. **61:**1501, 1973.

211. Lanzkowsky, P.: Watercress craving and iron deficiency, Unpublished observation, 1978.

212. Lanzkowsky, P.: Exudative enteropathy due to iron-deficiency anemia, Unpublished manuscript, 1978.

213. Lanzkowsky, P.: Iron supplementation of milk proposed to eliminate anemia, Pediatr. News **4**(9), 1970.

214. Lanzkowsky, P.: Radiological features of iron-deficiency anemia, Am. J. Dis. Child. **116:**16, 1968.

215. Lanzkowsky, P.: Hematologic values in healthy infants and children in three racial groups in Cape Town, J. Pediatr. **61:**620, 1962.

216. Lanzkowsky, P.: The influence of maternal iron-deficiency anaemia on the haemoglobin of the infant, Arch. Dis. Child. **36:**205, 1961.

217. Lanzkowsky, P.: The effect of intramuscular iron-dextran complex administered to women during pregnancy on their haematological values and on the haemoglobin levels of their infants, J. Obstet. Gynecol. Br. Cwlth. **68:**52, 1961.

218. Lanzkowsky, P.: The effect of intramuscular iron-dextran complex on iron-deficiency anemia in otherwise ill infants and pre-school children, Acta Pediatr. Scand. **50:**25, 1961.

219. Lanzkowsky, P.: Carcinogenic risks of iron-dextran complex, S. Afr. Med. J. **34:**351, 1960.

220. Lanzkowsky, P.: Effects of early and late clamping of umbilical cord on infant's haemoglobin level, Br. Med. J. **2:**1777, 1960.

221. Lanzkowsky, P.: Investigation into the aetiology and treatment of pica, Arch. Dis. Child. **34:**140, 1959.

222. Lanzkowsky, P.: Iron-deficiency anaemia in infants and pre-school children in three racial groups in Cape Town, M.D. thesis, University of Cape Town, Cape Town, South Africa, 1959.

223. Lanzkowsky, P.: Aetiology of pica, Lancet **2:**619, 1959.

224. Lanzkowsky, P., Karayalcin, G., Betkerur, U., and Shende, A.: Unreliability of the oral iron absorption test, J. Pediatr. **90:**494, 1977.

225. Lanzkowsky, P., Karayalcin, G., and Kazi, A.: Reversibility of cellular changes in iron-deficient postweaning rats, Pediatr. Res. **11:**474, 1977.

226. Lanzkowsky, P.: Iron deficiency anemia, Pediatr. Ann. **3:**6, 1974.

226a. Lanzkowsky, P.: Iron deficiency: a public health problem, Evansville, Ind., 1975, Mead Johnson.

226b. Lanzkowsky, P.: Iron metabolism in the newborn infant, Clin. Endocrinol. Metab. **5:**149, 1976.

227. Layrisse, M., Cook, J. D., Martinez, C., Roche, M., et al.: Food iron absorption: A comparison of vegetable and animal foods, Blood **33:**430, 1969.

228. Letsky, E. A., Miller, F., Worwood, M., and Flynn, D. M.: Serum ferritin in children with thalassaemia regularly transfused, J. Clin. Pathol. **27:**652, 1974.

229. Leventhal, B., and Stohlman, F., Jr.: Regulation of erythropoiesis. XVII. The determinants of red cell size in iron-deficiency states, Pediatrics **37:**62, 1966.

230. Linman, J. W., and Pierre, R. V.: Experimental observations on stimulation of thrombopoiesis by human factors, J. Lab. Clin. Med. **60:**994, 1962.

231. Low, J. A., Kerr, N. D., and Cochon, A. R.: Plasma and blood volume of the normal newborn infant and patterns of adjustment in initial 24 hours of the neonatal period, Am. J. Obstet. Gynecol. **86:**886, 1963.

232. Luke, C. G., David, P. S., and Deller, D. J.: Changes in gastric iron-binding protein (Gastroferrin) during iron-deficiency anaemia, Lancet **1:**926, 1967.

233. Magotra, M. L., Tondon, B. N., and Saraya, A. K.: Small bowel in iron-deficiency anaemia, Indian J. Med. Res. **59:**1788, 1971.

234. Macdougall, L. G.: Red cell metabolism in iron-deficiency anemia. III. The relationship between glutathione peroxidase catalase, serum vitamin E, and susceptibility of iron-deficiency red cells to oxidative hemolysis, J. Pediatr. **80:**775, 1972.

235. Macdougall, L. G.: A simple test for detection of iron in stools, J. Pediatr. **76:**764, 1970.

236. Macdougall, L. G.: Red cell metabolism in iron-deficiency anemia, J. Pediatr. **72:**303, 1968.

237. Macdougall, L. G., Anderson, R., McNab, G. M., and Katz, J.: The immune response in iron-deficient children: impaired cellular defense mechanisms with altered humoral components, J. Pediatr. **86:**833, 1975.

238. Macdougall, L. G., Jadisch, J. M., and Mistry, S. B.: Red cell metabolism in iron-deficiency anemia. II. The relationship of red cell survival and alterations in red cell metabolism, J. Pediatr. **76:**660, 1970.

239. MacKay, H. M. M.: Anemia in infancy: prevalence and prevention, Arch. Dis. Child. **3:**117, 1928.

240. Marks, J. W.: Lettuce craving and iron deficiency, Ann. Intern. Med. **79:**612, 1973.

241. Marner, F.: Haemoglobin, erythrocytes, and serum iron values in normal children 3-6 years of age, Acta Paediatr. Scand. **58:**363, 1969.

242. Marsh, A., Long, M., and Stierwalt, E.: Comparative hematologic response to iron fortification of a milk formula for infants, Pediatrics **24:**404, 1959.

243. Masawe, A. E. J., Muindi, J. M., and Swai, G. B. R.: Infections in iron-deficiency and other types of anaemia in the tropics, Tech. Rep. Ser. W.H.O. **405:**13, 1968.

244. Masawe, A. E. J., Muindi, J. M., and Swai, G. B. R.: Infections in iron deficiency and other types of anaemia in the tropics, Lancet **2:**314, 1974.

245. Masson, P. L., Heremans, J. P., and Dive, C. L.: An iron binding protein common to many external secretions, Clin. Chim. Acta **14:**735, 1966.

246. Masson, P. L., Heremans, J. F., and Schonne, E.: Lactoferrin, an iron binding protein in neutrophilic leukocytes, J. Exp. Med. **130:**643, 1969.

247. McDonald, R., and Marshall, S. R.: The value of iron therapy in pica, Pediatrics **34:**558, 1964.

248. McKay, H. M. M.: Nutritional anaemia in infancy with special reference to iron-deficiency anaemia, Med. Res. Counc. Spec. Rep. Ser. **157:**1, 1931.

249. McLaurin, L. P., Jr., and Cotter, J. R.: Placental transfer of iron, Am. J. Obstet. Gynecol. **98:**931, 1967.

250. Mecheles, T. F., Maldonado, N., Barquet-Chediak, A., and Allen, D. M.: Homozygous erythrocyte glutathione-peroxidase deficiency: clinical and biochemical studies, Blood **33:**164, 1969.

251. Meehl, P.: Nuisance variables and ex post facto design, Minnesota Symposium on the Philosophy of Science, 1972, University of Minnesota Press.

252. Melhorn, D. K., Gross, S., and Childers, G.: Vitamin E-dependent anemia in the premature infant. II. Relationships between gestational age and absorption of vitamin E, J. Pediatr. **79:**581, 1971.

253. Melhorn, D. K., Gross, S., and Childers, G.: Vitamin E-dependent anemia in the premature infant. I. Effects of large doses of medicinal iron, J. Pediatr. **79:**569, 1971.

254. Melhorn, D. K., Gross, S., Lake, G. A., and Leu, J. A.: The hydrogen peroxidase fragility test and serum tocopherol level in anemias of various etiologies, Blood **37:**438, 1971.

255. Millican, F. K., et al.: The prevalence of ingestion and mouthing of nonedible substances by children, Clin. Proc. Child Hosp. Wash. **18:**207, 1962.

256. Misenheimer, H. R.: Fetal hemorrhage associated with amniocentesis, Am. J. Obstet. Gynecol. **94:**1133, 1966. 1966.

257. Moe, P. J.: Normal red blood picture during the first three years of life, Acta Pediatr. Scand. **54:**69, 1965.

258. Moeschlin, S., et al.: Increased absorption of radioiron in gastrectomized patients by the addition of hydrochloric acid, Acta Haematol. **33:**200, 1965.

259. Mohan, M., Agarwal, K. N., and Bhutt, I., and Khanduja, P. C.: Iron therapy in pica, J. Indian M. Assoc. **51:**16, 1968.

260. Mollison, P. L., Veall, N., and Cutbush, M.: Red cell and plasma volume in newborn infants, Arch. Dis. Child. **25:**242, 1950.

261. Montrevil, J., and Spik, G.: Comparative studies of carbohydrate and protein moieties of human serotransferrin and lactotransferrin. In Crichton, R. R., ed.: Proteins of iron storage and transport in biochemistry and medicine, Amsterdam, North Holland Publishing Co., 1975.

262. Moore, C. B., Arrowsmith, W. R., Welch, J., and Minnich, V.: Studies in iron transportation and metabolism: observations on the absorption of iron from the gastrointestinal tract, J. Clin. Invest. **18:**553, 1939.

263. Moore, C. V.: The importance of nutritional factors in the pathogenesis of iron-deficiency anemia, Am. J. Clin. Nutr. **3:**3, 1955.

264. Moore, C. V.: The importance of nutritional factors in the pathogenesis of iron-deficiency anemia, Scand. J. Clin. Lab. Invest. **9:**292, 1957.

265. Moore, C. V.: Iron metabolism and nutrition, Harvey Lect. Ser. **55:**67, 1959-1960.

266. Moore, C. V.: The importance of nutritional factors in the pathogenesis of iron-deficiency anemia. In International Symposium on Iron Metabolism, Berlin, 1964, Springer Verlag.

267. Moore, C. V.: Iron nutrition and requirements, Ser. Haematol. **6:**1, 1965.

268. Moore, C. V., et al.: Absorption of ferrous and ferric radioactive iron by human subjects and by dogs, J. Clin. Invest. **23:**755, 1944.

269. Moore, C. V., and Dubach, R.: Metabolism and requirements of iron in the human, J.A.M.A. **162:**197, 1958.

270. Moores, R. R., Stohlman, F., Jr., and Brecher, G.: Humoral regulation of erythropoiesis. XI. The pattern of response to specific therapy in iron-deficiency anemia, Blood **22:**286, 1963.

271. Morgan, E. H.: Transferrin and transferrin iron. In Jacobs, A., Worwood, M., eds.: Iron in biochemistry and medicine, London, 1974, Academic Press, Ltd.

272. Munday, B., Shepherd, M. L., Emerson, L., et al.: Hemoglobin differences in healthy white and Negro infants, Am. J. Dis. Child. **55:**776, 1938.

273. Murray, M. J., and Stein, N.: Contribution of maternal iron stores to fetal iron in maternal iron deficiency and overload, J. Nutr. **101:**1583, 1971.

274. Murray, M. J., and Stein, N.: The integrity of the stomach as a requirement for maximal iron absorption, J. Lab. Clin. Med. **70:**673, 1967.

275. Murray, M. J., and Stein, N.: The effect of achylia gastrica in rats on the absorption of dietary iron, Proc. Soc. Exp. Biol. Med. **133:**183, 1970.

276. Murray, M. J., and Stein, N.: The contribution of maternal iron stores to fetal iron in rats, J. Nutr. **100:**1023, 1970.

277. Nadas, A. S.: Pediatric cardiology, Philadelphia, 1957, W. B. Saunders, Co.

278. Naiman, J. L., Oski, F., Diamond, L. K., Vawter, G. F., and Schwachman, H.: The gastrointestinal effects of iron-deficiency anemia, Pediatrics **33:**83, 1964.

279. Nalder, B. N., Mahoney, A. W., Ramakrishnan, R., and Hendriks, D. G.: Sensitivity of the immunologic response to the nutritional status of rats, J. Nutr. **102:**535, 1972.

280. Nebesky, O.: Beitrag zur Nabelschurzerreissung intra partum, Arch. Gynäkol. **100:**601, 1913.

281. Neffgen, J. F., and Korecky, B.: Cellular hyperplasia and hypertrophy in cardiomegalies induced by anemia in young and adult rats, Circul. Res. **30:**104, 1972.

282. Niccum, W. L., Jackson, R. L., and Stearns, G.: Use of ferric and ferrous iron in the prevention of hypochromic anemia in infants, Am. J. Dis. Child. **86:**553, 1953.

283. Nist, R. T., Bhardwaj, B., and Lanzkowsky, P.: Prevalence and pathogenetic factors of anemia in children in New York City, Paper presented to American Pediatric Ambulatory Care Society, Atlantic City, N.J., April, 1968.

284. Noldeke, H.: Geburtskomplikationen bei insertio velamentosa, Zentralbl. Gynäkol. **58:**351, 1934.

285. Novak, F.: Posthemorrhagic shock in newborns during labor and after delivery, Acta Med. Iugoslavia **7:**280, 1953.

286. Ogunbode, E., Oluboyede, O., Ayeni, O., and Abioye, A. A.: The treatment of iron-deficiency anaemia with a new intramuscular iron preparation (Ferastral), Scand. J. Haematol. Suppl. **32:**364, 1977.

287. Oppe, T. E., et al.: The health of the colored child in Great Britain, Proc. Roy. Soc. Med. **57:**321, 1964.

288. Osgood, E. E.: Development and growth of hematopoietic tissues, Pediatrics **15:**733, 1955.

288a. Owen, G. M., Nelson, C. E., and Garry, P. J.: Nutritional status of preschool children: hemoglobin, hematocrit and plasma iron values, J. Pediatr. **76:**761, 1970.

289. Pearson, H. A.: Iron-fortified formulas in infancy, J. Pediatr. **79:**557, 1971.

290. Pearson, H. A., and Abrams, I., Fernbach, D. J., Gyland, S. P., and Hahn, D. A.: Anemia in preschool children in the United States of America, Ped. Res. **1:**169, 1967.

291. Pearson, H. A., McLean, F. W., and Brigety, R. E.: Anemia related to age: Study of a community of young black americans, J.A.M.A. **215:**1982, 1971.

292. Pinkerton, P. H.: Control of iron absorption by the intestinal epithelial cell, Ann. Intern. Med. **70:**401, 1969.

293. Piomelli, S., Brickman, A., and Carlos, E.: Rapid diagnosis of iron deficiency by measurement of free erythrocyte prophyrins and hemoglobin: The FEP/hemoglobin ratio, Pediatrics **57:**136, 1976.

294. Piomelli, S., and Davidow, B.: Free erythrocyte protoporphyrin concentration: a promising screening test for lead poisoning, Pediatr. Res. **6:**366, 1972.

295. Pollack, S., et al.: A search for a mucosal iron carrier, J. Lab. Clin. Med. **80:**322, 1972.

296. Pollitt, E., and Leibel, R. L.: Iron deficiency and behavior, J. Pediatr. **88:**372-381, 1976.

297. Pollycove, M.: Iron metabolism and kinetics: the functions, distribution, and properties of iron compounds in humans, Sem. Haematol. **3:**235, 1966.

298. Pollycove, M., and Mortimer, R.: The quantitative determination of iron kinetics and hemoglobin synthesis in human subjects, J. Clin. Invest. **40:**753, 1961.

299. Pollycove, M., and Mortimer, R.: The quantitative determination of iron kinetics and hemoglobin synthesis in human subjects, International Symposium on Iron Metabolism, Berlin, 1964, Springer Verlag, p. 148.

300. Pommerenke, W. T., Hahn, P. F., Bale, W. F., and Balfour, W. M.: Transmission of radioactive iron to the human fetus, Am. J. Physiol. **137:**164, 1942.

301. Prasad, A. S., Halsted, J. A., and Nadimi, M.: Syndrome of iron deficiency, hepatosplenomegaly, hypogonadism, dwarfism, and geophagia, Am. J. Med. **31:**532, 1961.

302. Pribilla, W., Bothwell, T., and Finch, C. A.: Iron transport to the fetus in man. In Wallerstein, R. O., and Mettier, S. R., eds.: Iron in clinical medicine, Los Angeles, 1958, University of California Press.

303. Prichard, J. A., Whalley, P. J., and Scott, D. E.: The influence of maternal folate and iron deficiencies on intrauterine life, Am. J. Obstet. Gynecol. **104:**388, 1969.

304. Puragganan, H. B., and Naiman, J. L.: Exchange transfusion in severe iron-deficiency anemia prior to emergency surgery, J. Pediatr. **69:**804, 1966.

305. Putnam, F. W.: Transferrin. In Putnam, F. W., ed.: The plasma proteins, structure, function, and genetic control, ed. 2, vol. 1, New York, 1975, Academic Press, Inc.

306. Ramachandran, M., and Iyer, G. Y. N.: NADH-Methaemoglobin reductase of human erythrocytes in iron-deficiency anaemia, Clin. Chim. Acta **43:**101, 1973. 1973.

307. Rasch, C. A., et al.: Blood loss as a contributing factor in iron-lack anemia of infancy, Am. J. Dis. Child. **100:**627, 1960.

308. Ratten, G. J.: Spontaneous haematoma of the umbilical cord, Aust. N. Z. J. Obstet. Gynecol. **9:**125, 1969.

309. Rausen, A. R., Seki, M., and Strauss, L.: Twin transfusion syndrome: A review of 19 case studies at one institution, J. Pediatr. **66:**613, 1965.

310. Rausen, A. R., Gerald, P. S., and Diamond, L. K.: Genetical evidence for synthesis of transferrin in the foetus, Nature **192:**182, 1961.

311. Rawson, A., Rosenthal, F. D.: The mucosa of the stomach and small intestine in iron deficiency, Lancet **1:**730, 1960.

312. Report of committee on nutrition: On the feeding of solid foods to infants, Pediatrics **21:**685, 1958.

313. Reynolds, R. D., Binder, M. J., Miller, M. B., Chang, W. W. Y., and Moran, S.: Pagophagia and iron-deficiency anemia, Ann. Intern. Med. **69:**435, 1968.

314. Riose, E., Lipschitz, D. A., Cook, J. D., and Smith, N. J.: Relationship of maternal and infant iron stores as assessed by determination of plasma ferritin, Pediatrics **55:**694, 1975.

315. Rios, E., Lipschitz, D. A., Cook, J. D., Smith, N. J., and Finch, C. A.: The absorption of iron as supplements in infant cereal and infant formulas, Pediatrics **55:**686, 1975.

316. Robinson, S. H., and Koeppel, E. J.: Preferential hemolysis of immature erythrocytes in experimental iron-

deficiency anemia. Source of erythropoietic bilirubin formation, J. Clin. Invest. **50:**1847, 1971.

317. Robscheit-Robbins, F. S., and Whipple, G. H.: Infection and intoxication: their influence on hemoglobin production in experimental animals, J. Exp. Med. **63:**767, 1936.

318. Rodvien, R., Gillum, A., and Weintraub, L. R.: Decreased glutathione peroxidase activity secondary to severe iron deficiency: a possible mechanism responsible for the shortened life span of the iron-deficient red cell, Blood **43:**281, 1974.

319. Rothman, R. H., Klemer, J. S., and Toton, J. J.: The effect of iron-deficiency anemia on fracture healing, Clin. Orthop. **77:**276, 1971.

320. Roselle, H. A.: Association of laundry starch and clay ingestion with anemia in New York City, Arch. Intern. Med. **125:**57, 1970.

321. Ross Conference: Iron Nutrition in Infancy. In Sixty-second Conference on Pediatric Research, Columbus, Ohio, 1970, Ross Laboratories.

322. Rudolph, A. M., Nadas, A. S., and Borges, W. H.: Hematologic adjustments to cyanotic congenital heart diseases, Pediatrics **11:**454, 1953.

323. Russell, S. J. M.: Blood volume studies in healthy children, Arch. Dis. Child. **24:**88, 1949.

324. Russo, G., Musumeci, S., and Mazzone, D.: Iron binding by gastric juice, Lancet **1:**258, 1969.

325. Saarinen, U. M., Siimes, M. A., and Dallman, P. R.: Iron absorption in infants: high bioavailability of breast milk iron as indicated by the extrinsic tag method of iron absorption and by the concentration of sreum ferritin, J. Pediatr. **91:**36, 1977.

326. Saha, T. K., Chatterjea, J. B., Chaudhuri, R. N.: Jejunal mucosa in iron-deficiency anemia, Bull. Calcutta Sch. Trop. Med. **13:**6, 1965.

327. Samuels, L. D.: Leukemoid reaction to parenteral iron-dextran complex: a case report, J.A.M.A. **182:**1334, 1962.

328. Schachter, D., et al.: Active transport of ^{59}Fe by everted segments of rat duodenum, Am. J. Physiol. **198:**609, 1960.

329. Schacter, D., et al.: Active transport of iron by intestine: features of the two-step mechanism, Am. J. Physiol. **203:**73, 1962.

330. Schacter, D., et al.: Active transport of iron by intestine: mucosal iron pools, Am. J. Physiol. **207:**893, 1964.

331. Schade, A. L., and Caroline, L.: A iron-binding component in human blood plasma, Science **104:**340, 1946.

332. Schade, A. L., and Caroline, L.: Raw hen egg white and the role of iron in growth inhibition of *Shigella dysenteriae, Staphylococcus aureus, Saccharomyces cerevisiae,* Science **100:**14, 1944.

333. Schade, S. G., Felsher, B. F., Bernier, G. M., et al.: Interrelationship of cobalt and iron absorption, J. Lab. Clin. Med. **75:**435-441, 1970.

334. Schloesser, L. L., Kipp, M. A., and Wenzel, F. J.: Thrombocytosis in iron-deficiency anemia, J. Lab. Clin. Med. **66:**107-114, 1965.

335. Schubert, W. K.: Frequency of iron deficiency. In Iron nutrition in infancy, report of the Sixty-second Ross Conference on Pediatric Research, Columbus, Ohio, 1970, Ross Laboratories.

336. Schulman, I.: Iron requirements in infancy, J.A.M.A. **175:**118, 1961.

337. Schulman, I., and Smith, C. H.: Studies on the anemia of prematurity. III. The mechanism of anemia, Am. J. Dis. Child. **88:**582, 1954.

338. Schulz, J., and Smith, N. J.: A quantitative study of the absorption of food iron in infants and children, Am. J. Dis. Child. **95:**109, 1958.

339. Schulze, H. V., and Morgan, A. F.: Relation of ascorbic

340. Seely, J. R., Humphrey, G. B., and Matter, B. J.: Copper deficiency in a premature infant fed on iron-fortified formula, N. Engl. J. Med. **286:**109, 1972.

341. Segond, A.: De la gastro-enterit chronique chez les negres vulgairement appelée mal d'estomac, Tr. Med. Paris **13:**156, 1833.

342. Seip, M., and Halvorsen, S.: Erythrocyte production and iron stores in premature infants during the first months of life, Acta Paediatr. **45:**600, 1956.

343. Seltzer, C. C., Wenzel, B. J., and Mayer, J.: Serum iron and iron-binding capacity in adolescents. I. Standard values, Am. J. Clin. Nutr. **13:**343, 1963.

344. Shafer, A. W., and Marlow, A. A.: Toxic reaction to intramuscular injection of iron, N. Engl. J. Med. **260:**180, 1959.

345. Shahidi, N. T., and Diamond, L. K.: Skull changes in infants with chronic iron-deficiency anemia, N. Engl. J. Med. **262:**137, 1960.

346. Shahidi, N. T., Nathan, D. G., and Diamond, L. K.: Iron-deficiency anemia associated with an error of iron metabolism in two siblings, J. Clin. Invest. **43:**510, 1964.

347. Sharpe, I. M., et al.: The effect of phytate and other food factors on iron absorption, J. Nutr. **41:**433, 1950.

348. Sheehan, R. G., and Frenkel, E. P.: The control of iron absorption by the gastrointestinal mucosal cell, J. Clin. Invest. **51:**224, 1972.

349. Shepherd, M. K., Weatherall, D. J., and Conley, C. L.: Semiquantitative estimation of distribution of fetal hemoglobin in red cell populations, Bull. Johns Hopkins Hosp. **110:**293, 1962.

350. Siimes, M. A., Addiego, J. E., and Dallman, P. R.: Ferritin in serum: diagnosis of iron deficiency and iron overload in infants and children, Blood **43:**581, 1974.

351. Sisson, T. R. C., and Lund, C. J.: The influence of maternal iron deficiency on the newborn, Am. J. Dis. Child. **94:**525, 1957.

352. Sisson, T. R. C., Whalen, L. E., and Lelek, A.: The blood volume of infants. II. The premature infant during the first year of life, J. Pediatr. **54:**430, 1959.

353. Slawsky, P., and Desforges, J. F.: Erythrocyte 2,3-diphosphoglycerate in iron deficiency, Arch. Intern. Med. **129:**914-917, 1972.

354. Smith, C. H., Schulman, I., and Morgenthau, J. E.: Iron metabolism in infants and children; serum iron and iron-binding protein; diagnostic and therapeutic implications. In Levine, S. Z., ed.: Advances in peditrics, vol. 5, Chicago, 1952, Year Book Medical Publishers, Inc.

355. Smith, N. J.: Considerations of iron metabolism in early infancy, J. Pediatr. **54:**654, 1959.

356. Smith, N. J.: Iron as a therapeutic agent in pediatric practice, J. Pediatr. **53:**37, 1958.

357. Smith, N. J., Rosello, S., Say, M. B., and Yeya, K.: Iron storage in the first five years of life, Pediatrics **16:**166, 1955.

358. Smith, N. J., and Rios, E.: Iron metabolism and iron deficiency in infancy and childhood. In Schulman, I., ed.: Advances in Pediatrics, vol. 21, Chicago, 1974, year book Medical Publishers.

359. Smith, P. M.: Gastric iron binding in hemochromatosis, Lancet **2:**1143, 1968.

360. Sorbie, J., Olatunbosum, D., Corbett, W. E. N., et al.: Cobalt excretion test for the assessment of body iron stores, Can. Med. Assoc. J. **104:**777, 1971.

361. Sourkes, T. L.: Psychopharmacology. In Albers, R. W., Siegel, G. J., Katzman, R., and Agranoff, B. W., eds.: Basic neurochemistry, Boston, 1972, Little, Brown & Co.

362. Strikantia, S. G., Prasad, J. S., Bhaskaram, C., and

Krishnamachari, K. A. V. R.: Anemia and immune response, Lancet **1:**1307, 1976.

363. Stavem, P., Saltvedt, E., Elgjo, K., and Rootwelt, K.: Congenital hypochromic-microcytic anemia with iron overload of the liver and hyperferraemia, Scand. J. Haematol. **10:**153, 1973.

364. Steinberg, M. H., and Necheles, T. F.: Erythrocyte glutathione peroxidase deficiency: biochemical studies on the mechanisms of drug-induced hemolysis, Am. J. Med. **50:**542, 1971.

365. Stockman, J. A., Weiner, L. B., Stuart, M. J., and Oski, F. A.: The micromeasurement of free erythrocyte porphyrin (FEP) as a means of screening for β-thalassemia minor in subjects with microcytosis, Blood **42:**990, 1973.

366. Sturgeon, P.: Studies of iron requirements in infants and children. In Wallerstein, R. O., and Mettier, S. A., editors: Iron in clinical Medicine, Los Angeles, 1958, University of California Press.

367. Sturgeon, P.: Iron metabolism: a review, Pediatrics **18:**267, 1956.

368. Sturgeon, P.: Studies of iron requirements in infants and children. I. Normal values for serum iron, copper, and free erythrocyte protoporphyrin, Pediatrics **13:**107, 1954.

369. Sulzer, J. L., Wesley, H. H., and Leonig, F.: Nutrition and behavior in head start children: results from the Tulane study. In Kallen, D. J., ed.: Nutrition, development, and social behavior. No. (NIH)73-242, U.S. Department of Health, Education, & Welfare, 1973.

370. Swarup, S., Ghosh, S. K., and Chatterjea, J. B.: Aconitase activity in iron deficiency, Acta Haematol. **37:**53, 1967.

371. Swedberg, B.: A clinical investigation of an iron-poly (sorbitol-gluconic acid) complex, Ferastral, for the treatment of iron-deficiency anaemia, Scand. J. Haematol., Suppl. **32:**260, 1977.

372. Symes, A. L., Sourkes, T. L., Youdim, M. B. H., et al.: Decreased monamine oxidase activity in liver of iron-deficient rats, Can. J. Biochem. **47:**999, 1969.

373. Reference deleted in proofs.

374. Reference deleted in proofs.

375. Thomas, F. B., et al.: Effect of phenobarbital on the absorption of inorganic and hemoglobin iron in the rat, Gastroenterology **62:**590, 1972.

376. Thomson, A. B. R., Shaver, C., Lee, D. J., et al.: Effect of varying iron stores on site of intestinal absorption of cobalt and iron, Am. J. Physiol. **220:**674, 1971.

377. Thorbecke, G. J., et al.: Sites of formation of the serum proteins transferrin and hemopexin, J. Clin. Invest. **52:**725, 1973.

378. Tosatti, C.: Gaz. Osp. Clin. **28:**154, 1907.

379. Tunnessen, W. W., Smith, C., Oski, F. A.: Beeturia: a sign of iron deficiency, Am. J. Dis. Child. **117:**424, 1969.

380. Turnbull, A., et al.: Iron absorption of hemoglobin iron, J. Clin. Invest. **41:**1897, 1962.

381. Turnbull, A., Giblett, E. R.: The binding and transport of iron by transferrin variants, J. Lab. Clin. Med. **57:**450, 1961.

382. Usher, R., and Lind, J.: Blood volume of the newborn premature infant, Acta. Paediatr. Scand. **54:**419, 1965.

383. Usher, R., Shepard, M., and Lind, J.: The blood volume of the newborn infant and placental transfusion, Acta Paediatr. **52:**497, 1963.

384. Vahlquist, B.: Das serumeisen: Eine pädiatrisch-klinische und experimentelle Studie, Acta Paediatr. **28:**1, 1941.

385. Valbert, L. S., Ludwig, J., and Olatunbosun, D.: Alteration in cobalt absorption in patients with disorders of iron metabolism, Gastroenterology **56:**241, 1969.

386. Valbert, L. S., Sorbie, J., Corbett, W. E. N., and Lud-

wig, J.: Cobalt test for the detection of iron-deficiency anemia, Ann. Intern. Med. **77:**181, 1972.

387. Vitale, J. J., Restrepo, A., Valez, H., Riker, J. B., and Hellerstein, E. E.: Secondary folate deficiency induced in the rat by dietary iron deficiency, J. Nutr. **88:**315, 1966.

388. Viteri, F. W.: Physical fitness and anemia. In Abstracts of international symposium on malnutrition and blood cells, Kyoto, 1972, U.S.-Japan Medical Science Program.

389. Voorhess, M. C., Stuart, M. J., Stockman, J. A., and Oski, F. A.: Iron-deficiency anemia and increased urinary norepinephrine excretion, J. Pediatr. **86:**542, 1975.

390. Vosburgh, G. J., and Flexner, L. B.: Maternal plasma as a source of iron for the fetal guinea pig, Am. J. Physiol. **161:**202, 1950.

391. Vossough, P., Leikin, S., and Purugganan, G.: Evaluation of parameters of folic acid and vitamin B_{12} deficiency in patients with iron-deficiency anemia, Ped. Res. **2:**179, 1968.

392. Walters, G. O., Miller, F., and Worwood, M.: Serum ferritin concentration and iron stores in normal subjects, J. Clin. Pathol. **26:**770, 1973.

393. Webb, T. E., and Oski, F. A.: Behavioral status of young adolescents with iron-deficiency anemia, J. Spec. Ed. **8:**153, 1974.

394. Webb, T. E., and Oski, F. A.: Iron-deficiency anemia and scholastic achievement in young adolescents, J. Pediatr. **82:**827, 1973.

395. Webb, T. E., and Oski, F. A.: The effect of iron-deficiency anemia on scholastic achievement, behavioral stability, and perceptual sensitivity of adolescents, Pediatr. Res. **7:**294, 1973.

396. Weintraub, L. R., et al.: The role of a heme-splitting substance in the intestinal mucosa, J. Clin. Invest. **47:** 531, 1968.

397. Werkman, S., Shifman, L., and Shelly, T.: Psychosocial correlates of iron deficiency in early childhood, Psychosom. Med. **26:**125, 1964.

398. Wheby, M. S.: Regulation of iron absorption, Gastroenterology **50:**888, 1966.

399. Wheby, M. S., et al.: Role of transferrin in iron absorption, J. Clin. Invest. **42:**1007, 1963.

400. Wheby, M. S., et al.: Studies on iron absorption: intestinal regulatory mechanisms, J. Clin. Invest. **43:**1433, 1964.

401. Wheby, M. S., et al.: The gastrointestinal tract and iron absorption, Blood **22:**416, 1963.

402. Wheby, M. S., et al.: Effect of transferrin saturation on iron absorption in man, N. Engl. J. Med. **271:**1391, 1964.

403. Wheby, M. S., et al.: Role of transferrin in iron absorption, J. Clin. Invest. **42:**1007, 1963.

404. Wheby, M. S., et al.: Studies on iron absorption: intestinal regulatory mechanisms, J. Clin. Invest. **43:**1433, 1964.

405. Wheby, M. S., et al.: The gastrointestinal tract and iron absorption, Blood **22:**416, 1963.

406. Wheby, M. S., et al.: Studies on iron absorption, N. Engl. J. Med. **271:**1391, 1964.

407. Wheby, M. S., et al.: The role of bile in the control of iron absorption, Gastroenterology **42:**310, 1962.

408. Whipple, G. H., Sisson, T. R. C., and Lund, C. J.: Delayed ligation of the umbilical cord: its influence on the blood volume of the newborn, Am. J. Obstet. Gynecol. **10:**603, 1957.

409. Widdowson, E. N., and Spray, C. M.: Chemical development in utero, Arch. Dis. Child. **26:**205, 1951.

410. Wilson, J. F., Heiner, D. C., and Lahey, M. E.: Studies on iron metabolism. IV. Milk-induced gastrointestinal

bleeding in infants with hypochromic-microcytic anemia, J.A.M.A. **189:**568, 1964.

411. Wilson, J. F., Lahey, M. E., and Heiher, D. C.: Studies on iron metabolism. V. Further observations on cow's milk-induced gastrointestinal bleeding in infants with iron-deficiency anemia, J. Pediatr. **84:**335, 1974.

412. Wintrobe, M. M.: Clinical hematology, Philadelphia, 1974, Lea & Febiger.

413. Wintrobe, M. M.: Factors and mechanisms in the production of red corpuscles, Harvey Lect. Ser. **45:**87, 1949-1950.

414. Wipple, G. H., and Robscheit-Robbins, F. S.: Iron and its utilization in experimental anemia, Am. J. Med. Sci. **191:**11, 1936.

415. Woodruff, C. W.: The utilization of iron administered orally, Pediatrics **27:**194, 1961.

416. Woodruff, C. W.: Multiple causes of iron deficiency in infants, J.A.M.A. **167:**715, 1958.

417. Woodruff, C. W., and Bridgeforth, E. B.: Relationship between the hemogram of the infant and that of the mother during pregnancy, Pediatrics **12:**681, 1953.

418. Woodruff, C. W., and Clark, J. L.: The role of fresh cow's milk in iron deficiency. I. Albumin turnover in infants with iron-deficiency anemia, Am. J. Dis. Child. **124:**18, 1972.

419. Woodruff, C. W., Latham, C., and McDavid, S.: Iron nutrition in the breast-fed infant, J. Pediatr. **90:**36, 1977.

420. Woodruff, C. W., Wright, S. W., and Wright, R. P.: The role of fresh cow's milk in iron deficiency. II. Comparison of fresh cow's milk with a prepared formula, Am. J. Dis. Child. **124:**26, 1972.

421. World Health Organization: Nutritional anemias, Geneva, 1968, Tech. Rep. Ser., No. 405.

422. World Health Organization: Nutritional anemias, Geneva, 1972, Tech. Rep. Ser., No. 503.

423. Worwood, M., and Jacobs, A.: The subcellular distribution of ^{59}Fe in small intestinal mucosa, Br. J. Haematol. **20:**587, 1971.

424. Worwood, M., and Jacobs, A.: The subcellular distribution of ^{59}Fe in small intestinal mucosa, Br. J. Haematol. **22:**265, 1972.

425. Yao, A. C., Moinian, M., and Lind, J.: Distribution of blood between infant and placenta after birth, Lancet **2:**871, 1969.

426. Zachau-Christiansen, B., Hoff-Jorgensen, E., and Kristensen, H. P.: The relative haemoglobin, iron, vitamin B_{12}, and folic acid values in the blood of mothers and their newborn infants, Danish Med. Bull. **9:**157, 1962.

427. Ziai, M.: Anemia and increased intracranial pressure in an infant, Clin. Pediatr. **12:**59, 1973.

428. Zipursky, A., Pollock, J., Neelands, P., Chown, B., and Israels, L. G.: The transplacental passage of foetal red blood cells and the pathogenesis of Rh immunisation during pregnancy, Lancet **2:**489, 1963.

7 □ Megaloblastic anemias and other nutritional anemias

Philip Lanzkowsky

Megaloblastic anemias are characterized by the presence of megaloblasts in the marrow and macrocytes in the blood. The megaloblast is bigger than the normoblast at a similar stage of development, the nuclear chromatin is more finely divided and the parachromatin more prominent, and the cytoplasm of the megaloblast is more intensely basophilic. There are also morphologic changes in the white cells and megakaryocytes, a reflection of intracellular biochemical abnormalities.

Megaloblasts may be considered the morphologic result of any biochemical defect resulting in slowed deoxyribonucleoprotein (DNA) synthesis. The resulting "nuclear-cytoplasmic dissociation," or asynchrony, is caused by relatively slow DNA synthesis in relation to relatively normal RNA synthesis and is manifested morphologically in all proliferating tissues, such as bone marrow, by large cells containing slowly maturing and dividing nuclear DNA surrounded by more normal-appearing cytoplasmic RNA. There is an inability to double the amount of nuclear DNA (DNA synthesis phase) for the cell to divide. These biochemical abnormalities may be the result of rare inborn errors of metabolism, and occasionally they may occur in association with some other blood dyscrasias, but usually they are the result of a relative or absolute deficiency of certain substances necessary for normal hematopoiesis. These deficiencies can arise from a variety of causes, such as defective dietary intake, defective absorption, increased losses, increased requirements, and the presence of antagonists, acting either singly or in combination. The two deficiencies that produce megaloblastic anemia in more than 95% of cases are folate and vitamin B_{12} deficiencies. In addition it has been claimed that deficiencies of ascorbic acid, tocopherol, and thiamine may be related to megaloblastic anemia.

Both vitamin B_{12} and folic acid (pteroylglutamic acid) are essential for normal metabolic processes. A comparison of the two is summarized in Table 7-1. These two substances function as coenzymes in the synthesis of nucleoproteins. A deficiency of either substance causes a megaloblastic type of anemia associated with abnormalities in the maturation of granulocytes and megakaryocytes and gives rise to macrocytosis in the mucosa of the mouth, stomach, intestine, and vagina; an inadequate amount of vitamin B_{12} also leads to serious derangements of the nervous system. A deficiency of either vitamin B_{12} or folic acid usually is most apparent in the cells involved in erythropoiesis. The delay in cell division and maturation is reflected in the appearance of the nuclei of erythro-

Table 7-1. Some characteristics of vitamin B_{12} and folate

	Vitamin B_{12}	Folate
Parent form	Cyanocobalamin	Pteroylglutamic acid (folic acid)
Molecular weight	1,355 daltons	441 daltons
Natural forms	Methylcobalamin, deoxyadenosyl-cobalamin, hydroxycobalamin	Reduced, methylated, or formylated pteroylpolyglutamates
Foods	Animal origin only (liver, meat, fish, daily produce)	Yeast, liver, green vegetables, nuts, cereals, fruit, etc.
Effect of cooking	Little or no effect	May destroy completely
Adult daily requirements	1-2 μg	100 μg
Normal daily intake	3-30 μg	600-700 μg
Body stores	3-5 mg (2-4 years' supply)	6-20 mg (4 months' supply)
Site of absorption	Ileum	Duodenum and jejunum
Mechanism	Gastric intrinsic factor	Deconjugation, reduction, and methylation
Enterohepatic circulation	Yes	Yes

cyte precursors; the chromatin pattern of the nucleus remains dispersed while the cytoplasm enlarges and hemoglobinization progresses. These morphologic abnormalities and the known importance of DNA and RNA metabolism in cell growth and division suggest that a main function of these vitamins is concerned with DNA and RNA metabolism. Biochemically, when the defect is in the folate- and vitamin B_{12}–dependent pathway of DNA-thymine synthesis, it may be easily uncovered by the "dU suppression test," which measures radioactive iododeoxyuridine or tritiated thymidine incorporation into DNA.[55,125]

The causes of megaloblastosis are as follows.

A. Vitamin B_{12} deficiency
B. Folate deficiency
C. Miscellaneous
   1. Congenital disorders in DNA synthesis
      a. Orotic aciduria (uridine-responsive)
      b. Thiamine-responsive megaloblastic anemia
      c. Congenital familial megaloblastic anemia requiring massive doses of vitamin B_{12} and folate
      d. Congenital dyserythropoietic anemia
      e. Lesch-Nyhan syndrome (adenine-responsive) (?)
   2. Acquired defects in DNA synthesis
      a. Liver disease
      b. Sideroblastic anemias
      c. Leukemia, especially acute myeloid leukemia
      d. Aplastic anemia (constitutional or acquired)
      e. Di Guglielmo's disease
      f. Refractory megaloblastic anemia
   3. Drug-induced megaloblastosis
      a. Purine analogs (6-mercaptopurine, 6-azathioprine, thioguanine, etc.)
      b. Pyrimidine analogs (5-fluorouracil, 6-azauridine)
      c. Inhibitors of ribonucleotide reductase (cytosine arabinoside, hydroxyurea)

VITAMIN B_{12}
Biochemistry

Vitamin B_{12} is the largest of the vitamins; cyanocobalamin has a molecular weight of 1,355 daltons, and B_{12} coenzymes have slightly higher molecular weights.[63] Vitamin B_{12} has been shown to be essential for a number of biochemical reactions in nature, most of them involving an intramolecular rearrangement of hydrogen or carbon.[12] These include the reduction of ribonucleotides (in some bacteria), biosynthesis of methionine (in mammals), isomerization of methylmalonate to succinate (in mammals), isomerization of β-methyl aspartate to glutamate (in *Clostridium tetanomorphum*), and conversion of aldehydes to diols (in some bacteria). Of these reactions the ones known to occur in humans include the biosynthesis of methionine and the isomerization of methylmalonate to succinate. The role of vitamin B_{12} in the metabolism of formiminoglutamate and aminoimidazole carboxamide may be indirect via an effect on folate metabolism.[56]

Methionine synthesis. The enzyme concerned in methionine synthesis is N^5-methyltetrahydrofolate homocysteine methyltransferase and the reactions require 5-methyltetrahydrofolate as methyl donor, S-adenosylmethionine, and a reducing agent ($FADH_2$) as well as methylcobalamin as coenzyme (Fig. 7-1). Methylfolate probably donates the methyl groups to methylcobalamin bound to the protein apoenzyme, which then passes the methyl group to homocysteine.

The main importance of vitamin B_{12}–dependent methionine synthesis is probably in the regeneration of tetrahydrofolate from methyltetrahydrofolate.

Isomerization of methylmalonyl CoA to succinyl CoA. The conversion of propionate to succinate involves three enzymes. Carboxylation of propionyl CoA to D-methylmalonyl CoA by propionyl carboxylase requires biotin. The enzyme methylmalonyl CoA racemase converts the inactive D-isomer to the active L-enantiomorph. The third reaction, which uses two molecules of deoxyadenosylcobalamin (coenzyme B_{12}) per molecule of apoenzyme as prosthetic group, consists of the isomerization of L-methylmalonyl CoA to succinyl CoA.[23] The amount of vitamin B_{12} normally present is probably sufficient for this reaction and

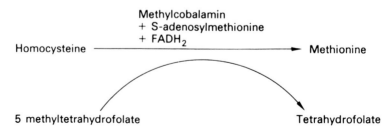

Fig. 7-1. Conversion of homocysteine to methionine. This is the only known biochemical reaction that requires both vitamin B_{12} and folate. (From Hardisty, R. M., and Weatherall, D. J.: Blood and its disorders, Oxford, 1974, Blackwell Scientific Publications, Ltd.)

is not normally rate limiting.[71] This reaction is therefore part of a route by which cholesterol and odd-chain fatty acids, as well as a number of amino acids and thymine, may be used for energy requirements via the Krebs cycle, for gluconeogenesis, or to form δ-aminolevulinic acid (Fig. 7-2). The importance of these reactions in humans is best illustrated by the syndromes that have recently been described in infants suffering from inborn errors of metabolism involving them.

Metabolism

Dietary sources. A normal Western diet contains between 3 and 30 μg of vitamin B_{12} daily, usually 5 to 10 μg. Vitamin B_{12} is synthesized exclusively by microorganisms, and these are the source of the vitamin found in food. The highest concentrations are found in liver (which contains about 1 μg/gm), kidney, shellfish, muscle meats, fowl, and dairy products including milk, which in humans has 0.1 μg/100 gm. There is probably no vitamin B_{12} in fruits, vegetables, nuts, and cereals unless they have been contaminated by bacteria. Soil and natural waters also contain vitamin B_{12} from bacterial contamination. In general vitamin B_{12} is not destroyed by cooking, but under alkaline conditions and in the presence of vitamin C some may be lost at high temperatures (e.g., in boiling fresh milk); severe heating of meat and meat products may also partly degrade vitamin B_{12}.

Stores and requirements. Estimates of total human adult body vitamin B_{12} stores by microbiologic and isotope dilution techniques have ranged from 2 to 11 mg, with a mean usually in the range of 3 to 5 mg.[46,114] The highest concentration (about 1 μg/gm) is in liver, with about a fifth this level in kidney, adrenal glands, and pancreas and lower levels in other organs. The cere-

brospinal fluid contains only 30 pg/ml. Most liver vitamin B_{12} and vitamin B_{12} in other cells is in mitochondria as the deoxyadenosyl form. Small amounts of methylcobalamin are present in cells, and this is the main form in plasma.

Despite the competitive advantage for B_{12} demonstrated by the fetus in utero,[15] total body stores at birth are probably reduced. Fetal liver contains only one-third the concentration of vitamin B_{12} found in adult liver.[105] Liver stores average about 25 μg in the newborn and are rarely depleted before 1 year of age.

Daily requirements are thought to be about 2 to 3 μg, although a smaller dose (between 0.1 and 1 μg) will produce an optimal hematologic response in a patient with megaloblastic anemia caused by vitamin B_{12} deficiency. The daily requirement in infants is probably less than 0.1 μg/day.[8] Losses occur mainly in the urine and in feces, but the human body does not seem able to degrade vitamin B_{12}. In practice it takes from 2 to 4 years for megaloblastic anemia to develop following total gastrectomy, which causes sudden cessation of vitamin B_{12} absorption.

Absorption. Both active and passive mechanisms exist for the absorption of vitamin B_{12}. The active process is dependent on intrinsic factor and an intact ileum receptor site, and it is of primary importance in the absorption of physiologic (2 μg or less) amounts of vitamin B_{12}. The passive mechanism, probably diffusion, occurs in the entire small intestine and becomes important only for pharmacologic amounts of the vitamin. Dietary vitamin B_{12} is released from protein and peptide complexes in the stomach and duodenum and normally attaches to intrinsic factor. This is a glycoprotein of molecular weight 44,000 to 48,000 daltons[3] with about 15% carbohydrate, which is

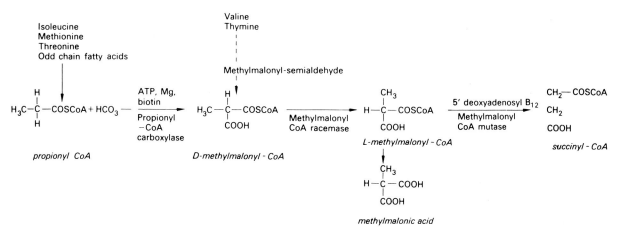

Fig. 7-2. Metabolism of propionate to succinate. The exact site at which valine and thymine feed into the pathway is unknown. (From Hardisty, R. M., and Weatherall, D. J.: Blood and its disorders, Oxford, 1974, Blackwell Scientific Publications, Ltd.)

secreted by the parietal cells of the body and fundus of the stomach in humans, the cells that also secrete hydrochloric acid.[60]

An essential property of intrinsic factor is its ability to bind vitamin B_{12} avidly. This occurs readily over a wide pH range, including the normal acid milieu of the stomach. Vitamin B_{12} in beef muscle and other proteins is bound loosely at acid pH,[29] and therefore intrinsic factor competes favorably in the stomach for vitamin B_{12} bound to food proteins. One molecule of intrinsic factor binds one molecule of vitamin B_{12}.

One unit of intrinsic factor is defined as the amount that binds 1 ng of vitamin B_{12}. Intrinsic factor and acid are present in the gastric secretions of neonates on the day of birth. Although outputs of intrinsic factor and hydrochloric acid are low the first day of life, a gradual and sustained increase in production of these glandular secretory components begins immediately, so that at 2 to 3 months of age infants have levels of intrinsic factor comparable to those observed in older children and adults.[1] Furthermore, by the second week the average infant has intrinsic factor output sufficient to ensure absorption of an adequate amount of vitamin B_{12}. Basal secretion by young men is about 3,000 units/hour, or about 36 units/ml; women secrete a similar concentration but about half the total amount. Following histamine, betazole, gastrin, pentagastrin, or insulin stimulation, secretion increases to 16,000 units/hour or to 100 units/ml in concentration in young men. There is a relationship between the amounts of acid and intrinsic factor secreted, except in the first 15 minutes after stimulation, when intrinsic factor secretion rises disproportionately, probably the result of release of preformed intrinsic factor. Intrinsic factor has two receptor sites, one for vitamin B_{12} and the other for ileal intestinal microvilli, which specifically requires a neutral pH and the presence of free calcium.

The relatively stable intrinsic factor–vitamin B_{12} (IF-B_{12}) complex is then carried to the ileum, where the absorption of vitamin B_{12} occurs in humans.[18] Vitamin B_{12} is absorbed mainly in the distal portion of the ileum, at a roughly neutral pH; both intrinsic factor and calcium ions are necessary for the absorption of physiologic amounts, but the mechanism by which intrinsic factor promotes absorption is uncertain. The IF-B_{12} complex is resistant to digestion, a binding that may prevent utilization of the vitamin by the bacteria of the intestine before absorption occurs. The absorption of vitamin B_{12} is accomplished by some interaction between the mucosal cell and the IF-B_{12} complex. The role of calcium ions appears to be the attachment of intrinsic factor to mucosal cells; vitamin B_{12} first attaches to one of the active sites of the

intrinsic factor and then the other active site of the intrinsic factor attaches to the mucosal cell. The receptor is located on the microvilli of the ileal cells. The attachment of the IF-B_{12} complex to the brush border (microvilli) of the ileal cell does not appear to require metabolic energy,[34] although the subsequent intracellular movement of B_{12} may be energy dependent.[126] Although it has been suggested that the intrinsic factor molecule enters the mucosal cell by pinocytosis or by other means, the evidence indicates that the intrinsic factor is not absorbed as vitamin B_{12} enters the cell. Intrinsic factor does not pass through the mucosal cells into the portal blood,[102] but whether it is digested off at the brush border or enters the mitochondria is uncertain.[78,115]

Vitamin B_{12} enters the mitochondria of the cell and remains there during a period of mucosal delay (about 6 hours), the peak blood level being reached only 8 to 12 hours after an oral dose.[17,101] Thereafter vitamin B_{12} is transferred to the portal blood, where it attaches mainly to transcobalamin II[50] and possibly also to transcobalamins I and III.[30] Cyanocobalamin enters plasma largely or completely unchanged in humans.[19]

Only 0.5% to 1.5% of a single oral dose of the order of 30 to 300 μg of vitamin B_{12} is absorbed in humans without intrinsic factor. This absorption occurs through the duodenum and jejunum (or nasal, buccal, or respiratory tract mucosa) and is rapid, with a rise in serum level in 1 hour.

Enterohepatic circulation. Variable estimates have been given of the amount of vitamin B_{12} in the bile, ranging from less than 1 μg to as high as 43 μg/day. Further vitamin B_{12} enters the gut lumen from gastric, pancreatic, and intestinal secretions and from sloughed intestinal cells. In patients with malabsorption of vitamin B_{12} this is all lost in feces; in normal persons and vegans a large proportion of this vitamin B_{12} is presumably reabsorbed.

Transport. Vitamin B_{12} is present in plasma as a methylcobalamin, 5'-deoxyadenosylcobalamin, or hydroxocobalamin bound to at least two proteins.[49] Transcobalamin I and II bind vitamin B_{12} stoichiometrically. Newly absorbed vitamin B_{12} emerging from ileal cells into the portal blood becomes bound to transcobalamin II. Portions may also bind to other serum binding proteins, e.g., transcobalamin I.

Transcobalamin I. Transcobalamin I, an α_1-globulin, carries nearly all the vitamin B_{12} normally present in serum and is capable on the average of binding another 200 to 300 pg/ml, being 50% to 70% saturated. It is the serum and intracellular storage protein for vitamin B_{12}; it binds the vitamin avidly and gives up vitamin B_{12} only slowly to tissues. Absence of this binder from plasma, noted in two brothers, has been reported to cause a low level of vitamin B_{12} in serum but no clinical abnormality.[25] It has been postulated that the leukocytes are the source of transcobalamin I, which appears to be the mechanism for transport of covitamin B_{12}, methylocobalamin, in the plasma and in its passage from cells.

Transcobalamin II. The second vitamin B_{12}–binding protein in plasma is a weak binder and has a molecular weight of 36,000. Electrophoresis shows it to be a β-globulin and it is probably synthesized in the liver.[128] It is responsible for the delivery of vitamin B_{12} to the cell. The protein normally carries less than 20 pg/ml of vitamin B_{12} but is capable of binding about 1,000 pg/ml and, being unsaturated, binds most of the vitamin B_{12} added to plasma in vitro. It facilitates the entry of vitamin B_{12} into cells, and it probably serves this physiologic function.[27,49] Uptake of vitamin B_{12} from transcobalamin II by hematopoietic cells appears to require Ca^{++} or Mg^{++} ions, to require active cellular protein synthesis, and to be reduced if cells are vitamin B_{12} deficient but normal or increased if cells are folate deficient.[62,110] Congenital deficiency of transcobalamin II causes the development of megaloblastic anemia at a few weeks of age because of inability to transfer vitamin B_{12} from either the intestine or tissues to the marrow.[48] An antibody to transcobalamin II has been described in patients receiving long-term therapy with a depot vitamin B_{12} preparation of hydroxocobalamin, and such patients show extremely high (>10 ng/ml) serum vitamin B_{12} levels.[121]

Differences in the serum binders of vitamin B_{12} in newborn infants have been reported.[72] In addition to the two normal carrier proteins for B_{12}, transcobalamin I and II, a third, or "fetal," binder has been noted. This binder is the same size as transcobalamin I, but it does not contain endogenous B_{12} nor does it transfer B_{12} to HeLa cells. The significance of the "fetal" binder is presently unclear.

Disturbances of vitamin B_{12}–binding proteins in disease. Changes in concentrations in serum of the vitamin B_{12}–binding proteins may occur in a variety of diseases and may or may not be associated with changes in the serum vitamin B_{12} level.[52] The most common abnormality is a rise in transcobalamin I, which occurs in chronic granulocytic leukemia and also in other myeloproliferative diseases such as myelosclerosis, polycythemia vera, and acute myeloid leukemia (particularly with promyelocytic differentiation). The serum vitamin B_{12} level in chronic granulocyte leukemia is usually in the range of 1,000 to 10,000 pg/ml. There is some evidence that the binder in these conditions may be qualitatively abnormal, since it may bind vitamin B_{12} so firmly that the serum vita-

min B_{12} level remains normal even if the patient also develops pernicious anemia with megaloblastic anemia.[20] Benign diseases with a leukocytosis were not thought to cause a rise in the vitamin B_{12}–binding capacity,[89] but mild rises in patients with chronic leukocytosis caused by infections occasionally associated with a rise in the serum vitamin B_{12} level have recently been reported.[24]

High serum vitamin B_{12} levels occur when the liver cells are breaking down, such as in acute hepatitis, active cirrhosis, liver abscess, hepatoma, and other forms of acute liver damage, and can be used to follow the response to therapy. Part of the vitamin B_{12} may be free, but increased levels of both β- and α-globulin binders have also been described, as well as a variant of transcobalamin I in children with hepatoma.[133] In untreated pernicious anemia there is an increase in unsaturated vitamin B_{12}–binding capacity but a decrease in total vitamin B_{12}–binding capacity caused by a fall in the level of transcobalamin II.[74] In pregnancy, on the other hand, there is an increase in transcobalamin II. The serum vitamin B_{12} level and vitamin B_{12}–binding capacity may also be increased in chronic renal failure.

Detailed study of patients with congenital defects of vitamin B_{12} absorption and transport has provided the following summary of the concepts of plasma transport of vitamin B_{12}.

A. Intrinsic factor
   1. Is required for B_{12} absorption and postnatal survival. (Congenital intrinsic factor lack [congenital pernicious anemia] at birth is normal.)
   2. Is needed for B_{12} metabolism postabsorption.
B. Transcobalamin II
   1. Carries plasma B_{12} immediately postabsorption.
   2. Carries plasma B_{12} from one tissue to another.
   3. Is necessary for survival.
C. Transcobalamin I
   1. May have no true transport function.
   2. Cannot substitute for deficient transcobalamin II.
D. Neither intrinsic factor nor fetal transcobalamin II is essential for the fetus.

Excretion. The main excretion route of vitamin B_{12} is through the bile, and about 40 μg passes into the jejunum each day. The enterohepatic circulation results in most of this being reabsorbed in the ileum by the intrinsic factor mechanism. Small amounts of vitamin B_{12} also enter the intestine from gastric, pancreatic, and intestinal secretions. Unabsorbed vitamin B_{12} passes into the feces and together with that derived from bacterial synthesis in the colon amounts to 3 to 6 μg daily, depending on the size of the body stores.

Urinary excretion by glomerular filtration of

vitamin B_{12} unbound to protein varies from 0 to 0.25 μg/day, the total loss from the body being 2 to 5 μg daily.

Causes of vitamin B_{12} deficiency

The causes of vitamin B_{12} deficiency can be summarized as follows.

A. Inadequate intake
   1. Dietary (<1 mg/day): food fads, veganism, malnutrition
   2. Maternal deficiency
B. Defective absorption
   1. Failure to secrete intrinsic factor
      a. Congenital pernicious anemia (gastric mucosa normal) (intrinsic factor deficiency)
         (1) Quantitative
         (2) Qualitative (biologically inert)*
      b. Juvenile pernicious anemia (gastric atrophy)
      c. Juvenile pernicious anemia with endocrinopathies
      d. Juvenile pernicious anemia with IgA deficiency
      e. Gastric mucosal disease
         (1) Corrosives
         (2) Gastrectomy (partial/total)
   2. Failure of absorption in small intestine
      a. Specific vitamin B_{12} malabsorption
         (1) Abnormal intrinsic factor*
         (2) Abnormal ileal uptake (Imerslund-Gräsbeck syndrome)
         (3) Ingestion of chelating agents (phytates, EDTA)
      b. Intestinal disease causing generalized malabsorption including vitamin B_{12} malabsorption
         (1) Intestinal resection
         (2) Regional ileitis
         (3) Tuberculosis of terminal ileum
         (4) Lymphosarcoma of terminal ileum
         (5) Pancreatic insufficiency
         (6) Zollinger-Ellison syndrome
         (7) Celiac disease
         (8) Other less specific malabsorption syndromes
      c. Competition for vitamin B_{12}
         (1) Small-bowel bacterial overgrowth
            (a) Small bowel diverticulosis
            (b) Anastomoses and fistulas
            (c) Blind loops and pouches
            (d) Multiple strictures
            (e) Scleroderma
            (f) Achlorhydria
            (g) Gastric trichobezoar
         (2) *Diphyllobothrium latum*
C. Defective transport
   1. Congenital deficiency of transcobalamin II
   2. Transient deficiency of transcobalamin II
   3. Partial deficiency of transcobalamin I

D. Disorders of vitamin B_{12} metabolism
   1. Congenital
      a. Specific inability to form adenosylcobalamin (vitamin B_{12}–responsive methylmalonic aciduria)
      b. Defect in methylmalonyl-CoA mutase apoenzyme (vitamin B_{12}–nonresponsive methylmalonic aciduria)
      c. Failure to form both adenosylcobalamin and methylcobalamin (methylmalonic aciduria and homocystinuria)
      d. Abnormality of N^5-methyltetrahydrofolate homocysteine methyltransferase apoenzyme
   2. Acquired
      a. Liver disease
      b. Protein malnutrition (kwashiorkor, marasmus)
      c. Drugs (and usages) associated with impaired absorption and/or utilization
         (1) Para-aminosalicylic acid (PAS): tuberculosis
         (2) Colchicine: gout
         (3) Neomycin: antibiotic
         (4) Ethanol: societal
         (5) Oral contraceptive agents (?): contraception
         (6) Metformin: diabetes

Inadequate intake

Infants. Breast milk contains vitamin B_{12} in about the same concentration as serum.[9] Therefore children born of vitamin B_{12}–deficient mothers, if fed solely on maternal milk, may develop vitamin B_{12} deficiency. This produces a syndrome occurring in the first 2 years of life and characterized by developmental retardation or regression, megaloblastic anemia, central nervous system involvement, and (at least in Indian infants) hyperpigmentation of the skin and mucosae.[124]

This hyperpigmentation is not specific for vitamin B_{12} deficiency but has also been observed in megaloblastic anemia associated with folate deficiency.[37] All these abnormalities are reversible on treatment with oral vitamin B_{12}, although if treatment is delayed central nervous system damage may become irreversible.

Pathak and Gadwin[99] have found low serum vitamin B_{12} levels at 40 days of age in fourteen of twenty-four premature infants. This results from low dietary intake coupled with increased demand by the prematurely born infants.

Children. Although serum vitamin B_{12} levels in vegetarians are lower than in nonvegetarians[88] frank megaloblastic anemia caused by defective dietary intake of vitamin B_{12} occurs only occasionally.[58,103] Even in South India where, because of the largely vegetarian diet, the intake of vitamin B_{12} is low, pure dietary deficiency is an uncommon cause of megaloblastic anemia.[7]

Individuals who for religious and often eco-

---

*Same condition.

nomic reasons avoid all animals foods such as meat, fish, and dairy products develop vitamin B_{12} deficiency. The main fall in serum vitamin B_{12} levels occurs within the first two years on a vegan diet. A further decrease may not occur even after many years, and persons may remain in perfect health. Possibly the intact enterohepatic circulation reduces losses of vitamin B_{12} when stores are low and minute quantities of vitamin B_{12} eaten maintain hematopoiesis at an adequate level.

Defective absorption (Table 7-2)

Failure to secrete intrinsic factor

CONGENITAL PERNICIOUS ANEMIA (INTRINSIC FACTOR DEFICIENCY). Children with congenital pernicious anemia are born with congenital absence of intrinsic factor and no other abnormalities.[90] The stomach is normal on biopsy and tests of gastric acid and pepsin secretion. There are no antibodies to parietal cell or intrinsic factor.[86] The disease is transmitted as an autosomal recessive disorder; five definite pairs of siblings and four other possible cases have been recorded. In several cases the parents were related. These children usually present with megaloblastic anemia or neuropathy between the fourth and twenty-eighth month of life, but some are teenagers.

The serum B_{12} level is below normal and intrinsic factor is absent or altered. In earlier studies the diagnostic criteria usually included demonstration of decreased absorption of low, physiologic doses of B_{12} that was restored to normal by addition of normal human intrinsic factor or hog intrinsic factor. More recently immunologic methods have been utilized that in general depend on the ability of anti–intrinsic factor antibodies to bind either to intrinsic factor, and thereby prevent its combination with cobalamin, or to the cobalamin–intrinsic factor complex. Absence of intrinsic factor activity in such assays does not necessarily imply the complete absence of intrinsic factor, since a structurally abnormal intrinsic factor that had lost its ability to bind cobalamin would not be detected.[69]

Waters and Murphy[132] reported two cases of pernicious anemia and refer to another case of anemia probably present in a third brother who had died previously. Both parents and five other siblings absorbed subnormal or borderline amounts of a test dose of labeled vitamin B_{12}. It was concluded that both parents carried the gene for the deficient secretion of intrinsic factor as heterozygotes and that the affected children were presumably homozygous for the gene, having inherited it from both parents. In several studies it was shown that relatives of patients with pernicious anemia have been reported to have a deficiency of intrinsic factor[22] and defective vitamin B_{12} absorption.[87] Typical congenital pernicious anemia may result therefore

Table 7-2. Features of congenital and acquired defects of vitamin B_{12} absorption

| Types of anemia | Age of onset (years) | Stomach | | | Schilling test | | Serum antibodies | | Associated features |
		Histology	Intrinsic factor	HCl acid	Without intrinsic factor	With intrinsic factor	Intrinsic factor	Parietal cell	
Congenital pernicious anemia	Under 3	Normal	Absent	Normal	Decreased	Normal	Absent	Absent	None
Juvenile pernicious anemia	Over 10	Atrophy	Absent	Achlorhydria	Decreased	Normal	Present	Present	Occasional SLE,[85] IgA deficiency, moniliasis, endocrinopathy in siblings
Juvenile pernicious anemia and endocrinopathies	Over 10	Atrophy	Absent	Achlorhydria	Decreased	Normal	Present	Present	Hypothyroid, hypoparathyroid, Addison's disease, moniliasis
Specific vitamin B_{12} malabsorption	Infancy	Normal	Present	Normal	Decreased	Decreased	Absent	Absent	Benign proteinuria, aminoaciduria
Generalized malabsorption	Any age	Normal	Present	Normal	Decreased	Decreased	Absent	Absent	Malabsorption syndrome
Acquired intestinal lesions	Any age	Normal	Present	Normal	Decreased	Decreased	Absent	Absent	Findings of associated disease/surgery

Familial incidence column (between Age of onset and Stomach): Autosomal inheritance; Absent; Absent; Present; Absent; Absent from the homozygous inheritance of a gene responsible for the deficient secretion of intrinsic factor. The adult form is explained on the basis of an inherited heterozygous defect of intrinsic factor secretion, on which is superimposed an atrophic lesion of the mucosa.

One patient[68] was found to have immunologically normal but biologically inert intrinsic factor. Apparently, as in the hemophilias,[106] there can be a disabling congenital defect in the structure of the protein as well as congenital deficiency in the amount of the protein.

JUVENILE PERNICIOUS ANEMIA (AUTOIMMUNE). A form of pernicious anemia resembling that in adults may occur in children. These children show gastric atrophy with achlorhydria and absent intrinsic factor; there are a high incidence of intrinsic factor antibody (90%) and a low incidence of parietal cell antibody (10%) in serum.

JUVENILE PERNICIOUS ANEMIA (AUTOIMMUNE) WITH ENDOCRINOPATHIES. One form of pernicious anemia resembles that in adults and also has associated endocrinopathy such as hypoparathyroidism, myxedema, or Addison's disease, which may present before or after the anemia.* Siblings may show an endocrinopathy such as myxedema, hypoparathyroidism, or adrenal atrophy, and some patients and siblings have suffered from moniliasis and steatorrhea.[134] These children thus have a genetically determined tendency to develop organ-specific antibodies that is similar but more marked than in adults with pernicious anemia.

A case of pernicious anemia has been reported in a 10-year-old girl with familial Addison's disease, idiopathic hypoparathyroidism, and moniliasis.[104] Pernicious anemia was diagnosed by the demonstration of a megaloblastic anemia, achlorhydria, gastric atrophy, absence of intrinsic factor, antibodies against human intrinsic factor, and response to vitamin B_{12} therapy. Several other cases of pernicious anemia associated with one or the other of these endocrinopathies have been previously reported.

JUVENILE PERNICIOUS ANEMIA WITH IgA DEFICIENCY. Seven cases of achlorhydric juvenile pernicious anemia with selective IgA deficiency have been reported. The anemia responded to vitamin B_{12} therapy, but IgA deficiency persisted following B_{12} therapy.† There does not appear to be a direct relationship between the inheritance of the two abnormalities.

The features of congenital and juvenile pernicious anemia are summarized in Table 7-2.

GASTRIC MUCOSAL DISEASE. Severe vitamin B_{12} deficiency caused by lack of intrinsic factor is the inevitable result of total gastrectomy, the peak incidence of megaloblastic anemia or neuropathy being from 2 to 8 years after the operation. Serum vitamin B_{12} levels have been found to fall steeply a few months after the operation, but definitely subnormal levels are usually reached later. Vitamin B_{12} deficiency might also occur following partial gastrectomy; the most important factor determining the incidence of vitamin B_{12} deficiency is size of the resection.

Failure of absorption in small intestine

SPECIFIC VITAMIN B_{12} MALABSORPTION. Receptors for intrinsic factor exist in the small intestine and play a vital role in the absorption of physiologic amounts of vitamin B_{12}. Patients have been described who have congenital absorptive defects of the ileum for vitamin B_{12}.

ABNORMAL INTRINSIC FACTOR. Katz et al.[68] have succeeded in demonstrating an abnormal, structurally altered intrinsic factor protein in a patient with congenital vitamin B_{12} malabsorption. A 3-year-old boy who was the child of a consanguineous marriage presented with megaloblastic anemia and was found to have all the characteristics of congenital intrinsic factor deficiency except that intrinsic factor was detectable in normal adult levels (60 units/ml) in the gastric juice by radioimmunoassay. This abnormal intrinsic factor was found to behave chromatographically and by isoelectric focusing electrophoresis exactly like normal human intrinsic factor, and it appeared normal in vitamin B_{12} binding, molecular weight, total amino acid and carbohydrate composition, and results of immunodiffusion. The patient presumably had an abnormal intrinsic factor in at least one antigenic determinant, and this was theoretically caused by an amino acid substitution at the ileal rather than the vitamin B_{12} binding site. The probable basis for the malabsorption was demonstrated by the failure of the patient's IF-B_{12} complex to bind normally to human ileal mucosal homogenates.

These results demonstrate that the B_{12} and ileal binding sites of the intrinsic factor molecule reside in different regions of the protein and that structural abnormalities may affect one function without affecting the other. Further investigations of patients with intrinsic factor abnormalities may reveal a variety of functional changes in intrinsic factor, each of which might lead to malabsorption. In addition to those already mentioned, such abnormalities might include increased susceptibility of the IF-B_{12} complex to proteolysis,[69] failure of the complex to protect vitamin B_{12} from utilization by intestinal bacteria,[35] and defects in the release of B_{12} from the complex with intrinsic factor, a process that might occur after binding of the complex to ileal receptors during the passage into or through the mucosal cell.[69]

---

*References 65, 66, 76, 86, 104, 107.
†References 41, 122, 129, 130.

ABNORMAL ILEAL UPTAKE. In 1960 Imerslund[67] and Gräsbeck et al.[44] independently described children with familial malabsorption of vitamin B_{12} that appeared to be caused by abnormalities in the ileal uptake of vitamin B_{12}. In these patients gastric biopsy, gastric acid, secretion, and intrinsic factor secretion are normal but IF-B_{12} complex is not absorbed, and thus an ileal defect is thought to be present.[91] The ileum appears normal, however, by both light and electron microscopy and in one case took up the complex normally in vitro.[81] Absorption of other substances and small bowel roentgenograms are normal. More than eighty cases of this sort have now been reported.[13,45,81]

Proteinuria, which is mild (25 to 150 mg/dl of urine), nonspecific (mainly albumin), and benign, is present in nearly all cases, though three have not shown this feature. The urinary tract is usually normal, though Imerslund[67] found congenital abnormalities of the kidneys and ureters and a mild aminoaciduria in some cases, albeit from a highly inbred community. Two patients had increased excretion of alanine, glycine, glutamine, serine, valine, tyrosine, and phenylalanine. Urinary amino acids have been identified by either high-voltage electrophoresis or paper chromatography. Two patients described by Spurling et al.[123] demonstrated increases in taurine, ethanolamine, and histidine. Mohamed et al.[91] found aminoaciduria in four of sixteen patients and incidental cystinuria in one patient. Rubin et al.[117] described a case of selective malabsorption of vitamin B_{12} with elevated excretion or clearance of threonine, alanine, tyrosine, histidine, glycine, serine, and leucine before and after therapy; this finding supports the concept of an associated distinct renal tubular defect separate from vitamin B_{12}–dependent metabolic pathways.

The characteristic picture is the development of early megaloblastic anemia. The patients remain well on maintenance vitamin B_{12} therapy and failure to provide this results in relapse. These patients possess normal intrinsic factor and normal serum vitamin B_{12}–binding proteins. There is no generalized malabsorption, although nonspecific malabsorption may occur secondarily when the patients are severely B_{12} deficient.[131] The specificity of the absorptive defect is thus best demonstrated after appropriate treatment with parenteral vitamin B_{12}. It is assumed that in each of these patients a specific defect is present in the intestinal mucosa that prevents the normal absorption of vitamin B_{12}. Ben-Bassat et al.[13] were unsuccessful in correcting the malabsorption of cyanocobalamin following the administration of normal intestinal juice in eleven of thirteen patients with a specific defect in absorption of cyanocobalamin. The possible sites for such defects are many: (1) in the ileal membrane receptor for the IF-B_{12} complex, (2) in the

release of vitamin B_{12} from binding to intrinsic factor, (3) in the movement of vitamin B_{12} through the mucosal cell, and (4) in the release of vitamin B_{12} into the bloodstream. However, in no single patient has any of these mechanisms been demonstrated. Biopsies of the ileal mucosa have been normal by light and electron microscopy.[45,81] Attempts to demonstrate abnormalities in the release of cobalamin from its complex with intrinsic factor have been inconclusive.[45] In a family study, MacKenzie et al.[81] showed that attachment of intrinsic factor–cobalamin complex to ileal mucosal homogenates was not altered.[81] It was postulated that the defect was in a stage of transport beyond the cell surface but before plasma transport. Further investigations may reveal genetic heterogeneity among different families with this type of vitamin B_{12} malabsorption as well as define the normal processing of cobalamin during ileal uptake.

INTESTINAL DISEASE CAUSING GENERALIZED MALABSORPTION. Small intestinal disease affecting the ileum may lead to vitamin B_{12} malabsorption and megaloblastic anemia. The symptoms related to B_{12} deficiency and the anemia resemble those of pernicious anemia, with additional complaints and findings related to the underlying small intestinal disorder.

Resection of the ileum removes the physiologic site of absorption of vitamin B_{12} in humans.[16] Thus patients who have had ileal resection (for congenital stenosis, intussusception, volvulus, trauma, etc.) become B_{12} deficient if not given B_{12} parenterally. Regional ileitis (Crohn's disease) and tuberculosis of the ileum are inflammatory disorders that destroy the ileal mucosa, thus impairing B_{12} absorption. Other granulomatous diseases and malignant lesions affecting the ileum (e.g., lymphosarcoma of the terminal ileum) are rare causes of vitamin B_{12} malabsorption. Chronic diarrheal syndromes may be associated with B_{12} malabsorption. The cause may be impairment of function of the ileal mucosa rather than hypermotility.

Malabsorption of vitamin B_{12} has been described in patients with severe chronic pancreatitis and ascribed to lowered pH in the ileum and to lowered calcium ion concentration caused by the formation of insoluble calcium soaps. Zollinger-Ellison syndrome may be associated with vitamin B_{12} malabsorption caused by lowered pH in the ileum. Defective absorption of vitamin B_{12} is found in some patients with celiac disease. The vitamin B_{12} absorptive defect is not influenced by giving extra intrinsic factor nor is it influenced by the administration of antibiotics.[92] The absorptive defect must therefore be related to an interference with the normal ileal mechanism of vitamin B_{12} absorption caused by the toxic action of wheat gluten.[116] As a result of the vitamin B_{12} malabsorption, serum vitamin B_{12} levels may be low in some patients, but pure vitamin B_{12}–deficiency megaloblastic anemia is rare.[92]

COMPETITION FOR VITAMIN B_{12}

SMALL BOWEL BACTERIAL OVERGROWTH. In the blind loop syndrome symptoms of diarrhea, steatorrhea, weight loss, and abdominal cramps may occur. This syndrome consists of vitamin B_{12} deficiency and anemia associated with anatomic abnormalities of the small intestine, including single or multiple diverticula of the small bowel,[28] small intestinal anastomoses, ileotransverse colostomy, and intestinal strictures.[2,19,51] The blind loop syndrome appears to be caused at least partly by intestinal stasis with bacterial overgrowth in the small intestine, resulting in utilization of ingested B_{12} by intestinal bacteria. There is a good clinical and hematologic response to tetracycline or other broad-spectrum antibiotic drugs.

TRICHOBEZOAR. Gastric trichobezoar was described by Bernstein et al.[14] in a 6-year-old child with megaloblastic anemia from vitamin B_{12} deficiency. In addition, hyperfolatemia and hypoalbuminemia were demonstrated. A combination of low B_{12} and markedly elevated serum folate levels in the presence of megaloblastic anemia suggests bacterial overgrowth within the upper small bowel. Although it is an unusual cause of megaloblastic anemia in childhood, trichobezoar should be considered when low vitamin B_{12} levels and hyperfolatemia are present together with a gastric mass. The occurence of this combination suggests that bacterial overgrowth is present within the upper small bowel and that the bezoar therefore probably extends into the small bowel.

DIPHYLLOBOTHRIUM LATUM INFESTATION. The parasite *Diphyllobothrium latum* competes with the host for the available vitamin B_{12} in the intestinal lumen and is able to take up free B_{12} or B_{12} bound to intrinsic factor. Fish tapeworm anemia occurs most frequently in the Scandinavian countries, Japan, and the Great Lakes region of the United States and Canada where raw freshwater fish are consumed. In Finland, where up to 20% of the population may harbor the parasite, only 3% or fewer of the carriers develop anemia. Many persons with fish tapeworm anemia have hydrochloric acid in their gastric secretion. The increased incidence of pernicious anemia in the families of persons with fish tapeworm anemia suggests that a predisposition to gastric atrophy may exist in certain persons because of a basic constitutional factor. Symptoms and complications of the B_{12} deficiency are similar to those of pernicious anemia. After expulsion of the worm B_{12} absorption improves and the anemia remits. Parenteral B_{12} therapy with or without expulsion of the worm is also effective.

Defective transport

Abnormalities of transcobalamin II. Transcobalamin II deficiency is a serious and potentially fatal defect in early infancy if massive doses of vitamin B_{12} are not administered; this clearly indicates that transcobalamin II is the principal transport system of vitamin B_{12}. The deficiency is inherited as an autosomal recessive trait.

In 1971 Hakami et al.[48] reported the first cases of transcobalamin II deficiency in two siblings who were seen at 3 and 5 weeks of age with failure to thrive, vomiting and diarrhea, progressive pancytopenia, and megaloblastic bone marrow changes. Levels of serum vitamin B_{12} were normal. This indicates that adequate vitamin B_{12} was available to the children in utero, since they did not have any signs of B_{12} deficiency at birth. Vitamin B_{12} transport in utero may have been mediated by a fetal type of transport protein that normally disappears after the first few weeks of life. An alternative and more likely explanation is a transplacental transfer of maternal transcobalamin II to the fetus followed by development of megaloblastic anemia on the decay of this protein shortly after birth.

An additional case has been reported from Switzerland by Hitzig et al.[59] Born of consanguineous parents, the child early in life manifested severe malabsorption resulting from atrophy of the small intestinal mucosa. He was unable to form specific antibodies and plasma and had pancytopenia caused by bone marrow insufficiency. In each of these cases the progressive life-threatening course was relieved by large doses of vitamin B_{12}. Subsequent investigations revealed that there was virtually no serum protein capable of binding vitamin B_{12} and migrating with transcobalamin II during chromatography or polyacrylamide gel electrophoresis. Gimpert et al.[40] failed to detect the presence in the serum of any substance that was immunologically cross reactive with antibody to normal transcobalamin II, so by this criterion transcobalamin II appeared to be absent rather than present in an altered form incapable of binding B_{12}. Transcobalamin I was present in the sera of all three patients, although somewhat decreased in those studied by Hakami et al., and certain other B_{12}–binding proteins of the so-called secondary or fetal types were also demonstrated.[40,48]

A transient deficiency of transcobalamin II has been reported by Lawrence[75] in a patient with pernicious anemia whose level of transcobalamin II became normal with vitamin B_{12} therapy. Similar observations have been made by Carmel and Herbert[25] about another patient with pernicious anemia.

Partial deficiency of transcobalamin I. Partial deficiency of transcobalamin I has been reported in only two adult brothers. Transcobalamin I deficiency was discovered in the index case during investigation of a subnormal serum B_{12} concentration 3 years after subtotal gastrectomy for gastric ulcer. Serum B_{12} concentrations were persistently low, and repeated transcobalamin I concentrations ranged from 25% to 54% of the mean normal concentration. Transcobalamin II concentrations were also slightly low, with means of 71% and 78% of the mean normal value. No specific clinical abnormalities could be associated with these findings.[25] Since the decrease in transcobalamin I was incomplete, for the moment no conclusion is warranted with respect to the effects of a more complete deficiency of this protein. The entity has not been reported in children.

Disorders of metabolism

Congenital disorders. Once vitamin B_{12} has been taken up into cells, it must be converted to the correct, coenzymatically active derivative, located in the proper subcellular compartment, to act as a cocatalyst with vitamin B_{12}–dependent apoenzymes.

In humans the two enzymes that are known to depend for activity on cobalamin derivatives are methylmalonyl-CoA mutase, which requires adenosylcobalamin, and N^5-methyltetrahydrofolate homocysteine methyltransferase, which requires methylcobalamin (Figs. 7-1 and 7-2). Genetic conditions have been described that involve an abnormality in the activity of one or both of these enzymes.

Methylmalonyl-CoA mutase catalyzes the conversion of methylmalonyl-CoA to succinyl-CoA. A decreased activity of methylmalonyl-CoA mutase is reflected by the excretion of elevated amounts of methylmalonic acid. Investigation of patients with various genetically determined forms of methylmalonic aciduria has been proceeding rapidly in recent years.[111,112]

SPECIFIC INABILITY TO FORM ADENOSYLCOBALAMIN. A group of patients has been distinguished who suffer from specific inability to form adenosylcobalamin. Clinically these children usually have life-threatening or fatal ketoacidosis in the first few weeks or months of life. The acidosis is often accompanied by hypoglycemia and hyperglycinemia. Failure to thrive or developmental retardation may be a consequence of the acidosis and is reversed by relief of the ketoacidosis. Serum cobalamin concentrations are normal.

Studies from these patients have shown that intact cells fail to oxidize propionate normally.[113] Methylmalonyl-CoA arises chiefly through the carboxylation of propionate, which in turn is derived largely from degradation of valine, isoleucine, methionine, and threonine.

DEFECTS IN METHYLMALONYL-CoA MUTASE APOENZYME FORMATION. Another group of patients with methylmalonic aciduria results from defects in the formation of methylmalonyl-CoA mutase apoenzyme. The clinical picture in untreated patients with this disorder resembles that in untreated patients with cobalamin A or B mutations. Methylmalonic aciduria is accompanied by life-threatening or fatal ketoacidosis. The techniques for demonstration of defects in methylmalonyl-CoA mutase are relatively straightforward. Intact cells are generally unable to oxidize propionate. Tissue extracts fail to convert methylmalonyl-CoA to succinyl-CoA, and this failure is not relieved by the addition of supplemental adenosylcobalamin.[93]

Patients with defects of mutase apoenzyme encountered to date have not been responsive to vitamin B_{12} therapy.

FAILURE TO FORM BOTH ADENOSYLCOBALAMIN AND METHYLCOBALAMIN. A metabolic abnormality has been described that resulted in an inability to maintain normal tissue concentrations of the two coenzyme forms of vitamin B_{12}, methylcobalamin and adenosylcobalamin (Figs. 7-1 and 7-2). Lack of methylcobalamin leads to deficient activity of N^5-methyltetrahydrofolate homocysteine methyltransferase with reduced ability to methylate homocysteine resulting in homocysteinuria. Lack of adenosylcobalamin results in deficient activity of methylmalonyl-CoA mutase, which accounts for the methylmalonic aciduria. Both these enzyme activities are defective in whole cells. In suitable extracts the activities could be restored by addition of the cobalamin derivative in question. Most directly the tissues and cultured fibroblasts of these patients contain far less than normal amounts of both adenosylcobalamin and methylcobalamin.[33,79,84,95]

Such patients therefore have both methylmalonic aciduria and homocysterinuria as a result of failure to form both adenosylcobalamin and methylcobalamin. Only four such patients have been described. Two of the patients died at 7 weeks and 7 years of age with severe illnesses that included mental and developmental retardation, recurrent megaloblastic anemia, and susceptibility to infections.[33,77] At autopsy one of these patients had pulmonary fibrosis and the brain showed lesions typical of those seen in subacute combined degeneration of the cord. Two other patients are brothers, approximately 19 and 8 years old. They are much less severely affected,[43] although the older brother is mildly mentally retarded and in the past few years has had recurrent episodes of thrombophlebitis.[42]

ABNORMALITY OF N^5-METHYLTETRAHYDROFOLATE HOMOCYSTEINE METHYLTRANSFERASE APOENZYME. A defect in the apoenzyme has been reported only in a single patient, a mentally retarded girl studied when she was 6 months old by Arakawa et al.[6]

This child had megaloblastic anemia and abnormally high total folate activity in the serum. Assays of liver extracts showed that the activities of a number of enzymes involved in folate metabolism were not decreased but that there was a partial decrease in the specific activity of N^5-methyltetrahydrofolate homocysteine methyltransferase measured in the presence of cyanocobalamin. The activity in the extract of the patient's liver was 32% to 45% of that observed in control liver extracts. It is of interest that this patient was not homocystinuric.

Subsequent work on this patient by Mudd[96] indicated that the preliminary data were inconclusive, since severe generalized defects of N^5-methyltetrahydrofolate homocysteine methyltransferase are likely to be accompanied by homocystinuria. The child may have had a partial primary defect in the methyltransferase apoenzyme, expressed chiefly in the liver. An alternative possibility is that this child may have an undefined primary defect at another step in folate metabolism. Methyltransferase defects would then be epiphenomenal.

Acquired disorders. Impaired utilization of vitamin B_{12} has been reported in protein malnutrition (kwashiorkor, marasmus) and liver disease. Certain drugs (p. 178) are associated with impaired absorption and/or vitamin B_{12} utilization.

Clinical manifestations of vitamin B_{12} deficiency

Many cases of vitamin B_{12} deficiency are detected during the first 2 years of life, whereas others become manifest during childhood until puberty. The onset is insidious, and pallor, apathy, fatigability, anorexia are early symptoms. A beefy, red, sore tongue; papillary atrophy; and other features of recurrent glossitis are common.

Parasthesias also are common, even in patients without objective evidence of neuropathy. Episodic or continuous diarrhea may occur. Pigmentation of the skin (mild jaundice), which together with pallor gives the patient a "lemon yellow" tint, and a mild fever are common findings. The spleen is palpable in about half the severely anemic patients.

Signs of subacute dorsolateral degeneration of the spinal cord occur infrequently.[108] Patients may present with neurologic disease as well as, or instead of, anemia. The usual symptoms are parasthesias in the hands or feet, difficulty in walking, and, more rarely, difficulty with use of the hands. The symptoms arise because of a peripheral neuropathy, associated in some cases with degeneration of the posterior and lateral tracts of the spinal cord. The basic pathologic process is demyelination, which in more severe cases is accompanied by degeneration of axis cylinders.[47] The legs are nearly always more severely affected than the arms. Loss of vibration and position sense, ataxic gait, and positive Romberg's sign are features of posterior column and peripheral nerve loss. Spastic paresis with knee and ankle reflexes increased by lateral tract loss may occur, but flaccid weakness with loss of these reflexes and presence of an extensor Babinski response may also occur. The biochemical basis for the neuropathy is obscure, although attempts have been made to relate it to disturbed fatty acid metabolism secondary to a block in propionate metabolism.[39]

Laboratory findings

Peripheral blood. Peripheral blood values vary according to the severity of anemia. When the hemoglobin level is low (4 to 6 gm/dl), there is a marked variation in size and shape of red cells with many oval macrocytes, cell fragments, and distorted cells (Fig. 7-3). The number of red cells is reduced to a greater extent than the hemoglobin, and the MCV is raised to levels between 110 and 140 fl. The higher the MCV, the more likely is megaloblastic anemia to be present. When iron-deficiency and megaloblastic anemia are combined, however, the MCV may be normal; nevertheless, the blood and bone marrow still show some of the morphologic characteristics of megaloblastic anemia. Howell-Jolly bodies and punctate basophilia are present and reticulocytes are in normal proportion. The red cells are well hemoglobinized, the macrocytes stain deeply, and the MCHC is normal. The leukocyte count is reduced to 1.5 to 4.0 × 10⁹/liter by a fall in both neutrophils and lymphocytes; a proportion of the neutrophils show hypersegmented nuclei, i.e., more than five lobes (with an average of more than 3.42 lobes per cell); and eosinophils show more than two lobes. Very large neutrophils with eight or more lobes (macropolycytes) may be present. The platelet count is moderately reduced, usually to levels of 50 to 150 × 10⁹/liter. Patients with leukocyte counts less than 1 × 10⁹/liter and platelet counts of 15 × 10⁹/liter or less have been described, and the condition may be mistaken for aplastic anemia or acute leukemia. Megaloblasts and myelocytes may be found in the peripheral blood, particularly if buffy coat films are examined.

When anemia is less severe, macrocytosis is still the main feature but the distortion of red cells and the decrease in leukocytes and platelets are less marked. In mildly anemic or nonanemic patients only a few macrocytes and hypersegmented neutrophils and a raised MCV may suggest the diagnosis. Macrocytosis may also occur in patients with myxedema, aplastic anemia, leukoerythroblastic anemia, acquired sideroblastic anemia, and

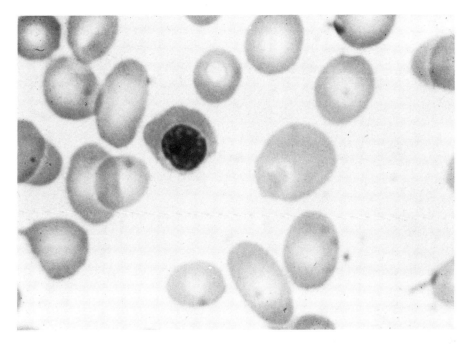

Fig. 7-3. Typical blood smear in megaloblastic anemia.

liver disease and in any patient with an increased reticulocyte count, e.g., as a result of hemolytic anemia or acute hemorrhage. Hypersegmented neutrophils are also seen in renal failure and as a familial disorder.

The blood appearance is the same in all megaloblastic anemias, whether caused by vitamin B_{12} or folate deficiencies.

Bone marrow. The bone marrow in the severely anemic patient is hypercellular, usually with a lowered or reversed myeloid:erythroid ratio. The extent of hemopoietic marrow is increased, particularly in younger subjects, and red marrow may be found in the tibias and bones of the forearm. There is an increased proportion of early cells (pronormoblasts and myeloblasts), and the erythroid cells at all stages take on a megaloblastic appearance. The cells are large, and the nucleus has an open, stippled, or lacy appearance. The cytoplasm is comparatively more mature than the nucleus, and this dissociation (nuclear-cytoplasmic dissociation) is best seen in the later cells, since fully orthochromic cells may be present with nuclei that are still not fully condensed (Fig. 7-4). Mitoses are frequent and sometimes abnormal, and nuclear remnants, Howell-Jolly bodies, binucleated and trinucleated cells, and dying cells are evidence of gross dyserythropoiesis.

There is an increased number and size of siderotic granules in the developing erythroblasts, and marrow iron stores usually appear normal or increased if associated iron deficiency is not a complicating factor. The abnormalities of granulocyte precursors are best seen in the metamyelocytes, which are abnormally large (giant) with a horseshoe-shaped nucleus. Hypersegmented polymorphs may be seen, and the megakaryocytes show an increase in nuclear lobes. Iron deficiency may partly mask the changes in the red cells but not those in the white cells.

The severity of megaloblastic change is related to the degree of anemia. In less anemic patients hypercellularity of the marrow with an increased proportion of early and erythroid cells is less marked or absent. The main features are the abnormal nuclear pattern and dissociation between nuclear and cytoplasmic development of the red cells and the giant metamyelocytes. The megaloblastic changes in less anemic patients may be described as intermediate, early, mild, or transitional.[32] The term "megaloblastoid" is best avoided altogether, as it has been used in several ways—to denote mild changes, changes not responsive to vitamin B_{12} or folate, or changes of which the observer is not sure.

Other abnormalities. Aminoimidazolecarboxamide excretion in the urine is increased in patients with vitamin B_{12} deficiency.[80] However, it is also increased in some patients with pure folate deficiency[53,54]; therefore this test is of no value in distinguishing between the two deficiency states.

Methylmalonic acid excretion in the urine is increased in vitamin B_{12} deficiency.[10,31] In pure folate deficiency the excretion of methylmalonic

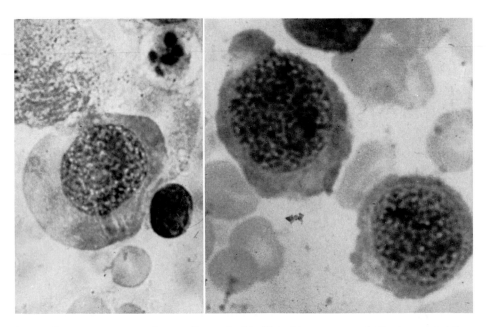

Fig. 7-4. Bone marrow smear from a 13-month-old child with severe megaloblastic anemia. Note three typical megaloblasts and in upper left a hypersegmented neutrophil.

acid has been reported as being normal.[21] Methylmalonic acid excretion measures a specific biochemical defect induced by vitamin B_{12} deficiency. The urinary excretion of methylmalonic acid returns slowly to normal after vitamin B_{12} treatment. The abnormality does not respond to folic acid in doses high enough to cause a hematologic response, and it has not been found in folate deficiency.

There is shortened red cell survival and ineffective erythropoiesis. Red cell survival is reduced by both intracorpuscular and extracorpuscular defects. The serum bilirubin level is usually in the range of 1.0 to 3.0 mg/dl with an increase mainly in the prehepatic (unconjugated) component. Stercobilinogen excretion is increased relative to the circulating hemoglobin mass. The plasma methemalbumin level is high with a positive Schumm's test in more than 50% of severe cases. Hemosiderinuria is uncommon, but absence of haptoglobin is usual. The serum lactic dehydrogenase level is raised to 1,000 to 10,000 IU[57] mainly by an increase in the first and second (heat-stable) isoenzymes. The rise has been attributed to an increase in enzyme level in individual megaloblasts as well as to increased cell destruction, but this is not established. Levels of serum γ-hydroxybutyric dehydrogenase, SGOT, phosphohexose isomerase, aldolase, isocitric dehydrogenase, and malic dehydrogenase, among other enzymes, may also be increased and there is a moderate rise in the level of serum lysozyme (muramidase).[100] The activities of many enzymes in red cells increase in megaloblastic anemia and decrease with specific therapy. There is generally a higher level of amino acids in blood and urine and increased urea excretion, although serum levels of methionine are low and of valine normal.[98] The serum cholesterol level is reduced.

C_3 hypocomplementemia has been observed in vitamin B_{12} deficiency as a consequence not of immune mechanisms but of altered synthesis of C_3.[64] C_3 levels return to normal after vitamin B_{12} treatment.

The serum iron level is increased to the range of 150 to 250 μg/dl in more anemic patients. Plasma iron clearance is rapid, iron turnover is increased, but incorporation into red cells is reduced.[36] The maturation time of red cells as studied by ^{59}Fe incorporation is prolonged.[97]

Diagnosis

The blood smear and bone marrow indicate a macrocytic megaloblastic anemia. Tests of serum vitamin levels determine whether the megaloblastic anemia is caused by folic acid or vitamin B_{12} deficiency. These tests include measurement of the serum B_{12} level by microbiologic assays with *Euglena gracilis*,[5] *Lactobacillus leishmannii*,[119] or *Ochromonas malhamensis*[38] or by isotope dilution techniques using protein-coated charcoal.[73] Although several methods are available, the most popular at present is the hemoglobin-coated charcoal radioassay of Lau et al.[73] Folic acid is measured classically by microbiologic assay[127] or by radioimmunoassay.

In vitamin B_{12} deficiency the serum vitamin B_{12} level is low (<100 pg/ml) and the serum folate level usually is normal or high. Normal values range from 200 to 800 pg/ml (10^{-12} gm/ml); overt deficiency is unlikely when levels are greater than 100 pg/ml. A deficiency of both vitamins may be seen in patients with small bowel malabsorption. One third of patients with folate deficiency may have low or borderline serum B_{12} levels that return to normal levels within 1 to 3 weeks after institution of therapy with folic acid. The reason for these low levels of B_{12} is obscure, but they probably do not reflect a depletion of tissue B_{12} stores. Therefore both serum vitamin levels should be measured, and the physician should be aware of these variations in interpreting serum vitamin levels. The presence of antibiotics in the patient's serum may affect the microbiologic assays for serum B_{12}[11,109] and folate. The isotope dilution assays are not affected by antibiotics or nonspecific growth factors in serum.

Vitamin B_{12} absorption tests are useful in establishing whether there is a defect in vitamin B_{12} absorption. After the oral administration of vitamin B_{12} labeled with radioactive cobalt, its appearance may be measured in the feces, urine, plasma, or liver, or its retention in the whole body may be ascertained. Direct measurement of body retention of the labeled vitamin by a whole body counter is undoubtedly the most sensitive method available and requires minimal patient cooperation. However, facilities for whole body counting are still available only in very specialized centers.

The urinary excretion test described by Schilling is widely used in the differential diagnosis of megaloblastic anemia.[118] The test is performed by administering 0.5 to 2.0 μg of radioactive vitamin B_{12} orally. This is followed in 2 hours by intramuscular injection of 1,000 μg of nonradioactive vitamin B_{12} to saturate the vitamin B_{12}–binding proteins and allow the subsequently absorbed oral radioactive vitamin B_{12} to be excreted in the urine. All urine is collected for 24 hours and may be collected for a second 24 hours, especially if there is renal disease. Normal subjects excrete 10% to 35% of the administered dose, and those with severe malabsorption of vitamin B_{12} because of lack of intrinsic factor or intestinal malabsorption excrete less than 3%.

The Schilling test measures both the availability of intrinsic factor and the intestinal phase of vitamin B_{12} absorption. The test results are therefore abnormal in any type of vitamin B_{12} malabsorption. The test is repeated with commerical intrinsic factor (usually hog) administered with the oral radioactive vitamin B_{12}. In pernicious anemia the defect is bypassed by the addition of intrinsic factor, and the vitamin B_{12} is absorbed. Vitamin B_{12} malabsorption will persist despite the addition of intrinsic factor if the cause is intestinal malabsorption. When bacterial competition (blind loop syndrome) is suspected, the test may be repeated after treatment with tetracycline and results often revert to normal.

The Schilling test correlates well with vitamin B_{12} malabsorption and it is a sensitive test of ileal function. The results may be abnormal when the ileum appears morphologically normal, as has been observed in cases of early tropical sprue.[26] However, the use of the Schilling test requires administration ot pharmacologic amounts of vitamin B_{12} and thus should be done only after serum is obtained for testing of vitamin B_{12} and folate levels. Abnormal Schilling test results that are not corrected by intrinsic factor must still be considered, since patients with untreated pernicious anemia have concomitant intestinal malabsorption of vitamin B_{12} that is reversed by vitamin B_{12} replacement. To establish the diagnosis in this situation, it is necessary to assess the gastric phase (i.e., gastric acidity, intrinsic factor content, and serum antibodies to intrinsic factor).

It should be emphasized that the demonstration of vitamin B_{12} malabsorption does not necessarily imply vitamin B_{12} deficiency, since the time taken to develop deficiency depends on the body stores of the vitamin and on the duration and severity of the absorptive defect.

Assays for intrinsic factor in gastric juice, antibodies to parietal cells, and antibodies to intrinsic factor provide additional diagnostic tools. Absence of acid in gastric secretions after histamine stimulation may be helpful in distinguishing between the two forms of pernicious anemia in children, and a gastric biopsy provides additional information.

The presence of ileal disease should be sought by barium studies as well as studies of gastrointestinal absorption, e.g., fat balance.

Disorders of vitamin B_{12} metabolism should be excluded by urinary examination for excessive methylmalonic acid and homocysteine as well as other sophisticated enzymatic assays.

Megaloblastic anemias produced by deficiencies of folic acid or vitamin B_{12} must be distinguished from the rare disorder of pyrimidine biosynthesis, hereditary orotic aciduria.

Approach to investigation of the patient

It is essential to establish whether the anemia is caused by vitamin B_{12} or folate deficiency and to ascertain the exact cause of the deficiency in every case. The tests needed include, first, those to establish the diagnosis of megaloblastic anemia: full blood count (including red and white cells, platelets, and reticulocytes) and examination of blood film; bone marrow aspiration and examination, including iron stain; and testing of serum iron, bilirubin, proteins, LDH, urea, and electrolytes. The second group of tests is to differentiate vitamin B_{12} and folate deficiency: tests of serum vitamin B_{12} and serum and red cell folate levels; methylmalonic acid excretion in urine; and therapeutic trial. Finally, there are tests to establish the cause of the deficiencies. In all cases there should be a barium meal and follow-through examination of the small intestine, chest x-ray examination, urinalysis, and diet and drug history. If appropriate, the following tests should also be conducted: determinations of antibodies to parietal cells, intrinsic factor, thyroid, reticulin, and immunoglobulins in serum; tests of vitamin B_{12} absorption with and without intrinsic factor; tests of gastric secretion of acid and intrinsic factor; gastric biopsy; jejunal biopsy; determinations of xylose absorption and fecal fat; as well as tests for other suspected diseases.

The tests in the first two groups should be performed before treatment is started, since rapid reversal of the blood and biochemical changes occur with therapy. Measurement of the serum vitamin B_{12} level is particularly important and should always be carried out in suspected cases of vitamin B_{12} neuropathy regardless of the hematologic findings. Tests for the cause of the deficiencies can be delayed, if necessary, until treatment has started and the patient's condition has improved.

Treatment

Prevention. In conditions in which there is a risk of developing vitamin B_{12} deficiency, e.g., total gastrectomy or ileal resection, prophylactic administration of vitamin B_{12} should be prescribed.

Active treatment. Most patients with vitamin B_{12} deficiency require treatment throughout life. Optimal doses for children are not as well defined as those for adults. When the diagnosis is firmly established, several daily doses of 25 to 100 μg may be used to initiate therapy. Alternatively, in view of the ability of the body to store vitamin B_{12} for long periods, maintenance therapy can be started with the first of a series of monthly intramuscular injections. Doses ranging between 50 and 1,000 μg have been successfully employed.

Patients with defects affecting the intestinal absorption of cobalamin, because of abnormalities either of intrinsic factor or of ileal uptake, respond to parenteral vitamin B_{12} administration. Such a therapeutic maneuver completely bypasses the defective step and is the chief means by which these patients are managed currently.

Patients with complete transcobalamin II deficiency respond only to large amounts of vitamin B_{12}. For example, one patient required 1,000 μg intramuscularly twice weekly.[48] In a second patient 1,000 μg given intramuscularly three times a week or taken each day orally appeared to maintain adequate control.[59] The exact mechanism of this response remains to be defined.

Patients with methylmalonic aciduria with defects in the synthesis of cobalamin coenzymes are likely to benefit from massive doses of vitamin B_{12}. These children may require 1 mg[113] to 2 mg[82] of vitamin B_{12} parenterally daily. However, not all patients in this group respond to vitamin B_{12}. Morrow et al. recently reported eight patients whose cultured fibroblasts were specifically unable to form adenosylcobalamin. Two of the eight were clinically unresponsive to vitamin B_{12} therapy.[70,93]

It may be possible to treat vitamin B_{12}-responsive patients antenatally. In utero diagnosis of congenital methylmalonic aciduria has been accomplished by measurements of methylmalonate in amniotic fluid or maternal urine.[4,83,94] More detailed definition of the type of mutation can be achieved by studies of cultured amniotic cells.[4,83] One vitamin B_{12}-responsive fetus has been so identified, and the increasing maternal excretion of methylmalonate responded to large doses of vitamin B_{12}.[4] Whether such treatment is beneficial will be known only when the effects of methylmalonate accumulation during prenatal life have been evaluated.[4]

In vitamin B_{12}-responsive megaloblastic anemia the numbers of reticulocytes begin to increase on the third to fourth day, rise to a maximum on the sixth to eighth day, and fall gradually to normal about the twentieth day.[159] The amount of increase in the reticulocyte count is inversely proportional to the degree of anemia. Beginning bone marrow reversal from megaloblastic to normoblastic cells is obvious within 6 hours, and cells are completely normoblastic in 72 hours.

Prompt hematologic responses are also obtained with the use of oral folic acid. Folic acid is, however, contraindicated because it has no effect on neurologic manifestations and has been known to precipitate or accelerate their development. Indeed, megaloblastic anemia should never be treated before a serum folic acid or vitamin B_{12} assay has determined the precise cause so that correct treatment can be administered. Iron administration is occasionally required for a patient with a generally inadequate diet that is deficient in iron.

FOLIC ACID
Biochemistry

In 1941 Mitchell et al.[230] isolated a substance from spinach leaves ("folic acid") that stimulated

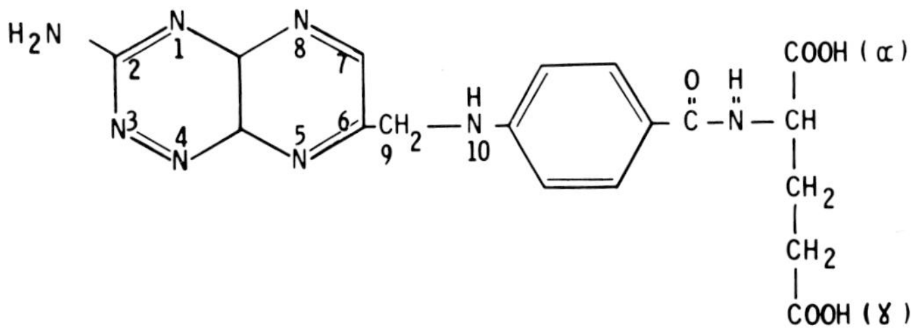

Fig. 7-5. Structural formula of folic acid (pteroylglutamic acid). Dietary folates may contain (1) additional hydrogen atoms at positions 7 and 8 of the pteridine moiety (dihydrofolate) or positions 5, 6, 7, and 8 (tetrahydrofolate), (2) a formyl group (CHO) at N^5 or N^{10} or a methyl group (CH$_3$) at N^5 or another single carbon unit, or (3) additional glutamate moieties attached to the γ-carboxyl group of the glutamate moiety. (From Hardisty, R. M., and Weatherall, D. J.: Blood and its disorders, Oxford, 1974, Blackwell Scientific Publications, Ltd.)

the growth of mutant strains of *Streptococcus faecalis* and *Lactobacillus casei*.

Folic acid (pteroylglutamic acid) is the parent compound of a large group of naturally occurring structurally related compounds collectively called folates. Folic acid itself has a molecular weight of 441.4; forms yellow, spear-shaped crystals; and is sparingly soluble in water but dissolves readily in dilute alkali. The molecule consists of three portions: pteridine, para-aminobenzoic acid, and *l*-glutamic acid (Fig. 7-5). The natural folate compounds differ from folic acid in three respects: (1) three states of reduction of the pteridine ring can occur, (2) six different one-carbon units may be present at position N^5 or N^{10} or both, and (3) a chain of variable length consisting of additional *l*-glutamic acid residues may be linked in series by γ-peptide bonds to the glutamic acid. The polyglutamyl side chain is usually three, five, or seven residues in length, but the exact number varies from one tissue to the next and within a given tissue many different chain lengths may be present. The form in human plasma and cerebrospinal fluid is 5-methyltetrahydrofolate (5-methyl THF),[187] but in liver 75% to 80% of the folates are pteroylpolyglutamates. Mature leukocytes contain from 40 to 120 ng/ml packed cells,[196] of which about 85% is pteroylpolyglutamates,[271] and red cells contain at least 90% pteroylpolyglutamates.[235]

Action. Folates in the tetrahydro form act as coenzymes in all mammalian metabolic systems in which there is a transfer of a one-carbon unit. These are (1) the formylation of glycinamide ribonucleotide and 5-amino-4-imidazole carboxamide ribonucleotide in early purine synthesis, (2) the methylation of deoxymandylic acid to thymidylic acid in pyrimidine nucleotide biosynthesis, (3) amino acid conversions, and (4) the generation and utilization of formate.

The amino acid conversions are (1) serine to glycine (this also requires pyridoxine), (2) histi-

dine to glutamic acid through formiminoglutamic acid (FIGLU), and (3) homocysteine to methionine, which also requires cobalamin as a coenzyme. Here there is a transfer of methyl group from N^5-methyltetrahydrofolic acid to cobalamin to form methylcobalamin and a subsequent transfer of the methyl group to homocysteine to form methionine.

Metabolism

Dietary sources. Folates are widely distributed in nature. The total folate in a "normal" diet, as determined by *L. casei* assay, is in the range of 1.0 to 1.2 mg. *L. casei* in the presence of ascorbate and other reducing substances can utilize a broad spectrum of folate derivatives[182] and is therefore more reliable as a test organism than *S. faecalis,* which does not grow on all folate forms. Foods having the highest concentrations of folate include liver, kidney, nuts, fresh green and yellow leafy vegetables, legumes, citrus fruits, and berries. Liver is a particularly rich source and contains about 300 μg/100 gm; other meat products, fresh vegetables, whole grain cereals, and dried beans are also adequate sources, with 10 to 100 μg/100 gm.

Milk is a poor source of folate. Breast milk or pasteurized cow's milk contains approximately 35 μg/liter (3.5 μg/100 gm), below the amount present in most foods and near the minimum required to sustain rapid growth in infancy. Heat treatment lowers the folate content of milk further. Thus sterilization of formula by boiling halves the folate content, and reconstituted evaporated milk has less than 20 μg/liter. Cooking, canning, or other processing may destroy 50% to 95% of food folates. Folates may be easily destroyed, in large volumes of water and, if food is reheated (when the protective effect of food ascorbate is lost), 90% to 100% of the folate may be lost.

Folic acid is readily absorbed from the gastrointestinal tract. In its synthesized form it is known as pteroylglutamic acid. For its metabolically active form it must be converted from its conjugated state to folinic acid (citrovorum factor) or to tetrahydrofolic acid.

Requirements and stores. The minimal daily requirement for folate has not been clearly established. Recent studies using hematologic criteria suggest that the daily requirement for folic acid (pteroylmonoglutamic acid) is in the range of 50 to 75 μg in adults[185,269] and 25 to 50 μg in infants.[270] In pregnant women and patients with hemolytic anemias the folate requirement may be increased three to six times.[137,283]

The folate requirement also increases in patients with malignant disease,[200] hyperthyroidism,[214] acute intermittent porphyria,[175] paroxysmal nocturnal hemoglobinuria,[237] myelofibrosis with myeloid metaplasia,[201] and leukemia.[252]

Total body stores are from 6 to 20 mg, situated mainly in the liver, which contains an average of approximately 10 μg/gm.[153] Thus stores are sufficient for only a few months and, indeed, a person can develop early megaloblastic anemia in 4 months on an experimental diet lacking folate.[183]

Absorption. Folate absorption occurs mainly through the duodenum and jejunum. Ingested folates probably enter the portal blood as a single compound, 5-methyltetrahydrofolate.[241] At least three biochemical reactions are needed to convert the natural forms to this compound: (1) deconjugation, (2) reduction, and (3) methylation (Fig. 7-6).

Deconjugation is brought about by "folate conjugase," which is present in the small intestinal mucosa. The amounts in the lumen of the small intestine are low, and it seems possible that deconjugation of dietary folate occurs partly in the lysosomes of the mucosal cells.[198]

The greater the number of glutamate residues in the chain, the less well the compound is absorbed.[146,150] Dietary folates are well absorbed (>50%) at low doses (e.g., 200 μg), but at higher doses the proportion absorbed falls to less than 50%.[191] The rate-limiting step is probably transfer of the compounds across the luminal surface membrane of the cell, rather than deconjugation.

Dietary dihydrofolate or nonreduced compounds are converted to the tetrahydrofolate derivative by the enzyme dihydrofolate reductase. Formylated and other nonmethylated compounds are all converted to the 5-methyl derivative.[241] Folic acid itself is a poor substrate for dihydrofolate reductase and, except in small physiologic doses, is largely transferred across the intestinal mucosa unchanged.[280]

Plasma transport. Specific physiologic plasma binders of folate have not been identified. When large amounts of folate are added to plasma, up to two thirds is bound loosely to albumin.[204] Serum folates in normal individuals tend to remain relatively constant over a period of weeks to months, suggesting that some endogenous mechanisms regulate plasma folate levels. Measurements of normal plasma levels of folate by *L. casei* assay vary among laboratories but generally range from 3 to 20 ng/ml. When folic acid in a dose of 15 μg/kg is injected intravenously into a normal subject, it is cleared from the plasma rapidly; by the end of 4 to 6 hours serum folate returns to preinjection levels.[154]

Storage. Mild folate deficiency is common in pregnant women. As in the case of iron, there is a placental gradient favorable to the fetus. The folate level in the cord blood is normally more than twice as high as that in the mother. After birth there is an exponential drop in both blood and serum folate content, and a period of marginal folate nutrition follows.* By the age of 2 weeks the stores established during fetal life become depleted, as reflected by mean values for blood and serum folate, which are slightly below those of the normal adult.

---

*References 149, 224-226, 247, 257.

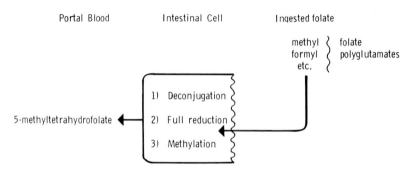

Fig. 7-6. Steps involved in absorption of dietary folates. (From Hardisty, R. M., and Weatherall, D. J.: Blood and its disorders, Oxford, 1974, Blackwell Scientific Publications, Ltd.)

These remain somewhat depressed throughout the first year of life and then return toward adult values. In premature infants the depression of blood and serum folate below adult values is even more marked, especially between 1 and 3 months of age, when 68% of infants who weighed less than 1,700 gm at birth are reported to have low serum folate levels. These values suggest that the folate intake of the infant is marginal and is likely to be deficient if heat-treated or evaporated milk forms the bulk of the diet.

The total content of folate in the body is about 70 mg, of which about a third is in the liver (5 to 15 μg/gm).

Folate is incorporated in red cells during erythropoiesis, and the folate content decreases only slightly during their life span. The folate is largely in polyglutamate form but is rapidly broken down in hemolysates at acid pH by plasma conjugases. Red cell folate is a useful indicator of body folate status. The average level is 300 ng/ml whole blood, corrected to a hematocrit of 45% with a range of 160 to 640 ng/ml. The levels are higher in neonates and they fall during the first year of life. Premature infants have still higher levels, but the rate of fall is more rapid, particularly at 4 to 8 weeks.

Liver folate levels fall to approximately 1.5 μg/gm in 130 days on a folate-deficient diet; megaloblastic changes also occur. A diet containing as much as 200 μg daily is necessary to prevent such changes. During pregnancy an additional 100 μg daily is required.

The sequential pattern of developing folic acid deficiency was demonstrated in a hematologist kept on a very low folic acid intake (5 μg daily).[184] A low serum folic acid level, the first evidence of the deficiency, appeared at 3 weeks and was followed by the presence of hypersegmented neutrophils at 7 weeks, high urinary FIGLU excretion after histidine loading at 13 weeks, megaloblastic bone marrow changes at 19 weeks, and anemia at 19½ weeks.

Fig. 7-7 shows the sequence of biochemical and hematologic events during the development of folate deficiency.[184]

Excretion. Approximately 5 μg of folate is excreted daily in the urine of normal persons and an unknown quantity appears in the bile. Evidence exists for an enterohepatic circulation of folate in humans.[145] The small daily urinary excretion is much increased after an oral dose when the tissues are saturated. Some folate is lost in sweat and saliva. In the newborn infant the average daily loss of folate per unit surface area was nearly eight times greater in the first few days of life than in the adult.[215]

When 5 mg of folic acid is injected or ingested by normal subjects, 2 to 3 mg appears in the urine in 24 hours, whereas in folate-deficient subjects less than 1.5 mg is excreted.

Interrelationships of folic acid and vitamin B$_{12}$. Folic acid is closely associated with vitamin B$_{12}$ in the synthesis of nucleic acids, acting as catalysts at different stages of this process.[233] There is evidence also that a balance exists between folic acid and vitamin B$_{12}$ and that a deficiency of one increases the requirement for the other.[244,279] There is a close relationship between vitamin B$_{12}$ and folate metabolism, and it is possible that vitamin B$_{12}$ deficiency produces megaloblastic anemia by a secondary effect on folate metabolism. The most

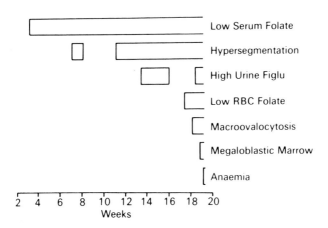

Fig. 7-7. Sequence of biochemical and hematologic events in development of folate deficiency. At first only a low serum folate level indicates a negative folate balance, and the red blood cell folate content starts to fall. Only after the latter becomes subnormal do megaloblastic changes and anemia develop. (From Herbert, V.: Trans. Assoc. Am. Phys. **745**:307, 1962.)

attractive hypothesis is the methyltetrahydrofolate trap.[188,236] In *E. coli* the following reaction requires a vitamin B_{12} coenzyme[181]:

$$\text{homocysteine} + N^5\text{-methyltetrahydrofolate} \rightarrow$$
$$\text{methionine} + \text{tetrahydrofolate}$$

A similar system has been demonstrated in mammalian liver[216] but not so far in humans. In vitamin B_{12} deficiency it is postulated that there is a block in the folate cycle, an accumulation of N^5-methyltetrahydrofolate, and therefore a deficiency of other forms of folate such as those necessary for nucleotide synthesis. This hypothesis, however, makes several assumptions and cannot explain all the accumulated experimental data.[234] It is clear that further studies are needed in this complex field.

Causes of folic acid deficiency

Folic acid deficiency is caused by inadequate intake, defective absorption (congenital and acquired), increased requirements, disorders of folic acid metabolism (congenital and acquired), and increased excretion.

The following outline lists the causes of folic acid deficiency.

A. Inadequate intake
   1. Poverty, ignorance, fadism
   2. Method of cooking (sustained boiling)
   3. Goat's milk feeding
   4. Malnutrition (marasmus, kwashiorkor)
   5. Special diets for phenylketonuria or maple syrup urine disease
B. Defective absorption
   1. Congenital: congenital malabsorption of folate
   2. Acquired
      a. Idiopathic steatorrhea
      b. Tropical sprue
      c. Partial or total gastrectomy
      d. Multiple diverticula of small intestine
      e. Jejunal resection
      f. Regional ileitis
      g. Whipple's disease
      h. Intestinal lymphoma
   3. Drugs (and usages) associated with impaired absorption and/or utilization[266]
      a. Phenytoin (Dilantin): anticonvulsant
      b. Primidone: anticonvulsant
      c. Barbiturates: sedative
      d. Oral contraceptive agents: contraception
      e. Cycloserine: tuberculosis
      f. Metformin: diabetes
      g. Ethanol: societal
      h. Dietary amino acids (glycine, methionine): societal
      i. Nitrofurantoin (?): antibiotic
      j. Glutethimide (?): sedative
C. Increased requirements
   1. Rapid growth, e.g., prematurity, pregnancy
   2. Chronic hemolytic anemia

   3. Malignancy
   4. Hypermetabolic states, e.g., infection, hyperthyroidism
   5. Extensive skin disease
   6. Cirrhosis
D. Disorders of metabolism
   1. Congenital
      a. Dihydrofolate reductase deficiency
      b. Glutamate formiminotransferase deficiency
      c. Pyridoxine–folic acid–responsive formiminotransferase deficiency
      d. N^5-Methyltetrahydrofolate homocysteine methyltransferase deficiency
      e. Pyridoxine treatment of homocystinuria
   2. Acquired: impaired utilization of folate
      a. Folate antagonists
      b. Vitamin B_{12} deficiency
      c. Alcoholism
      d. Liver disease (acute and chronic)
      e. Drugs (and usages) that are dihydrofolate reductase inhibitors[266]
         (1) 4-Amino-4-deoxyfolates, i.e., methotrexate: chemotherapy, immunosuppression, psoriasis
         (2) 2,4-Diaminopyrimidine, i.e., pyrimethamine: malaria, toxoplasmosis
         (3) Triamterene: diuretic
         (4) Diamidine compounds, i.e., pentamidine isethionate: *Pneumocystis carinii*, protozoacidal
         (5) Trimethoprim: antibacterial
E. Increased excretion
   1. Chronic dialysis
   2. Vitamin B_{12} deficiency
   3. Liver disease
   4. Heart disease

Inadequate intake. Breast milk from a folate-replete mother contains about 25 μg of folate/liter[226] and presumably provides enough folate for the normally developing child. However, many processed milks and any milk subjected to boiling may have less folate, and the continued use of such milks may result in folate-deficiency anemia.[170] Heating of milk results in a 40% loss of folate, and reheating of pasteurized milk destroys 80% of the folate content.

Even though the red cell folate levels in premature infants are higher than those in full-term infants,[277] premature infants seem more prone to develop megaloblastic anemia.[268] Birth removes the maternal source of folate and, since it is usually the custom to give premature infants sterilized milk, the dietary folate intake may be inadequate to provide for the needs of the rapidly growing child. It appears that all premature children fed heat-sterilized or artificial diets should be given folate supplements.

Goat's milk anemia is a type of nutritional folate deficiency that has been described in Germany, Italy, New Zealand, the United States, and other countries. It occurs in infants fed goat's milk, which has only one-sixth the folate content of cow's milk (6 μg folate/liter versus 35 μg/liter). As in other megaloblastic anemias of infancy, an infection often precipitates the onset of clinical symptoms.

Since folates are widely distributed in many foodstuffs, after the age of weaning pure dietary folate deficiency—in the absence of other complicating factors—occurs only in those living on very restricted diets, whether for preference, as prescribed by physicians, or for reasons of poverty or ignorance. The diagnosis of dietary folate deficiency is often one of exclusion, eliminating other known possible causes.

A dietary lack of folate generally results from a loss of the vitamin during cooking rather than from its deficiency in food. Folate deficiency is most common in circumstances in which the requirement for folate is increased, e.g., rapid body or cell growth. This is most dramatic in premature infants, during pregnancy, and in severe chronic hemolytic states.[152,213]

Kwashiorkor, or protein-calorie malnutrition, is usually accompanied by multiple deficiency states. Since the basic diet differs in different parts of the world, it is not surprising that the reported prevalence of various deficiencies in patients with kwashiorkor should also differ. Thus megaloblastosis in kwashiorkor has been found in from 10% to 14%[262] to 60% to 70%[177,239] of affected children. This megaloblastosis is nearly always associated with folate deficiency and/or responds to treatment with folate.* The factors involved in the pathogenesis of the folate deficiency may be multiple. Undoubtedly decreased dietary intake plays a major role, but frequently these children also have an infection that may increase folate requirements.[262] Furthermore, in kwashiorkor intestinal epithelial changes may occur,[148] and it is possible that there may be some interference with the absorption of food folate.

Megaloblastic anemia caused by failure to provide folate supplementation in the dietary treatment of phenylketonuria has been described.[253] Similarly infants on diets for maple syrup urine disease have also developed megaloblastic anemia.[212]

Defective absorption
Congenital disorders
CONGENITAL MALABSORPTION OF FOLATE. Folic acid deficiency arising as a result of a congenital isolated defect in folic acid absorption has only rarely been recorded.

In 1961 Luhby et al.[220] described a child who had relapsing megaloblastic anemia starting at 3

months of age as a result of a specific defect in the gastrointestinal absorption of folic acid. There was no defect in the gastrointestinal absorption of fat, glucose, or vitamin A, and roentgenographic examination of the gastrointestinal tract did not reveal any abnormalities. Folic acid absorption studies showed a peak folate level of 5.2 ng/ml after the oral administration of 10 mg of folic acid for 10 days. In a follow-up of this case in 1965 and 1967 Luhby et al.[218,219] described a sister of this patient who had the same disorder and stated that both children had megaloblastic anemia, ataxia, mental retardation, and convulsions. They demonstrated a severe isolated defect in the transport of folic acid across the intestinal and spinal cord membranes in both children. Hematologic normalcy could be maintained by 15 mg folic acid given orally or 100 μg folic acid given intramuscularly.

In 1969 Lanzkowsky et al.[211] described a unique girl who had folic acid deficiency and megaloblastic anemia as a result of an isolated defect in the gastrointestinal absorption of physiologic amounts of folic acid associated with a defect in the transport of folic acid from the plasma into the cerebrospinal fluid. She had mental retardation, seizures, and punctate calcification of the basal ganglia, particularly of the caudate nucleus.

Fig. 7-8 shows plasma, red cells, and cerebrospinal fluid folate levels; white cell count; Arneth count; hemoglobin level; platelet count; and reticulocyte count of this patient on the following diet: folic acid 40 mg daily orally, ordinary ward diet for 17 weeks, folic acid 250 μg orally daily for 12 days, and folic acid 250 μg intramuscularly daily for 48 days. It is seen that the folate levels and hematologic values in this patient were maintained only on folic acid 40 mg daily orally and on 250 μg daily intramuscularly.

A specific defect in absorption of folic acid in its naturally occurring form as pteroylpolyglutamic acid as well as pteroylmonoglutamic, pteroyldiglutamic, and pteroyltriglutamic acid and N^5-formyl- and N^5-methyltetrahydrofolic acid and an inability normally to transfer folic acid from the blood into the cerebrospinal fluid were demonstrated. Absorption was not enhanced in the presence of normal human duodenal juice, lyophilized calf jejunum, or lyophilized calf pancreas (Table 7-3).

In addition, impaired renal tubular reabsorption of folate was demonstrated by increased 24-hour urinary folate excretion while the patient was receiving folate intramuscularly.[210]

In 1973 Santiago-Borrero et al.[254] described an 11-year-old girl who had had severe megaloblastic anemia since the age of 3 months; the anemia was a result of impaired intestinal absorption of both

---

*References 135, 177, 208, 239, 263.

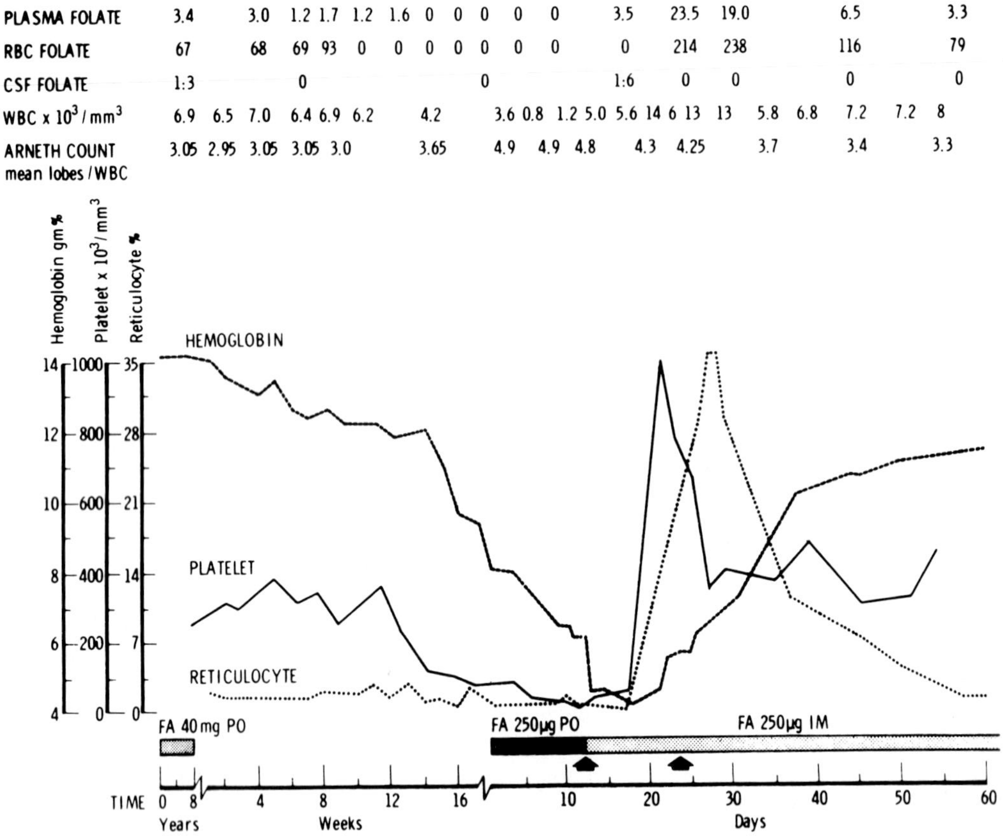
PLASMA FOLATE 3.4 3.0 1.2 1.7 1.2 1.6 0 0 0 0 0 3.5 23.5 19.0 6.5 3.3
RBC FOLATE 67 68 69 93 0 0 0 0 0 0 0 0 214 238 116 79
CSF FOLATE 1:3 0 0 1:6 0 0 0 0
WBC x 10³/mm³ 6.9 6.5 7.0 6.4 6.9 6.2 4.2 3.6 0.8 1.2 5.0 5.6 14 6 13 13 5.8 6.8 7.2 7.2 8
ARNETH COUNT mean lobes/WBC 3.05 2.95 3.05 3.05 3.0 3.65 4.9 4.9 4.8 4.3 4.25 3.7 3.4 3.3
Hemoglobin gm%
Platelet x 10³/mm³
Reticulocyte %
HEMOGLOBIN
PLATELET
RETICULOCYTE
FA 40 mg PO
FA 250µg PO
FA 250µg IM
TIME
Years
Weeks
Days

Fig. 7-8. Folate levels and hematologic data in patient on an ordinary ward diet for 17 weeks and receiving folic acid, 250 µg/day orally for 12 days and 250 µg/day intramuscularly. (From Lanzkowsky, P.: Am. J. Med. **48:**580, 1970.)

Table 7-3. Peak plasma folate levels in absorption tests in patient and controls following ingestion of various folic acid compounds*

Folic acid compounds administered orally	Peak plasma folate level (ng/ml)†	
	Patient	Controls
Pteroylmonoglutamic acid (PGA) 3.0 mg	6.8	42-175
PGA 3.0 mg + 3 ml normal duodenal juice	7.3	—
PGA 3.0 mg + lyophilized calf jejunum	2.5	—
PGA 3.0 mg + lyophilized calf pancreas	6.5	—
Pteroyldiglutamic acid 4.2 mg	6.5	29.5-59.5
Pteroyltriglutamic acid 5.4 mg	4.6	55-600
N^5-Formyl tetrahydrofolic acid (folinic acid) 5.0 mg	7.1	
N^5-Methyltetrahydrofolic acid 5.0 mg	2.9	—

*From Lanzkowsky, P.: Am. J. Med. **48:**580, 1970.
†*L. casei* microbiologic assay.

physiologic and pharmacologic doses of pteroylglutamic acid. A prompt hematologic response to intramuscular folic acid occurred.

The precise defect in folate transport has not been elucidated in these cases. Despite the phenotypic similarities of these patients with defects in folate transport, there are sufficient differences clinically to suggest that these various entities might represent different defects of folic acid transport at the molecular level; for this reason they should not presently be considered as the same disorder at the biochemical level.

Acquired disorders. Folate deficiency caused by malabsorption is common in such chronic diarrheal states as tropical sprue, gluten intolerance, and idiopathic steatorrhea, particularly in infancy. A combination of factors is likely to be responsible. First, there is apparently a loss of intestinal conjugase activity in these conditions, since a small dose of monoglutamic folate produces a prompt therapeutic response, whereas large doses of the polyglutamic folates that are present in food are poorly absorbed. Second, loss of intestinal flora through use of broad-spectrum antibiotics or through diarrhea may reduce the contribution of bacteria as a supplementary source of folate. Finally, diarrhea may interfere with the absorption and normal enterohepatic circulation of folate through an excessively rapid intestinal passage. Folate deficiency has been reported to develop in some patients with multiple diverticula of the small intestine. The deficiency appears to be caused by utilization of folate by the large numbers of intestinal bacteria in competition with the host. This disorder responds to therapy with broad-spectrum antibiotics or folic acid.[206]

After extensive resection of the jejunum, folate absorption may be impaired and folate deficiency may develop because of an inadequate absorptive area of the small intestine. Folate deficiency occurs in most patients with active Crohn's disease on the basis of poor diet and increased requirements for folate as well as possible mild malabsorption. Salicylazosulfapyridine (sulfasalazine) therapy may also cause malabsorption of folate.[165] The deficiency is unusual when the disease is quiescent.[200] In extreme cases megaloblastic anemia may occur but, in these cases the anemia, which is partly caused by the inflammatory disease itself and sometimes by iron deficiency, is not completely corrected by folic acid therapy alone.[199]

Mild folate deficiency is common following partial gastrectomy, but severe folate deficiency is unusual and mainly of dietary origin.[160]

Folate deficiency and megaloblastic anemia in patients on long-term therapy with phenytoin (Dilantin) for seizure disorders have been shown to be the result of inhibition of folate conjugase activity in the intestine.[195] Food polyglutamyl folates are not deconjugated to the absorbable monoglutamyl forms in the presence of this drug. In addition, when careful dietary histories have been taken from patients who developed megaloblastic anemia while taking phenytoin, they were found to have small or marginal amounts of folate in their diets.[163] The estrogen-progestin oral contraceptive agents are associated with an increased frequency of folate deficiency, and megaloblastic anemia has resulted from inhibition of folate conjugase activity in the intestine.[267] Withdrawal of the phenytoin or the oral contraceptive has been followed by hematologic recovery (reticulocytosis, rise in hemoglobin level, etc.) with or without folate supplementation.

Increased requirements

Infancy. Folate deficiency in infancy is a result of dietary intake being insufficient to meet demands, particularly if intake is reduced or demands are increased for any reason. Newborn infants show serum and red cell folate levels two to three times those of adults.[176] These fall exponentially to normal levels over the first few weeks of life.[276]

The folate content of breast milk is approximately 50 μg/liter, but powdered milk, particularly if it is boiled, may contain much less than this[164] and provide insufficient folate for newborn infants, whose demands have been estimated to be ten times those of adults on a body-weight basis.

Premature infants show marked diminution of folate levels during the first few weeks of life, probably as a result of consumption of folate during growth, poor folate stores as compared to full-term infants, and also perhaps excess urinary folate excretion.[257,277] The average daily loss of folate per unit of surface area is greatest in the first few days of life.[215] This could account for the fall in plasma folate activity that occurs at this time. Shojania and Hornady,[258] on the other hand, have shown rapid clearance of folic acid from plasma and diminished urinary excretion of folic acid in newborns and have suggested that this demonstrates an increased demand for folic acid in the neonatal period and early infancy, a demand not met by dietary folate. Boiling milk to ensure sterility destroys its folate content. A proportion of premature infants, particularly those of lowest birth weight, actually develop megaloblastic anemia at about 6 to 10 weeks of age.[268] Infants who have infections, feeding difficulties, or exchange transfusions are particularly prone to this complication, and prophylactic folic acid administration is worthwhile for all such infants.[173]

Nutritional megaloblastic anemia in full-term infants usually occurs later (6 months to 3 years), typically in generally malnourished children who develop infections of the respiratory or urinary tract and childhood viral infections.[225,286] In some cases this anemia may be associated with scurvy or kwashiorkor.

Pregnancy. Folate deficiency during pregnancy has been the subject of several major studies.[155,284] The incidence of megaloblastic anemia in pregnancy varies from about 0.5% in Western countries to 50% in Southern India. Requirements for folate are thought to increase by about 100 to 300 μg daily, owing to folate transfer to the fetus, which causes a fall in serum and red cell folate. This decrease is most marked in the last trimester, when low serum folate levels may occur in 50% of patients and low red cell folate levels in about 30%.

Severe folate deficiency in pregnancy is more common in patients who are also iron deficient, in those with twin pregnancies, in those with low serum and red cell folate levels in early pregnancy, and in multiparas as compared to primiparas. Megaloblastic anemia may also be precipitated by infection, usually of the urinary tract, in which case megaloblastic "arrest" of hematopoiesis has been described. Folate is lost during lactation, and this may be an additional drain on already depleted stores.[254]

Hemolytic anemia. Folate deficiency is likely to occur in most types of hemolytic anemia, but particularly in those with ineffective erythropoiesis, since primitive cells contain and utilize more folate than mature cells. The deficiency may produce an aplastic crisis that can be diagnosed by bone marrow examination.[203] In a few cases of megaloblastic anemia daily doses of folic acid larger than the usual adult requirements have been required to produce a response.[213]

Very low serum folate levels have been found in a quarter and positive FIGLU tests were present in sixteen of twenty-two patients with sickle cell anemia[238]; the deficiency is common in other major hemoglobinopathies such as Hb H disease, Hb SC disease, and thalassemia major.[192] The deficiency is also frequent in warm-type autoimmune hemolytic anemia,[152] in which 40% of patients recently studied had serum folate levels below 3.0 ng/ml,[192] and also in mechanical, drug-induced, and microangiopathic hemolytic anemia.[192] Megaloblastic anemia caused by folate deficiency has been recorded in hereditary spherocytosis on a number of occasions but is probably less common in this disease. The deficiency is even less common in patients with pyruvate kinase deficiency and in paroxysmal nocturnal hemoglobinuria, in which, indeed, folate clearance is usually slower than normal.

Infections. Various infective states may be associated with folate-deficiency megaloblastic anemia. Since normal persons have adequate stores of folate for several months, this most often occurs in patients with chronic infections such as pulmonary tuberculosis. However, the relative roles of the infection per se and the effects of any treatment need to be distinguished.

In children with gastrointestinal, pulmonary, and other infections, folate-deficiency megaloblastic anemia is not uncommon, and this is particularly so in children from poorer socioeconomic groups.[205,217,222] However, without a prospective study it is impossible to determine whether the infection has precipitated the folate deficiency or whether folate deficiency has predisposed to or aggravated the infection.

Malignancy. The demand for folic acid in proliferating tissue of white cell origin may also account for megaloblastic anemia in patients with lymphoma and leukemia. The increased demands of rapidly growing neoplastic tissue for folic acid may be associated with a deficiency of this vitamin caused by malabsorption.[242] Megaloblastic changes in myeloid leukemia and erythroleukemia that are refractory to folic acid and vitamin B_{12} therapy may also occur. Vitamin therapy for megaloblastic anemia associated with leukemia is contraindicated.

Skin diseases. Patients with extensive skin disease may develop megaloblastic changes in the bone marrow caused by folate deficiency. Thus Shuster et al.[259] found megaloblastic bone marrow in five of nine patients, and Fry et al.[166] found mild megaloblastic changes in five of thirteen patients with dermatitis herpetiformis.

The pathogenesis of the folate deficiency in these patients may be related to the increased cell turnover in the skin (as in some cases of hemolytic anemia), but it should be noted that patients with skin disease may also have intestinal changes[166,223] that may produce folate malabsorption.

Disorders of metabolism
Congenital disorders
DIHYDROFOLATE REDUCTASE DEFICIENCY. Dihydrofolate reductase is the enzyme responsible for the conversion of folic acid to tetrahydrofolic acid. In 1967 a boy with evidence of a partial deficiency of dihydrofolate reductase was described.[278] Anemia was discovered at the age of 6 weeks and subsequently became megaloblastic. He did not respond to small doses of oral or parenteral pterolymonoglutamic acid (100 μg) but did respond to a similar dose of folinic acid (N^5-formyltetrahydrofolic acid).

A Schilling test gave normal results and produced a transient improvement in the hematologic findings. An abnormal histidine loading test with urinary excretion of excessive amounts of formiminoglutamate was interpreted as suggesting an abnormality of folic acid metabolism. Dihydrofolate reductase activity in a single biopsy sample of the patient's liver was more than two standard deviations lower than samples obtained at autopsy in seven subjects with no known liver disease. This finding, along with the therapeutic response to physiologic doses of the reduced folate, 5-formyltetrahydrofolate, but not to unreduced folic acid, suggested a deficiency of dihydrofolate reductase.[278] Oral administration of 5 mg of folic acid daily produced a complete hematologic remission, which was sustained for 3 years; a relapse occurred when the folic acid was discontinued. Subsequently this patient manifested sociopathic behavior resulting in repeated incarcerations and is considered to have mild mental retardation.

Recent studies of extracts of his cultured skin fibroblasts show dihydrofolate reductase activity that is normal in amount, kinetic values, and heat stability. Similarly the cells in culture require normal levels of folic acid for growth. Thus it seems possible either that this patient's abnormalities are not the result of dihydrofolate reductase deficiency or that dihydrofolate reductase deficiency is indeed present but is not expressed in the skin.[161] The failure to respond to parenteral folic acid makes congenital malabsorption of folate unlikely. The reported absence of homocystinuria and the normal serum folate level at a time when megaloblastosis and pancytopenia were present are evidence against a functional deficiency of reduced folates. Yet the hematologic and biochemical remissions in response to physiologic doses of reduced but not unreduced folate are difficult to explain by any single defect other than dihydrofolate reductase deficiency.

Tauro et al.[272] reported two unrelated neonates with severe megaloblastic anemia caused by an abnormality of the enzyme dihydrofolate reductase. An older sibling of each patient had died, apparently from a similar disease. Autosomal recessive inheritance is probably the mode of transmission. Both patients had abnormal deoxyuridine suppression tests, corrected to normal by 5-formyltetrahydrofolic acid, and satisfactory clinical response occurred in both patients following parenteral therapy with 5-formyltetrahydrofolic acid.

GLUTAMATE FORMIMINOTRANSFERASE DEFICIENCY. The first inborn error to be attributed to deficiency of a specific folate enzyme was described in 1963 by Arakawa,[138] who subsequently identified five affected Japanese patients, two of whom were siblings.[141,144] Although the findings in the original group of patients included severe mental retardation, subsequent reports have suggested that this may well be a benign biochemical abnormality. All the patients have had markedly elevated urinary levels of formiminoglutamate, the natural substrate of the enzyme glutamate formiminotransferase, usually while on a normal diet but consistently after the oral dose of *l*-histidine, a metabolic precursor of formiminoglutamate. Serum vitamin B_{12} levels have consistently been normal. Of the five patients originally described by Arakawa, mental and physical retardation were prominent features in all except possibly one. Four patients showed marked cortical atrophy on pneumoencephalography, with dilatation of the cerebral ventricles noted in three. All had abnormal electroencephalograms, and several had frank seizure disorders. All patients except one[144] showed a striking elevation of serum folate levels, the average from repeated determinations being five to twelve times greater than the normal upper limit; this suggests its possible usefulness for screening. In addition to high urinary formiminoglutamate levels, the metabolic block in histidine degradation was confirmed by the decreased appearance of $^{14}CO_2$ in exhaled air after intravenous injection of *l*-^{14}C-histidine in the two patients tested.

Glutamate formiminotransferase activity of crude liver extracts ranged from 14% to 54% of controls, whereas the formiminotransferase ac-

tivity of red cell lysates was 35% to 37% of normal in the three patients tested. In contrast, the activities of seven other folate enzymes variously tested in liver or erythrocytes from one or more patients were reportedly normal.

Five additional persons, including two pairs of siblings, have been reported to have some of the features of formiminotransferase deficiency as described by Arakawa but differing in important ways.* One of these had subtle megaloblastic bone marrow changes with mild anemia, normal intelligence, and no malabsorption; this patient's condition improved with combined folate therapy and a reduction in dietary carbohydrate.[190]

PYRIDOXINE–FOLIC ACID–RESPONSIVE FORMIMINO-TRANSFERASE DEFICIENCY. Arakawa et al.[143] described an infant with formiminotransferase deficiency syndrome associated with megaloblastic anemia, probably of congenital origin, responsive to pyridoxine and folic acid. The anemia was found soon after birth, and both ringed sideroblasts and megaloblastoid cells were found in bone marrow smears. In this case the megaloblastic pyridoxine–folic acid–responsive anemia appeared as one of the prominent clinical manifestations, and mental retardation, although present, was much less severe even though dilatation of cerebral ventricles and cortical atrophy were demonstrated on pneumoencephalograms. The occurrence of megaloblastic pyridoxine–folic acid–responsive anemia was not observed in two cases of formiminotransferase deficiency syndrome previously reported by Arakawa et al.[141,142]

N^5-METHYLTETRAHYDROFOLATE HOMOCYSTEINE METHYLTRANSFERASE DEFICIENCY. One case of mental retardation and megaloblastic anemia associated with hyperfolicacidemia and low levels of N^5-methyltetrahydrofolate homocysteine methyltransferase activity in the liver has been described.[140] Deficiency of this enzyme would interfere with folate metabolism and cause a relative deficiency of folate similar to that seen in some cases of severe vitamin B_{12} deficiency. However, although the administration of pteroylmonoglutamic acid in large doses produced a reticulocyte response, the marrow apparently remained megaloblastic, suggesting that there was some other factor influencing DNA synthesis apart from a relative folate deficiency.

PYRIDOXINE TREATMENT OF HOMOCYSTINURIA. Patients with homocystinuria show a lowering of folate levels while they are receiving pyridoxine, and administration of folic acid caused further biochemical improvement in pyridoxine-responsive patients and subjective clinical improvement in all. In no case was the hypofolatemia associated with

---

*References 139, 190, 232, 240.

hematologic changes. The mechanism for lowering of folate levels during pyridoxine administration may depend on removal of substrate inhibition of the enzyme N^5-methyltetrahydrofolate homocysteine methyltransferase by pyridoxine-induced lowering of the substrate homocysteine. It is suggested that patients with homocystinuria should be given a long trial with pyridoxine and that folic acid should be given in all cases in which pyridoxine in used.[282]

Acquired. Folate analogs, such as methotrexate, pyrimethamine, pentamidine isethionate, and trimethoprim, react with dihydrofolate reductase and interfere with the conversion of dihydrofolate substrates to the active tetrahydro forms. Consequently hypersegmentation of neutrophils and megaloblastic changes in the bone marrow and peripheral blood are common concomitants of this form of antimetabolite therapy. The hematopoietic effect of these drugs is dose related and presumably is also influenced by initial body folate stores and dietary folate intake.

Alcohol in amounts consumed daily by heavy drinkers suppresses the hematologic response to 75 μg of folic acid and reinduces megaloblastic changes in the marrow of partially treated folate-deficient patients. With folic acid therapy normal reticulocytosis is suppressed and the leukocyte and platelet counts rise. Removal of alcohol is followed by hematologic recovery. Leukopenia[227] and thrombocytopenia[243] have also been reported in folate-deficient alcoholic subjects. Thrombocytopenia has been shown to be the result of impairment of thrombopoiesis by alcohol, with diminution of megakaryocyte number and impairment of megakaryocyte maturation in the marrow. The effects of alcohol on the erythroid and megakaryocytic cells of the marrow are ameliorated in part by larger amounts of folic acid or by alcohol withdrawal. Alcoholism is not a major pediatric problem.

Folate deficiency has been described in all forms of liver disease, but it is particularly common in alcoholics and in patients with hemochromatosis.[189] The occurrence of a macrocytic anemia with a megaloblastic type of erythropoiesis has been observed in hemochromatosis. Its causation is related to the associated cirrhosis hindering the storage of folic acid. In a patient with hemochromatosis with megaloblastic anemia there was a striking response to folic acid but not to vitamin B_{12}.[171]

Megaloblastic anemia associated with certain drugs such as phenytoin, primidone, and phenobarbital derivatives have been reported. Nearly all the patients who developed the anemia had been taking the drugs for long periods, usually for years, but it has been reported after only 6 months of treatment. The peripheral blood is characterized by a macrocytic anemia, leukopenia with multisegmented granulocytes, and thrombocytopenia. Subnormal serum folate levels have been found in 50% of epileptic children being treated with anticonvulsants. Although slight macrocytosis was found in one fifth, megaloblastic anemia was not seen in any. Red cell indices and Arneth counts were not significantly different from those found in a control group of children.[229]

Although the pathogenesis of the syndrome is not entirely understood, several explanations have been suggested. The anemia may be a manifestation of folate deficiency produced by the drug acting as a competitive inhibitor of some enzyme system normally involving folic acid as a cofactor. Another theory is that the drug displaces folate from its plasma carrier; a third suggestion is that the drug by inhibiting intestinal conjugases in some way interferes with absorption of folate. In any event an inadequate dietary intake, particularly of folic acid and ascorbic acid, may be a contributing factor.

Increased excretion. The loss of folate from plasma into dialysis fluid in patients who are undergoing hemodialysis for renal disease has been demonstrated,[178] although deficient dietary folate intake appears to play a primary role in the development of folate deficiency in these patients.[281]

Rook et al.[251] have incriminated heart disease as another producer of folate deficiency in children. In adults with congestive heart failure folate deficiency has been ascribed to excessive urinary folate losses (100 μg or more each day), presumably through release of folate from "sick" liver cells.[246] Rook et al. found raised FIGLU excretion in six of twenty children with congenital or rheumatic heart disease, including two without either heart failure or secondary polycythemia. The exact meaning of these findings is uncertain, however, since the serum and red cell folate levels were normal in all six children and a positive FIGLU test can be caused by abnormalities other than folate deficiency. The hematologic responses to folic acid reported in two of the children were not clear-cut.

Clinical manifestations

The symptoms of anemia caused by folate deficiency are similar to those of megaloblastic anemia caused by vitamin B_{12} deficiency. Apart from possible minor mental changes or depression, folate deficiency has not been proved to cause a neuropathy.

Folic acid deficiency may adversely affect fetal and postnatal growth. In a study of infants with erythroblastosis Gandy and Jacobson[167] have shown a strong correlation between maternal and cord serum folate and the incidence of small-for-date infants. In addition, during the first year of life there was a strong correlation between serum folate levels of 8 μg/liter or more and rising weight percentiles and 5 μg/liter or less and falling percentiles. It is suggested that in some erythroblastotic infants a shortage of folic acid may be a limiting factor for a normal growth rate.[167-169]

A recent study has found evidence suggesting that maternal folate deficiency during pregnancy may be deleterious to the development of the central nervous system of the fetus and infant.[173]

In some patients an underlying condition such as celiac disease, epilepsy with anticonvulsant therapy, or pregnancy is known to be present, but in other patients the underlying disease is first diagnosed clinically or by laboratory tests only when megaloblastic anemia occurs. In all patients, however, it is unsafe to assume the deficiency is caused by folate deficiency rather than vitamin B_{12} deficiency unless appropriate laboratory tests have been carried out.

It has been shown that cell-mediated immunity is depressed in megaloblastic anemia caused by folate deficiency and that this depression is reversed by folate treatment.[174] The depressed cell-mediated immunity has been shown using dinitrochlorobenzene skin tests, phytohemagglutinin-stimulated lymphocyte transformation, and rosette inhibition by antilymphocyte globulin.

Laboratory findings

Peripheral blood and bone marrow. The peripheral blood and bone marrow changes are identical to those found in vitamin B_{12} deficiency and in general give a good indication of the severity of folate deficiency, since the more severe the anemia (and thus the morphologic changes in the blood and marrow), the greater the degree of folate deficiency measured biochemically. In patients who develop the anemia rapidly the blood film may show surprisingly little change, apart from pancytopenia, even though anemia is marked and the marrow shows florid megaloblastosis. The fall in white cell and platelet counts is usually in keeping with the degree of anemia, but occasional patients may show relatively severe degrees of leukopenia or thrombocytopenia. This may occur when there is arrest of hematopoiesis by methotrexate, alcohol, or other antifolate drugs or by infection.

Hypersegmentation of the neutrophils in peripheral blood is the single most useful laboratory aid to early diagnosis. It is often evident, even in mixed deficiency states with an iron and protein lack, whereas red cell indices and serum folate levels are less reliable. An average of more than 3.42 lobes/cell in 100 neutrophils is considered abnormal. More frequently hypersegmentation is a subjective impression that prompts confirmation of the diagnosis by serum studies, bone marrow aspiration, or a therapeutic trial.

Serum folate. Serum folate is measured microbiologically with a mutant strain of *Lactobacillus casei*, which grows well on 5-methyltetrahydrofolic acid, the predominant form of serum folate. This assay is accurate, reproducible, and available in most diagnostic laboratories. However, it is tedious and may be invalidated by previous administration of folic acid or by antibiotics such as penicillin, chloramphenicol, and tetracycline in the patient's serum.[245] The normal ranges for serum folate show a wide variation, but most laboratories would agree that levels below 3.0 ng/ml are low, 3.0 to 5.0 borderline, and levels about 5.0 or 6.0 ng/ml definitely normal.[231] The upper limit of normal is also poorly defined, and values between 7.0 and 31.0 ng/ml have been quoted. Elevated serum folate levels (>20 ng/ml) may be found in one third of vitamin B_{12}–deficient patients and in patients with blind loop syndrome (folate-producing microorganisms).

The serum folate assay is a sensitive, reliable guide to the presence of folate deficiency and remains the best way of confirming early folate deficiency. The results are subnormal in all patients with the deficiency and normal or high in vitamin B_{12}–deficient patients who are not also folate deficient. The serum folate level gives little guide to the severity of folate deficiency, since it may be equally low in gross megaloblastic anemia and in patients with normoblastic hematopoiesis. The level falls when a normal subject takes a folate-free diet for a few days and is extremely low after a few weeks of such a diet.[251] The rapid fall has been attributed to lack of displacement of liver folate, the normal source of serum folate, by recently ingested folate. Raised serum folate levels are not only found in some patients with vitamin B_{12} deficiency but may also be found in the intestinal stagnant loop syndrome, in liver damage, and in renal failure as well as in patients receiving folate or in bacterially contaminated sera.

Red cell folate. Red cell folate levels are measured in the same way as serum folate, with *L. casei*. The normal range is from 160 to 640 ng/ml and the result is subnormal in patients with megaloblastic anemia caused by folate deficiency (particularly in the most anemic patients) and in patients with significant tissue depletion of folate without megaloblastic anemia. The level is normal in patients with normoblastic hemopoiesis, even if the serum folate level is low.[197] Unfortunately the red cell folate level is subnormal in about 60% of patients with megaloblastic anemia caused by vitamin B_{12} deficiency, and this is particularly so

Table 7-4. Serum and red cell folate levels in the first year of life*

	Red cell (ng/ml)	Serum (ng/ml)
Neonate	598 (196-1,256)	24.5 (3-59)
3-4 months	283 (110-489)	12.2 (5-30)
6-8 months	247 (100-466)	7.7 (3.5-16)
12 months	277 (74-995)	9.3 (3-35)

*From Vanier, T. M., and Tyas, J. F.: Arch. Dis. Child. **41:** 658, 1966.

in the most anemic patients.[157,179,197] Reticulocytes contain more folate than mature cells, and high red cell folate levels may occur in patients with a reticulocytosis from any cause such as hemolysis or hemorrhage; the overall red cell folate level may be normal in these conditions, despite the presence of megaloblastic anemia.[197] Normal red cell folate levels may also occur in patients with severe folate deficiency who have received transfusions in the weeks before blood is taken for assay, since the folate in mature red cells is not released until the cell dies.

Changes in serum and red cell folate levels in the first year of life are shown in Table 7-4.[276] These values show that in the first year of life there is a rapid fall in the whole blood and serum folate levels in the first six weeks, and values are halved by 3 months of age.

FIGLU excretion. Formiminoglutamic acid (FIGLU), a normal intermediate product of the metabolism of histidine, requires active tetrahydrofolic acid for further degradation to glutamic acid (Fig. 7-9). When tetrahydrofolic acid is insufficient, FIGLU accummulates, and its excretion in the urine thus serves as a useful indicator of clinical folic acid deficiency.[217,265] Metabolic cor-

rection of the deficiency following administration of folic acid can be shown by the elimination of the increased urinary FIGLU.

Histidine is normally metabolized to FIGLU and then to glutamic acid through interaction with tetrahydrofolic acid. To increase the sensitivity of the test for FIGLU excretion when folic acid deficiency is suspected, loading doses of *l*-histidine are given orally to the patient. Normal persons excrete less than 2 mg of FIGLU in an hour (usually a trace or none). In folic acid deficiency excretion is greater than 3.5 mg/hour, with especially large amounts (30 to 80 mg) in idiopathic steatorrhea.[158]

The test is no longer widely used, since positive results are also obtained in 50% to 60% of patients with severe vitamin B_{12} deficiency,[206,285] as well as in many patients with liver disease, carcinoma, tuberculosis, sarcoidosis, polyarteritis nodosa, scleroderma, myelosclerosis, and thyrotoxicosis in the absence of folate deficiency or out of proportion to the degree of folate deficiency.[151,207,228]

It has also been claimed that the large doses of histidine in the loading test may be unphysiologic and account for overlapping results noted in folic acid deficiency, vitamin B_{12} deficiency, and other hematologic states.[183,186]

Moreover, the FIGLU test may be negative despite severe folate deficiency in pregnancy[156] and in patients with severe protein deficiency (kwashiorkor), in which lack of urocanase causes a block in FIGLU production from urocanic acid with an increased excretion of urocanic acid itself.[136,194] Urocanic acid excretion is also increased in liver disease and in conditions that cause liver dysfunction, e.g., carcinoma and tuberculosis, but probably bears no relation to folate deficiency in these diseases.

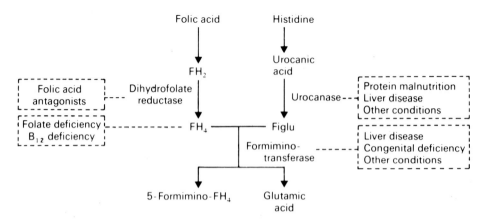

Fig. 7-9. Histidine metabolic pathway and sites of blockade. Tetrahydrofolate is a necessary acceptor of formimino groups produced by histidine metabolism. In folate deficiency or metabolic blockade unaltered FIGLU is excreted in the urine after a histidine load. (From Today's tests, Br. Med. J. **2:**100, 1969.)

Folic acid clearance test. Folic acid clearance may be measured microbiologically using *L. casei.*[154] Blood samples are taken at 3-, 15-, 30-, and 60-minute intervals after the intravenous administration of folic acid. Clearance is increased in patients with severe folate deficiency and, in the absence of folate deficiency, in patients with conditions of increased cell turnover such as pregnancy or hemolytic anemia.[193,213] The test is cumbersome and is not now used for routine clinical purposes.

Therapeutic trial. Therapeutic trial has not been used widely to establish the etiology of megaloblastic anemia since the development of faster, less cumbersome means of evaluation. However, when appropriately used, it is reliable when other clinical and laboratory tests are not available. Its successful use depends on the following conditions: (1) absence of critical illness in the patient and freedom from significant infection, renal disease, inflammatory disorder, or malignancy, (2) availability of frequent reticulocyte counts, (3) ability to maintain the patient on a basal diet with avoidance of foods high in folate content (e.g., red meats, liver, kidney, other organ meats, fresh leafy green and yellow vegetables, and citrus fruits and juices), and (4) administration of daily physiologic doses of vitamin B_{12} (1 to 5 μg parenterally) or folic acid (50 to 100 μg orally or parenterally) for therapeutic trial.

A positive therapeutic trial depends on the development of a prompt reticulocyte response that is specific to either vitamin B_{12} or folic acid in the aforementioned dosages. Since nonspecific responses can be obtained with larger doses, the smaller doses indicated must be used in a therapeutic trial.

Diagnosis

The first step is suspicion that megaloblastic anemia or vitamin B_{12} or folate deficiency is present. A dietary history may suggest that an individual could be suffering from vitamin B_{12} or folate deficiency, e.g., the breast-fed child, the child fed on goat's milk, the strict vegetarian, or the food faddist. A previous history of intestinal surgery or a history of chronic diarrhea may suggest the presence of an anatomic lesion of the intestine or some other intestinal disease. The prolonged use of alcohol or drugs, especially anticonvulsants, may suggest the presence of a folate-deficiency anemia.

Suspicion may arise because of symptoms of anemia, neuropathy, or gastrointestinal disease or other conditions that may predispose to one or other deficiency (Table 7-3). Examination of the patient may not only reveal pallor but may also show evidence of underlying disease that is the cause of folate deficiency, e.g., celiac disease or a chronic inflammatory or malignant disease. The next step is a close examination of the blood film; a blood count including hemoglobin estimation and red cell, white cell, and platelet counts; and, if necessary, examination of the bone marrow, which not only establishes whether megaloblastosis is present but also reveals the iron status of the patient. If the clinical and hematologic features suggest a deficiency, assays of serum vitamin B_{12} and folate, red cell folate, and possibly urine methylmalonic acid after valine loading, and a therapeutic trial in patients with uncomplicated megaloblastic anemia can establish whether vitamin B_{12} or folate deficiency or both are present. Further tests are then necessary to determine the cause of the deficiency. In either case a diet history and barium meal and follow-through x-ray examination are needed. Gastric function and vitamin B_{12} absorption studies, tests for parietal cell and intrinsic factor antibodies in serum, and gastric or jejunal biopsy if sprue is suspected are valuable for elucidating the cause of vitamin deficiency. Tests for the cause of folate deficiency include jejunal biopsy; xylose, folate, and fat absorption tests; and tests for underlying hematologic, inflammatory, or malignant disease, although these are usually obvious when severe folate deficiency occurs.

Mild folate deficiency is far more common than megaloblastic anemia caused by the deficiency. The decision whether a patient with, for instance, a subnormal serum folate level has a deficiency severe enough to warrant full investigation and treatment is determined largely by the blood and bone marrow findings and, if this is measured, on the red cell folate level. On the other hand, a subnormal serum vitamin B_{12} level is a highly significant finding that always requires proper investigation and more often than not necessitates lifelong vitamin B_{12} therapy.

In a patient with megaloblastic anemia a low serum vitamin B_{12} level with a normal or high serum folate level indicates vitamin B_{12} deficiency as the cause of the condition, and a normal serum vitamin B_{12} level with a low serum and red cell folate level indicates folate deficiency. However, when both the serum vitamin B_{12} and the serum folate levels are low, the result is more difficult to interpret since this combination can be found in patients with pure folate deficiency, pure vitamin B_{12} deficiency, and combined deficiencies. In such cases the relative severity of the reduction in serum levels, evidence of increased methylmalonic acid excretion, and the therapeutic response to treatment may be helpful in differentiating the relative roles of vitamin B_{12} and folate deficiency in the production of the anemia. Finally it must be remembered that low serum vitamin B_{12} and/or low serum and red cell folate concentrations does not necessarily imply that the bone marrow is megaloblastic, there being no absolute correlation between morphology and these concentrations.

Treatment

Successful treatment of patients with folate deficiency involves (1) correction of the folate deficiency, (2) amelioration of the underlying disorder, if possible, (3) improvement of the diet to increase folate intake, and (4) follow-up evaluations at intervals to monitor the patient's clinical status.

An optimal response occurs in most patients with 100 to 200 μg folic acid daily. Nevertheless, it is usual to treat deficient patients with 1 to 5 mg daily. Smaller doses are in fact usually adequate, but the commercially available tablets contain 1 or 5 mg. To reduce the folate content would probably not significantly reduce the cost, and since pteroylmonoglutamic acid rarely produces side effects except in patients with vitamin B_{12} deficiency, there is little reason to reduce the dose. Further, a smaller oral dose might not always be effective in patients with folate malabsorption. In most patients, 5 to 15 mg of folic acid daily for 7 to 14 days induces a maximal hematologic response and significant replenishment of body stores. This may be given orally because, even in those with severe malabsorption, sufficient folate is absorbed from this dose to replenish stores. Before folic acid is given (in these large doses) it is always necessary to ensure that vitamin B_{12} deficiency is not present.

The clinical and hematologic response to folic acid is prompt. Within 1 to 2 days the patient's appetite improves (often becoming voracious) and a sense of well-being returns, with increased energy and interest in surroundings. There is a fall in serum iron content (often to low levels) in 24 to 48 hours, an increase in reticulocytes in 2 to 4 days that reaches a peak at 4 to 7 days, and a return of hemoglobin levels to normal in 2 to 6 weeks. The leukocytes and platelets increase with the reticulocytes and the megaloblastic changes in the marrow diminish within 24 to 48 hours, but large myelocytes, metamyelocytes, and band forms may be present for several days. A few hypersegmented neutrophils may still be found 6 to 8 weeks after institution of folate therapy, although the hemoglobin level and leukocyte and platelet counts are normal.

It is uncertain how long initial folic acid therapy should be continued, although it is usual to give the vitamin for several months until a new population of red cells has been formed. Folinic acid is reserved for combating the toxic effects of dihydrofolate reductase inhibitors such as methotrexate and pyrimethamine.

It is often possible to correct the cause of the deficiency and thus to prevent recurrence of the deficiency, e.g., by an improved diet, a gluten-free diet in celiac disease, or treatment of an inflammatory disease such as tuberculosis or Crohn's disease. In these cases there is no need to continue folic acid administration for life. In other situations, however, it is advisable to give folic acid continually to prevent the recurrence of deficiency, e.g., in chronic hemolytic anemia such as thalassemia or in patients with malabsorption who do not respond to a gluten-free diet.

MEGALOBLASTIC ANEMIA NOT CAUSED BY FOLATE OR VITAMIN B₁₂ DEFICIENCY
Congenital disorders

Orotic aciduria. Orotic aciduria is a rare but well-characterized syndrome in which there is a congenital defect in all tissues of the body of one or two enzymes (orotidylic pyrophosphorylase and orotidylic decarboxylase) concerned in pyrimidine synthesis. The condition is inherited as a Mendelian recessive trait, heterozygotes having enzyme levels intermediate between those of normal persons and homozygotes.[250]

The metabolic pathway of orotic acid is shown in the following diagram:

$$\text{orotic acid} \xrightarrow{\substack{\text{orotidylic} \\ \text{pyrophosphorylase}}} \text{orotidylic acid} \xrightarrow{\substack{\text{orotidylic} \\ \text{decarboxylase}}}$$

$$\text{uridylic acid} \longrightarrow \text{nucleic acids}$$
$$\uparrow$$
$$\text{uridine}$$

The disease appears in the first year or two of life with failure to thrive, mental retardation, and megaloblastic anemia unresponsive to vitamin B_{12} or folate.[162,250,261] It is characterized by severe megaloblastic changes in the bone marrow, hypochromic macrocytes and microcytes, anisocytosis, poikilocytosis, multisegmented neutrophils and giant platelets in the peripheral blood, and the excretion of large amounts of orotic acid in the urine. The orotic acid crystalluria is caused by a congenital defect in the pathway of synthesis of pyrimidine nucleotides. In a recent review of eight cases Smith[260] demonstrated a marked decrease in the activities of both orotidylic pyrophosphorylase and orotidylic decarboxylase in the erythrocytes of seven patients (type I orotic aciduria). Leukocytes, liver cells, and cultured fibroblasts were also deficient. One patient's red cells lacked orotidylic decarboxylase only (type II).

Investigation of parents and siblings indicates a heterozygous state without clinical abnormalities and a minimal decrease in urinary excretion of orotic acid. Thus an autosomal recessive mode of inheritance was demonstrated. The relatively high frequency of heterozygotes suggests that some affected fetuses die in utero.[248]

The condition should be suspected in a child with megaloblastic anemia with unexplained crystalluria or when mental retardation and anemia coexist. Vitamin B_{12} and folic acid serum levels are normal, and the megaloblastic anemia is resistant to vitamin B_{12}, folic acid, pyridoxine, iron, and ascorbic acid therapy.

The diagnosis of hereditary orotic aciduria is made by finding crystals of orotic acid in the urine. A urinary screening test has been described.[248] The test is based on the conversion of orotic acid to barbituric acid by the action of saturated bromine water and subsequent reduction by ascorbic acid. The excretion of orotic acid reaches 6 gm/24 hours owing to failure of orotic acid utilization and to excessive orotic acid synthesis from failure of product inhibition by uridine. Specific enzyme assays should be performed to differentiate type I from type II disease.

Hematologic remission is induced by the ingestion of a mixture of uridylic and cytidylic acid. The first child diagnosed died,[202] but in subsequent cases treatment with uridine in large oral doses (e.g., 300 mg five times daily) has been successful.[261] A reticulocyte response is usually noted within 48 hours.

Thiamine-responsive megaloblastic anemia. Only one child with thiamin-responsive megaloblastic anemia has been described. Megaloblastic anemia appeared to be caused by excess thiamine utilization.[249] The child showed no clinical evidence of thiamine deficiency and the cellular levels of three enzymes known to require thiamine were normal. The biochemical basis for the anemia is unknown. The patient was an 11-year-old white girl with megaloblastic anemia refractory to folate and vitamin B_{12} therapy but responsive to treatment with thiamine. Withdrawal of supplemental vitamins resulted in a relapse within 3½ months. When the implicated vitamins were given sequentially, a reticulocytosis followed the administration of thiamine. Anemia again recurred 4 months after vitamin supplementation was discontinued. On this occasion the anemia was corrected by 20 mg oral thiamine daily. The patient therefore appeared to have a thiamine-dependent megaloblastic anemia. Additional abnormalities included diabetes mellitus, aminoaciduria, and sensorineural deafness.

Congenital familial megaloblastic anemia. Two sisters with megaloblastic anemia, presenting at 3 and 7 weeks of age, have been described by Lampkin et al.[209] The anemia responded well to vitamin B_{12} and folic acid given together in large doses, even though normal serum levels of both folic acid and vitamin B_{12} had been demonstrated

while they were receiving no therapy. The anemia relapsed if either vitamin was discontinued. The older sister had severe mental retardation. The site of the biochemical defect is unknown, but thymidylate synthesis and orotic acid excretion were both normal. The optimal hemoglobin response after administration of both vitamins suggests that both folic acid and vitamin B_{12} may be necessary at some other preliminary step in DNA synthesis.

Congenital dyserythropoietic anemia. Megaloblastic anemia unresponse to vitamin B_{12} and folate therapy has been described in congenital dyserythropoietic anemia. (See Chapter 8.)

Lesch-Nyhan syndrome. Lesch-Nyhan syndrome consists of mental retardation, self-mutilation, and gout; it is a result of a congenital defect of the enzyme hypoxanthine-guanine phosphoribosyltransferase, which is concerned with purine synthesis. There is no adequately documented case of megaloblastic anemia in this syndrome, but a case with megaloblastic anemia that apparently responded to adenine was briefly reported.[274,275]

Acquired disorders

Blood dyscrasias. Patients with various blood dyscrasias such as sideroblastic anemia,[221] hemachromatosis,[273] leukemia, and DiGuglielmo's syndrome (erythroleukemia)[255] may have a megaloblastic bone marrow that is unresponsive to therapy with any known hematinic. Approximately 10% of patients with pyridoxine-responsive anemia have megaloblastic marrow morphology.[180] The megaloblastosis may be caused by associated folate deficiency in a few, it may respond to pyridoxine in others, and in other patients it persists after hematologic improvement with pyridoxine therapy. The mechanism of megaloblastosis in the second and third groups is obscure. Most of the reported patients with pyridoxine-response anemia and megaloblastosis have been female.

In aplastic anemia with hypocellular marrow, approximately 15% of the patients have variable degrees (usually mild or moderate) of megaloblastosis in the few erythroid cells present in the marrow. The megaloblastosis may improve or persist despite remissions of the anemia (spontaneous or induced by testosterone therapy). The term "refractory megaloblastic anemia" refers to a syndrome of marrow hyperplasia with megaloblastosis and anemia, usually occurring in elderly individuals. Variable degrees of leukopenia, thrombocytopenia, or pancytopenia may be present. The hematologic course in a few patients evolves into myeloblastic or erythroblastic leukemia. The syndrome of refractory megaloblastic anemia undoubtedly represents a heterogenous group of disorders yet to be delineated. Such patients presumably have an unidentified metabolic block in DNA

Table 7-5. Drugs capable of producing megaloblastosis

Drug	Use
Purine antagonists	
6-Mercaptopurine (6-MP)	Chemotherapy, immunosuppression
Thioguanine	Chemotherapy, immunosuppression
Azothioprine	Immunosuppression
Pyrimidine antagonists	
5-Fluorouracil (5-FU)	Chemotherapy
6-Azauridine	Chemotherapy, psoriasis
Inhibitors of ribonucleotide reductase	
Cytosine arabinoside	Chemotherapy, antiviral
Hydroxyurea	Chemotherapy, psoriasis
Mechanism unknown	
Benzene	Solvent
L-Asparaginase	Chemotherapy
Azulfidine	Ulcerative colitis
Arsenic	Poison

synthesis. Patients with these dyscrasias may also develop a relative or absolute folate deficiency and so have folate-responsive megaloblastic anemia.

Drugs. A number of antipyrimidine drugs (as well as dihydrofolate reductase inhibitors) (notably cytosine arabinoside, which inhibits DNA polymerase; 5-fluorouracil, which inhibits thymidylate synthetase; hydroxyurea, which inhibits ribonucleotide reductase; and azauridine, which inhibits orotodylic decarboxylase) cause megaloblastosis without interfering directly with folate or vitamin B_{12} metabolism. Antipurine drugs, e.g., 6-mercaptopurine, azathioprine, and thioguanine, cause megaloblastosis less frequently, whereas drugs that interfere with DNA metabolism other than synthesis, e.g., chelating agents, do not cause megaloblastosis.

Table 7-5 provides a list of drugs capable of producing megaloblastosis.

REFERENCES
Vitamin B_{12}

1. Agunod, M., Yamaguchi, N., Lopez, R., et al.: Correlative study of hydrochloric acid, pepsin, and intrinsic factor secretion in newborns and infants, Am. J. Dig. Dis. **14:**400, 1969.
2. Ainley, N. J., and Lamb, D. C.: Megaloblastic anemia following operations on the small intestine, Br. J. Surg. **48:**608, 1961.
3. Allen, R. H., and Mehlman, C. S.: Isolation of gastric vitamin B_{12}-binding proteins using affinity chromatography. I. Purification and properties of human intrinsic factor, J. Biol. Chem. **248:**3660, 1973.
4. Ampola, M. G., Mahoney, M. J., Nakamura, E., et al.: Prenatal therapy of a patient with vitamin-B_{12}-responsive methylmalonic acidemia, N. Engl. J. Med. **293:**313, 1975.
5. Anderson, B. B.: Investigation into the Euglena method for the assay of vitamin B_{12} in serum, J. Clin. Pathol. **17:**14, 1964.
6. Arakawa, T., Narisawa, K., Tanno, K., et al.: Megaloblastic anemia and mental retardation associated with hyperfolic-acidemia: probably due to N^5-methyltetrahydrofolate transferase deficiency, Tohoku J. Exp. Med. **93:**1, 1967.
7. Baker, S. J.: Tropical megaloblastic anemia, Lancet **2:**337, 1965.
8. Baker, S. J.: Human vitamin B_{12} deficiency, World Rev. Nutr. Diet. **8:**62, 1967.
9. Baker, S. J., Jacob, E., Rajan, K. T., and Swaminathan, S. P.: Vitamin B_{12} deficiency in pregnancy and the puerperium, Br. Med. J. **1:**1658, 1962.
10. Barness, L. A., Young, D., Mellman, W. J., et al.: Methylmalonate excretion in a patient with pernicious anemia, N. Engl. J. Med. **268:**144, 1963.
11. Beard, M. E., and Allen, D. M.: Effect of antimicrobial agents on the *Lactobacillus casei* folate assay, Am. J. Clin. Pathol. **48:**401, 1967.
12. Beck, W. S.: The metabolic functions of vitamin B_{12}, N. Engl. J. Med. **266:**708, 1962.
13. Ben-Bassat, I., Feinstein, A., and Ramot, B.: Selective vitamin B_{12} malabsorption with proteinuria in Israel, Isr. J. Med. Sci. **5:**62, 1969.
14. Bernstein, L. H., Gutstein, M. D., Efron, G., et al.: Trichobezoar: an unusual cause of megaloblastic anemia and hypoproteinemia in childhood, Dig. Dis. **18:**67, 1973.
15. Boger, W. P., Bayne, G. M., Wright, L. D., and Beck, G. D.: Differential serum vitamin B_{12} concentrations in mothers and infants, N. Engl. J. Med. **256:**1085, 1957.
16. Booth, C. C.: The metabolic effects of intestinal resection in man, Postgrad. Med. J. **37:**725, 1961.
17. Booth, C. C., and Mollin, D. L.: Plasma, tissue and urinary radioactivity after oral administration of ^{56}Co-labelled vitamin B_{12}, Br. J. Haematol. **2:**223, 1956.
18. Booth, C. C., and Mollin, D. L.: The site of vitamin B_{12} absorption in man, Lancet **1:**18, 1959.
19. Booth, C. C., and Mollin, D. L.: The blind loop syndrome, Proc. R. Soc. Med. **53:**658, 1960.
20. Britt, R. P., and Rose, D. P.: Pernicious anemia with a normal serum vitamin B_{12} level in a case of chronic granulocytic leukemia, Arch. Intern. Med. **117:**32, 1966.
21. Brozovic, M., Hoffbrand, A. V., Dimitriadou, A., and Mollin, D. L.: The excretion of methylmalonic acid and succinic acid in vitamin B_{12} and folate deficiency, Br. J. Haematol. **13:**1021, 1967.
22. Callender, S. T., and Denborough, M. A.: A familial study of pernicious anaemia, Br. J. Haematol. **3:**88, 1957.
23. Cannata, J. J. B., Focesi, A., Jr., Mazumder, R., et al.: Metabolism of propionic acid in animal tissues. XII. Properties of mamalian methylmalonyl coenzyme A mutase, J. Biol. Chem. **240:**3249, 1965.
24. Carmel, R.: Vitamin B_{12}-binding protein abnormality in subjects without myeloproliferative disease. I. Elevated serum vitamin B_{12}-binding capacity levels in patients with leucocytosis, Br. J. Haematol. **22:**43, 1972.
25. Carmel, R., and Herbert, V.: Deficiency of vitamin B_{12}-binding alpha globulin in two brothers, Blood **33:**1, 1969.
26. Carmel, R., Waxman, S., Epstein, B., et al.: Acquired(?) selective malabsorption of B_{12} in a family. Simultaneous sessions, Twelfth congress of the International Society of Hematology, New York, 1969. (Abstract.)
27. Chikkapa, G., Corcino, J., Greenberg, M. L., and Her-

bert, V.: Correlation between various blood white cell pools and the serum B_{12}-binding capacities, Blood **37**:142, 1971.

28. Cooke, W. T., et al.: The clinical and metabolic significance of jejunal diverticula, Gut **4**:115, 1963.

29. Cooper, B. A., and Castle, W. B.: Sequential mechanisms in the enhanced absorption of vitamin B_{12} by intrinsic factor in the rat, J. Clin. Invest. **39**:199, 1960.

30. Cooper, B. A., and White, J. J.: Absence of intrinsic factor from human portal plasma during ^{57}Co-B_{12} absorption in man, Br. J. Haematol. **14**:73, 1968.

31. Cox, E. V., and White, A. M.: Methylmalonic acid excretion: an index of vitamin B_{12} deficiency, Lancet **2**:853, 1962.

32. Dacie, J. V., and White, J. C.: Erythropoiesis with particular reference to its study by biopsy of human bone marrow: a review, J. Clin. Pathol. **2**:1, 1949.

33. Dillon, M. J., England, J. M., Gompertz, D., et al.: Mental retardation, megaloblastic anaemia, methylmalonic aciduria and abnormal homocysteine metabolism due to an error in vitamin B_{12} metabolism, Clin. Sci. Mol. Med. **47**:43, 1974.

34. Donaldson, R. M., MacKenzie, I. L., and Trier, J. S.: Intrinsic-factor mediated attachment of vitamin B_{12} to brush borders and microvillous membranes of hamster intestine, J. Clin. Invest. **46**:1215, 1967.

35. Ellenbogen, L.: Absorption and transport of cobalamin. Intrinsic factor and the transcobalamins. In Babior, B. M., ed.: Cobalamin, biochemistry and pathophysiology, New York, 1975, John Wiley & Sons, Inc.

36. Finch, C. A., Coleman, D. H., Motulsky, A. G., et al.: Erythrokinetics in pernicious anemia, Blood **11**:807, 1956.

37. Flemming, A. F., and Dawson, I.: Pigmentation in megaloblastic anaemia, Br. Med. J. **2**:236, 1972.

38. Ford, J. E.: The microbiological assay of "vitamin B_{12}": the specificity of the requirement of *Ochromonas malhamensis* for cyanocobalamin, Br. J. Nutr. **7**:299, 1953.

39. Frenkel, E. P.: Abnormal fatty acid metabolism in peripheral nerves of patients with pernicious anemia, J. Clin. Invest. **52**:1237, 1973.

40. Gimpert, E., Jakob, M., and Hitzig, W. H.: Vitamin B_{12} transport in blood. I. Congenital deficiency of transcobalamin II, Blood **45**:71, 1975.

41. Ginsberg, A., and Mullinax, F.: Pernicious anemia and monoclonal gammopathy in a patient with IgA deficiency, Am. J. Med. **48**:787, 1970.

42. Goodman, S. I.: Personal communication, U.S.-Japan Cooperative Medical Science Program, Sendai, Japan, December 2-3, 1976.

43. Goodman, S. I., Moe, P. G., Hammond, K. B., et al.: Homocystinuria with methylmalonic aciduria: two cases in a sibship, Biochem. Med. **4**:500, 1970.

44. Gräsbeck, R., Gordin, R., Kantero, I., et al.: Selective vitamin B_{12} malabsorption and proteinuria in young people, Acta Med. Scand. **167**:289, 1960.

45. Gräsbeck, R., and Kvist, G.: Defecto congenito y selectivo de absorcion de la vitamina B_{12} con proteinuria, Rev. Clin. Esp. **106**:448, 1967.

46. Gräsbeck, R., Nyberg, W., and Reizenstein, P.: Biliary and fecal vitamin B_{12} excretion in man, an isotope study, Proc. Soc. Exp. Biol. Med. **97**:780, 1958.

47. Greenfield, J. G., and Meyer, A.: Vitamin B_{12} neuropathy (subacute combined degeneration of the spinal cord). In Blackwood, W., ed.: Greenfield's neuropathy, London, 1963, Edward Arnold (Publishers), Ltd.

48. Hakami, N., Nieman, P. E., Canellos, G. P., and Lazerson, J.: Neonatal megaloblastic anemia due to inherited transcobalamin II deficiency in two siblings, N. Engl. J. Med. **285**:1163, 1971.

49. Hall, C. A.: Vitamin B_{12}-binding proteins of man, Ann. Intern. Med. **75**:297, 1971.

50. Hall, C. A., and Finkler, A. E.: The dynamics of transcobalamin II: a vitamin B_{12}-binding substance in plasma, J. Lab. Clin. Med. **65**:459, 1965.

51. Halsted, J. W., Lewis, P. M., and Gasster, M.: Absorption of radioactive vitamin B_{12} in the syndrome of megaloblastic anemia associated with intestinal stricture or anastomosis, Am. J. Med. **20**:42, 1956.

52. Herbert, V.: Diagnostic and prognostic values of measurement of serum vitamin B_{12}-binding proteins, Blood **32**:305, 1968.

53. Herbert, V., Streiff, R. R., Sullivan, L. W., and McGeer, P. L.: Deranged purine metabolism manifested by aminoimidazole-carboxamide excretion in megaloblastic anaemias, haemolytic anaemia, and liver disease, Lancet **2**:45, 1964.

54. Herbert, V., Streiff, R., Sullivan, L., and McGreer, P. L.: Accumulation of a purine intermediate (aminoimidazolecarboxamide) (AIC) in megaloblastic anemias associated with vitamin B_{12} deficiency, folate deficiency with alcoholism, and liver disease, Fed. Proc. **23**:188, 1964.

55. Herbert, V., Tisman, G., Go, L. T., et al.: The dU suppression test using I^{125} UdR to define biochemical megaloblastosis, Br. J. Haematol. **24**:711, 1973.

56. Herbert, V., and Zalusky, R.: Interrelations of vitamin B_{12} and folic acid metabolism: folic acid clearance studies, J. Clin. Invest. **41**:1263, 1962.

57. Hess, B., and Gehm, E.: Über die milchsäurehydrogenase und menschlichen serum, Klin. Wochenschr. **33**:91, 1955.

58. Hines, J. D.: Megaloblastic anemia in an adult vegan, Am. J. Clin. Nutr. **19**:260, 1966.

59. Hitzig, W. H., Dohmann, U., Pluss, H. J., et al.: Hereditary transcobalamin II deficiency: clinical findings in a new family, J. Pediatr. **85**:622, 1974.

60. Hoedemaeker, P. J., Abels, J., Wachters, J. J., et al.: Further investigations about the site of production of Castle's gastric intrinsic factor, Lab. Invest. **15**:1163, 1966.

61. Hoffbrand, A. V.: Vitamin-B_{12} and folate metabolism: the megaloblastic anaemias and related disorders. In Hardisty, R. M., and Weatherall, D. J., eds.: Blood and its disorders, Oxford, 1974, Blackwell Scientific Publishers, Ltd.

62. Hoffbrand, A. V., Tripp, E., and Das, K. C.: Uptake of vitamin B_{12} by phytohaemagglutinin-transformed lymphocytes, Br. J. Haematol. **24**:147, 1973.

63. Hogenkamp, H. P. C.: Structure and chemical reactions of the cobamide coenzymes, Ann. N.Y. Acad. Sci. **112**:552, 1964.

64. Horton, M. A., and Burman, J. F.: Reversible C_3 hypocomplementaemia in megaloblastic anaemia due to vitamin B_{12} deficiency, Br. J. Haematol. **36**:23, 1977.

65. Hung, W., Migeon, C. J., and Parrott, R. H.: A possible autoimmune basis for Addison's disease in three siblings, one with idiopathic hypoparathyroidism, pernicious anemia and superficial moniliasis, N. Engl. J. Med. **269**:658, 1963.

66. Hurwitz, L. J.: Spontaneous hypoparathyroidism with megaloblastic anaemia, Lancet **1**:234, 1956.

67. Imerslund, O.: Idiopathic chronic megaloblastic anaemia in children, Acta Pediatr. **49**(suppl.):119, 1960.

68. Katz, M., Lee, S. K., and Cooper, B. A.: Vitamin B_{12} malabsorption due to biologically inert intrinsic factor, N. Engl. J. Med. **287**:425, 1972.

69. Katz, M., Mehlman, C. S., and Allen, R. H.: Isolation

and characterization of an abnormal human intrinsic factor, J. Clin. Invest. **53:**1274, 1974.

70. Kaye, C. I., Morrow, G., III, and Nadler, H. L.: In vitro "responsive" methylmalonic acidemia: a new variant, J. Pediatr. **85:**55, 1974.
71. Kerwar, S. S., Spears, C., McAuslan, B., and Weissbach, H.: Studies on vitamin B_{12} metabolism in Hela cells, Arch. Biochem. Biophys. **142:**231, 1971.
72. Kumento, A.: The serum binders of vitamin B_{12} in newborn infants, Acta Paediatr. Scand. **58:**553, 1969. (Abstract.)
73. Lau, K. S., et al.: Measurement of serum vitamin B_{12} using radioisotope dilution and coated charcoal, Blood **26:**202, 1965.
74. Lawrence, C.: The binding of vitamin B_{12} by serum proteins in normal and B_{12}-deficient subjects, Br. J. Haematol. **12:**569, 1966.
75. Lawrence, C.: B_{12}-binding protein deficiency in pernicious anemia, Blood **27:**389, 1966.
76. Lee, F. I., Jenkins, G. C., Hughes, D. T. D., et al.: Pernicious anaemia, myxoedema and hypogammaglobulinaemia: a family study, Br. Med. J. **1:**598, 1964.
77. Levy, H. L., Mudd, S. H., Schulman, J. D., et al.: A derangement in B_{12} metabolism associated with homocystinemia, cystathioninemia, hypomethioninemia and methylmalonic aciduria, Am. J. Med. **48:**390, 1970.
78. Linnell, J. C., Hoffbrand, A. V., Peters, T. J., and Matthews, D. M.: Chromatographic and bioautographic estimation of plasma cobalamins in various disturbances of vitamin B_{12} metabolism, Clin. Sci. **40:**1, 1971.
79. Linnell, J. C., Matthews, D. M., Mudd, S. H., et al.: Cobalamins in fibroblasts cultured from normal control subjects and patients with methylmalonic aciduria, Pediatr. Res. **10:**179, 1976.
80. Luhby, A. L., and Cooperman, J. M.: Aminoimidazolecarboxamide excretion in vitamin B_{12} and folic-acid deficiencies, Lancet **2:**1381, 1962.
81. MacKenzie, I. L., Donaldson, R. M., Trier, J. S., and Mathan, V. I.: Ileal mucosa in familial selective vitamin B_{12} malabsorption, N. Engl. J. Med. **286:**1021, 1972.
82. Mahoney, J. J., and Rosenberg, L. E.: Inborn errors of cobalamin metabolism. In Babior, B. M., ed.: Cobalamin, biochemistry and pathophysiology, New York, 1975, John Wiley & Sons, Inc.
83. Mahoney, M. J., Rosenberg, L. E., Lindblad, B., et al.: Prenatal diagnosis of methylmalonic aciduria, Acta Pediatr. Scand. **64:**44, 1975.
84. Mahoney, M. J., Rosenberg, L. E., Mudd, S. H., et al.: Defective metabolism of vitamin B_{12} in fibroblasts from children with methylmalonicaciduria, Biochem. Biophys. Res. Commun. **44:**375, 1971.
85. Mauer, H. S., Chio, H. S., Forman, E. N., and Honig, G. R.: Pernicious anemia with persistent malabsorption of vitamin B_{12} in a child, J. Pediatr. **83:**832, 1973.
86. McIntyre, O. R., Sullivan, L. W., Jeffries, G. H., and Silver, R. H.: Pernicious anemia in childhood, N. Engl. J. Med. **272:**981, 1965.
87. McIntyre, P. A., Hahn, R., Conley, C. L., and Glass, B.: Genetic factors in predisposition to pernicious anemia, Bull. Johns Hopkins Hosp. **104:**309, 1959.
88. Mehta, B. M., Rege, D. V., and Satoskar, R. S.: Serum vitamin B_{12} and folic acid activity in lactovegetarian and non vegetarian healthy adult Indians, Am. J. Clin. Nutr. **15:**77, 1964.
89. Meyer, L. M., Bertcher, R. W., Cronkite, E. P., et al.: Co^{60} vitamin B_{12} binding capacity of serum in persons with hematologic disorders, various medical diseases and neoplasms, Acta Med. Scand. **169:**557, 1961.
90. Miller, D. R., Bloom, G. E., Streiff, R. R., et al.: Juvenile "congenital" pernicious anemia, N. Engl. J. Med. **275:**978, 1966.

91. Mohamed, S. D., McKay, E., and Galloway, W. H.: Juvenile familial megaloblastic anaemia due to selective malabsorption of vitamin B_{12}, Q. J. Med. **35:**433, 1966.
92. Mollin, D. L., Booth, C. C., and Chanarin, I.: The pathogenesis of deficiency of vitamin B_{12} and folic acid in idiopathic steatorrhoea. In Proceedings of the World Congress of Gastroenterology, Baltimore, 1958, The Williams & Wilkins Co.
93. Morrow, G., III, Mahoney, M. J., Matthews, C., et al.: Studies of methylmalonyl coenzyme A carbonylmutase activity in methylmalonic acidemia. I. Correlation of clinical, hepatic, and fibroblast data, Pediatr. Res. **9:**641, 1975.
94. Morrow, G., III, Schwarz, R. H., Hallock, J. A., et al.: Prenatal detection of methylmalonic acidemia, J. Pediatr. **77:**120, 1970.
95. Mudd, S. H.: Homocystinuria and homocysteine metabolism: selected aspects. In Nyhan, W. H., ed.: Heritable disorders of amino acid metabolism, ed. 2, New York, 1974, John Wiley & Sons, Inc.
96. Mudd, S. H.: Cobalamin-responsive genetic disorders, Paper presented at the International Symposium on Nutritional Deficiency Secondary to Inborn Errors of Metabolism, U.S.-Japan Cooperative Medical Science Program, Sendai, Japan, December 1976.
97. Nathan, D. G., and Gardner, F. H.: Erythroid cell maturation and hemoglobin synthesis in megaloblastic anemia, J. Clin. Invest. **41:**1086, 1962.
98. Parry, T. E.: Serum valine and methionine levels in pernicious anaemia under treatment, Br. J. Haematol. **16:**22, 1969.
99. Pathak, A., Godwin, H. A., and Prudent, L. M.: Vitamin B_{12} and folic acid values in premature infants, Pediatrics **50:**584, 1972.
100. Perillie, P. E., Kaplan, S. S., and Finch, S. C.: Significance of changes in serum muramidase activity in megaloblastic anemia, N. Engl. J. Med. **277:**10, 1967.
101. Peters, T. J., and Hoffbrand, A. V.: Absorption of vitamin B_{12} by the guinea-pig. I. Subcellular localization of vitamin B_{12} in the ileal enterocyte during absorption, Br. J. Haematol. **19:**369, 1970.
102. Peters, T. J., and Hoffbrand, A. V.: Absorption of vitamin B_{12} by the guinea-pig. The role of the ileal mitochondrion. In Arnstein, H. R. V., and Wrighton, R. J., ed.: The cobalamins, a Glaxo symposium, Edinburgh, 1971, Churchill-Livingstone.
103. Pollycove, M., Apt, L., and Colbert, M. J.: Pernicious anemia due to dietary deficiency of vitamin B_{12}, N. Engl. J. Med. **255:**164, 1956.
104. Quinto, M. G., Leikin, S. L., and Hung, W.: Pernicious anemia in a young girl associated with idiopathic hypoparathyroidism, familial Addison's disease, and moniliasis, J. Pediatr. **64:**241, 1964.
105. Rappazzo, M. E., Salmi, H. A., and Hall, C. A.: The content of vitamin B_{12} in adult and foetal tissue: a comparative study, Br. J. Haematol. **18:**425, 1970.
106. Ratnoff, O. D.: Progress of hemostasis and thrombosis. In Spaet, T. H., ed.: Molecular basis of hereditary clotting disorder, New York, 1972, Grune & Stratton, Inc.
107. Reisner, D. J., and Ellsworth, R. M.: Coexistent idiopathic hypoparathyroidism and pernicious anemia in a young girl: case report, Ann. Intern. Med. **43:**1116, 1955.
108. Reisner, E. H., Jr., Wolff, J. A., McKay, R. J., Jr., and Doyle, E. F.: Juvenile pernicious anemia, Pediatrics **8:**88, 1951.
109. Reizenstein, P.: Errors and artefacts in serum folic acid assays, Acta Med. Scand. **178:**133, 1965.
110. Retief, F. P., Gottlieb, C. W., and Herbert, V.: Mecha-

nism of vitamin B_{12} uptake by erythrocytes. J. Clin. Invest. **45:**1907, 1966.

111. Rosenberg, L. E.: Disorders of propionate, methylmalonate and cobalamin metabolism. In Stanbury, J. B., Wyngaarden, J. B., and Fredrickson, D. S., eds.: The metabolic basis of inherited disease, ed. 4, New York, 1976, McGraw-Hill Book Co.

112. Rosenberg, L. E.: Vitamin-responsive inherited metabolic disorders. In Harris, H., and Hirschhorn, K., eds.: Advances in human genetics, Vol. 6, New York, 1976, Plenum Publishing Corp.

113. Rosenberg, L. E., Lilljeqvist, A. C., and Hsia, Y. E.: Methylmalonic aciduria: metabolic block localization and vitamin B_{12} dependency, Science **162:**805, 1968.

114. Ross, G. I. M., and Mollin, D. L.: Vitamin B_{12} in tissues in pernicious anaemia and other conditions. In Heinrich, H. C., ed.: Vitamin B_{12} and intrinsic factor. I. Europäiches symposion, Stuttgart, 1956, Ferdinand Enke Verlag.

115. Rothenberg, S. P., Weisberg, H., and Ficarra, A.: Evidence for the absorption of immunoreactive intrinsic factor into the intestinal epithelial cell during vitamin B_{12} absorption, J. Lab. Clin. Med. **79:**587, 1972.

116. Rubin, C. E., Brandborg, L. L., Flick, A. L., et al.: Studies of celiac sprue. III. The effect of repeated wheat installation into the proximal ileum of patients on a gluten free diet. Gastroenterology **43:**621, 1962.

117. Rubin, H. M., Giorgio, A. J., MacDonald, R. R., and Linarelli, L. G.: Selective malabsorption of vitamin B_{12}: report of a case with metabolic studies, Am. J. Dis. Child. **127:**713, 1974.

118. Schilling, R. F.: Intrinsic factor studies. II. The effect of gastric juice on the urinary excretion of radioactivity after the oral administration of radioactive vitamin B_{12}, J. Lab. Clin. Med. **42:**860, 1953.

119. Skeggs, H. R.: Lactobacillus leishmannii assay for vitamin B_{12}. In Kavanaugh, F., ed.: Analytical microbiology, New York, 1963, Academic Press, Inc.

120. Skouby, A. P., Hippe, E., and Olesen, H.: Antibody to transcobalamin II and B_{12} binding capacity in patients treated with hydroxocobalamin, Blood **38:**769, 1971.

121. Smith, L. H., Jr.: Pyrimidine metabolism in man, N. Engl. J. Med. **288:**764, 1973.

122. Spector, J. I.: Juvenile achlorhydric pernicious anemia with IgA deficiency: a family study, J.A.M.A. **228:**334, 1974.

123. Spurling, C. L., Sacks, M. S., and Jiji, R. M.: Juvenile pernicious anemia, N. Engl. J. Med. **271:**995, 1964.

124. Srikantia, S. G., and Reddy, V.: Megaloblastic anaemia of infancy and vitamin B_{12}, Br. J. Haematol. **13:**949, 1967.

125. Stebbins, R., Scott, J., and Herbert, V.: Therapeutic trial in the test tube: the "dU suppression test" using "physiologic" doses of B_{12} and folic acid to replace therapeutic trial in vivo for diagnosis of B_{12} and folate deficiency, Blood **40:**927, 1972.

126. Strauss, E. W., and Wilson, T. H.: Factors controlling B_{12} uptake by intestinal sacs in vitro, Am. J. Physiol. **198:**103, 1960.

127. Sullivan, L. W.: Differential diagnosis and management of the patient with megaloblastic anemia, Am. J. Med. **48:**609, 1970.

128. Tan, C. H., and Hansen, H. J.: Studies on the site of synthesis of transcobalamin II. Proc. Soc. Exp. Biol. Med. **127:**740, 1968.

129. Tomkin, G. H., Mawhinney, H., and Nevin, N. C.: Isolated absence of IgA with autosomal dominant inheritance, Lancet **2:**124, 1971.

130. Twomey, J. J., et al.: The syndrome of immunoglobulin deficiency and pernicious anemia, Am. J. Med. **47:**340, 1969.

131. Walters, T. R., and Koch, H. F.: Generalize malabsorption, failure to thrive and megaloblastic anemia: result of cyanocobalamin deficiency, Am. J. Dis. Child. **124:**766, 1972.

132. Waters, A. H., and Murphy, M. E. B.: Familial juvenile pernicious anaemia: a study of hereditary basis of pernicious anaemia, Br. J. Haematol. **9:**1, 1963.

133. Waxman, S., and Gilbert, H.: A tumor related vitamin B_{12}-binding protein in juvenile hepatoma, N. Engl. J. Med. **289:**1053, 1973.

134. Wuepper, K. D., and Fudenberg, H. H.: Moniliasis "autoimmune" polyendocrinopathy and immunologic family study, J. Clin. Exp. Immunol. **2:**71, 1967.

Folic acid

135. Adams, E. B., Scragg, J. N., Naidoo, B. T., et al.: Observations on the aetiology and treatment of anaemia in kwashiorkor, Br. Med. J. **3:**451, 1967.

136. Allen, D. M., and Whitehead, R. G.: The excretion of urocanic acid and formiminoglutamic acid in megaloblastosis accompanying kwashiorkor, Blood **25:**283, 1965.

137. Alperin, J. B.: Folic acid deficiency complicating sickle cell anemia, Arch. Intern. Med. **120:**298, 1967.

138. Arakawa, T.: Congenital defects in folate utilization, Am. J. Med. **48:**594, 1970.

139. Arakawa, T., Fujii, M., and Ohara, K.: Erythrocyte formiminotransferase activity in formiminotransferase deficiency syndrome, Tohoku J. Exp. Med. **88:**195, 1966.

140. Arakawa, T., Narisawa, K., Tanno, K., et al.: Megaloblastic anemia and mental retardation associated with hyperfolic acidemia: probably due to N^5 methyltetrahydrofolate transferase deficiency, Tohoku J. Exp. Med. **93:**1, 1967.

141. Arakawa, T., Ohara, K., Kudo, Z., et al.: "Hyperfolicacidemia with formiminoglutamic-aciduria following histidine loading": suggested for a case of congenital deficiency in formiminotransferase, Tohoku J. Exp. Med. **80:**370, 1963.

142. Arakawa, T., Ohara, K., Takahashi, Y., et al.: Formiminotransferase deficiency syndrome: a new inborn error of folic acid metabolism, Ann. Pediatr. **205:**1, 1965.

143. Arakawa, T., Tamura, T., Higashi, O., et al.: Formiminotransferase deficiency syndrome associated with megaloblastic anemia responsive to pyridoxine or folic acid, Tohoku J. Exp. Med. **94:**3, 1968.

144. Arakawa, T., Yoshida, T., Konno, T., et al.: Defect of incorporation of glycine-1-^{14}C into urinary uric acid in formiminotransferase deficiency syndrome, Tohoku J. Exp. Med. **106:**213, 1972.

145. Baker, S. J., Kumar, S., and Swaminathen, S. P.: Excretion of folic acid in bile, Lancet **1:**685, 1965.

146. Baugh, C. M.: Studies on the absorption and metabolism of folic acid. I. Folate absorption in the dog after exposure of violated intestinal segments to synthetic pteroylpolyglutamates of various chain lengths, J. Clin. Invest. **50:**2009, 1971.

147. Becroft, D. M. O., and Phillips, L. I.: Hereditary orotic aciduria and megaloblastic anaemia: a second case with response to uridine, Br. Med. J. **1:**547, 1965.

148. Brusner, O., Reid, A., Monckeberg, F., Maccioni, A., and Contreras, I.: Jejunal biopsies in infant malnutrition with special reference to mitotic index, Pediatrics **38:**605, 1966.

149. Burland, W. L., Simpson, K., et al.: Response of low birthweight infants to treatment with folic acid, Arch. Dis. Child. **46:**189, 1971.

150. Butterworth, C. E., Jr., Bauch, C. M., and Krumdieck, C.: A study of folate absorption and metabolism in man utilizing carbon-14-labelled polyglutamates synthesized

by the solid phase method, J. Clin. Invest. **48:**1131, 1969.

151. Carter, F. C., Heller, P., Schaffner, G., and Korn, R. J.: Formiminoglutamic acid (FIGLU) excretion in hepatic cirrhosis, Arch. Int. Med. **108:**41, 1961.
152. Chanarin, I., Dacie, J. V., and Mollin, D. L.: Folic-acid deficiency in haemolytic anaemia, Br. J. Haematol. **5:**245, 1959.
153. Chanarin, I., Hutchinson, M., McLean, A., and Moule, M.: Hepatic folate in man, Br. Med. J. **1:**396, 1966.
154. Chanarin, I., Mollin, D. L., and Anderson, B. B.: The clearance from the plasma of folic acid injected intravenously in normal subjects and patients with megaloblastic anaemia, Br. J. Haematol. **4:**435, 1958.
155. Chanarin, I., Rothman, D., Ward, A., and Perry, J.: Folate status and requirement in pregnancy, Br. Med. J. **2:**390, 1968.
156. Chanarin, I., Rothman, D., and Watson-Williams, E. J.: Normal formiminoglutamic acid excretion in megaloblastic anaemia of pregnancy. Studies of histidine metabolism in pregnancy, Lancet **1:**1068, 1963.
157. Cooper, B. A., and Lowenstein, L.: Relative folate deficiency of erythrocytes in pernicious anemia and its correction with cyanocobalamin, Blood **24:**502, 1964.
158. Dacie, J. V., and Lewis, S. M.: Practical haematology, ed. 3, New York, 1963, Grune & Stratton, Inc.
159. DeGruchy, G. C.: Clinical haematology in medical practice, Springfield, Ill., 1958, Charles C Thomas, Publisher.
160. Deller, D. J., Ibbotson, R. N., and Crompton, B.: Metabolic effect of partial gastrectomy with special reference to calcium and folic acid. II. The contribution of folic acid deficiency to the anaemia, Gut **5:**225, 1964.
161. Erbe, R. W.: Inborn errors of folate metabolism, N. Engl. J. Med. **293:**807, 1975.
162. Fallon, H. J., Smith, L. H., Graham, J. B., and Burnett, C. H.: A genetic study of hereditary orotic aciduria, N. Engl. J. Med. **270:**878, 1964.
163. Flexner, J. M., and Hartmann, R. C.: Megaloblastic anemia associated with anticonvulsant drugs, Am. J. Med. **28:**386, 1960.
164. Ford, J. E., and Scott, K. J.: The folic acid activity of some milk foods for babies, J. Dairy Res. **35:**85, 1968.
165. Franklin, J. L., and Rosenberg, N. H.: Impaired folic acid absorption in inflammatory bowel disease: effects of salicylazosulfapyridine (azulfidine), Gastroenterology **64:**517, 1973.
166. Fry, L., Keir, P., McMinn, R. M. H., Cowan, J. D., and Hoffbrand, A. V.: Small intestinal structure and function and haematological changes in dermatitis herpetiformis, Lancet **2:**729, 1967.
167. Gandy, G., and Jacobson, W.: Influence of folic acid on birthweight and growth of the erythroblastotic infant. I. Birthweight, Arch. Dis. Child. **52:**1, 1977.
168. Gandy, G., and Jacobson, W.: Influence of folic acid on birthweight and growth of the erythroblastotic infant. II. Growth during the first year, Arch. Dis. Child. **52:**7, 1977.
169. Gandy, G., and Jacobson, W.: Influence of folic acid on birthweight and growth of the erythroblastotic infant. III. Effect of folic acid supplementation, Arch. Dis. Child. **52:**16, 1977.
170. Ghitis, J.: The labile folate of milk, Am. J. Clin. Nutr. **18:**452, 1966.
171. Granville, N., and Dameshek, W.: Hemochromatosis with megaloblastic anemia responding to folic acid, N. Engl. J. Med. **258:**586, 1958.
172. Gray, O. P., and Butler, E. B.: Megaloblastic anaemia in premature infants, Arch. Dis. Child. **40:**53, 1965.
173. Gross, R. L., Newberne, P. M., and Reid, J. V. O.: Adverse effects of infant development associated with maternal folic acid deficiency, Nutr. Rep. Int. **10:**241, 1974.
174. Gross, R. L., Reid, J. V. O., Newberne, P. M., et al.: Depressed cell-mediated immunity in megaloblastic anemia due to folic acid deficiency, Am. J. Clin. Nutr. **28:**225, 1975.
175. Gross, S.: Hematologic studies on erythropoietic porphyria: a new case with severe hemolysis, chronic thrombocytopenia, and folic acid deficiency, Blood **23:**762, 1964.
176. Grossowicz, N., Aronovitch, J., Rachmilewitz, I., et al.: Folic and folinic acid in maternal and foetal blood, Br. J. Haematol. **6:**296, 1960.
177. Halsted, C. H., Sourial, N., Guindi, S., et al.: Anemia of kwashiorkor in Cairo: deficiencies of protein, iron and folic acid, Am. J. Clin. Nutr. **22:**1371, 1969.
178. Hampers, C. L., et al.: Megaloblastic hematopoiesis in uremia and in patients on long-term hemodialysis, N. Engl. J. Med. **276:**551, 1967.
179. Hansen, H. A., and Weinfeld, A.: Metabolic effects and diagnostic value of small doses of folic acid and B_{12} in megaloblastic anemias, Acta Med. Scand. **172:**427,
180. Harris, J. W., Price, J. M., Whittington, R., et al.: Pyridoxine responsive anemia in the adult human, J. Clin. Invest. **35:**709, 1956.
181. Hatch, F. T., Larrabee, A. R., Cathou, R. E., and Buchanan, J. M.: Enzymatic synthesis of the methyl group of methionine. I. Identification of the enzymes and cofactors involved in the system isolated from *Escherichia coli,* J. Biol. Chem. **236:**1095, 1961.
182. Herbert, V.: The assay and nature of folic acid activity in human serum, J. Clin. Invest. **40:**81, 1961.
183. Herbert, V.: The evaluation of assay methods in folic acid deficiency, Blood **17:**368, 1961.
184. Herbert, V.: Experimental nutritional folate deficiency in man, Trans. Assoc. Am. Phys. **75:**307, 1962.
185. Herbert, V.: Minimal daily adult folate requirement, Arch. Intern. Med. **110:**649, 1962.
186. Herbert, V., Baker, H., Frank, O., et al.: The measurement of folic acid activity in serum: a diagnostic acid in the differentiation of the megaloblastic anemias, Blood **15:**223, 1960.
187. Herbert, V., Larabee, A. R., and Buchanan, J. M.: Studies on the identification of a folate compound of human serum, J. Clin. Invest. **41:**1134, 1962.
188. Herbert, V., and Zalusky, R.: Interrelations of vitamin B_{12} and folic acid metabolism: folic acid clearance studies, J. Clin. Invest. **41:**1263, 1962.
189. Herbert, V., Zalusky, R., and Davison, C. S.: Correlation of folate deficiency with alcoholism and associated macrocytosis, anemia, and liver disease, Ann. Intern. Med. **58:**977, 1963.
190. Herman, R. H., Rosensweiz, N. S., Stifel, F. B., et al.: Adult formiminotransferase deficiency: a new entity, Clin. Res. **17:**304, 1969.
191. Hoffbrand, A. V.: Folate absorption, J. Clin. Pathol. **24**(suppl.):66, 1971.
192. Hoffbrand, A. V.: The red cell folate assay, D.M. thesis, Oxford, 1972, University of Oxford.
193. Hoffbrand, A. V., Chanarin, I., Kremenchuzky, S., et al.: Megaloblastic anaemia in myelosclerosis, Q. J. Med. **37:**493, 1968.
194. Hoffbrand, A. V., Neale, G., Hines, J. D., and Mollin, D. L.: The excretion of formiminoglutamic acid and urocanic acid after partial gastrectomy, Lancet **1:**1231, 1966.
195. Hoffbrand, A. V., and Necheles, T. F.: Mechanisms of folate deficiency in patients receiving phenytoin, Lancet **2:**538, 1968.

196. Hoffbrand, A. V., and Newcombe, B. F. A.: Leucocyte folate content in vitamin B$_{12}$ and folate deficiency in leukemia, Br. J. Haematol. **13:**954, 1967.
197. Hoffbrand, A. V., Newcombe, B. F. A., and Mollin, D. L.: Method of assay of red cell folate and the value of the assay as a test for folate deficiency, J. Clin. Pathol. **19:**17, 1966.
198. Hoffbrand, A. V., and Peters, T. J.: Recent advances in clinical and biochemical aspects of folate, Schwiez. Med. Wochenschr. **100:**1954, 1970.
199. Hoffbrand, A. V., Stewart, J. S., Booth, C. C., and Mollin, D. L.: Folate deficiency in Crohn's disease: Incidence, pathogenesis and treatment, Br. Med. J. **2:**71, 1968.
200. Hoffbrand, A. V., et al.: Incidence and pathogenesis of megaloblastic erythropoiesis in multiple myeloma, J. Clin. Pathol. **20:**699, 1967.
201. Hoffbrand, A. V., et al.: Megaloblastic anemia in myelosclerosis, Q. J. Med. **37:**493, 1968.
202. Huguley, C. M., Bain, J. A., Rivers, S. L., and Scoggins, R. B.: Refractory megaloblastic anemia associated with the excretion of orotic acid, Blood **14:**615, 1959.
203. Jandl, J. H., and Greenberg, M. S.: Bone marrow failure due to relative nutritional deficiency in Cooley's haemolytic anemia, N. Engl. J. Med. **260:**461, 1959.
204. Johns, D. G., Sperti, S., and Burger, A. S. V.: The metabolism of tritiated folic acid in man, J. Clin. Invest. **40:**1684, 1961.
205. Kho, L. K., and Odang, O.: Megaloblastic anemia in infancy and childhood in Djakarta, Am. J. Dis. Child. **97:**209, 1959.
206. Klipstein, F. A.: Folate deficiency secondary to disease of the intestinal tract, Bull. N.Y. Acad. Med. **42:**638, 1966.
207. Kohn, J., Mollin, D. L., and Rosenbach, L. M.: Conventional voltage electrophoresis for formiminoglutamic-acid determination in folic acid deficiency, J. Clin. Pathol. **14:**345, 1961.
208. Kondi, A., MacDougall, L., Foy, H., et al.: Anaemias of marasmus and kwashiorkor in Kenya, Arch. Dis. Child. **38:**267, 1963.
209. Lampkin, B. C., Pyesmany, A., Hyman, C. B., and Hammond, D.: Congenital familial megaloblastic anemia, Blood **37:**615, 1971.
210. Lanzkowsky, P.: Congenital malabsorption of folate associated with mental retardation, Paper presented at the International Symposium on Nutritional Deficiency Secondary to Inborn Errors of Metabolism, U.S.-Japan Cooperative Medical Science Program, Sendai, Japan, December 1976.
211. Lanzkowsky, P., Erlandson, M. E., and Bezan, A.: Isolated defect of folic acid absorption associated with mental retardation and cerebral calcification, Blood **34:**452, 1969.
212. Levy, H. L., Truman, J. T., Ganz, R. N., and Littlefield, J. W.: Folic acid deficiency secondary to a diet for maple syrup urine disease, J. Pediatr. **77:**294, 1970.
213. Lindenbaum, J., and Klipstein, F. A.: Folic acid deficiency in sickle cell anemia, N. Engl. J. Med. **269:**875, 1963.
214. Lindenbaum, J., and Klipstein, F. A.: Folic acid clearances and basal serum folate levels in patients with thyroid disease, J. Clin. Pathol. **17:**666, 1964.
215. London, M. J., and Hey, E. N.: Renal loss of folate in the newborn infant, Arch. Dis. Child. **49:**292, 1974.
216. Loughlin, R. E., Elford, H. L., and Buchanan, J. M.: Enzymatic synthesis of the methyl group of methionine. VII. Isolate of a cobalamin containing transmethylase (5-methyl-tetra-hydrofolate-homocysteine) from mammalian liver, J. Biol. Chem. **239:**2888, 1964.

217. Luhby, A. L.: Megaloblastic anemia in infancy: clinical considerations and analysis, J. Pediatr. **54:**617, 1959.
218. Luhby, A. L., and Cooperman, J. M.: Congenital megaloblastic anemia and progressive central nervous system degeneration. Further clinical and physiological characterization and therapy of syndrome due to inborn error of folate transport, Paper presented at the annual meeting of American Pediatric Society, Inc., Atlantic City, N.J., April 1967.
219. Luhby, A. L., Cooperman, J. M., and Pesci-Bourel, A.: A new inborn error of metabolism: folic acid responsive megaloblastic anemia, ataxia, mental retardation and convulsions, Paper presented at the annual meeting of American Pediatric Society, Inc., Philadelphia, May 1965.
220. Luhby, A. L., Eagle, F. J., Roth, E., and Cooperman, J. M.: Relapsing megaloblastic anemia in an infant due to a specific defect in gastrointestinal absorption of folic acid, Am. J. Dis. Child. **102:**482, 1961.
221. MacGibbon, B. H., and Mollin, D. L.: Sideroblastic anaemia in man; observations on 70 cases, Br. J. Haematol. **11:**59, 1965.
222. MacIver, J. E.: Megaloblastic anemias, Pediatr. Clin. North Am. **9:**727, 1962.
223. Marks, J., Shuster, S., and Watson, A.: Small-bowel changes in dermatitis herpetiformis, Lancet **2:**1280, 1966.
224. Matoth, Y., Pinkas, A., Zamir, R., et al.: Studies on folic acid in infancy. I. Blood levels of folic and folinic acid in healthy infants, Pediatrics **33:**507, 1964.
225. Matoth, Y., Pinkas, A., Zamir, R., et al.: Studies on folic acid in infancy. II. Folic and folinic acid blood levels in infants with diarrhea, malnutrition and infection, Pediatrics **33:**694, 1964.
226. Matoth, Y., Pinkas, A., Zamir, R., et al.: Studies on folic acid in infancy. III. Folates in breast-fed infants and their mothers, Am. J. Clin. Nutr. **16:**356, 1965.
227. McFarland, W., and Libre, E. P.: Abnormal leukocyte response in alcoholism, Ann. Int. Med. **59:**865, 1963.
228. Merrit, A. D., Rucknegal, D. L., Silverman, M., and Gardiner, R. C.: Urinary urocanic acid in man: the identification of urocanic acid and the comparative excretions of urocanic acid and N-formiminoglutamic acid after oral histidine in patients with liver disease, J. Clin. Invest. **41:**1472, 1962.
229. Miller, D. R.: Serum folate deficiency in children receiving anticonvulsant therapy, Pediatrics **41:**630, 1968.
230. Mitchell, H. K., Snell, E. E., and Williams, R. J.: The concentration of folic acid, J. Am. Chem. Soc. **63:**2284, 1941.
231. Mollin, D. L., and Hoffbrand, A. V.: The diagnosis of folate deficiency, Ser. Haematol. **3:**1, 1965.
232. Niederwieser, A., Giliberti, P., Matasovic, A., et al.: Folic acid non-dependent formiminoglutamic aciduria in two siblings, Clin. Chim. Acta **54:**293, 1974.
233. Nieweg, H. O., Faver, J. G., de Vries, J. A., and Kroese, W. F. S.: Relationship of vitamin B$_{12}$ and folic acid in megaloblastic anemias, J. Lab. Clin. Med. **44:**118, 1954.
234. Nixon, P. F., and Bertino, J. R.: Interrelationships of vitamin B$_{12}$ and folate in man, Am. J. Med. **48:**555, 1970.
235. Noronha, J. M., and Aboobaker, V. S.: Studies on the folate compounds of human blood, Arch. Biochem. Biophys. **101:**445, 1963.
236. Noronha, J. M., and Silverman, M.: On folic acid, vitamin B$_{12}$, methionine and formiminoglutamic acid metabolism, in vitamin B$_{12}$ and intrinsic factor. In Heinrich, H. C., ed.: 2nd Europäisches symposion, Stuttgart, 1962, Ferdinand Enke Verlag.

237. Pavlic, G. J., and Bouroncle, B. A.: Megaloblastic crisis in paroxysmal nocturnal hemoglobinuria, N. Engl. J. Med. **273:**789, 1965.

238. Pearson, H. A., and Cobb, W. T.: Folic acid studies in sickle-cell anemia, J. Lab. Clin. Med. **64:**913, 1964.

239. Pereira, S. M., and Baker, S. J.: Hematologic studies in kwashiorkor, Am. J. Clin. Nutr. **18:**413, 1966.

240. Perry, T. L., Applegarth, D. A., Evans, M. E., et al.: Metabolic studies of a family with massive formimino-glutamic aciduria, Pediat. Res. **9:**117, 1975.

241. Perry, J., and Chanarin, I.: Intestinal absorption of reduced folate compounds in man, Br. J. Haematol. **18:**329, 1970.

242. Pitney, W. R., Joske, R. A., and Mackinnon, N. L.: Folic acid and other absorption tests in lymphosarcoma, chronic lymphocytic leukaemia and some related conditions, J. Clin. Pathol. **13:**440, 1960.

243. Post, R. M., and DesForges, J. F.: Thrombocytopenia and alcoholism, Ann. Intern. Med. **68:**1230, 1968.

244. Reisner, E. H., Jr.: The nature and significance of megaloblastic blood formation, Blood **13:**313, 1958.

245. Reizenstein, P.: Errors and artefacts in serum folic acid assays. Effects of age, food, drugs, and radiation, Acta Med. Scand. **178:**133, 1965.

246. Retief, F. P., and Huskisson, Y. J.: Serum and urinary folate in liver disease, Br. Med. J. **2:**150, 1969.

247. Roberts, P. M., Arrowsmith, D. E., et al.: Folate state of premature infants, Arch. Dis. Child. **44:**637, 1969.

248. Rogers, L. E., and Porter, F. S.: Hereditary orotic aciduria. II. A urinary screening test, Pediatrics **42:**423, 1968.

249. Rogers, L. E., Porter, F. S., and Sidbury, J. B., Jr.: Thiamine-responsive megaloblastic anemia, J. Pediatr. **74:**494, 1969.

250. Rogers, L. E., Warford, L. R., Patterson, R. B., and Porter, F. S.: Hereditary orotic aciduria. 1. A case with family studies, Pediatrics **42:**415, 1968.

251. Rook, G. D., Lopez, R., Shimizu, N., and Cooperman, J. M.: Folic acid deficiency in infants and children with heart disease, Br. Heart J. **35:**87, 1973.

252. Rose, D. P.: Folic acid deficiency in leukemia and lymphomas, J. Clin. Pathol. **19:**29, 1966.

253. Royston, N. J. W., and Parry, T. E.: Megaloblastic anemia complicating dietary treatment of phenylketonuria in infancy, Arch. Dis. Child. **37:**430, 1962.

254. Santiago-Borrero, P. J., Santini, R., Perez-Santiago, E., et al.: Congenital isolated defect of folic acid absorption, J. Pediatr. **82:**450, 1973.

255. Scott, R. B., Ellison, R. R., et al.: A clinical study of 20 cases of erythroleukemia (Di Guglielmo's syndrome), Am. J. Med. **37:**162, 1964.

256. Shapiro, J., Alberts, H. W., Welch, P., and Metz, J.: Folate and vitamin B_{12} deficiency associated with lactation, Br. J. Haematol. **11:**498, 1965.

257. Shojania, A. M., and Gross, S.: Folic acid deficiency and prematurity, J. Pediatr. **64:**323, 1964.

258. Shojania, A. M., and Hornady, G.: Folate metabolism in newborns and during early infancy. II. Clearance of folic acid in plasma and excretion of folic acid in urine by newborns, Pediatr. Res. **4:**422, 1970.

259. Shuster, S., Marks, J., and Chanarin, I.: Folic acid deficiency in patients with skin disease, Br. J. Dermatol. **79:**398, 1967.

260. Smith, L. H., Jr.: Pyrimidine metabolism in man, N. Engl. J. Med. **288:**764, 1973.

261. Smith, L. H., Jr., Huguley, C. M., Jr., and Bain, J. A.: Hereditary orotic aciduria. In Stanbury, J. B., Wyngaarden, J. B., and Fredrickson, D. S., eds.: The metabolic basis of inherited disease, New York, 1972, McGraw-Hill Book Co.

262. Spector, I., and Metz, J.: Folate and vitamin B_{12} metabolism in weanling rats given a maize diet, Am. J. Clin. Nutr. **19:**187, 1966.

263. Spector, I., and Metz, J.: Giant myeloid cells in the bone marrow of protein malnourished infants: relationship to folate and vitamin B_{12} nutrition, Br. J. Haematol. **12:**737, 1966.

264. Spray, G. H., Fourman, P., and Witts, L. J.: The excretion of small doses of folic acid, Br. Med. J. **2:**202, 1951.

265. Spray, G. H., and Witts, L. J.: Excretion of formiminoglutamic acid as an index of folic acid deficiency, Lancet **2:**702, 1959.

266. Stebbins, R., Scott, J., and Herbert, V.: Drug-induced megaloblastic anemias, Semin. Hematol. **10:**235, 1973.

267. Streiff, R. R.: Malabsorption of polyglutamic folic acid secondary to oral contraceptives, Clin. Res. **17:**71, 1969.

268. Strelling, M. K., Blackledge, G. D., Goodall, H. B., and Walker, C. H. M.: Megaloblastic anaemia and whole blood folate levels in premature infants, Lancet **1:**898, 1966.

269. Sullivan, L. W., and Herbert, V.: Suppression of hematopoiesis by ethanol, J. Clin. Invest. **43:**2048, 1964.

270. Sullivan, L. W., Luhby, A. L., and Streiff, R. R.: Studies on the daily requirement for folic acid in infants and the etiology of folate deficiency in goat's milk megaloblastic anemia, Am. J. Clin. Nutr. **18:**311, 1966.

271. Swendseid, M. E., Bethell, F. H., and Bird, O. D.: The concentration of folic acid in leucocytes: observations in normal subjects and persons with leukemia, Cancer Res. **11:**864, 1951.

272. Tauro, G. P., Danks, D. M., Rowe, P. B., et al.: Dihydrofolate reductase deficiency causing megaloblastic anemia in two families, N. Engl. J. Med. **294:**466, 1976.

273. Toghill, P. J.: Megaloblastic anaemia in haemochromatosis, Postgrad. Med. J. **41:**86, 1965.

274. Van der Zee, S. P. M., Lommen, E. J. P., Trijbels, J. M. F., et al.: The influence of adenine on the clinical features and purine metabolism in the Lesch-Nyhan syndrome, Acta Paediatr. Scand. **59:**259, 1970.

275. Van der Zee, S. P. M., Schretlen, E. D. A. M., and Monnens, L. A. H.: Megaloblastic anemia in the Lesch-Nyhan syndrome, Lancet **1:**1427, 1968.

276. Vanier, T. M., and Tyas, J. F.: Folic acid status in normal infants during the first year of life, Arch. Dis. Child. **41:**658, 1966.

277. Vanier, T. M., and Tyas, J. F.: Folic acid status in premature infants, Arch. Dis. Child. **42:**57, 1967.

278. Walters, T.: Congenital megaloblastic anemia responsive to N^5-formyl tetrahydrofolic acid administration, J. Pediatr. **70:**686, 1967.

279. Welch, A. D., and Heinle, R. W.: Hematopoietic agents in macrocytic anemias, Pharmacol. Rev. **3:**345, 1951.

280. Whitehead, V. M., and Cooper, B. A.: Absorption of unaltered folic acid from the gastro-intestinal tract in man, Br. J. Haematol. **13:**679, 1967.

281. Whitehead, V. M., et al.: Homeostasis of folic acid in patients undergoing maintenance hemodialysis, N. Engl. J. Med. **279:**970, 1968.

282. Wilcken, B., and Turner, B.: Homocystinuria: reduced folate levels during pyridoxine treatment, Arch. Dis. Child. **48:**58, 1973.

283. Willoughby, M. L. N.: An investigation of folic acid requirements in pregnancy, Br. J. Haematol. **13:**503, 1967.

284. Willoughby, M. L. N., and Jewell, F. J.: Investigation of folic acid requirements in pregnancy, Br. Med. J. **2:**1568, 1966.
285. Zalusky, R., and Herbert, V.: Failure of formiminoglutamic acid (FIGLU) excretion to distinguish vitamin B_{12} deficiency from nutritional folic acid deficiency, J. Clin. Invest. **40:**1091, 1961.
286. Zuelzer, W. W., and Ogden, F. N.: Megaloblastic anemia in infancy, Am. J. Dis. Child. **71:**211, 1946.

8 □ Erythropoiesis and hypoplastic anemias

Denis R. Miller

Normal erythropoiesis

Erythropoiesis, the production of erythrocytes, is intimately related to the primary function of the red blood cell, namely the delivery of oxygen to and the removal of carbon dioxide from the tissues. The factors that modulate erythrocyte production (Fig. 8-1) consist of a finely tuned circuit of stimulators and inhibitors, including the circulating red cell mass and its precursors in the bone marrow, the quantity and functional characteristics of hemoglobin, the intraerythrocyte environment (which influences the affinity of hemoglobin for oxygen), the functional capacity of the cardiovascular and pulmonary systems, and the hormonal regulator of erythropoiesis (erythropoietin). The essential kinetic and physiologic aspects of normal erythropoiesis are considered in the first section of this chapter; clinical disorders of erythropoiesis are discussed in the second section.

THE ERYTHRON AND CELLULAR KINETICS OF ERYTHROPOIESIS

The term "erythron"[13] refers to the tissues that comprise the circulating red blood cells and their precursors in the bone marrow. It conveys a sense of functional unity to a series of morphologically recognizable cells, ranging from the early pronormoblast to the nonnucleated red corpuscle. However, a discussion of the erythron (one of the committed compartments of hematopoiesis) must begin with an overview of the multipotential hematopoietic stem cell.

Metcalf[98] has proposed that hematopoietic populations are organized in a sequence of four functional compartments, each of which is larger and less capable of self-replication than the preceding one. In a steady state the compartments consist of the following:

1. *Stem cells* comprise 0.2% of the population and are capable of self-replication. They are multipotential and undifferentiated morphologically; most are in a resting, or G_0, state.
2. *Progenitor cells* comprise about 1.0% of the population. They are possibly capable of self-replication, are uni- or bipotential, and are undifferentiated morphologically; 70% to 80% of these cells are in DNA synthesis (S phase).
3. *Proliferating differentiated cells* comprise about 2% to 10% of the population. These cells are possibly capable of limited self-replication, are unipotential, and are morphologically differentiated and in continuous cell cycle.
4. *Maturing and end cells* comprise about 90% of the population and are incapable of division; most are mature end cells.

Little was known until recently about the dynamic interrelationship between the multipotential stem cells and the erythron. Stem cells have never been identified morphologically, although recent studies suggest that they are small lymphocyte-like or transitional cells[31] that form a heterogeneous population within the bone marrow. The study of hematopoietic stem cells was revolutionized by the introduction of the spleen colony technique of Till and McCulloch[134] in which hematopoietic cells are injected intravenously in lethally irradiated compatible mice, migrate to the spleen, and then proliferate to form discrete colonies of hematopoietic cells. Splenic colonies produced by a single stem cell, or colony-forming unit (CFU), are comprised of pure populations of erythroid or myeloid cells, megakaryocytes, or mixtures of two or more of these cells. By using marker chromosomes it was shown that each colony or clone is derived from a single stem cell.[8] Three features of spleen colonies prove that the cells initiating colony formation are stem cells:

1. Most colonies contain stem cells, indicating that the cells originating the colony are capable of self-maintenance.
2. Stem cells in any one colony are multipotential and able to generate colonies of all morphologic types.
3. On continued growth most colonies contain erythroid, myeloid, and megakaryocytic cells, reemphasizing the multipotential nature of the stem cell.

The exact number of hematopoietic stem cells in human bone marrow is unknown but Schofield and Lajtha[120] have calculated that in the mouse

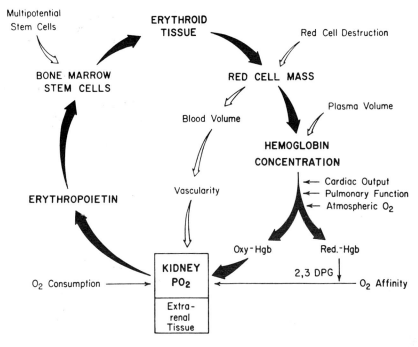

Fig. 8-1. Updated feedback circuit with the incorporation of blood volume and hemoglobin oxygen affinity in the oxygen-transporting direction, with the kidney and a hypothetical extrarenal tissue as the oxygen-sensing organ, and with the unipotential bone marrow stem cell as the target cell for erythropoietin. (From Erslev, A. J.: In Nakao, K., Fisher, J. W., and Takaku, F., eds.: Erythropoiesis, Tokyo/Baltimore, 1974, University of Tokyo Press/University Park Press.)

2×10^5 cycling stem cells give rise to about 4.5×10^8 red cells daily. In humans the daily production of red blood cells is 3×10^9 cells/kg.[32] The bone marrow erythropoietic pool (normoblasts plus reticulocytes) is approximately 7.95×10^9 cells/kg.

Recently a population of large lymphocytes without T or B cell characteristics has been separated from human peripheral blood mononuclear cells; on culture in vivo in diffusion chambers this population has proliferated and differentiated into erythrocytic, granulocytic, and megakaryocytic progeny, marking the first clear demonstration of hematopoietic stem cells in humans. The presence of these cells in the peripheral blood is not surprising since they may be in transit from one hematopoietic site to another. Pluripotential progenitor cells have not yet been separated, isolated, and unequivocally identified in human bone marrow.[6]

Previously it was thought that stem cells differentiated directly into pronormoblasts. More recent studies demonstrated the presence of an intermediate compartment of erythroid-committed precursors (ECPs) or progenitor cells.[82]

These cells precede the cells that synthesize hemoglobin and proceed through five to ten doublings before entering the recognizable erythron.

This compartment of erythroid-committed precursors acts as an amplifier of the erythron and produces a continuous excess of cells in normal and abnormal conditions, whether or not a demand for differentiated cells exists. Cells in the later stages of the compartment are sensitive to the differentiating effect of erythropoietin and have been termed erythropoietin-sensitive or erythropoietin-responsive cells (ESCs or ERCs).[120]

The third functional stage of erythropoiesis is the recognizable erythron itself, which consists of proliferating differentiated erythroid precursors (pronormoblasts and basophilic and early polychromatophilic normoblasts) and the maturing erythroid precursors, the late polychromatophilic and orthochromic normoblasts, and the reticulocytes. In steady state conditions the maturation time from pronormoblast to erythrocyte is about 4 to 6 days, with cells remaining in each stage of maturation for approximately 1 day.[32,83] The generation times, the times from one mitosis to another for the proliferating erythroid precursors, are 0.83 day for the pronormoblasts and basophilic normoblasts and 1.25 days for polychromatophilic normoblasts.[32,78] The period of DNA synthesis is 12 to 16 hours and of mitosis 30 to 40 minutes. During this period three to four mitotic divisions occur, so that one pronormoblast produces eight to sixteen mature erythrocytes. Normally approximately 10% to 15% of the erythroid precursors die after cell division; therefore a smaller number of cells is the product of skipped mitotic divisions. Increased intramedullary destruction of red blood cell precursors is termed ineffective erythropoiesis.

In the absence of stress reticulocytes remain in the bone marrow for 1 to 2 days.[38] Their physical characteristics of stickiness and nondeformability impede their release from the bone marrow.[84] They remain in the circulation as reticulocytes for another day. The distribution of cells in the erythropoietic pool and their generation and turnover times are listed in Table 8-1.

Theoretically, on the basis of this kinetic concept of erythropoiesis, a number of mechanisms exist whereby red blood cell production can be increased. These mechanisms include (1) shortening of generation time, (2) acceleration of maturation by omission of one or more intermediate mitotic divisions, (3) diminution of ineffective erythropoiesis, and (4) acceleration of maturation of the nondividing erythroid precursors. Autoradiographic studies show that cell cycle time may be shortened in response to hypovolemia and hemolysis.[4,63,143] In stress erythropoiesis mitotic divisions may be skipped and polychromatophilic reticulocytes may be released prematurely into the circulation where maturation occurs (rather than in the bone marrow). The major mechanism of increasing erythropoiesis, however, is to amplify the number of erythroid-committed precursors that, under the stimulation of erythropoietin, will become differentiated, proliferating pronormoblasts and, in 4 days, mature erythrocytes.

In vitro techniques have been developed recently that permit the growth and differentiation of erythroid colonies in cultures implanted in plasma clots,[124] on methylcellulose,[27,72] or in fluid suspension.[50] The precursor cells from which these colonies arise have been called CFU-Es (erythroid colony forming units); they are extremely sensitive to erythropoietin and do not form erythroid colonies in its absence. These cells are considered to be late erythropoietin-responsive cells of the erythroid-committed precursor. A second erythroid colony-producing cell produces "bursts" of erythroid colonies and has been termed BFU-E (erythroid burst forming unit). The BFU-Es are ten times less sensitive to erythropoietin than CFU-Es and are probably precursors of the CFU-Es. Recent studies suggest that BFU-Es are null cells and require T cells for proliferation.[247]

These in vitro techniques have greatly advanced our understanding of the cellular kinetics of erythroid differentiation and are now being applied to clinical disorders of hematopoiesis.

ROLE OF MICROENVIRONMENT IN ERYTHROPOIESIS

Normal erythropoiesis requires three factors: (1) hematopoietic stem cells, (2) specific hormonal regulators, and (3) a microenvironment consisting of supporting stroma and cell-to-cell interactions that permit differentiation, proliferation, and transformation of stem cells into committed erythroid precursors.[95,102] It is unlikely that proliferation and differentiation from the progenitor stage onward through the erythron requires microenvironmental influences because of the ability to grow erythroid colonies in vitro. However, considerable existing evidence supports the role of a hospitable and inductive microenvironment that permits the initial conversion of a multipotential hematopoietic stem cell to a committed erythroid progenitor. In the spleen colony system employed by Trentin[136] areas or microenvironments exist with specific inductive capacities that commit the cell to one specific pathway of differentiation by selectively derepressing part of the genome, initiating proliferation of stem cells, and leading to the generation of an expanding clone of progeny cells of one cell line (erythroid, myeloid, or megakaryocytic). When bone was implanted in the white pulp of the spleen of lethally irradiated animals, granulocytic differentiation occurred ad-

Table 8-1. Distribution of cells and cellular kinetics of the erythron*

Cell type	No. of cells/kg body weight (×10⁹)	Relative No. of cells	Generation time (days)	Turnover time (days)
Nucleated red blood cells	5.0	1.5	4-6	
Pronormoblasts	0.10		0.83	
Basophilic normoblasts	0.48		0.83	
Polychromatophilic normoblasts	1.47		1.25	
Orthochromic normoblasts	2.95			2.07
Reticulocytes (bone marrow)	5.0	1.5		1.67
Reticulocytes (peripheral blood)	3.3	1.0		1-3
Mature erythrocytes	330.0	100.0		120

*Data from Donohoe et al.[32] and Lajtha and Oliver.[83]

jacent to bone spicules, whereas the red pulp favored erythropoiesis.

The best experimental illustration of the importance of the microenvironment is provided by cross-transplantation studies in two strains of genetically anemic mice. The first, *Sl/Sl*^{d}, has normal hematopoietic stem cells but a defective splenic microenvironment, which does not support erythropoiesis.[94] The second, *W/W*^{v}, has a normal microenvironment but an abnormal multipotential stem cell.[93] Cross-exchange of cell or organ grafts between these strains of mice restores normal erythropoiesis.

PHYSIOLOGY OF OXYGEN DELIVERY

The interrelated factors affecting oxygen delivery to the tissues are presented schematically in Fig. 8-2. Hemoglobin becomes fully saturated with oxygen at the pulmonary capillary Po_2 of 100 mm Hg. Oxygen delivery to the tissues can be represented by the differences between the saturation of arterial and venous blood. This difference is determined by the amount of oxygen released by hemoglobin during tissue perfusion. In the case of

normally structured hemoglobin this process is influenced by the Pco_2 and pH of the blood, the MCHC, and the concentration of erythrocyte organic phosphate compounds (primarily 2,3-DPG and secondarily ATP).

The influence of pH on the oxygen dissociation curve (Bohr effect) is a result of the reciprocal binding of oxygen and hydrogen ion by deoxyhemoglobin. Acidosis decreases and alkalosis increases the affinity of hemoglobin for oxygen. In addition to the effect of pH on oxyhemoglobin concentration, a marked decrease in blood pH can reduce the glycolytic activity of erythrocytes and the synthesis of 2,3-DPG and ATP, thereby affecting the affinity of hemoglobin for oxygen. The dissociation of oxygen from hemoglobin at the tissue level is facilitated by increased intraerythrocytic 2,3-DPG and ATP as a result of their preferential binding to deoxyhemoglobin. In the absence of a change in the red blood cell mass or rate of blood flow, oxygen delivery by a normal molecule of hemoglobin can be altered by changes in Pco_2 and in the concentrations of blood hydrogen ions or red cell organic phosphates.

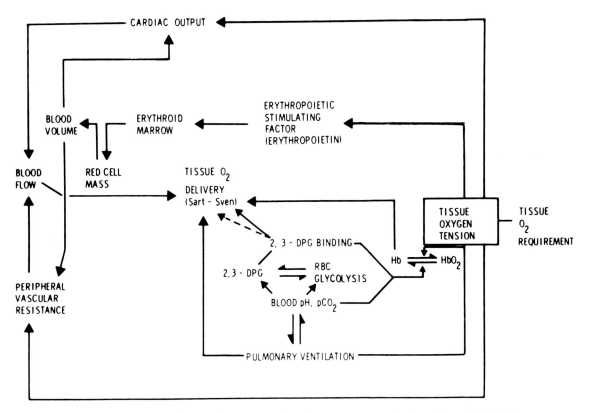

Fig. 8-2. Interrelated regulators of oxygen tension. Compensatory mechanisms for anemia include increase in cardiac output and alterations in peripheral resistance, resulting in redistribution of blood flow to organs. Modifications of intracellular metabolism increase the level of 2,3-DPG, which aids in maximum peripheral oxygen delivery. (Modified from Miller, D. R., and Lichtman, M. A.: In Weed, R. I., ed.: Hematology for internists, Boston, 1971, Little, Brown & Co.)

Cardiovascular compensation can result in increased blood flow in response to a decreased oxygen flow to tissues as a result of a reduction in blood volume or in hemoglobin and red cell mass. The cardiovascular compensatory mechanisms include an increase in cardiac output and alterations in peripheral resistance, resulting in a redistribution of blood flow to vital organs (brain, heart, and liver). This sequence of events is usually a manifestation of acute blood loss and has been studied thoroughly in animals made acutely hypovolemic by reduction in blood volume. In mild to moderate anemia of gradual development cardiac output does not increase.

In addition, in the absence of renal disease and in the presence of a normally responsive marrow, renal chemoreceptors respond to a decreased flow of oxygen by elaborating the hormonal regulator of erythropoiesis, erythropoietin, which acts on erythropoietin-responsive cells of the erythroid-committed precursor compartment and leads to the eventual restoration of hemoglobin and red cell mass.

ERYTHROPOIETIN

Nearly a century ago Bert[9] discovered that high altitude caused polycythemia. Seventy years later Grant and Root[56] showed that hypoxia provides the primary stimulus for erythropoiesis (as evidenced by polycythemia in chronic hypoxic states) and that erythropoiesis is suppressed when oxygen concentration is increased by hyperoxia or hypertransfusion. It was hypothesized that bone marrow hypoxia provided the primary stimulus for erythropoiesis, but this was disproved by direct measurements of the oxygen concentration within the bone marrow. Accordingly an alternative hypothesis, that lowered oxygen tension stimulated bone marrow erythroid activity by mediation of a humoral factor, received more attention. The ability of the serum and plasma of bled animals to induce an increase in reticulocytes, red blood cells, and hemoglobin when injected into normal animals gives support to the presence of such a humoral factor, the existence of which was originally postulated in 1906 by Carnot and Deflandre.[16] Reismann[113] presented the first convincing evidence for the existence of a humoral factor by elegantly demonstrating similar erythroid hyperplasia of the bone marrow in a pair of parabiotic rats following chronic hypoxia induced in only one partner. Erslev et al.[35,36,57] stimulated further interest in this mechanism by the bioassay of large amounts of plasma from bled rabbits and monkeys that had induced reticulocytosis and ^{59}Fe incorporation into newly formed red blood cells in normal animals. Bonsdorff and Jalavist[11] introduced the term "erythropoietin" in 1948.

Biochemistry of erythropoietin

A millionfold purification of erythropoietin from the plasma of anemic sheep has been achieved. The final recovery was small (0.36%), but the purity was high (9,200 units/mg). When erythropoietin was purified from the urine of anemic animals and man, the recovery was fiftyfold greater than that from plasma. Depending on the purification procedure, the molecular weight of erythropoietin is 60,000 to 70,000 daltons and the sedimentation coefficient is 5S to 6S.[51] More recent studies suggest that the molecular weight is lower (40,000 to 62,000 daltons).[79] Chemical analysis revealed that erythropoietin is a glycoprotein in a single polypeptide chain. Thirty percent of the molecule is carbohydrate, of which one third is sialic acid. Biologic activity in vivo was lost after treatment with neuraminidase (which removes sialic acid), but the ability of erythropoietin to stimulate the synthesis of hemoglobin in vitro is unaffected. The proteases trypsin, chymotrypsin, pepsin, and papain also inactivated the hormone by cleaving lysine and/or arginine bonds of the polypeptide.[123] Millipore filtration[137] also destroyed the activity of erythropoietin, but *p*-chloromercuribenzoate[51] (which inactivates sulfhydryl groups), fluorescein isothiocyanate, iodination, acetylation, and esterification of carboxyl groups had no destructive effect.[79]

The biologic assay of erythropoietin employs mice in which polycythemia has been induced and erythropoiesis has been suppressed by hypertransfusion[47] or hypoxia[28] or both. The test material of erythropoietin is injected subcutaneously and is followed a few days later by the intravenous injection of ^{59}Fe. The amount of ^{59}Fe incorporated into the newly formed erythrocytes (induced by the injected erythropoietin) is measured 1 to 3 days later. The international standard (standard B) against which erythropoietin is assayed has been derived from human urine. An international unit of erythropoietin is defined as the activity present in 1.48 mg of standard B. Assay procedures with immunologic methods, although theoretically and practically less tedious and time consuming than the assay using the exhypoxic polycythemic mouse, are dependent on a pure antibody to pure erythropoietin. Thus these methods suffer from imprecision and nonspecificity. Normal levels in humans are more accurately determined in urine. Males excrete 2.8 to 4.0 units/day and females 0.9 ± 0.4 units (SD)/day.[2]

Biogenesis of erythropoietin

The kidneys are the major but not the sole site of production of erythropoietin. Approximately 90% of the capacity to increase erythropoietin production in response to anemia and hypoxia resides in the kidneys as demonstrated by studies of erythropoiesis in anephric humans and animals subjected to bilateral nephrectomy. The mechanism by which renal hypoxia stimulates the increased synthesis of erythropoietin is unknown. The perfusion of kidneys with hypoxic blood[81] and with cobalt[43] and renal ischemia induced by constriction of the renal artery[45] all resulted in increased production of erythropoietin. About 10% of erythropoietin is produced in presently unknown extrarenal sites. As demonstrated in patients with severe renal failure, the extrarenal site or sites are responsive to testosterone, which increases erythropoietin levels in patients with severe renal failure.[101] Recent studies of Peschle et al.[111,112] suggest that the reticuloendothelial system (RES) is associated with extrarenal production of erythropoietin. In anephric rats a correlation was observed between hyperplasia of the RES and the potentiation of the erythropoietin response to hypoxia. Kupfer cells seemed to have an important role since subtotal hepatectomy prevented the production of erythropoietin.[46] Thus it is conceivable that extrarenal sites become activated when the renal sites are shut off or destroyed.

The precursor of biologically active erythropoietin (renal erythropoietic factor, REF) appears to be synthesized in the light mitochondrial fraction of the renal cortex, medulla, glomeruli, and tubules.[52] Recent studies with fluorescent antibody indicate that the hormone may be synthesized in the visceral epithelial cells of the glomerular tuft.[15]

The biogenesis of erythropoietin has not yet been completely elucidated. Gordon et al.[52] proposed that biologically active erythropoietin required the interaction of a renal enzyme (REF) or erythrogenin with a serum substrate or precursor, possibly synthesized by the liver. Supporting this hypothesis are studies by Zanjani et al.,[148] who showed that the incubation of REF with hypoxic serum rendered devoid of erythropoietin by prior incubation with antierythropoietin resulted in the generation of large amounts of erythropoietin.

Apparently two types of REF, REF I and REF II, exist. REF I is biologically inactive when administered by itself but REF II possesses erythropoietic activity, which is not further enhanced by incubation with serum. Some preparations containing a mixture of REF I and II possess erythropoietic activity that is enhanced on incubation with normal serum. Immunologic studies performed by Peschle and Condorelli[111] using REF II, antierythropoietin antibody, and goal antirabbit γ-globulin, showed that the erythropoietic activity of REF II was neutralized by antierythropoietin and that REF II, immunologically and biologically indistinct from erythropoietin, is equivalent to circulating, biologically active erythropoietin. REF I is

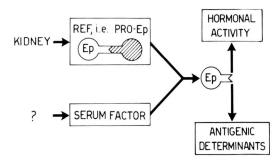

Fig. 8-3. Scheme for the biogenesis of erythropoietin. Renal erythropoietic factor (REF I), or proerythropoietin (PRO-Ep), is a precursor molecule produced in the kidney and activated by a serum factor to become REF II, which is biologically active, possesses antigenic determinants, and is inactivated by anti-Ep antiserum. (From Peschle, C., and Condorelli, M.: In Congenital disorders of erythropoiesis, Ciba Foundation symposium 37 [new series], New York, 1976, American Elsevier Publishing Co., Inc.)

not inhibited by antierythropoietin but appears to be a proerythropoietin molecule.

In summary recent evidence suggests that a precursor molecule, REF I, produced in the kidney, is activated by a serum factor of undetermined origin (Fig. 8-3). The active material, REF II, is erythropoietin. This system has obvious similarities to the proinsulin-insulin model. Since REF I is not inactivated by antierythropoietin antibody, the antigenic determinants are masked by the carrier molecule, preventing recognition of the proerythropoietin or REF I by the antibody.

Metabolism of erythropoietin

Although the rate of production of erythropoietin in humans is unknown, mice require 0.4 units/day to maintain normal red cell production. However, urinary levels of erythropoietin reflect serum levels, and a direct relationship between the two exists. Although both the liver and the bone marrow may be sites of hormone inactivation and degradation, the exact role of these organs is uncertain. The half-disappearance time of erythropoietin is 7 to 43 hours in humans with erythroid hypoplasia and only a few hours in the presence of erythroid hyperplasia.[62] That the plasma or serum erythropoietin level is influenced by the functional state of the erythroid tissues of the marrow, as well as the severity of the hypoxic stimulus, is suggested by the high plasma values noted in refractory anemias and the relatively low values in most hemolytic disorders.[125] Erythropoietin is preferentially utilized by a hyperplastic rather than an aplastic or hypoplastic marrow. The plasma erythropoietin level is therefore related to the degree of erythroid activity of the marrow. Plasma erythropoietin levels reflect the balance between the erythropoietin produced in response to hypoxia and that utilized by the bone marrow. Any condition that leads to a decrease in bone marrow production of red cells would therefore permit an accumulation of erythropoietin in the plasma by virtue of decreased utilization.

Just as hypoxemia is the stimulus for increased production of REF by the kidney, hypertransfusion causes a marked inhibition of REF activity and a reduction in erythropoietin.[53] It is not yet clear whether this inhibition is a result of the presence of erythropoietic inhibiting factors[80,141] or merely the consequence of increased hemoglobin and red cell mass with resultant increased delivery of oxygen to the kidneys.[132]

Mechanism of action

As previously stated, erythropoietin acts on the erythropoietin-responsive cells (ERCs), inducing them to enter the erythron. The erythroid response to erythropoietin is modulated by the size and the proliferative rate of the committed erythroid precursors.[120] Erythropoietin-induced differentiation does not deplete the number of cells in this self-sustaining compartment but induces the ERCs to differentiate into the population of cells synthesizing hemoglobin. Without erythropoietin stimulation the cells are lost to this pathway (Fig. 8-4). In the presence of large amounts of erythropoietin (such as may normally be produced in anemia) extra amplification of younger population cells, the immediate precursors of ERCs, occurs. Under the influence of erythropoietin the population of erythroid-committed precursor cells acts as an amplifying compartment to convert a relatively small number of stem cells into a large number of erythroblasts. This amplification is elastic and is modified and modulated by various humoral and cellular factors such as androgenic steroids that increase the production of erythropoietin and the number of CFU-Es. Normally erythropoietin is not necessary for the maturation of erythroblasts to erythrocytes. The observed phenomena of decreased transit time of erythroblasts in the marrow of anemic humans,[66] reduced cell cycle time of erythroblasts in anemic animals[129] and increased mitotic index of erythroblasts when marrow cells are incubated in vitro with erythropoietin,[106] early denucleation of basophilic or polychromatophilic normoblasts,[127] and increase in macrocytic reticulocytes in the blood 24 hours after the administration of erythropoietin[106] may reflect an increased rate of erythropoiesis. With severe stress or with markedly increased levels of erythropoietin, however, the hormone may directly effect erythroblast maturation.

A number of lipid-soluble substances possess erythropoietic activity. These include steroids,[55] a nonsteroid lipid, batyl alcohol,[90] and sphingolipid extractable from rabbit leukocytes.[22] The latter agent produced an increased number of basophilic erythroblasts (pronormoblasts) in vitro but should not be confused with erythropoietin since its action appears to be on differentiated erythroid precursors and not on the ERCs.

Intracellularly erythropoietin exerts a number of effects. In sequence these effects include (1) an increase in specific fractions of DNA-dependent RNA, i.e., ribosomal precursor RNA, ribosomal RNA, transfer RNA, and probably messenger RNA[59]; (2) an increase in the synthesis of non-hemoglobin protein[110]; (3) an increase in the syn-

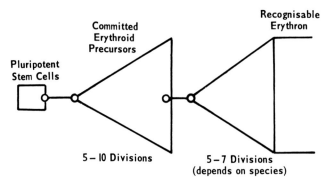

Fig. 8-4. Three functionally different stages of erythropoiesis. One of the progeny of the pluripotent stem cell is the cell destined to become an erythrocyte if it completes its potential differentiative course. If the late committed erythroid precursor is stimulated by erythropoietin, it moves into the erythron, or hemoglobin-synthesizing population, recognizable morphologically in the bone marrow; this population inevitably develops into erythrocytes. (From Schofield, R., and Lajtha, L. G.: In Congenital disorders of erythropoiesis, Ciba Foundation symposium 37 [new series] New York, 1976, American Elsevier Publishing Co., Inc.)

thesis of DNA[33]; (4) an increase in the accumulation of intracellular iron and an increase in the synthesis of ferritin and nonferritin protein[70]; (5) synthesis of new marrow cell stroma and receptors[34]; (6) synthesis of hemoglobin[70]; and (7) alteration of the hemotopoietic microenvironment.[136]

In the stressed bone marrow this effect of erythropoietin on hemoglobin synthesis may be responsible for the presence of macrocytes. Nucleic acid synthesis is shut off at a cytoplasmic hemoglobin concentration of 20%.[91] With accelerated hemoglobin synthesis and a constant generation time this critical cytoplasmic hemoglobin concentration is reached earlier, terminal divisions of the polychromatophilic normoblast are skipped, and polychromatophilic macrocytes or stress reticulocytes are produced. Conversely, because of the low critical cytoplasmic hemoglobin concentration in iron-deficiency erythropoiesis, microcytes occur because of additional divisions of the normoblasts.

Chang et al.[18] have identified an erythropoietin receptor on the surface of the ERCs and suggest that cells of the hematopoietic system become ERCs and capable of being induced to differentiate, eventually to become erythrocytes by virtue of possessing receptors for erythropoietin. They have also proposed that the stimulation of RNA synthesis by erythropoietin is mediated by a cyto-plasmic protein that is found in ERCs after their interaction with erythropoietin. This factor (marrow cytoplasmic factor) then interacts with the nucleus of the ERCs, triggering erythroid differentiation and hemoglobin synthesis (Fig. 8-5).

Stimulators and inhibitors

There are a number of agents that increase or decrease the production of erythropoietin.[79]

A. Stimulators
  1. Vasoconstrictors
     a. Angiotensin
     b. Epinephrine
     c. Serotonin, tryptamine
     d. Histamine
     e. Vasopressin
  2. Cobalt
  3. Dimethylnitrosamine
  4. Dibutyryl cyclic AMP, prostaglandins E_1 and A
  5. Androgenic hormones
     a. 5-β-H testosterone
     b. Fluoxymesterone
     c. Oxymetholone
  6. Pituitary hormones
     a. ACTH
     b. Growth hormone
     c. Prolactin
  7. Other hormones
     a. Human placental lactogenic hormone

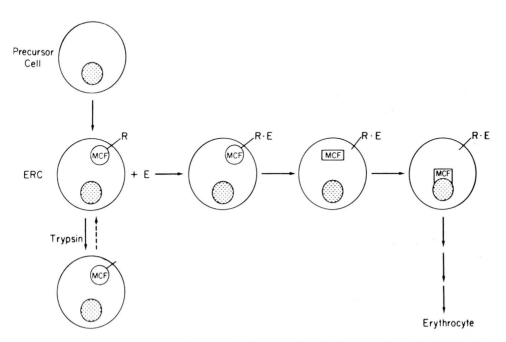

Fig. 8-5. Scheme for the action of erythropoietin on erythropoietin-responsive cells (ERCs). *R,* Erythropoietin receptor; *E,* erythropoietin; *MCF,* marrow cytoplasmic factor. Shaded circle represents the cell nucleus; the change in shape of MCF represents the formation of the active factor that can interact with the cell nucleus. (From Chang, S. C.-S., Sikkema, D., and Goldwasser, E.: Biochem. Biophys. Res. Commun. **57:**399, 1974.)

b. Thyroid hormone
c. Hydrocortisone
B. Inhibitors
1. Diuretics
a. Meralluride
b. Triamterene
c. Mercaptomerin
d. Bendroflumethiazide
2. β_2-Adrenergic blockers
a. *dl*-Propranolol
b. Butoxamine
3. Actinomycin D
4. Chlorambucil, thio-TEPA
5. Uranyl nitrate
6. Estrogens
7. Methylprednisolone

Stimulators of erythropoietin production include vasoconstrictors that constrict the afferent renal blood vessels, such as angiotensin, epinephrine, serotonin and vasopressin; cobalt, which decreases kidney respiration, oxidative phosphorylation, and renal blood flow; androgenic hormones, hydrocortisone, dibutyryl cyclic AMP, and prostaglandin E; pituitary hormones, ACTH and growth hormone; and other hormones, such as prolactin, human placental lactogenic hormone, and thyroid hormone. Dimethylnitrosamine, a nephro- and hepatotoxin, increases erythropoietin by either increasing the production or decreasing the catabolism of the hormone.

Erythropoietin is decreased by diuretics (meralluride and mercaptomerin); actinomycin D; uranyl nitrate, which causes damage to the proximal tubules; chlorambucil and thio-TEPA, alkylating agents that are highly concentrated in the kidney; estrogens; and methylprednisolone. Different amounts of these agents will often decrease erythropoietin either by suppressing production or by inhibiting the measurable response to hypoxia.

Nonhematologic conditions associated with increased erythropoietin levels. Elevated levels of erythropoietin have been demonstrated in a number of neoplastic[138] and paraneoplastic disorders,[131] the most common being renal tumors* (adenoma, carcinoma, Wilms' tumor), hydronephrosis and renal cysts, hepatomas,[54] uterine[109,146] and esophageal leiomyomas,[48] meningiomas[135] and cerebellar hemangioblastomas, and cystadenomas.[76] The tumor or diseased organ is the source of erythropoietin, and in many of these disorders elevated levels of erythropoietin have been detected in the serum, plasma or urine or extracted from the affected tissues. Erythrocytosis may or may not be an associated finding, and the erythropoietic material isolated from the various tumors may not be identical. In some cases the levels of erythropoietin correlated well with the

response to surgery, radiation therapy, and/or chemotherapy.[104]

FETAL AND NEONATAL ERYTHROPOIESIS
Erythropoietin production in the fetus

Erythropoietin is actively involved in fetal erythropoiesis[42,147] and has been detected in the plasma and urine of human fetuses by the thirty-second week of gestation and in the amniotic fluid.[40] Measurable erythropoietin in fetal blood increases with gestational age and increased amounts are found in the cord blood at term. The level of hormone in the cord blood and amniotic fluid is significantly higher in anemic than in normal fetuses and in the offspring of anemic mothers. Thus the fetus is capable of responding to hypoxemia whether the cause is the fetus itself (anemia), the placenta (reduced perfusion), or the mother (anemia and hypoxemia).

Thus erythropoietin production in the fetus is regulated by the relative availability of oxygen to fetal tissues but fetal kidneys, unlike those of the adult, are not the sole or major site of erythropoietin production.[121] Because erythropoiesis antedates renal development, an extrarenal source of erythropoietin must be available. In an unusual experiment of nature, normal erythropoiesis was observed in a human fetus with bilateral renal agenesis and cyanotic congenital heart disease.[60] In fetal goats bilateral nephrectomy did not inhibit the production of erythropoietin in response to bleeding, even in the absence of maternal kidneys, indicating that the source of erythropoietin is a nonrenal site in the fetus; erythropoietin does not cross the placenta.[147]

Further evidence for fetal production of erythropoietin was provided by experiments in which fetal erythropoiesis was completely abolished by the administration of adult antierythropoietin antibodies and subsequent neutralization of circulating erythropoietin in the fetus.[121] These findings also suggest that the biologic activity and the antigenic determinants of adult and fetal erythropoietin are similar.

Sites of action

Erythropoietin induces cultures of fetal mouse hepatic erythroblasts to synthesize hemoglobin with normal α- and β-chains.[19] Thus the type of hemoglobin synthesis stimulated by erythropoietin in extramedullary sites in the fetus is indistinguishable from normal hemoglobin.

As in the mature organism, the principal effect of erythropoietin is on immature erythroid precursor cells, which persist in the presence of the hormone and maintain their capacity to replicate and to differentiate into erythroblasts. In the absence of the hormone committed erythroblasts

---

*References 77, 103-105, 133.

continue their development but erythropoiesis is not sustained. Thus the target cell in the fetus is similar as well.[79] In humans fetal liver erythropoiesis is also sensitive to erythropoietin. Erythropoietin has no effect on the initial site of erythropoiesis, the yolk sac.[24]

Neonatal and postnatal erythropoiesis

The polycythemia of the newborn infant is a response to intrauterine hypoxia. During the first week of life of the normal newborn, erythropoiesis decreases markedly.[60] After the second day of life erythropoietin can no longer be detected in the serum or in the urine until 6 to 8 weeks of age.[21] This suppression of erythropoiesis is most likely related to improved oxygenation, a cessation of erythropoietin production, and perhaps, as suggested by some investigators, the presence of an erythropoiesis-inhibiting factor in the plasma and in urine.* The nature of the inhibitor awaits further study although recent work has ruled out estrogens.[20]

Despite the fact that erythropoietin is indetectable in the neonatal period by currently available and admittedly insensitive methods and that markedly depressed erythropoiesis continues, albeit at a low or basal rate, full-term and premature neonates are capable of producing erythropoietin in response to hypoxic stimuli.[96] Infants with cyanotic congenital heart disease and premature infants with severe respiratory distress have high levels of erythropoietin during the first weeks of life. In infants, living at high altitude (corresponding to an aterial oxygen saturation of 89%) has no appreciable effect on the postnatal decline of hemoglobin. At 3 to 4 months of age erythropoiesis is activated and, as expected, the levels of hemoglobin are significantly higher in infants residing at an altitude of 2,400 meters than in those living at sea level.[128] In response to anemic hypoxia alone, however, the level of hemoglobin or packed cell volume at which erythropoietin production is switched on is much lower from birth to 3 months of age than in later infancy, childhood, and adult life. An increase in erythroid activity in the marrow and reticulocytes in the peripheral blood is not seen until the hemoglobin level reaches a nadir of 6 to 8 gm/dl.[107] In a group of sixteen anemic but otherwise healthy premature infants (mean birthweight, 1,272 gm; mean gestational age, 32 weeks; mean postdelivery age, 51 days) no erythropoietin was detected, whereas erythropoietin levels were raised in all of a group of older children with a similar degree of anemia.[14]

The apparently impaired erythropoietin response to anemia in the first few months of life signifies

either an adequate delivery of oxygen to the tissues or an increased sensitivity to erythropoietin. The progressive rightward shift of the oxygen dissociation curve, related to a decreased concentration of fetal hemoglobin and an increase in the effective 2,3-DPG fraction (the product of 2,3-DPG and Hb A), provides sufficient oxygen to the tissues.[30,108] In fact at 2 months of age an infant with a hemoglobin level of 12 gm/dl delivers an amount of oxygen equivalent to that delivered by a newborn infant with a hemoglobin level of 17 gm/dl (Fig. 8-6). These normal compensatory and physiologic alterations provide sufficient oxygen delivery and lead to decreased production of erythropoietin and decreased erythropoiesis until the second to third months of life. After this period, increased erythropoietin levels are again detected, erythropoiesis resumes, and the hemoglobin and red blood cell mass rises in response to hypoxia.

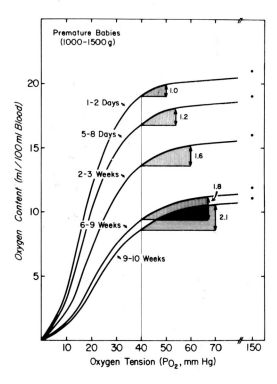

Fig. 8-6. Oxygen equilibrium curves of blood from premature infants at different postnatal ages. Double arrows represent the oxygen-unloading capacity between a given arterial and venous P_{O_2}. Points corresponding to 150 mm Hg on the abscissa are the oxygen capacities. Each curve represents the mean value of the infants studied in each group. Oxygen-unloading capacity is 2.1-fold greater at 9 to 10 weeks than at 1 to 2 days, balancing the decreased hemoglobin and oxygen content in older infants. (From Stockman, J. A., III: In Oski, F. A., Jaffé, E. R., and Miescher, P., eds.: Current problems in pediatric hematology, New York, 1975, Grune & Stratton, Inc. Used by permission.)

---

*References 20, 25, 88, 89, 122.

In premature infants the level of hemoglobin at which erythropoiesis resumes is lower and may be related in part to the shorter survival of premature red blood cells.

Ineffective erythropoiesis and dyserythropoiesis

The concept of ineffective erythropoiesis or dyserythropoiesis applies to the production of defective erythrocytes, which are destroyed either as precursors of mature cells within the marrow or almost immediately on release into the peripheral blood.[65,145] Although occurring normally to a slight degree, significant ineffective erythropoiesis is characteristic of a number of anemias in which the bone marrow shows marked erythroblastic hyperplasia with a peripheral anemia—notably thalassemia major, pernicious anemia, and congenital dyserythropoietic anemia.[67,87] In the case of pernicious anemia the total activity of the erythroid marrow may be increased to three times normal, but only one third of the cells produced enter the circulation, where the rate of survival is decreased.[38,49] Others are presumably defective and are destroyed at birth, either as end cells or as precursors capable of further division and maturation. Ineffective erythropoiesis or dyserythropoiesis implies a qualitative, quantitative, or combined disturbance of red blood cell production and may also be associated with states of bone marrow hypoplasia, aplasia, or leukemic infiltration. Profound morphologic abnormalities of nucleated and mature red cells and disturbed erythrokinetics are the hallmarks of dyserythropoiesis. A classification of anemias associated with dyserythropoiesis is precented here*:

A. Primary dyserythropoiesis
 1. Congenital dyserythropoietic anemias
  a. Type I
  b. Type II (HEMPAS)
  c. Type III
  d. Type IV
  e. Atypical cases
 2. Aquired dyserythropoietic anemias
B. Secondary dyserythropoiesis
 1. Known etiology
  a. Defects of nuclear DNA
   (1) Vitamin B_{12} deficiency
   (2) Folate deficiency
  b. Defects of heme and/or globin synthesis
   (1) Thalassemia
   (2) Iron-deficiency anemia
   (3) Sideroblastic anemias
   (4) Infection

---

*Modified from Lewis, S. M., and Verwilghen, R. L.: In Brown, E. B., ed.: Progress in hematology, vol. 8, New York, 1973, Grune & Stratton, Inc.

 2. Obscure etiology
  a. Aplastic anemia
  b. Myelosclerosis
  c. Erythroleukemia and other leukemias

Laboratory evaluation of erythropoiesis

The effectiveness or ineffectiveness of erythropoiesis can be quantified by a number of laboratory procedures that permit a total evaluation of erythrokinetics. Patterns that emerge from these studies include (1) normal or increased destruction or loss of hemoglobin and red blood cell mass, (2) decreased stimulation of the marrow, (3) decreased responsiveness of the marrow to normal stimulation, (4) increased marrow response or proliferation with effective erythropoiesis, (5) increased marrow proliferation with ineffective erythropoiesis, and (6) decreased marrow proliferation with ineffective erythropoiesis and increased destruction of hemoglobin and red cell mass.

The following are theoretical erythrokinetic data for a normal 30 kg child.

A. Assumptions
 1. Blood volume: 2,100 ml
 2. Venous hematocrit: 41%
 3. Mean body hematocrit: 38%
B. Calculated values
 1. Red cell mass: 800 ml
 2. Hemoglobin mass: 264 gm
 3. Circulating iron mass: 892 mg
 4. Circulating pyrrole pigment: 9.05 gm
C. Daily turnover (0.83% to 1.0%) (total/day and total/kg body weight):
 1. Red blood cells: 6.6 to 8.0 ml (0.22 to 0.26 ml/kg)
 2. Hemoglobin: 2.19 to 2.64 gm (0.07 to 0.09 gm/kg)
 3. Iron: 7.40 to 8.92 mg (0.25 to 0.30 mg/kg)
 4. Urobilinogen: 76.9 to 92.7 mg (2.56 to 3.09 mg/kg)
D. Normal conversion constants
 1. Body hematocrit factor: 0.92 × venous hematocrit
 2. MCHC: 33 gm/dl
 3. MCV: 87 fl
 4. Iron/gm hemoglobin: 3.38 mg
 5. Daily red cell breakdown: $1/120$ or 0.83%
 6. Protoporphyrin molecular weight: 566
 7. Stercobilinogen molecular weight: 580
 8. Hemoglobin molecular weight: 66,000

Reticulocyte count and production index. The uncorrected reticulocyte count is a crude measure of erythropoiesis. However, a more accurate estimate of total erythropoiesis is obtained in the reticulocyte count is expressed as the absolute number of reticulocytes per liter of blood (the product of the reticulocyte percentage and the red blood cell count); the normal value is 50 to 100 × 10^9/liter or if the reticulocyte count is corrected

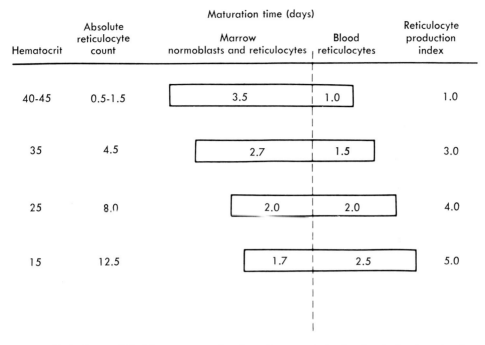

Hematocrit	Absolute reticulocyte count	Maturation time (days)		Reticulocyte production index
		Marrow normoblasts and reticulocytes	Blood reticulocytes	
40-45	0.5-1.5	3.5	1.0	1.0
35	4.5	2.7	1.5	3.0
25	8.0	2.0	2.0	4.0
15	12.5	1.7	2.5	5.0

Fig. 8-7. Reticulocyte shift. Marrow maturation times (iron transit time) and reticulocyte maturation times (absolute reticulocyte count divided by PIT production index) are shown for specific levels of phlebotomy-induced anemia. The total maturation period remains relatively constant, while marrow reticulocytes are delivered prematurely to circulation. This prolongs the blood reticulocyte maturation time and results in falsely high absolute reticulocyte counts. A corrected reticulocyte production index is obtained by dividing the absolute count by the approximate maturation time of blood reticulocytes. (From Hillman, R. S., and Finch, C. A.: Semin. Hematol. **4:**327, 1967. Used by permission.)

for a normal hematocrit (observed reticulocyte count × observed hematocrit ÷ normal hematocrit. The normal *corrected reticulocyte count,* or *reticulocyte index,* is 1. An index greater than 1 indicates increased erythropoiesis; a value of less than 1 indicates decreased or ineffective erythropoiesis.

A second correction takes into account the marrow maturation time of normoblasts and reticulocytes under circumstances of normal or stressed erythropoiesis. The maturation time progressively shortens as the degree of anemia, measured by the hematocrit, increases. The normal marrow maturation time of 3.5 days shortens to 2.7 days at a hematocrit of 35%, 2.0 days at a hematocrit of 25%, and 1.7 days at a hematocrit of 15%. The maturation time of the reticulocytes in the peripheral blood increases progressively from 1.0 to 1.5 days, 2.0 days, and 2.5 days at the respective values of hematocrit[67] (Fig. 8-7). Dividing the corrected reticulocyte count by the blood maturation time yields the *reticulocyte production index,* a value that agrees almost perfectly with ferrokinetic measurements of effective erythropoiesis.[114] The formulas for reticulocyte production are summarized here:

Calculations for corrected reticulocyte count and reticulocyte production index*

Absolute reticulocyte count (cells × 10^9/liter):

Observed reticulocyte count (%) × red blood cell count
NORMAL VALUE: 50 to 100 × 10^9/liter

Corrected reticulocyte count (%) or reticulocyte index:

$$\text{Observed reticulocyte count (\%)} \times \frac{\text{observed hematocrit}}{\text{normal hematocrit for age}}$$
NORMAL VALUE: 1

Reticulocyte production index:

$$\frac{\text{Corrected reticulocyte count (\%)}}{\text{Blood reticulocyte maturation time}}$$
NORMAL VALUE: 1

Blood reticulocyte maturation time (plasma iron turnover production index):

$$\frac{\text{Patient's PIT}}{0.65}$$
NORMAL PIT: 0.65 mg/dl whole blood

*From Hillman, R. S.: Characteristics of marrow production and reticulocyte maturation in normal man in response to anemia, J. Clin. Invest. **48:**443, 1969.

It has been estimated that the maximal rate of red blood cell production is seven to eight times normal.[29] Iron supply plays a critical role in erythropoiesis.[69] Whereas orally administered or reticuloendothelial iron is sufficient to increase erythropoiesis to more than two to three times the normal rate, the increased iron supply from nonviable red cells, hemolysis, or iron-dextran infusions permits marrow production to increase four to eight times normal. In extreme cases associated with severe chronic hemolytic anemia and ectopic bone marrow, erythropoiesis churned at ten to twenty times the normal rate.

Bone marrow. The normal ratio of nucleated erythroid:myeloid cells in the normal bone marrow obtained by aspiration or biopsy is approximately 1:3, a figure that varies with different ages in infancy and childhood (Chapter 2). The ratio

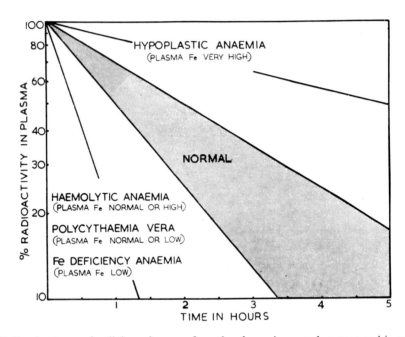

Fig. 8-8. Usual patterns of radioiron clearance from the plasma in normal persons and in patients with various blood disorders. (From Bothwell, T. H., et al.: Br. J. Haematol. **2:**1, 1956.)

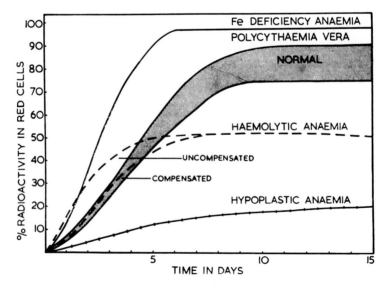

Fig. 8-9. Patterns of red cell utilization in normal persons and in patients with various blood disorders.

provides only a rough qualitative estimate of total erythropoietic activity. The presence of morphologic abnormalities in the erythroid precursors (e.g., megaloblastosis and multinuclearity) suggests dyserythropoiesis. Marrow cellularity can best be evaluated in samples obtained by biopsy, particularly in hypoplastic or aplastic states. The proliferative activity can be evaluated morphologically by determination of the mitotic index or autoradiographically with tritiated thymidine by the quantification of the labeling index and cell cycle times.[10,37,99] Nucleic acid metabolism and synthesis can be evaluated with radiochemical and histochemical techniques.[26] As discussed previously, recently developed techniques of in vitro bone marrow culture and erythroid colony formation offer useful information regarding the hematopoietic stem cells and erythroid progenitors.[97,130]

Ferrokinetics. Ferrokinetic studies with ^{52}Fe or ^{59}Fe measure the amounts of and rates at which iron is cleared from the plasma and incorporated into newly formed erythrocytes and the anatomic sites of iron delivery, accumulation, and utilization. Distinct patterns of plasma clearance, utilization, and organ uptake of iron are seen in disorders associated with increased, decreased, or ineffective dyserythropoieses. Generally, rapid plasma clearance is seen in hemolytic and iron-deficiency anemias and prolonged plasma clearance is observed in aplastic or hypoplastic states (Fig. 8-8). Normally 80% of the ^{59}Fe reappears in newly formed circulating red cells by 10 to 14 days. Decreased utilization is observed in compensated and uncompensated hemolytic anemias, reflecting increased peripheral destruction of red cells, and in hypoplastic anemias, reflecting the decreased

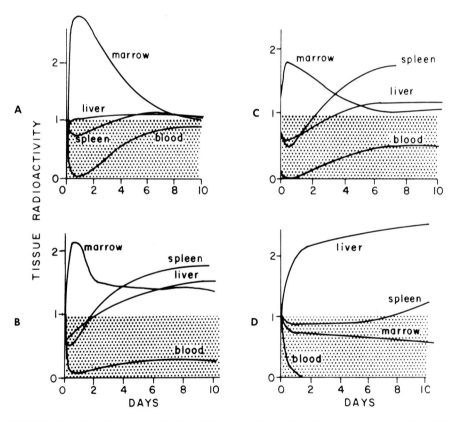

Fig. 8-10. Profiles of radioiron distribution. A tissue radioactivity of 1 represents the radioactivity in the individual tissue immediately after the injection of transferrin-bound radioiron. **A,** In the normal individual, as radioiron leaves the plasma, there is a corresponding rise in marrow activity, which falls as radioiron is incorporated into newly formed erythrocytes. **B,** In hereditary spherocytosis iron turnover is increased and initially radioiron is concentrated in the marrow. With the release of tagged cells, activity increases in the spleen, a result of sequestration and destruction. **C,** In ineffective erythropoiesis initial localization is in the marrow, but most of the radioiron becomes secondarily fixed in the spleen, liver, and marrow, indicating early destruction of tagged cells. **D,** In asplastic anemia no localization in the marrow occurs and, instead, iron is taken up by the parenchymal cells of the liver. (From Hillman, R. S., and Finch, C. A.: Semin. Hematol. **4:**327, 1967. Used by permission.)

erythroid activity of the marrow. Supernormal values of utilization with an earlier peak are observed in iron-deficiency anemia and polycythemia vera[12] (Fig. 8-9).

The time sequence and profile of radioiron distribution obtained by surface counting over the sacrum, heart, liver, and spleen provide useful information concerning active sites of erythropoiesis, of iron deposition, and of red cell sequestration and destruction (Fig. 8-10).[67] Normally after clearance from the plasma radioactivity rapidly appears in the bone marrow (sacrum) and after 8 to 10 days reappears in the blood (heart) with little if any change in the counts over the liver or spleen. In aplastic anemia early concentration in the marrow does not occur and the bulk of the iron is deposited in hepatic parenchymal cells. In ineffective erythropoiesis counts over the sacrum remain high, indicating retention of radioactivity in the bone marrow. The appearance of radioactivity in the liver and spleen is related to early destruction of newly formed erythrocytes in these organs.

Whole body scanning with ^{59}Fe is another useful technique for evaluating the body distribution of erythropoietic marrow, splenic sequestration of red cells, and hepatic deposition of iron.[118] Using ^{52}Fe (which has a much shorter half-life than ^{59}Fe) and the positron scintillation camera, or γ-camera, only sites of erythropoiesis can be determined.[5] The whole body scanning techniques serve as a useful check on the data obtained from external monitoring, the accuracy of which depends on positioning of the probes and extrapolation to zero time. Extramedullary erythropoiesis (e.g., in myeloid metaplasia) or paravertebral ectopic erythropoiesis (in thalassemia major) can be detected with whole body scanning as well.

Bilirubin, stercobilin, and urobilinogen. Unconjugated hyperbilirubinemia in the absence of an equivalent degree of hemolysis in the peripheral blood suggests ineffective erythropoiesis. It is impossible to determine the source of the bilirubin, bone marrow, or circulating erythrocytes unless radioisotopic studies are performed. Bilirubin pigment is formed in the monocyte-macrophage elements of the bone marrow, liver, spleen, and lymph nodes. About 10% to 20% of total bile pigment is derived from precursors other than hemoglobin of circulating erythrocytes[92] such as heme not used in the synthesis of hemoglobin, myoglobin, and heme-containing enzymes in the liver such as cytochrome, peroxidase, and catalase.[116] The early appearance of labeled stercobilin (the "early labeled peak")[7] after the administration of 2-^{14}C-glycine in patients with ineffective erythropoiesis is caused by the destruction of abnormal erythrocytes within the bone marrow.[73,115]

Bile pigments in human serum range from 0.5 to 0.8 mg/dl of blood and are derived from the breakdown of heme. The porphyrin portion of hemoglobin (exclusive of iron) constitutes 3.5% by weight of the hemoglobin molecule. Theoretically all of the porphyrin of catabolized hemoglobin is converted to bilirubin, most of which is excreted in the stool as urobilinogen. Thus quantitative estimates of urobilinogen excretion are an index of hemoglobin breakdown. It has been estimated that 1 mg of urobilinogen is derived from approximately 29 mg of destroyed hemoglobin and that the daily turnover of hemoglobin is 7 to 9 mg/kg (0.13% to 1.0% of the total hemoglobin mass). The normal daily range for fecal urobilinogen is 2.7 to 3.2 mg/kg. Calculation of heme turnover from the excretion of fecal bile pigment has been erratic, unaesthetic, and unpredictable. Degradation of urobilinogen to unidentifiable products or alternate pathways in heme catabolism, bypassing urobilinogen, often lead to an underestimation of heme turnover. This discrepancy is noted in an older study[100] in which the normal daily mean value for fecal urobilinogen ranged from 3.8 mg in infants younger than 1 year of age to 45.2 mg in children from 10 to 14 years of age. These values are far less than the theoretical levels of urobilinogen production.

Carbon monoxide generation. Endogenous carbon monoxide (CO) production arising from the degradation of hemoglobin at the α-methene bridge of the porphyrin ring can be used as a measure of heme catabolism.[23] Using glycine-2-^{14}C as a precursor of heme, Coburn et al. found that the early labeled peak of stercobilin accompanies the "early labeled" peak of ^{14}CO and that endogenous CO is markedly increased in patients with ineffective erythropoiesis.[142] The CO peaks preceded maximal labeling of circulating heme, indicating the premature death of erythroid cells within the bone marrow.

Red blood cell survival. Erythrokinetic studies in patients with disordered erythropoiesis have demonstrated associated increased rates of erythrocyte destruction.[86,116] Radioactive sodium chromate (^{51}Cr) can be satisfactorily used to measure the circulating red cell mass, blood volume, and red cell survival and to localize the site of red cell destruction.[71,75]

Enzyme markers of disordered erythropoiesis. The presence of stress erythropoiesis is associated with the liberation of a number of intracellular enzymes into the plasma. Of these enzymes, aldolase and lactic dehydrogenase have been used as markers of ineffective erythropoiesis.[58,64] Raised levels of nucleoside deaminase in the mouse[119] and formyltetrahydrofolic acid synthetase in humans[144] are other markers of erythropoietic stress and not merely a reflection of a younger population of erythrocytes. The activity of these enzymes remains elevated for the full life span of erythrocytes formed during stress and represents a biochemical difference between normal red cells and the cells produced under conditions of accelerated erythropoiesis. An alteration in a human red cell membrane antigen—the emergence of i antigens, usually a characteristic feature of fetal cells—is also associated with marrow stress.[68]

Erythropoietin. Assays of erythropoietin and inhibitors of erythropoietin aid in determining whether an anemia is related to decreased stimulation of the marrow (decreased erythropoietin or erythropoietin inhibitors) or to decreased, ineffective responsiveness of the marrow to normal stimulation (normal or increased erythropoietin). Significantly decreased concentrations of erythropoietin are observed in patients with renal failure,[126] infection, and chronic inflammation,[149] and raised levels of erythropoietin have been noted in congenital hypoplastic anemia, aplastic anemia, acute and chronic leukemia, and hemolytic conditions.[74] Thalassemic patients with hemoglobin levels between 15 and 7 gm/dl showed no increase in erythropoietin. The rise in erythropoietin in the serum and urine was abrupt and increased markedly as the patients' hemoglobin decreased to lower than 7 gm/dl.[3]

Erythropoietin levels in the anemia of chronic disorders. The anemia of chronic disorders (Chapter 16) is characterized by decreased plasma iron level and iron-binding capacity, despite increased stores of iron in the reticuloendothelial cells in the marrow.[17] Other features include an impairment of release of iron into the plasma from the RES, a slight decrease in red cell survival, and failure to increase erythropoiesis adequately or sufficiently to compensate for the increased rate of red blood cell destruction. The compromised erythropoiesis may result from (1) failure of the anemia to elicit an increase in the production of erythropoietin (infection, inflammation, and renal disease), (2) inhibition of the biologic activity of erythropoietin (renal failure),[139,150] and (3) defective bone marrow response to erythropoietin (advanced malignancy without marrow infiltration). In patients with iron-deficiency anemia, primary hematopoietic disease (aplastic and hypoplastic anemia, refractory sideroblastic anemia, and leukemia), and malignancy, the level of erythropoietin correlates with the degree of anemia (Fig. 8-11). In chronic infection and inflammation the levels of erythropoietin are significantly lower and there is no correlation with anemia.[140,149,150] The response of the bone marrow to erythropoietin is diminished in patients with malignancy but is normal in those with infection or inflammation.[149]

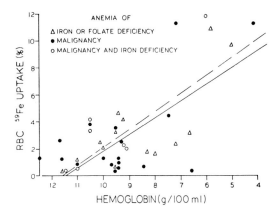

Fig. 8-11. Correlation of serum level of erythropoietin with the venous hemoglobin concentration. The solid line indicates the slope for patients with iron deficiency and folate deficiency and the dashed line for patients with malignancy.

Functional and erythrokinetic classification of anemia. In Chapter 5 two classifications of the anemias, physiologic and morphologic, were presented. On the basis of a fuller understanding of erythropoiesis and improved methods of evaluation, abnormal erythropoiesis may be classified erythrokinetically, i.e., according to the phase of red cell development in which the disorder occurs. In this regard three major types of defects can be recognized: (1) defects affecting proliferation, (2) defects affecting maturation, and (3) defects affecting the survival of the circulating red blood cell. Erythropoiesis may be effective or ineffective or the marrow may be unresponsive to erythropoietin (marrow failure) or there may be a deficiency or inhibitor of erythropoietin. Overlapping occurs in many disorders in which ineffective erythropoiesis is associated with increased destruction of mature erythrocytes. This classification* considers hematopoietic stem cells and erythroid precursors, the microenvironment of the marrow, and nutritional and humoral factors that are required for and stimulate erythropoiesis as well as intrinsic hereditary or acquired disorders affecting red blood cell production and destruction. These clinical disorders are considered in the second part of this chapter.

    A. Proliferative defects
       1. Erythropoietin
          a. Inadequate production
             (1) Renal disease
             (2) Infection, inflammation, or malignancy
             (3) Endocrine disorders

*Modified from Hillman, R. S., and Finch, C. A., Semin. Hematol. **4:**327, 1967.

    b. Inhibitors
      (1) Renal disease
      (2) "Physiologic anemia" of infancy(?)
  2. Erythroid marrow
    a. Marrow damage
      (1) Idiopathic: immune or genetic(?)
        (a) Congenital hypoplastic anemia
        (b) Pure red cell anemia
        (c) Aplastic anemia
      (2) Radiation, chemical, drugs
    b. Marrow replacement
    c. Defective response to erythropoietin
      (1) Malignancies
  3. Iron-deficiency anemia
B. Maturation defects with dyserythropoiesis
  1. Nuclear
    a. Vitamin B_{12}, folate deficiency
    b. Orotic aciduria
    c. Congenital dyserythropoietic anemias
  2. Cytoplasmic
    a. Heme synthesis
      (1) Sideroblastic anemias
      (2) Erythroblastic porphyria
      (3) Lead poisoning
      (4) Iron-deficiency anemia
    b. Globin synthesis
      (1) Thalassemia syndromes
      (2) Unstable hemoglobin hemolytic anemias
C. Peripheral defects with effective erythropoiesis
  1. Hemorrhage
  2. Hemolysis
    a. Hereditary: membrane, hemoglobin, or metabolic
    b. Acquired: immune, microangiopathic

Clinical disorders of erythropoiesis

GENERAL CONSIDERATIONS

The hypoplastic and dysplastic anemias constitute a heterogenous group of anemias that include several well-defined entities and a larger number of still obscure or emerging disorders reflecting degrees of suppressed or ineffective erythropoiesis. In either event an inadequate number of normally functioning red blood cells are delivered to the circulation and often those that reach the circulation are destined to an early demise. These anemias are not caused by excessive hemolysis, by blood loss, or in the majority of instances by space-occupying infiltrations of the bone marrow but result from a failure of red cell production and hemoglobin synthesis to compensate for the normal or increased rate of blood destruction. Erythropoiesis alone is significantly decreased in the disorders to be discussed in this chapter. The defect may extend to the granulocytes and platelets, resulting in a peripheral pancytopenia. (See Chapter 17 for discussion of aplastic anemia.)

Bone marrow aspiration or biopsy reveals the anticipated erythroid hypoplasia or a specimen varying from normal cellularity to hypercellularity[221,288] with or without morphologic evidence of dyserythropoiesis. Previously the difficulties of reconciling the state of the bone marrow with the peripheral blood picture and the resistance of many of these disorders to all forms of therapy except transfusions had prompted their designation as refractory anemias.[159,260] With the recent application of advanced kinetic, immunologic, and biochemical techniques to the study of these disorders, more rational and effective therapy should be available.

The anemias are usually normocytic and normochromic, occasionally macrocytic with moderate anisocytosis, and distinguished from other blood dyscrasias by a diminished number of reticulocytes and other evidences of inadequate erythropoiesis. The absence of enlargement of lymph nodes, liver, and spleen in patients with the major anemias of this group is of diagnostic importance.

In keeping with the functional and erythrokinetic classification of anemia, congenital defects of erythroid proliferation involving primary abnormalities of the bone marrow, those associated with dyserthropoiesis, and acquired anemias related to inadequate production of or inhibitors to erythropoietin are presented in this chapter. The reader is referred to Chapters 6 (defects of iron metabolism), 7 (megaloblastic anemias), 10 (immune hemolysis), 11 (membrane defects), 12 (metabolic defects), 13 to 15 (defects of heme and globin synthesis), 16 (anemias of systemic disease), and 17 (aplastic anemia) for a fuller presentation of other clinical disorders of erythropoiesis.

DEFECTS OF ERYTHROID MARROW
Congenital hypoplastic anemia

Definition. Congenital hypoplastic anemia (Diamond-Blackfan syndrome) has also been called chronic congenital arregenerative anemia, congenital pure red cell aplasia, primary erythroid hypoplasia, and erythrogenesis imperfecta. The term "congenital hypoplastic anemia" refers to a congenital anemia confined to a failure of erythropoiesis without an equivalent depression of the white blood cells or platelets.[171,217] The bone marrow is characterized by a complete or almost complete absence of morphologically recognizable cells of the erythroid series with normally proliferating cells of the granulocytic series and megakaryocytes. Congenital hypoplastic anemia should be distinguished from pure red cell aplasia (an acquired condition, more common in adults, in which a sudden cessation of erythropoiesis occurs) or from transitory states of erythroid hypoplasia caused by exposure to drugs, toxins, or chemicals or associated with infections, autoimmune and allergic states, or crises occurring with other hereditary hemolytic syndromes.

Historical perspective. Anemia resulting from isolated erythroid hypoplasia or aplasia in young infants was first described by Josephs in 1936.[217] In 1938 Diamond and Blackfan[171] described four cases of congenital hypoplastic anemia in childhood, a syndrome now called Diamond-Blackfan anemia. Since then more than 200 cases have been described in the literature, which has been thoroughly reviewed recently.[173,198]

Etiology. The exact etiology of congenital hypoplastic anemia is uncertain, but most current evidence implicates a failure in the end-organ, the erythroid stem cell. Previous theories[155] suggesting that a disturbance of tryptophan metabolism was responsible for the anemia have been discredited by the demonstration that the abnormal excretion of metabolites of tryptophan is nonspecific and occurs in a variety of anemias.[196,257] Increased levels of erythropoietin in the plasma and urine mitigates against decreased stimulation as a cause of end-organ failure.[195] An inhibitor of erythropoiesis measured by heme synthesis was detected in the sera of four patients with congenital hypoplastic anemia,[250] but others were unable to demonstrate an erythropoietic inhibitory effect of sera from five patients either in vivo in animals or in vitro with normal human bone marrow.[189] Freedman et al.[182] found that patients with anemia and diminished recognizable erythroid precursors had reduced or absent erythropoietin-stimulated heme synthesis but that, even in the absence of erythroid precursors, erythroid colonies (CFU-Es) grew in vitro.[183] No inhibitors of erythropoiesis or antibodies to erythropoietin were detected. The summation of this recent study is that the erythropoietic failure in Diamond-Blackfan syndrome is not caused by an absence of erythroid stem cells, their unresponsiveness to erythropoietin, an abnormal or deficient erythropoietin, or a serum inhibitor to erythropoiesis. Recent studies by Hoffman et al.[207] have detected a lymphocyte-mediated inhibitor of erythroid colony formation in vitro, suggesting that the defect in steroid-refractory patients with congenital hypoplastic anemia may be at a cellular or microenvironmental level involving lymphocyte (T cell) erythroid precursor interaction. Freedman and Saunders[184] have proposed that two types of Diamond-Blackfan anemias exist, the first steroid responsive and without lymphocyte suppressors and the second steroid refractory and with demonstrable lymphocyte-mediated suppression. Nathan et al.[247] could not detect cell-mediated inhibition of erythroid colony formation in steroid-resistant, transfusion-dependent patients with Diamond-Blackfan syndrome.

Genetics. A congenital factor in the etiology of the Diamond-Blackfan syndrome is suggested by its early onset, the associated minor congenital anomalies and chromosomal defects, and the occurrence in parents, siblings, and identical twins.[294] Both autosomal dominant* and autosomal recessive[162,271] patterns of inheritance have been described, but relatively few familial cases have been reported, making a definitive statement concerning genetics impossible.

Congenital malformations have been recorded in about 25% of the patients. Skeletal anomalies involving the radial aspect of the upper extremity, particularly triphalangeal thumbs, have been reported most frequently.[151,214,245] Other birth defects include cleft lip and palate, peculiar facies,[163] retinopathy, webbed neck, ventricular septal defect,[204] hypocalcemia,[281] hypogammaglobulinemia,[161] and minor chromosomal abnormalities.[204,281] The relationship between these anomalies and erythroid hypoplasia is uncertain but obviously prenatal factors are operative.

Clinical and laboratory findings. Congenital hypoplastic anemia has an insidious onset with progressive pallor, irritability, listlessness, anorexia, and anemia, which are usually apparent at the age of 2 to 3 months or later in the first year. Anemia is present at birth in about 15% of the patients but most infants appear healthy and general growth and development proceed normally. Rarely the onset of the disease may be delayed; such a delay has been reported in a child 6 years old.[197]

Except for pallor and associated congenital malformations, there are few abnormalities to be observed at physical examination. A phenotype resembling Turner's syndrome has been reported.[173] In some patients a particular type of facies has been described,[163] consisting of two-colored hair, snub nose, thick upper lips, rather wide-set eyes, and an intelligent expression. Jaundice is absent, there are no manifestations of bleeding, and the liver, spleen, and lymph nodes are not enlarged; mild hepatosplenomegaly may be present as a result of congestive heart failure or transfusion hemosiderosis. Chronic transfusion therapy results in increased pigmentation of the skin resulting from excessive melanin formation.[228] Cardiac enlargement, multiple arrhythmias, and refractory heart failure are frequently inevitable consequences in patients who are unresponsive to corticosteroid therapy.

The outstanding laboratory feature is an aregenerative anemia in which there is a striking absence of nucleated erythroid cells in the marrow without a simultaneous depression of granulocytes, platelets, and their precursors. The marrow myeloid:

*References 179, 180, 194, 210, 226, 244, 291.

erythroid ratio may be as high as 50:1. The anemia is normochromic, but macrocytosis and an increased MCV (>90 fl) have been noted in many patients either at diagnosis or in remission. The reticulocytes are low in number or absent. Without supportive transfusions or response to therapy the hemoglobin level falls as low as 2 to 4 gm/dl. The fetal hemoglobin level may be increased.

The number of platelets and leukocytes and the differential counts are normal. Lymphocytosis in the peripheral blood and bone marrow inappropriate for the patient's age has been observed rarely. Later, marked leukopenia and moderate depression of platelets occur in rare instances of hypersplenism; the bone marrow in such patients shows normal myeloid activity and a normal number of megakaryocytes. In a 13-year-old girl under our observation platelet counts remained intermittently low following splenectomy. The bone marrow frequently contains varying numbers of primitive cells previously termed hematogones[274,289] that are thought to represent progenitors of the erythroid series. Although such cells are smaller than mature lymphocytes, they resemble them closely in size and morphology. They possess a dense homogeneous matlike nucleus and a narrow rim of nongranular basophilic cytoplasm. In a patient reported by Miale and Bloom[241] the number of lymphocytes in the marrow decreased and the number of erythroid precursors and thymidine-labeled lymphoid cells increased after initiation of corticosteriod therapy.

In rare cases the cells in the marrow are heavily vacuolated. Their significance is unknown, but with corticosteroid treatment the vacuoles disappear. The serum iron level is elevated and with prolonged transfusion therapy transferrin becomes completely saturated. Ferrokinetic studies reveal a markedly delayed rate of clearance from plasma of ^{59}Fe, a markedly decreased rate of reappearance of ^{59}Fe into peripheral red cells, and liver uptake but little localization of radioactivity over the sacrum. In addition to the macrocytosis and increased but heterogeneously distributed HbF, the circulating erythrocytes in Diamond-Blackfan syndrome have additional characteristics of fetal red cells: i antigen and raised levels of G-6-PD, glyceraldehyde-3-phosphate dehydrogenase, enolase, and lactate dehydrogenase.[237]

Differential diagnosis. Significant erythroid hypoplasia with intact granulopoiesis and platelet production differentiates congenital hypoplastic anemia from aplastic anemia and is the sine qua non for the diagnosis. In a typical case the disease is fully established in the first 6 months of life but the initial diagnosis may be obscured if steroids have been given for any prolonged period. The bone marrow may show erythroid hyperplasia and

the reticulocyte count may be elevated. Elimination of all therapy may be necessary before a diagnosis can be established. Occasionally congenital hypoplastic anemia follows erythroblastosis fetalis[275] and is mistaken for the protracted depression of erythropoiesis that sometimes accompanies the latter disorder. Acute transitory erythroblastopenia is an acquired disorder of older infants and children. Hypoplasia of the erythroid marrow may be extreme, but spontaneous recovery occurs in 1 to 2 weeks after onset. This condition may complicate an underlying hemolytic disorder and can be differentiated from Diamond-Blackfan syndrome by the absence of macrocytosis, normal levels of Hb F, and low or normal activities of glycolytic enzymes.[238]

Pathologic findings. The essential feature is widespread hemosiderosis, at times associated with hemochromatosis. In patients who die of heart failure, postmortem examination reveals the typical syndrome of transfusional hemochromatosis, including diabetes mellitus and skin pigmentation. The heart is greatly enlarged. Many of the myocardial fibers are hypertrophied, vacuolated, and necrotic; contain iron pigments; and show scanty interstitial mycocardial fibrosis. Other patients with severe hepatitis have massive liver necrosis and generalized hemosiderosis with fibrosis of the liver, pancreas, thyroid, parathyroid, and gonads.

Treatment. Major therapy consist of corticosteroids, transfusions, and in selected cases splenectomy.

Corticosteroids. The adrenocorticosteroids (prednisone and prednisolone) and similar synthetic substances are given primary consideration since they represent a potent form of therapy.* The overall response rate to corticosteroids is about 67%. Corticosteroids should be started as expeditiously as possible after a definitive diagnosis is made. In Allen and Diamond's study, the response rate was 100% when therapy was started within 3 months of the onset of anemia. The response rate decreased to 67% if therapy was delayed from 3 to 12 months, and the rate was reduced to 0% if 3 years or more transpired between onset of anemia and initiation of therapy or if hemosiderosis occurred after prolonged transfusion therapy.[188] The dosage of prednisone (or prednisolone) is 2 mg/kg/day given in divided doses every 6 to 8 hours. In the responsive patient evidence of bone marrow and peripheral blood remission should be manifested in 1 to 3 weeks. Erythroid hyperplasia, reticulocytosis, and increased hemoglobin level, hematocrit, and red blood cell count are the hallmarks of a favorable

---

*References 154, 172, 187, 253.

response. If and when the patient responds, the dosage should be slowly tapered to a maintenance level. This amount varies with the individual patient but should be the lowest dose possible to maintain an acceptable level of hemoglobin. Intermittent therapy is given to reduce the hazard of growth retardation. In this case dosages of 2.5 mg of prednisone twice weekly, 2.5 mg every other day, or 5 mg once weekly are not unusual despite their seeming homeopathic levels. Most clinicians have been reluctant to discontinue the drug entirely.

If there is no response to corticosteroids after 3 to 4 weeks, therapy should be tapered and discontinued and the patient should be started on transfusion therapy. Testosterone and other androgenic steroids recommended for the treatment of aplastic anemia are without proven value in congenital hypoplastic anemia.[171]

Transfusions. Supportive transfusions to maintain the hemoglobin at levels compatible with freedom from symptoms constitute a basic need for steroid-unresponsive patients. The use of washed or frozen-thawed packed cells is recommended if these products are available. Usually patients do not require transfusions until hemoglobin levels fall to 7 to 7.5 gm/dl, at which point clinical symptoms appear, including anorexia, listlessness, apathy, and incipient signs of heart failure. The onset of hemosiderosis is to be expected following repeated transfusions. Accordingly these patients should receive chelation therapy with desferrioxamine in an effort to delay the inevitable appearance of transfusional hemosiderosis. A current regimen utilizes desferrioxamine in a dosage of 20 mg/kg/day subcutaneously as a continuous or 8 hour infusion administered via an automatic syringe.[193,258]

Splenectomy. When transfusions are required at increasingly frequent intervals to maintain a physiologically sufficient, although reduced, level of hemoglobin, it is postulated that an extracorpuscular hemolytic component, presumably located in the spleen, has developed. Accelerated destruction can be confirmed by labeling normal donor red cells with ^{51}Cr and determining their shortened survival rate and site of destruction. Splenectomy, frequently recommended only as a last resort, has nevertheless proved effective on occasion in reducing the number of transfusions and in improving the white blood cell and platelet counts in patients with hypersplenism. In one large study[177] of patients with congenital hypoplastic anemia the hazards of infection after splenectomy were demonstrated in three patients who died 3 months, 18 months, and 4 years after splenectomy. Two died of pneumococcal sepsis and pneumonia and one died of varicella, with

complications including massive pericardial effusion and pneumonia.

Prognosis. Prior to corticosteroid therapy the course of congenital hypoplastic anemia was one of chronic and progressive anemia with a fatal outcome. It had been known, however, that in selected patients supportive transfusion therapy could maintain a concentration of hemoglobin compatible with health. It had also been observed that spontaneous recovery was possible.

In a long-term study of thirty patients with Diamond-Blackfan syndrome[172] eighteen required regular transfusions for varying periods of time. Six of the eighteen patients developed spontaneous remissions after periods ranging from 8 months to 13 years. Four of the six were alive at the time of the report, two patients having died while in a state of remission.

An important factor in evaluating therapy and prognosis is the possibility of spontaneous remission. Such recovery occurred in three of twelve patients cited by Diamond and in others reported by Palmen and Vahlquist[252] and by Hardisty.[198] Remission can occur at any period from early childhood to adolescence with stabilization at a lower level of hemoglobin. One of Diamond's steroid-unresponsive patients had received more than 400 transfusions from 2 months to 14½ years of age, when a spontaneous remission occurred. At 16 years of age the patient was in surprisingly good clinical condition with a hemoglobin level of 13 gm/dl and a normal bone marrow. She relapsed again 14 years later and died of acute myeloblastic anemia.[293] Although leukemia is known to occur in patients with acquired pure red cell aplasia,[268] idiopathic aplastic anemia, and Fanconi's aplastic anemia,[157] this association with congenital hypoplastic anemia is unique.

Of the thirty patients in Diamond's series, twenty-two had been given one or more trials of therapy with corticosteroids.[154] Twelve of the twenty-two patients developed a steroid-induced remission and three of these were well without medication at the time of the report, having been treated for 11 months, 1 year, and 6 years, but intermittent therapy was mandatory in the others. The only side effect of therapy was growth retardation. Data from reported studies suggest that a more favorable response to steriod therapy is related to a lesser degree of erythroid hypoplasia, but early onset of disease and prompt initiation of therapy appear to be the key.

Patients who fail to respond to steroids have extremely guarded prognoses. Long-term transfusions carry the hazards of hemosiderosis and hemochromatosis. Death results from cardiac failure, hepatitis during the course of transfusions, and overwhelming infection and sepsis. One patient died at 25 years of age of hepatocellular carcinoma that developed in a hemochromatotic liver.[278] Unlike others who developed hepatocellular carcinoma in idiopathic or Fanconi's aplastic anemia, the patient was not treated with androgenic steroids.[236]

Future perspectives. The ability to grow erythroid colonies in vitro and recent results suggesting that an immunologic basis underlies this disorder have provided new approaches to the pathogenesis and therapy of the Diamond-Blackfan syndrome. The mechanism of action of corticosteroids is unknown in patients responding to this form of therapy and their continued response to miniscule doses is equally as baffling. Techniques of in vitro bone marrow culture may elucidate the nature on the stem cell defect and provide useful prognostic information if a relationship between CFU-E, age, and response to therapy can be demonstrated. The development of more effective chelation therapy either with the prolonged use of desferrioxamine or with orally administered chelating agents should add years to the lives of transfusion-dependent patients. Finally, bone marrow transplantation may be a viable alternative approach for the patient who has not responded to all other therapy. Early diagnosis and initiation of corticosteroid therapy still offer the best promise for children with Diamond-Blackfan syndrome.

Acquired hypoplastic anemia

Pure red cell aplasia

Definition. Pure red cell aplasia, an acquired defect of erythropoiesis, is currently considered to be an autoimmune condition and is characterized by absent erythropoiesis and the presence of serum inhibitors to erythropoiesis.* This group of disorders is distinct from congenital hypoplastic anemia, aplastic anemia, and transitory erythroblastopenia associated with hemolytic anemia or toxic, infectious, drug-induced, or allergic causes, although all share the finding of isolated absence or suppression of erythropoiesis.

Classification. Three types of pure red cell aplasia have been identified.[254] The first, type I, is characterized by the presence in the serum or plasma of elevated levels of erythropoietin and an IgG inhibitor of erythropoiesis acting at the marrow level. Type II pure red cell aplasia is characterized by the absence or near absence of erythropoietin activity in the serum and the presence of a serum IgG antibody to circulating erythropoietin. Both type I and type II respond to immunosuppressive therapy with disappearance of the inhibitor after remission is induced. In patients with

*References 212, 221, 222, 224.

type III pure red cell aplasia serum IgG inhibitors of erythroid precursors or erythropoietin are absent. Patients in this group may be in a preleukemic state because of the progression of pure red cell aplasia to acute myeloid leukemia in some patients.[254]

Drug-induced pure red cell aplasia forms a second major category of these acquired disorders of the erythroid marrow, but the mechanism of action of these agents is toxic or allergic rather than immune.[259]

Incidence. Pure red cell aplasia primarily affects adults[174] although a few cases in adolescents[268] have been reported, some of whom may have had Diamond-Blackfan syndrome with spontaneous remission and later relapse. The incidence of thymoma in adults with erythroid aplasia is about 50%, and 5% of patients with thymoma develop pure red cell aplasia.[206,263] The spindle cell type of tumor predominates and almost all are benign. The association of pure red cell aplasia and thymoma in children has not been reported.

Etiology and pathogenesis. There is little doubt that non-drug-induced pure red cell aplasia is caused by an immunologic abnormality. Clinical evidence includes the high incidence of thymoma, with remission occurring in 25% to 30% of patients after thymectomy; the frequent association of immune or autoimmune conditions such as hypo- or agammaglobulinemia,[174,232] paraproteinemia,[222] lupus erythematosis,[222] autoimmune hemolytic anemia, multiple myeloma, and anti-muscle antibodies; myasthenia gravis; and the response to corticosteroids and other immunosuppressive agents.

The studies of Krantz and Kao[222] and Peschle's group[254,255] have defined and established the immunologic basis of pure red cell aplasia. Plasma from patients with pure red cell aplasia greatly inhibited in vitro heme synthesis of normal or patients' marrow cells, but normal plasma did not, ruling out a histocompatibility factor. IgG purified from the plasma of affected patients inhibited heme synthesis, but following treatment with the immunosuppressive drugs 6-mercaptopurine or cyclophosphamide or with steroids, the IgG inhibitor of heme synthesis disappeared from the plasma. More recent studies[221] suggested that (1) the IgG was cytotoxic to erythroblasts,[224] (2) the reaction was complement dependent, and (3) the cytotoxic factor is an antibody or an immune complex. Although Peschle's experimental results in vivo and in vitro were similar in their demonstration of an IgG inhibitor of erythropoiesis, his conclusions were at variance with those of Krantz. Because of the absence or near absence of recognizable erythroid precursors in the marrows of patients with pure red cell aplasia, Peschle proposed that the primary target of the inhibitor is an earlier erythroid precursor that has been differentiated from the erythroid-responsive cell compartment by erythropoietin.

One of seven patients in Peschle's series[254] had indetectable levels of erythropoietin and a serum IgG inhibitor (antibody) to circulating erythropoietin. Erythropoietin levels returned to normal after immunosuppressive therapy induced a remission in this patient. Animal models for both types of pure red cell aplasia have been established and further support the contention that an autoantibody plays a major role in pathogenesis. Other researchers[213,218,305] have also identified IgG inhibitors of erythropoiesis in the plasma and urine of patients with pure red cell aplasia.

Clinical and laboratory features. The disease has an insidious onset and affects males and females equally. The hematologic findings are similar to those in congenital hypoplastic anemia except for the coexistence of autoimmune diseases or thymoma in some patients.

Differential diagnosis. Acquired pure red cell aplasia may be caused by infection, malnutrition (kwashiorkor), drugs, toxins, renal failures, hemolytic syndromes, riboflavin deficiency, carcinoma, or leukemia and these precipitating causes or associated conditions must be excluded. It is unlikely that congenital hypoplastic anemia has its onset after the first few years of life; thus late onset cases of hypoplastic anemia are best considered pure red cell aplasia pending immunologic studies.

Treatment and prognosis. Conventional therapy with cobalt,[290] corticosteroids, androgens, splenectomy, and thymectomy have been disappointing, with about 25% to 30% responding to the latter procedure. Recent success has been achieved with the long-term administration of immunosuppressive therapy, notably cyclophosphamide, azathioprine, and 6-mercaptopurine alone or in combination with prednisone.[223,266,284] Patients failing to respond to cyclophosphamide may achieve remission after splenectomy or combined immunosuppressive therapy with cyclophosphamide and antilymphocyte globulin.[220,234] Because of the rarity of pure red cell anemia and thymoma in children, thoracic exploration is not recommended in patients without radiographic evidence of mediastinal widening. Prior to the introduction of immunosuppressive therapy the prognosis was poor. A mortality of about 40% had been observed, with death occurring about 3 years after diagnosis. Spontaneous remissions are uncommon and occur in 10% of the patients. The encouraging results with cyclophosphamide and other immunosuppressive drugs make these agents the initial treatment of choice.

Transitory hypoplastic anemias

Anemia caused by infections, drugs, chemicals, toxins, and allergic states. Under the heading of acute erythroblastopenias Gasser[188] described temporary and occasionally recurrent aregenerative crises of 1 week's duration as a result of toxic, infectious, or allergic causes. This acquired type of pure red cell aplasia was noted in patients who had been given drugs such as penicillin, chenopodium, and barbiturates and in those patients with infections including mumps, atypical pneumonia, and bacterial sepsis caused by meningococcus and staphylococcus. Allergic manifestations were common among these patients and their relatives. A case of acute transitory erythroid aplasia and vascular purpura in an otherwise hematologically normal child has been reported.[190] During the period of aplasia, bone marrow aspiration revealed the presence of giant pronormoblasts and an almost complete depletion of all other erythroid elements. Severe anemia never developed, either during the period of reticulocytopenia or in the recovery phase.

In addition to the drugs mentioned by Gasser a number of other agents have been associated with hypoplastic anemia, although the evidence implicating some is circumstantial. These drugs include phenytoin (Dilantin) in children[304] and isoniazid,[191] sulfathiazole,[280] arsphenamine,[272] tolbutamide, chlorpropamide,[259] glutethimide, colchicine, aspirin, aminosalicylic acid, and heparin in adults.* Although the mechanism of action of many of these drugs is unknown, phenytoin exerts its toxic effects by specifically inhibiting DNA synthesis in erythroid cells at the site of deoxyribotide formation.[304]

Idiopathic transitory erythroblastopenia. Transient anemia (symptomatic and more severe than in the aplasia described by Gasser), reticulocytopenia, and virtual absence of erythroid precursors in an otherwise normal marrow have been described.[233,302,303] Many but not all patients had preceding viral or bacterial infections and erythropoietin was present. Recovery was spontaneous and occurred within a few weeks of diagnosis. The inevitable spontaneous remissions and older age at onset differentiate transient erythroblastopenia from Diamond-Blackfan syndrome. The absence of giant pronormoblasts and relapses differentiates this disorder from Gasser's syndrome. The MCV is usually low (<80 fl), Hb F is normal, and i antigen is not increased,[237] findings that further differentiate the transient from the congenital disorder. An intermediate disorder with severe anemia, reticulocytopenia, and a matura-

---

*According to a tabulation of reports compiled by the Panel on Hematology of the AMA.

tion arrest at the pronormoblast stage without giant erythroid precursors was reported by Wranne et al.[303] The patient was treated with corticosteroids and 6-mercaptopurine and had a complete remission within 4 months after onset.

Transient erythroid aplasia in hemolytic anemia. Hypoplastic crises occur in patients with a number of hemolytic conditions. The acute form of erythroblastopenia was originally described by Owren[251] as a cause of sudden, severe anemia in hereditary spherocytosis. Aplastic crises have also been reported in sickle cell anemia,* thalassemia major,[211] other hemoglobinopathies, nonspherocytic hemolytic anemia,[208] G-6-PD deficiency,[166] hereditary elliptocytosis, and autoimmune hemolytic anemia.[177,269] Crises in these conditions are not hyperhemolytic, as was originally thought, but instead hypoplastic. The bone marrow shows a complete absence of erythropoiesis, the occasional presence of proerythroblasts, and occasionally a relative increase in immature granulocytic precursors and a decrease of megakaryocytes. Serum iron and percent saturation of transferrin increase and bilirubin and urobilinogen levels usually decrease during the crisis. The condition lasts only a few days and is followed by an erythroblastic hyperplasia and a rise in reticulocyte count and hemoglobin level. The severity of the anemia is aggravated by the fact that the aplasia occurs in patients with preexisting hemolytic disease in which the life span of the red cell is already reduced.[156,167]

Factors that contribute to erythroid aplasia in patients with an underlying hemolytic condition include infections[165] and folic acid deficiency.[215] Serum or cell-mediated inhibitors of erythropoiesis or to erythropoietin have not been detected in these disorders.

Characteristically patients have a syndrome of fever, anorexia, nausea, vomiting, headache, abdominal pain, rapidly falling hematocrit, and reticulocytopenia. The aplasia is self-limited with recovery beginning in 10 to 14 days. Therapeutic measures include treatment of any underlying infection and supportive transfusions. Rarely folic acid deficiency coexists with the crisis, requiring replacement therapy.

Erythroid hypoplasia in nutritional deficiencies

Riboflavin deficiency. Pure red cell aplasia has been observed in the course of galactoflavin-induced human riboflavin deficiency.[153,225] The anemia was normochromic and normocytic and in some cases levels of hemoglobin fell as much as 9 gm/dl. No changes in the white cell and platelet counts were noted. Serial marrow examina-

tions revealed a gradual reduction in basophilic and polychromatophilic normoblasts. The administration of riboflavin resulted in prolonged reticulocytosis, erythroid hyperplasia of the bone marrow, and correction of the anemia, despite the continuation of a riboflavin-deficient diet and galactoflavin administration. Although experimental riboflavin deficiency induces erythroid hypoplasia, its clinical significance is less certain because isolated riboflavin deficiency in the malnourished patient does not occur.

Protein-calorie malnutrition (kwashiorkor). Transient red cell aplasia commonly occurs during the treatment phase of kwashiorkor, beginning after 3 weeks of treatment and spontaneously remitting in about 10 days.[152,219,292] Multiple nutritional deficiencies including folate, iron, vitamin E, and riboflavin deficiencies have been implicated, but riboflavin given from the onset of therapy did not prevent the crisis.[181]

Erythroid hypoplasia and megaloblastic anemia have also been observed in patients with malnutrition and either folate or vitamin B_{12} deficiency.[256]

Anemia resulting from suppressive effect of multiple transfusions on erythropoiesis. The suppressive effect of multiple transfusions on erythropoiesis, which has been demonstrated in connection with thalassemia major,[276] probably extends also to the hypoplastic anemias in which transfusions are required therapy.

Congenital dyserythropoietic anemia

Definition. The term "congenital dyserythropoietic anemia" (CDA) refers to a group of hereditary disorders of erythropoiesis characterized by ineffective erythropoiesis, multinuclearity of erythroblasts, and secondary hemochromatosis.

Classification. On the basis of results of electron microscopic and serologic studies, four types of congenital dyserythropoietic anemia have been identified although there is considerable overlap between and variation within the types[229,270] (Table 8-2). The distinguishing features of the four types are as follows.

Type I is characterized by macrocytosis, megaloblastoid changes, and frequent internuclear chromatin bridges.

Type II (hereditary erythroblastic multinuclearity with positive acid-serum test [HEMPAS]) is characterized by binuclearity, multinuclearity, pluripolar mitoses, karyorrhexis, and the presence of abnormal antigens on the red cells.

Type III is characterized by multinuclearity with as many as twelve nuclei, gigantoblasts, and macrocytosis.

Type IV resembles type II morphologically but without the serologic abnormalities of type II.

---

*References 164, 215, 227, 273.

Table 8-2. Characteristics of congenital dyserythropoietic anemias

	Type I	Type II (HEMPAS)	Type III	Type IV
Incidence				
No. of reported cases	21	84	23	7
Percent of all cases	16	62	17	5
Inheritance	Autosomal recessive	Autosomal recessive	Autosomal dominant	Autosomal dominant (?)
Age at diagnosis (range)	Birth to 32 yr	Birth to 30 yr	2 mo to 72 yr	19 mo to 51 yr
Red cell morphologic features	Macrocytosis, aniso-poikilocytosis, shistocytosis	Anisopoikilo-cytosis, anisochromasia, shistocytosis	Macrocytosis	Normocytic normo-chromic of aniso-poikilocytosis
Marrow erythroid features	Megaloblastoid changes	Binuclearity, multi-nuclearity, Gaucher-like RE cells	Gigantoblasts, multi-nuclearity (12 nuclei)	Multinuclearity (29%-36%)
Electron microcopy	Nonspecific	Nonspecific, "double" cyto-plasmic membrane	Nonspecific	Nonspecific, "double" mem-brane
Serologic tests				
Acid hemolysis	Negative	Positive	Negative	Negative
Anti-I agglutination	Normal	Positive	Positive	Normal
Anti-i agglutination	Normal	Positive	Positive	Normal

Historical perspective. The first cases of congenital dyserythropoietic anemia (non–type III) were described in 1951 by Wolff and von Hofe.[301] In the early 1960s other cases of atypical congenital hemolytic anemia[169] associated with erythroblast multinuclearity and ineffective erythropoiesis appeared in the literature as "familial erythroid multinuclearity,"[301] "hereditary benign erythroreticulosis,"[158] "erythroblastic endopolyploidy,"[170] "haemolytic anaemia with multinucleated normoblasts,"[261] "ineffective erythropoiesis with morphologically abnormal erythroblasts and unconjugated hyperbilirubinemia,"[287] and "constitutional anemia with abnormality of nuclear division of the erythroblasts."[267] The term "congenital dyserythropoietic anemia" was used for the first time by Wendt and Heimpel in 1967.[203,299] Crookston et al.[168] identified the serologic abnormalities associated with Type II and coined the acronym "HEMPAS" to differentiate this type from the others. Recently, Lewis and Frisch[229] have clarified the common and distinguishing ultrastructural features of congenital dyserythropoietic anemia. The reader is referred to other excellent reviews.[231,286]

Incidence. The majority (62%) of the reported cases are of the type II variety. Of the others 16% are type I, 17% are type III, and only 5% are type IV.

Etiology and pathogenesis. Although a variety of biochemical disturbances, defects of the nuclear membrane, and defects of the plasma membrane have been described, the primary disturbance in congenital dyserythropoietic anemia has not been clarified. In vitro colony formation (CFU-C and CFU-E)[243] progresses normally but multinuclearity is present (Fig. 8-12). Abnormalities in granulocytes and megakaryocytes[298] have been detected by electron microscopy. Despite the perturbation in mitosis, the chromosomes themselves are normal.[201] The proliferation and nuclear structure of early erythroid precursors, erythroblasts, and basophilic normoblasts are also normal. However, increased cellular death[160,202] and decreased content of DNA[178] have been observed at the polychromatophilic and orthochromic normoblast stages. Electron microscopic studies have uncovered a number of anomalies of the nuclear membrane and pore complex[229] that are vital to DNA and RNA transport and polyribosome formation.[168,199] If such a defect were primary, the outcome would be failure of nuclear division and multinuclearity at the morphologic level and failure of DNA and RNA synthesis, RNA transport, disintegration of polyribosomes, and altered synthesis of hemoglobin at the biochemical level.[209,239]

A third mechanism, a defect in the plasma membrane, is suggested by the specific presence of the "HEMPAS antigen" on red cells in type II. The increased susceptibility of these cells involves an IgM anti-HEMPAS antibody (present in about 33% of all normal sera) and the binding of the fourth component of complement (C4).[168,265] A primary defect in the plasma membrane may block

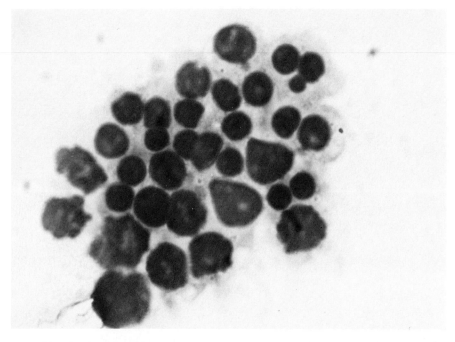

Fig. 8-12. Binuclearity and multinuclearity of erythroid colonies cultured in vitro from bone marrow of a patient with congenital dyserythropoietic anemia.

cytoplasmic cleavage with resultant secondary nuclear and biochemical abnormalities. Other membrane and cytoplasmic alterations such as (1) increased agglutinability in the presence of anti-i, (2) increased mitochondrial iron, (3) autophagocytic vacuoles in the cytoplasm,[298] and (4) increased red cell lipids[297] are nonspecific abnormalities that may be present in other states associated with dyserythropoiesis (such as thalassemia major, megaloblastic anemia, and sideroblastic anemia).

Genetics. On the basis of adequate family studies the mode of inheritance of types I and II is autosomal recessive. Type III appears to be inherited as an autosomal dominant characteristic. The inheritance pattern in type IV is uncertain because of the atypical nature of this variant and the small number of cases described to date.

Clinical and laboratory features. The onset and severity of symptoms in congenital dyserythropoietic anemia are variable. Although the disorders are congenital, the diagnosis in most cases is delayed until the second decade of life or later.[267] Intermittent jaundice, dark urine, mild to moderately severe anemia, splenomegaly, variable degrees of hepatomegaly, and cholelithiasis are the usual but nonspecific clinical findings. Hemosiderosis and hemochromatosis with nonfamilial diabetes mellitus, hypogonadism, hypothyroidism, and delayed secondary sexual maturation have been reported in older patients. Although few patients are transfusion dependent, iron overload appears to be related to increased gastrointestinal iron absorption, a result of marked erythroid hyperplasia.

The general laboratory features of dyserythropoiesis (p. 222) are present and include a low reticulocyte count relative to the anemia, particularly when corrected for hematocrit and maturation time, indirect hyperbilirubinemia, increased urobilinogen, and a ferrokinetic pattern of dyserythropoiesis with rapid ^{59}Fe clearance, decreased utilization (25% to 50%), and uptake over the bone marrow. The serum iron is normal or elevated and the percent saturation is high. Macrocytosis is characteristic of types I and III, but anisocytosis; poikilocytosis; schistocytes; irregularly contracted, fragmented, and crenated cells; polychromasia; and basophilic stippling are also seen in films of peripheral blood.

Nonspecific erythrocyte enzymatic abnormalities have been observed in types I and II, as well as in other dyserythropoietic states (chronic refractory anemia, folate deficiency, preleukemia and overt leukemia, juvenile chronic granulocytic anemia, and paroxysmal nocturnal hemoglobinuria).* Generally the values for phosphofructokinase, glutathione peroxidase, adenylate kinase, ribose phosphate pyrophosphokinase, adenine-phosphoribosyl transferase, and acetylcholine esterase were lower

*References 176, 242, 262, 283.

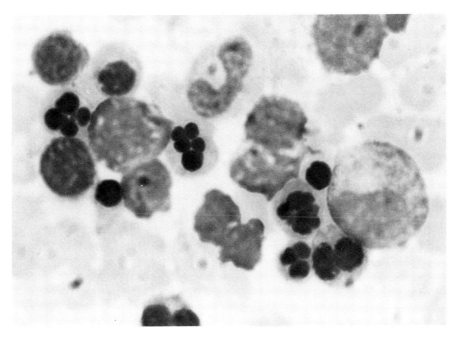

Fig. 8-13. Bone marrow findings in congenital dyserythropoietic anemia with erythroid hyperplasia, binuclearity, and multinuclearity of polychromatophilic and orthochromic normoblasts.

than expected for the degree of reticulocytosis and were similar to values obtained in cord blood erythrocytes.[246,282,283] The activity of pyruvate kinase was below the mean of cord red cells, a characteristic seen in many other acquired chronic refractory anemias.[283] Other features shared with fetal erythropoiesis include a high level of HbF,[175,235,295] γ-chain glycine:alanine ratio of fetal blood,[262,264] presence of i antigen,[205] and a cord blood lactic dehydrogenase isoenzyme pattern.[277,279]

Red blood cell survival has varied from normal to moderately decreased. Splenic sequestration is not usually seen although it has been documented in type III.[192]

No distinctive pattern of red blood cell lipids has emerged from four reported studies. Both increased[216,297] and decreased[249,270] total phospholipids and increased[297] and normal cholesterol levels[270] have been reported. Abnormalities in the distribution of phospholipid classes has been observed as well with reports of increased phosphatidylcholine (lecithin),[216,270,297] decreased[270,297] and increased[249] sphingomyelin, and decreased phosphatidylethanolamine levels.[249] The significance of these diverse findings is uncertain and may merely reflect underlying hepatic dysfunction or red blood cell destruction.

The bone marrow findings are characteristic with marked erythroid hyperplasia, binuclearity, multinuclearity (up to twelve nuclei per giant nor-

moblasts in type III), and internuclear bridging (Fig. 8-13). Gaucher-like histocytes containing birefringent crystalline inclusions have been seen in type II. Reticuloendothelial iron content is increased as are sideroblasts and siderocytes.

A number of ultrastructural abnormalities have been described.* These include persistent cytoplasmic bridges and microtubules, alterations in structure and density of chromatin, abnormalities of the nuclear envelope (with loss of integrity and myelinization of one or both layers of the nuclear membrane), widened nuclear pores, intranuclear intrusion by organelles such as mitochondria, intranuclear and cytoplasmic annulate lamellae, and various intracytoplasmic inclusions, notably membrane residues and cisternal structures (Fig. 8-14). The latter structures simulate the so-called double-membrane when they are opposed to the plasma membrane and represent an unusual persistence of endoplasmic reticulum. Ribosomes may be absent or distributed abnormally, mitochondria are laden with iron, and the plasma membrane itself is altered by vacuolization, myelinization, and disintegration. Autophagocytic vacuoles containing mitochondria and other cellular debris are also seen. Lewis and Frisch[229] have raised a justifiable note of caution concerning the over-interpretation of electron microscopic findings. Whereas previously specific ultrastructural fea-

---

*References 185, 186, 230, 285.

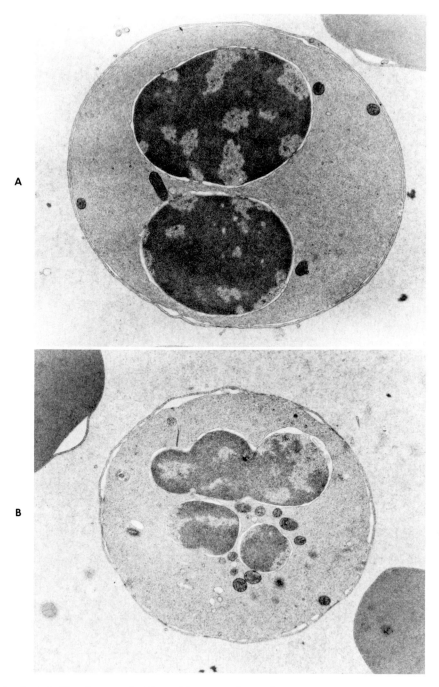

Fig. 8-14. A, Binucleate erythroblast with uneven chromatin condensation. There is focal apparent breakdown of the nuclear envelope and widening of the perinuclear cisternae. The peripheral cistern is prominent. (×10,000.) **B,** Erythroblast showing multiple nuclei with distention of perinuclear cisternae and spongy chromatin. Mitochondria contain iron. Note peripheral cistern. (×7,200.)

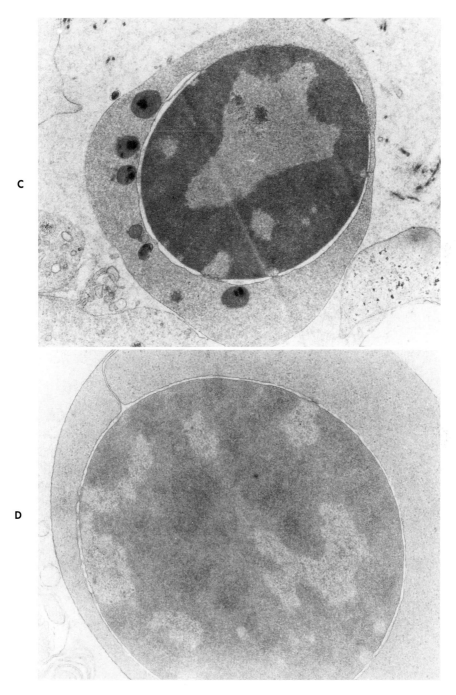

Fig. 8-14, cont'd. C, Erythroblast showing uneven chromatin condensation and spongy change in nucleus. There is distention of perinuclear cistern. Note iron-laden mitochondria. (×15,200.) **D,** Erythroblast showing uneven chromatin condensation, distention of the perinuclear cistern, and continuity between peripheral and perinuclear cisternae. (×21,600.)

Continued.

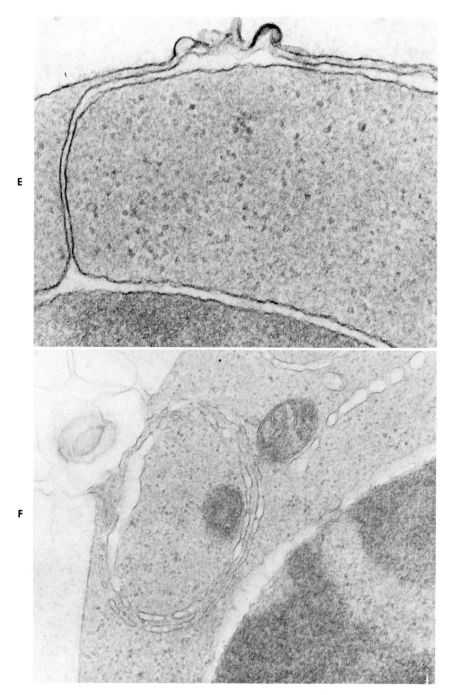

Fig. 8-14, cont'd. E, Portion of erythroblast showing continuity between peripheral and perinuclear cisternae. Note myelinization of plasma membrane. This is a higher magnification of a portion of **D.** (×84,000.) **F,** Erythroblast showing spongy nuclear chromatin and distention of perinuclear cistern. Note annulate lamellae in cytoplasm and myelinization of plasma membrane. (×40,000.) (Courtesy Philip Lieberman, M.D., Memorial Sloan-Kettering Cancer Center, New York.)

tures were ascribed to the different types of congenital dyserythropoietic anemia (e.g., internuclear bridges in type I and double plasma membrane in type II), more recent studies have demonstrated that these aberrations are characteristic of dyserythropoiesis in general. Some or all of these ultrastructural features have been seen in each of the congenital dyserythropoietic anemias and in other disorders of erythropoiesis (including thalassemia major, aplastic anemia, and lymphosarcoma).

The abnormal and distinguishing serologic studies are summarized in Table 8-2. The acidified-serum hemolysis (Ham's) test is positive in only two conditions, congenital dyserythropoietic anemia type II (HEMPAS) and paroxysmal nocturnal hemoglobinuria (PNH). Unlike paroxysmal nocturnal hemoglobinuria, however, the sucrose hemolysis test is negative in HEMPAS. Lysis and agglutination of erythrocytes by anti-I cold antibody is seen in types II and III congenital dyserythropoietic anemia; enhanced i-antigen activity with increased lysis and agglutination by anti-i is seen in types II and III but not in types I and IV.

Although a number of atypical syndromes have been reported, one interesting variant with features of both congenital dyserythropoietic anemia and β-thalassemia deserves special mention. Weatherall et al.[296] described six members of a family and Hruby et al.[209] reported a single case of apparent congenital dyserythropoietic anemia with autosomal dominant transmission, a clinical picture of anemia, jaundice and splenomegaly, 2% to 4% multinucleated erythroblasts, increased Hb F, and a negative acidified serum hemolysis test. Red blood cell indices were normal and *the morphology of the erythrocytes was not characteristic of thalasemia.* Weatherall's patients had moderate agglutination with anti-i, whereas Hruby's did not. The significant finding was unbalanced globin chain synthesis with α-chain production exceeding that of β-chain. In the patient with type IV the ratio of α-chain:β-chain was normal and no imbalance of chain synthesis was noted.[242] Furthermore, the concentration of fetal hemoglobin was normal. Excessive synthesis of β-chains relative to α-chains has been reported in sideroblastic anemia, an acquired form of dyserythropoietic anemia.[300]

Differential diagnosis. It is necessary to differentiate congenital dyserythropoietic anemia from a number of other hematologic disorders associated with varying degrees of dyserythropoiesis. Dyserythropoiesis in these disorders (p. 241) is a secondary event related to marrow failure (e.g., aplastic anemia, leukemia, erythroleukemia, and myelosclerosis), defects of nucleoprotein synthesis (e.g., vitamin B_{12} or folate deficiency), or defects of heme or globin synthesis (e.g., thalas-

semia syndromes, iron deficiency, sideroblastic anemias, lead poisoning, and infections). Serologic studies help distinguish type II from paroxysmal nocturnal hemoglobinuria. Because of the evolving heterogeneity of congenital dyserythropoietic anemia and the lack of distinguishing ultrastructural features among the various types, it may be difficult to categorize certain cases into specific types.

Treatment and prognosis. Most patients are not transfusion dependent and remain in generally good health. Splenectomy may be of benefit to patients with severe anemia who require chronic transfusion therapy. Deaths related to overwhelming infection in the postsplenectomy state have been reported and accordingly prophylactic penicillin is recommended. Cholelithiasis and chronic hepatic dysfunction have occurred and a number of patients have required gallbladder surgery, sometimes antedating a definite diagnosis. Hematinics such as folate, vitamin B_{12}, pyridoxine, vitamin E, and corticosteroids have been ineffective in modifying the anemia or the morphologic abnormalities of these disorders.

Future perspectives. Specific therapy of these disorders must await a better understanding of the molecular and cellular pathology. Advanced techniques of high-resolution electron microscopy may help determine a causal relationship between the nuclear, cytoplasmic, and membrane anomalies, and dyserythropoiesis, not only in congenital dyserythropoietic anemia but in secondary disorders as well. Another important area of investigation is to determine where in hematopoietic differentiation the lesion of dyserythropoiesis is located, i.e., in the stem cell or erythroid committed precursor. Finally, more definitive techniques may yield abnormalities of chromosomes such as partial trisomies and inversions.

REFERENCES
Normal erythropoiesis

1. Adamson, J. W., Alexanian, R., Martinez, C., and Finch, C. A.: Erythropoietin excretion in normal man, Blood **28:**354, 1966.
2. Alexanian, R.: Urinary excretion of erythropoietin in normal men and women, Blood **28:**344, 1966.
3. Alexanian, R., and Alfrey, C.: Erythropoiesis in anemia of bone marrow failure, J. Clin. Invest. **49:**1986, 1970.
4. Alpen, E. L., and Cranmore, D.: Observations on the regulation of erythropoiesis and cellular dynamics by Fe[59] autoradiography. In Stohlman, F., Jr., ed.: The kinetics of cellular proliferation, New York, 1959, Grune & Stratton, Inc.
5. Anger, H. O., and Van Dyke, D. C.: Human bone marrow distribution shown in vivo by iron-52 and the positron scintillation camera, Science **144:**1587, 1964.
6. Barr, R. D., Whang-Peng, J., and Perry, S.: Hematopoietic stem cells in human peripheral blood, Science **190:**284, 1975.
7. Barret, P. V. D., Cline, M. J., and Berlin, N. I.: The

association of the urobilin "early peak" and erythropoiesis in man, J. Clin. Invest. **45:**1657, 1966.

8. Becker, A. J., McCulloch, E. A., and Jell, J. E.: Cytological demonstration of the clonal nature of spleen colonies derived from transplanted mouse marrow cells, Nature **197:**452, 1963.

9. Bert, P., cited by Krantz, S., and Graber, S. E.: Erythropoietin. In Root, W. S., and Berlin, N. I.: Physiological pharmacology, Vol. 5, Blood, New York, 1974, Academic Press, Inc.

10. Bond, V. P., Odartchenko, N., Cottier, H., et al.: The kinetics of the more mature erythropoietic precursors studied with tritiated thymidine. In Jacobson, L. O., and Doyle, M., eds.: Erythropoiesis, New York, 1962, Grune & Stratton, Inc.

11. Bonsdorff, E., and Jalavisto, E.: Humoral mechanism in anoxic erythrocytosis, Acta Physiol. Scand. **16:**150, 1948.

12. Bothwell, T. H., Callender, S., Mallett, B., and Witts, L. T.: Study of erythropoiesis using tracer quantities of radioactive iron, Br. J. Haematol. **2:**1, 1956.

13. Boycott, A. E.: The blood as a tissue: hypertrophy and atrophy of the red corpuscles, Proc. R. Soc. Med. **23:**15, 1929.

14. Buchanan, G. R., and Schwartz, A. D.: Impaired erythropoietin response in anemic premature infants, Blood **44:**347, 1974.

15. Busuttil, R. W., Roh, B. L., and Fisher, J. W.: The cytological localization of erythropoietin in the human kidney using the fluorescent antibody technique, Proc. Soc. Exp. Biol. Med. **137:**327, 1971.

16. Carnot, P., and Deflandre, C.: Sur l'activité hémopoiétique du serum, Compt. Rend. Acad. Sc. **143:**384, 1906.

17. Cartwright, G. E.: The anemia of chronic disorders, Semin. Hematol. **3:**351, 1966.

18. Chang, S. C.-S., Sikkema, D., and Goldwasser, E.: Evidence for an erythropoietin receptor protein on rat bone marrow cells, Biochem. Biophys. Res. Commun. **57:**399, 1974.

19. Chui, D. H., Djaldetti, M., Marks, P. A., and Rifkind, R. A.: Erythropoietin effects on fetal mouse erythroid cells. I. Cell population and hemoglobin synthesis, J. Cell. Biol. **51:**585, 1971.

20. Clark, A. C. L.: Erythropoiesis in the newborn. III. Urinary inhibitor—is it an oestrogen? Aust. Paediatr. J. **10:**270, 1974.

21. Clark, A. C. L., and Roche, D. A.: Erythropoiesis in the newborn. I. Urinary erythropoietin assays, Aust. Paediatr. J. **9:**121, 1973.

22. Clayton, R. B., Cooper, J. M., Boorsook, H., et al.: Stimulation of erythroblast maturation in vitro by sphingolipids, J. Lipid Res. **15:**557, 1974.

23. Coburn, R. F., Williams, W. J., White, P., and Kahn, S. B.: The production of carbon monoxide from hemoglobin in vivo, J. Clin. Invest. **46:**346, 1967.

24. Cole, R. J., and Paul, J.: The effect of erythropoietin on haemsynthesis in mouse yolk sac and cultured foetal liver cells, J. Embryol. Exp. Morphol. **15:**245, 1966.

25. Collins, R. B., Clark, A. C. L., and Patterson, B.: Erythropoiesis in the newborn. II. Urinary inhibitor of erythropoiesis, Aust. Paediatr. J. **9:**129, 1973.

26. Cooper, E. H., and Wickramasinghe, S. N.: Quantitative cytochemistry in the study of erythropoiesis, Ser. Haematol. II. **4:**65, 1969.

27. Cooper, M. D., Levy, J., Cantor, L. N., et al.: Effect of erythropoietin on colonial growth of erythroid precursors in vitro, Proc. Natl. Acad. Sci. U.S.A. **71:**1677, 1974.

28. Cotes, P. M., and Bangham, D. R.: Bio-assay of erythropoietin in mice made polycythaemic by exposure to air at a reduced pressure, Nature **191:**1065, 1961.

29. Crosby, W. H.: The limits of erythropoiesis: how much can the marrow produce with total recruitment? Blood Cells **1:**497, 1975.

30. Delivoria-Papadopoulos, M., Roncevic, N. P., and Oski, F. A.: Postnatal changes in oxygen transport in term, premature, and sick infants: the role of red cell 2,3-diphosphoglycerate and adult hemoglobin, Pediatr. Res. **5:**235, 1971.

31. Dicke, K. A., van Noord, M. J., and Van Bekkum, D. W.: Attempts at morphological identification of the hematopoietic stem cells in rodents and primates, Exp. Haematol. **1:**36, 1973.

32. Donohoe, D. M., Reiff, R. H., Hanson, M. L., et al.: Quantitative measurement of the erythrocytic and granulocytic cells of the marrow and blood, J. Clin. Invest. **37:**1571, 1958.

33. Dukes, P. P.: In vitro studies of DNA synthesis of bone marrow cells stimulated by erythropoietin, Ann. N.Y. Acad. Sci. **149:**437, 1968.

34. Dukes, P. P., and Goldwasser, E.: On the mechanism of erythropoietin-induced differentiation. III. The nature of erythropoietin action on (14C) glucosamine incorporation by marrow cells in culture, Biochem. Biophys. Acta **108:**447, 1965.

35. Erslev, A. J.: Humoral regulation of red cell production, Blood **8:**349, 1953.

36. Erslev, A. J., and Lavietes, P. H.: Observations on the nature of the erythropoietic serum factor, Blood **9:**1055, 1954.

37. Faille, A. Najean, Y., and Dresch, C.: Kinetic pattern of erythropoiesis in fourteen cases of "ineffective erythropoiesis" with morphologic abnormalities of erythroblasts and multinuclearity, Nouv. Rev. Fr. Hematol. **12:**631, 1972.

38. Finch, C. A.: Some quantitative aspects of erythropoiesis, Ann. N.Y. Acad. Sci. **77:**410, 1959.

39. Finch, C. A., Coleman, D. H., Motulsky, A. G., et al.: Erythrokinetics in pernicious anemia, Blood **11:**807, 1956.

40. Finne, P. H.: Erythropoietin levels in the amniotic fluid, particularly in Rh-immunized pregnancies, Acta Paediatr. Scand. **53:**269, 1964.

41. Finne, P. H.: Erythropoietin levels in cord blood as an indicator of intrauterine hypoxia, Acta Paediatr. Scand. **55:**478, 1966.

42. Finne, P. H., and Halvorsen, S.: Regulation of erythropoiesis in the fetus and newborn, Arch. Dis. Child. **47:**683, 1972.

43. Fisher, J. W., and Langston, J. W.: Effects of testosterone, cobalt, and hypoxia on erythropoietin production in the isolated perfused dog kidney, Ann. N.Y. Acad. Sci. **149:**75, 1968.

44. Fisher, J. W., Moriyama, Y., and Lertora, J. J. L.: Mechanisms of androgen stimulated erythropoiesis and inhibitors of heme synthesis in uremia, Blood Cells **1:**573, 1975.

45. Fisher, J. W., Samuels, A. I., and Langston, J.: Effects of angiotensin, norepinephrine, and renal artery constriction on erythropoietin production, Ann. N.Y. Acad. Sci. **149:**308, 1968.

46. Fried, W.: The liver as a source of extrarenal erythropoietin production, Blood **40:**671, 1972.

47. Fried, W., Plzak, L. F., Jacobson, L. O., and Goldwasser, E.: Studies on erythropoietin. III. Factors controlling erythropoietin production, Proc. Soc. Exp. Biol. Med. **94:**237, 1957.

48. Fried, W., Ward, H. P., and Hopeman, A. R.: Leiomyoma and erythrocytosis: A tumor producing a factor which increases erythropoietin production, report of a case, Blood **31:**813, 1968.

49. Giblett, E. R., Coleman, D. H., Perzio-Beroli, G., et al.:

Erythrokinetics: Quantitative measurements of red cell production and destruction in normal subjects and patients with anemia, Blood **11**:291, 1956.

50. Golde, D. W.: Regulation of human erythropoiesis in liquid culture. In Nakao, K., Fisher, J. W., and Takaku, F., eds.: Erythropoiesis, Baltimore, 1975, University Park Press.

51. Goldwasser, E., and Kung, C. K. H.: Progress in the purification of erythropoietin, Ann. N.Y. Acad. Sci. **149**:49, 1968.

52. Gordon, A. S., Cooper, G. W., and Zanjani, E. D.: The kidneys and erythropoiesis, Sem. Hematol. **4**:337, 1967.

53. Gordon, A. S., Katz, R., Zanjani, E. D., et al.: Renal mechanisms underlying actions of androgens and hypoxia on erythropoiesis, Proc. Soc. Exp. Biol. Med. **123**:475, 1966.

54. Gordon, A. S., Zanjani, E. D., and Zalusky, R.: A possible mechanism for the erythrocytosis associated with hepatocellular carcinoma in man, Blood **35**:171, 1970.

55. Granick, S., and Kappas, A.: Steroid control of porphyrin and heme biosynthesis: A new biological function of steroid hormone metabolites, Proc. Nat. Acad. Sci. U.S.A. **57**:1463, 1967.

56. Grant, W. C., and Root, W. S.: Fundamental stimulus for erythropoiesis, Physiol. Rev. **4**:449, 1952.

57. Gray, D. F., and Erslev, A. J.: Reticulocytosis induced by serum from hypoxic animals, Proc. Soc. Exp. Biol. Med. **94**:283, 1957.

58. Griffiths, W. J., and Lothian, E. J.: Erythropoiesis, red-cell and plasma aldolase activity in anaemia in the rabbit and man, Br. J. Haematol. **17**:477, 1969.

59. Gross, M., and Goldwasser, E.: On the mechanism of erythropoietin-induced differentiation. V. Characterization of the ribonucleic acid formed as a result of erythropoietin action, Biochemistry **8**:1795, 1969.

60. Halvorsen, K., Haga, P., and Halvorsen, S.: Regulation of erythropoiesis in the fetus and neonate. In Nakao, K., Fisher, J. W., and Takaku, F., eds.: Erythropoiesis, Proceedings of Fourth International Conference on Erythropoiesis, Baltimore, 1975, University Park Press.

61. Halvorsen, S.: Plasma erythropoietin levels in cord blood and in blood during the first week of life, Acta Paediatr. Scand. **52**:425, 1963.

62. Hammond, D., and Ishikawa, A.: In Jacobson, L. B., and Doyle, M., eds.: Erythropoiesis, New York, 1962, Grune & Stratton, Inc.

63. Hanna, I. R. A., Spicer, S. S., Green, W. B., and Horn, R. G.: Shortening of the cell-cycle time of erythroid precursors in response to anaemia, Br. J. Haematol. **16**:381, 1969.

64. Hansen, N. E., and Anderson, V.: Lactate dehydrogenase of human marrow in the study of haemopoiesis, Acta Med. Scand. **183**:581, 1968.

65. Haurani, F. I., and Tocantins, L. M.: Ineffective erythropoiesis, Am. J. Med. **31**:519, 1961.

66. Hillman, R. S.: Characteristics of marrow production and reticulocyte maturation in normal man in response to anemia, J. Clin. Invest. **48**:443, 1969.

67. Hillman, R. S., and Finch, C. A.: Erythropoiesis: Normal and abnormal, Semin. Hematol. **4**:327, 1967.

68. Hillman, R. S., and Giblett, E. R.: Red cell membrane alteration associated with "marrow stress," J. Clin. Invest. **44**:1730, 1965.

69. Hillman, R. S., and Henderson, P. A.: Control of marrow production by levels of iron supply, J. Clin. Invest. **48**:454, 1969.

70. Hrinda, M. E., and Goldwasser, E.: On the mechanism of erythropoietin-inducted differentiation. VI. Induced accumulation of iron by marrow cells, Biochem. Biophys. Acta **195**:165, 1969.

71. Hughes-Jones, N. C., and Szur, L.: Determination of the sites of red-cell destruction using ^{51}Cr-labelled cells, Br. J. Haematol. **3**:320, 1957.

72. Iscove, N. N., Sieber, F., and Winterhalter, K. H.: Erythroid colony formation in cultures of mouse and human bone marrow: Analysis of the requirement for erythropoietin by gel filtration and affinity chromatography on agarose-concanavalin, Am. J. Cell. Physiol. **83**:309, 1974.

73. Israels, L. G., Skanderberg, J., Guyda, H., et al.: A study of the early-labelled fraction of bile pigment: the effects of altering erythropoiesis on the incorporation of (2-^{14}C) glycine into haem and bilirubin, Br. J. Haematol. **9**:50, 1963.

74. Ishikawa, A., and Hammond, G. D.: Erythropoietin in serum and urine in Cooley's anemia, Am. J. Dis. Child. **102**:592, 1961.

75. Jandl, J. H., Greenberg, M. S., Yonemoto, R., et al.: Clinical determination of the sites of red cell sequestration in hemolytic anemias, J. Clin. Invest. **35**:842, 1956.

76. Kawafuchi, J., Shirakura, T., Ozuma, M., et al.: Hematologic study on a case with cerebellar hemangioblastoma associated with erythrocytosis, with special reference to a erythropoiesis-stimulating activity present in the fluid of the cyst of tumor, Blut **20**:69, 1970.

77. Kenny, G. M., Mirand, E. A., Staubitz, W. J., et al.: Erythropoietin levels in Wilms tumor patients, J. Urol. **104**:758, 1970.

78. Killman, S. A., Cronkite, E. P., Fliedner, T. M., and Bond, V. P.: Mitotic indices of human bone marrow cells. III. Duration of some phases of erythrocytic and granulocytic proliferation computed from mitotic indices, Blood **24**:267, 1964.

79. Krantz, S. B., and Graber, S. E.: Erythropoietin. In Root, W. S., and Berlin, N. I., eds.: Physiological pharmacology, Vol. 5, Blood, New York, 1974, Academic Press, Inc.

80. Krzymowski, T., and Krzymowski, H.: Studies on the erythropoiesis inhibiting factor in the plasma of animals with transfusion polycythemia, Blood **19**:38, 1962.

81. Kuratowska, Z., Lewartowski, B., and Michalak, E.: Studies on the production of erythropoietin by isolated perfused organs, Blood **18**:527, 1961.

82. Lajtha, L. G., Gilbert, C. W., and Guzman, E. E.: Kinetics of haematopoietic colony growth, Br. J. Haematol. **20**:343, 1971.

83. Lajtha, L. G., and Oliver, R.: Studies on the kinetics of erythropoiesis: A model of the erythron. In Wolstenholme, G. E. W., and O'Connor, M., eds.: Ciba Foundation Symposium on Haemopoiesis, New York, 1966, Academic Press, Inc.

84. Leblond, P. F., LaCelle, P. L., and Weed, R. I.: Cellular deformability: a possible determinant of the normal release of maturing erythrocytes from the bone marrow, Blood **37**:40, 1971.

85. Lewis, J. P., Alford, D. A., Moores, R. R., et al.: Dialysis as a tool in the study of erythropoietin, J. Lab. Clin. Med. **73**:154, 1969.

86. Lewis, S. M.: Red cell abnormalities and haemolysis in aplastic anaemia, Br. J. Haematol. **8**:322, 1962.

87. Lewis, S. M., and Verwilghen, R. L.: Annotation: dyserythropoiesis and dyserythropoietic anaemias, Br. J. Haematol. **23**:1, 1972.

88. Lindemann, R.: Urinary excretion of erythropoietin and erythropoiesis inhibitors in the neonatal period, Acta Paediatr. Scand. **63**:764, 1974.

89. Lindemann, R.: Erythropoietin and erythropoiesis inhibitors in the neonatal period, In Nakao, K., Fisher, J. W., and Takaku, F., eds.: Erythropoiesis, Proceedings of Fourth International Conference in Erythropoiesis, Baltimore, 1975, University Park Press.

90. Linman, J. W., Long, M. J., Korst, D. R., et al.: Studies on the stimulation of hemopoiesis by batyl alcohol, J. Lab. Clin. Med. **54:**335, 1959.

91. London, I. M., Favill, A. S., Vanderhoff, G. A., et al.: Erythroid cell differentiation and the synthesis and assembly of hemoglobin, Dev. Biol. (suppl.) **1:**227, 1967.

92. London, I. M., West, R., Shemin, D., and Rittenberg, D.: On the origin of bile pigment in normal man, J. Biol. Chem. **184:**351, 1950.

93. McCulloch, E. A., Siminovitch, L., and Till, J. E.: Spleen colony formation in anemic mice of genotype WW^v, Science **144:**844, 1964.

94. McCulloch, E. A., Siminovitch, L., Till, J. E., et al.: The cellular basis of the genetically determined hemopoietic defect in anemic mice of genotype S1/S1^d, Blood **26:**299, 1965.

95. McCulloch, E. A., and Till, J. E.: Control of hematopoiesis at the cellular level. In Gordon, A. S., ed.: Regulation of hematopoiesis, New York, 1970, Appleton-Century-Crofts.

96. McIntosh, S.: Erythropoietin excretion in the premature infant, J. Pediatr. **86:**202, 1975.

97. McLeod, D. L., Shreeve, M. M., and Axelrad, A. A.: Improved plasma culture system for production of erythrocytic colonies in vitro: Quantitative assay method for CFU-E, Blood **44:**517, 1974.

98. Metcalf, D.: Hematopoietic stem cells. In Root, W. S., and Berlin, N. I., eds.: Physiological pharmacology, Vol. 5, Blood, New York 1974, Academic Press, Inc.

99. Meuret, G., Boll, I., Graf Keyserlingk, G., and Heissmeyer, H.: Morphologasche und kinetische befunde bei einer kongenitalen dyserythropoietischen Anaemie, Blut **21:**341, 1970.

100. Mills, S. D., and Mason, H. L.: Values for fecal urobilinogen in childhood, Am. J. Dis. Child. **84:**322, 1952.

101. Mirand, E. A., and Murphy, G. P.: Erythropoietin alterations in patients with uremia, renal allografts, or without kidneys. J.A.M.A. **209:**392, 1969.

102. Miura, Y., Suzuki, S., Mizoguchi, H., and Takaku, F.: Role of microenvironments in erythropoiesis. In Erythropoiesis, Proceedings of Fourth International Conference on Erythropoiesis, Baltimore, 1975, University Park Press.

103. Murphy, G. P., Mirand, E. A., Johnston, G. S., et al.: Erythropoietin release associated with Wilms' tumor, Johns Hopkins Med. J. **120:**26, 1967.

104. Murphy, G. P., Mirand, E. A., Johnston, G. S., et al.: Erythropoietin alterations in human genitourinary disease states: correlation with experimental observations, J. Urol. **99:**802, 1968.

105. Murphy, G. P., Allen, J. E., Staubitz, W. J., et al.: Erythropoietin levels in patients with Wilms' tumor, N.Y. State J. Med. **72:**487, 1972.

106. Necheles, T. F., Sheehan, R. G., and Meyer, H. J.: Studies on the control of hemoglobin synthesis: nucleic acid synthesis and normoblast proliferation in the presence of erythropoietin, Ann. N.Y. Acad. Sci. **149:**449, 1968.

107. O'Brien, R. T., and Pearson, H. A.: Physiologic anemia of the newborn infant, J. Pediatr. **79:**132, 1971.

108. Oski, F. A., and Stockman, J. A.: Anaemia in early infancy, Br. J. Haematol. **27:**195, 1974.

109. Ossias, A. L., Zanjani, E. D., Zalusky, R., et al.: Case report: studies on the mechanism of erythrocytosis associated with uterine fibromyoma, Br. J. Haematol. **25:**179, 1973.

110. Paul, J., and Hunter, J. A.: Synthesis of macromolecules during induction of haemoglobin synthesis by erythropoietin, J. Mol. Biol. **42:**31, 1969.

111. Peschle, C., and Condorelli, M.: Regulation of fetal and adult erythropoiesis. In Congenital disorders of erythropoiesis, Ciba Foundation symposium 37 (new series), New York, 1976, American Elsevier Publishing Co., Inc.

112. Peschle, C., Sasso, G. F., Rappaport, I. A., and Condorelli, M.: Extrarenal erythropoietin production: possible role of the renal erythropoietic factor, J. Lab. Clin. Med. **79:**950, 1972.

113. Reismann, K. R.: Studies on the mechanism of erythropoietic stimulation in parabiotic rats during hypoxia, Blood **5:**372, 1950.

114. Rhyner, K., and Ganzoni, A.: Erythrokinetics: evaluation of red cell production by ferrokinetics and reticulocyte counts, Eur. J. Clin. Invest. **2:**96, 1972.

115. Robinson, S. H., Lester, R., Crigler, J. F., Jr., et al.: Early-labeled peak of bile pigment in man; studies with glycine-^{14}C and delta-aminolevulinic acid-^{3}H, N. Engl. J. Med. **277:**1323, 1967.

116. Robinson, S. H., and Tsong, M.: Hemolysis of "stress" reticulocytes: a source of erythropoietic bilirubin formation, J. Clin. Invest. **49:**1025, 1970.

117. Robinson, S. H., Tsong, M., Brown, B. W., and Schmid, R.: The sources of bile pigment in the rat: studies of the "early labeled" fraction, J. Clin. Invest. **45:**1569, 1966.

118. Ronai, P., Winchell, H. S., Anger, H. O., and Lawrence, J. H.: Whole-body scanning of ^{59}Fe for evaluating body distribution of erythropoietic marrow, splenic sequestration of red cells, and hepatic deposition of iron, J. Nucl. Med. **10:**469, 1969.

119. Rothman, I. K., Zanjani, E. D., Gordon, A. S., and Silber, R.: Nucleoside deaminase: an enzymatic marker for stress erythropoiesis in the mouse, J. Clin. Invest. **49:**2051, 1970.

120. Schofield, R., and Lajtha, L. G.: Cellular kinetics of erythropoiesis. In Congenital disorders of erythropoiesis, Ciba Foundation symposium 37 (new series), New York, 1976, American Elsevier Publishing Co., Inc.

121. Schooley, J. C., Garcia, J. F., Cantor, L. N., and Havens, V. W.: A summary of some studies in erythropoiesis using anti-Ep immune serum, Ann. N.Y. Acad. Sci. **149:**266, 1968.

122. Skjaelaaen, P., and Halvorsen, S.: Inhibition of erythropoiesis by plasma from newborn infants, Acta Paediatr. Scand. **60:**301, 1971.

123. Slaunwhite, W. R., Jr., Mirand, E. A., and Prentice, T. C.: Probable polypeptidic nature of erythropoietin, Proc. Soc. Exp. Biol. Med. **96:**616, 1957.

124. Stephensen, J. R., Axelrad, A. A., McLeod, D. L. and Shreeve, M. M.: Induction of colonies of hemoglobin-synthesizing cells by erythroipoietin in vitro, Proc. Nat. Acad. Sci. U.S.A. **68:**1542, 1971.

125. Stohlman, F., Jr.: Observations on physiology of erythropoietin and its role in regulation of red cell production, Ann. N.Y. Acad. Sci. **77:**710, 1959.

126. Stohlman, F., Jr.: The kidney and erythropoiesis, N. Engl. J. Med. **279:**1437, 1968.

127. Stohlman, F., Jr., Beland, A., and Howard, D.: Mechanism of macrocytic response to erythropoietin, J. Clin. Invest. **42:**984, 1963.

128. Tafari, N., and Habte, D.: "Physiologic anaemia" of infancy at high altitude, Acta Paediatr. Scand. **61:**706, 1972.

129. Tarbutt, R. G.: Cell population kinetics of the erythroid system in the rat: the response to protracted anaemia and to continuous α irradiation, Br. J. Haematol. **16:**9, 1969.

130. Tepperman, A. D., Curtis, J. E., and McCulloch, E. A.:

Erythropoietic colonies in cultures of human marrow, Blood **44:**659, 1974.

131. Thorling, E. B.: Paraneoplastic erythrocytosis and inappropriate erythropoietin production, Scand. J. Haematol. Suppl. 17, 1972.

132. Thorling, E. B., and Erslev, A. J.: The "tissue" tension of oxygen and its relation to hematocrit and erythropoiesis, Blood **31:**332, 1968.

133. Thurman, W. G., Grabstald, H., and Lieberman, P. H.: Elevation of erythropoietin levels in association with Wilms' tumor, Arch. Intern. Med. **117:**280, 1966.

134. Till, J. E., and McCulloch, E. A.: A direct measurement of the radiation sensitivity of normal mouse bone marrow cells, Radiat. Res. **14:**213, 1961.

135. Toyama, K., Fujiyama, N., Chan, T. P., et al.: Erythrocytosis associated with various tumors: with a case report of meningioma associated with erythrocytosis. In Nakao, K., Fisher, J. W., Takaka, F., eds.: Erythropoiesis, Proceedings of Fourth International Conference on Erythropoiesis, Baltimore, 1975, University Park Press.

136. Trentin, J. J.: Influence of hemopoietic organ stroma (hematopoietic inductive microenvironments) on stem cell differentiation. In Gordon, A. S., ed.: Regulation of hematopoiesis, New York, 1970, Appleton-Century-Crofts.

137. Van Dyke, D. C.: In Jacobson, L. O., and Doyle, M., eds.: Erythropoiesis, New York, 1962, Grune & Stratton, Inc.

138. Waldmann, T. A., Rosse, W. F., and Swerm, R. L.: The erythropoiesis stimulating factors produced by tumors, Ann. N.Y. Acad. Sci. **149:**509, 1968.

139. Wallner, S. F., Ward, H. P., Vautrin, R., et al.: The anemia of chronic renal failure: in vitro response of bone marrow to erythropoietin, Proc. Soc. Exp. Biol. Med. **149:**939, 1975.

140. Ward, H. P., Kurnick, J. E., and Pisarczyk, M. J.: Serum level of erythropoietin in anemias associated with chronic infection, malignancy, and primary hematopoietic disease, J. Clin. Invest. **50:**332, 1971.

141. Whitcomb, W. H., and Moore, M.: The physiologic significance of an erythropoietic factor appearing in plasma subsequent to hypertransfusion, Ann. N.Y. Acad. Sci. **149:**462, 1968.

142. White, P., Coburn, R. F., Williams, W. J., et al.: Carbon monoxide production associated with ineffective erythropoiesis, J. Clin. Invest. **46:**1986, 1967.

143. Wickramasinghe, S. N.: Human bone marrow, Oxford, 1975, Blackwell Scientific Publications, Ltd.

144. Wilmanns, W., Sauer, H., and Gelinsky, P.: Beiziehungen zwischen enzymatischer Formiataktivierung und Erythrozytenlebensdauer, Blut **19:**457, 1969.

145. Witts, L. J.: Some aspects of the pathology of anaemia. I. Theory of maturation arrest, Br. Med. J. **2:**325, 1961.

146. Wrigley, P. F. M., Malpas, J. S., Turnbull, A. L., et al.: Secondary polycythaemia due to a uterine fibromyoma producing erythropoietin, Br. J. Haematol. **21:**551, 1971.

147. Zanjani, E. D., Peterson, E. N., Gordon, A. S., and Wasserman, L. R.: Erythropoietin production in the fetus: role of the kidney and maternal anemia, J. Lab. Clin. Med. **83:**281, 1974.

148. Zanjani, E. D., McLaurin, W. D., Gordon, A. S., et al.: Biogenesis of erythropoietin: role of the substrate for erythrogenin, J. Lab. Clin. Med. **77:**751, 1971.

149. Zucker, S., Friedman, S., and Lysik, R. M.: Bone marrow erythropoiesis in the anemia of infection, inflammation, and malignancy, J. Clin. Invest. **53:**1132, 1974.

150. Zucker, S., and Lysik, R.: Bone marrow erythropoiesis in anemia of inflammation, J. Lab. Clin. Med. **84:**620, 1974.

Clinical disorders of erythropoiesis

151. Aase, J. M., and Smith, D. W.: Congenital anemia and triphalangeal thumb: a new syndrome, J. Pediatr. **74:**471, 1969.

152. Adams, E. B.: Anemia associated with protein deficiency, Sem. Hematol. **7:**55, 1970.

153. Alfrey, C. P., and Lane, M.: The effect of riboflavin deficiency on erythropoiesis, Sem. Hematol. **7:**49, 1970.

154. Allen, D. M., and Diamond, L. K.: Congenital (erythroid) hypoplastic anemia: cortisone treated, Am. J. Dis. Child. **102:**416, 1961.

155. Altman, K. I., and Miller, G.: A disturbance of tryptophan metabolism in congenital hypoplastic anemia, Nature **172:**868, 1953.

156. Bauman, A. W., and Swisher, S. N.: Hyporegenerative processes in hemolytic anemia, Sem. Hematol. **4:**265, 1967.

157. Beard, M. E. J.: Fanconi's anaemia. In Congenital disorders of erythropoiesis, Ciba Foundation symposium 37 (new series), New York, 1976, American Elsevier Publishing Co. Inc.

158. Bergstrom, I., and Jacobsson, L.: Hereditary benign erythroreticulosis, Blood **19:**296, 1962.

159. Bomford, R. R., and Rhoads, C. P.: Refractory anaemia, Quart. J. Med. **34:**175, 1941.

160. Breton-Gorius, J., Daniel, M., Clauvel, J., and Dreyfus, B.: Anomalies ultrastructurales des erythroblastes dans six cas de dyserythropoiese congenitale, Nouv. Rev. Fr. Hematol. **13:**23, 1973.

161. Brookfield, E. G., and Singh, P.: Congenital hypoplastic anemia associated with hypogammaglobulinemia, J. Pediatr. **85:**529, 1974.

162. Burgert, E. O., Kennedy, R. L. J., and Pease, G. L.: Congenital hypoplastic anemia, Pediatrics **13:**218, 1954.

163. Cathie, I. A. B.: Erythrogenesis imperfecta, Arch. Dis. Child. **25:**313, 1950.

164. Charney, E., and Miller, G.: Reticulocytopenia in sickle cell disease, Am. J. Dis. Child. **107:**450, 1964.

165. Choremis, C. B., Megas, H. A., Liaromati, A. A., and Michael, S. C.: Aplastic crisis in the course of infectious diseases: report of 10 cases, Helv. Paediatr. Acta **16:**134, 1961.

166. Cloutier, M. D., and Burgert, E. O., Jr.: Congenital nonspherocytic hemolytic disease secondary to glucose-6-phosphate dehydrogenase deficiency: report of three cases, Mayo Clin. Proc. **41:**316, 1966.

167. Conklin, G. T., George, J. N., and Sears, D. A.: Transient erythroid aplasia in hemolytic anemia: a review of the literature with two case reports, Tex. Rep. Biol. Med. **32:**2, 1974.

168. Crookston, J. H., Crookston, M. C., Burnie, K. L., et al.: Hereditary erythroblastic multinuclearity associated with a positive acidified serum test: a type of congenital dyserythropoietic anaemia, Br. J. Haematol. **17:**11, 1969.

169. Dacie, J. V., Mollison, P. L., Richardson, N., et al.: Atypical congenital heamolytic anaemia, Quart. J. Med. **22:**79, 1953.

170. DeLozzio, C. B., Valencia, J. I., and Acame, E. A.: Chromosomal study in erythroblastic endopolyploidy, Lancet **1:**1004, 1962.

171. Diamond, L. K., and Blackfan, K. D.: Hypoplastic anemia, Am. J. Dis. Child. **56:**464, 1938.

172. Diamond, L. K., Allen, D. M., and Magill, F. B.: Congenital (erythroid) hypoplastic anemia: a 25 year study, Am. J. Dis. Child. **102:**403, 1961.

173. Diamond, L. K., Wang, W. C., and Alter, B. P.: Congenital hypoplastic anemia. In Schulman I., ed.: Ad-

vances in pediatrics, Vol. 22, Chicago, 1976, Year Book Medical Publishers, Inc.

174. DiGiacomo, J., Furst, S. W., and Nixon, D. D.: Primary acquired red cell aplasia in the adult, J. Mt. Sinai Hosp. N.Y. **33:**382, 1966.

175. Dreyfus, B., Rochant, H., and Sultan, C.: Anémies réfractaires: enzymopathies acquises des cellules souches hématopoiétiques, Nouv. Rev. Fr. Hématol. **9:**65, 1969.

176. Dreyfus, B., Sultan, C., Rochant, H., et al.: Anomalies of blood group antigens and erythrocyte enzymes in two types of chronic refractory anaemia, Br. J. Haematol. **16:**303, 1969.

177. Eisenmann, G., and Dameshek, W.: Splenectomy for "pure red-cell" hypoplastic (aregenerative) anemia associated with autoimmune hemolytic disease, N. Engl. J. Med. **251:**1044, 1954.

178. Faille, A., Najean, Y., and Dresch, C.: Cinétique de l'érythropoièse dans 14 cas "d'érythropoièse inefficace" avec anomalies morphologiques des érythroblastes et polynucléarité, Nouv. Rev. Fr. Hématol. **12:**631, 1972.

179. Falter, M. L., and Robinson, M. G.: Autosomal dominant inheritance and aminoaciduria in Blackfan-Diamond anaemia, J. Med. Genet. **9:**64, 1972.

180. Förare, S. A.: Pure red cell aplasia in step siblings, Acta Paediatr. Scand. **52:**159, 1963.

181. Foy, H., Kondi, A., and MacDougall, L.: Pure red-cell aplasia in marasmus and kwashiorkor treated with riboflavin, Br. Med. J. **1:**937, 1961.

182. Freedman, M. H., Amato, D., and Saunders, E. F.: Haem synthesis in the Diamond-Blackfan syndrome, Br. J. Haematol. **31:**515, 1975.

183. Freedman, M. H., Amato, D., and Saunders, E. F.: Erythroid colony growth in congenital hypoplastic anemia, J. Clin. Invest. **57:**673, 1976.

184. Freedman, M. H. and Saunders, E. F.: Diamond-Blackfan syndrome: types 1 and 2, Clin. Res. **25:**339A, 1977.

185. Freeman, A. I., Edwards, J. A., Cohen, M., and Sinks, L. F.: Morphological studies in a recently described dyserythropoietic state, Blood **40:**473, 1972.

186. Frisch, B., Lewis, S. M., and Sherman, D.: The ultrastructure of dyserythropoiesis in aplastic anaemia, Br. J. Haematol. **29:**545, 1975.

187. Gasser, C.: Aplastische Anämie (chronische Erythroblastophthise) und Cortison, Schweiz. Med. Wochenschr. **81:**1241, 1951.

188. Gasser, C.: Aplasia of erythropoiesis, acute and chronic erythroblastopenias or pure (red cell) aplastic anemias in childhood, Pediatr. Clin. North Am. **4:**445, 1957.

189. Geller, G., Krivit, W., Zalusky, R., and Zanjani, E. D.: Lack of erythropoietic inhibitory effect of serum from patients with congenital pure red cell aplasia, J. Pediatr. **86:**198, 1975.

190. Ginsberg, S. M.: Acute erythroid aplasia (erythroblastopenia and vascular purpura) in an otherwise hematologically normal child, Ann. Intern. Med. **55:**317, 1961.

191. Goodman, S. B., and Block, M. H.: A case of red cell aplasia occurring as a result of antituberculosis therapy, Blood **24:**616, 1964.

192. Goudsmit, R., Beckers, D., DeBruijne, J. I., et al.: Congenital dyserythropoietic anaemia, type III, Br. J. Haematol. **23:**97, 1972.

193. Graziano, J. H., Markenson, A. L., Miller, D. R., et al.: Chelation therapy in iron overload. I. Intravenous and subcutaneous desferrioxamine, J. Pediatr. **92:**648, 1978.

194. Hamilton, P. J., Dawson, A. A., and Galloway, W. H.: Congenital erythroid hypoplastic anaemia in mother and daughter, Arch. Dis. Child. **49:**71, 1974.

195. Hammond, D., and Keighley, G.: The erythrocyte-stimulating factor in serum and urine in congenital hypoplastic anemia, Am. J. Dis. Child. **100:**466, 1960.

196. Hankes, L. V., Brown, R. R., Schiffer, L., and Schmaeler, M.: Tryptophan metabolism in humans with various types of anemias, Blood **32:**649, 1968.

197. Hansen, H. G.: Ueber die essentielle Erythroblastopenie, Acta Haematol. **6:**335, 1951.

198. Hardisty, R. M.: Diamond-Blackfan anemia. In Congenital disorders of erythropoiesis, Ciba Foundation symposium 37 (new series), New York, 1976, American Elsevier Publishing Co., Inc.

199. Harris, J. R., Price, M. R., and Willison, M.: A comparative study on rat liver and hepatoma nuclear membranes, J. Ultrastruct. Res. **48:**17, 1974.

200. Hathaway, W. E., and Githens, J. H.: Pancytopenia with hyperplastic marrow, Am. J. Dis. Child. **102:**389, 1961.

201. Heimpel, H.: Congenital dyserythropoietic anaemia type I: clinical and experimental aspects. In Congenital disorders of erythropoiesis, Ciba Foundation symposium 37 (new series), New York, 1976, American Elsevier Publishing Co. Inc.

202. Heimpel, H., Forteza-Vila, J., Queisser, W., and Spiertz, E.: Electron and light microscopic study of the erythropoiesis of patients with congenital dyserythropoietic anemia, Blood **37:**299, 1971.

203. Heimpel, H., and Wendt, F.: Congenital dyserythropoietic anemia with karyorrhexis and multinuclearity of erythroblasts, Helv. Med. Acta **34:**103, 1968.

204. Heyn, R., Kurczynski, E., and Schmickel, R.: The association of Blackfan-Diamond syndrome, physical abnormalities, and an abnormality of chromosome 1, J. Pediatr. **85:**531, 1974.

205. Hillman, R. S., and Giblett, E. R.: Red cell membrane alteration associated with "marrow stress," J. Clin. Invest. **44:**1730, 1965.

206. Hirst, E., and Robertson, T. I.: The syndrome of thymoma and erythroblastopenic anemia: a review of 56 cases including 3 case reports, Medicine **46:**225, 1967.

207. Hoffman, R., Zanjani, E. D., Vila, J., et al.: Diamond-Blackfan syndrome: lymphocyte-mediated suppression of erythropoiesis, Science **193:**899, 1976.

208. Horsfall, W. R.: A case of congenital nonspherocytic haemolytic anaemia presenting with an aplastic crisis, Med. J. Aust. **2:**340, 1956.

209. Hruby, M. A., Mason, R. G., and Honig, G. R.: Unbalanced globin chain synthesis in congenital dyserythropoietic anemia, Blood **42:**843, 1973.

210. Hunter, R. E., and Hakami, N.: The occurrence of congenital hypoplastic anemia in half brothers, J. Pediatr. **81:**346, 1972.

211. Jandl, J. H., and Greenberg, M. S.: Bone-marrow failure due to relative nutritional deficiency in Cooley's hemolytic anemia, N. Engl. J. Med. **260:**461, 1959.

212. Jepson, J. H., and Lowenstein, L.: Inhibition of erythropoiesis by a factor present in the plasma of patients with erythroblastopenia, Blood **27:**425, 1966.

213. Jepson, J. H., and Vas, M.: Decreased in vivo and in vitro erythropoiesis induced by plasma of ten patients with thymoma, lymphosarcoma, or idiopathic erythroblastopenia, Cancer Res. **34:**1325, 1974.

214. Jones, B., and Thompson, H.: Triphalangeal thumb associated with hypoplastic anemia, Pediatrics **52:**609, 1973.

215. Jonnson, U., Roath, O. S., and Kirkpatrick, C. I. F.: Nutritional megaloblastic anemia associated with sickle cell states, Blood **15:**535, 1959.

216. Joseph, K. C., Gockerman, J. P., and Alving, C. R.: Abnormal lipid composition of the red cell membrane in congenital dyserythropoietic anemia type II (HEMPAS), J. Lab. Clin. Med. **85:**34, 1975.

217. Josephs, H. W.: Anaemia of infancy and early childhood, Medicine **15**:307, 1936.

218. Kawada, K., Sakurai, T., Kudo, H., et al.: Erythropoiesis inhibiting factor(s) in patients with erythroid hypoplasia. In Nakao, K., Fisher, J. W., and Takaku, F., eds.: Erythropoiesis, Proceedings of Fourth International Conference on Erythropoiesis, Baltimore, 1975, University Park Press.

219. Kho, L. K., Odang, O., Thajeb, S., and Markum, A. H.: Erythroblastopenia (pure red cell aplasia) in childhood in Djakarta, Blood **19**:168, 1962.

220. Krantz, S. B.: Studies on red cell aplasia. III. Treatment with horse anti-human thymocyte gamma globulin, Blood **39**:347, 1972.

221. Krantz, S. B.: Pure red-cell aplasia, N. Engl. J. Med. **291**:345, 1974.

222. Krantz, S. B., and Kao, V.: Studies in red cell aplasia. I. Demonstration of a plasma inhibitor to heme synthesis and an antibody to erythroblast nuclei, Proc. Natl. Acad. Sci. U.S.A. **58**:493, 1967.

223. Krantz, S. B., and Kao, V.: Studies on red cell aplasia. II. Report of a second patient with an antibody to erythroblast nuclei and remission after immunosuppressive therapy, Blood **34**:1, 1969.

224. Krantz, S. B., Moore, W. H., and Zaentz, S. D.: Studies on red cell aplasia. V. Presence of erythroblast cytotoxicity in γ-globulin fraction of plasma, J. Clin. Invest. **52**:324, 1973.

225. Lane, M., and Alfrey, C. P., Jr.: The anemia of human riboflavin deficiency, Blood **25**:432, 1965.

226. Lawton, J. W. M., Aldrich, J. E., and Turner, T. L.: Congenital erythroid hypoplastic anaemia: autosomal dominant transmission, Scand. J. Haematol. **13**:276, 1974.

227. Leikin, S. L.: The aplastic crisis of sickle-cell disease, Am. J. Dis. Child. **93**:128, 1957.

228. Lerner, A. B.: Melanin pigmentation, Am. J. Med. **19**:902, 1955.

229. Lewis, S. M., and Frisch, B.: Congenital dyserythropoietic anaemias: electron microscopy. In Congenital disorders of erythropoiesis, New York, 1976, American Elsevier Publishing Co. Inc.

230. Lewis, S. M., Nelson, D. A., and Pitcher, C. S.: Clinical and ultrastructural aspects of congenital dyserythropoietic anaemia type I, Br. J. Haematol. **18**:465, 1970.

231. Lewis, S. M., and Verwilghen, R. L.: Dyserythropoietic anemias. In Brown, E. B., and Moore, C. V., eds.: Progress in hematology, vol. 8, New York, 1973, Grune & Stratton, Inc.

232. Linsk, J. A., and Murray, C. K.: Erythrocyte aplasia and hypogammaglobulinemia: response to steroids in a young adult, Ann. Intern. Med. **55**:831, 1961.

233. Lovric, V. A.: Anaemia and temporary erythroblastopenia in children, Aust. Ann. Med. **1**:34, 1970.

234. Marmont, A., and Peschle, C.: Anti-lymphocyte globulin (ALG): an additional therapeutical tool in adult pure red cell aplasia (PRCA). In Nakao, K., Fisher, J. W., and Takaku, F., eds.: Erythropoiesis, Proceedings of Fourth International Conference on Erythropoiesis, Baltimore, 1975, University Park Press.

235. Mauer, H. S., Vida, L. N., and Honig, G. R.: Similarities of the erythrocytes in juvenile chronic myelogenous leukemia to fetal erythrocytes, Blood **39**:778, 1972.

236. Meadows, A. T., Naiman, J. L., and Valdes-Dapena, M.: Hepatoma associated with androgenic therapy for aplastic anemia, J. Pediatr. **84**:109, 1974.

237. Mentzer, W. C., Wang, W. C., and Diamond, L. K.: Differentiation of congenital hypoplastic anemia from transient erythroblastopenia, J. Pediatr. **88**:783, 1976.

238. Mephan, R. H., and Lane, G. R.: Nucleopores and polyribosome formation, Nature **22**:288, 1969.

239. Meuret, G., Tschan, P., Schlüter, G., et al.: DNA-, histone-, RNA-, hemoglobin-content and DNA-synthesis in erythroblasts in a case of congenital dyserythropoietic anemia: type I, Blut **24**:32, 1972.

240. Meyer, L. M., and Bertcher, R. W.: Acquired hemolytic anemia and transient erythroid hypoplasia of bone marrow, Am. J. Med. **28**:606, 1960.

241. Miale, T. D., and Bloom, G. E.: The significance of lymphocytosis in congenital hypoplastic anemia, J. Pediatr. **87**:550, 1975.

242. Miller, D. R., Baehner, R. L., and Diamond, L. K.: Paroxysmal nocturnal hemoglobinuria in childhood and adolescence, Pediatrics **39**:675, 1967.

243. Miller, D. R., Sitarz, A. L., Liberman, P. H., et al.: Congenital dyserythropoietic anaemia, Type IV, Pediatr. Res. **11**:477, 1977.

244. Mott, M. G., Apley, J., and Raper, A. B.: Congenital (erythroid) hypoplastic anaemia: modified expression in males, Arch. Dis. Child. **44**:757, 1969.

245. Murphy, S., and Lubin, B.: Triphalangeal thumbs and congenital erythroid hypoplasia: report of a case with unusual features, J. Pediatr. **81**:987, 1972.

246. Murphy, S., and Oski, F. A.: Congenital dyserythropoietic anemia, Type II: report of two cases and a review of the literature, Pediatrics **50**:858, 1972.

247. Nathan, D. G., Chess, L., Hillman, D., et al.: Erythroid burst forming units are null cells, but their growth in vitro requires helper T-cells, Blood **50**(suppl. 1):133, 1977.

248. Oliner, H. L., and Heller, P.: Megaloblastic erythropoiesis and acquired hemolysis in sickle-cell anemia, N. Engl. J. Med. **261**:19, 1959.

249. O'Regan, S., Melhorn, D. K., Newman, M. S., and Graham, R. C.: Erythrocyte lipids and vitamin E in type II congenital dyserythropoietic anemia, J. Pediatr. **84**:355, 1974.

250. Ortega, J. A., Shore, N. A., and Dukes, P. P.: Erythropoietic inhibitory effect of serum from patients with congenital hypoplastic anemia, Blood **45**:83, 1975. (Abstract.)

251. Owren, P. A.: Congenital hemolytic jaundice: pathogenesis of "hemolytic crisis," Blood **3**:231, 1948.

252. Palmen, K., and Vahlquist, B.: Stationary hypoplastic anemia, Acta Haematol. **4**:273, 1950.

253. Pearson, H. A., and Cone, T. E., Jr.: Congenital hypoplastic anemia, Pediatrics **19**:192, 1957.

254. Peschle, C.: Regulation of erythropoiesis and its defects, Br. J. Haematol. **31**(suppl.):69, 1975.

255. Peschle, C., Marmont, A. M., Marone, G., et al.: The IgG serum inhibitor in adult pure red cell aplasia (PRCA): assay techniques and mechanism of action. In Nakao, K., Fisher, J. W., and Takaku, F., eds.: Erythropoiesis, Proceedings of Fourth International Conference on Erythropoiesis, Baltimore, 1975, University Park Press.

256. Pezzimenti, J. F., and Lindenbaum, J.: Megaloblastic anemia associated with erythroid hypoplasia, Am. J. Med. **53**:748, 1972.

257. Price, J. M., Brown, R. R., Pfaffenbach, E. C., and Smith, N. J.: Excretion of urinary tryptophan metabolites by patients with congenital hypoplastic anemia (Diamond-Blackfan syndrome), J. Lab. Clin. Med. **75**:316, 1970.

258. Propper, R. O., Cooper, B., Rufo, R. R., et al.: Continuous subcutaneous administration of deferoxamine in patients with iron overload, N. Engl. J. Med. **297**:418, 1977.

259. Recker, R. R., and Hynes, H. E.: Pure red blood cell

aplasia associated with chlorpropamide therapy, Arch. Intern. Med. **123**:445, 1969.

260. Rhoads, C. P., and Miller, D. K.: Histology of the bone marrow in aplastic anemia, Arch. Pathol. **26**:648, 1938.

261. Roberts, P. D., Wallis, P. G., and Jackson, A. D. M.: Haemolytic anaemia with multinucleated normoblasts in the marrow, Lancet **1**:1186, 1962.

262. Rochant, H., Dreyfus, B., Bouguerra, M., and Hoi, T-H.: Hypothesis: refractory anemia, preleukemic conditions, and fetal erythropoiesis, Blood **39**:721, 1972.

263. Roland, A. S.: The syndrome of benign thymoma and primary aregenerative anemia: an analysis of forty-three cases, Am. J. Med. Sci. **247**:719, 1964.

264. Rosa, J., Beuzard, Y., Brun, B., and Toulgoat, N.: Evidence for various types of synthesis of human γ chains of haemoglobin in acquired haematological disorders, Nature (New Biol.) **233**:111, 1971.

265. Rosse, W. F., Logue, G. L., Adams, J., and Crookston, J. H.: Mechanisms of immune lysis of the red cells in hereditary erythroblastic nuclearity with a positive acidified serum test and paroxysmal nocturnal hemoglobinuria, J. Clin. Invest. **53**:31, 1974.

266. Safdar, S. H., Krantz, S. B., and Brown, E.: Successful immunosuppressive treatment of erythroid aplasia appearing after thymectomy, Br. J. Haematol. **19**:435, 1970.

267. Schärer, K., and Bauman, T.: Konstitutionelle Anämie mit kernteilungstörung der Erythroblasten, Schweiz. Med. Wochenschr. **94**:1322, 1964.

268. Schmid, J. R., Kiely, J. M., Pease, G. L., and Hargraves, M. M.: Acquired pure red cell agenesis, Acta Haematol. **30**:255, 1963.

269. Seip, M.: Aplastic crisis in a case of immunohemolytic anemia, Acta Med. Scand. **153**:137, 1955.

270. Seip, M., Skrede, S., Bjerve, K. S., et al.: Congenital dyserythropoietic anemia with features of both Type I and Type II, Scand. J. Haematol. **15**:272, 1975.

271. Seligmann, M., Bernard, J., Chassigneux, J., and Dresch, C.: Anemie hypoplastic famiale, Nouv. Rev. Fr. Hématol. **3**:209, 1963.

272. Sharff, O., and Neumann, H.: Ueber Cine Seltene Form von Knochenmarkschadigung durch Salvarsan, Med. Klin. **40**:500, 1944.

273. Singer, K., Molutsky, A. G., and Wile, S. A.: Aplastic crisis in sickle cell anemia: a study of its mechanism and its relationship to other types of hemolytic crises, J. Lab. Clin. Med. **35**:721, 1950.

274. Smith, C. H.: The anemias of early infancy, J. Pediatr. **16**:375, 1940.

275. Smith, C. H.: Chronic congenital aregenerative anemia (pure red-cell anemia) associated with iso-immunization by the blood group factor "A," Blood **4**:697, 1949.

276. Smith, C. H., Schulman, I., Ando, R. E., and Stern, G. S.: Studies in Mediterranean (Cooley's) anemia: the suppression of hematopoiesis by transfusion, Blood **10**:707, 1955.

277. Starkweather, W. H., Spencer, H. H., and Schoch, H. K.: The lactate dehydrogenases of hemopoietic cells, Blood **28**:860, 1966.

278. Steinherz, P. G., Canale, V. C., and Miller, D. R.: Hepatocellular carcinoma, transfusion-induced hemochromatosis, and congenital hypoplastic anemia (Diamond-Blackfan syndrome), Am. J. Med. **60**:1032, 1976.

279. Stewart, A. G., and Birbeck, J. A.: The activities of lactate dehydrogenase, transaminase, and glucose-6-phosphate dehydrogenase in the erythrocytes and plasma of newborn infants, J. Pediatr. **61**:395, 1962.

280. Strauss, A. M.: Erythrocyte aplasia following sulfathiazole, Am. J. Clin. Pathol. **13**:249, 1943.

281. Tartaglia, A. P., Propp, S., Amarose, A. P., et al.: Chromosome abnormality and hypocalcemia in congenital erythroid hypoplasia, Am. J. Med. **41**:990, 1966.

282. Valentine, W. N., Crookston, J. H., Paglia, D. E., and Konrad, P. N.: Erythrocyte enzymatic abnormalities in HEMPAS (hereditary erythroblastic multinuclearity with a positive acidified-serum test), Br. J. Haematol. **23**:107, 1972.

283. Valentine, W. N., Konrad, P. N., and Paglia, D. E.: Dyserythropoiesis, refractory anemia, and "preleukemia": metabolic features of the erythrocytes, Blood **41**:857, 1973.

284. Velan, J., Rhyner, K., and Ganzoni, A. M.: Pure red cell aplasia: successful treatment with cyclophosphamide, Blut **26**:27, 1974.

285. Verwilghen, R. L.: Congenital dyserythropoietic anemia type II (Hempas). In Congenital disorders of erythropoiesis, Ciba Foundation Symposium 37 (new series), New York, 1976, American Elsevier Publishing Co., Inc.

286. Verwilghen, R. L., Lewis, S. M., Dacie, J. V., et al.: HEMPAS: congenital dyserythropoietic anaemia (Type II), Quart. J. Med. (new series) **27**:257, 1973.

287. Verwilghen, R., Verhaegen, H., Waumans, P., et al.: Ineffective erythropoiesis with morphologically abnormal erythroblasts and unconjugated hyperbilirubinaemia, Br. J. Haematol. **17**:27, 1969.

288. Vilter, R. W., Jarrold, T., Will, J. J., et al.: Refractory anemia with hyperplastic bone marrow, Blood **15**:1, 1960.

289. Vogel, P., and Bassen, F. A.: Sternal marrow of children in normal and in pathological states, Am. J. Dis. Child. **57**:245, 1939.

290. Voyce, M. A.: A case of pure red-cell aplasia successfully treated with cobalt, Br. J. Haematol. **9**:412, 1963.

291. Wallman, I. S.: Hereditary red cell asplasia, Med. J. Aust. **2**:488, 1956.

292. Walt, F. J., Taylor, E. D., Magill, F. B., and Nestadt, A.: Erythroid hypoplasia in kwashiorkor, Br. Med. J. **1**:73, 1962.

293. Wasser, J., Yolken, R. H., Miller, D. R., and Diamond, L. K.: Congenital hypoplastic anemia (Diamond-Blackfan syndrome) terminating in acute myeloblastic leukemia, Blood **51**:991, 1978.

294. Waterkotte, G. W., and McElfresh, A. E.: Congenital pure red cell hypoplasia in identical twins, Pediatrics **54**:646, 1974.

295. Weatherall, D. J., Edwards, J. A., and Donohoe, W. T. A.: Haemoglobin and red cell enzyme changes in juvenile myeloid leukemia, Br. Med. J. **1**:679, 1968.

296. Weatherall, D. J., Clegg, J. B., Knox-Macaulay, H. H. M., et al.: A genetically determined disorder with features both of thalassemia and congenital dyserythropoietic anaemia, Br. J. Haematol. **24**:681, 1973.

297. Weatherly, T. L., Flannery, E. P., Doyle, W. F., et al.: Congenital dyserythropoietic (CDA) with increased red cell lipids, Am. J. Med. **57**:912, 1974.

298. Weiss, S., Gaftu, U., Van der Lyn, E., and Djaldetti, M.: Congenital dyserythropoietic anaemia with peculiar nuclear abnormality, Scand. J. Haematol. **15**:261, 1975.

299. Wendt, F., and Heimpel, H.: Kongenitale dyserythropoietische Anaemie bei einem Zwillingsparr, Med. Klin. **62**:172, 1967.

300. White, J. M., Brain, M. C., and Ali, M. A. M.: Globin synthesis in sideroblastic anemia. I. α and β peptide chain synthesis, Br. J. Haematol. **20**:263, 1971.

301. Wolff, J. A., and von Hofe, F. H.: Familial erythroid multinuclearity, Blood **6**:1274, 1951.

302. Wranne, L.: Transient erythroblastopenia in infancy and childhood, Scand. J. Haematol. **7:**76, 1970.
303. Wranne, L., Bonnevier, J. O., Killander, A., and Killander, J.: Pure red-cell anaemia with pro-erythroblast maturation arrest, Scand. J. Haematol. **7:**73, 1970.
304. Yunis, A. A., Arimura, G. K., Lutcher, C. L., et al.: Biochemical lesion in dilantin-induced erythroid aplasia, Blood **30:**587, 1967.
305. Zalusky, R., Zanjani, E. D., and Gidari, A. S.: Site of action of a serum inhibitor of erythropoiesis, J. Lab. Clin. Med. **81:**867, 1973.

9 □ Hemolytic anemias: general considerations

Howard A. Pearson

Red blood cells normally live for 100 to 120 days in the circulation. In the steady state about 1% of senescent red cells are removed from the bloodstream each day and replaced by an equal number of newly fabricated red cells released from the bone marrow. The fundamental basis of the hemolytic anemias is a reduced survival rate of red blood cells in the circulation. Biochemical and hematologic features of hemolytic states can be explained by increased red cell destruction and the compensatory processes marshalled by the body in response to this.

Reduced to its simplest expression, the red blood cell count (or hemoglobin level) represents a balance between red cell production and destruction or loss of red cells; schematically:

$$RBC = \frac{production}{destruction \ or \ loss}$$

A decreased red blood cell count or hemoglobin level can therefore result from either underproduction or a rate of destruction that exceeds the synthetic capacity of the bone marrow.

In the hemolytic anemias red cell destruction is increased to varying degrees from a nearly normal to a remarkably increased rate. In compensation the bone marrow increases its output of red cells, a response mediated by increased production of erythropoietin, the erythropoietic stimulating hormone produced by the kidney in response to tissue hypoxia. In adults with hereditary spherocytosis it has been estimated that the bone marrow can increase the basal output of red cells six- to eightfold.[19] With this kind of maximal response, red cell survival can be reduced to only 20 to 30 days without resultant anemia (compensated hemolysis).

The limits of red cell production in many other hemolytic states have not been determined, particularly for infants and children. It is likely that the capacity of young infants to increase red cell production is less than that of adults, as reflected by the observation that the degree of anemia in children with congenital hemolytic anemias is often more severe during the first years of life than later. This may occur because there is little yellow marrow during infancy, precluding compensatory hypertrophy; however, with increasing age and concomitant growth of the skeleton the actual medullary space simultaneously increases, permitting red marrow expansion.

Suspected hemolytic processes may be documented in a number of ways. Red cell destruction can be measured directly by red cell survival studies or indirectly by measuring increased levels of the chemical by-products or consequences of hemolysis. Alternatively a hemolytic process may be inferred by documentation of the increase in red cell production that usually accompanies hemolytic states.

Destruction of red cells may occur within the circulation (intravascular) or within phagocytic elements of the reticuloendothelial elements of liver, spleen, and bone marrow (extravascular). Depending on the loci of destruction as well as the magnitude and rate of hemolysis, characteristic biochemical changes are noted.

In conditions associated with intravascular hemolysis, free hemoglobin is liberated into the general circulation. Within the circulation it is rapidly oxidized into methemoglobin. Dissociation into hemoglobin dimers ($\alpha\beta$) and into free heme and globin also occurs.[12]

The concentration of hemoglobin normally found in the plasma is less than 5 mg/dl. This small amount of hemoglobin is believed to result from a normal rate of red cell physiologic destruction taking place within the cells of the reticuloendothelial tissues caused by a small but finite leakage of free hemoglobin out of the RE cell into the plasma. The absence of increased hemoglobinemia in patients with many types of hemolytic disease indicates that hemolysis principally occurs extravascularly as in hereditary spherocytosis and other hereditary hemolytic anemias. Mildly elevated levels of plasma hemoglobin are characteristic of sickle cell anemia and thalassemia major. In severe intravascular hemolysis the concentration of plasma hemoglobin increases and, if it exceeds the renal threshold for hemoglobin (100 to 150 mg/dl), the pigment appears in the urine.[18,20] In patients with marked hemoglobinemia the plasma is red or brown. Extreme hemoglobinemia occurs in patients with autoimmune hemolytic anemia, hemolytic transfusion reactions, and drug-induced hemolysis in G-6-PD deficiency. Hemoglobinuria accompanies marked hemoglobinemia when the red cell destruction is considerably rapid and severe and primarily takes place in the circulating blood. Depending on the degree, the urine may be pink, red, brown, or almost black. Hemoglobin in the urine can be detected by benzidine or guaiac reactions.

In patients with chronic hemoglobinemia, brownish granules of hemosiderin appear in the urine, and testing of the urine with acidified potassium ferrocyanide reveals the presence of the Prussian blue hemosiderin.[18] Hemosiderinuria is a characteristic finding in patients with paroxysmal nocturnal hemoglobinuria and in patients with hemolysis secondary to intravascular prostheses such as Starr-Edwards valves.[44]

HAPTOGLOBIN

The haptoglobins (Hp) are α_2-glycoproteins found in the serum that function as specific transport proteins for hemoglobin. The haptoglobin molecule is comprised of two sets of polypeptide chains designated α and β, respectively; genetic variants have been described in both chains. One molecule of haptoglobin is capable of irreversibly binding with two half molecules of hemoglobin ($\alpha\beta$ dimers).

Starch gel electrophoresis of serum from normal individuals may reveal as many as twelve different genetically determined haptoglobin bands.[65,66] Autosomal allelic genes, Hp^1 and Hp^2, in the homozygous state are responsible for the Hp^1/Hp^1 and the Hp^2/Hp^2 genotypes. The Hp^1/Hp^1 genotype is characterized by a single haptoglobin band. The Hp^2/Hp^2 genotype has several components as a result of polymeric forms. The heterozygous genotype Hp^1/Hp^2 also results in several haptoglobin bands caused by polymeric combinations that are separated by the sieving activity of the gel.[64,67] The genetically determined congenital absence of haptoglobin resulting from a gene designated Hp^0 has been described, but it is not associated with clinical or hematologic abnormalities.[43] When haptoglobin combines with hemoglobin, the complex is irreversibly cleared from the plasma by the reticuloendothelial system with a rapid half-time.[36] If the capacity of the liver to synthesize haptoglobin is exceeded by its clearance from the plasma, the level of serum haptoglobin decreases to undetectable levels. Thus low levels of haptoglobin or anhaptoglobinemia are characteristic of many hemolytic states.[11,35] This is true even when hemolysis is occurring predominantly extravascularly. The large molecular weight of the haptoglobin-hemoglobin complex prevents its passage into the urine. Hemoglobinuria does not occur until the amount of plasma hemoglobin exceeds the binding power of the free circulating haptoglobin.

Haptoglobin is an acute phase reactant, and in patients with acute infections, inflammation, or malignancy or those receiving corticosteroid therapy the levels of serum haptoglobin may be normal or even elevated despite active hemolysis.[72] If the level of serum haptoglobin is to be used as an indicator of hemolysis, its level should be correlated with other acute phase reactants. Liver disease may be associated with a decreased synthesis of haptoglobin independent of rates of hemolysis.

Haptoglobins can be demonstrated in cord blood or in the early neonatal period in less than 10% of cases; however, they appear by the end of the first or second week of life.[4,53,63] Their low level in early life is at least in part caused by the short survival of the fetal red blood cell, resulting in their utilization. After the first months of life the normal level of serum haptoglobin is 30 to 160 mg/dl, expressed as the hemoglobin-binding capacity of serum.[47]

HEMOPEXIN

Hemopexin, a β_1-globulin, is the major transport protein of heme. In plasma, hemopexin combines with heme forming a red complex consisting of one mole of hemopexin to one of heme.[31] The mean hemopexin level in adults is 77 mg/dl with a range of 60 to 100 mg/dl. The mean level in the newborn is 18 mg/dl with a range of 6.5 to 25 mg/dl.

In states of excessive intravascular hemolysis plasma heme complexes with hemopexin, and the combination is cleared more rapidly from the plasma than it is synthesized. Accordingly during acute hemolytic episodes plasma hemopexin concentrations are reduced.[28,58] The plasma hemopexin concentration is not decreased without a concomitant reduction of haptoglobin level, although the converse is frequently observed.[45] There is considerable overlap in hemopexin concentration between newborn infants with and without evident hemolysis. Hemopexin quantitative determinations are therefore of limited value in supporting a diagnosis of hemolysis in the newborn period.[39]

METHEMALBUMIN

When large amounts of hemoglobin are released into the plasma by severe intravascular red cell destruction, as occurs in hemolytic transfusion reaction, hematin combines with albumin to form methemalbumin. Schumm's test is commonly used to detect methemalbuminemia.[21] Serum is covered with a layer of ether and a $^1/_{10}$ volume of saturated yellow ammonium sulfide is added. This results in the formation of hemochromagen with an intense,

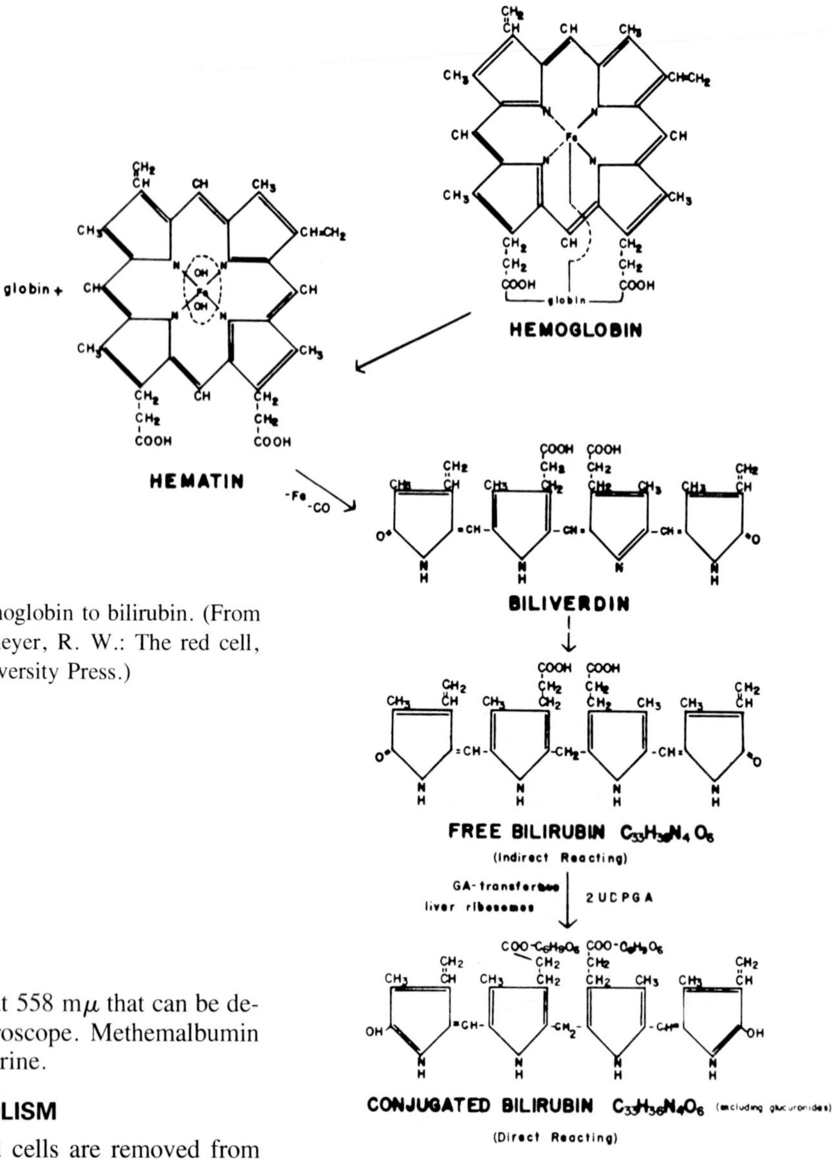

Fig. 9-1. Conversion of hemoglobin to bilirubin. (From Harris, J. W., and Kellermeyer, R. W.: The red cell, Boston, 1970, Harvard University Press.)

narrow absorption band at 558 mμ that can be detected with a hand spectroscope. Methemalbumin is not excreted into the urine.

HEMOGLOBIN CATABOLISM

Effete or damaged red cells are removed from the circulation by the active phagocytic activity of reticuloendothelial elements of the spleen, liver, and bone marrow (extravascular hemolysis). Within RE cells hemoglobin is converted to bilirubin by the series of enzymatic steps outlined in Fig. 9-1.[27] First, globin is split from the hemoglobin molecule and the protein is rapidly catabolized to amino acids. The remaining porphyrin complex is designated hematin. This is cleaved at an α-methane bridge by the enzyme heme oxygenase.[68] This cleavage results in formation of one molecule of carbon monoxide, and at the same time the iron molecule of hemoglobin is released for ultimate reutilization in hemoglobin synthesis. The resulting straight chain molecule, designated biliverdin, is enzymatically reduced by the enzyme biliverdin reductase to free or unconjugated bilirubin, the indirect bilirubin of the classical van den Bergh reaction. Unconjugated bilirubin has a strong affinity for lipids and is insoluble in aqueous solutions. Even when markedly increased plasma levels are present, it is not excreted in the urine, so-called acholuric jaundice.

Unconjugated bilirubin is transported through the plasma to the liver tightly bound to albumin in a molecular ratio of 2:1. Hepatic parenchymal cells extract bilirubin from the plasma by means of an active process involving cytoplasmic proteins designated the Y and Z proteins.[38] Once within the parenchymal cell, bilirubin is successively conjugated with two molecules of glucuronic acid by the enzyme glucuronyl transferase.[57] Bilirubin diglucuronide, or conjugated bilirubin, the direct or immediate fraction of the van den Bergh reaction, is water soluble. When present in increased levels in the plasma, it is excreted in the urine, producing the dark yellow urine and positive foam test characteristic of obstructive jaundice.

Conjugated bilirubin is actively secreted into the bile and then excreted into the duodenum. A small amount of this intestinal bilirubin is reabsorbed into the blood, a pathway that constitutes the enterohepatic circulation.[37] Most of the intestinal bilirubin is acted on by intestinal bacteria forming various derivatives that are designated urobilinogins. These colorless compounds have characteristic chemical reactivities with specific analytic reagents.[70] Although almost all of the intestinal urobilinogen is eliminated in the feces; a small amount is reabsorbed from the gut and subsequently excreted in the urine.

CARBON MONOXIDE EXCRETION AND CARBOXYHEMOGLOBIN LEVELS

In the initial step of heme catabolism a molecule of carbon monoxide is generated, which is transported through the plasma as carboxyhemoglobin and is ultimately excreted in the expired air by the lungs.[15] Because this reaction constitutes the only endogenous source of carbon monoxide and because hemoglobin degradation is the major source (85%), measurement of expired carbon monoxide as well as levels of carboxyhemoglobin in the blood have been used to assess red cell destruction.[16,24] Measurement of carboxyhemoglobin and expired carbon monoxide is somewhat difficult to standardize, but despite these difficulties these techniques have been used for the study of rates of hemolysis in newborn infants.[42,48]

HYPERBILIRUBINEMIA AND JAUNDICE

The level of serum bilirubin reflects both the rate of hemolysis and the capacity of the liver to remove the pigment from the plasma. During the first week of life, because of hepatic immaturity of enzyme systems, the conjugation of bilirubin is limited, resulting in the physiologic jaundice of the newborn. Thereafter the liver is usually able to conjugate large amounts of bilirubin.

In patients with chronic hemolytic anemias the plasma bilirubin level usually ranges between 1 to 3 mg/dl and rarely exceeds 5 mg/dl. Levels of conjugated bilirubin greater than about 5 mg/dl are almost always indicative of concomitant hepatic dysfunction. Clinical jaundice usually can be perceived when the serum bilirubin level exceeds 2.5 mg/dl, but in newborns clinical jaundice may not be manifested until the serum level exceeds about 7.0 gm/dl. It should be emphasized that jaundice is not a sine qua non of hemolysis.

UROBILINOGEN EXCRETION

Increased blood destruction results in excessive urobilinogen excretion. Although elevated fecal urobilinogen excretion is indicative of increased hemolysis, its measurement is an unaesthetic and tedious determination that is seldom used today. Only small amounts of urobilinogen are excreted by the kidneys; therefore the urine levels are not reliable or consistent indicators of hemolysis.

DISORDERS OF BILIRUBIN METABOLISM

A number of genetically determined disorders of bilirubin metabolism and excretion are manifested as clinical jaundice. These disorders may be superficially mistaken for hemolytic states but are not usually associated with accelerated cell destruction.

A recessively inherited deficiency of the enzyme glucuronyl transferase is the basis of the syndrome of congenital nonhemolytic unconjugated hyperbilirubinemia and kernicterus, or Crigler-Najjar syndrome.[1] Affected infants have onset of severe hyperbilirubinemia in the neonatal period and frequently develop kernicterus. Some patients with this probably heterogenous syndrome have responded to phenobarbital therapy with decreased serum bilirubin levels, presumably caused by microsomal enzyme induction of glucuronyl transferase.[74] The Gunn rat is an animal model of this syndrome.

A dominantly inherited abnormality of the mechanisms that effect the clearance of bilirubin from the plasma into hepatocytes plus a possible mild defect in glucuronidization are believed to be the basis of Gilbert's disease, or familial nonhemolytic jaundice.[7] Affected patients have recurrent episodes of jaundice frequently provoked by infections. Serum unconjugated bilirubin levels fluctuate and may increase to 5 to 6 mg/dl, but no anemia or reticulocytosis is present. Minimally shortened red cell survival is present in some patients.

The active secretion of bilirubin diglucuronide into the bile is believed to involve active transport mechanisms. Inherited defects in these mechanisms are the basis of syndromes characterized by conjugated hyperbilirubinemia such as Rotor and Dubin-Johnson syndromes.[22,67]

RED CELL SURVIVAL STUDIES

The life span of the circulating red cells can be measured directly in several ways. Cohort methods involve incorporation of an isotopically labeled compound into a small population of red cells of uniform age within the bone marrow, which can then be serially followed for the duration of their span. Cohort labels used for red cell survival studies include glycine-^{14}C, [55]Fe, and ^{59}Fe, all of which can be actively incorporated into hemoglobin by red cell precursors in the bone marrow.[5,6] When the originally labeled cohort of red cell reaches the end of its life span and if reincorporation of the label can be prevented, an abrupt decrease in circulating radioactivity gives an accurate indication of the red cell life span. Despite their potential accuracy, cohort methods are cumbersome and difficult and are rarely employed in clinical situations.

The alternative method involves following survival of a population of red cells of differing ages. The classical Ashby technique for determining red cell survival capitalizes on differences in red cell antigens, such as ABO or MN, between donor and recipient.[2] Following infusion of a relatively large volume of donor red cells, serial blood samples are obtained from the recipient. The recipient's red cells are agglutinated from these samples using an appropriate antiserum against antigen that is lacking in the donor red cells but present in those of the recipient. Serial counts of these unagglutinated (donor) red cells provide a survival curve from which red cell life span can be determined. There are major limitations of the Ashby method. It cannot be used to determine survival of the patient's red cells in his own body. Furthermore, it is technically difficult and has been extensively replaced by radioactive techniques.

The most widely used radioactive labeling method utilizes the isotope [51]Cr.[23,33] A small sample of peripheral blood is incubated with a tracer dose of Na_2-[51]CrO_4. [51]Cr enters the red cell and attaches preferentially to the β-chains of hemoglobin.[50] These labeled red cells can then be injected into a patient's circulation and serial measurements of radioactivity in the blood may provide an indication of red cell survival.

The graphic plot of the disappearance of ^{51}Cr activity from the blood does not follow a straight line. In addition to the steady decrease resulting from the removal of labeled red cells from the circulation, there is also nonspecific elution of radiochromium from the red cells.[60] The ^{51}Cr survival curve represents a combination of both red cell destruction and elution. Elution rates are relatively constant at about 1%/day. In significant hemolytic anemias with short survival times the contribution of elution to the ^{51}Cr survival curve is relatively unimportant.

The normal red cell [51]Cr T½ is 25 to 35 days, corresponding to a true half-life of about 60 days. A T½ of less than 20 days indicates a significant shortening of the red cell life span. Because of its technical ease, the ^{51}Cr method has become the most frequently employed method for red cell survival studies.

Additional important information may be obtained from ^{51}Cr red cell survival studies. External counting for ^{51}Cr activity with scintillation probes positioned over the liver and spleen can be used to determine major sites of red cell destruction. A disproportionately large number of counts over the spleen compared to the liver may indicate that splenectomy is likely to ameliorate a hemolytic process.[13] The amount of blood being lost into the gastrointestinal tract from various lesions can also be precisely quantitated by labeling a patient's red blood cells with ^{51}Cr and subsequently measuring fecal radioactivity.[73]

Other isotopic methods for determination of red cell survival involve the use of diisopropylflourophosphate (DFP) labeled with ^{32}P or [3]H. DFP irreversibly attaches to red cell acetylcholinesterase and other red cell components.[14] This method is technically difficult because it involves a Geiger-Müller counter as opposed to a scintillation counter. In addition, the isotopic compounds are expensive.

EVIDENCE OF INCREASED RED CELL PRODUCTION

With development of anemia and reduced delivery of oxygen to the tissues an increase of red cell production is mediated by increased production of erythropoietin. When a sustained increase in production of red cells is documented, increased destruction or loss of red cells can be reasonably inferred.

ERYTHROID MARROW HYPERPLASIA

In the bone marrow of older normal children and adults approximately 20% of the marrow tissue is comprised of fat. The medullary spaces of the long bones are filled with fatty ''yellow'' marrow. Hyperplasia of any marrow element results in reduction of marrow fat and extension of ''red,'' or hematopoietic, marrow into the entire medullary space. In infants and young children there is proportionately much less fat in hematopoietic tissues.

Marked hypertrophy of the erythroid marrow may have structural consequences. The marrow space becomes expanded, particularly in the small bones of the hands and feet and in the skull. Osseous changes are seen in the most extreme form in thalassemia major but occur to a lesser degree in sickle cell anemia and other hemoglobinopathies as well as congenital hemolytic states such as hereditary spherocytosis. Moderate skeletal changes may also occur in infants with acquired anemias such as iron-deficiency anemia. In young children extramedullary hematopoiesis may develop in response to hemolysis. This is seen most frequently in thalassemia major and occurs to a lesser degree in other chronic hemolytic states.

The ratio of erythroid to myeloid precursors in the bone marrow is designated the M:E ratio. In childhood, this ratio averages 2:1 to 3:1. In chronic hemolytic states and conditions in which erythroid hyperplasia is a characteristic finding, the M:E ratio may be 1:1 or even reversed. A reduction of myeloid elements may also result in an alteration of the M:E ratio.

RETICULOCYTES

At the time of their release into the circulation from the bone marrow, red cells contain RNA and are able to synthesize hemoglobin. The RNA imparts a purplish color (polychromasia) to red cells stained with Wright stain. In addition, RNA is precipitated by supravital stains such as methylene blue as a blue mesh within the reticulocyte. Reticulocytes can be enumerated and expressed as a percentage of red cells in the blood. In hemolytic anemias reticulocytes are almost always increased, both in absolute numbers and in percentage of red cells. A sustained reticulocytosis accompanying a steady hemoglobin level almost always indicates hemolysis. Reticulocytes are relatively large and so reticulocytosis may be associated with relative macrocytosis with an MCV of more than 90 fl.

In some young infants and younger children with severe hemolytic anemias nucleated red cells may occur in the peripheral blood. These may come from extramedullary erythropoietic sites.

A low reticulocyte count in patients with various hemolytic anemias may be indicative of an "aplastic crisis."[49,61] Because the hemoglobin level in hemolytic anemias is maintained by marrow hyperactivity, any factor that compromises compensation will result in rapidly worsening anemia. A variety of viral infections may interfere with erythropoiesis and result in a virtual cessation of erythropoiesis. The observation of aplastic crises in members of a family is further evidence of an infectious origin.[30]

During aplastic crises, the degree of anemia rapidly increases. Reticulocytosis or deepening jaundice is absent. Examination of the bone marrow reveals a paucity of red cell precursors with M:E ratios of 7:1 to 20:1. Occasionally huge, abnormal red cell precursors (gigantoblasts) are noted.[27] Aplastic crises usually terminate spontaneously in 10 to 14 days, and after a period of extraordinary erythroid activity with marked reticulocytosis the blood count returns to its usual state.

CLASSIFICATION OF HEMOLYTIC DISORDERS

The hemolytic disorders may be conveniently classified into two groups on the basis of whether shortened red cell survival is a result of (1) an in-

trinsically abnormal red cell or (2) an extrinsic abnormality acting on a normal red cell.

Hemolytic anemias resulting from intrinsic defects are generally inherited abnormalities of the membrane, hemoglobin, or intracellular enzymes of the red cell. Nutritional deficiencies are also associated with intrinsically abnormal red cells with shortened life spans. In contrast extrinsic disorders are usually acquired and result from forces or agents within the circulation that chemically, mechanically, or physically damage the red blood cell.

These two categories are not mutually exclusive and some hemolytic disorders are caused by a combination of both intrinsic and extrinsic mechanisms.

A. Intrinsic red cell defects leading to hemolysis
  1. Disorders of red cell membrane
     a. Hereditary spherocytosis
     b. Hereditary hemolytic ovalocytosis
     c. Stomatocytosis
     d. Blood group "null"
  2. Disorders of hemoglobin
     a. Hemoglobinopathies (S, C, D, etc.)
     b. Thalassemias
     c. Congenital Heinz body anemias
  3. Disorders of red cell enzymes
     a. Deficiency of glycolytic enzymes (pyruvate kinase, hexokinase, etc.)
     b. Deficiencies of pentose phosphate pathway enzymes and compounds (G-6-PD, 6-PGD, GSH, etc.)
  4. Nutritional deficiencies (iron, vitamin B_{12}, folic acid, Vitamin E, etc.)
B. Extracorpuscular defects
  1. Immune
     a. Isoantibodies (erythroblastosis fetalis, transfusion reactions)
     b. Autoimmune hemolytic anemia (warm and cold antibodies)
     c. Drug associated: methyldopa (Aldomet), penicillin
  2. Chemical damage: snake venoms, acetyl phenyhydrazine
  3. Parasitism: bartonella malaria
  4. Microangiopathic hemolytic anemia
     a. DIC
     b. Intravascular prostheses
     c. Hemolytic uremic syndrome and thrombotic thrombohemolytic purpura
  5. Hypersplenism

THE PORPHYRIAS

The porphyrias are a group of uncommon metabolic diseases characterized by excessive production, usually with urinary excretion, of various types of porphyrins. They are classified into two general groups, depending on whether the majority of excessive porphyrin production occurs in the liver or in the bone marrow. In some of these conditions anemia may be present. Recent studies have indicated that enzyme deficiencies in the heme biosynthetic pathway underlie the biochemical abnormalities that characterize the porphyrias.[8]

The metabolic sequence of heme synthesis and the involved enzymes are outlined in Fig. 9-2.[10] The first step involves the condensation of glycine and succinyl CoA to form δ-aminolevulinic acid (ALA) through the activity of the mitochondrial enzyme ALA synthetase.[59] Vitamin B_6, pyridoxine, is a cofactor in this crucial reaction. The four subsequent intermediate reactions occur in the cytoplasm. Two molecules of ALA condense to form porphobilinogen (PBG), a monopyrrolic compound. Four molecules of PBG are then complexed together to form a ring tetrapyrrolic compound designated uroporphyrinogen III (UROgen III). UROgen III is successfully converted to coproporphyrinogen III (COPROgen III) by a series of oxidation and decarboxylation reactions. The reaction then reenters the mitochondria where protoporphyrinogen III (PROTOgen IX) is formed. Protoporphyrinogen III is subsequently oxidized to protoporphyrin IX (PROTO IX), which directly combines with iron to form heme.

Except for protoporphyrinogen III, the other porphyrin compounds formed by oxidation of porphyrinogens are catabolic by-products of heme synthesis. Porphyrinogen compounds are colorless, whereas porphyrins are red, fluorescent compounds capable of inducing intense tissue reactions.

Heme synthesis primarily occurs in the bone marrow and the liver, and the porphyrias are conveniently grouped into hepatic and erythropoietic varieties.

Hepatic porphyrias

Acute intermittent porphyria. Acute intermittent porphyria is associated with increased urinary excretion of the porphyrin precursors, ALA and PBG. These compounds result in a urine that becomes brownish red on standing, and the presence of PBG can be demonstrated by the Watson-Schwartz reaction. There is a strong female predominance of the disease. Patients with this

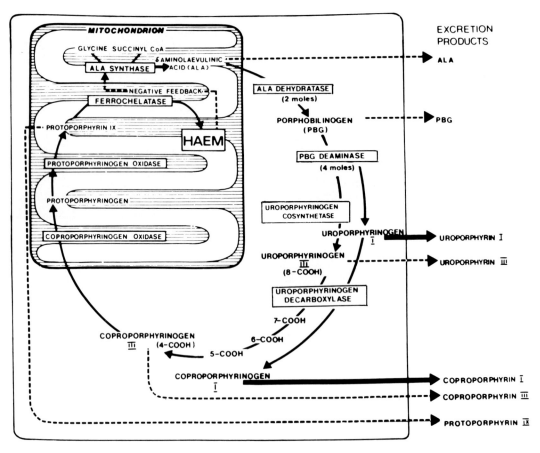

Fig. 9-2. Metabolic sequence of heme synthesis. (From Brodie, M. J., Moore, M. R., and Goldberg, A.: Lancet **2:**699, 1977.)

disease do not usually develop symptoms until early in adult life when intermittent attacks begin; they are manifested as severe abdominal pain resembling a surgical abdomen caused by autonomic neuropathy. Severe constipation is usually present. Death from respiratory paralysis may occur. Neuropsychiatric disorders including psychoses are prominent. The attacks may be precipitated by many drugs, especially barbiturates. Skin photosensitivity is not noted. A deficiency of uroporphyrinogen I synthetase, the enzyme responsible for conversion of PBG to uroporphyrinogen has been found in liver, cultured fibroblasts, and red cells of these patients.[46]

Variegate porphyria. Variegate porphyria occurs predominantly in South Africa and Sweden. The signs and symptoms are similar to those of acute intermittent porphyria, but in addition cutaneous photosensitivity occurs. Urinary excretion of coproporphyrin PBG, and ALA can be documented. A defect of the enzyme ferrochelatase has been found in some cases.[3]

Porphyria cutanea tarda. Porphyria cutanea tarda is an acquired defect whose major manifestation is cutaneous photosensitivity. Although a genetic predisposition appears to be present, alcoholism and liver disease are also operative in most cases. Uroporphyrin, ALA, and PBG are excreted in the urine. A defect of hepatic uroporphyrinogen decarboxylase has been demonstrated.[34]

Acquired porphyrias. Rare instances of syndromes of acquired porphyria have been associated with hepatoma. An epidemic of acquired porphyria in association with ingestion of grain treated with hexachlorobenzene has been described.[56]

Erythropoietic porphyrias

Congenital erythropoietic porphyria. Congenital erythropoietic porphyria is a rare autosomal recessive disease that results from excess production of uroporphyrin. A deficiency of the enzyme uroporphyrinogen cosynthetase has been demonstrated in cells from these patients.[54] Uroporphyrin accumulates in the tissues and binds with teeth (and bones) producing discolored teeth that fluoresce under Wood's light. The urine is pink or deep red resembling port wine. Porphyrins in the skin undergo photooxidation when exposed to the light, evoking blistering and tissue breakdown. The blisters break down and often become infected, producing scarring and mutilation of the fingers, nose, and ears. Many of the bone marrow normoblasts when examined by ultraviolet microscopy show intense fluorescence. A hemolytic anemia with significant splenomegaly often develops and splenectomy may be required.

Erythropoietic protoporphyria. Erythropoietic protoporphyria is a dominantly inherited condition associated with an accumulation of protoporphyrin in red cells and tissues. No abnormal urinary excretion of porphyrins is noted. The primary clinical manifestation is cutaneous sensitivity, rash, and blistering in response to exposure to the sun (hydroa aestivale). In one case a hemolytic anemia was benefited by splenectomy.[51] Reduced levels of ferrochelatase have been found in skin fibroblasts and livers.[9]

SIDEROBLASTIC ANEMIAS

Sideroblastic anemias are uncommon syndromes manifested as hypochromic microcytic anemias, iron overload, and the presence of large numbers of ringed sideroblasts in the bone marrow. These characteristic cells are polychromatophilic and acidophilic normoblasts with Prussian blue–staining, siderotic granules arranged in a perinuclear necklace-like pattern. By electron microscopy these granules can be shown to be iron-laden mitochondria. Sideroblastic anemias may be classified as hereditary or acquired.

Hereditary sideroblastic anemia

Hereditary sideroblastic anemia is inherited as an X-linked recessive disease; there is a strong male predominance.[29,32,58] Anemia is occasionally noted in infancy, but the onset is most often in young adulthood.[71] Female carriers often show a mixed population of circulating red cells, some being hypochromic and microcytic, the rest being normal.[71] This is thought to represent a morphologic expression of random X-chromosome inactivation (Lyon hypothesis).[40]

Affected patients have severe anemia with marked hypochromia, microcytosis, and anisocytosis. In contrast to iron-deficiency anemia, free erythrocyte porphyrin levels are not elevated. Serum iron is high, with increased saturation of transferrin, and erythropoiesis is markedly ineffective.[62]

A deficiency of ALA synthetase has been suggested in some children with this disease.[69] Because pyridoxine is a cofactor for this enzymatic reaction, a hematologic response may be produced in some cases with pharmacologic doses (50 to 250 mg/day) of oral pyridoxine.[52] Other cases of elevated levels of free erythrocyte coproporphyrin suggest a deficiency of coproporphyrin oxidase.[25] This enzyme does not require pyridoxine as a cofactor; therefore these patients do not respond to treatment.

Congenital sideroblastic anemia with vacuolization of bone marrow precursors and pancreatic fibrosis

I have seen three children and am aware of two others with a previously undescribed congenital sideroblastic syndrome. The features included early onset of severe, transfusion-dependent anemia, neutropenia, and variable thrombocytopenia. The bone marrow was hypercellular and was remarkable for prominent, degenerative, cytoplasmic vacuolization of both red cell and granulocyte precursors. A marked increase of iron and ringed sideroblasts were also present in the bone marrow. Two children died in the first 3 years of life, and postmortem examination revealed marked fibrosis of the exocrine pancreas. Three other children who are still living are less seriously affected but also have abnormal exocrine pancreatic function.

Acquired sideroblastic anemias

Sideroblastic anemia may occur in association with a variety of malignancies and inflammatory and endocrine diseases. However, this complication rarely if ever is encountered in childhood.[41]

A number of drugs and toxic materials have also been reported to induce sideroblastic anemia. The most important of these toxins in childhood is lead (Chapter 16).

REFERENCES

1. Arias, I. M., Gartner, L. M., et al.: Chronic nonhemolytic unconjugated hyperbilirubinemia with glucuronyl transferase deficiency: clinical, biochemical pharmacologic, and genetic evidence of heterogeneity, Am. J. Med. **47:**395, 1969.
2. Ashby, W.: The span of life of the red blood cells: a resume, Blood **3:**486, 1948.
3. Becker, D. M., Viljoen, J. D., Katz, J., Kramer, S.: Reduced ferrochelatase activity: a defect common to porphyria variagata and protoporphyria, Br. J. Haematol. **36:**171, 1977.
4. Bergstrand, C. C., Czar, B., and Tarokosk, P. H.: Serum haptoglobin in infancy, Scand. J. Clin. Invest. **13:**576, 1961.
5. Berlin, N. I., Beeckmans, M., Elmlinger, P. J., and Lawrence, J. H.: Comparative study of the Ashby differential agglutination: carbon 14 and iron 59 methods for determination of red cell life span, J. Lab. Clin. Med. **50:**558, 1957.
6. Berlin, N. I., Waldmann, T. A., and Weissman, S. M.: Life span of the red blood cell, Physiol. Rev. **39:**577, 1959.
7. Black, M., and Billing, B. H.: Hepatic bilirubin UDP glucuronyl transferase activity in liver disease and Gilbert's syndrome, N. Engl. J. Med. **280:**1266, 1969.
8. Bloomer, J. R.: The hepatic porphyrias, Gastroenterology **71:**689, 1976.
9. Bonkowsky, J. L., Bloomer, J. R., Ebert, P. S., and Mahoney, M. J.: Heme synthetase deficiency in human protoporphyria, J. Clin. Invest. **56:**1139, 1975.
10. Brodie, M. J., Moore, M. R., and Goldbert, A.: Enzyme abnormalities in the porphyrias, Lancet **2:**699, 1977.
11. Brus, I., and Lewis, S. M.: The haptoglobin content of serum in haemolytic anemia, Br. J. Haematol. **5:**348, 1959.
12. Bunn, H. F.: Erythrocyte destruction and hemoglobin catabolism, Semin. Hematol. **9:**3, 1972.
13. Cline, M. J., and Berlin, N. I.: The red cell chromium elution rates in patients with some hematologic diseases, Blood **21:**63, 1963.
14. Cline, M. J., and Berlin, N. I.: An evaluation of DFP[32]

15. Coburn, R. F.: Endogenous carbon monoxide production, N. Engl. J. Med. **282:**207, 1970.
16. Coburn, R. F., Williams, W. J., and Kahn, S. B.: Endogenous carbon monoxide production in patients with hemolytic anemia, J. Clin. Invest. **45:**460, 1966.
17. Connell, G. E., Dixon, G. H., and Smithies, O.: Subdivision of the three common haptoglobin types based on hidden differences, Nature **193:**505, 1962.
18. Crosby, W. H.: The hemolytic states, Bull. N.Y. Acad. Med. **30:**27, 1954.
19. Crosby, W. H., and Akeroyd, J. H.: The limit of hemoglobin synthesis in hereditary hemolytic anemia: its relation to the excretion of bile segment, Am. J. Med. **13:**273, 1952.
20. Crosby, W. H., and Dameshek, W.: The significance of hemoglobinemia and associated hemosiderinuria with particular reference of various types of hemolytic anemia, J. Lab. Clin. Med. **38:**829, 1951.
21. Davidsohn, I., and Stern, K.: Diagnosis of hemolytic transfusion reactions, Am. J. Clin. Pathol. **25:**381, 1955.
22. Dubin, I. N.: Chronic idiopathic jaundice, Am. J. Med. **24:**268, 1958.
23. Ebaugh, F. G., Jr., Emerson, C. P., and Ross, J. F.: The use of radioactive chromium SI as an erythrocyte tagging agent for the determination of red cell survival in vivo, J. Clin. Invest. **32:**1260, 1953.
24. Engel, R., Berk, P. D., Rodkey, F. L., Howe, R. B., and Berlin, N. I.: Estimation of hemeturnover and erythrocyte survival in man from clearance of bilirubin ^{14}C and from carbon monoxide production, Clin. Res. **17:**325, 1969.
25. Garby, L.: Chronic refractory hypochronic anemia with disturbed haem-metabolism, Br. J. Haematol. **3:**55, 1957.
26. Gartner, L. M., and Arias, I. M.: Formation, transport, metabolism and execution of bilirubin, N. Engl. J. Med. **280:**1339, 1969.
27. Gasser, C.: Aplasia of erythropoiesis, Pediatr. Clin. North Am. **4:**445, 1957.
28. Hanstein, A., and Muller-Eberhard, U.: Concentration of serum hemopexin in healthy children and adults and those with a variety of hematological disorders, J. Lab. Clin. Med. **71:**232, 1968.
29. Harris, J. W., and Horrigan, D. L.: Pyridoxine-responsive anemia, Adv. Intern. Med. **12:**103, 1964.
30. Harris, J. W., and Kellermeyer, R. W.: The red cell, Boston, 1970, Harvard University Press.
31. Heide, K., Haupt, H., Storiko, K., and Schultze, H. E.: On the heme-binding capacity of hemopexin, Clin. Chimica Acta **10:**460, 1964.
32. Hines, J. D., and Grasso, J. A.: The sideroblastic anemia, Semin. Hematol. **7:**86, 1970.
33. ICHS Panel on diagnostic applications of radioisotopes in haematology: Recommended methods for radioisotope red cell survival studies: a report, Br. J. Haematol. **21:**241, 1971.
34. Kuchner, J. B., Barbuto, A. J., and Lee, G. R.: An inherited enzymatic defect in prophyria cutaneatarda: decreased uroporphyrinogen decarboxylase activity, J. Clin. Invest. **58:**1089, 1976.
35. Lathem, W., and Jensen, W. N.: Plasma hemoglobin-binding capacity in sickle cell disease, Blood **14:**1047, 1959.
36. Laurell, C. B., and Nyman, M.: Studies on the serum haptoglobin level in hemoglobinemia and its influence on renal excretion of hemoglobins, Blood **12:**493, 1957.
37. Lester, R., Schumer, W., and Schmid, R.: Intestinal absorption of bile pigments. IV. Urobilinogen absorption in man. N. Engl. J. Med. **272:**939, 1965.

38. Levi, A. J., Gatmaitan, A., and Arias, I. M.: Two hepatic cytoplasmic protein fractions Y and Z and their possible role in the hepatic uptake of bilirubin, sulfobromophthalien and other anions, J. Clin. Invest. **48:**2156, 1969.
39. Lundh, B., Oski, F. A., and Gardner, F. H.: Plasma hemopexin and haptoglobin in hemolytic diseases of the newborn, Acta Paediatr. Scand. **59:**121, 1970.
40. Lyon, M. F.: Sex chromatin and gene action in the mammalian x-chromosome, Am. J. Hum. Gen. **14:**135, 1962.
41. MacGibbon, B. H., and Mollin, D. L.: Sideroblastic anaemia in man: observations on seventy cases, Br. J. Haematol. **11:**59, 1965.
42. Maisels, M. J., Pathak, A., Nelson, N. M., Nathan, D. G., and Smith, C. A.: Endogenous production of carbon monoxide in normal and erythroblastic newborn infants, J. Clin. Invest. **50:**1, 1971.
43. Mehta, S. R., and Jensen, W. N.: Haptoglobins in haemoglobinopathy: a genetic and clinical study, Br. J. Haematol. **6:**250, 1960.
44. Miller, M. L., Pearson, H. A., Wheat, M. W., White, A. W., and Schiebler, G. L.: Delayed onset of hemolytic anemia in a child: an indicator of ball variance of aortic valve prosthesis, Circulation **40:**55, 1969.
45. Muller-Eberhard, U., Liem, H. H., Hanstein, A., and Hanna, M.: Plasma concentrations of hemopexin, haptoglobin, and heme in patients with various hemolytic disease, Blood **32:**811, 1968.
46. Myer, U. A.: Hepatic prophyrias: new findings on the nature of metabolic defects, Prog. Liver Dis. **5:**280, 1976.
47. Nyman, M.: Serum haptoglobin, Scand. J. Clin. Lab. Invest. **11**(suppl. 39):87, 1959.
48. Oski, F. A., and Altman, A. A.: Carbohemoglobin levels in hemolytic disease of the newborn, J. Pediatr. **61:**709, 1962.
49. Owen, P. A.: Congenital hemolytic jaundice: pathogenesis of the hemolytic crises, Blood **3:**231, 1948.
50. Pearson, H. A., and Vertrees, K. M.: The site of binding of chromium⁵¹ to haemoglobin, Nature **189:**1019, 1961.
51. Porter, F. S., and Lowe, B. A.: Congenital erythropoietic protoporphyna. I. Case reports, clinical studies, and porphyrin analysis in two brothers, Blood **22:**521, 1963.
52. Raob, S. O.: Pyridoxine-responsive anemia, Blood **18:**285, 1961.
53. Rausen, A. R., Gerald, P. S., and Diamond, L. K.: Haptoglobin patterns in cord blood serums, Nature **191:**717, 1961.
54. Romeo, G., Glenn, B. L., and Levin, E. Y.: Uroporphyrinogen III cosynthetase in asymptomatic carriers of congenital erythropoietic porphyria, Biochem. Genet. **4:**719, 1970.
55. Rundles, R. W., and Falls, H. F.: Hereditary (7 sex linked) anemia, Am. J. Med. Sci. **211:**641, 1946.
56. Schmid, R.: Direct-reacting bilirubin, bilirubin glucuronide, in serum bile and urine, Science **124:**76, 1956.
57. Schmid, R.: Cutaneous prophyria in Turkey, N. Engl. J. Med. **263:**397, 1960.
58. Sears, D. A.: Plasma heme-binding in patients with hemolytic disorders, J. Lab. Clin. Med. **71:**484, 1968.
59. Shemin, D.: The succinate glycine cycle in porphyrin biosynthesis and metabolism. Ciba Foundation Symposium No. 30, Edinburgh, 1955, Churchill-Livingstone.
60. Shenk, W. G., Jr., and Bow. T. M.: Post-transfusion erythrocyte survival, Arch. Surg. **82:**391, 1961.
61. Singer, K., and Molulsky, A. G.: Aplastic crises in sickle cell anemia: a study of its mechanism and its relationship to other types of hemolytic crises, J. Lab. Clin. Med. **35:**74, 1950.
62. Singh, A. K.: Ferrokinetic abnormalities and their significance in persons with sideroblastic anemia, Br. J. Haematol. **18:**67, 1970.
63. Sklavurw-Zurukzoglu, S., and Malaka, K.: Serum haptoglobins in childhood, Lancet **2:**722, 1961.
64. Smithies, O.: An improved procedure for starch gel electrophoresis: further variation in the serum proteins of normal individuals, Biochem. J. **71:**585, 1959.
65. Smithies, O.: Zone electrophoresis on starch gels: group variations in the serum proteins of normal human adults, Biochem. J. **61:**629, 1955.
66. Smithies, O., and Walker, N. F.: Notation for serum protein groups and the genes controlling their inheritance, Nature **178:**694, 1956.
67. Sprinz, H., and Nelson, R. S.: Persistent non-hemolytic hyperbilirubinemia associated with lipochrome-like pigment in liver cells: report of four cases, Ann. Intern. Med. **41:**952, 1954.
68. Tenhunen, R., and Morver, H. H.: The enzymatic conversion of heme to bilirubin by microsomal heme oxygenase, Proc. Nat. Acad. Sci. **61:**748, 1968.
69. Vogler, W. R., and Mingioli, E. S.: Heme synthesis in pyridoxine responsive anemia, Blood **32:**979, 1968.
70. Watson, C. J.: Gold from dross: the first century of the urabilinoids, Ann. Intern. Med. **70:**839, 1969.
71. Weatherall, D. J., Pembrey, M. E., Hall, E. G., Sanger, R., Tippet, P., and Gavin, J.: Familial sideroblastic anaemia: problem of X_g and x chromosome inactivation, Lancet **2:**744, 1970.
72. Whitten, C. F.: Studies on serum haptoglobin: a functional inquiry, N. Engl. J. Med. **266:**529, 1962.
73. Wilson, J. F., Herner, D. C., and Lahey, M. E.: Studies on iron metabolism. IV. Milk induced gastrointestinal bleeding in infants with hypochromic, microcytic anemia, J.A.M.A. **189:**568, 1964.
74. Yaffee, S. G., Levy, G., Metsuzawa, T., and Ballah, T.: Enhancement of glucuronide conjugating capacity in a hyperbilirubinemic infant to apparent enzyme induction by phenobarbital, N. Engl. J. Med. **275:**1461, 1966.

10 □ Hemolytic anemia: immune defects

Martin R. Klemperer

Immune hemolysis

Immune hemolysis constitutes a pathophysiologic mechanism in which erythrocyte survival is decreased as a result of the deposition of specific antibody, immunoglobulin, on the cell surface. Such antibody is most frequently of the IgG or IgM class. Occasionally autoantibodies may be IgA. In general IgG antibodies do not agglutinate erythrocytes in vitro and have a thermal optimum of 37° C. They therefore are termed incomplete or warm-type antibodies. IgM antibodies frequently cause in vitro agglutination of erythrocytes and bind most firmly at temperatures below 20° C. They are called complete or cold-type antibodies. Most frequently the binding of antibody to the erythrocyte membrane does not cause intravascular lysis but leads to its destruction through adherence to and phagocytosis by cells of the fixed macrophage system, the reticuloendothelial system.

The sine qua non of immune hemolysis is the demonstration of increased amounts of antibody or complement components, C3 and C4, bound to the erythrocyte membrane. This is accomplished through the use of the direct antiglobulin Coombs test or modifications of this procedure. It must be stressed that the binding of immunoglobulin or complement to the erythrocyte membrane does not lead invariably to shortened survival.

The concept of antibody-mediated hemolysis as an autoimmune disease was initiated in 1938 by the observations of Dameshek and Schwartz of hemolytic antibody in the sera of patients with acquired acute hemolytic anemia.[25] Autoagglutination of erythrocytes and the presence of hemolysins in the sera of patients had been documented systematically in the first decade of this century.[14,132] By 1940 Dameshek and Schwartz[26] had reported that approximately 100 cases of acquired hemolytic anemia had been described in the literature. It was, however, the discovery of the antiglobulin test by Coombs et al.[16,17] in 1945 that introduced the modern era in the diagnosis of immune hemolytic disorders. It was through the application of the direct Coombs test that acquired hemolytic anemia could be separated accurately

from entities such as hereditary spherocytosis. It has been therefore the fusion of the disciplines of hematology and immunology that has led to the present understanding of immune hemolysis.

ETIOLOGY

Acquired immune hemolytic disease constitutes a diverse spectrum of disease entities in which the target cell is the erythrocyte. The following is a classification of immune hemolytic disease.

A. Idiopathic: no definable cause or underlying disease (usually warm-type antibody)
B. Postinfectious or postimmunization
  1. Warm-type antibody
    a. Cytomegalovirus
    b. Hepatitis
    c. Immunization
      (1) DPT
      (2) Poliomyelitis
      (3) Typhoid
  2. Cold-type antibody
    a. *M. pneumoniae* pneumonia
    b. Infectious mononucleosis (EB virus)
  3. Biphasic hemolysins
    a. Measles
    b. Mumps
    c. Chickenpox
    d. Infectious mononucleosis
    e. Congenital syphilis
C. Drug-related
  1. Warm-type antibody
    a. Immune complex disease (stibophen type)
    b. Erythrocyte binding (penicillin type)
    c. Antibody induction type (α-methyldopa type)
D. Secondary with associated noninfectious disease
  1. Warm-type antibody
    a. Immune connective tissue disease
    b. Malignancy
    c. Immunodeficiency
  2. Cold-type antibody: lymphoreticular malignancy

In general terms it may be subdivided into three categories[22]: (1) a disease in which the morbid process involves the erythrocyte predominantly and in which there is no demonstrable underlying or precipitating disease (such cases have been termed primary or idiopathic hemolytic anemias);

(2) diseases in which the erythrocyte is but one of several targets in a clearly defined underlying morbid process (such cases have been termed secondary or symptomatic hemolytic anemias); and (3) cases in which there is a well-documented association with a drug or chemical.

Although this classification is conceptually useful, it is quite likely that the distinction between "primary" and "secondary" hemolytic anemias will disappear as the techniques for detecting immunologic aberrations become more sophisticated. All forms of autoimmune hemolytic disease imply a perturbation of the affected individual's immune system and are therefore "secondary" to a more generalized process.[70,85] The evidence supporting this concept as applied to humans consists of (1) documented reports of the familial occurrence of autoimmune hemolytic disease,* (2) the occurrence of autoimmune hemolytic anemia in families with aberrations of immunoglobulins,[38,114] and (3) the report of an increased incidence of the histocompatibility antigens HLA-A1 and HLA-B8 in individuals with autoimmune disease.[23]

The reasons for an individual's development of autoimmune disease at a given time remain for the most part obscure. The inciting agent is defined most clearly in drug-related hemolytic disease. Postulated and documented mechanisms for immune hemolytic diseases are as follows:

1. Spontaneous derepression of a clone of immunocytes through the postulated effect of a viral agent.
2. Alteration of erythrocyte membrane antigens by a viral agent or a drug. Such an altered antigen would not be recognized as "self" by the individual's immune system.
3. Possible cross-reacting antibodies induced by an infectious organism.
4. Binding of a drug or a metabolite of the drug to the erythrocyte membrane.
5. Antigen-antibody complex deposition on the erythrocyte membrane. The erythrocyte is an "innocent bystander."
6. Drug-induced, but with the antibody directed against the Rh antigen complex, and not against the drug.
7. Secondary to an underlying or associated disease.

PATHOGENESIS
Derepression or modification of suppressor T cells

The pathogenesis of "idiopathic" immune hemolytic disease is obscure. Two hypotheses have been suggested as possible biologic mechanisms. No evidence exists that they are relevant to human

*References 18, 29, 68, 97, 98, 121.

disease. Fundamental to the individual's biologic integrity is that it be able to recognize "self."[126] It has been proposed that, through the effect of a viral agent or other factors, a clone of immunocytes escapes from normal immunologic suppression.[10] A virus or pharmacologic agent may in some way alter an erythrocyte antigen so that it is no longer recognized as self. Tolerance is broken by the altered antigen, and antibodies are produced that are capable of reacting with the unmodified antigen. Immune responses could be triggered through alterations in B cell–T cell interaction. A population of T cells (thymus-derived cells) specifically suppresses B cell (non-thymus-derived) function.[93] The interation of such suppressor T cells with B cells could be altered by a viral agent or drug.[130] It is beyond the scope of this chapter to discuss self-recognition, tolerance, clonal deletion, or specific T cell–mediated immune suppression. (See Chapter 20 for a discussion of lymphocyte function.)

Alteration of red cell membrane or stimulation of cross-reacting antibodies by infective agent

Frequently immune hemolytic disease is associated in time with an acute infectious episode or immunization. The specific mechanism of induction of a pathologic immune process remains unclear, but two broad mechanisms have been proposed: (1) the infectious agent contains an immunogen that evokes a normal antibody response, and the resulting antibody cross-reacts with an autologous red cell antigen and (2) the infectious agent alters an erythrocyte membrane antigen so that it becomes antigenic.

Infections with *Mycoplasma pneumoniae* are associated with an increased titer of anti-I. The immunogenic relationship between the production of anti-I and the antigens of *M. pneumoniae* are unclear. Some investigators have reported antigens related to human I antigens to be present in certain strains of *Mycoplasma*.[19,74] However, others have been unable to demonstrate any immunologic relationship between anti-I and *M. pneumoniae,* since (1) exposing serum to *M. pneumoniae* does not decrease the titer of anti-I, (2) there is no correlation between the titer of anti-I and antibodies to *M. pneumoniae,* and (3) individuals with chronic hemolytic disease caused by anti-I do not have demonstrable antibody against *M. pneumoniae*.[36] However, it is of interest that these investigators produced cold agglutinins in rabbits that were challenged with *M. pneumoniae*–treated human erythrocytes. They concluded that a reaction product of *M. pneumoniae* and the red cell might be immunogenic.[37]

The connection between infection and autoimmune hemolytic disease is uncertain. Zuelzer et al.[139] have postulated that basic to the pathogenesis is an "immunologic handicap" that predisposes an individual to occult viral infections. Such infections induce antibody production against erythrocyte antigens in a way that is still undefined.

Drug administration

Drug-associated immune hemolytic disease is extremely uncommon in children and will not be emphasized for this reason. It has two basic mechanisms: (1) the antibody is directed against the drug or metabolic products. The antigen-antibody complex may bind to the erythrocyte surface, or the antibody may react to the antigen, which is bound to the red cell membrane. (2) The antibody produced is specific for a normally present red cell antigen that has no chemical relationship to the drug.

Immune complex–induced hemolysis. The mechanism underlying immune complex–induced hemolysis is the formation of a drug–plasma protein complex in which the protein acts as a carrier and the drug as a hapten. This complex is immunogenic and most frequently leads to the production of IgG or IgM antibodies. The resulting antigen-antibody complex is deposited nonspecifically on the erythrocyte membrane and frequently activates complement. The resulting red cell destruction is rapid and occurs intravascularly. Since the affinity of the drug-protein complex for the red cell membrane is weak, there is significant dissociation in vitro. The optimal in vitro detection occurs when drug, patient's fresh serum, and erythrocytes are incubated together. Immune complex hemolytic anemia was first described in 1954 by Harris[51] in a patient exposed to stibophen for a second time. Immune complex hemolytic anemia has been associated with an increasing number of drugs, including phenacetin, antihistamines, sulfonamides, insulin, quinine, and other agents.[20,95]

Erythrocyte binding. Drugs or their metabolites may become immunogenic through their binding to the erythrocyte membrane. This has been well documented for penicillin and its major haptenic determinant, the benzyipenicilloyl (BPO) group.[94] The incidence of sensitization varies directly with the administered dose of penicillin. Thirty percent of patients given 1.2 to 2.4 million units daily and 100% of patients given 10 million or more units daily had demonstrable erythrocyte-bound penicillin.[72] The binding of penicillin or its metabolites to the erythrocyte membrane does not result in shortened red cell survival. However, hemolytic disease occurs in those individuals who develop significant levels of antibody to penicillin. This antibody then reacts with the penicillin bound to the erythrocyte membrane. These antibodies are generally of IgG class and do not activate complement. The destruction of erythrocytes is rarely intravascular, although fulminant intravascular hemolysis and complement binding have been reported.[102]

Other agents that have been documented to cause hemolytic anemia or to yield positive direct Coombs reactions through antibody directed against erythrocyte-bound drugs are cephalosporins[40,47] and carbromal.[124]

Drug-induced hemolytic disease. Several drugs have been reported to induce positive direct Coombs reactions and autoimmune hemolytic disease through the stimulation of antibodies that react directly with the red cell membrane and have no reactivity against the drugs or their degradation products. Such antibodies almost invariably have specificity for the Rh antigen and are of IgG class. The best-documented agent inducing this type of hemolytic disease is α-methyldopa.[134] Although 15% of patients taking this drug develop a positive direct antiglobulin test, less than 1% developed hemolytic disease.[13,135] L-Dopa has been reported to be associated frequently with a positive direct Coombs test.[46,52] However, immune hemolytic disease associated with this drug is rare.[127] One other agent, mefenamic acid, has been implicated as an infrequent cause of immune hemolytic disease.[35,104,120] It is possible that the effect of these agents is to affect T cell–B cell interaction, which leads to the production of antibody against the Rh complex.[130]

"Secondary" or "symptomatic" immune hemolytic disease

The occurrence of immune hemolytic disease in association with a well-defined underlying disease is well documented. Certainly immune hemolytic disease is a common manifestation of systemic lupus erythematosus.[85,128] In adults malignant lymphoma,[64] chronic lymphocytic leukemia[123] and Hodgkin's disease[32] have been reported to be associated with immune hemolytic disease. Immune hemolytic disease has been reported in association with solid malignancies such as ovarian dermoid cysts and teratomas[3,27] and thymoma.[109] In children immune hemolytic disease has been reported in association with neuroblastoma[39] and immunoblastic lymphadenopathy.[12] An interesting series of case reports describes immune hemolytic disease occurring in children with immune deficiency states, i.e., congenital X-linked agammaglobulinemia,[103] thymic dysplasia,[116] dysgammaglobulinemia,[115,125] and Wiskott-Aldrich syndrome.[111] The observations of an increased incidence of autoantibody production in first-degree relatives of individuals with immune hemolytic disease[41] give additional strength to the concept that immune hemolytic disease may be a manifestation of a basic immunologic aberration.

CLINICAL FEATURES
Incidence and sex and age distribution

Pirofsky[99] has estimated the minimum annual incidence of immune hemolytic disease to be 1 case/80,000 population in the Northwestern United States and, from Letman's data,[71] 1/75,000 in Denmark. The incidence in childhood is much lower since the majority of patients are over 40 years of age, with a peak in the sixth to eighth decade of life.[22,99] In childhood the disease is most common in the first 5 years of life, with a significant incidence in children younger than 1 year old (Table 10-1). Children may be affected within the first month of life,[99,139] and one case has been reported in a 7-day-old infant.[60] Such cases are most unusual. In childhood, boys appear to be affected more frequently than girls with a male:female ratio of 1.4:1. In the adult population women are affected more frequently than men.

Course and prognosis

The course of immune hemolytic disease is exceedingly variable in onset and duration. There is some degree of correlation clinically between acute onset and short duration of overt disease and insidious onset and more protracted disease. However, exceptions do occur.

Acute immune hemolytic disease is associated frequently with a well-defined episode of infectious disease or with immunization.[48,140] It is characterized by the sudden onset of significant symptoms and physical findings. Pallor, tachycardia, fever, jaundice, and hemoglobinuria are frequent findings. Patients may present with a picture of shock, diarrhea, vomiting, abdominal pain, and dehydration. Splenomegaly is a common finding but is rarely massive. Since severe anemia may develop rapidly, cardiac decompensation may result. Renal failure is seen rarely and requires the occurrence of significant intravascular hemolysis.

Table 10-1. Age at diagnosis and duration of immune hemolytic disease*

Age at diagnosis	No. of cases	Duration	
		<3 mo	>3 mo
<1 year	35	19	16
1-5 years	57	29	28
6-10 years	35	13	22
>10 years	25	1	24
TOTAL	152	62	90

*Data from Habibi et al.,[48] Zuelzer et al.,[139] and Zupánska et al.[140]

The direct cause of renal failure is uncertain, since experimentally both hemoglobin[6] and stroma from incompatible erythrocytes[117] have produced renal failure in humans.

The course of immune hemolytic disease may be limited to a few weeks and to a single episode. More protracted illness may be marked by periods of quiescence and exacerbation of the hemolytic process. Frequently exacerbations are linked to infectious episodes. Such episodes may be associated with increased antibody production, since the direct Coombs test may become more strongly positive. They may also be associated with activation of fixed macrophages resulting in increased erythrophagocytosis.

Chronic hemolytic disease is most common in children older than 10 years of age. Association with a well-defined acute infection is uncommon. The clinical course is characterized by insidious onset, pallor, mild jaundice, and minimal to moderate splenomegaly. Hemoglobinuria is infrequent. The disease may be characterized by episodes of increased erythrocyte destruction and by "aplastic" crises. Such crises may be life threatening since red cell production may decrease precipitously. If the red cell survival is significantly decreased, severe anemia may develop extremely rapidly.

Paroxysmal cold hemoglobinuria is most frequently an acute disease characterized by dark brown urine following exposure to the cold. The degree of exposure required to precipitate an attack varies from individual to individual. A few minutes to several hours after exposure, the patient may complain of leg or back pain, abdominal pain, cramps, nausea, vomiting, and diarrhea. Chills and fever usually precede the episode of hemoglobinuria. Paroxysmal cold hemoglobinuria is seen in children following infectious diseases such as chickenpox, mumps, measles, infectious mononucleosis, or the "flu."[15,22,90] The disease usually is self-limited, ending within a few weeks. Protection from the cold is the only measure usually required.

The prognosis for children with immune hemolytic disease is related to a great extent to any underlying disease. In several published series reporting observations restricted to childhood disease mortality ranged from 9% to 28%.[9,48,139,140] It is unclear whether there is any significant difference in the mortality rates in acute disease or chronic disease. It must be noted, however, that if the disease occurs as an acute episode in a previously healthy child who has no demonstrable underlying disease, the prognosis is excellent. This form of immune hemolytic disease may be considered to be the red cell counterpart of thrombocytopenic purpura of childhood.

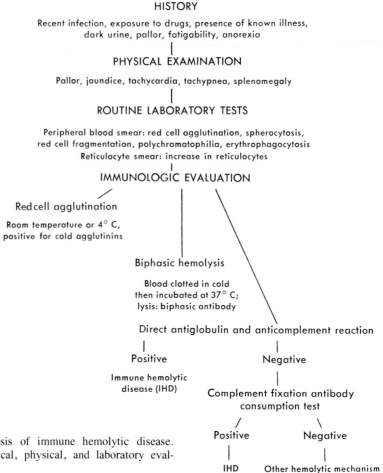

HISTORY

Recent infection, exposure to drugs, presence of known illness,
dark urine, pallor, fatigability, anorexia

PHYSICAL EXAMINATION

Pallor, jaundice, tachycardia, tachypnea, splenomegaly

ROUTINE LABORATORY TESTS

Peripheral blood smear: red cell agglutination, spherocytosis,
red cell fragmentation, polychromatophilia, erythrophagocytosis
Reticulocyte smear: increase in reticulocytes

IMMUNOLOGIC EVALUATION

Red cell agglutination

Room temperature or 4° C,
positive for cold agglutinins

Biphasic hemolysis

Blood clotted in cold
then incubated at 37° C;
lysis: biphasic antibody

Direct antiglobulin and anticomplement reaction

Positive   Negative

Immune hemolytic
disease (IHD)

Complement fixation antibody
consumption test

Positive Negative

IHD Other hemolytic mechanism

Fig. 10-1. Diagnosis of immune hemolytic disease. Schema of historical, physical, and laboratory evaluations.

DIFFERENTIAL DIAGNOSIS (Fig. 10-1)

The criterion for the diagnosis of immune hemolytic disease is the demonstration of immunoglobulin or complement components on the red cell surface. This criterion distinguishes these entities from other inborn or acquired lesions leading to decreased red cell survival. Conditions to be considered are hereditary spherocytosis; paroxysmal nocturnal hemoglobinuria; enzyme deficiencies such as G-6-PD deficiency; copper intoxication, both extrinsic, e.g., $CuSo_4$ ingestion, and intrinsic, e.g., Wilson's disease; and microangiopathic and macroangiopathic anemias.

LABORATORY EVALUATION
Peripheral blood

The initial procedure in the evaluation of any child suspected of having immune hemolytic disease is the examination of the peripheral blood. The hematocrit, red cell count, and hemoglobin value vary from individual to individual depending on the rate of red cell destruction and the compensatory capacity of the bone marrow. Usually there is an increase in the absolute reticulocyte count, which may reach 900×10^{12}/liter. Because of the reticulocytosis, the MCV is frequently in the macrocytic range. However, the absolute reticulocyte count may be normal or even low at the time of diagnosis. The white cell count is extremely variable but is within the normal range in the majority of patients. The platelet count is extremely variable but is usually within the normal range. Thrombocytopenia in association with immune hemolytic disease is known as Evans' syndrome.[33]

Study of the peripheral blood smear reveals that the majority of cells are normochromic and normocytic. Polychromasia and macrocytosis are evidence of the degree of reticulocytosis. In stressed individuals nucleated red blood cells may be present. The most constant morphologic abnormality of the red blood cells is the presence of spherocytes. Erythrocyte fragmentation is seen but is less striking than that present in micro- or macroangiopathic hemolytic anemia. Erythrophagocytosis is occasionally seen on direct blood smears,[28] and the phenomenon may be enhanced by making smears of the buffy coat after incubation at 37° C for 2 to 3 hours.[138] Examination of the buffy coat may also reveal rosette formation involving erythrocytes and lymphocytes.[42] Agglutination of red cells may be seen in the smears of patients with cold agglutinin disease.

Bone marrow

The bone marrow at the time of diagnosis most frequently reveals erythroid hyperplasia. In some patients a general increase in cellularity is noted. Infrequently the marrow may be found to be normal, and in about 10% of patients a decrease in the erythroid series is noted. Megaloblastic changes in the erythroid series may be present, although serum levels of folate and vitamin B_{12} are usually normal.[99] Diagnostically the marrow is of little importance.

Immunologic evaluation

The most important criterion for establishing the diagnosis of immune hemolytic disease is the demonstration of antibody or complement components on the red cell membrane. In the majority of cases the presence of the antibody on the red cell surface does not produce any immediately observable event. Therefore the demonstration of antibody or complement binding requires methods that translate such binding into observable and quantifiable reactions.

Agglutination. Agglutination of red cells suspended in a medium is affected by the surface charge and by the ionic field immediately surrounding them. These charge effects are termed the "zeta potential" of the cell and may be altered by enzymatic treatment of the red cell or by the addition of colloid to the suspended medium.[89,100] Antibodies of the IgM type are macromolecular and are comprised of five identical monomeric units linked together. Because of their size and high avidity, IgM antibodies can overcome these repulsive forces and directly agglutinate red cells in saline suspension. The most commonly occurring agglutinating antibodies in children with immune hemolytic disease are cold agglutinins of anti-I specificity. Cold agglutinins, which cause agglutination of red cells best at 0° to 4° C and agglutinate red cells poorly at temperatures above 32° C, are most frequently antibodies of IgM type. Occasionally cold agglutinins of IgG type have been noted in children.[105]

The cold agglutinins in postinfectious states such as after *M. pneumoniae* pneumonia charac-

teristically have anti-I specificity and agglutinate adult erythrocytes more strongly than fetal erythrocytes. Cold agglutinins developing in the course of infectious mononucleosis are usually of anti-i specificity[107] and agglutinate fetal cells more strongly than adult erythrocytes. Cold agglutinins may be of anti-SP$_1$ specificity.[80] Such agglutinins react equally well against all human cells, adult and fetal. Cold agglutinins developing after infections are usually polyclonal in nature. They have broad electrophoretic mobility and contain both κ and λ light chains.[49] In adults with chronic cold agglutinin disease, the cold agglutinin is almost invariably of one light chain and has restricted electrophoretic mobility.[119] Because of the antibody homogeneity in the chronic disease form, it can be considered to be an aberration of a single clone of immunocompetent cells.

Drug-induced hemolytic disease associated with the deposition of immune complexes is at times associated with visible in vitro red cell agglutination. In such instances the antibody may be of either the IgM or IgG class and requires the presence of the inducing drug, serum, and red cells. In adults cold agglutinins of the IgA type have been reported,[136] although most are IgG and IgM.

Hemolysis. The great majority of cold agglutinins are of the IgM type and have the capacity of activating serum complement. Since the thermal optimal zone for the binding of antibody to the red cell may be very narrow, dissociation may occur at a temperature at which complement-mediated hemolysis does not occur. Those sera containing antibodies that remain bound at a temperature of 10° C or higher effect hemolysis.[119]

Perhaps the most widely known hemolytic antibody is the Donath-Landsteiner (D-L) antibody described in 1904.[30] In this classic paper the authors reported that paroxysmal cold hemoglobinuria was caused by an antibody that binds to erythrocytes at low temperatures and that together with heat-labile factors effects the lysis of the persensitized cells when the temperature is raised. Red cell antibodies of this type are termed "biphasic hemolysins" because of the initial binding of antibody and C1 in the cold and the subsequent activation of the eight other complement components at higher temperatures, optimally at 37° C, which causes cell lysis. Biphasic hemolysins are almost invariably of the IgG type and are usually directed against antigens of the P antigen system.[73]

Antiglobulin and anticomplement reactions. In the majority of instances of immune hemolytic disease in children there is no direct evidence in vitro of antibody–red cell interaction. Such cases involve the action of IgG-type antibody, which binds firmly at 37° C and does not cause agglutination. It is for these reasons that such an antibody is termed warm reacting or incomplete antibody. The binding of antibody and/or complement components to the red cell can be demonstrated by the use of heterologous (rabbit) antibodies to human immunoglobulins or complement components, usually C3. The presence of these proteins bound to the red cell surface is demonstrated by agglutination of the persensitized erythrocytes by the heterologous antibody. The exposure of the washed persensitized human red cells and the rabbit antibody is called the direct Coombs test or direct antiglobulin test. If antibody to human IgG is employed, the test is termed a γ-Coombs test. Cell-bound C3 is detected by using a "non-γ" Coombs reagent. Such terminology is vague and imprecise. Since reagents are available against IgG, IgM, IgA, C3, and C4, the antibody reagent used should be designated. The use of anticomplement reagents (anti-C3) is of great importance since immunoglobulin may dissociate from the red cell membranes under the conditions in which a direct Coombs test is performed. If complement were activated by the antibody–red cell antigen interactions, complement components would be bound to the erythrocyte membrane and remain bound even when the antibody-antigen complex dissociated. One molecule of antigen-bound IgM or two molecules of IgG in close approximation will activate serum complement and lead to the stable binding of C1, C4, and C3 on the membrane. C3 is present on the membrane in the greatest quantity[50,77] and therefore is the complement component usually detected by the direct Coombs test when anti-C3 and anti-C4 reagents are used.[112]

The pattern of reactions obtained with antibody reagents has some correlation with the clinical course of the disease. There is a high incidence of "mixed-type" reactions, red cells being agglutinated with anti-IgG antisera and with anti-C3 antisera, in children with chronic disease.[48] Reactions limited to anti-complement sera only are seen most commonly in children who have acute hemolytic disease. However, there are enough exceptions to these generalizations to make one hesitant in their application in individual cases of immune hemolytic disease.

The direct Coombs test yields information only about whether or not immunoglobulin or complement components are bound to the red cell membrane. It does not give any information relevant to the antigenic specificity of the antibody. This information can be obtained by employing the indirect Coombs test, or indirect antiglobulin test. This assay is performed by incubating red cells with the patient's serum, which may have free antibody, or with an eluate prepared from red cells that have demonstrable bound antibody. After incubation with serum or eluate the red cells are washed and exposed to antisera to immunoglobulins and complement, and microscopic or macroscopic agglutination is sought. When a panel of red cells of defined antigenic specificities is employed, the antigenic specificity of the antibody can be determined by employing the indirect antiglobulin test and correlating the reaction patterns with the red cell antigens.

"Coombs-negative" hemolytic anemia. The limitation of the antiglobulin test is its sensitivity. Depending on the quality of the antisera used and on the spatial distribution of immunoglobulin on the red cell surface, a minimum of 250 to 500 molecules of IgG is required for a positive reaction.[31] Thus there is a population of patients who have specific erythrocyte-bound antibody but negative results in the Coombs test. At times such antibody may be detected by incubating enzyme-treated red cells with the patients' serum and then performing an indirect antiglobulin test.[112] However, patients may have insufficient antibody in their serum for it to be demonstrated by such procedures.

Small amounts of cell-bound IgG may be detected accurately by the complement-fixing antibody consumption test introduced by Gilliland et al.[43,44] In this test an accurately determined quantity of red blood cells is incubated with a standardized antihuman IgG. The amount of antibody per cell is determined by the decrease in complement fixation when the antihuman IgG is then reacted with carefully standardized IgG. Normally less than 40 molecules of IgG per red cell are bound nonspecifically, and the demonstration of 40 to 250 molecules of IgG/cell is diagnostic for an immune hemolytic process.

Other test systems of exquisite sensitivity are those employing hexadimethrine bromide (Polybrene), a positively charged antiheparin agent; polyvynal pyrrolidine (PVP), or assays employing radioisotope-labeled antibody or antigen (radioimmunoassay, RAI).[69] Any of these tests can be used to detect quantities of cell bound antibody below the sensitivity of the direct antiglobulin test.

PATHOPHYSIOLOGY

The ultimate fate of the antibody-coated red cell is clearance by the fixed phagocytic cells of the reticuloendothelial system. In most instances immune hemolysis does not result from the intravascular lysis of red cells, but when this does occur the erythrocyte stroma rather than persensitized red cells are removed by cells of the fixed macrophage system. Phagocytosis of antibody-coated particles is an efficient process because of the presence of receptors for the Fc portion of IgG and for C3 on phagocytic cells.[5,8,76] IgG and C3 have therefore been termed heat-stable and heat-labile opsonins. Since phagocytic cells do not possess any receptors for the heavy chain of IgM, this type of immunoglobulin does not promote phagocytosis and is not an opsonin.

The binding of nonlytic, or nonagglutinating, antibody to the red cell membrane results in a decrease in the negative surface charge but does not induce any detectable structural alteration. The effect of such antibody binding in red cell destruction is mediated through the Fc portion of the heavy chain and by nonlytic complement activation. Both fixed macrophages and neutrophils possess Fc and C3 receptors. Of the four subclasses of IgG in humans only two, IgG1 and IgG3, possess Fc regions that are opsonic.[1,59] When IgG reacts specifically with a red cell membrane antigen, the Fc region of the heavy chain undergoes conformational change, which increases its avidity for the Fc receptors of phagocytic cells.[8] If the density of membrane antigen is high, the effective valency of Fc increases and it will bind more firmly to the Fc receptor.[96] Since free plasma IgG1 and IgG3 compete for the Fc receptor sites of phagocytic cells, erythrocytes that have a high density of bound antibody will adhere more strongly than will erythrocytes with a low density of membrane-bound antibody.[8,57] The interrelation of antibody density and fluid phase immunoglobulin has been demonstrated. The binding of phagocytic cells of Rh-positive (D) red cells that are coated with anti-D is inhibited significantly by free IgG1 and IgG3.[8] There is, however, a relatively direct relationship between the amount of bound antibody and the rate of removal of sensitized cells from the circulation.[83]

The deposition of complement components on the red cell membrane is most frequently nonlytic. Complement activation leads most commonly to the fixation of C3b, a cleavage product of C3,[86] on the cell surface. Since phagocytic cells possess receptors for C3b, their interaction with persensitized erythrocytes is increased. The opsonic effect of cell-bound C3b is not inhibited by free, uncleaved C3 but is inhibited by free C3b. The phagocyte receptor sites for Fc and C3b are present in each cell but are distinct entities.[58,79] Cell-bound C3b is cleaved rapidly to C3c and C3d by a plasma protein called C3b inactivator or KAF (conglutinogen activating factor). The opsonic activity of the cleavage product, C3d, which remains cell bound, is not known. However, some phagocytic cells do possess C3d receptors.[101]

The in vivo effect of antibody and complement persensitization of red blood cells leads to their decreased survival through extravascular destruction by cells of the fixed macrophage system predominantly in the liver and spleen (Fig. 10-2). It is this red cell–macrophage interaction that results in the production of the spherocyte, the morphologic characteristic of immune hemolytic disease (Fig. 10-3).

The circulation of antibody-coated red cells through the spleen results in their exposure and adherence to fixed macrophages, particularly in the cords of Billroth.[7] This adherence causes red cell damage through loss of the membrane and fragmentation.[75] If the amount of IgG on the red cell surface is high, the liver becomes an important site for erythrocyte destruction.[61,110,111] The majority of deformed red cells recirculate as spherocytes. Since such cells are less deformable and have a higher volume:surface ratio than do normal erythrocytes, they are osmotically labile and susceptible to splenic trapping.[129]

The binding of C3b to the red cell membrane leads to the adhesion of phagocytic cells in vivo. The erythrocyte-phagocyte adhesion does not appear firm and occurs primarily in the liver.[81,118] Phagocytosis does not appear to be increased significantly by membrane fixed C3b alone,[5,113] and

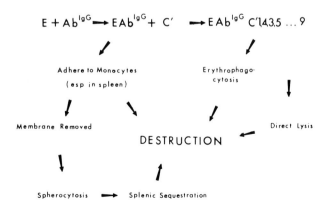

Fig. 10-2. Principal mechanism of red cell destruction by IgG antibodies. (From Rosse, W. F.: Prog. Hematol. **8:**51, 1973. Used by permission.)

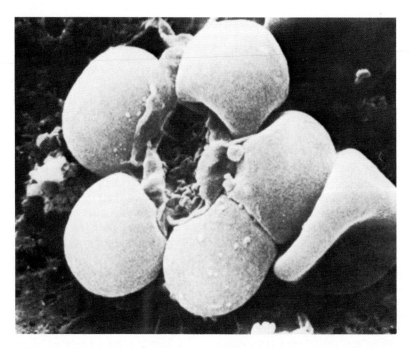

Fig. 10-3. Scanning electron photomicrograph of a monocyte surrounded by complement-coated red cells. (From Logue, G., and Rosse, W.: Semin. Hematol. **13:**277, 1976. Used by permission.)

the majority of sequestered red cells are released to the circulation after several hours.[8,118] Erythrocytes persensitized by C3b alone appear to have a normal survival after reappearance in the circulation.[118] Since most cases of autoimmune hemolytic disease in children are characterized by both IgG and C3b binding on the red cell surface, the kinetics of C3b-mediated red cell destruction may not be of great clinical significance. However, the rate of adherence mediated by erythrocyte-bound C3b is much more rapid than that mediated by IgG, and extravascular hemolysis may be more efficient in the presence of both opsonins.[76]

Cold agglutinins in children are almost invariably of the IgM type. Red cell destruction mediated by IgM antibodies appears to be effected primarily in two distinct ways:

1. *Hepatic sequestration:* Human red cells persensitized with anti-A hemagglutinins or with anti-I are cleared from the circulation and sequestered in the liver.[21,34,61,62]

2. *Complement-mediated hemolysis:* At times the complement system may be activated rapidly and to an extent that permits C3 to be hemolytically active for a period of time to effect activation of C5 to C9.[76] In this condition red cell destruction occurs intravascularly and the stroma are cleared by fixed macrophages. The reasons why this mode of red cell destruction does not occur more frequently are unclear.

Biphasic hemolysins are IgG antibodies that have been associated with paroxysmal cold hemoglobinuria. Hemolysis is intravascular and complement dependent. Antibody binds to the red cell in the cold, e.g., in an exposed extremity or the face. C1 is bound to the red cell surface at low temperatures and its binding possibly increases the binding of antibody.[53,54] When the cells are warmed the remaining complement components are "fixed," and hemolysis is effected.

Immunocytes of the B cell type have been demonstrated to have both Fc receptors[4] and C3b and C3d receptor[106] and to be able to effect antibody-dependent cell-mediated cytotoxicity.[93] Another subpopulation of lymphocytes, K cells, have been demonstrated to be effector cells in this immunologic reaction,[78,81] which requires IgG. The precise role of this form of antibody-dependent, nonphagocytic hemolysis in the pathogenesis of immune hemolysis in humans remains to be demonstrated. It is, however, another example of IgG Fc-dependent cytolysis.

THERAPY

Therapy of immune hemolytic disease in children has two objectives: (1) support of cardiovascular function and (2) decreasing the rate of red cell destruction through decreasing erythrophagocytosis and antibody synthesis. Obviously a scrupulous effort must be made to detect the presence of any underlying disease or any previous therapy with drugs so that specific therapy may be instituted or drug exposure terminated. It must be remembered that the majority of cases of immune hemolytic disease in childhood follow a definable infectious episode or have no demonstrable cause. In most cases the disease is mediated through IgG, "warm-reacting" antibody.

Transfusion therapy

The transfusion of red cells is necessary if there are objective signs of cardiovascular decompensation or anoxia. The unnecessary transfusion of red cells should be avoided, since there is poor red cell survival, risk of severe transfusion reactions, and the possibility of sensitizing the patient to red cell antigens present on the donor erythrocytes. Transfusion therapy is required most frequently in the initial phase of therapy before the effects of drug therapy have altered the course of the disease.

Obtaining truly compatible blood for transfusion may present major problems. There is a risk of mistyping the patients' red cells because the bound IgG may "block" specific typing sera or may lead to agglutination in high-colloid media.[106] In almost all cases of warm hemolytic disease, antibody specificity is directed against an antigenic determinant that is basic to the Rh complex[131] or perhaps to an antigen complex that includes components not defined by specific Rh alloantibodies used in red cell typing.[69] The antibody reacts against all red cells bearing Rh antigenic material and is negative only to Rh_{null} red cells. Occasionally specificity for an Rh antigen can be demonstrated; in the majority of cases it is directed against e (hr").[106]

In most instances compatible blood cannot be obtained for the patient and the "least incompatible" red cells are used for transfusion therapy. "Least incompatible" blood is determined empirically by cross matching several units of blood against the patient's serum and selecting that which has the weakest in vitro reactivity. There is no guarantee, however, that red cells having the least reactivity in vitro will have the longest survival in vivo. Rosenfield and Jagathambal[106] have noted that red cell survival in the sensitized individual is described by an exponential curve. The rate of destruction is a percentage of the cells present at any given time. The greater the volume of transfusate, the greater the absolute number of erythrocytes destroyed. Therefore small periodic transfusions are preferable to single large transfusions for two reasons: (1) cardiac decompensation is a common occurrence in rapidly developing severe anemia, and anemic individuals frequently have an increased blood volume, and (2) the destruction of a large quantity of red cells may

cause severe transfusion reactions. Packed cells, if available, should be the only blood product used. It is advised to limit the volume of packed red cells to 50 ml/m² per transfusion and to transfuse only when indicated clinically.

In the uncommon instances in which the patient has immune hemolytic disease mediated by a cold agglutinin or biphasic antibody an additional precaution must be taken. Severe hemolytic reactions may occur if chilled blood or blood at room temperature is administered. A controlled-temperature blood warmer for administering blood at 37° C must be used.

Drug therapy

Drug therapy is instituted to reverse the pathophysiologic processes mediated by specific antibody on the erythrocyte surface, to reverse phagocytosis and fragmentation by the cells of the fixed macrophage system, and possibly to decrease antibody production. Since IgG has a half-life of approximately 21 days,[84] the dramatic initial clinical improvement that is noted frequently in patients treated with steroids must be caused by effects other than decreased antibody synthesis.

Corticosteroids. Ever since the reporting in 1951[24] of their effectiveness in immune hemolytic disease, corticosteroids have been the primary agent in the treatment of immune hemolytic disease of the warm antibody type and always should be used initially. Acutely ill patients should be treated with intravenous preparations such as hydrocortisone at a dose of 200 mg/m² for the first 24 to 48 hours or until an oral agent such as prednisone can be tolerated. Oral therapy should be started before intravenous therapy is discontinued. Less severely ill children can be treated solely with an oral agent such as prednisone in a total dosage of 40 to 60 mg/m²/day in four divided doses. After 4 to 7 days prednisone can be given as a single daily dose. The high dose of prednisone should be continued until the hemoglobin value stabilizes at 10 gm/dl or higher and there is a decrease in the reticulocyte index. At this point the dose can be decreased by 50% and slow tapering over a 2-month period attempted. Recrudescence of activity is managed by increasing the prednisone dose until improvement occurs. To decrease side effects, children who require prolonged prednisone administration should be given the drug every other day whenever possible. The success rate in children with hemolytic disease of all types treated with corticosteroids has been reported to be 32% to 77%.[9,48,139,140]

Of all the agents used in treating immune hemolytic disease, corticosteroids have the most diverse physiologic effects, which may decrease the rate of red cell destruction. Four effects of steroid administration have been postulated to result in the clinical improvement observed.

1. Adrenal corticoids inhibit the sequestration of antibody-coated red cells by organs of the fixed macrophage system.[66]
2. Adrenal corticoids may affect the binding of antibody, resulting in a dissociation from the red cell membrane.[111]
3. Adrenal corticosteroids decrease IgG synthesis.[11]
4. Adrenal corticosteroids produce lymphocytopenia in humans[137] and thus affect antibody production and possibly affect antibody-dependent cell-mediated cytolysis.

Immunosuppressive agents. The reported use of immunosuppressive agents in the treatment of steroid-unresponsive immune hemolytic disease in children is limited. Johnson and Abildgaard[63] have reviewed seventeen reported cases in which nine patients derived clinical benefits. Azathioprine was used as a single agent in five cases and with either 6-mercaptopurine or chlorambucil in three cases. The most detailed reports by Hitzig and Massimo[56] recommended decreasing steroid administration only after 4 to 8 weeks of azathioprine therapy. If steroids can be stopped completely, azathioprine therapy should be continued for an additional 3 to 4 months. The usual dose for azathioprine is 2.5 mg/kg/day. Twice this dose can be administered if necessary, if white cell counts and platelet counts are obtained once or twice weekly.

Chronic cold agglutinin disease is extremely rare in children. In adults treatment with adrenal corticosteroids or splenectomy has not been very successful.[88] However, in a small number of individuals therapy with immunosuppressive agents such as cyclophosphamide[119] or chlorambucil[56] has been reported to be quite successful.

Splenectomy

Since splenectomy is an irreversible procedure that is associated with a significantly increased incidence of sepsis and death,[122] immunosuppressive agents should be used before a splenectomy is performed. If combined steroid and immunosuppressive therapy fails or produces excessive toxicity or side effects, splenectomy should be considered. Because of the possible long-term consequences of immunosuppressive agents, many authorities do not advocate their routine use in nonmalignant disorders such as autoimmune hemolytic anemia.

As a general rule the spleen is the primary site for destruction of red cells sensitized with IgG antibody. Two factors affect splenic destruction of antibody-coated cells: (1) macrophage receptors for the Fc fragment and C3b, which leads to erythrophagocytosis, and (2) filtration of fragmented cells, which have decreased deformability.[7,129]

The use of ^{51}Cr-labeled red cells to quantify the uptake of red cells in the spleen and liver has led to a more scientific approach to splenectomy, since there is a correlation between uptake and the results of splenectomy.[45] If the ratio of splenic to hepatic uptake is 2.3:1 or greater at 50% ^{51}Cr survival, significant splenic sequestration is present.[2] However, there is enough disparity between splenic ^{51}Cr red cell uptake and the results of splenectomy that the decision for splenectomy is essentially clinical. Success in children is probably less than 50%.

Because of the risk of children developing postsplenectomy sepsis and death, the use of prophylactic penicillin is recommended. This antibiotic probably gives some protection against pneumococcal infections, but controlled studies in splenectomized children have not been performed. Better protection may be afforded through immunization to pyogenic organisms such as *S. pneumoniae, N. meningococcus,* and *H. influenzae*.

Thymectomy

Thymectomy at this time remains the final form of immunologic intervention in children with autoimmune hemolytic anemia. Reports are available on five children who were subjected to this procedure.* Success as marked by a cessation or a decrease in the hemolytic process was obtained in three cases.[65,67,133]

Hemolytic disease of the newborn

In the previous section immune hemolysis has been described as a consequence of a perturbation of the immune process. This section describes the consequences of immune hemolysis occurring in the fetus as a result of the transplacental passage of maternal antibody directed against a fetal red cell antigen that is not shared by the mother. The antibody is the product of the normal immune response to a foreign substance and is invariably of the IgG type. Although hemolytic disease of the newborn caused by ABO incompatibility always has been more common than that caused by Rh incompatibility, ABO hemolytic disease is usually less severe and has not been associated with fetal and neonatal death or significant sequelae to the extent that has Rh hemolytic disease.

The spectrum of pathology resulting from the immune destruction of red cells in the fetus and the newborn infant ranges from minimal anemia or hyperbilirubinemia to hydrops fetalis. The recognition by Diamond et al.[161] that these diverse clini-

---

*References 63, 65, 67, 91, 133.

cal syndromes constituted one basic pathophysiologic entity was fundamental to the present understanding of isoimmune hemolytic disease. The immunologic basis of erythroblastosis was not ascertained until 1939, when Levine and Stetson[184] described a red cell agglutinin of unknown specificity in a mother with an affected infant, and 1940 when Landsteiner and Weiner[181] noted their findings on the agglutination of human red cells by an antibody raised against rhesus monkey red cells. The introduction in 1945 of the direct antiglobulin test by Coombs et al. enabled the laboratory detection of sensitized individuals, which was followed closely by the introduction and widespread use of exchange transfusion for the treatment of hemolytic disease of the newborn.* Although such treatment for severe hemolytic disease of the newborn significantly decreased the incidence of neurologic sequelae and of postpartum mortality, it did not alter fetal wastage or prevent maternal sensitization. The salvage of some severely affected infants through the use of intrauterine transfusions[186] was made possible through the realization that the quantification in amniotic fluid of pigmented breakdown products of fetal red cells could predict the severity of hemolytic disease in utero.[145,148,186] It was, however, the ability to prevent sensitization to the Rh factor in Rh-negative mothers bearing Rh-positive infants that brought a solution to the enormous problems of Rh sensitization.[164,171,172]

Prior to the effective prevention of Rh sensitization, hemolytic disease of the newborn caused 10,000 deaths annually in the United States.[165] The passive immunization using high-titered Rh immunoglobulin (RhoGAM†) of Rh-negative women eventually should eradicate Rh hemolytic disease. However, this success is leading to a complacency in diagnosing and following antepartum women who are sensitized to other Rh antigens, e.g., C and E. Although the number of affected infants is low, hemolytic disease of the newborn caused by non-D (Rh$_0$) antigens is becoming a principal cause of severe disease.

Rh hemolytic disease of the newborn remains the model for isoimmune hemolytic disease. The major part of the following discussion is devoted to this entity.

ETIOLOGY AND PATHOGENESIS

Although the placenta constitutes a significant barrier to the entrance of fetally derived products into the maternal circulation, it is not totally impervious. If the fetus and mother are incompatible for one or more red cell antigens, the potential for hemolytic disease of the newborn exists. Rh

*References 163, 176, 197, 219.
†Ortho Diagnostics, Raritan, N.J.

disease is most significant clinically because of its severity, although ABO hemolytic disease is about twice as common.[141] About 2% to 3% of cases of hemolytic disease of the newborn are caused by other blood group incompatibilities such as hr′ (c), rh′ (C), hr″ (e), rh″ (E), Kell (K), Duffy (Fy^a), and Kidd (Jk^a).[140]

The passage of fetal red cells across the placenta into the maternal circulation may result in the production of antibodies against fetal red cell antigens recognized by the mother as "not self." Evidence that fetal cells enter the maternal circulation was reported by Chown[154] in 1954. The reported case was one of a fetal-maternal hemorrhage in which approximately 160 ml of blood entered the maternal circulation. Such massive losses of fetal blood are unusual causes of maternal sensitization. The introduction of a sensitive acid elution technique for identifying fetal cells by the demonstration of intracellular Hb F enabled the detection of 0.05 ml of fetal blood in the maternal circulation.[180] Under the conditions of the Kleihauer-Betke technique adult hemoglobin is soluble and escapes from red blood cells. Fetal hemoglobin is insoluble and remains intracellular. Cells containing fetal hemoglobin stain intensely, whereas cells containing adult hemoglobin remain as ghosts. The ratio of Hb F–containing cells to non–Hb F–containing cells is determined and the amount of fetal blood can be calculated. If the fetus and mother differ in ABO blood groups so that the mother has isohemagglutinins against fetal red blood cells, these cells are removed rapidly from the circulation and therefore are not detected by the acid elution technique.

Using the acid elution technique Cohen et al.[156] demonstrated that fetal cells in one of fifteen women examined were present in the maternal circulation by the third month of gestation and that 50% of mothers who were ABO compatible had demonstrable circulating fetal cells at term. Zipursky et al.[225] noted the presence of fetal red cells at 9 weeks of gestation. The interpretation of an increased number of cells containing Hb F in early pregnancy as evidence for the passage of fetal red cells into the maternal circulation has been challenged by Pembrey et al.,[201] who noted an increase in the amount of circulating Hb F during the first trimester in 17% of thirty-nine women. Evidence that this Hb F was of maternal origin was obtained by analysis of the γ^{15}-peptide. The glycine:alanine ratio was in the adult Hb F range rather than the fetal range. Additional evidence was obtained through in vitro hemoglobin synthesis studies employing ^{14}C-labeled L-leucine. Maternal reticulocytes synthesized both Hb A and Hb F in ratios present in the peripheral blood. In early pregnancy Hb F–specific activity generally was greater than that of Hb A. The gestational age at which fetal-maternal transplacental leakage of red cells begins is therefore uncertain. The volume of fetal blood that at any one time enters the maternal circulation during a normal pregnancy is small, probably less than 0.1 ml. It is during delivery that larger boluses, greater than 0.2 ml, enter the maternal circulation.[212] It is these larger fetal-maternal hemorrhages that stimulate the production of antibody. Immunologic fetal-maternal bleeds may occur in spontaneous or induced abortions,[205,208] ectopic pregnancy,[179,185] cesarian section,[225] and manual removal of the placenta.[207] The risk of sensitization is related to the volume of the fetal-maternal bleeding.[222,223] However, investigations involving human volunteer subjects have demonstrated that a significant number of Rh-negative individuals do not produce Rh antibodies after repeated immunizations with Rh-positive blood.[195]

In 1943 Levine[183] reported a decreased incidence of ABO-incompatible matings among the parents of offspring with Rh hemolytic disease; he believed that such major blood group incompatibilities protected against Rh isosensitization through the destruction of fetal cells in the maternal circulation by anti-A or anti-B. Later studies confirmed this observation by demonstrating both a decrease in the incidence of circulating fetal red cells in ABO-incompatible mothers and a reduction in the amount of transplacental bleeding.[155,221] Woodrow and Donahoe[221] evaluated peripheral blood samples obtained from 2,000 ABO-compatible and 417 ABO-incompatible primagravidas within 72 hours of delivery. Fifty-six percent of the ABO-compatible and 24.7% of the ABO-incompatible blood contained circulating fetal red cells. There was a significant difference in the size of the transplacental hemorrhage in the two groups: 18.5% of the ABO-compatible mothers had 0.2 ml or more fetal blood, whereas only 1.9% of the incompatible mothers had fetal bleeding of this magnitude. Sera were screened for anti-D 6 months after delivery. Sixty-one of 760 (8.03%) sera from ABO-compatible pregnancies were positive, whereas 2 of 208 (0.96%) of the incompatible sera were positive for anti-D.

In general the larger the fetal-maternal hemorrhage, the greater the incidence of demonstrable sensitization. Since sensitization occurs most frequently during birth, the most accurate indicator for sensitization is the demonstration of maternal antibodies during the succeeding pregnancy. The incidence of sensitization at the end of the second pregnancy is about 17% in ABO-compatible mothers. Thus about half of the women sensitized are not detected after the first pregnancy.

The maternal antibody response to the fetal Rh_0-bearing red cells is of primary importance to the pathogenesis of hemolytic disease of the newborn. The production of IgM anti-D does not constitute any threat to the fetus, since antibodies of this class do not cross the placenta. Usually IgM anti-D is detected early in sensitization, is of low titer, and is present for a short period.[220] Most frequently the switch to the production of IgG antibody occurs rapidly. It is the IgG antibody response that is persistent and basic to the development of hemolytic disease of the newborn. IgG is the only immunoglobulin of maternal origin that is present in the fetus, since it is transported actively across the placenta.[169]

The zygosity of the father for Rh is a major determinant of maternal sensitization, since approximately 83% of the white population is Rh positive. However, approximately 42% are homozygous and 58% are heterozygous.[195] In each heterozygous mating the chance of having an Rh-positive fetus is 50%; if the father is homozygous, the chance is 100%. The effects of Rh zygosity and ABO compatibility are given in Table 10-2.

CLINICAL FEATURES

All of the clinical manifestations of hemolytic disease of the newborn are the result of the rate of red cell destruction and the degree of compensatory erythrocyte production by the fetus. The balance between red cell destruction and production determines if the disease is characterized by a low-grade hemolytic process or hydrops fetalis terminating in intrauterine death. In general the more severe the anemia, the more severe the clinical manifestations and the higher the risk for central nervous system damage caused by hyperbilirubinemia.

Jaundice

Most infants with hemolytic disease of the newborn are not jaundiced at birth because the placenta is an effective organ for clearing bilirubin.[209] Jaundice is noted within the first 24 hours after birth and in untreated infants reaches maximum

Table 10-2. Effect of ABO compatibility and Rh dose on the risk of sensitization by pregnancy in Rh-negative women*

| Husband's zygosity for Rh | ABO compatibility of husband | | ABO type of husband unknown (%) |
	Incompatible (%)	Compatible (%)	
Heterozygous	1	3	2
Homozygous	4-5	11	9
Zygosity unknown	2-3	7-8	5

*From Allen, F. H., Jr., and Diamond, L. K.: Erythroblastosis fetalis, Boston, 1958, Little, Brown & Co.

levels by the third to fifth day. Any infant who becomes jaundiced in the first day of life must be suspected of having hemolytic disease of the newborn, and serologic studies to establish this diagnosis must be performed. Jaundice is most detectable in daylight or under white fluorescent lamps. Blanching the skin by stretching it between two fingers or compressing it with a glass slide may help the examiner detect minimal jaundice. The development of jaundice is caused by the infant's inability to excrete bilirubin derived from red cell breakdown. Since each gram of degraded hemoglobin yields approximately 35 mg of bilirubin, the severity of the hyperbilirubinemia is related to the degree of hemolysis. Once separated from the placenta, the newborn is not capable of excreting a significant bilirubin load. Bilirubin is excreted primarily as a conjugate with glucuronic acid.[146] Conjugation is a function of the normal liver and is dependent on glucuronyl transferase, a microsomal enzyme. Newborn infants, particularly premature infants, have low levels of glucuronyl transferase activity.[149] In addition, the fetal liver is also deficient in two transport proteins, X and Y, which are required for the active transport of bilirubin from the hepatocyte to the biliary canaliculus.[142]

Immune hemolysis and anemia

Immune hemolysis is present in each affected infant. The degree of anemia is the result of the balance between the hemolytic process and capability of the bone marrow to produce red cells. In most cases red cell production is sufficient to maintain a normal or only slightly decreased red cell mass. At birth most infants appear relatively normal with minimal anemia and slight enlargement of the liver and spleen. As the severity of anemia increases, the degree of hepatic and splenic enlargement increases. In cases of profound anemia congestive heart failure develops associated with massive hepatosplenomegaly, edema, ascites, and pleural effusion. Some patients with hydrops are not profoundly anemia but are severely hypoproteinemic.[170] The cause of the hypoproteinemia is obscure. This form of erythroblastosis is known as hydrops fetalis and is associated with poor survival since most infants die within hours after birth. Frequently infants with severe hydrops fetalis die in utero.

Some infants with hemolytic disease of the newborn become progressively more anemic after the immediate newborn period. Such late anemia occurs most frequently after exchange transfusion. A consistent, gradual decrease in red cell mass occurs, which results in a hemoglobin level as low as 5 or 6 gm/dl at 4 to 6 weeks of life.[200] Delayed anemia may occur also in infants with mild hemolytic disease who did not require therapeutic ex-

change transfusion. Progressive anemia may become severe enough to require transfusion of red cells and if overlooked has resulted in death.

Encephalopathy (kernicterus)

In terms of chronic disease the encephalopathy caused by the effects of unconjugated bilirubin on the central nervous system constitutes the major complication of hemolytic disease of the newborn. The term "kernicterus" relates to the yellow staining by bilirubin of the basal ganglia and cerebellum. The clinical manifestations of kernicterus usually become evident during the first week of life but may appear at any time in infancy. Since the encephalopathy is the direct result of hyperbilirubinemia, it may be sequela of metabolic defects such as Crigler-Najjar syndrome or infections such as neonatal hepatitis or bacterial sepsis. Kernicterus presents initially with lethargy, poor feeding, and hypotonia.[215] With increasing severity of central nervous system involvement the infant develops a high-pitched cry, spasticity, and opisthotonus. In its most severe form kernicterus is characterized by irregular respirations, pulmonary hemorrhage, and death.

Infants who survive the episode of acute bilirubin encephalopathy suffer permanent residua. In general the severity of the central nervous system sequelae is related to the degree of hyperbilirubinemia. The most common residua are sensorineural deafness, dyslexia, and speech defects.[217] More severe neurologic effects include cerebral palsy with mental retardation, ataxia, and athetosis.

Other clinical features

Purpura associated with thrombocytopenia is common in severely affected infants. The mechanism of thrombocytopenia is unclear. Recent studies have indicated that the pathogenesis of hemorrhage may be more complex than isosensitization to blood platelets and that hemorrhage is a result of disseminated intravascular coagulation.[153,157,173]

Hypoglycemia is frequently noted in severely affected infants.[177] It is associated with elevated plasma insulin levels, and hypertrophy of the islet cells of the pancreas is a common finding.[197]

Rh disease is a form of isoimmune hemolytic disease mediated by IgG antibody. The section discussing IgG-mediated immune hemolysis is applicable to Rh disease in the newborn.

LABORATORY EVALUATION
Peripheral blood

Evidence for increased red cell destruction is the principal finding in the peripheral blood. The degree of anemia, reticulocytosis, and normoblastosis is proportional to the severity of the hemo-

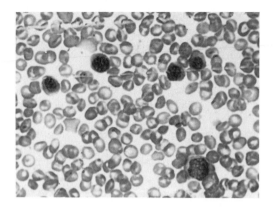

Fig. 10-4. Peripheral blood smear in Rh hemolytic disease of the newborn. Four nucleated red blood cells and one lymphocyte are present. Spherocytes are not present. (Courtesy J. Shafer, University of Rochester Medical Center.)

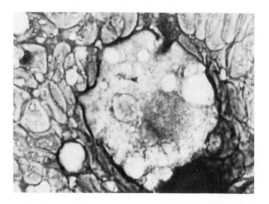

Fig. 10-5. Bone marrow touch preparation in erythrophagocytosis. The remains of several ingested red blood cells are present in the cytoplasm of the macrophage. (Courtesy J. Shafer, University of Rochester Medical Center.)

lytic process. Initial determinations from the cord blood, although accurately reflecting the severity of the hemolytic process, may not be good predictors of the degree of hyperbilirubinemia that may develop. Normal hemoglobin levels, 14 gm/dl or more, may be present because of adequate marrow erythroid production. Since these red cells are at risk for immune extravascular destruction, a significant amount of biliribin will be produced.

The peripheral smear reveals polychromasia and anisocytosis in addition to normoblastosis (Fig. 10-4). In hemolytic disease caused by Rh incompatibilities spherocytes are an uncommon finding. Intense leukocytosis may be seen in severely affected infants and may show a marked shift to the left, an increase in immature forms.

Bone marrow

Bone marrow for examination is usually obtained at postmortem examination. Erythroid hyperplasia is invariably present. At times the marrow is hyperplastic in all series. Rarely erythrophagocytosis is seen (Fig. 10-5).

Immunologic evaluation

The findings in Rh hemolytic disease of the newborn are identical to those of autoimmune hemolytic disease mediated by IgG antibody. The discussion in the previous section is applicable to the evaluation of the newborn, with one exception. Since hemolytic disease of the newborn is caused by an antibody response *by the mother*, the best source of antibody is maternal serum and not the affected newborn's serum. Thus all evaluations involving serum should make use of maternal serum if it is available. Cord blood or the infant's blood is used for typing and for the direct antiglobulin test. The diagnosis is established if red cells from an Rh-positive infant born to an Rh-negative mother give a positive direct antiglobulin test.

Serum bilirubin

The major threat to survival and to normal neurologic function in the erythroblastotic infant is the degree of diffusible unconjugated bilirubin. Because in vitro unconjugated bilirubin is actively transported across the placenta,[210] cord bilirubin levels are not high and levels in excess of 4 mg/dl are evidence of severe disease.[200] After birth the level of bilirubin may rise precipitously because the effective clearance by the placenta is lost.

The level of unconjugated, indirect-reacting bilirubin must be followed closely, since both the rate of increase and the absolute levels are important predictors of risk for developing kernicterus. Serum samples should not be exposed to light for prolonged periods, and hemolyzed samples are unsatisfactory for spectrophotometric analysis.

Unconjugated bilirubin is bound by serum proteins, principally by albumin. The binding to albumin is dependent on blood pH (acidosis causes a dissociation[212]) and on the presence of a number of drugs such as salicylates, sulfonamides, vitamin K, hydrocortisone, gentamycin, and other agents.[213] These findings have lead to the development of methods to quantify the level of free bilirubin in the plasma by gel filtration chromatography[211] or to estimate the bilirubin binding reserve of albumin by quantifying the binding of specific dyes such as PSP, which is decreased if bilirubin is bound to albumin.[190] Although these more sophisticated methods may be more reliable in predicting the risk of kernicterus than are determinations of unconjugated bilirubin, infants with demonstrated free dye binding sites on albumin have developed kernicterus,[190] as have infants whose serum level of unconjugated bilirubin was kept below 20 mg/dl, an accepted "safe" level.[178]

PATHOPHYSIOLOGY
Hemolysis

The destruction of IgG-coated red cells in the fetus and newborn with isoimmune Rh hemolytic disease is identical to that which occurs in immune hemolytic disease mediated by IgG immunoglobulin. This has been discussed in the section on immune hemolysis.

Bilirubin metabolism and toxicity

Bilirubin that is derived from the degradation of hemoglobin is lipid soluble and can cross cell membranes freely. Clearance from the plasma of free, lipid-soluble, unconjugated bilirubin is dependent on hepatocellular uptake. It has been demonstrated that two specific bilirubin-binding proteins are present in hepatocytes. These proteins have been termed Y and Z, or liganden.[142,188] In newborn monkeys levels of these proteins have been reported to be decreased.[182] The decreased levels of hepatocellular bilirubin-binding proteins would lessen the diffusion of bilirubin across the cell membrane, which would result in higher plasma levels.

Free unconjugated bilirubin is conjugated primarily with glucuronic acid[146] after uptake of hepatocytes. Conjugated bilirubin is water soluble and lipid insoluble and is excreted in the bile and urine. Since the conjugated form is lipid insoluble, it does not diffuse into the central nervous system and has not been implicated in central nervous system damage.

The deleterious effects of bilirubin on the central nervous system are most probably related directly to the levels of free unconjugated plasma bilirubin. Factors such as pH and albumin-bound drugs affect the level of free bilirubin. It has been demonstrated that brain damage such as anoxia contributes to bilirubin neurotoxicity.[160] The development of kernicterus is therefore the result of several factors.

THERAPY
Prevention of Rh isosensitization

The problems presented by Rh hemolytic disease have been obviated by the introduction and routine administration of Rh immune globulin to all unsensitized Rh-negative mothers who have given birth to an Rh-positive infant or who have had a spontaneous or induced abortion. Since the introduction of Rh immune globulin in the early 1960s there has been a steady decrease in the incidence of isosensitization to D (Rh$_0$) in Rh-negative mothers and as a result a corresponding decrease in the incidence of Rh hemolytic disease[166] (Figs. 10-6 and 10-7). The success observed with its use is further evidence that in most instances Rh sensitization occurs through significant fetal transplacental hemorrhage at the time of delivery. Prior to the use of Rh immune globulin approximately 13% to 16% of Rh-negative women delivered of an Rh-positive infant developed anti-D antibodies. With its use the incidence is less than 1%.[166]

The accepted method of preventing isosensitization to D is the administration of 300 μg of Rh immune globulin intravenously to all unsensitized Rh-negative women within 72 hours of the delivery of an Rh-positive infant. In cases in which Rh immune globulin has not been given within 72 hours, it should be administered late rather than withheld. Although the incidence of Rh sensitization is decreased significantly in ABO-incompatible maternal-fetal pairs, Rh immune globulin should be given to all women at risk.[224]

Treatment of the affected infant

The decreasing incidence of Rh isosensitization is a heartening advance in clinical perinatology. However, a significant number of women of childbearing age exist who are isoimmunized to Rh$_0$. For these individuals the administration of Rh immune globulin serves no purpose and its use should be avoided. The severity of Rh hemolytic disease in the offspring of such women will vary from mild to severe. The treatment of the affected offspring is governed by the severity of disease and has two major objectives: (1) the prevention of intrauterine fetal death and (2) the prevention of bilirubin encephalopathy in the live-born infant.

Prevention of intrauterine fetal death. Since maternal anti-D antibody is transported actively across the placenta, it can lead to destruction of D-positive red cells early in pregnancy. The developing fetus is at risk from severe anemia, not from hyperbilirubinemia, since the placenta effectively clears this substance. Therapy of the severely affected fetus is directed therefore solely toward correcting the severe anemia. The prediction in utero of the severely affected fetus becomes essential to the institution of therapy and to possible fetal salvage.

Past predictors for the extent of intrauterine Rh hemolytic disease had been relatively imprecise. The generalization that the severity of disease increased in successive pregnancies and that a severely affected or stillborn infant predicted a similar outcome in succeeding pregnancies had sufficient exceptions to make one hesitant to govern therapy on history alone. Maternal antibody titer

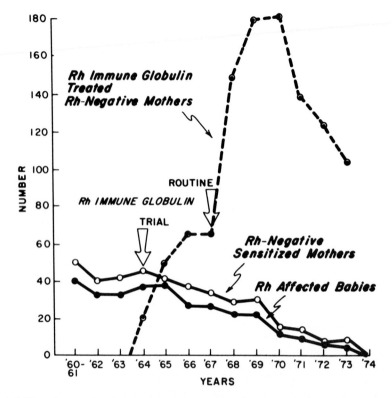

Fig. 10-6. Effect of preventive therapy with Rh immune globulin on the incidence of maternal sensitization and Rh hemolytic disease of the newborn. (From Freda, V., et al.: N. Engl. J. Med. **292:** 1014, 1975. Reprinted by permission.)

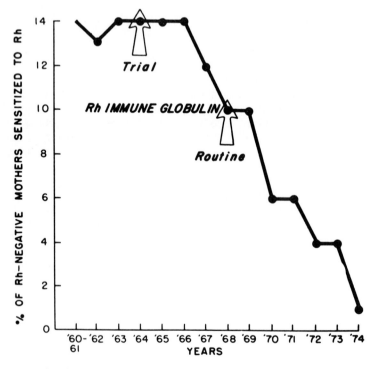

Fig. 10-7. Decreasing incidence of sensitized Rh-negative mothers seen at the Rh Antepartum Clinic, Columbia-Presbyterian Medical Center, from 1960 to 1974. (From Freda, V., et al.: N. Engl. J. Med. **292:**1014, 1975. Reprinted by permission.)

has been used as a quantitative guide of fetal disease. Although a correlation does exist between maternal antibody titers and severity of disease, enough exceptions occur to preclude relying on this parameter alone.[219] However, the obstetric history and maternal antibody titer combined can serve as guides for the performance of amniocentesis to assess accurately the severity of intrauterine disease.

There are no absolute criteria for performing amniocentesis. Since amniocentesis is associated with significant risks to the mother and the fetus,[174] it should be limited to cases in which the history and antibody titer indicate a high risk of stillbirth. Rh-negative women should be evaluated for isosensitization on their first prenatal visit. Any found to have anti-D antibodies should be followed closely with frequent quantification of

antibody titers. Should the titer reach the critical level (the titer associated with intrauterine or neonatal death), amniocentesis is indicated. The critical level varies among laboratories and must be established for each laboratory and each time new reagents are used for determining antibody titers.

Amniotic fluid is normally colorless or of a pale straw hue. When the fetus is affected with hemolytic disease, pigments derived from heme degradation enter the amniotic fluid by an as yet unknown mechanism.[213] The pigment is mainly bilirubin, which is cleared very slowly from the amniotic fluid.[152] The amount of pigment correlates with the severity of the hemolytic process and is predictive of the degree of anemia at birth.[148,186] The amniotic fluid is analyzed spectrophotometrically from 350 mμ to 700 mμ, and the optical density rise at 450 mμ is determined.[148] This peak

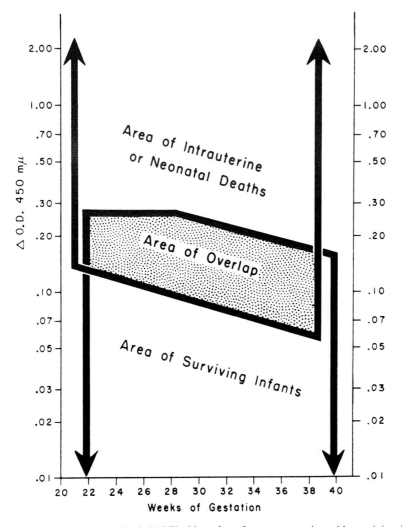

Fig. 10-8. Distribution of amniotic fluid bilirubin values from pregnancies with surviving infants and pregnancies resulting in death in utero or in the neonatal period. The area of overlap is critical to the following of amniotic fluid bilirubin levels during pregnancy. (From Queenan, J. T., and Goetschel, E.: Obstet. Gynecol. **32:**120, 1968.)

correlates with the amount of bilirubin present. Since bilirubin levels as low as 0.2 mg/dl can be associated with significant hemolytic disease, spectrophotometric analysis rather than a chemical method is used.[216] In normal pregnancy the value for the 450 mμ peak falls steadily from 26 weeks to term. When the fluid is analyzed the 450 mμ value is plotted on a graph (Fig. 10-8), which defines degrees of fetal risk.[204] No matter where the initial value falls, another sample must be obtained to verify a poor prognostic value or to establish a rising, falling, or horizontal trend.[204]

Since great significance is placed on the analysis of amniotic fluid, it must not have prolonged exposure to light, which oxidizes the pigments, resulting in a falsely low optical density. The specimen must not contain fetal or maternal blood or meconium, which yields a falsely high optical density.[187]

If the analysis of the amniotic fluid is indicative of severe disease, intrauterine transfusion should be considered. Transfusion earlier than 24 weeks of gestation is difficult because of the small size of the fetus. Success has been limited in this age group, which has a 90% (fifty-eight of sixty-four) fetal death rate.[203] In general intrauterine transfusion is most applicable in treating fetuses between 26 and 34 weeks of gestation. The risk per transfusion for intrauterine fetal death at this age ranges between 6% and 24% in several series.[147] Premature labor prior to 35 weeks of gestation occurs in 30% of the pregnancies, and neonatal death occurs in 15% of live births.[147] In intrauterine transfusion fresh packed red cells are introduced into the peritoneal cavity of the fetus. The red cells enter the circulation through diaphragmatic lymph channels. Volumes of transfused cells vary from 25 ml at 22 weeks to 125 ml at 33 weeks. Usually intrauterine transfusions are repeated at 2- to 3-week intervals until delivery.

Maternal complications of intrauterine transfusion include infection,[203] hepatitis,[192] placental separation,[192] and central nervous system embolization.[143] Fetal complications are much more numerous. Perforations of various structures such as bowel, stomach, bladder, thorax, spinal cord and cranium, and pericardium have been reported.[167] Possible graft versus host disease from lymphocytes in the transfusate has been reported.[198]

Prevention of bilirubin encephalopathy. Exchange transfusion remains the major effective means of managing hyperbilirubinemia in the affected newborn. The objectives of exchange transfusions are (1) to remove antibody-coated red cells, which are a potentially lethal source of bilirubin, and to replace them with red cells compatible to the mother, (2) to remove bilirubin, and (3) to remove antibody that would combine with any new red cells produced by the infant.

Since both IgG and bilirubin have significant extravascular distributions in the body, the effectiveness of exchange transfusions depends on their rate of equilibration with the intravascular space.

The exchange transfusion employs fresh whole blood that is ABO and Rh compatible with the mother. Most commonly group O Rh-negative blood is used. Theoretically the use of group O Rh-negative red cells suspended in fresh AB plasma would constitute a "universally acceptable whole blood" for exchange transfusion, since the plasma lacks isohemagglutinins. However, there is probably no practical advantage of this blood product over properly cross matched blood compatible with the mother. The risk of serum hepatitis is doubled when "universally acceptable whole blood" is used.

The volume of an exchange transfusion is usually calculated at two times the blood volume of the exchanged infant, or about 160 ml/kg. Since most of the effective removal of red cells occurs during the exchange of the first 80 ml/kg,[214] the volume of exchange is limited to one unit of whole blood or less in small infants. A two-volume exchange replaces approximately 90% of the circulating red cells.

The removal of bilirubin and IgG anti-D is not as effective as the removal of red cells, since both are distributed significantly extravascularly. Approximately 50% of albumin, to which bilirubin is bound, and IgG is extravascular. Both these proteins equilibrate rapidly with the intravascular compartment, so that exchange transfusion does decrease the extravascular pool. However, a two-volume exchange decreases the serum bilirubin level to 55% of its original level.[214] The postexchange "rebound," or increase in serum bilirubin levels, is mainly a result of the equilibration with the extravascular pool. Some contribution to the "rebound" hyperbilirubinemia is made by the destruction of residual or newly formed Rh-positive red cells since anti-D, though decreased, is still present.

The administration of albumin prior to or during the exchange transfusions has been advocated.[158,199] The usual dose is 1.0 gm/kg. Theoretically albumin administered 1 to 2 hours before exchange transfusions is more completely equilibrated with free bilirubin than when it is given in the transfusate.

The basics of exchange transfusion have remained unchanged for over 20 years and are described completely in the monograph by Allen and Diamond.[141] Use of ACD (acid-citrate-dextrose) blood creates potential hazards to the infant.

1. Since citrate binds to calcium, exchange transfusions may produce hypocalcemia. To avoid symptomatic hypocalcemia, calcium gluconate is administered intermittently dur-

ing the exchange transfusion. The usual dose is 1 ml of 10% calcium gluconate/100 to 150 ml exchanged volume.

2. Fresh blood, preferably obtained within the previous 24 hours, should be used to lessen the risk of hyperkalemia. Since stored red cells leak potassium, blood stored for more than 4 days should not be used.
3. The pH of freshly drawn ACD blood is less than 7.4 and decreases during storage. During the exchange transfusion a fall in the infant's blood pH has been reported.[151] Blood pH values below 7.0 have been observed during the exchange procedure.[202] Small premature infants have the most significant fall in blood pH.[151] It is recommended therefore that sodium bicarbonate be added to donor blood during the exchange transfusion.[168]
4. Thrombocytopenia and neutropenia are a direct result of exchange transfusions. The degree of thrombocytopenia is lessened if fresh blood is used.

Use of CPD as the preferred anticoagulant for blood transfusion obviates some of these potential hazards. The acid load of CPD is much less than that of ACD whole blood. Also, because it preserves 2,3-DPG, CPD assures favorable oxygen transport and exchange by transfused red cells. (See Chapter 4.)

The use of heparinized blood has been advocated because it reduces the potential for hypocalcemia and acidosis. Heparinized blood can be stored for only 24 hours. Because of this it is a guaranteed source of fresh whole blood. This short storage requirement makes most blood banks reluctant to supply heparinized blood.

The infant with hydrops fetalis, although possibly hyperbilirubinemic, suffers frequently from life-threatening anemia and congestive heart failure. The first priority is to increase the oxygen-carrying capacity of the blood. This is effected by the exchange of a small volume of packed red cells that are compatible with the mother. A full exchange transfusion is not the initial therapeutic choice. Albumin should never be administered to these infants, since it would increase the circulating blood volume.

The decision of when to perform an exchange transfusion is not based on firm criteria. Table 10-3 lists a suitable guide for exchange.[194] Newer techniques in the management of hyperbilirubinemia are stimulating controlled studies to establish firm criteria, particularly in mildly affected, nonerythroblastotic infants. None of the following manipulations has gained general acceptance in the treatment of hemolytic disease of the newborn.

1. *Prophylactic phenobarbital:* Phenobarbital stimulates several hepatic enzyme systems, including that of glucuronyl transferase. The increase is not immediate and an induction period is required. When given to mothers at a dose of 30 to 60 mg/day for 2 to 3 weeks prior to delivery, or to newborn infants at 5.0 mg/kg/day, one of fifty-six premature infants required exchange transfusions for hyperbilirubinemia, whereas eleven of fifty-six control infants required exchange.[163]

Table 10-3. Guidelines for exchange transfusion for Rh hemolytic disease of the newborn*

Findings	Observe	Consider exchange	Do exchange
At birth			
History or cause of action in previous offspring	No exchange transfusion	Exchange transfusion was necessary or kernicterus was observed	Death or near death from erythroblastosis
Maternal Rh antibody titer	<1:64	>1:64	
Clinical situation	Apparently normal	Induced or spontaneous delivery of premature infant	Jaundice, fetal hydrops
Cord hemoglobin	>14 gm/dl	12-14 gm/dl	<12 gm/dl
Cord bilirubin	<4 mg/dl	4-5 mg/dl	>5 mg/dl
After birth			
Capillary blood hemoglobin	>12 gm/dl	<12 gm/dl	<12 gm/dl and falling in first 24 hours
Serum bilirubin	<18 mg/dl	18-20 mg/dl	20 mg/dl in first 48 hours or 22 mg/dl on two successive determinations at 6- to 8-hour intervals after 48 hours. Clinical signs suggesting kernicterus at any time or at any bilirubin level

*From McKay, R. J.: Pediatrics **33**:763, 1964.

2. *Phototherapy:* Phototherapy with fluorescent lights that yield energy at 450 to 460 mμ has been demonstrated to break down bilirubin in vivo into products that are water soluble and excretable in the urine and bile.[150] Phototherapy has been most successful in decreasing the rate of exchange transfusion in the hyperbilirubinemia of prematurity or in instances in which the rate of increase in serum bilirubin is slow.[189,191] Phototherapy has been associated with minor side effects such as bronze skin, diarrhea, fever, and skin rashes.[144] No long-term sequelae have been reported.[144]

The greatest risk of nonexchange transfusion procedures is that they delay the initiation of an effective therapy for severe jaundice in the newborn. Although there is no proved benefit of immediate or early exchanges in the treatment of hyperbilirubinemia, all infants receiving therapy other than exchange transfusion must be monitored and observed repeatedly with bilirubin determinations obtained each 4 to 8 hours. If an exchange transfusion is not performed, the risk of developing late anemia is significant and therefore these infants must be observed continuously until endogenous red cell production becomes effective.

ABO HEMOLYTIC DISEASE OF THE NEWBORN

ABO hemolytic disease of the newborn has been reported to be the cause of about two thirds of the cases of hemolytic disease of the newborn.[141] It differs from Rh hemolytic disease primarily in the degree of severity. Severe hyperbilirubinemia is unusual and hydrops fetalis extremely rare. The pathophysiology of ABO hemolytic disease is identical to that of Rh disease. The antibody causing the immune destruction is of the IgG class, since IgM anti-A or anti-B cannot cross the placenta.

ABO hemolytic disease is restricted almost totally to group A or B infants born to group O mothers. It is most unusual in incompatible infants born to group A or B mothers. The most reasonable assumption to explain this clinical observation is the fact that IgG anti-A and, to a lesser degree, anti-B occurs spontaneously and simultaneously with IgM isohemagglutinins in a high percentage of group O individuals.[195] The naturally occurring isohemagglutinins in type A and type B individuals are almost exclusively of the IgM class. Since incompatible fetal cells entering the maternal circulation are removed rapidly through the binding and agglutination by IgM anti-A or anti-B, the chances for isosensitization in mothers who are not group O is minimal.

Since approximately 15% of group O pregnancies are AB incompatible, one could expect a much higher incidence of hemolytic disease than is noted clinically. The reasons for the lack of clinical disease are not known completely. However, certain factors may affect the interaction of anti-A with A cells in the fetus and newborn: (1) the antigenic density of A sites on fetal cells is much less than in adult cells[195] and (2) soluble blood group substances (A and B) are present in the plasma and extravascular compartment and may combine with the maternal anti-A, thereby inhibiting its reaction with the infants' red blood cells.[159]

Diagnosis

The diagnosis of ABO hemolytic disease is not as well defined as is that of Rh hemolytic disease. For it to be considered, the hyperbilirubinemic infant must almost always be type A or type B and be born to a type O mother. ABO hemolytic disease in type A or B mothers is rare but does occur. The following characteristics are found in the majority of cases:

1. Spherocytosis is the most prominent feature of ABO hemolytic disease. Significant spherocytosis is not seen in Rh hemolytic disease. Significant anemia, normoblastosis, reticulocytosis, and polychromasia are noted most commonly in Rh hemolytic disease but may be noted in ABO hemolytic disease.
2. A weakly positive direct antiglobulin test on cord blood or newborn blood may be found. A strongly positive test is unusual in ABO hemolytic disease.
3. Free anti-A or anti-B may be demonstrated in the serum of the newborn. This study must be carried out within the first few days of life since free antibody disappears rapidly from the neonate's serum.[175]
4. Confirmatory evidence is the presence of IgG anti-A or anti-B in the maternal serum. However, IgG anti-A or anti-B occurs in a high proportion of type O individuals. The finding of only IgM isohemagglutinins would exclude ABO hemolytic disease. Mothers of affected children usually have high titers of IgG anti-A or anti-B.[195]

Thereapy of severe ABO hemolytic disease is similar to that of Rh hemolytic disease. In the frequently occurring mild cases phototherapy or phenobarbital therapy has been successful in decreasing the need for exchange transfusions.[188]

HEMOLYTIC DISEASE CAUSED BY "MINOR" BLOOD GROUP ANTIBODIES

Hemolytic disease of the newborn is associated with Rh sensitization or ABO incompatibility in 98% or more of cases. Theoretically maternal isoantibody or IgG of any specificity can cause hemolytic disease of the newborn. Most commonly ''minor'' blood group hemolytic disease of the newborn is caused by antibodies to antigens of the Rh complex such as c, C, E, or e and other blood group antigenic systems such as Kell or Duffy.

For isosensitization to be suspected the infant must have a positive direct antiglobulin reaction with his or her red cells. Identification of the antibody specificity is accomplished most easily by using maternal serum against a panel of cells of known antigenic constitution. Identification of very rare, or ''private,'' antigen isoimmunization requires the use of paternal cells and maternal serum.

The list of possible causes of neonatal jaundice other than isoimmune disease is extensive. The major categories and specific diseases are as follows.

A. Antibody-mediated immune hemolysis: autoimmune anemia in the mother, e.g., systemic lupus erythematosus
B. Intrinsic red cell defects
  1. Hereditary deficiencies manifest by abnormal structure
    a. Spherocytosis
    b. Stomatocytosis
    c. Elliptocytosis
  2. Hereditary enzyme deficiencies
    a. G-6-PD deficiency
    b. Pyruvate kinase deficiency
    c. Others
  3. Vitamin E deficiency
C. Oxidant drugs
  1. Vitamin K
  2. Sulfonamides
  3. Thiazide diuretics
D. Infection
  1. Bacterial
    a. Gram-negative: *E. coli*
    b. Gram-positive: *Staphylococcus*
  2. Viral: rubella, cytomegalovirus, herpes simplex, hepatitis
  3. Protozoal: toxoplasmosis
  4. Spirochetal: syphilis
E. Enclosed hemorrhage, e.g., subcapsular hematoma
F. Metabolic disorders
  1. Galactosemia
  2. Hypothyroidism
  3. Crigler-Najjar syndrome
  4. Secondary to breast feeding
  5. Maternal hyperbilirubinemia
G. ''Physiologic'' jaundice

REFERENCES
Immune hemolysis

1. Abramson, N., Gelfand, E. W., Jandl, J. H., and Rosen, F. S.: The interaction between human monocytes and red cells: specificity for IgG subclasses and IgG fragments, J. Exp. Med. **132:**1207, 1970.
2. Algood, J. W., and Chaplin, N.: Idiopathic acquired autoimmune hemolytic anemia, Am. J. Med. **43:**254, 1967.
3. André, R., et al.: Anémie hémolytique autoimmune et tumeur maligne de l'ovaire, Presse Med. **77:**2133, 1969.
4. Bastrin, A., Miller, J. F. A. P., Sprent, J., and Dye, J.: A receptor for antibody on β lymphocytes. I. Method of detection and functional significance, J. Exp. Med. **135:**610, 1972.
5. Bianco, C., Griffen, F. M., Jr., and Silverstein, S. C.: Studies of the macrophage complement receptor: alteration of receptor function upon macrophage activation, J. Exp. Med. **141:**1278, 1975.
6. Blackburn, C. R. B., Hensley, W. J., Grant, D. K., and Wright, F. B.: Studies on intravascular hemolysis in man: the pathogenesis of the initial stages of acute renal failure, J. Clin. Invest. **33:**825, 1954.
7. Bowdler, A. J.: The role of the spleen and splenectomy in auto-immune hemolytic disease, Semin. Hematol. **13:**335, 1976.
8. Brown, D. L.: The behavior of phagocytic cell receptors in relation to allergic red cell destruction, Ser. Haematol. **7:**348, 1974.
9. Buchanan, G. R., Boxer, L. A., and Nathan, D. G.: The acute and transient nature of idiopathic immune hemolytic anemia in childhood, J. Pediatr. **88:**780, 1976.
10. Burnet, M.: Auto-immunity and auto-immune disease: a survey for physician or biologist, Philadelphia, 1972, F. A. Davis Co.
11. Butler, W. T.: Corticosteroids and immunoglobulin synthesis, Transplant. Proc. **7:**49, 1975.
12. Canale, V. C., and Smith, C. H.: Chronic lymphadenopathy simulating malignant lymphoma, J. Pediatr. **70:**891, 1967.
13. Carstairs, K. C., et al.: Incidence of positive direct Coombs' test in patients on alpha-methyldopa, Lancet **2:**133, 1966.
14. Chauffard, M. A., and Troisier, J.: Anémie grave avec hémolysine dans la sérum ictere hémolysinique, Sem. Med. **28:**94, 1908.
15. Colley, E. W.: Paroxysmal cold haemoglobinuria after mumps, Br. Med. J. **1:**1552, 1964.
16. Coombs, R. R. A., Mourant, A. E., and Race, R. R.: A new test for the detection of weak and ''incomplete'' Rh agglutinins, Br. J. Exp. Pathol. **26:**255, 1945.
17. Coombs, R. R. A., Mourant, A. E., and Race, R. R.: Detection of weak and ''incomplete'' Rh agglutinins: a new test, Lancet **2:**15, 1945.
18. Cordova, M. S., et al.: Acquired hemolytic anemia with positive antiglobulin (Coombs' test) in mother and daughter, Arch. Intern. Med. **117:**692, 1966.
19. Costea, N., et al.: Inhibition of cold agglutinins (anti-I) my *M. pneumoniae* antigens, Proc. Soc. Exp. Biol. Med. **139:**476, 1972.
20. Croft, J. D., Jr., et al.: Coombs'-test positivity induced by drugs. Mechanisms of immunologic reactions and red cell destruction, Ann. Intern. Med. **68:**176, 1968.
21. Cutbush, M., and Mollison, P. L.: Relation between characteristics of blood group antibodies in vitro and associated patterns of red cell destruction in vivo, Br. J. Haematol. **4:**115, 1958.
22. Dacie, J. V.: The hemolytic anaemias, congenital and acquired, part II, ed. 2, New York, 1962, Grune & Stratton, Inc.
23. DaCosta, J. A. G., et al.: Increased incidence of HL-A1 and 8 in patients showing IgG or complement coating on their red cells, J. Clin. Pathol. **27:**353, 1974.
24. Dameshek, W., Rosenthal, M. C., and Schwartz, L. I.: The treatment of acquired hemolytic anemia with adrenocorticotropic hormone (ACTH), N. Engl. J. Med. **244:**117, 1951.

25. Dameshek, W., and Schwartz, S. O.: The presence of hemolysins in acute hemolytic anemia, N. Engl. J. Med. **218:**75, 1938.

26. Dameshek, W., and Schwartz, S. O.: Acute hemolytic anemia (acquired hemolytic icterus, acute type), Medicine **19:**231, 1940.

27. DeBruyère, M., et al.: Autoimmune hemolytic anemias, Prog. Hematol. **6:**82, 1966.

28. deGruchy, G. C.: The diagnosis and management of acquired haemolytic anemia, Aust. Ann. Med. **3:**106, 1954.

29. Dobbs, C. E.: Familial autoimmune hemolytic anemia, Arch. Intern. Med. **116:**273, 1965.

30. Donath, J., and Landsteiner, K.: Über paroxysmale hemoglobinurie, Munich Med. Wochenschr. **51:**1590, 1904.

31. Dupuy, M. E., Elliot, M., and Masouredis, S. P.: Relationship between red cell bound antibody and agglutination in the antiglobulin reaction, Vox Sang. **9:**40, 1964.

32. Eisner, E., Ley, A. B., and Mayer, K.: Coombs'-positive hemolytic anemia in Hodgkins' disease, Ann. Intern. Med. **66:**258, 1967.

33. Evans, R. S., et al.: Primary thrombocytopenic purpura and acquired hemolytic anemia, Arch. Intern. Med. **87:**48, 1951.

34. Evans, R. S., et al.: Chronic hemolytic anemia due to cold agglutinins: the mechanism of resistance of red cells to complement haemolysis by cold agglutinins, J. Clin. Invest. **46:**1461, 1967.

35. Farid, N. R., Johnson, R. J., and Law, W. T.: Haemolytic reaction to mefenamic acid, Lancet **2:**382, 1971. (Letter.)

36. Feizi, T., and Taylor-Robinson, D.: Cold agglutinin anti-I and *Mycoplasma pneumoniae,* Immunology **13:**405, 1967.

37. Feizi, T., et al.: Cold agglutinin production in rabbits immunized with *Mycoplasma pneumoniae*–treated human erythrocytes, Clin. Res. **17:**366, 1969.

38. Fialkow, P. J., Fudenberg, H., and Epstein, W. V.: ''Acquired'' antibody hemolytic anemia and familial aberrations in gamma globulins, Am. J. Med. **36:**188, 1964.

39. Finklestein, J. V.: Personal communication, 1977.

40. Forbes, C. D., et al.: Acute intravascular hemolysis associated with cephalexin therapy, Postgrad. Med. J. **48:**186, 1972.

41. Fudenberg, H. H.: Immunologic deficiency, autoimmune disease and lymphomas: observations, implications, and speculations, Arthritis Rheum. **9:**464, 1966.

42. Gelfand, E. W., Abramson, H., Segel, G. B., and Nathan, D. G.: Buffy coat observations and red cell antibodies in acquired hemolytic anemia, N. Engl. J. Med. **284:**1250, 1971.

43. Gilliland, B. C., Baxter, E., and Evans, R. S.: Red-cell antibodies in acquired hemolytic anemia with negative antiglobulin serum tests, N. Engl. J. Med. **285:**252, 1971.

44. Gilliland, B. C., Leddy, J. P., and Vaughan, J. H.: The detection of cell-bound antibody on complement-coated red cells, J. Clin. Invest. **49:**898, 1970.

45. Goldberg, A., Hutchison, H. E., and MacDonald, E.: Radiochromium in the selection of patients with haemolytic anemia for splenectomy, Lancet **1:**109, 1966.

46. Goldberg, L. S., and Bluestone, R.: Studies on serologic abnormalities induced by L-dopa, Vox Sang. **24:**171, 1973.

47. Gralnick, H. R., et al.: Hemolytic anemia associated with cephalothin, J.A.M.A. **217:**1193, 1971.

48. Habibi, B., Homberg, J. C., Schaison, G., and Salmon, C.: Autoimmune hemolytic anemia in children. A review of 80 cases, Am. J. Med. **56:**61, 1974.

49. Harboe, M., and Deverill, J.: Immunochemical properties of cold agglutinins, Scand. J. Haematol. **1:**223, 1964.

50. Harboe, M., et al.: Identification of the components of complement participating in the antiglobulin reaction, Immunology **6:**412, 1963.

51. Harris, J. W.: Studies on the mechanism of a drug-induced hemolytic anemia, J. Lab. Clin. Med. **44:**809, 1954.

52. Henry, R. E., et al.: Serologic abnormalities associated with L-dopa therapy, Vox Sang. **20:**306, 1971.

53. Hinz, C. F., Jr., Picken, M. E., and Lepow, I. H.: Studies on immune hemolysis. II. The Donath-Landsteiner reaction as a model system for studying the mechanism of action of complement and the role of C'1 and C'1 esterase, J. Exp. Med. **113:**193, 1961.

54. Hinz, C. F., Jr., and Mollner, A. M.: Studies on immune hemolysis. III. Rise of 11S component in initiating the Donath-Landsteiner reaction, J. Immunol. **91:**512, 1964.

55. Hippe, E.: Chlorambucil treatment of patients with cold agglutinin syndrome, Blood **35:**68, 1970.

56. Hitzig, W. H., and Massimo, L.: Treatment of autoimmune hemolytic anemia in children with azathioprine (Imuran), Blood **28:**840, 1966.

57. Hoyer, L. W., and Trabold, N. C.: The significance of erythrocyte antigen site density. II. Hemolysis, J. Clin. Invest. **50:**1840, 1971.

58. Huber, H., et al.: Human monocytes: distinct receptor sites for the third complement of complement and for immunoglobulin G, Science **162:**1281, 1968.

59. Huber, H., et al.: IgG subclass specificity of human monocyte receptor sites, Nature **229:**419, 1970.

60. Iafusco, F., and Buffa, V.: Autoimmune hemolytic anemia in a newborn infant, Pediatria **70:**1256, 1962.

61. Jandl, J. H., and Kaplan, M. E.: The destruction of red cells by antibodies in man. III. Quantitative factors influencing the patterns of hemolysis in vivo, J. Clin. Invest. **39:**1145, 1960.

62. Jandl, J. H., and Tomlinson, A. S.: The destruction of red cells by antibodies in man. II. Pyrogenic, leukocytic and dermal responses to immune hemolysis, J. Clin. Invest. **37:**1202, 1958.

63. Johnson, C. A., and Abildgaard, C. F.: Treatment of idiopathic autoimmune hemolytic anemia in children: Review and report of two fatal cases in infancy, Acta Paediatr. Scand. **65:**375, 1976.

64. Jones, S. E.: Autoimmune disorders and malignant lymphoma, Cancer **31:**1092, 1973.

65. Jorppla, V., et al.: Splenectomy and thymectomy for autoimmune anemia in infants, Acta Paediatr. Jap. **74:**513, 1970.

66. Kaplan, M. E., and Jandl, J. H.: Inhibition of red cell sequestration by cortisone, J. Exp. Med. **114:**921, 1961.

67. Karaklis, A., Valaes, T., Pantelakis, S. N., and Doxiadis, S. A.: Thymectomy in an infant with autoimmune haemolytic anemia, Lancet **2:**778, 1964.

68. Kissmeyer-Nielson, F., Bent-Hansen, K., and Kieler, J.: Immunohemolytic anemia with familial occurrence, Acta Med. Scand. **144:**35, 1952.

69. Lalezari, P.: Serologic profile in autoimmune disease: Pathophysiologic and clinical interpretations, Semin. Hematol. **13:**291, 1976.

70. LePetit, J. C.: Expression of genetic marker of erythrocyte immunoglobulin G autoantibodies in autoimmune hemolytic anemia, Vox Sang. **183:**31, 1976.

71. Letman, H.: Red cell destruction in the anemias, thesis,

Copenhagen, 1959. Quoted in Pirofsky, B.: Clinical aspects of autoimmune hemolytic anemia, Semin. Hematol. **13**:251, 1976.

72. Levine, B. B., and Redmond, A.: Immunochemical mechanisms of penicillin induced Coombs' positive and hemolytic anemia in man, Int. Arch. Allergy Appl. Immunol. **31**:594, 1967.

73. Levine, P., Celano, M. J., and Fiakowski, F.: The specificity of the antibody in paroxysmal cold hemoglobinuria (PCN), Transfusion **3**:278, 1963.

74. Lind, K.: Production of cold agglutinins in rabbits injected by *Mycoplasma pneumoniae, Listeria monocytogenes* or *Streptococcus* MG, Acta Pathol. Microbiol. Scand. (B) **81**:487, 1973.

75. LoBuglio, A. F., et al.: Red cells washed with immunoglobulin G: binding and sphering by mononuclear cells in man, Science **158**:1582, 1967.

76. Logue, G., and Rosse, W.: Immunologic mechanisms in autoimmune hemolytic disease, Semin. Hematol. **13**:277, 1976.

77. Logue, G. L., et al.: Measurement of the third complement of complement bound to red blood cells in patients with cold agglutinin syndrome, J. Clin. Invest. **52**:493, 1973.

78. MacLennon, I. C. M.: Antibody in the induction and inhibition of lymphocyte cytotoxicity, Transplant. Rev. **13**:67, 1972.

79. Mantovani, B., Rabinovitch, M., and Nussenzweig, V.: Phagocytosis of immune complexes by macrophages. Different roles of the macrophage receptor site for complement (C3) and for immunoglobulin (IgG), J. Exp. Med. **135**:780, 1972.

80. Marsh, W. L., and Jenkins, W. J.: Anti-Sp₁: the recognition of a new cold antibody, Vox Sang. **15**:177, 1968.

81. McDonald, H. R., Bonnar, A. D., Sordat, S., and Zawodnik, S. A.: Antibody-dependent cell-mediated cytotoxicity: heterogenicity of effector cells in human peripheral blood, Scand. J. Immunol. **4**:487, 1975.

82. Mollison, P. L.: The role of complement in antibody-mediated red-cell destruction, Br. J. Haematol. **18**:249, 1970.

83. Mollison, P. L., et al.: Rate of removal from the circulation of red cells sensitized with different amounts of antibody, Br. J. Haematol. **11**:461, 1965.

84. Morell, A., Terry, W. D., and Waldman, T. A.: Metabolic properties of IgG subclasses in man, J. Clin. Invest. **49**:673, 1970.

85. Morgan, E. S., et al.: Direct antiglobulin (Coombs) reaction in patients with connective tissue disorders, Arthritis Rheum. **10**:502, 1967.

86. Müller-Eberhard, H. J.: Complement, Ann. Rev. Biochem. **44**:667, 1975.

87. Muller-Eckhardt, C.: Reappraisal of the clinical and etiologic significance of immunoglobulin deviations in autoimmune hemolytic anemia ("warm type"), Blut **34**:39, 1977.

88. Murphy, S., and LoBuglio, A. F.: Drug therapy of autoimmune hemolytic anemia, Prog. Hematol. **13**:323, 1976.

89. Neber, J., and Damashek, W.: The improved demonstration of circulating antibodies in hemolytic anemia by the use of a bovine albumin medium, Blood **2**:371, 1947.

90. O'Neill, J., and Marshall, W. C.: Paroxysmal cold haemoglobinuria and measles, Arch. Dis. Child. **42**:183, 1967.

91. Oski, F. A., and Abelson, N. M.: Autoimmune hemolytic anemia in an infant: report of a case treated unsuccessfully with thymectomy, J. Pediatr. **67**:752, 1965.

92. Pangburn, M. K., Schrieber, R. D., and Muller-Eberhard, H. J.: Human complement C3b inactivator: isolation characterization and demonstration of an absolute requirement for the serum protein R1H for cleavage of C3b and C4b in solution, J. Exp. Med. **106**:257, 1977.

93. Parish, C. R.: Separation and functional analysis of subpopulations of lymphocytes bearing complement and Fc receptors, Transplant. Rev. **25**:98, 1975.

94. Petz, L. D., and Fudenberg, H. H.: Coombs-positive hemolytic anemia caused by penicillin administration, N. Engl. J. Med. **274**:171, 1966.

95. Petz, L. D., and Fudenberg, H. H.: Immunologic mechanisms in drug-induced cytopenias. In Brown, E. B., ed.: Progress in hematology, vol. 9, New York, 1975, Grune & Stratton, Inc.

96. Philips-Quagliata, J. M., Levine, B. B., Quagliata, F., and Uhr, J. W.: Mechanisms underlying binding of immune complexes to macrophages, J. Exp. Med. **133**:589, 1971.

97. Pirofsky, B.: Hereditary aspects of autoimmune hemolytic anemia: a retrospective analysis, Vox Sang. **14**:334, 1968.

98. Pirofsky, B.: Autoimmunization and autoimmune hemolytic anemias, Baltimore, 1969, The Williams & Wilkins Co.

99. Pirofsky, B.: Clinical aspects of autoimmune hemolytic anemia, Semin. Hematol. **13**:251, 1976.

100. Pollack, W., et al.: A study of forces involved in the second stage of hemagglutination, Transfusion **5**:158, 1965.

101. Reynolds, H. Y., Atkinson, J. P., Newball, H. H., and Frank, M. M.: Receptors for immunoglobulin and complement on human alveolar macrophages, J. Immunol. **114**:1813, 1975.

102. Ries, C. A., et al.: Penicillin-induced immune hemolytic anemia: occurrence of massive intravascular hemolysis, J.A.M.A. **233**:432, 1975.

103. Robbins, J. B., Skinner, R. G., and Pearson, H. A.: Autoimmune hemolytic anemia in a child with congenital X-linked hypogammaglobulinemia, N. Engl. J. Med. **280**:75, 1969.

104. Robertson, J. H., Kennedy, C. C., and Hill, C. M.: Haemolytic anemia associated with mefenamic acid, Irish J. Med. Sci. **140**:226, 1971.

105. Roekke, D., et al.: IgG-type cold agglutinins in children and corresponding antigens: detection of a new Pr antigen: Prₐ, Vox Sang. **20**:218, 1971.

106. Rosenfield, R. E., and Jagathambal: Transfusion therapy for autoimmune hemolytic anemia, Semin. Hematol. **13**:311, 1976.

107. Rosenfield, R. E., Schmidt, P. J., Calvo, R. C., and McGuiniss, M. H.: Anti-i, a frequent cold agglutinin in infectious mononucleosis, Vox Sang. **10**:631, 1965.

108. Ross, G. D., and Polley, M. J.: Specificity of human lymphocyte complement receptors, J. Exp. Med. **141**:1163, 1975.

109. Ross, J. F., Finch, S. C., Street, R. B., and Strieder, J. W.: The simultaneous occurrence of benign thymoma and refractory anemia, Blood **9**:935, 1954.

110. Rosse, W. F.: Quantitative immunology of immune hemolytic anemia. I. The fixation of C1 by autoimmune antibody and heterologous anti-IgG antibody, J. Clin. Invest. **50**:727, 1971.

111. Rosse, W. F.: Quantitative immunology of immune hemolytic anemia. II. The relationship of cell-bound activity to hemolysis and the effect of treatment, J. Clin. Invest. **50**:734, 1971.

112. Rosse, W. F.: The detection of small amounts of antibody on the red cell in autoimmune hemolytic anemia, Ser. Haematol. **7**:358, 1974.

113. Rosse, W. F., de Borsfleury, A., and Bessis, M.: The

interaction of phagocytic cells and red cells modified by immune reactions: comparison of antibody and complement coated red cells, Blood Cells **1**:345, 1975.

114. Roth, P., et al.: Familiäre autoimmunhämolytische anämie (AIHA) mit negativem Coombs-test, Lymphozytopenie und Hypogammaglobulinamie, Schweiz. Med. Wochenschr. **105**:1584, 1975.

115. Sandler, S. G., et al.: IgA deficiency and autoimmune hemolytic disease, Arch. Intern. Med. **136**:93, 1976.

116. Schaller, J., et al.: Hypergammaglobulinemia, antibody deficiency, autoimmune hemolytic anemia and nephritis in an infant with a familial lymphopenic immune defect, Lancet **2**:825, 1966.

117. Schmidt, P. J., and Holland, P. V.: Pathogenesis of the acute renal failure associated with incompatible transfusion, Lancet **2**:1169, 1967.

118. Schreiber, A. D., and Frank, M. M.: Role of antibody and complement in the immune clearance and destruction of erythrocytes. I. In vivo effects of IgG and IgM complement fixing sites, J. Clin. Invest. **51**:575, 1972.

119. Schubothe, H.: The cold agglutinin disease, Semin. Hematol. **3**:27, 1966.

120. Scott, G. L., Myles, A. B., and Bacon, P. A.: Autoimmune haemolytic anemia and mefenamic acid therapy, Br. Med. J. **3**:534, 1968.

121. Shapiro, M.: Familial autohemolytic anemia and runting syndrome with Rh$_0$-specific auto-antibody, Transfusion **7**:281, 1967.

122. Singer, D. B.: Postsplenectomy sepsis. In Rosenberg, H. S., and Bolande, R. P., eds.: Perspective in pediatric pathology, vol. 1, Chicago, 1973, Year Book Medical Publishers, Inc.

123. Steinkamp, R. C., et al.: Long term experiences with the use of P-32 in the treatment of chronic lymphocytic leukemia, J. Nucl. Med. **4**:92, 1963.

124. Stephanini, M., and Johnson, N. L.: Positive anti-human globulin test in patients receiving carbromal, Am. J. Med. Sci. **259**:49, 1970.

125. Stoelinga, G. B., and vanMunster, P. J.: Antibody deficiency syndrome and autoimmune hemolytic anaemia in a boy with isolated IgM deficiency dysgammaglobulinemia type 5, Acta Paediatr. Scand. **58**:352, 1969.

126. Tauber, J. W.: "Self": standard of comparison for immunological recognition of foreignness, Lancet **2**:291, 1976.

127. Territo, M. C., Peters, R. W., and Tanaka, K. R.: Autoimmune hemolytic anemia due to levodopa therapy, J.A.M.A. **226**:1347, 1973.

128. Videbaek, A.: Auto-immune haemolytic anemia in systemic lupus erythematosus, Acta Med. Scand. **171**:187, 1962.

129. Weed, R. I., and Reed, C. F.: Membrane alterations leading to red cell destruction, Am. J. Med. **41**:681, 1966.

130. Weens, J. H., and Schwartz, R. S.: Etiologic factors in autoimmune hemolytic anemia, Ser. Haematol. **7**:303, 1974.

131. Weiner, W., and Vos, G. H.: Serology of acquired hemolytic anemias, Blood **22**:606, 1963.

132. Widal, F., Abrami, P., and Brulé, M.: Hémolyse par fragilité globulaire et hémolyse par action plasmatique, Bull. Soc. Biol. **63**:346, 1907.

133. Wilmers. M. J., and Russell, R. A.: Autoimmune haemolytic anemia in an infant treated by thymectomy, Lancet **2**:915, 1963.

134. Worlledge, S. M., Carstairs, K. C., and Dacie, J. V.: Autoimmune haemolytic anemia associated with α-methyldopa therapy, Lancet **2**:135, 1966.

135. Worlledge, S. M.: Immune drug-induced haemolytic anemias, Semin. Hematol. **6**:181, 1969.

136. Worlledge, S. M., and Blajchmann, M. A.: The autoimmune haemolytic anemias, Br. J. Haematol. **23**(suppl.): 61, 1972.

137. Yu, D. T. Y., et al.: Human lymphocyte subpopulations. Effects of corticosteroids, J. Clin. Invest. **53**:565, 1974.

138. Zinkham, W. H., and Diamond, L. K.: In vitro erythrophagocytosis in acquired hemolytic anemia, Blood **7**: 592, 1952.

139. Zuelzer, W. W., et al.: Autoimmune hemolytic anemia: natural history and viral-immunologic interactions in childhood, Am. J. Med. **49**:80, 1970.

140. Zupańska, B., et al.: Autoimmune haemolytic anaemia in children, Br. J. Haematol. **34**:511, 1976.

Hemolytic disease of the newborn

141. Allen, F. H., Jr., and Diamond, L. K.: Erythroblastosis fetalis, Boston, 1958, Little, Brown & Co.

142. Arias, I.: The pathogenesis of physiologic jaundice of the newborn. In Symposium on bilirubin metabolism: birth defects, Original article series, vol. 6, 1970, The National Foundation, The Williams & Wilkins Co.

143. Barnes, P. H., McInnis, A. C., Friesen, R. F., and Bowman, J. M.: Maternal mishap following fetal transfusion, Can. Med. Assoc. J. **92**:1277, 1965.

144. Berman, R. E.: Preliminary report of the committee on phototherapy in the newborn infant, J. Pediatr. **84**:135, 1974.

145. Bevis, D. C. A.: Blood pigments in haemolytic disease of the newborn, J. Obstet. Gynaecol. Br. Cwlth. **63**:68, 1956.

146. Billing, B. H., and Lathe, G. H.: The excretion of bilirubin as an ester glucuronide, giving the direct van der Bergh reaction, Biochem. J. **63**:6p, 1956. (Abstract.)

147. Bowes, W. A., Jr.: Intrauterine transfusion: indications and results, Obstet. Gynecol. **14**:561, 1971.

148. Bowman, J. M., and Pollock, J. M.: Amniotic fluid spectoscopy and early delivery in the management of erythroblastosis fetalis, Pediatrics **35**:815, 1965.

149. Brown, A. K., and Zuelzer, W. W.: Studies on the neonatal development of the glucuronide conjugating system, J. Clin. Invest. **37**:332, 1958.

150. Callahan, E., et al.: Phototherapy of severe unconjugated hyperbilirubinemia. Pediatrics **48**:841, 1970.

151. Callandine, M., and Gaudner, D.: Acid-base changes following exchange transfusion with citrated blood, Arch. Dis. Child. **40**:626, 1965.

152. Cherry, S. H., et al.: Mechanism of accumulation of amniotic fluid pigment in erythroblastosis fetalis, Am. J. Obstet. Gynecol. **106**:297, 1970.

153. Chessels, J. M., and Wigglesworth, J. S.: Hemostasis failure in rhesus immunization, Pediatr. Res. **5**:95, 1971. (Abstract.)

154. Chown, B.: Anemia from bleeding of the fetus into the mother's circulation, Lancet **1**:1213, 1954.

155. Cohen, F., and Zuelzer, W. W.: Mechanisms of isoimmunization. II. Transplacental passage and postnatal survival of fetal erythrocytes in heterospecific pregnancies, Blood **30**:796, 1967.

156. Cohen, F., Zuelzer, W. W., Gustafson, D. C., and Evans, M. M.: Mechanisms of isoimmunization. I. The transplacental passage of fetal erythrocytes in homospecific pregnancies, Blood **23**:621, 1964.

157. Cole, V. A., Normand, I. C. S., Reynolds, E. O. R., and Rivers, R. P. A.: Pathogenesis of haemorrhagic pulmonary oedema and massive pulmonary hemorrhage in the newborn, Pediatrics **51**:175, 1973.

158. Comley, A., and Wood, B.: Albumin administration in exchange transfusion for hyperbilirubinemia, Arch. Dis. Child. **43**:151, 1968.

159. Denborough, M. A.: Serum blood group substances and

ABO hemolytic disease, Br. J. Haematol. **16:**103, 1969.

160. Diamond, I., and Schmid, R.: Experimental bilirubin encephalopathy. The mode of entity of bilirubin-C^{14} into the central nervous system, J. Clin. Invest. **45:**678, 1966.

161. Diamond, L. K., Blackfan, K. D., and Baty, J. M.: Erythroblastosis fetalis and its association with universal edema of fetus, icterus gravis meonatorum, and anemia of the newborn, J. Pediatr. **1:**269, 1932.

162. Diamond, L. K., et al.: Erythroblastosis fetalis: treatment with exchange transfusion, N. Engl. J. Med. **244:**39, 1951.

163. Doxiadis, S.: Phenobarbital prophylaxis for neonatal jaundice, Hosp. Prac. **5:**115, 1970.

164. Finn, R., et al.: Experimental studies on the prevention of Rh hemolytic disease, Br. Med. J. **1:**1486, 1961.

165. Freda, V. J.: Rh immunization: experience with full term pregnancies, Clin. Obstet. Gynecol. **14:**594, 1971.

166. Freda, V. J., Gorman, J. G., Pollack, W., and Bowe, E.: Prevention of Rh hemolytic disease: ten years' clinical experience with Rh immune globulin, N. Engl. J. Med. **292:**1014, 1975.

167. Friesen, R. F.: Complications of intrauterine transfusions, Clin. Obstet. Gynecol. **14:**572, 1971.

168. Gaudy, G., Partridge, J. W., and Gairdner, D.: Control of acidosis during exchange transfusion with citrated blood, Arch. Dis. Child. **43:**147, 1968.

169. Gitlin, D., Kumate, J., Urrusti, J., and Morales, C.: The selectivity of the human placenta in the transfer of plasma proteins from mother to fetus, J. Clin. Invest. **43:**1938, 1964.

170. Gordon, H.: The diagnosis of hydrops fetalis, Clin. Obstet. Gynecol. **14:**548, 1971.

171. Gorman, J. G., Freda, V. J., and Pollack, W.: Intramuscular injection of a new experimental gammaglobulin preparation containing high levels of Rh antibody as a means of preventing sensitization to Rh, Proc. Ninth Cong. Int. Soc. Hematol. **2:**545, 1962.

172. Gorman, J. G., Freda, V. J., and Pollack, W.: Prevention of Rh haemolytic disease, Lancet **2:**181, 1965.

173. Gross, S., and Melhorn, D. K.: Exchange transfusion with citrated whole blood for disseminated intravascular coagulation, J. Pediatr. **78:**415, 1971.

174. Grove, C. S., Crombetta, G. C., and Amstey, M. S.: Fetal complications of amniocentesis, Am. J. Obstet. Gynecol. **115:**1154, 1973.

175. Gunson, H. H.: An evaluation of the immunological tests used in the diagnosis of AB hemolytic disease, Am. J. Dis. Child. **94:**123, 157.

176. Hart, A. P.: Familial icterus of the newborn and its treatment, Can. Med. Assoc. J. **15:**1008, 1925.

177. Hey, E. N.: Hypoglycaemia in haemolytic disease of the newborn, Arch. Dis. Child. **48:**79, 1973.

178. Johnson, L. H., and Boggs, T. R.: Failure of exchange transfusions to prevent minimal cerebral damage when employed so as to maintain serum bilirubin concentrations below 18 and 20 mg/100 ml, Pediatr. Res. **4:**481, 1970. (Abstract.)

179. Katz, J., and Marcus, R. G.: The risk of Rh isoimmunization in ruptured tubal pregnancy, Br. Med. J. **2:**667, 1972.

180. Kleihauer, E., Braun, H., and Betke, K.: Demonstration von fetalem hamoglobin in den erythrocyten einen blatausstrichs, Klin. Wochenschr. **35:**637, 1957.

181. Landsteiner, K., and Weiner, A. S.: Agglutinable factor in human blood recognized by immune sera for rhesus blood, Proc. Soc. Exp. Biol. Med. **43:**223, 1940.

182. Levi, A. J., et al.: Deficiency of hepatic organic anion-binding protein, impaired organic anion uptake by liver and "physiologic" jaundice in newborn monkeys, N. Engl. J. Med. **283:**1136, 1970.

183. Levine, P. A.: Serological factors as possible causes of spontaneous abortion, J. Hered. **34:**71, 1943.

184. Levine, P., and Stetson, R. E.: Unusual cases of intra-group agglutination, J.A.M.A. **113:**126, 1939.

185. Liedholm, P. C.: Feto-maternal hemorrhage in ectopic pregnancy, Acta Obstet. Gynecol. Scand. **50:**367, 1971.

186. Liley, A. W.: Liquor amnii analysis in the management of pregnancy complicated by Rhesus sensitization, Am. J. Obstet. Gynecol. **82:**1359, 1961.

187. Liley, A. W.: Errors in the assessment of hemolytic disease from amniotic fluid, Am. J. Obstet. Gynecol. **86:**485, 1963.

188. Litwack, G., et al.: Ligandin: a hepatic protein which binds steroids, bilirubin, carcinogens and a number of exogenous organic amines, Nature **234:**466, 1971.

189. Lucey, J. F.: Changing concepts regarding exchange transfusions and neonatal jaundice, Clin. Obstet. Gynecol. **14:**586, 1971.

190. Lucey, J. F., et al.: Serum albumin reserve PSP dye-binding capacity in infants with kernicterus, Pediatrics **39:**876, 1967.

191. Maisils, M. J.: Bilirubin: on understanding and influencing its metabolism in the newborn infant, Pediatr. Clin. North Am. **19:**447, 1972.

192. Mandelbaum, B.: Fetal transfusions, Int. J. Gynaecol. Obstet. **7:**71, 1969.

193. Mandelbaum, B., and Robinson, A. R.: Amniotic fluid pigment in erythroblastosis fetalis, Obstet. Gynecol. **28:**118, 1966.

194. McKay, R. J.: Current status of exchange transfusion in newborn infants, Pediatrics **33:**763, 1964.

195. Mollison, P. L.: Blood transfusion in clinical medicine, ed. 5, Oxford, 1972, Blackwell Scientific Publications.

196. Mollison, P. L., and Cutbush, M.: Exchange transfusion, Lancet **2:**522, 1948.

197. Molsted-Pedersen, L., Trautner, H., and Jorgensen, K. R.: Plasma insulin and K values during intravenous glucose tolerance tests in newborn infants with erythroblastosis foetalis, Acta Paediatr. Scand. **62:**11, 1973.

198. Naiman, J. L., et al.: Possible graft-versus-host reaction after intrauterine transfusion, N. Engl. J. Med. **281:**697, 1969.

199. Odel, G. B., Cohen, S. N., and Gordes, E. H.: Administration of albumin in the management of hyper-bilirubinemia by exchange transfusions, Pediatrics **30:**613, 1962.

200. Oski, F. A., and Naiman, J. L.: Hematologic problems in the newborn. In Major problems in clinical pediatrics, vol. 1, Philadelphia, 1966, W. B. Saunders Co.

201. Pembrey, M. E., Weatherall, D. J., and Clegg, J. B.: Maternal synthesis of haemoglobin F in pregnancy, Lancet **2:**489, 1973.

202. Povey, M. S. C.: pH changes during exchange transfusion, Lancet **2:**339, 1964.

203. Queenan, J. T.: Intrauterine transfusions: a collaborative study, Am. J. Obstet. Gynecol. **104:**397, 1969.

204. Queenan, J. T.: Amniotic fluid analysis, Clin. Obstet. Gynecol. **14:**505, 1971.

205. Queenan, J. T., Gadow, E. C., and Lopes, A. C.: Role of spontaneous abortions in Rh-immunization, Am. J. Obstet. Gynecol. **110:**128, 1971.

206. Queenan, J. T., and Goetschel, E.: Amniotic fluid analysis for erythroblastosis fetalis, Obstet. Gynecol. **32:**120, 1968.

207. Queenan, J. T., and Nakamoto, J.: Postpartum immunization: the hypothetical hazard of manual removal of the placenta, Obstet. Gynecol. **23:**392, 1964.

208. Queenan, J. T., Shah, S., Kubarych, S. F., and Holland, B.: Role of induced abortion in Rh-immunization, Lancet **2:**815, 1971.

209. Schenker, S., et al.: Bilirubin metabolism in the fetus, J. Clin. Invest. **43:**32, 1964.

210. Schier, R. W., et al.: Bilirubin transfer across the human placenta, Am. J. Obstet. Gynecol. **111:**677, 1971.

211. Schiff, D., Chan, G., and Stern, L.: Sephadex G-25 quantitative estimation of free bilirubin potential in jaundiced newborn infants' sera: a guide to the prevention of kernicterus, J. Lab. Clin. Med. **80:**455, 1972.

212. Schmid, R.: Bilirubin metabolism in man, N. Engl. J. Med. **287:**703, 1972.

213. Stern, L.: Drugs in the newborn infant and the binding of bilirubin to albumin, Pediatrics **49:**916, 1972.

214. Valaes, T.: Bilirubin distribution and dynamics of bilirubin removal by exchange transfusion, Acta Paediatr. Scand. **149**(suppl.):1, 1963.

215. VanPraagh, R.: Diagnosis of kernicterus in the neonatal period, Pediatrics **28:**870, 1961.

216. Walker, W.: Haemolytic anemia in the newborn, Clin. Haematol. **4:**145, 1975.

217. Walker, W., et al.: A follow-up study of survivors of Rh haemolytic disease, Dev. Med. Child Neurol. **16:**592, 1974.

218. Wallerstein, H.: Treatment of severe erythroblastosis by simultaneous removal and replacement of the blood by the newborn infant, Science **103:**583, 1956.

219. Walsh, R. J., and Ward, H. K.: Haemolytic disease of the newborn. An analysis of family histories and serologic findings, Aust. Ann. Med. **8:**262, 1959.

220. Ward, H. K.: The persistence of antibodies in the absence of antigenic stimulus, Aust. J. Exp. Biol. Med. Sci. **35:**499, 1957.

221. Woodrow, J. C., and Donohoe, W. T. A.: Rh-immunization by pregnancy: results of a survey and their relevance to prophylactic therapy, Br. Med. J. **4:**139, 1968.

222. Woodrow, J. C., and Finn, R.: Transplacental haemorrhage, Br. J. Haematol. **12:**297, 1966.

223. Zipursky, A.: Preventing Rh immunization, Postgrad. Med. **43:**100, 1968.

224. Zipursky, A.: The universal prevention of Rh immunization, Clin. Obstet. Gynecol. **14:**869, 1971.

225. Zipursky, A., et al.: The transplacental passage of foetal red blood cells and the pathogenesis of Rh immunization during pregnancy, Lancet **2:**489, 1963.

11 □ Hemolytic anemia: membrane defects

Henry Chang
Denis R. Miller

An approach to understanding the properties of the red cell membrane involves consideration of each of its components: protein, lipid, carbohydrate, and the combinations of these. Such molecular species are not static during the life span of the red cell but undergo dynamic change with membrane synthesis, accretion, loss, and destruction. This chapter presents some fundamental concepts of the normal erythrocyte membrane and then deals with the pathogenesis of disorders leading to membrane failure and hemolysis.

MEMBRANE BIOCHEMISTRY
Current model of erythrocyte membrane

The structure of the red cell membrane is at present better understood than the mechanisms involved in its various physiologic functions. These subjects are covered in several reviews.[27,35,45] The currently accepted model for the red cell membrane is the fluid-mosaic model proposed by Wallach[51] and Singer and Nicolson.[47] The membrane consists of approximately 50% protein, 40% lipid, and 10% carbohydrate. In this model the lipids are arranged in a bilayer with their hydrophilic moieties oriented externally and their hydrophobic regions internally (Fig. 11-1). The proteins are either partially embedded in this bilayer or extend transmurally to the outer surface. The carbohydrate groups are attached to either the lipids (glycolipids) or proteins exposed on the exterior of the cell (glycoproteins). Each of these components will be discussed in more detail.

Membrane proteins

Although the distinction between true membrane proteins and those that are merely adsorbed to the surface seems arbitrary in some respects, the former have hydrophobic areas that allow relatively stronger association with the lipid bilayer. This property also makes it difficult to study these molecules experimentally because they aggregate unless an organic solvent or detergent is used to solubilize them. A common technique is to electrophorese membrane proteins that have been dissociated with an ionic detergent, sodium dodecyl sulfate, through polyacrylamide gels (SDS-PAGE). Because a relatively constant proportion of SDS binds to protein (1.4 gm SDS/gm protein),[49] the

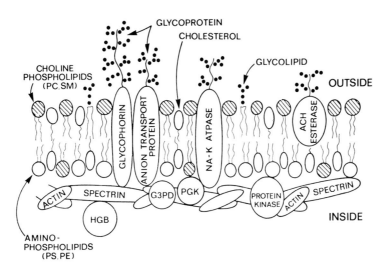

Fig. 11-1. Current model of erythrocyte membrane. Hypothetical cross section of a lipid bilayer, showing the disposition of membrane proteins. (Courtesy Dr. Samuel Lux.)

mobility of a protein through this gel is inversely proportional to the log of its molecular weight.[53] Membrane proteins can be separated into seven to ten classes by this method[12] (Fig. 11-2). The presence of large polysaccharide groups to which SDS does not bind will cause glycoproteins to migrate more slowly and appear to have a higher than the true molecular weight. Similarly the protein stain Coomassie blue binds poorly to carbohydrate-rich molecules, which then must be visualized by some other technique, such as the periodic acid–Schiff (PAS) method. It should be emphasized that each band may be quite heterogeneous and variations in gel pattern may result from proteolysis, aggregation, or altered mobility, depending on the extent of glycosylation.

The disposition of these components in the membrane has been studied by a variety of biochemical techniques (Table 11-1). The results of these experiments indicate that, whereas most proteins are situated on the cytoplasmic surface, band 3 and the PAS bands (the most prominent one called glycophorin) consist of transmembrane proteins (Fig. 11-1). The estimated number of these molecules correlates with the presence of membrane-associated particles seen in freeze-fracture electron micrographs in which the bilayer is split into two leaves.[55] However, similar studies on red cells lacking the major glycoprotein have failed to reveal any gross deficiency in such particles.[2] In a later section evidence is presented for the role of the transmembrane proteins in cellular transport whereas other proteins on the cytoplasmic surface, i.e., bands 1 and 2 (the spectrins) and band 5 ("actin"), are thought to have a different function, providing the structural framework for the red cell.

During erythropoiesis membrane proteins such as those in bands 1, 2, and 3 are made asynchronously.[4] The current hypothesis is that their synthesis begins on ribosomes that are free in the cytoplasm, but as nonpolar amino acids are added to the polypeptide chain, the complex becomes bound to membrane vesicles. The degree of insertion of the protein into the bilayer depends on the hydrophobicity of this "signal sequence."[3,35] Glycosylation may take place within the vesicles, which then fuse with the plasma membrane, but some proteins may also reach the cytoplasmic surface by diffusion.

Insight into the distribution of particles over the membrane may be afforded by an experiment in which unlike cells were fused with Sendai virus.[15] Antibodies to each cell type labeled with separate fluorescent markers were added. Initially each of the dyes was localized over distinct halves of the heterokaryon, but after 40 minutes their colors had become mixed over the entire cell surface. The process was not affected by metabolic inhibitors, as is the "capping" phenomenon of lymphocytes or fibroblasts,[11] but was delayed by cooling and may have been related to membrane viscosity. Recently the rate of lateral mobility of integral membrane proteins has been measured in the erythrocyte.[14]

Membrane lipids

Phospholipid structures and cholesterol in a molar ratio of 1.25 constitute the major membrane lipids (Table 11-2). The former consist of two fatty acid chains linked to a glycerol backbone in which

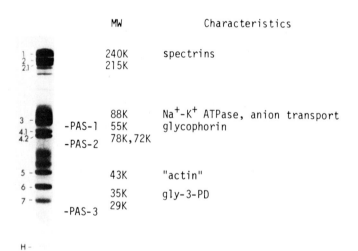

Fig. 11-2. Pattern of red cell membrane proteins as seen after polyacrylamide gel electrophoresis in sodium dodecyl sulfate (SDS-PAGE). Proteins may be visualized by Coomassie blue and glycoproteins by PAS stain (the latter not shown). The components are labeled in order of decreasing molecular weight and their roles in the membrane are given if known.

Table 11-1. Methods for study of membrane structure

Component	Technique	Manipulation	Result
Protein	Elution studies	Low ionic strength	Elute spectrins (bands 1 and 2) and "actin" (band 5)
		Nonionic detergents	Triton X-100 releases bands 3, 4.2, 6 and all PAS
	Surface labels	Alkyl sulfonic acids, diazonium compounds, pyridoxal phosphate + NaB^3H_4	Nonpenetrating reagents label primary amino groups on exterior of intact cells
		Lactoperoxidase + $Na^{125}I$	Tyrosine and histidine residues labeled
		Antibodies	Show surface markers by electron microscopy
	Cross-linking reagents	Formaldehyde, glutaraldehyde, oxidizing agents, suberimidates, adipimidates, acetimidates	Establish proximity of adjacent molecules
	Controlled proteolysis	Trypsin, chymotrypsin	Localization of proteins by digestion of inside-out or right-side-out vesicles or intact cells
Lipid	Lipid exchange	Assay for phospholipid bound to proteins or cholesterol bound to vesicles	Suggests preferential association between lipids and other membrane components
	Controlled lipolysis	Phospholipases	Used in studies of lipid asymmetry
Carbohydrate	Surface labels	Lectins, galactose oxidase + NaB^3H_4	Specific labeling of surface sugars
	Enzymatic digestion	Neuraminidase	Cleaves terminal sialic acid residues

Table 11-2. Lipid composition of the normal red cell membrane

Molar concentration (μmoles/10^{10} cells)	Lipids*	Concentration by weight (mg/10^{10} cells)
4.0	Phospholipids	(1.7-3.2)
1.2	Phosphatidylcholine	1.0
1.1	Phosphatidylethanolamine	0.9
1.0	Sphingomyelin	0.8
0.6	Phosphatidylserine	0.4
	Neutral lipids	
3.2	Cholesterol	(1.1-1.4)
7.4	TOTAL LIPIDS	(3.9-5.2)

*The lipid composition by molar concentration is shown to the left of zero, the concentration by weight to the right.

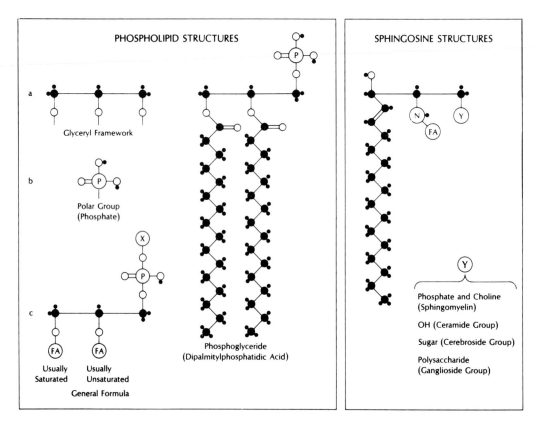

Fig. 11-3. Lipid structures of the red cell membrane. (From Chapman, D.: Hosp. Prac. **8**:79, 1973, and Weissmann, G., and Claiborne, R., eds.: Cell membranes: biochemistry, cell biology and pathology, New York, 1975, HP Publishing Co., Inc. Used with permission of HP Publishing Co., Inc.)

the third position is occupied by a phosphate. Various amine groups are attached to the latter, thereby altering the polarity of the molecules. Slight variations in bonding of the fatty acids and alternatives to the phosphate group such as mono- or polysaccharides give rise to similar structures called the sphingolipids (Fig. 11-3). De novo synthesis of fatty acids does not occur in the mature red cell, which lacks acetyl CoA carboxylase, but condensation and cleavage reactions with the phospholipid backbone may be carried out via acyltransferases and phospholipases.[44]

In model systems phospholipids may assume either a micellar or a lamellar configuration. The former arrangement consists of phospholipids with their hydrophobic chains directed toward the center of the micelles (hexagonal packing, type 1), but as they become more closely packed and fuse, their polar groups become oriented about aqueous channels (hexagonal packing, type 2).[50] Various environmental and compositional factors may influence these structural transitions, which may play a role in membrane permeability,[26] although membrane proteins are thought to be important as well.

At the secondary and tertiary levels of molecular structure, phospholipids are not fixed within the membrane but engage in a variety of motions as determined by electron spin resonance[22] and nuclear magnetic resonance[39] spectroscopy. The vibration or side-to-side "waggle" of the fatty acid chains (10^8 to 10^9/second)[28] and their lateral diffusion (1.8×10^{-8} cm^2/second at room temperature[8]) are relatively fast, whereas the inversion or "flip-flop" of the phospholipid from the inner to the outer aspect of the bilayer is rather slow (10^4 to 10^5 seconds).[36] In general the mobility of a phospholipid is directly proportional to its degree of unsaturation and inversely related to its chain length.[9]

The composition of lipids, unlike that of proteins, may be modified in the adult red cell by exchange with plasma (Fig. 11-4). Half of membrane cholesterol, which stabilizes the proximal part of the fatty acid chains, is replaced every 6 hours, whereas phospholipid turnover is more than ten times slower. Accumulation of membrane cholesterol may occur in hypercholesterolemic states or when its binding to low-density β-lipoproteins of the plasma is diminished. Decreased conversion of cholesterol to its plasma esters may also

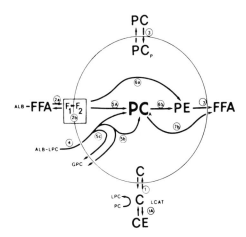

Fig. 11-4. Lipid exchange and conversion reactions in the mature red cell membrane. Pathways of lipid acquisition and turnover in the mature red cell membrane: *C,* cholesterol; *CE,* cholesterol ester; *PC,* phosphatidyl choline (lecithin); *LPC,* lysophosphatidyl choline; *PE,* phosphatidyl ethanolamine; *LPE,* lysophosphatidyl ethanolamine; *FFA,* free fatty acid; *Alb,* albumin; *GPC,* glycerylphosphoryl choline; *LCAT,* lecithin-cholesterol acyltransferase. Reactions and pathways: *1,* exchange of cholesterol with plasmic lipoprotein; *1a,* LCAT reaction; *2a,* transfer of FFA from albumin to membrane; *2b,* penetration of FFA to a metabolically active site; *3,* exchange of PC with plasma lipoprotein; *4,* transfer of LPC from albumin to membrane; *5a,* LPC + FFA → PC; *5b,* 2LPC → FFA + GPC; *5c,* LPC → FFA + GPC; *6a,* LPE + FFA → PE; *6b,* PC + LPE → LPC + PE; *7,* PE → LPE + FFA; *7b,* PC → LPC + FFA. (From Shohet, S. B.: N. Engl. J. Med. **286:**577, 1972. Reprinted by permission.)

result in its accretion. This situation arises when the enzyme lecithin-cholesterol acyltransferase (LCAT) is deficient or when its activity is inhibited by excess bile salts.[45]

Although seemingly passive in their behavior, lipids have important interactions with one another and with proteins. For example, at certain temperatures phospholipids convert from solid to liquid states and vice versa. Since this transition temperature is different for each molecular structure, a mixture of phospholipids has a temperature range over which the solid and fluid states coexist. The addition of cholesterol will broaden this range and stabilize the intermediate phase.[34] In their interaction with proteins the alkyl chains of fatty acids probably stabilize the hydrophobic sequences of proteins and protect them from binding to other molecules in the absence of a specific reaction. Furthermore, lipids may influence the lateral mobility of proteins[14] and their rotation within the plane of the membrane, as well as the extent of their projection perpendicular to the membrane surface.

Recent evidence indicates that phospholipids are not distributed uniformly over the membrane. *Cis*

asymmetry has been demonstrated by the partition of a spin marker into lipid patches.[42] *Trans* asymmetry is exhibited by the greater proportion of phosphatidylcholine (choline phosphoglyceride in the new international nomenclature) and sphingomyelin in the outer half of the bilayer. The more unsaturated phosphatidylethanolamine and phosphatidylserine (ethanolamine and serine phosphoglyceride, respectively) are located in greater quantity on the inner side,[19] are less accessible to phospholipases,[5] and exchange poorly with the medium.

As further evidence of membrane asymmetry, certain drugs bind to the external surface in preference to the internal surface of the membrane and cause red cell crenation[7]; they include anionic and strongly cationic amphipathic compounds (e.g., free fatty acids, barbiturates, and quaternary amines). Other drugs penetrate and cause membrane invagination; they consist of weakly cationic amphipathic drugs (e.g., procaine and other local anesthetics, chlorpromazine, quinidine, and other tertiary amines).[41] The effect of anesthetic agents on membrane expansion may involve proteins as well as lipids.[40]

Membrane carbohydrates

Carbohydrates are present in the membrane as glycoproteins or glycolipids. They are poorly understood because of the many possible permutations of polysaccharide bonding, but some data from partial hydrolysis and hemagglutination inhibition studies have been obtained.[52] Several generalizations about their structure can be made.[33] First, if the carbohydrate group is considered to resemble a tree, its "root" consists of specific sugars bound to certain amino acids or sphingosine (see outline below). Second, despite all the bonding positions available, each sugar in the chain can give rise to only two branches. Finally, separate polysaccharide chains are similar in sequence but present at different stages of completion. They are synthesized by glycosyltransferases within vesicles or located on cell surfaces.[46]

Basic principles of glycoprotein structure

1. Only five sugars may be bound to only five amino acids. (Those found in the red cell are italicized.)

Sugar	Bond	Amino acid
C_6: Glucose	?—S—O—	
Galactose	—C—O—	Hydroxylysine
Mannose		
Xylose	—C—O—	Serine
C_5: *Fucose*		
Arabinose	—C—O—	Hydroxyproline
NAc-D-glucosamine	—C—N—	Asparagine
-D-galactosamine	—C—O—	Serine or threonine
Neuraminic (sialic) acid		

2. Each sugar may give rise to only a single branch point for two polysaccharide chains.
3. Separate polysaccharide chains have an overlapping sequence of structures that are similar to each other but in different stages of completion.

The addition of carbohydrates to the membrane is an important modification. In the red cell it amplifies surface diversity and antigenicity. Residues such as sialic acid contribute to the negative charge, which keeps cells apart and helps to maintain membrane asymmetry. A similar phenomenon may occur to keep glycoproteins and glycolipids dispersed on the surface of the membrane by repulsive forces. The effect of covalently linked carbohydrates on ion transport is as yet unclear.

Membrane function

The primary importance of the cell membrane is to separate the milieu intérieur from the more random external environment. As a semipermeable barrier, it allows some substances to penetrate unhindered but regulates the passage of others. The former process is basically diffusion with two definable parameters, the rate and the equilibrium conditions. Factors such as molecular size, density of the medium, and temperature primarily influence the rate of diffusion, whereas osmotic forces affect mainly the equilibrium conditions. Concentration gradients, their alteration by intracellular reactions, and charge distribution play a role in determining both.

The active transport function of the membrane is characterized by specificity for a given substrate that is moved unidirectionally against a gradient.

The mechanism also exhibits the properties of saturation kinetics, specific inhibition (either competitive or noncompetitive), and energy dependence. Several methods have been used to study these phenomena. A common problem is to examine membrane integrity as reflected in its permeability to sodium and potassium. Rate or flux studies may be carried out by washing red cells free of the ion of interest and photometrically measuring its loss from the cells or its accumulation in the medium with time. Radioactive isotopes may also be used to quantitate how quickly given ions enter or leave cells.

The relationship of active transport to cellular metabolism was suggested by Harris,[21] who found that the potassium content of red cells was maintained by glucose and ATP and was dependent on temperature. Glynn[18] showed that for every 3 Na^+ ions expelled from the red cell, 2 K^+ ions were carried inward. This process consumed 1 molecule of ATP, and Skou[48] demonstrated that its hydrolysis was performed by an ATPase that required not only K^+ but also Na^+ and Mg^{++}. This was unusual because most K^+-dependent enzymes were thought to be inhibited by Na^+. Furthermore, the ATPase could be blocked by the addition of ouabain, which had been known to inhibit Na^+ and K^+ transport in intact cells.[37] Later it was shown using erythrocyte ghosts resealed with ATP and varying ionic concentrations that the consumption of ATP occurred only when the membranes were loaded with Na^+ and bathed in a medium containing K^+.[56] Under these circumstances ion transport took place to shift Na^+ out of the ghosts and K^+ into them.

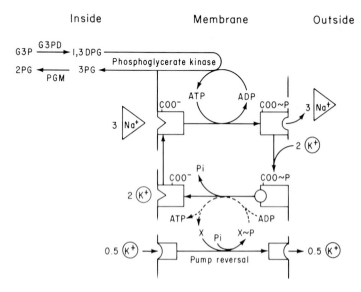

Fig. 11-5. Mechanism for cation transport operating via Na^+-K^+ ATPase and sustained by glycolytic generation of ATP. (See text.)

Furthermore, ATP added externally was not metabolized, and if the internal or external media contained only Na^+ or K^+, little ATP was consumed, showing that both ions were linked in the process. Further studies of the reaction have shown that in the presence of Na^+ and Mg^{++} the γ-^{32}P label from radioactive ATP is transferred to the enzyme, but when K^+ is added the $^{32}P_i$ is cleaved.[6,32] Additional evidence cited in three reviews indicates that reversal of the pump mechanism such as in Na^+-Na^+ or K^+-K^+ exchange may result in net synthesis of ATP,[10,31,38] and thus also supports the coupling of this substrate to transport. A recent report suggests that an enzyme complex of phosphoglycerate kinase (PGK), glyceraldehyde-3-phosphate dehydrogenase (G-3-PD), and phosphoglycerate mutase (PGM) may serve as the metabolic link to transport.[13] The entire sequence of events is diagrammed in Fig. 11-5.

The brain and kidney have the most active ATPase; the activity in red cells is several thousand times less. It has been estimated that the human erythrocyte contains only 250 sites inhibitable by ouabain, which account for more than 70% of the cationic flux. A minor component sensitive to ethacrynic acid may be responsible for the remainder under certain conditions (Table 11-3). Other ATPases, including one dependent on calcium,[23] have also been identified, but their characteristics may vary under different conditions.[1]

There is another form of transport, often referred to as facilitated diffusion, which is passively mediated. This mechanism operates to transport substances against a gradient by sharing a common carrier with another substrate whose flux does not require energy. For example, in this manner the movement of Na^+ down a gradient into the cell is accompanied pari passu by the facilitated diffusion of glucose to allow its concentration against a gradient. This system of cotransport also may hold for certain amino acids. The means by which

reactive species such as oxygen can freely diffuse through the membrane remains enigmatic.

Correlation of membrane function with structure has been difficult because the methods generally used to isolate and identify membrane components may interfere with their activity. Furthermore, the experimental conditions are extremely important and may explain differences between laboratories.[1] Since phosphorylation is an important step for the major Na^+-K^+ ATPase described above, incubation of red cells with γ-AT^{32}P results in the incorporation of radioactivity into membrane bands 2 and 3. This corresponds with a total molecular weight of 250,000 for the complex (band 2), consisting of two large 100,000-dalton subunits (band 3) and one small 50,000-dalton subunit, which is not labeled. The rate of turnover can be obtained from data on incorporation and depletion of radioactivity if the latter studies are carried out after inhibiting glycolysis.[17]

Compounds that simultaneously block and label membrane pores may be used to identify the anion channel (e.g., fluorodinitrobenzene, sulfonates, and sulfanilates) and the glucose transport protein (cytochalasin B, glucosyl isothiocyanate, dextran, or glutathione maleimide) which are found in band 3. Although it is important to be careful that these proteins are not nonspecifically labeled, the result is not surprising since band 3 consists of a group of transmembrane proteins. Most recent attempts to correlate structure with function involve incorporation of membrane components into liposomes. Such techniques will permit the study of isolated processes followed by analysis of the molecules responsible for performing them.

Cell deformability

Since active transport and metabolism are interdependent, they share a common goal: the maintenance of cellular deformability so that erythrocytes may pass through the microvasculature and

Table 11-3. Cation transport systems in the red cell membrane*

	Pump I	Pump Ia	Pump II	
			Na-Na exchange	K-K exchange
Cation requirements				
Internal medium	Na^+, Mg^{++}		Mg^{++}?	K^+
External medium	K^+	Na^+	Na^+	
Energy source	ATP	ATP		ATP
Inhibitors	Ouabain, Ca^{++}, oligomycin	Ouabain	Ethacrynic acid, external K^+	Ouabain
Percent total net flux	50-70	20-30		

*Normal ion content of red cells: Na, 5-12 mEq/liter of cells, or 7-17 mEq/liter of cell water (red cells contain 69% to 72% water); K, 90-103 mEq/liter of cells, or 128-147 mEq/liter of cell water.[136]

the interstices of the spleen without destruction. It has been shown that as aging and defective cells become depleted of ATP, they swell into a spherical shape.[29] They also gain sodium, lose potassium, and accumulate calcium in their membranes, making them rigid (Gardos effect).[16] Although the spectrin-actin lattice (complexes of bands 1, 2, and 5) is hypothesized to be responsible for membrane shape, it binds only some of the calcium. The bulk of the cation is bound by other components,[30] other proteins, or perhaps lipids with calcium "soap" formation.

The physical property of cellular deformability has been measured in several ways:

1. *Whole cell:* passage through 3 μ polycarbonate filters[20] or 3 to 12 μ capillaries[54]
2. *Whole membrane:* elasticity tested with 0.8 μ pipette[24]
3. *Internal fluidity or microviscosity:* spin label movements[22] or rotation of fluorescent probe[43]

Membrane failure

Membrane failure may result from defects that are either inherited or acquired. In the first category hemolysis may be secondary to an enzyme deficiency or a hemoglobinopathy (Chapters 12 and 13) or primarily as a result of an abnormal membrane component alone. Even though this latter condition has a genetic basis, it has not been possible to establish definitively whether a mutant molecule or its structural absence is the cause in many cases. Examples of intrinsic membrane defects are hereditary spherocytosis, elliptocytosis, stomatocytosis, Rh$_{null}$ red cells,[25] and those bearing the McLeod phenotype.[57]

Acquired membrane damage may be brought about by physical or chemical agents. In either case the insult may be severe enough to cause direct intravascular hemolysis or milder, resulting in removal of the erythrocyte by the reticuloendothelial system. Physical processes frequently produce cell fragmentation into small triangular schistocytes, helmet-shaped cells, and microspherocytes. Major causes are microangiopathy, trauma, and burns (Chapter 14).

Chemical agents such as drugs or toxins may cause extensive damage to the red cell membrane, again either indirectly through effects on hemoglobin or metabolism or by direct attack on the membrane. Oxidants, typified by certain drugs and peroxides; heavy metals, including lead and copper; and proteases and phospholipases *(Clostridium welchii)* are examples. Other biologically active molecules such as antibodies and complement are capable of causing cell lysis (Chapter 10). In some cases of dyserythropoiesis, such as paroxysmal nocturnal hemoglobinuria, there may be an intrinsic membrane defect as well.

MEMBRANE PATHOLOGY—INHERITED DEFECTS
Hereditary spherocytosis

Definition and history. Hereditary spherocytosis is a condition of abnormal red cell morphology seen microscopically as erythrocytes that have lost the central pallor characteristic of the biconcave disc shape. The cells are instead rounder, more fragile, and susceptible to extravascular hemolysis in the spleen. As a result patients with this disorder suffer from variable degrees of anemia, splenomegaly, and acholuric jaundice.

The closest description of this syndrome was first provided in 1871 by Vanlair and Masius,[109] who published drawings of the cells as microspherocytes and "globules atrophiques" headed for destruction. Subsequent observers such as Wilson and Stanley[112] and Minkowski[95] completed the picture by describing familial and congenital forms of this hemolytic anemia with jaundice. Chauffard[64] demonstrated increased osmotic fragility of the red cells, and Dacie and Mollison[71] showed that transfused hereditary spherocytosis cells survived only 14 days in a healthy recipient. According to Dacie's review of the history and clinical picture of hereditary spherocytosis,[70] the first splenectomy that cured this condition was performed unwittingly in 1887 for removal of an abdominal "tumor." By 1922 this had become accepted therapy. Since then excellent clinical studies have been performed by Race,[100] Young,[113] and others, and the membrane defect has been the subject of intense investigation.

Prevalence and genetics. Hereditary spherocytosis is a common cause of hemolytic anemia among whites of Northern European descent. In the United States the incidence is about 1 in 5,000[97] and has been diagnosed at all ages, from 30 hours[62,104] to 77 years. It has been found infrequently in blacks[96] and members of other racial groups.

The pattern of inheritance is autosomal dominant,[113] with 50% of siblings and offspring of the propositus being affected regardless of sex. However, sporadic instances have been reported in which neither parent was affected; this occurs in approximately 10% to 15% of all cases of hereditary spherocytosis. In one family homozygosity for the trait was proposed for all thirteen children, nine of whom were physically and mentally retarded, but the parents' putative genotype was unclear.[61]

Clinical picture. Although this chronic hemolytic anemia is congenital, the symptoms may be quite variable, depending on the severity of the defect and the degree of compensation. In some patients the membrane abnormality is readily detected by the spleen and results in marked hemolysis and splenomegaly. Unconjugated hyperbilirubinemia is produced, the level depending on the efficiency of conjugation by the liver. Because of both red cell fragility and hepatic enzyme immaturity, hereditary spherocytosis may cause significant neonatal jaundice and kernicterus. Suspicion of hereditary spherocytosis should be raised if jaundice occurs within 24 hours after birth, is over 12 mg/dl in term infants or 15 mg/dl in premature babies, and persists beyond the first week of life. Examination of the parents' smears should assist in the diagnosis, although concurrent sepsis and ABO hemolytic disease may confuse the picture.[107] In older children and adults chronic hemolysis often results in calcium bilirubinate cholelithiasis and cholecystitis.[76] Poor growth may be a consequence of persistent anemia.

Compensatory erythropoiesis by the bone marrow may result in expansion of the medullary cavities or the development of ectopic hematogenous masses.[67] On occasion, however, an acute aplastic crisis may occur, manifested by the lack of formed elements in the marrow, peripheral reticulocytopenia, leukopenia, and thrombocytopenia.[72,98] Although the cause of the aplasia is often unknown, a deficiency of folic acid necessary for DNA synthesis may be responsible in some cases.[87] Particularly during pregnancy, the requirements for this vitamin and the incidence of this complication are increased.[89] Hemolytic crises may also occur, sometimes associated with splenomegaly caused by infections.[88] However, it may be

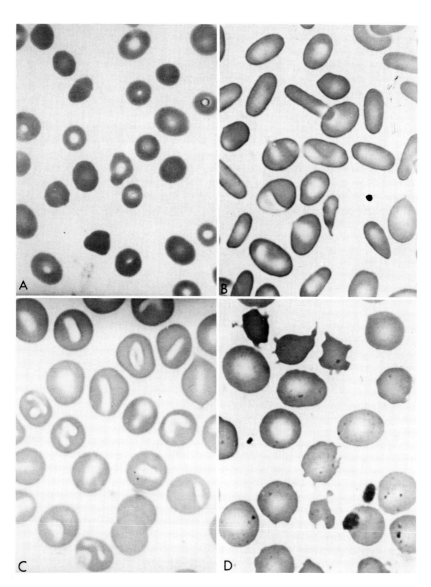

Fig. 11-6. Peripheral smears of patients with hemolytic anemias. **A,** Hereditary spherocytosis. **B,** Hereditary elliptocytosis. **C,** Hereditary stomatocytosis. **D,** Acanthocytosis. (From Miller, D. R.: Pediatr. Clin. North Am. **19:**865, 1972.)

hard to establish if the microbial agent first damages the red cells, which are then sequestered, or whether hypersplenism results from merely a response to inflammation. Other symptoms referable to leg ulcers,[105] epistaxis, hemochromatosis,[59] endocrine dysfunction,[74] neurologic problems,[69] acute renal failure secondary to hemolytic crisis,[80] and congenital anomalies[83] have been reported.

Laboratory manifestations. The cardinal feature of this disorder is the presence of numerous spherocytes on the peripheral smear. These are small, round erythrocytes that lack central pallor (Plate 3, *B,* and Fig. 11-6, *A*). Whereas the average size of these red cells may vary with the degree of reticulocytosis and folate depletion (MCV of 83 ± 8.5 fl in one series[94]), the MCHC is generally high (>35 gm/dl). The hemoglobin level is usually between 8 and 13 gm/dl but may be as low as 6 gm/dl. The reticulocyte count averages about 10%[93] but ranges from 2% to over 90%.[60] The bone marrow shows erythroid hyperplasia unless there is an aplastic crisis.

The other classical feature of this disease is an increase in osmotic fragility.[73] This phenomenon reflects the decreased surface:volume ratio of the cells. When red cells are placed in progressively hypotonic solutions of saline, they begin swelling (to macrospherocytes) until their surface area:volume ratio decreases further and they rupture. This is called the critical hemolytic volume. At a sodium chloride concentration of 0.45 gm/dl (half normal), about 50% of the hemoglobin has leaked from fresh normal erythrocytes. This point is reached earlier, at 0.6 gm/dl, for the metabolically stressed cell after a 24-hour incubation. In classical hereditary spherocytosis, however, a significantly greater proportion of cells hemolyze at either point, before or after an incubation that accentuates the defect. Under some circumstances the presence of only 1% to 2% spherocytes will generate an osmotically fragile "tail" on the hemolysis curve (Fig. 11-7, *B*). The glycerol lysis time is also shorter than normal for incubated cells.[79]

The autohemolysis test reveals spontaneous cell breakdown after incubation for 48 hours at 37° C. The normal value is less than 4% without additives or less than 0.6% with glucose. In hereditary spherocytosis the cells become metabolically depleted rather quickly with 10% to 50% hemolysis, but correction takes place with the addition of glucose.[102]

Mechanical fragility of the cells is also present. Serum haptoglobin and hemopexin are decreased, and the serum unconjugated (nonglucuronide) bilirubin is variably elevated. Paradoxically the red cell content of 2,3-DPG is low before splenectomy, perhaps as a result of the increased breakdown of this intermediate in the acid environment of the spleen.[99] However, the $P_{50}O_2$ in patients with compensated hemolysis is normal,[75] which suggests that tissue hypoxia is not overt in these patients.

Etiology and pathogenesis. The nature of the corpuscular defect in hereditary spherocytosis is not known. That it is an inherent erythrocyte abnormality is shown by cross-transfusion experiments in which hereditary spherocytosis cells survive poorly in normal recipients but normal cells

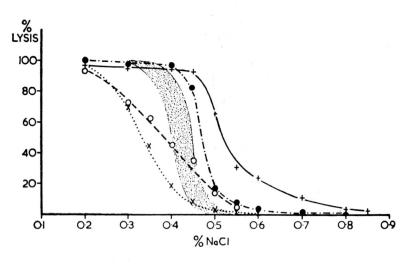

Fig. 11-7. Erythrocyte osmotic fragility. Curves of patients suffering from, **A,** sickle-cell disease (x. . . . . .x); **B,** thalassemia major (o------o); **C,** hereditary spherocytosis (•·····•); and **D,** idiopathic acquired hemolytic anemia (warm autoantibody) (+——+). The shaded area represents the normal range. (From Dacie, J. V.: The haemolytic anemias, congenital, and acquired. Part 1: the congenital anaemias, ed. 2, Edinburgh, 1960, Churchill Livingstone.)

survive well in hereditary spherocytosis patients.[71] No mutant hemoglobin is found, and glycolytic metabolism is normal[91] or even slightly overactive,[85] thus leaving the membrane as the probable cause.

The osmotically fragile membrane allows greater influx of Na^+ than normal,[85] and increased glycolytic generation of ATP is necessary to stimulate the compensatory mechanism for active extrusion of this ion. This is why autohemolysis is decreased after incubation of hereditary spherocytosis cells with glucose. Conversely stagnation of spherocytes in the spleen results in the depletion of nutrients from the environment and causes their destruction. Phospholipases are also present in the spleen,[77] and they may digest phospholipids that could play a role in transport.[84] The total lipid content of hereditary spherocytosis cells is lower than normal, even after splenectomy,[66] and turnover of all lipid classes is uniformly increased.[101] Two processes may be responsible: (1) consumption of lipid by increased metabolic activity in response to the permeability defect and (2) lipolytic attack, which aggravates this defect. Which factor is more important is uncertain; however, it is known that even though the Na^+ leak persists after splenectomy, the cells survive more normally.[111]

An increase in the membrane surface area of hereditary spherocytosis cells can be achieved by incubation in lipid-rich media, and their life span is prolonged when they are transfused into patients with obstructive jaundice.[65] However, in another study in which subjects were phlebotomized to make their erythrocytes hypochromic and flat, no improvement was seen.[68] The latter report involved patients with better red cell survival values in whom an uncorrectable residual defect may exist. Precursor cells in the bone marrow of patients with hereditary spherocytosis appear to be quite normal[90] but begin their transformation into spherocytes as they mature and enter the peripheral blood. Many of the cells are not truly round but may be stomatocytic in appearance.[110] This change may precede transformation into true spherocytes under certain conditions in vitro and may be part of the pathogenic mechanism.

Membrane proteins have been investigated extensively for the cause of the defect of hereditary spherocytosis. Deficiency of a particular species has been reported by some[78] but unconfirmed by others, probably because of the low resolving power of the techniques currently available. A more likely possibility is the presence of a mutant membrane component that resembles the normal molecule enough to competitively interfere with its function or that creates pathologic aggregates of other membrane proteins. In addition to the spectrins and actin, microfilamentous proteins are thought to be important in red cell structure, and defective microfilament formation has been observed.[86] Similarly, since protein kinase–mediated phosphorylation may affect the state and function of membrane proteins, it too has been examined and found to be diminished.[82] The basis for these abnormalities, however, is uncertain.[108]

Hereditary spherocytosis has also been described in the deer mouse[58] and the WBBF strain of mice. The latter's red cells are quantitatively deficient in spectrin.[81]

Differential diagnosis. Spherocytes are also found in other common states, such as dyserythropoiesis and various hemolytic anemias with hypersplenism. They may also be produced under severe toxic or oxidant stress of normal or G-6-PD-deficient red cells; however, they are not found in fresh blood in any significant proportion (>10%) except in patients with burns, hereditary spherocytosis, or immunohemolytic anemia. In immunohemolytic anemia negative family studies and a positive Coombs test should be diagnostic. Microspherocytes may also be seen in *Clostridium perfringens* sepsis,[133] severe hypophosphatemia,[84a] and hereditary pyropoikilocytosis.[145a,b]

Atypical cases may have only occasional spherocytes (<1% to 2%) on smear, questionably abnormal osmotic fragility before or after incubation, or autohemolysis that is not corrected by glucose. In the latter situation a more typical test result may be obtained after splenectomy.[114] Because of the variable expressivity in these cases, family studies should be pursued vigorously. However, if all investigations for hereditary spherocytosis prove to be negative, the diagnosis cannot be made with absolute certainty and the possibility of other occult causes of hemolysis should still be entertained.

Therapy. Transfusions should be given for hypoplastic crises and during the first year or two of life if the hemolytic anemia is not well compensated. Splenectomy is the treatment of choice because it generally prolongs red cell survival to almost 80% of normal.[63] The jaundice generally disappears within a few days; the anemia may take a few weeks to resolve depending on the initial hematocrit. The reticulocyte count decreases, but the spherocytes persist, with an abnormal osmotic fragility.[106] Leg ulcers may heal postoperatively.[105]

Because of the increased rate of infection in infants, splenectomy should be postponed until at least 5 years of age,[103] although some investigators have recommended earlier surgery.[62] This decision depends on the symptoms of the individual, but any further delay may interfere with the growth of the child. Even in the minimally symptomatic patient, gallstones are increasingly common after 10 years,[76] and the unpredictability of hemolytic and aplastic crises makes splenectomy almost mandatory. Folic acid should be administered until this operation is performed.

The complications of splenectomy—leukocytosis, thrombocytosis, and severe sepsis—are discussed in Chapter 21. Prophylactic maintenance penicillin should be given. Pneumococcal vaccine is also indicated but additional studies are necessary to determine whether polyvalent vaccine can replace penicillin.

Course and prognosis. As mentioned previously, the symptoms of this condition may be quite variable. In many cases chronic anemia affects the health of the child but can be compatible with long life.[100] Before splenectomy severe exacerbations may occur, resulting in death by cardiac failure or crisis. After surgery infection is also potentially life threatening, and the rare recurrence of hemolysis because of the presence of an accessory spleen has been reported.[92]

Hereditary elliptocytosis

Definition and history. Hereditary elliptocytosis is another genetically transmitted morphologic abnormality of the red cell in which more than 15% (usually 50% to 90%) of the erythrocytes are oval in shape.[117,125] This condition was first described by Dresbach[119] in 1904. Subsequently his observations were elaborated on by others, who divided the cases into three categories: those with no hemolysis, those with compensated hemolysis, and those with uncompensated hemolysis.

Prevalence and genetics. Hereditary elliptocytosis occurs in about 0.04% of the general population[117] and in all races.[123,128] It is transmitted as an autosomal dominant trait. Homozygosity has been proposed to be responsible for severe hemolysis in certain patients.[125] In some cases linkage with the Rh group exists; this is associated with the milder hemolytic states.[122]

Clinical picture. Unlike patients with hereditary spherocytosis, most individuals with hereditary elliptocytosis are asymptomatic. In about 12% there is evidence of increased hemolysis,[127] and these patients have clinical manifestations similar to those of hereditary spherocytosis. Anemia may or may not be present, depending on the degree of bone marrow compensation. Sporadic hemolytic episodes may occur in more than half of the patients[124]; an additional number probably go undetected. Severe anemia may occur rarely in infancy.[125]

Hereditary elliptocytosis has been found in association with G-6-PD deficiency,[128] glyoxalase II deficiency,[132] Hb S, Hb C,[134] thalassemia,[115] and hereditary hemorrhagic telangiectasia[127]; however, no cause-and-effect relationship between these conditions and hereditary elliptocytosis has been

worked out. Autoimmune hemolytic anemia and paroxysmal nocturnal hemoglobinuria have also been reported.[70]

Laboratory manifestations. The presence of a large proportion of elliptocytes (>15%)[121] in the peripheral blood is essentially pathognomonic (Plate 3, *C,* and Fig. 11-6, *B*). The cells are slightly smaller than normal and are on the average 1.5 times longer than they are wide.[125] However, the MCV can range from 50 fl to normal and the shape may be extremely elongated. Despite the wide range of variation from patient to patient, no morphologic differences can be seen between elliptocytes that have a normal life span and those that undergo accelerated destruction.[70] In infants the condition may first be recognized as pyknocytosis[116]; gradually the percentage of elliptocytes increases until about 3 to 4 months of age and then stabilizes.

The laboratory findings in hereditary elliptocytosis parallel the clinical symptoms: in the majority of patients, hemolysis is mild, with a hemoglobin value of greater than 12 gm/dl, reticulocyte count less than 4%, and approximately normal red cell survival. In about 10% to 15% of the patients hemolysis is severe, with a hemoglobin level ranging from 9 to 12 gm/dl, a reticulocyte count up to 20%, and an average red cell life span as short as 5 days.[131] In the severe cases the osmotic fragility of the red cells before and after incubation and autohemolysis without glucose or ATP is abnormal, but in patients without hemolysis these test results are usually normal.

Etiology and pathogenesis. That the primary defect is based in the membrane is again suggested by the lack of any abnormality found in hemoglobin or glycolytic enzymes.[118] As in hereditary spherocytosis, the oval shape is not present in nucleated erythroblasts, but becomes apparent in reticulocytes and is well established in mature red cells.[121,130] Even ghosts resulting from hypotonic lysis maintain their elliptical shape.[129] Incubation in various media or normal plasma has little effect on morphology.[130] This fact plus the mode of inheritance suggest that a membrane protein rather than a lipid is responsible, although cholesterol can be shown to be concentrated toward the poles of the cell.[126]

Hereditary elliptocytosis may be milder than hereditary spherocytosis in many cases because the elongated HE cell may not be trapped and stagnate in the spleen as easily or because the permeability defect and its metabolic demand are not as severe. Blood samples incubated in vitro show increased sodium flux and ATP depletion, but these studies correlate poorly with the degree of hemolysis.[133]

Elliptocytes are also found in camels and llamas. The red cells of the former have decreased osmotic fragility as compared to human corpuscles, which is thought to be a result of the higher protein: lipid ratio of these cells.[120] Avian erythrocytes are also elliptical but they are nucleated.

Differential diagnosis. Elliptocytes are present in a proportion of 1% to 15% in normal blood.[121] They may be increased in macrocytic (megaloblastic), microcytic, and myelophthisic anemias, hemoglobinopathies (especially thalassemia), and red cell enzyme deficiencies, but their numbers are not so striking as in hereditary elliptocytosis. Other morphologic features, e.g., of nutritional problems, may be superimposed on the basic red cell defect, and a mild degree of shape change may obscure the classical picture. In these cases family studies should be enlightening in distinguishing the patient with true hereditary elliptocytosis.

Therapy. If hemolysis is present, transfusion is palliative and splenectomy generally curative. As in hereditary spherocytosis, symptoms are relieved even though the erythrocyte abnormality persists.

Course and prognosis. Asymptomatic individuals are able to live a normal life span. Patients who respond to splenectomy also survive normally if the complications of the operation are avoided.

Hereditary stomatocytosis

Definition and history. Hereditary stomatocytosis is another disorder of red cell morphology in which the central pallor of the biconcave disc appears like an elongated slit resembling a mouth (hence the name) (Plate 3, *D,* and Fig. 11-6, *C*). The cells have also been described as uniconcave or cup shaped (Fig. 11-8). The hereditary form of this condition was first described in recent times by Lock et al.,[139] who studied two patients with increased osmotic fragility but poor response to splenectomy. Since then several other syndromes with stomatocytosis have been described.*

Prevalence and genetics. The incidence of the hereditary form of stomatocytosis is not known. Several types of red cell defect may produce this alteration in cells with or without hemolysis. Some families show an autosomal dominant pattern of transmission, but it is not known in severe cases whether another gene might be contributing to the membrane abnormality.

Clinical picture. Symptoms in this condition may be extremely variable, depending on pathogenesis. Patients with hemolysis from the hereditary defect have clinical problems similar to those in hereditary spherocytosis.

Laboratory manifestations. The peripheral blood smear is characteristic, generally with 10% to 50% stomatocytes. Anemia with unconjugated

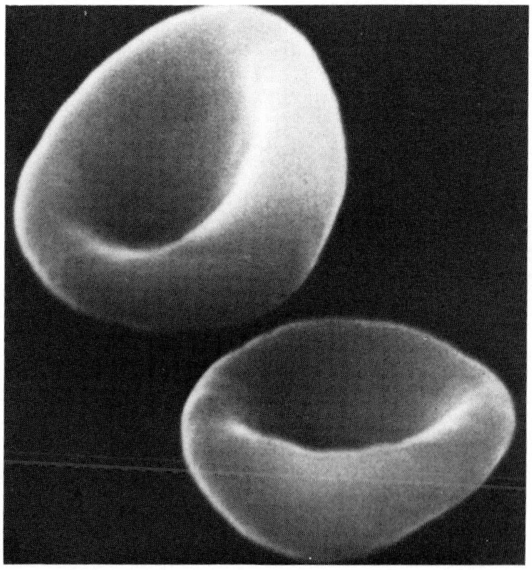

Fig. 11-8. Scanning electron micrograph of stomatocyte. (Courtesy Dr. Marcel Bessis.)

hyperbilirubinemia and reticulocytosis may be present in the severe cases. The osmotic fragility may be increased, normal, or decreased. Increased cation permeability to sodium and low intracellular potassium levels may be observed, accompanied by increased glucose consumption. Low levels of reduced glutathione have also been found.[141] In some cases, however, these values may be normal, perhaps partly as a result of cell populations of different ages in different patients. The reported findings are tabulated in Table 11-5.

Etiology and pathogenesis. From the variable clinical syndrome and laboratory studies it appears likely that several types of defect may cause stomatocytosis. Again, negative studies on hemoglobin and red cell metabolism suggest that the abnormality lies within the membrane. Since normal red cells can be made stomatocytic by the preferential binding of certain drugs to the inner aspect of the membrane, it is possible that a mutant gene product could do the same. Whereas the sodium influx in this disorder is accompanied by water to produce "hydrocytosis," another condition has been described in which potassium efflux was predominant and resulted in cellular dehydration or "xerocytosis."[136] It is uncertain whether the cation leak also includes an increased permeability to calcium, which could then accumulate and permanently deform the membrane. Stomatocytosis is also found in the dwarfed Alaskan malamute,[144] which may serve as an animal model for this disorder.

Differential diagnosis. The hereditary conditions should be distinguished from the acquired forms by the greater number of stomatocytes and

---

*References 135, 137, 138, 140-143, 145.

Table 11-5. Distinguishing characteristics of various syndromes of hereditary hemolytic anemia

Authors	Patients	Stomato-cytosis (%)	Reticulo-cytosis (%)	Osmotic fragility	Autohemolysis	Erythrocyte cation content (mM/liter RBCs)	Cation flux (Na:K)*	Other features
Lock et al.	2	10-30	12-33	Increased	Type I	—	—	G-6-PD deficiency; splenic sequestration in isologous study; stomatocytes in top layer
Miller et al.	1	"Many"	3-10	Increased	Type I; increased at 4° C	—	—	Decreased reduced glutathione; Polish
Zarkowsky et al.	1	"Numerous"	10-40	Increased	Increased; no change with glucose, ATP	Na, 91-108; K, 35-47	3:2	Increased cell water; normal enzymes, lipids, pore size; increased glycolysis; Hungarian
Oski et al.	3	1.8-19.7	1.2-1.8	Increased	Type I; normal at 4° C	Na, 39-53; K, 73-86	3:1	Early splenic, late hepatic sequestration; old cells (stomatocytes) at top; ATPase kinetics normal; German
Ducrou and Kimber	15	10-49	4-13	Normal	—	"Normal"	—	Splenomegaly, abdominal pain, splenic sequestration; Italian and Greek
Lo et al.	2	24-30	5-33	Increased	Increased; no change with glucose	Na, 65; K, 39	—	Decreased reduced glutathione; Swiss (?)
Meadow	1	30-40	11-34	Increased	Increased; type I	—	—	Jaundice, splenomegaly, psoriasis, ventricular septal defect
Miller et al.	3	16-35	11-35	Decreased	Increased; corr. with glucose, adenosine, inosine; normal at 4° C	Na, 20-21.5; K, 85-87	26:1	No specific sequestration; increased glycolysis, normal lipids, membrane protein; autosomal dominant; Swiss-German
Honig	7	—	0.2-0.9	Decreased	Type I	Na, normal; K, decreased	1:1	Red cell survival normal; Filipino

*Na, sodium efflux; K, potassium influx.

appropriate family studies. The morphologic abnormality may be seen in thalassemia trait, lead poisoning, hereditary spherocytosis, infectious mononucleosis, malignancies, glutathione peroxidase deficiency, glucose phosphate isomerase deficiency,[137a] liver disease, and Rh$_{null}$ red cells.[25] Various drugs including alcohol, chlorpromazine, and quinidine may also produce the defect.[7]

Therapy. In patients with moderate to severe hemolysis, transfusions are palliative. Splenectomy may be of benefit in some cases but only partially curative in others,[139,145] suggesting that hemolysis may occur in extrasplenic sites.

Course and prognosis. Asymptomatic individuals and patients responding to splenectomy lead normal lives. Those who continue to hemolyze suffer from symptoms of chronic anemia: fatigue, poor growth, jaundice, gallstones, and bone marrow expansion.

Hereditary pyropoikilocytosis

Definition and history. Hereditary pyropoikilocytosis is a congenital hemolytic anemia characterized by an abnormal susceptibility of the red cells to lysis by heat in vitro. It was described in three children by Zarkowsky et al.[145b] in 1975 and in three more by Walter et al.[145a] in 1977.

Clinical and laboratory manifestations. Pyropoikilocytosis is a rare disorder, probably autosomal recessive in inheritance. It is characterized by a moderate hemolytic anemia with splenomegaly, unconjugated hyperbilirubinemia, and occasionally obstructive jaundice. The hemoglobin level ranges from 7 to 9 gm/dl, with reticulocytosis and microspherocytes seen on the peripheral smear. The MCHC is high. The osmotic fragility and autohemolysis are increased.

Etiology and pathogenesis. That this is a membrane defect is suggested by the increased fragmentation of the red cells at 45° C, whereas normal erythrocytes vesiculate at 49° C. Also there is an increased ratio of cholesterol to phospholipid or membrane protein; cell deformability is decreased. Spectrin is also difficult to extract from these membranes.

Differential diagnosis. This condition may be distinguished from hereditary spherocytosis by the inheritance pattern, temperature sensitivity, decreased red cell deformability, and spectrin inextractibility. The thermal behavior of elliptocytes, however, may be similar. The microcytosis of thalassemia trait may be distinguished by the MCHC and osmotic resistance. Pyruvate kinase deficiency can also result in variations in cell size and shape and should be diagnosed by enzyme assay.

Course and prognosis. The patients reported have responded well to splenectomy with a rise in hemoglobin to about 12 gm/dl.

MEMBRANE PATHOLOGY—ACQUIRED DEFECTS
Acanthocytosis and spur cell anemia

Definitions and history. Acanthocytosis is a condition in which many spherical, irregularly spiculated red cells are present in the blood (Plate 3, *I*, and Figs. 11-6, *D*, and 11-9, *A*). It was first described by Bassen and Kornzweig[146] in a patient with atypical retinitis pigmentosa caused by a-β-lipoproteinemia. Subsequently morphologically

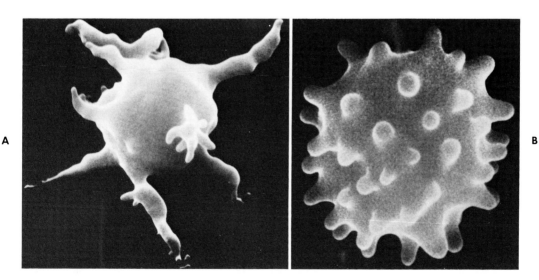

Fig. 11-9. Scanning electron micrograph of, **A,** acanthocyte and, **B,** echinocyte. (Courtesy Dr. Marcel Bessis.)

identical cells were seen in acquired cases of severe liver disease and also attributed to a lipid abnormality. These erythrocytes have been given a separate name and are called spur cells.[159,161]

Prevalence and genetics. As an inherited condition acanthocytosis is rare and usually found in association with the primary disorder of a-β-lipoproteinemia, which has an autosomal recessive mode of transmission. Several variants have been described in which the β-lipoproteins were not absent but low or normal in the presence of clinical symptoms and altered blood morphology. These cases may represent β-lipoprotein mutants.[152]

Clinical picture. In a-β-lipoproteinemia anemia is absent or mild, despite the large number of deformed cells. However, other symptoms of a lipid abnormality are evident. There is retarded growth; progressive ataxia involving the posterior columns, cerebellar pathways, and pyramidal tracts; retinitis pigmentosa with macular atrophy[157]; and steatorrhea without vitamin B_{12} malabsorption. Death generally occurs at an early age.[155]

In contrast, patients who have acquired the spur cell defect as a consequence of severe hepatic disease may have significant hemolysis and splenomegaly. In this setting additional factors such as dyserythropoiesis and poor nutrition may contribute to accelerated red cell destruction.

Acanthocytes or spur cells may be seen after splenectomy, in vitamin E deficiency, and in pyruvate kinase (PK) deficiency.[158]

Laboratory manifestations. Acanthocytes and spur cells possess about five to ten irregularly distributed spicules per cell. In recent years they have been distinguished from echinocytes or burr cells, which are crenated and have ten to thirty regularly spaced projections per cell (Fig. 11-9, *B*). The presence of acanthocytosis generally is not associated with marked shortening of the red cell life span, although hemolysis tends to be intermittent. Osmotic fragility, cation permeability,[153] and glycolysis[160] are usually normal, but autohemolysis is increased. Transfused cells acquire the acanthocytic shape, but reversion to normal morphology is incomplete.[149] In a-β-lipoproteinemia serum phospholipid, cholesterol, and triglyceride levels are low, secondary to a deficiency of low-density lipoproteins demonstrable by lipoprotein electrophoresis. Small intestinal biopsy reveals a picture compatible with inadequate fat absorption; lipid droplets of predominantly triglyceride are present within the mucosal cells but not in the intercellular spaces or lacteals.[154] In contrast, when spur cells are present hemolysis is moderate to marked and is accompanied by hyperbilirubinemia, elevated liver function tests, and high serum cholesterol levels.

Etiology and pathogenesis. In a-β-lipoproteinemia the molecular mechanism for transport of long-chain fatty acids from the intestine or for mobilization of triglyceride from the liver is defective. In addition, less phospholipid is available in the plasma for exchange with red cells, hence the low content of lecithin (phosphatidylcholine) in acanthocytes. The membrane sphingomyelin level, however, is elevated and the cholesterol level is high or normal.[148,162] Cases of acanthocytosis without plasma or red cell lipid abnormalities have been reported.[151]

Spur cells differ in that cholesterol is increased by 25% to 65% in the membrane but the phospholipid level is normal. This condition may result from an impairment of the esterifying serum enzyme LCAT, which is inhibited by excess bile salts accumulated in the plasma in liver disease.[147] The activity of this enzyme is also decreased in a-β-lipoproteinemia, but the significance of this finding is uncertain.[148] Perhaps the common denominator in the generation of acanthocytes and spur cells is the disproportionate excess of membrane cholesterol relative to phospholipid, whereas in target cells there is a balanced increase in these components. The spleen may also play a role in the loss of surface area from spur cells.[150]

Differential diagnosis. As mentioned previously, acanthocytes should be distinguished from crenated echinocytes, which are found in uremia, ulcer disease, carcinoma, and concurrent PK deficiency.[133] In this regard scanning electron microscopy may be helpful.[156] Membrane lipid composition tends to reflect that of the plasma and analysis of either should be revealing. Acanthocytes are also found in the hemolytic anemia associated with the McLeod phenotype in which the red cells of male patients lack the K_x (Kell) antigen.[57]

Therapy. There is no specific therapy for a-β-lipoproteinemia. Vitamin E deficiency may result from gastrointestinal malabsorption and replacement therapy should be given. In spur cell anemia, transfused cells may acquire the defect and hemolyze, so treatment of the underlying liver disease is essential.

Course and prognosis. Patients with a-β-lipoproteinemia generally die at a young age from neurologic sequelae. Those with spur cell anemia usually die of progressive hepatic decompensation within a few months.

Vitamin E deficiency

Definition and history. Hemolytic anemia may occur in vitamin E deficiency. In humans the fragility of erythrocytes was first demonstrated on incubation of the red cells with dilute solutions of hydrogen peroxide by Gordon and DeMetry[164] in 1952. Later more specific assays for vitamin E were developed[163] and it was shown that administration of this compound was accompanied by resolution of the hemolysis.[165]

Prevalence. Since vitamin E is fat soluble, a deficiency may occur in patients with malabsorption with steatorrhea or with biliary atresia and in premature infants at 6 to 10 weeks of age.[170] Therefore it is not uncommon, but there are no exact data on the prevalence of this condition.

Clinical picture. The vitamin E–deficient infant is generally underweight from prematurity or chronic disease such as malabsorption or biliary obstruction. There may be edema of the eyelids and extremities with muscle wasting.[171] Steatorrhea may be present.

Laboratory manifestations. The hemoglobin value usually ranges from 6 to 10 gm/dl with a mild to moderate reticulocytosis (reticulocyte count of about 10%). Most of the red cells are normocytic and normochromic, but the smear may show increased numbers of acanthocytes and irregularly contracted pyknocytes,[167] which are also found in normal infants. Bone marrow examination may reveal dyserythropoietic precursors with polyploid nuclei. The serum α-tocopherol level is less than 0.5 mg/dl, and hemolysis with hydrogen peroxide in vitro is greater than 30%.[172]

Etiology and pathogenesis. It is thought that vitamin E, being an antioxidant, prevents the peroxidation of membrane lipids. Since artificial infant formulas contain vegetable oil instead of milk fat, such diets increase the content of polyunsaturated fatty acids in membranes. The presence of unconjugated double bonds in these molecules increases the susceptibility to lipid peroxidation and therefore the requirement for vitamin E, which can trap free electrons. Other factors important in the pathogenesis of the membrane defect are the small body stores of tocopherol in the premature infant, oxygen therapy, the parenteral administration of oxidant drugs such as iron and ascorbic acid, physiologic deficiency of glutathione peroxidase, and malabsorption.

Vitamin E may also play a role in heme synthesis, and dyserythropoietic changes have been observed in animals and humans.[174]

Differential diagnosis. The morphologic abnormalities of the erythrocytes may be seen in infants with infantile pyknocytosis without vitamin E deficiency, and the peroxide hemolysis test may be positive in other hemolytic anemias. The serum level and a therapeutic trial should establish the diagnosis.

Therapy. The daily requirement for α-tocopherol is 0.4 mg/day for milk-fed infants and 1.5 mg/day for those on artificial formulas during the first year. The therapeutic maintenance dose is about 5 mg/day for infants, but as much as 30 mg/day has been given for short periods.

Course and prognosis. The outlook for the resolution of the anemia is good. Malabsorption may reduce the oral absorption of the vitamin, and the presence or absence of chronic disease determines the ultimate prognosis.

RARER MEMBRANE LIPID DISORDERS
Lecithin-cholesterol acyltransferase (LCAT) deficiency

LCAT deficiency is a rare condition in which the enzyme responsible for the conversion of cholesterol to its ester is absent.[169] Thus membrane cholesterol accumulates instead of being esterified and transported into the plasma. It has been reported as an autosomal recessive trait in Scandinavian families and is characterized by a moderate hemolytic anemia, renal disease, and corneal opacities. The blood contains numerous target cells, in contrast to the morphology of acanthocytosis, in which LCAT activity may be decreased but not absent. Both of these conditions have excess membrane; the erythrocytes in LCAT deficiency are also unusual for target cells because they are similar to spur cells in lipid composition, with high cholesterol but normal total phospholipid content. Obviously qualitative differences are important since red cells in LCAT deficiency have an elevated phosphatidylcholine but reduced phosphatidylethanolamine and sphingomyelin levels compared to acanthocytes. There is no specific therapy.

High-phosphatidylcholine hemolytic anemia

High-phosphatidylcholine hemolytic anemia is a rare cause of hemolysis accompanied by increased cation permeability. It has been transmitted as an autosomal dominant condition in a Dominican family.[166,173] The clinical manifestations are those of a mild hemolytic anemia. Occasional target cells are present in the peripheral blood and give rise to diminished osmotic fragility. The red cell life span is shortened, and autohemolysis is increased but correctable with glucose. Despite the absence of a plasma lipid abnormality, the red cell phosphatidylcholine level is higher than normal. It is believed that the defect resides in the faulty transfer of membrane fatty acids from phosphatidylcholine to the plasma. This is associated with increased cation permeability, which creates a greater metabolic demand on the red cell. Splenectomy is thought to be helpful in this disorder.

An elevated red cell phosphatidylcholine level also has been observed in patients with congenital dyserythropoietic anemia type IV.[168]

PAROXYSMAL NOCTURNAL HEMOGLOBINURIA (PNH)

Definition and history. PNH is an illness characterized classically by sporadic episodes of nighttime hemolysis in the renal parenchyma, producing hemoglobin in the urine. Although these are the classical symptoms, they are frequently absent. The hemolysis may be chronic without a nocturnal pattern and generalized or mild without hemoglobinuria. It is attributed to a membrane defect that makes PNH red cells unusually susceptible to lysis by complement.

The condition was first described in 1882 by Strübing,[210] who clearly defined the relationship of the hemoglobinuria to sleep and thought that it was a result of the accumulation of carbon dioxide or lactic acid. His observations were later elaborated on by Marchiafava[198] and Michell;[201] their names were given as an eponym to this syndrome. Since that time other observers such as van den Bergh,[194] Dacie,[70] and Ham[187] have described many cases in the literature and confirmed the variable manifestations of the defect. The history of PNH has been reviewed by Crosby.[180]

Prevalence and genetics. The exact incidence of PNH is not known, but it is relatively uncommon. It is most commonly found in adults between the second and fourth decades, but about 10% of cases occur in children and adolescents.[70,202] There is no familial tendency, and both males and females are affected. It has been reported in many racial groups.

Clinical picture. The diagnosis of PNH is often overlooked because only 21% of patients have hemoglobinuria.[183] Usually the disease is insidious in onset and patients complain of fatigue, sallow complexion, and other symptoms of anemia. In the uncomplicated case the usual signs are those of chronic hemolysis with slight jaundice and moderate splenomegaly with or without hepatic enlargement.

The severity of the disease ranges from a mild, indolent disorder to a debilitating, incapacitating one, but it tends to remain fairly constant for a given individual. Exacerbations in hemolysis do occur, however, precipitated by various stimuli, such as exercise,[175] iron injections,[70] whole blood transfusions,[188] infections,[70] vaccinations, operations,[70] and even menstruation.[70]

As in other hemolytic anemias, temporary aregenerative crises may occur, but PNH is often found in association with a more persistent hypoplastic or aplastic anemia, whether it is of the Fanconi,[182] drug-induced,[204] or idiopathic[196] type. The diagnosis of one condition may precede or follow the detection of the other. Since PNH is a manifestation of a dysplastic process, an abnormal clone of cells is present that is defective in membrane synthesis. Further involvement at the stem cell level may have occurred in cases of PNH reported in association with erythroleukemia,[176] myelofibrosis,[189] and acute myelocytic leukemia.[195]

Complications of PNH include infections, hemorrhage, and thrombosis. In patients with pancytopenia the white cell and platelet counts are low and these cells may be functionally abnormal. These cellular elements are susceptible to lysis similarly to the red cells and may liberate thromboplastic material. Intravascular coagulation then could result, the symptoms depending on the extent and organ of involvement. Abdominal pain should not be dismissed as a result of a hemolytic reaction, since mesenteric and portal venous thrombosis can occur. A common event is progressive diffuse hepatic venous thrombosis (Budd-Chiari syndrome) with or without hepatomegaly or ascites that is fatal within a few months.[203]

Thromboses may also occur in the extremities or brain. Neurologic signs and symptoms such as severe headache may be evident. The risk of thrombotic episodes is particularly high after surgery (e.g., splenectomy) and childbirth. About half of patients with PNH die of this complication.

Laboratory manifestations. The red cells in PNH are slightly larger than normal, but there is considerable anisocytosis. With excessive urinary iron loss, hypochromia and microcytosis may also be present. Poikilocytes are few, except in some cases of intravascular coagulation, when schistocytes may appear. Anemia is usually moderate to severe with a hemoglobin level of between 3 and 10 mg/dl, but the absolute reticulocyte count may be inappropriately low (range 0.1% to 66%), perhaps as a result of iron deficiency, marrow hypoplasia, or the early destruction of this cell population.

Leukopenia is often present (range 0.5 to 9 × 10^9/liter) with or without relative lymphocytosis. The neutrophil alkaline phosphatase level may be low or absent and the platelet count is often decreased (range 1 to 460 × 10^9/liter). Bone marrow examination generally shows erythroid hyperplasia in spite of the fact that there is peripheral pancytopenia; however, a hypoplastic or aplastic marrow also may be seen.

The hemoglobin type and osmotic fragility are normal and the direct Coombs test is negative, but autohemolysis may occur in the presence of complement. Studies carried out on plasma usually show a decrease in haptoglobin and an increase in unconjugated bilirubin as in other hemolytic anemias. The urine reveals the spectral presence of up to several grams of hemoglobin per day during exacerbations or a sediment chronically containing hemosiderin as shown by Prussian blue stain. Iron deficiency may develop if large amounts (as much as 20 mg/day) are excreted by this route.[197] Other findings (e.g., coagulation abnormalities) may be observed depending on the complications.

More specific tests for PNH are the acid lysis

(Ham[188,194]) and sucrose lysis[191] tests. The first is based on the susceptibility of PNH cells to lysis in fresh normal ABO-compatible serum at pH 6.8 to 7.0, but it has been subject to criticism because different sera have varying lytic potency. The second test is based on the fact that the attachment of complement to red cells is enhanced during incubation in isotonic sucrose. Thus when a small aliquot of citrated or defibrinated PNH blood is diluted with this solution and small amounts of normal serum, hemolysis takes place after 30 minutes at room temperature. Other tests that have been

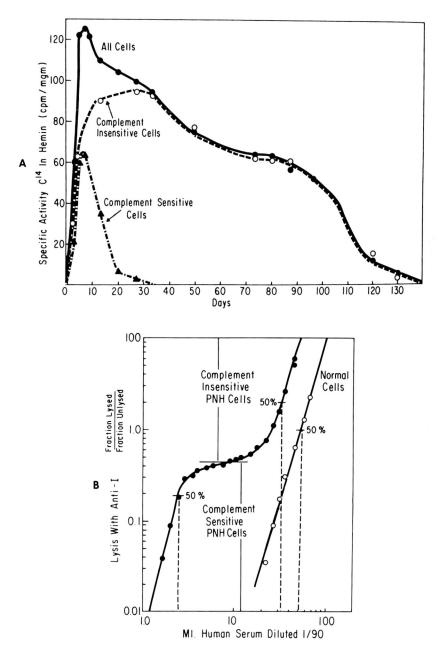

Fig. 11-10. A, Presence of two populations of cells in PNH as demonstrated by cohort labeling with ^{14}C-glycine. The cells were placed in serum that could lyse only complement-sensitive cells. **B,** Presence of two clones of PNH cells demonstrated by fractional lysis with anti-I and increasing amounts of complement in human serum. The 50% lysis point for each population is indicated by the broken line. o—o, normal donor; •—•, PNH patient with two populations of cells, complement sensitive and insensitive. (From Rosse, W. F.: In Williams, W. J., ed.: Hematology, New York, 1972, McGraw-Hill Book Co. Used with permission of McGraw-Hill Book Co.)

described are the thrombin,[179] hemolytic antibody,[207] and heat[193] tests.

Etiology and pathogenesis. PNH is thought to be caused by a population of cells that is unusually susceptible to lysis by complement. As part of a dyserythropoietic process an abnormal clone of precursors in the bone marrow is defective in some aspect of membrane synthesis. Thus PNH cells have a shortened life span when transfused into normal recipients, but normal erythrocytes survive normally in PNH patients.

Closer analysis of these erythrokinetic studies show two cohorts of PNH cells, one that is destroyed rapidly, with a half-life of about 6 days, and another that is hemolyzed more slowly.[206] The presence of at least two populations is confirmed by in vitro studies of complement sensitivity (Fig. 11-10). Only one-twelfth the amount of complement is necessary to lyse the sensitive PNH cells as normal cells. Occasionally there is a group of cells that can be demonstrated to lyse at intermediate concentrations. These hemolytic antibody tests are usually carried out with anti-I serum, but on occasion it is the fetal i-antigen that is expressed on the erythrocytes. The mechanism for complement activation is probably via the properdin pathway, since there is neither C3 nor antibody on the cells.

The membrane defect of PNH is apparent in the bone marrow and reticulocytes; both contain a higher proportion of complement-sensitive cells relative to the total number of mature red cells. The reticulocytes are probably destroyed soon after emergence from the marrow, a process that is compatible with increased medullary activity but decreased peripheral reticulocytosis. Thus the cells less sensitive to complement tend to be left in circulation and the percentage of these survivors correlates with the severity of the disease.

The temporal variation of the hemoglobinuria is more precisely correlated with sleep. It is thought that slight respiratory acidosis during sleep may exacerbate hemolysis, but prevention of carbon dioxide retention with a respirator failed to alter the pattern of hemoglobinuria.[181] More likely, local factors related to renal blood flow are also important.

The granulocytopenia and thrombocytopenia of PNH are probably related to defective membranes in these cellular elements as well. In addition to the red cells, leukocytes and platelets may also be sensitive to complement and lyse, releasing thrombogenic substances that trigger intravascular coagulation. Damaged platelet membranes and red cell stroma have been proposed as predisposing factors to a thrombotic event.[211] In addition to the complement sensitivity of leukocytes, their chemotactic response could be impaired if serum complement were consumed during severe hemolysis. These two factors may contribute to an increased risk of infection.

The biochemical nature of the membrane defect of the red cell is obscure. Both lipids and proteins have been suspected. Phospholatidylcholine (mainly in the outer half of the bilayer) has been reported to be decreased and phosphatidylserine (predominantly in the inner surface of the membrane) increased.[190] Fatty acids have been variably elevated or reduced, and an increased tendency to lipid peroxidation has been observed.[199]

Some investigators have shown a deficiency of membrane acetylcholinesterase and thus PNH cells label poorly with diisofluorophosphate 32 ($DF^{32}P$),[205] but this enzyme does not appear to be essential in maintaining the integrity of the membrane. Finally a decrease in surface thiol groups has been proposed to explain the defect in PNH, since treatment of normal erythrocytes with sulfhydryl-reactive compounds makes them complement sensitive.[186,208]

Differential diagnosis. PNH should be considered in any obscure situation of aplastic anemia and of hemolysis but must be distinguished from them by the appropriate serologic studies. For example, both paroxysmal cold hemoglobinuria and cold agglutinin disease are antibody mediated. The rarer congenital dyserythropoietic anemia type II, otherwise known as hereditary erythroblastic multinuclearity with positive acidified serum test (HEMPAS), is familial, and markedly abnormal bone marrow morphology is present.[178] Furthermore, HEMPAS cells do not lyse in the patient's own serum, and only in some but not all normal sera, and the sucrose lysis test is negative. The abnormal configuration of nuclei in this disorder strongly suggests that there is a disturbance of synthesis not only in the membrane but in other organelles as well (Chapter 8).

Treatment. Since the cause of the PNH defect is poorly understood, there is no definitive therapy. The need for palliative measures is dictated by the severity of the clinical symptoms.

Blood transfusions may be necessary in anemic patients and should be given as washed red cells to remove donor complement or other factors.[70] It is possible that any increased hemolysis, transfusion reaction, or leukoagglutination may result in thrombotic episodes. Splenectomy has been of no benefit. Iron deficiency should be treated, preferably by oral medication rather than parenterally, since free iron can catalyze lipid peroxidation and iron-dextran complexes may cause anaphylaxis.[200] A response to iron therapy, however, may increase the production of complement-sensitive cells and exacerbate hemolysis.

Steroids (1 to 2 mg/kg prednisone daily[184]) or

androgens[192] (1 to 2 mg/kg fluoxymesterone daily) may be tried for several weeks to determine if they are of any empirical benefit. Subsequently the dosage may be tapered for maintenance purposes.

Anticoagulants, both heparin and warfarin (Coumadin), have been tried both prophylactically and therapeutically for reducing the number and extent of thrombotic episodes. The results have been conflicting. They are contraindicated in thrombocytopenia, but in general it would be wise to anticipate situations of stress, e.g., immediately after surgical procedures, by anticoagulation with heparin, even though this drug has been implicated occasionally in causing thrombosis.[185]

Treatment with various medications, including the chemotherapeutic agent 6-mercaptopurine,[192] to suppress the abnormal cell population has been without success. Bone marrow transplantation has been performed with favorable outcome.[209]

Course and prognosis. PNH is a chronic disease with a median survival of 10 years, but the life span may be as long as 43 years after diagnosis.[177] Patients suffering from severe anemia caused by bone marrow hypoplasia and a high proportion of complement-sensitive cells do poorly. Hemolytic episodes may lead to thrombotic complications, and marrow aplasia often leads to infection and hemorrhage.

In mild cases patients are asymptomatic. Some may go into a temporary or even permanent remission with disappearance of all laboratory evidence of PNH.[177]

MEMBRANE DEFECTS CAUSED BY HEAVY METALS

Although lead poisoning primarily affects heme synthesis, membrane damage also occurs.[212] This is reflected in increased potassium loss with decreased membrane Na^+-K^+ ATPase. The osmotic fragility is diminished but the red cell life span may be shortened.

Copper deficiency may result in increased membrane cation permeability and osmotic fragility,[217] but more commonly copper excess may be responsible for hemolysis. Copper intoxication has been reported from ingestion of copper sulfate,[215] hemodialysis with fluid containing copper,[216] and release of hepatic copper in Wilson's disease.[214] In Wilson's disease anemia may be the presenting sign before hepatic and neurologic manifestations.[213] Increased autohemolysis may result from impairment of hexose monophosphate shunt enzymes, decreased glutathione, and Heinz body formation, but there may be a direct toxic effect of the metal on the membrane as well. The treatment in both cases is removal of the offending agent and reduction of toxic levels by chelation therapy.

REFERENCES
Membrane biochemistry

1. Avruch, J., and Fairbanks, G.: Phosphorylation of endogenous substrates by erythrocyte membrane protein kinases, Biochemistry **13**:5507, 1974.
2. Bachi, T., Whiting, K., Tanmer, M. J., et al.: Freeze fracture electron microscopy of human erythrocytes lacking the major membrane sialoglycoprotein, Biochem. Biophys. Acta **464**:635, 1977.
3. Blobel, G., and Dobberstein, J.: Transfer of proteins across membranes, J. Cell Biol. **67**:835, 1975.
4. Chang, H., Langer, P. J., and Lodish, H. F.: Asynchronous synthesis of erythrocyte membrane proteins, Proc. Nat. Acad. Sci. U.S.A. **75**:3206, 1976.
5. Colley, C. M., Zwaal, R. F., Roelofsen, B., and Van Deenen, L. L. M.: Lytic and non-lytic degradation of phospholipids in mammalian erythrocytes by pure phospholipases, Biochem. Biophys. Acta **307**:74, 1973.
6. Dahl, J. L., and Hokin, L. E.: The sodium-potassium adenosine triphosphatase, Ann. Rev. Biochem. **43**:327, 1973.
7. Deuticke, B.: Transformation and restoration of biconcave shape of human erythrocytes induced by amphophilic agents and changes of ionic environment, Biochim. Biophys. Acta. **163**:494, 1968.
8. Deveaux, P., and McConnell, H. M.: Lateral diffusion in spin-labeled phosphatidylcholine multibilayers, J. Am. Chem. Soc. **94**:4475, 1972.
9. Dowben, R. M.: Composition and structure of membranes. In Dowben, R. M., ed.: Biological membranes. Boston, 1969, Little, Brown & Co.
10. Dunham, P. B., and Gunn, R. B.: Adenosine triphosphatase and active cation transport in red blood cell membranes, Arch. Intern. Med. **129**:241, 1972.
11. Edidin, M., and Weiss, A.: Antigen cap formation in cultured fibroblasts, Proc. Nat. Acad. Sci. U.S.A. **69**:2456, 1972.
12. Fairbanks, G., Steck, T. L., and Wallach, D. F. H.: Electrophoretic analysis of the major polypeptides of the human erythrocyte membrane, Biochemistry **10**:2606, 1971.
13. Fossel, E. T., and Solomon, A. K.: Membrane mediated link between transport and metabolism in red blood cells, Biochim. Biophys. Acta. **464**:82, 1977.
14. Fowler, V., and Branton, D.: Lateral mobility of human erythrocyte integral membrane proteins, Nature **268**:23, 1977.
15. Frye, L. D., and Edidin, M.: The rapid intermixing of cell surface antigens after formation of mouse-human heterokaryons, J. Cell. Sci. **7**:319, 1970.
16. Gardos, G.: The role of calcium in the potassium permeability of human erythrocytes, Acta Physiol. Acad. Sci. Hung. **15**:121, 1959.
17. Gazitt, Y., Ohad, I., and Loyter, A.: Phosphorylation and dephosphorylation of membrane proteins as a possible mechanism for structural rearrangement of membrane components, Biochim. Biophys. Acta. **436**:1, 1976.
18. Glynn, I. M.: The ionic permeability of the red cell membrane, Prog. Biophys. **8**:241, 1957.
19. Gordesky, S. E., and Marinetti, G. V.: The asymmetric arrangement of phospholipids in the human erythrocyte membrane, Biochem. Biophys. Res. Commun. **50**:1027, 1973.
20. Gregersen, M. I., Bryant, C. A., Hammerle, W. E., et al.: Flow characteristics of human erythrocytes through polycarbonate sieves, Science **157**:825, 1967.
21. Harris, J. E.: The influence of the metabolism of human erythrocytes on their potassium content, J. Biol. Chem. **141**:579, 1941.
22. Keith, A. D., Sharnoff, M., and Cohn, G. E.: A sum-

mary and evaluation of spin labels used as probes for biological membrane structure, Biochim. Biophys. Acta. **300:**379, 1973.

23. Knauf, P. A., Proverbio, R., and Hoffman, J. F.: Electrophoretic separation of different phosphoproteins associated with Ca ATPase and Na K ATPase in human red cell ghosts, J. Gen. Physiol. **63:**324, 1974.

24. LaCelle, P. L.: Alteration of membrane deformability in hemolytic anemias, Semin. Hematol. **7:**355, 1970.

25. Levine, P., Tripodi, D., Struck, J., et al.: Hemolytic anemia associated with Rh null but not with Bombay blood, Vox Sang. **24:**417, 1973.

26. Lucy, J. A.: Ultrastructure of membranes: micellar organization, Br. Med. Bull. **24:**127, 1968.

27. Marchesi, V. T., Furthmayr, H., and Tomita, M.: The red cell membrane, Ann. Rev. Biochem. **45:**667, 1976.

28. McConnell, H. M., and McFarland, B. G.: The flexibility gradient in biological membranes, Ann. N.Y. Acad. Sci. **195:**207, 1972.

29. Nakao, M., Nakao, T., and Yamazoe, S.: Adenosine triphosphatase and maintenance of shape of human red blood cells, Nature **187:**945, 1960.

30. Palek, J., Church, A., and Fairbanks, G.: Transmembrane movements and distribution of calcium in normal and hemoglobin S erythrocytes. In Bolis, L., Hoffman, J. F., and Leaf, A., eds.: Membranes and disease, New York, 1976, Raven Press.

31. Parker, J. C., and Welt, L. G.: Pathological alterations of cation movements in red blood cells, Arch. Intern. Med. **129:**320, 1972.

32. Post, R. L., Merritt, C. R., Kinsolving, C. P., and Albright, C. D.: Membrane ATPase as a participant in the active transport of Na and K in the human erythrocyte, J. Biol. Chem. **235:**1796, 1960.

33. Roseman, S.: Sugars of the cell membrane, Hosp. Prac. **10:**61, 1975.

34. Rothman, J. E., and Engelman, D. M.: Molecular mechanism for the interaction of phospholipid with cholesterol, Nature (New Biol.) **237:**42, 1972.

35. Rothman, J. E., and Lenard, J.: Membrane asymmetry, Science **195:**743, 1977.

36. Rousselet, A., Guthmann, C., Matricon, J., et al.: Study of the transverse diffusion of spin labeled phospholipids in biological membranes, Biochim. Biophys. Acta **426:**357, 1976.

37. Schatzmann, H. J.: Herzglycoside als Hemmstoffe für den aktiven Kalium und Natrium Transport durch die Erythrocytenmembran, Helv. Phys. Pharm. Acta **11:**346, 1953.

38. Schwartz, A., Lindemayer, G. E., and Allen, J. C.: The sodium potassium adenosine triphosphatase: pharmacology, physiology, biochemical aspects, Pharmacol. Rev. **27:**3, 1975.

39. Seelig, J., and Niederberger, W.: Deuterium labeled lipids as structural probes in liquid crystalline bilayers, J. Am. Chem. Soc. **96:**2069, 1974.

40. Seeman, P.: The membrane actions of anesthetics and tranquilizers, Pharmacol. Rev. **24:**583, 1972.

41. Sheetz, M. P., and Singer, S. J.: Biological membranes as bilayer couples, Proc. Nat. Acad. Sci. U.S.A. **71:**4457, 1974.

42. Shimshick, E. J., and McConnell, H. M.: Lateral phase separation in phospholipid membranes, Biochemistry **12:**2351, 1973.

43. Shinitzky, M., and Inbar, M.: Microviscosity parameters and protein mobility in biological membranes, Biochim. Biophys. Acta **433:**133, 1976.

44. Shohet, S. B.: Hemolysis and changes in erythrocyte membrane lipids, N. Engl. J. Med. **286:**577, 1972.

45. Shohet, S. B., and Lux, S. E.: The red cell membrane and mechanisms of hemolysis. In Nathan, D. G. and

Oski, F. A., eds.: Hematology of infancy and childhood, Philadelphia, 1974, W. B. Saunders Co.

46. Shur, B. D., and Roth, S.: Cell surface glycosyltransferases, Biochim. Biophys. Acta **415:**473, 1975.

47. Singer, S. J., and Nicolson, G. L.: The fluid mosaic model of the structure of cell membranes, Science **175:**720, 1972.

48. Skou, J. C.: Enzymatic basis for active transport of sodium and potassium across cell membranes, Physiol. Rev. **45:**596, 1965.

49. Tanford, C., and Reynolds, J. A.: The gross conformation at protein-sodium dodecylsulfate complexes, J. Biol. Chem. **245:**5161, 1970.

50. Tinker, D. O., and Pinteric, L.: On the identification of lamellar and hexagonal phases in negatively stained phospholipid-water systems, Biochemistry **10:**860, 1971.

51. Wallach, D. F. H., and Zahler, P. H.: Protein conformations in cellular membranes, Proc. Nat. Acad. Sci. U.S.A. **56:**1552, 1966.

52. Watkins, W. M.: Blood group specific substances. In Gottschalk, A., ed.: Glycoproteins, vol. 5B, Amsterdam, 1972, Elsevier.

53. Weber, K., and Osborn, M.: The reliability of molecular weight determination by dodecyl sulfate-polyacrylamide gel electrophoresis, J. Biol. Chem. **244:**4406, 1969.

54. Weed, R. I., LaCelle, P. L., and Merrill, K. W.: Metabolic dependence of red cell deformability, J. Clin. Invest. **48:**795, 1969.

55. Weinstein, R. S.: The morphology of adult red cells. In Surgenor, D. M., ed.: The red blood cell, ed. 2, New York, 1974, Academic Press, Inc.

56. Whittam, R., and Wheeler, K. P.: Transport across cell membranes, Ann. Rev. Physiol. **32:**21, 1970.

57. Wimer, B. M., Marsh, W. L., Taswell, H. F., and Galey, W. R.: Hematological changes associated with the McLeod phenotype of the Kell blood group system, Br. J. Hematol. **36:**219, 1977.

Hereditary spherocytosis

58. Anderson, R., Huestis, R. R., and Motulsky, A. G.: Hereditary spherocytosis in the deer mouse, Blood **15:**491, 1960.

59. Barry, M., Schener, P. J., Sherlock, S., Ross, C. F., and Williams, R.: Hereditary spherocytosis with secondary haemochromatosis, Lancet **2:**481, 1968.

60. Baty, J. M.: A case of congenital hemolytic jaundice with an unusually high percentage of reticulocytes, Am. J. Med. Sci. **179:**546, 1930.

61. Bernard, I., Boiron, M., and Estager, J.: Une grande famille hemolytique, Semin. Hop. Paris **28:**3741, 1952.

62. Burman, D.: Congenital spherocytosis in infancy, Arch. Dis. Child. **33:**335, 1958.

63. Chapman, R. G.: Red cell life span after splenectomy in hereditary spherocytosis, J. Clin. Invest. **47:**2263, 1968.

64. Chauffard, M. A.: Pathogéne de l'ictère congenital de l'adulte, Semin. Med. **27:**25, 1907.

65. Cooper, R. A., and Jandl, J. H.: The role of membrane lipids in the survival of red cells in hereditary spherocytosis, J. Clin. Invest. **48:**736, 1969.

66. Cooper, R. A., and Jandl, J. H.: The selective and conjoint loss of red cell lipids, J. Clin. Invest. **48:**906, 1969.

67. Coventry, W. D., and LaBree, R. H.: Heterotopia of bone marrow simulating mediastinal tumor, Ann. Intern. Med. **53:**1042, 1960.

68. Crosby, W. H. and Conrad, M. F.: Hereditary spherocytosis: observations on hemolytic mechanisms and iron metabolism, Blood **15:**662, 1960.

69. Curschmann, H.: Funicular myelosis in hemolytic icterus, Dtsch. Z. Nervenheilkd. **122:**119, 1931.

70. Dacie, J. V.: The haemolytic anaemias, ed. 2, New York, Grune & Stratton, Inc.

71. Dacie, J. V., and Mollison, P. L.: Survival of normal erythrocytes after transfusion to patients with familial haemolytic anaemia (acholuric jaundice), Lancet 1:550, 1943.

72. Dameshek, W., and Bloom, M. L.: The events in the hemolytic crisis of hereditary spherocytosis, with particular reference to the reticulocytopenia, pancytopenia and an abnormal splenic mechanism, Blood 3:1381, 1948.

73. Emerson, C. P., Shen, S. C., Ham, T. H., et al.: Studies on the destruction of red blood cells, Arch. Intern. Med. 97:1, 1956.

74. Falconer, E. H.: Familial hemolytic icterus associated with endocrine dysfunction, Endocrinology 20:174, 1936.

75. Fernandez, L. A., and Erslev, A. J.: Oxygen affinity and compensated hemolysis in hereditary spherocytosis, J. Lab. Clin. Med. 80:780, 1972.

76. Gairdner, D.: Association of gallstones with acholuric jaundice in children, Arch. Dis. Child. 14:109, 1939.

77. Gallai-Hatchard, J. J., and Thompson, R. H.: Phospholipase A activity of mammalian tissues, Biochim. Biophys. Acta 98:128, 1965.

78. Gomperts, E. D., Metz, J., and Zail, S. S.: A red cell membrane protein abnormality in hereditary spherocytosis, Br. J. Haematol. 23:363, 1972.

79. Gottfried, E. L., and Robertson, N. A.: Glycerololysis time of incubated erythrocytes in the diagnosis of hereditary spherocytosis, J. Lab. Clin. Med. 84:746, 1974.

80. Grahl-Madsden, R., and Pallisgaard, G.: Acute renal failure in hereditary spherocytosis, Scand. J. Hematol. 5:41, 1968.

81. Greenquist, A. C., and Shohet, S. B.: Abnormal erythrocyte membrane properties of hereditary spherocytosis in mice, Blood 46:1005, 1975.

82. Greenquist, A. C., and Shohet, S. B.: Phosphorylation in erythrocyte membranes from abnormally shaped cells, Blood 48:877, 1976.

83. Hansen, K., and Klein, E.: Symptomatology and heredity of hemolytic jaundice, Dtsch. Arch. Klin. Med. 176:567, 1934.

84. Hokin, L. E., and Hokin, M. R.: Phosphatidic acid metabolism and active transport of sodium, Fed. Proc. 22:8, 1963.

84a. Jacob, H. S., and Amsden, T.: Acute hemolytic anemia with rigid red cells in hypophosphatemia, N. Engl. J. Med. 285:1446, 1971.

85. Jacob, H. S., and Jandl, J. H.: Increased cell membrane permeability in the pathogenesis of hereditary spherocytosis, J. Clin. Invest. 43:1703, 1964.

86. Jacob, H. S., Ruby, A., Overland, E. S., and Mazia, D.: Abnormal membrane protein of red blood cells in hereditary spherocytosis, J. Clin. Invest. 50:1800, 1971.

87. Jandl, J. H., and Greenberg, M. S.: Bone marrow failure due to relative nutritional deficiency in Cooley's hemolytic anemia: painful erythropoietic crises in response to folic acid, N. Engl. J. Med. 260:461, 1959.

88. Jandl, J. H., Jacob, H. S., and Daland, G. A.: Hypersplenism due to infection: a study of five cases manifesting hemolytic anemia, N. Engl. J. Med. 264:1063, 1961.

89. Kohler, H. G., Meynell, M. J., and Cooke, W. T.: Spherocytic anaemia, complicated by megaloblastic anaemia of pregnancy, Br. Med. J. 1:779, 1960.

90. Leblond, P. F., LaCelle, P. L., and Weed, R. I.: Cellular deformability: a possible determinant of the normal release of maturing erythrocytes from the bone marrow, Blood 37:40, 1971.

91. Loder, P. B., Babarczy, G., and deGruchy, G. C.: Red cell metabolism in hereditary spherocytosis, Br. J. Haematol. 13:95, 1967.

92. Mackenzie, F. A. F., Elliot, D. H., Eastcott, H. H.,

et al.: Relapse in hereditary spherocytosis with proven splenunculus, Lancet 1:1102, 1962.

93. MacKinney, A. A., Jr.: Hereditary spherocytosis, Arch. Intern. Med. 116:257, 1965.

94. MacKinney, A. A., Jr., Morton, N. E., Kosower, N. B., et al.: Ascertaining genetic carriers of hereditary spherocytosis by statistical analysis of multiple laboratory tests, J. Clin. Invest. 41:554, 1962.

95. Minkowski, O.: Uber eine hereditäre, unter dem Bilde eines chronischen Ikterus mit Urobilinurie, Splenomegalie und Nierensiderosis verlaufende Affection, Verh. Dtsch. Kongr. Inn. Med. 18:316, 1900.

96. Metz, J.: Hereditary spherocytosis in the Bantu. S. Afr. Med. J. 33:1034, 1959.

97. Morton, N. E., Mackinney, A. A., Kosower, N., et al.: Genetics of spherocytosis, Am. J. Hum. Genet. 14:170, 1962.

98. Owren, P. A.: Congenital hemolytic jaundice: the pathogenesis of the "hemolytic crisis," Blood 3:231, 1948.

99. Palek, J., Mircevova, L., and Brabec, V.: 2,3-DPG metabolism in hereditary spherocytosis, Br. J. Haematol. 17:59, 1969.

100. Race, R. R.: On the inheritance and linkage relations of acholuric jaundice, Ann. Eugen. 11:365, 1942.

101. Reed, C. F., and Swisher, S. N.: Erythrocyte lipid loss in hereditary spherocytosis, J. Clin. Invest. 45:777, 1966.

102. Selwyn, J. G., and Dacie, J. V.: Autohemolysis and other changes resulting from the incubation in vitro of red cells from patients with congenital hemolytic anemia, Blood 9:414, 1954.

103. Smith, C. H.: Blood diseases of infancy and childhood, ed. 3, St. Louis, 1972, The C. V. Mosby Co.

104. Stamey, C. C., and Diamond, L. K.: Congenital hemolytic anemia in the newborn, Am. J. Dis. Child. 94:616, 1957.

105. Taylor, E. S.: Chronic ulcer of the leg associated with congenital hemolytic jaundice, J.A.M.A. 113:1574, 1939.

106. Tileson, W.: Hemolytic jaundice, Medicine 1:355, 1922.

107. Trucco, J. I., and Brown, A. K.: Neonatal manifestations of hereditary spherocytosis, Am. J. Dis. Child. 113:263, 1967.

108. Valentine, W. N.: The molecular lesion of hereditary spherocytosis: a continuing enigma, Blood 49:241, 1977.

109. Vanlair, C., and Masius, L.: De la microcythemie, Bull. Acad. R. Med. Belg. 5(3rd series):515, 1871.

110. Weed, R. I.: Membrane structure and its relation to haemolysis, Clin. Haematol. 4:3, 1975.

111. Wiley, J. S.: Co-ordinated increase of sodium leak and sodium pump in hereditary spherocytosis, Br. J. Haematol. 22:529, 1972.

112. Wilson, C., and Stanley, D. A.: A sequel to some cases showing hereditary enlargement of the spleen, Trans. Clin. Soc. Lond. 26:163, 1893.

113. Young, L. E.: Hereditary spherocytosis, Am. J. Med. 18:486, 1955.

114. Young, L. E., Izzo, M. J., Altman, K. I., and Swisher, S. N.: Studies in spontaneous in vitro autohemolysis in hemolytic disorders, Blood 11:977, 1956.

Hereditary elliptocytosis

115. Aksoy, M. and Erdem, S.: Combination of hereditary elliptocytosis and heterozygous beta-thalassemia: a family study, J. Med. Genet. 5:298, 1968.

116. Austin, R. F., and Desforges, J. F.: Hereditary elliptocytosis: an unusual presentation of hemolysis in the newborn associated with transient morphologic abnormalities, Pediatrics 44:196, 1969.

117. Bannerman, R. M., and Renwick, J. H.: The hereditary elliptocytoses: clinical and linkage data, Ann. Hum. Genet. 26:23, 1962.

118. Cutting, H. O., McHugh, W. J., Conrad, F. G., and Marlow, A. A.: Autosomal dominant hemolytic anemia characterized by ovalocytosis, Am. J. Med. **39:**21, 1965.

119. Dresbach, M.: Elliptical human red corpuscles, Science **19:**469, 1904.

120. Eitan, A., Aloni, B., and Livne, A.: Unique properties of the camel erythrocyte membrane, Biochim. Biophys. Acta **426:**647, 1976.

121. Florman, A. L., and Wintrobe, M. M.: Human elliptical red corpuscles, Bull. Johns Hopkins Hosp. **63:**209, 1938.

122. Geerdink, R. A., Helleman, P. W., and Verloop, M. C.: Hereditary elliptocytosis and hyperhaemolysis: a comparative study of 6 families with 145 patients, Acta Med. Scand. **179:**715, 1966.

123. Haggitt, R. C., and Rising, J. A.: Hereditary elliptocytosis in a Chinese family, Arch. Pathol. **91:**225, 1971.

124. Jensson, O., Jonasson, T., and Olafsson, O.: Hereditary elliptocytosis in Iceland, Br. J. Haematol. **13:**844, 1967.

125. Lipton, E. L.: Elliptocytosis with hemolytic anemia: the effects of splenectomy, Pediatrics **15:**67, 1955.

126. Murphy, J. R.: Erythrocyte metabolism. VI. Cell shape and the location of cholesterol in the erythrocyte membrane, J. Lab. Clin. Med. **65:**756, 1965.

127. Penfold, J. B., and Lipscomb, J. M.: Elliptocytosis in man associated with hereditary haemorrhagic telangiectasia, Q. J. Med. **12:**157, 1943.

128. Pryor, D. S., and Pitney, W. R.: Hereditary elliptocytosis: a report of two families from New Guinea, Br. J. Haematol. **13:**126, 1967.

129. Rebuck, J. W., and Van Slyck, E. J.: An unsuspected ultrastructural fault in human elliptocytes, Am. J. Clin. Pathol. **49:**19, 1968.

130. Stephens, D. J., and Tatelbaum, A. J.: Elliptical human erythrocytes, J. Lab. Clin. Med. **20:**375, 1935.

131. Torlontano, G., Fontana, L., DeLaurenzi, A., et al.: Hereditary elliptocytosis, Acta Haematol. **48:**1, 1972.

132. Valentine, W. N., Paglia, D. E., Neerhout, R. C., and Konrad, P. N.: Erythrocyte glyoxalase II deficiency with coincidental hereditary elliptocytosis, Blood **36:**797, 1970.

133. Wintrobe, M. M.: Clinical hematology, Philadelphia, 1974, Lea & Febiger.

134. Wolman, I. J., and Ozge, A.: Studies on elliptocytosis, Am. J. Med. Sci. **234:**702, 1957.

Hereditary stomatocytosis

135. Ducrou, W., and Kimber, R. J.: Stomatocytes, haemolytic anaemia and abdominal pain in Mediterranean migrants: some examples of a new syndrome, Med. J. Aust. **2:**1087, 1969.

136. Glader, B. E., Fortier, N., Albala, M. M., and Nathan, D. G.: Congenital hemolytic anemia associated with dehydrated erythrocytes and increased potassium loss, N. Engl. J. Med. **291:**491, 1974.

137. Honig, G. R., Lacson, P. S., and Maurer, H. S.: A new familial disorder with abnormal erythrocyte morphology and increased permeability of the erythrocytes to sodium and potassium, Pediatr. Res. **5:**159, 1971.

137a. Kahn, A., Vives, J. L., Bertrand, O., et al.: Glucose phosphate isomerase deficiency due to a new variant (GPI Barcelona) and to a silent gene, Clin. Chim. Acta **66:**145, 1976.

138. Lo, S. S., Hitzig, W. H., and Marti, H. R.: Stomatozytose, Schweiz. Med. Wochenschr. **100:**1977, 1970.

139. Lock, S. P., Smith, R. S., and Hardisty, R. M.: Stomatocytosis: a hereditary red cell anomaly associated with haemolytic anemia, Br. J. Haematol. **7:**303, 1961.

140. Meadow, S. R.: Stomatocytosis, Proc. R. Soc. Med. **60:**13, 1967.

141. Miller, D. R., Rickles, F. R., Lichtman, M. A., et al.: A new varient of hereditary hemolytic anemia with stomatocytosis and erythrocyte cation abnormality, Blood **38:**184, 1971.

142. Miller, G., Townes, P. L., and MacWhinney, J. B.: A new congenital hemolytic anemia with deformed erythrocytes (?"stomatocytes") and remarkable susceptibility of erythrocytes to cold hemolysis in vitro. I. Clinical and hematologic studies, Pediatrics **35:**906, 1965.

143. Oski, F. A., Naiman, J. L., Blum, S. F., et al.: Congenital hemolytic anemia with high-sodium, low-potassium red cells: studies of three generations of a family with a new variant, N. Engl. J. Med. **280:**909, 1969.

144. Pinkerton, P. A., Fletch, S. M., Brueckner, P. J., and Miller, D. R.: Hereditary stomatocytosis with hemolytic anemia in the dog, Blood **44:**557, 1974.

145. Zarkowsky, H. S., Oski, F. A., Sha'afi, R., et al.: Congenital hemolytic anemia with high sodium, low potassium red cells. I. Studies of membrane permeability, N. Engl. J. Med. **278:**573, 1968.

Hereditary pyropoikilocytosis

145a. Walter, T., Mentzer, W., Greenquist, A., et al.: RBC membrane abnormalities in hereditary pyropoikilocytosis, Blood **50**(suppl.):72, 1977. (Abstract.)

145b. Zarkowsky, H. S., Mohandas, N., Speaker, C. B., and Shohet, S. B.: A congenital hemolytic anemia with thermal sensitivity of the erythrocyte membrane, Br. J. Haematol. **29:**537, 1975.

Acanthocytosis and spur cell anemia

146. Bassen, F. A., and Kornzweig, A. L.: Malformation of the erythrocytes in a case of atypical retinitis pigmentosa, Blood **5:**381, 1950.

147. Cooper, R. A.: Anemia with spur cells: a red cell defect acquired in serum and modified in the circulation, J. Clin. Invest. **48:**1820, 1969.

148. Cooper, R. A., and Gulbrandsen, C. L.: The relationship between serum lipoproteins and red cell membranes in abetalipoproteinemia: deficiency of lecithin: cholesterol acyltransferase, J. Lab. Clin. Med. **78:**323, 1971.

149. Cooper, R. A., and Jandl, J. H.: Acanthocytosis. In Williams, W. J., ed.: Hematology, New York, 1972, McGraw-Hill Book Co.

150. Cooper, R. A., Kimball, D. B., and Durocher, J. R.: Role of the spleen in membrane conditioning and hemolysis of spur cells in liver disease, N. Engl. J. Med. **290:**1279, 1974.

151. Estes, J. W., Morley, T. J., Levine, I. M., and Emerson, C. P.: A new hereditary acanthocytosis syndrome, Am. J. Med. **42:**868, 1967.

152. Gjone, E., Torsvik, H., and Norum, K. R.: Familial plasma cholesterol ester deficiency: a study of the erythrocytes, Scand. J. Clin. Lab. Invest. **21:**327, 1968.

153. Hoffman, J. F.: Cation transport and structure of the red cell plasma membrane, Circulation **26:**1201, 1962.

154. Isselbacher, K. J., Scheig, R., Plotkin, G. R., and Caulfield, J. B.: Congenital β-lipoprotein deficiency: an hereditary disorder involving a defect in the absorption and transport of lipids, Medicine **43:**347, 1964.

155. Kayden, H. J.: Abetalipoproteinemia, Ann. Rev. Med. **23:**285, 1972.

156. Kayden, H. J., and Bessis, M.: Morphology of normal erythrocyte and acanthocyte using Nomarski optics and the scanning electron microscope, Blood **35:**427, 1970.

157. Levine, I. M., Estes, J. W., and Looney, J. M.: Hereditary neurological disease with acanthocytosis, Arch. Neurol. **19:**403, 1968.

158. Nathan, D. G., Oski, F. A., Sidel, V. W., et al.: Studies of erythrocyte spicule formation in haemolytic anemia, Br. J. Haematol. **12:**385, 1966.

159. Silber, R., Amorosi, E., Lhowe, J., and Kayden, H. J.:

Spur-shaped erythrocytes in Laennec's cirrhosis, N. Engl. J. Med. **275**:639, 1966.

160. Simon, E. R., and Ways, P.: Incubation hemolysis and red cell metabolism in acanthocytosis, J. Clin. Invest. **43**:1311, 1964.

161. Smith, J. A., Lonergan, E. T., and Sterling, K.: Spur-cell anemia: hemolytic anemia with red cells resembling acanthocytes in alcoholic cirrhosis, N. Engl. J. Med. **271**:396, 1964.

162. Ways, P., Reed, C. F., and Hanahan, D. J.: Red-cell and plasma lipids in acanthocytosis, J. Clin. Invest. **42**:1248, 1963.

Vitamin E deficiency and rare membrane lipid disorders

163. Bunnell, R. H.: Modern procedures for the analysis of tocopherols, Lipids **6**:245, 1971.

164. Gordon, H. H., and DeMetry, J. P.: Hemolysis in hydrogen peroxide of erythrocytes of premature infants: effect of alpha-tocopherol, Proc. Soc. Exp. Biol. Med. **79**:446, 1952.

165. Horwitt, M. K., Century, B., and Zeman, A. A.: Erythrocyte survival time after tocopherol depletion in man, Am. J. Clin. Nutr. **12**:99, 1963.

166. Jaffe, E. R., and Gottfried, E. L.: Hereditary nonspherocytic hemolytic disease associated with an altered phospholipid composition of the erythrocytes, J. Clin. Invest. **47**:1375, 1968.

167. Keimowitz, R., and Desforges, J. F.: Infantile pycnocytosis, N. Engl. J. Med. **273**:1152, 1965.

168. Miller, D. R., Sitarz, A. L., Lieberman, P. H., et al.: Congenital dyserythropoietic anemia, type IV, American Society of Hematology, abstract no. 500, 1976.

169. Norum, K. R., Glomset, J. A., and Gjone, E.: Familial lecithin: cholesterol acyltransferase deficiency. In Stanbury, J. B., Wyngaarden, J. B., and Fredrickson, D. S., eds.: Metabolic basis of inherited diseases, New York, 1972, McGraw-Hill Book Co.

170. Oski, F. A., and Barness, L. A.: Vitamin E deficiency: a previously unrecognized cause of hemolytic anemia in the premature infant, J. Pediatr. **70**:211, 1967.

171. Ritchie, J. H., Fish, M. B., McMasters, V., and Grossman, M.: Edema and hemolytic anemia in premature infants, N. Engl. J. Med. **279**:1185, 1968.

172. Rose, C. S., and Gyorgy, P.: Specificity of hemolytic reaction in vitamin E deficiency erythrocytes, Am. J. Physiol. **168**:414, 1952.

173. Shohet, S. B., Livermore, B. M., Nathan, D. G., and Jaffe, E. R.: Hereditary hemolytic anemia associated with abnormal membrane lipids, Blood **38**:445, 1971.

174. Silber, R., and Goldstein, B. D.: Vitamin E and the hematopoietic system, Semin. Hematol. **7**:40, 1970.

Paroxysmal nocturnal hemoglobinuria

175. Blum, S. F., Sullivan, J. M., and Gardner, F. H.: The exacerbation of hemolysis in paroxysmal nocturnal hemoglobinuria by strenuous exercise, Blood **30**:513, 1967.

176. Carmel, R., Coltman, C. A., Yatteau, R. F., and Costanzi, J. J.: Association of paroxysmal nocturnal hemoglobinuria with erythroleukemia, N. Engl. J. Med. **283**:1329, 1970.

177. Charache, S.: Prolonged survival in paroxysmal nocturnal hemoglobinuria, Blood **3**:877, 1969.

178. Crookston, J. H., Crookston, M. C., Burnie, K. L., Francombe, W. H., Dacie, J. V., Davis, J. A., and Lewis, S. M.: Red cell abnormalities in HEMPAS, Br. J. Haematol. **23**:83, 1972.

179. Crosby, W. H.: Paroxysmal nocturnal hemoglobinuria, Blood **5**:843, 1950.

180. Crosby, W. H.: Paroxysmal nocturnal hemoglobinuria: plasma factors of the hemolytic system, Blood **8**:444, 1953.

181. Crosby, W. H.: Paroxysmal nocturnal hemoglobinuria: relation of the clinical manifestations to underlying pathogenetic mechanisms, Blood **8**:769, 1953.

182. Dacie, J. V., and Gilpin, A.: Refractory anaemia (Fanconi type): its incidence in three members of one family, with in one case a relationship to chronic haemolytic anemia with PNH, Arch. Dis. Child. **19**:155, 1944.

183. Dacie, J. V., and Lewis, S. M.: Paroxysmal nocturnal hemoglobinuria: clinical manifestations, haematology and nature of the disease. Ser. Haematol. **5**(3):3, 1972.

184. Firkin, F., Goldberg, H., and Firkin, B. G.: Glucocorticoid management of paroxysmal nocturnal hemoglobinuria, Aust. Ann. Med. **17**:127, 1968.

185. Fritsche, W., and Martin, H.: Properdin and hemolysis: heparin inhibition of erythrocyte hemolysis in patients with PNH, Klin. Wochenschr. **35**:1166, 1957.

186. Givone, S.: Considerazioni patogenetiche sull' emoglobinuria parossitica notturna, Minerva Pediatr. **13**:1074, 1961.

187. Ham, T. H.: Chronic hemolytic anemia with paroxysmal nocturnal hemoglobinuria, N. Engl. J. Med. **217**:915, 1937.

188. Ham, T. H.: Studies on destruction of red blood cells: I. Chronic hemolytic anemia with paroxysmal nocturnal hemoglobinuria: an investigation of the mechanism of hemolysis with observations in five cases, Arch. Intern. Med. **64**:1271, 1939.

189. Hansen, N. E., and Killman, S. A.: Paroxysmal nocturnal hemoglobinuria in myelofibrosis, Blood **36**:428, 1970.

190. Harris, I. M., Prankerd, T. A., and Westerman, M. P.: Abnormality of phospholipids in red cells of patients with paroxysmal nocturnal haemoglobinuria, Br. Med. J. **2**:1276, 1957.

191. Hartmann, R. C., Jenkins, D. E., and Arnold, A. B.: Diagnostic specificity of sucrose hemolysis test for PNH, Blood **35**:462, 1970.

192. Hartmann, R. C., and Kolhouse, J. F.: Viewpoints on the management of PNH, Ser. Haematol. **5**(3):42, 1972.

193. Hegglin, R., and Maier, C.: The "heat resistance" of erythrocytes: a specific test for the recognition of Marchiafava's anemia, Am. J. Med. Sci. **207**:624, 1944.

194. Hijmans van den Bergh, A. A.: Ictere hemolytique avec crises hemoglobinuriques, Rev. Med. **31**:63, 1911.

195. Kaufmann, R. W., Schechter, G. P., and McFarland, W.: Paroxysmal nocturnal hemoglobinuria terminating in acute granulocytic leukemia, Blood **33**:287, 1969.

196. Lewis, S. M., and Dacie, J. V.: The aplastic anemia-paroxysmal nocturnal haemoglobinuria syndrome, Br. J. Haematol. **13**:236, 1967.

197. Marchal, G., Leroux, M. E., and Duhamel, G.: Deficience en un profacteur plasmatique et serique de la thromboplastine (profacteur C?) su cours d'un syndrome Marchiafava-Micheli, Sangre **30**:181, 1959.

198. Marchiafava, E.: Anemie emolitica con emosiderinuria perpetua, Policlin. Sez. Med. **18**:241, 1931.

199. Mengel, C. E., Kann, H. E., and Meriweither, W.: Studies of paroxysmal nocturnal hemoglobinuria erythrocytes: increased lysis and lipid peroxide formation by hydrogen peroxide, J. Clin. Invest. **46**:1715, 1967.

200. Mengel, C. E., Kann, H. E., and O'Malley, B. W.: Increased hemolysis after intramuscular iron administration in patients with paroxysmal nocturnal hemoglobinuria: report of six occurrences in four patients, and speculations on a possible mechanism, Blood **26**:74, 1965.

201. Micheli, F.: Anemia emolitica con emosiderinuria perpetua, Policlin. Sez. Prat. **35**:2574, 1928.

202. Miller, D. R., Baehner, R. L., and Diamond, L. K.:

PNH in childhood and adolescence, Pediatrics **39:**675, 1967.

203. Peytermann, R., Rhodes, R. S., and Hartmann, R. C.: Thrombosis in paroxysmal nocturnal hemoglobinuria with particular reference to progressive, diffuse hepatic venous thrombosis, Ser. Haematol. **5**(3):115, 1972.

204. Quagliana, J. M., Cartwright, G. E., and Wintrobe, M. M.: Paroxysmal nocturnal hemoglobinuria following drug-induced aplastic anemia, Ann. Intern. Med. **6:**1045, 1964.

205. Rosse, W. F.: Paroxysmal nocturnal hemoglobinuria. In Williams, W. J., ed.: Hematology, New York, 1972, McGraw-Hill Book Co.

206. Rosse, W. F.: Variations in the red cells in paroxysmal nocturnal haemoglobinuria, Br. J. Haematol. **24:**327, 1973.

207. Rosse, W. F., and Dacie, J. V.: Immune lysis of normal human and paroxysmal nocturnal hemoglobinuria (PNH) red blood cells. I. The sensitivity of PNH red cells to lysis by complement and specific antibody, J. Clin. Invest. **45:**736, 1966.

208. Sircha, G., and Ferrone, S.: The laboratory substitutes of the red cells of PNH: PNH-like cells, Ser. Haematol. **5**(3):137, 1972.

209. Storb, R., Evans, R. S., Thomas, E. D., et al.: PNH and refractory marrow failure treated by marrow transplantation, Br. J. Haematol. **24:**743, 1973.

210. Strübing, P.: Paroxysmale Haemoglobinurie, Dtsch. Med. Wochenschr. **8:**1, 1882.

211. Zimmerman, T. S., Fierer, J., and Rothberger, H.: Blood coagulation and the inflammatory response, Semin. Hematol. **14:**391, 1977.

Membrane defects caused by heavy metals

212. Albahary, C.: Lead and hemopoiesis, Am. J. Med. **52:** 369, 1972.

213. Buchanan, G. R.: Acute hemolytic anemia as a presenting manifestation of Wilson disease, J. Pediatr. **86:**245, 1975.

214. Deiss, A., Lee, G. R., and Cartwright, G. E.: Hemolytic anemia in Wilson's disease, Ann. Intern. Med. **73:**413, 1970.

215. Fairbanks, V. F.: Copper sulfate-induced hemolytic anemia, Arch. Intern. Med. **120:**429, 1967.

216. Klein, W. J., Metz, E. N., and Price A. R.: Acute copper intoxication, Arch. Intern. Med. **129:**578, 1972.

217. Lynch, R. E., Lee, G. R., and Cartwright, G. E.: Copper and the red cell membrane, Blood **40:**963, 1972.

12 □ Hemolytic anemia: metabolic defects

Denis R. Miller

NORMAL ERYTHROCYTE METABOLISM

The hereditary hemolytic anemias are the result of inborn errors of metabolism involving any of the three main components of the red blood cell: the membrane, the hemoglobin molecule, or the intracellular enzymes and intermediates of cell metabolism. The red blood cell is one of nature's ultimate examples of an harmonious blending of structure and function. The mature, nonreplicating erythrocyte is incapable of synthesizing membrane protein, hemoglobin, or the enzymes of intracellular metabolism required to support its primary role —the delivery of oxygen to the tissues from the lungs and the transport of carbon dioxide in the reverse direction. The cell's metabolic machinery provides the energy required to sustain cation gradients, generate purine nucleotides that serve as cofactors to reduce the hemoglobin molecule, provide phosphorylated glycolytic intermediates that allosterically reduce the affinity of hemoglobin for oxygen, protect proteins against oxidative denaturation, and maintain the biconcave shape of the cell during its life span of 120 days and its intravascular journey of 175 miles.

In this chapter normal erythrocyte metabolism and those hereditary aberrations of red cell enzymes that are responsible for premature cell death are reviewed. The interrelationships of abnormal cell metabolism and function in the pathogenesis of these hereditary hemolytic anemias is stressed. Abnormalities of the membrane and of the hemoglobin molecule are discussed in Chapters 11 and 13, respectively. The following abbreviations are used throughout this chapter.

ADA	Adenosine deaminase
AK	Adenylate kinase
APRT	Adenine phosphoribosyl transferase
ATPase	Adenosine triphosphatase
DHAP	Dihydroxyacetone phosphate
1,3-DPG	1,3-Diphosphoglycerate
2,3-DPG	2,3-Diphosphoglycerate
2,3-DPGM	2,3-Diphosphoglycerate mutase
2,3-DPGP	2,3-Diphosphoglycerate phosphatase
E-4-P	Erythrose-4-phosphate
FAD	Flavine-adenine dinucleotide
FDP	Fructose diphosphate
F-3-P	Fructose-3-phosphate

F-6-P	Fructose-6-phosphate
GAPD	Glyceraldehyde phosphate dehydrogenase
Ga-3-P	Glyceraldehyde-3-phosphate
γ-GC	γ-Glutamyl cysteine
G-1,6-P	Glucose-1,6-phosphate
G-6-P	Glucose-6-phosphate
G-6-PD	Glucose-6-phosphate dehydrogenase
GPI	Glucose phosphate isomerase
GSH	Glutathione (reduced)
GSH-P	Glutathione peroxidase
GSSG	Glutathione (oxidized)
GSSG-R	Glutathione reductase
HGPRT	Hypoxanthine-guanine phosphoribosyl transferase
HK	Hexokinase
LDH	Lactate dehydrogenase
NAD	Nicotinamide adenine dinucleotide
NADH	Nicotinamide adenine dinucleotide (reduced)
NADPH	Nicotinamide adenine dinucleotide phosphate (reduced)
PEP	Phosphoenolpyruvate
PFK	Phosphofructokinase
1,3-PG	1,3-Phosphoglycerate
2-PG	2-Phosphoglycerate
3-PG	3-Phosphoglycerate
6-PG	6-Phosphogluconate
6-PGD	6-Phosphogluconic dehydrogenase
6-PGL	6-Phosphogluconolactone
PGK	Phosphoglycerate kinase
PGM	Phosphoglycerate mutase
Pi	Orthophosphate
PK	Pyruvate kinase
PRPP	5-Phosphoribosyl-1-pyrophosphate
R-5-P	Ribose-5-phosphate
RPK	Ribosephosphate pyrophosphokinase
Ru-5-P	Ribulose-5-phosphate
S-7-P	Sedoheptulose-7-phosphate
TPI	Triose phosphate isomerase
X-5-P	Xylulose-5-phosphate

Historical perspective

The metabolic importance of the red blood cell is a relatively recent discovery, considering the fact that van Leeuwenhoek provided the first accurate description of the erythrocyte in 1674. A century later Lavoisier discovered that red cells transported "oxygine" and "aeriform calcic acid" or carbon dioxide. In 1876, 200 years after the identification of the red cell, Bernard reported that erythrocytes utilize glucose.[165] The end product of glucose utilization, lactic acid, was discovered by Evans in 1922.[51] During the next decade the German biochemists Embden[50] and Meyerhof[97] and the Americans Guest and Rapoport[61] worked out many of enzymatic steps and intermediates of the anaerobic pathway of glycolysis, the Embden-Meyerhof pathway. The key phosphorylated intermediates ATP and 2,3-DPG were discovered in 1924 and 1925, respectively.[60,82] We now know that the Embden-Meyerhof pathway comprises eleven sequential reactions catalyzed by specific enzymes, that for each mole of glucose metabolized, 2 moles of lactic acid are produced, and that in the process 2 molecules of ATP are generated. The 2,3-DPG, or Rapoport-Luebering, cycle was discovered in 1950, but its role in modulating oxygen affinity awaited the simultaneous reports of Chanutin and Curnish[30] and Benesch and Benesch[11] in 1967.

The hexose monophosphate shunt, or aerobic pathway, was detected in 1935 and 1936 by Warburg and Christian,[155] whose enzyme "Zwischenferment," or G-6-PD, was discovered to be deficient in the exhaustive and painstaking studies of the group at the University of Chicago working on primaquine-sensitivity hemolytic anemia in the 1950s.[37] Although only 10% of glucose metabolism flows through the hexose monophosphate shunt, its protective function is vitally important.

Two other key functions of erythrocyte metabolism are the reduction of methemoglobin by NADH-dependent methemoglobin reductase, discovered by Gibson[57] in 1948, and cation transport, carried out by ATPase, an enzyme discovered by Post et al.[116] in 1960 and by Whittam[159] in 1962.

The elucidation of normal erythrocyte metabolism cleared the way for the identification of a number of inborn errors of erythrocyte metabolism that had languished under the catch-all term "congenital nonspherocytic hemolytic anemia" until the early 1960s.[33] Until the late 1950s and early 1960s hereditary hemolytic anemias were considered either "spherocytic" or "nonspherocytic," distinctions on the basis of morphology, the results of the autohemolysis test, and an incomplete understanding of the pathogenesis of hemolysis. In 1962 Tanaka et al.[146] defined the first of a number of inherited enzymopthies involving the Embden-Meyerhof pathway, PK-deficiency hereditary hemolytic anemia. At the present time seven other deficiencies of enzymes of the Embden-Meyerhof pathway, six involving the hexose monophosphate shunt, two associated with nucleotide metabolism, and one (ATPase) involving cation transport have been described in association with hereditary hemolytic anemia.[153]

Because the term "nonspherocytic hemolytic anemia" also included disorders now known to be caused by unstable hemoglobins and by membrane defects, its continued use today is meaningless and inappropriate, particularly since many of the so-called nonspherocytic hemolytic anemias are associated with some, albeit mild, spherocytosis. The spherocyte may be the morphologic representation in the final common pathway of cell destruction in many of the hereditary hemolytic anemias, particularly those characterized by deranged energy metabolism.

Developmental aspects

From the proerythroblast stage until maturation to an early polychromatophilic normoblast, the developing erythroid precursor possesses a complete biosynthetic capacity for replication, DNA and RNA synthesis, and the synthesis of proteins, purines, pyrimidines, lipids, and carbohydrates[52,59,89] (Table 12-1). Metabolic activity is represented by an active respiration chain and electron transfer system, the Krebs tricarboxylic acid (citrate) cycle, and the glycolytic Embden-Meyerhof and aerobic hexose monophosphate pathways.[62,118] The initial loss of biosynthetic function occurs at the late polychromatophilic normoblast stage coincident with the loss of DNA synthesis and the beginning degradation and loss of certain organelles such as mitochondria and ribosomes. With the extrusion of the nucleus the reticulocyte is no longer able to synthesize DNA or RNA but, by virtue of its having retained messenger, ribosomal, and transfer RNA as well as functional mitochondria and ribosomes, it is capable of synthesizing protein, particularly hemoglobin.

The metabolic transition from reticulocyte to erythrocyte occurs by way of complete degradation of ribosomes and mitochondria, selective decay of key enzymes of the organelles and the cytosol, and the partial breakdown of the membrane.[120,122,127] The enzymes involved in degradation are ribonuclease, phosphodiesterase, proteinase, and phospholipase.[136] Two protein inhibitors of respiration, inhibitors F[123,124,138] and C,[3,160] are iron proteins with sites of action on flavin enzyme-associated iron-sulfur proteins and cytochrome oxidase, respectively. The inhibitors of the electron transfer system are inactivated during the maturation of the reticulocyte and are not found in mature red cells.[128]

The ability of the reticulocyte to produce energy efficiently and abundantly is determined by the presence of mitochondria, the chief centers of cellular respiration. These cytoplasmic organelles are the cellular sites of various multienzyme metabolic processes, particularly the Krebs citric acid cycle, the oxygen-linked cytochrome system, and oxida-

Table 12-1. Comparison of metabolic pathways and capacities of erythroid cells during maturation

	Nucleated precursors	Reticulocytes	Erythrocytes
Biosynthetic capacity			
Replication	+*	0	0
DNA synthesis	+	0	0
RNA synthesis	+	0	0
RNA present	+	+	0
Protein synthesis	+	+	0†
Heme synthesis	+	+	0
Lipid synthesis	+	+‡	0
Purine synthesis (de novo)	+	+	0
Salvage pathway	+	+	+
Pyrimidine synthesis	+	+	0
Metabolic capacity			
Respiration (electron transfer and cytochrome system)	+	+	0
Krebs (citrate) cycle	+	+	0§
Embden-Meyerhof pathway	+	+	+
Hexose monophosphate shunt	+	+	+
Cation transport	+	+	+
Amino acid transport	+	+	+
Lipid exchange	+	+	+
Catabolic capacity			
Fatty acid breakdown	+	+	0
Amino acid catabolism	+	+	0

*Excluding late polychromatophilic and orthochromic normoblasts.
†Mature red blood cell synthesizes glutathione (γ-glutamyl cysteinyl glycine).
‡Weak.
§Residual enzymes present (malate dehydrogenase, fumarase).

Table 12-2. Comparative metabolic activities of young and old erythrocytes

Metabolic activity	Change with age of erythrocyte
Metabolic capacity[15]	
Glycolysis	Decrease
Oxygen utilization	Decrease
Nucleoside utilization	Decrease
Enzyme activity[9,22,27,32]	
HK	Decrease
GPI	Decrease
PFK	No change
Aldolase	Decrease
TPI	Decrease
GAPD	Little change
PGK	Decrease
PK	Decrease
LDH	Decrease
ATPase	Decrease
G-6-PD	Decrease
6-PGD	Decrease
GSSG-R	No change
Catalase	Decrease
NADH-methemoglobin reductase	Decrease
RPK	Decrease
Acetylcholinesterase	Decrease
Glyoxalase	Decrease
Glutamic oxaloacetic transaminase	Decrease
Intracellular contents	
Water[68]	Decrease
Methemoglobin[14,25,76]	Decrease
Lipids[129-131]	Decrease
Electrolytes[68]	
Sodium	Increase
Potassium	Decrease
Magnesium	Decrease
2,3-Diphosphoglycerate (2,3-DPG)	Decrease
GSH	No change
Functional characteristics	
Oxygen affinity[49]	Increase
Cation transport[68]	Decrease
Deformability[80]	Decrease
Osmotic fragility[34]	Increase
Density[132]	Increase

tive phosphorylation. They are present in all blood and lymphoid cells with the exception of the mature erythrocyte, which is unable to carry out these processes. The mitochondrial inner membrane is a specialized structure peculiar to this organelle. Its integrity is essential to the link between respiration and oxidative phosphorylation and ATP generation.

The metabolic capacity of the reticulocyte far exceeds that of the erythrocyte.[13,24] The reticulocyte utilizes as energy substrates amino acids from plasma, stromal proteins derived from mitochondrial ribosomes and other sources, and acetyl CoA derived from fatty acids. Its rate of oxygen consumption and glucose utilization are 60 and 7.5 times that of mature erythrocytes. Through oxidative phosphorylation the reticulocyte is able to produce 120 to 200 µmoles of ATP/ml cells/hour. The rate of lactate production through the anaero-

bic Embden-Meyerhof pathway reaches peak values of 100 µmoles/ml cells/hour, an increase 30 times greater than that achieved in mature erythrocytes. The activities of the enzymes of the Embden-Meyerhof pathway in reticulocytes are increased, accounting for this increased flux of glucose. In fact, the increased catalytic activity of a number of glycolytic enzymes is an accurate indicator of cell age.[1,15,84,90,117] Significantly higher activities of the following enzymes of the Embden-Meyerhof pathway are seen in reticulocytes and young mature erythrocytes: HK, GPI, TPI, PGK, PK, and LDH. A complete listing of metabolic differences and changes in young and old cells is presented in Table 12-2.

The decay in activity of certain enzymes may be related to the presence and ultimate inactivation of sensitive sulfhydryl groups. HK G-6-PD, PK, and δ-amino levulinic acid synthetase, the rate-limiting enzyme of heme synthesis, are examples of key enzymes possessing sulfhydryl groups susceptible to oxidant denaturation.

Reticulocytes formed under stress may contain up to 25 mg RNA/mg cells, have a high rate of respiration, and have increased activity of mitochondrial enzymes.[35] As the reticulocyte matures its content of RNA declines. When the intrareticulocyte content of RNA reaches 2 mg/ml cells, a sharp decline in mitochondrial enzymes occurs coincident with the appearance of inhibitor F.[127] Residual but nonfunctional activity of certain mitochondrial enzymes that survive the degradation of mitochondria is found in mature erythrocytes (e.g., glutamic oxaloacetic transaminase, fumarase, and malate dehydrogenase). A comparison of the metabolic capacity and constituents of reticulocytes and mature red cells is presented in Table 12-3.

Freed of a nucleus, organelles, and a complicated biosynthetic and metabolic capacity, the mature erythrocyte is launched into the peripheral blood with simplified metabolic pathways that permit it to perform its function of gas transport and at the same time protect it against hostile endogenous and exogenous factors capable of shortening its survival. Unlike the reticulocyte, the erythrocyte lacks a renewal system to replenish depleted or denatured constituents. Actually the red cell begins its irreversible process of aging when it loses the capacity to synthesize DNA. The finite life span of the red blood cell is determined by the gradual but inevitable deterioration of key enzymes of the two pathways of glycolysis—the Embden-Meyerhof pathway with generation of ATP, 2,3-DPG, and NADH and the hexose monophosphate shunt with the generation of NADPH and GSH.

Glycolysis and the Embden-Meyerhof pathway[121]

The enzyme reactions of the Embden-Meyerhof pathway account for about 90% of glycolysis within the mature red blood cell and are illustrated in Fig. 12-1. Theoretically each mole of glucose entering the Embden-Meyerhof pathway yields 2 moles of lactate and a net of 2 moles of ATP. One mole of ATP is used to phosphorylate glucose in the HK reaction, and another is used to convert F-6-P to FDP in the PFK reaction. The latter hexose phosphate is split into two triose phosphates, Ga-3-P and DHAP, at the aldolase step. Thus 2 moles of ATP are generated in the PGK reaction and another 2 at the PK step. In addition to being the sole source of ATP generation in the erythrocyte, the Embden-Meyerhof pathway has two other key functions: first, the generation of 2,3-DPG through the DPG, or Rapoport-Luebering, cycle and, second, the generation of NADH at the GAPD step. This pyridine nucleotide is the primary cofactor for the enzymatic reduction of methemoglobin, a reaction catalyzed by NADH-dependent methemoglobin reductase.

Although the in vitro activities of the thirteen enzymes of the Embden-Meyerhof pathway have been quantified under optimal conditions (Table 12-4), it is impossible to determine from this information which steps are rate limiting, i.e., which enzyme reactions control glycolysis. Three orders of magnitude separate the enzyme with greatest activity (TPI) from HK, aldolase, and 2,3-DPGP, the enzymes with the lowest activity (Fig. 12-2).

A second method of evaluating glycolytic activity of erythrocytes is provided by the measurement of glycolytic intermediates and nucleotides in steady state conditions of temperature and pH.[8,102,103,140] Such determinations have provided critical information concerning the change in free energy at the various steps of glycolysis and, as a corollary, point out those reactions that control or regulate glycolysis. Normal values for these intermediates of glycolysis are provided in Table 12-5.

Table 12-3. Comparison of metabolic capacity and constituents of reticulocytes and erythrocytes

Constituent	Reticulocyte	Erythrocyte
RNA (mg/ml)	4-25	0.3
Hemoglobin (mg/ml)	200-300	330
Nonhemoglobin protein (mg/ml)	45	15
Lipid (mg/ml)	9	5
ATP (μmoles/ml cells)	3.0	1.0-1.5
Metabolic capacity		
Oxygen consumption (μmoles/ ml cells/hr)	25-70	0.4-1.2
Glucose utilization (μmoles/ml cells/hr)	11-15	1.5-2.0
Lactate production (μmoles/ml cells/hr)		
Aerobic	30	0
Anaerobic	100	3-4
ATP production (moles/mole glucose consumed)	38	2
Oxidative phosphorylation (μmoles/ml cells/hr)	120-200	0
Aerobic glycolysis (μmoles/ ml cells/hr)	0-30	0

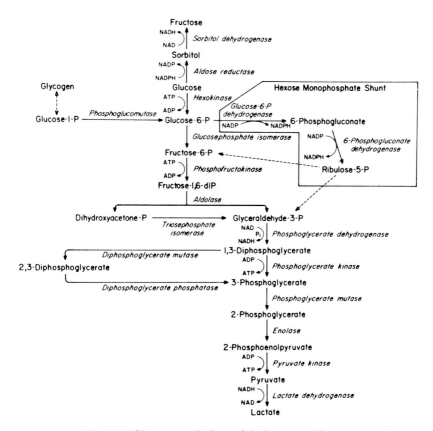

Fig. 12-1. Glucose metabolism of the human erythrocyte.

Table 12-4. Activities of glycolytic enzymes of the Embden-Meyerhof pathway

Enzyme	Mean activity			
	μmoles substrate/ hr/ml RBCs*	μmoles substrate/ hr/liter RBCs†	μmoles substrate/ min/10^{11} RBCs‡	μmoles substrate/ min/gm Hb
HK	5	10	1.7	0.6
GPI	151	900	89.0	28.4
PFK	82	200	24.8	12.6
Aldolase	31	40	5.0	3.2
TPI	5,100	16,000	2,160	1,441.0
GAPD	800	2,000	278	56.7
PGK	1,910	3,000	352	160.0
DPGM	—	20	1.1	—
DPGP	—	2	—	—
PGM	228	800	54.5	23.3
Enolase	95	200	19.5	7.6
PK	158	250	24.5	5.4
LDH	1,257	2,000	270	142.0

*Data from Chapman et al.[31]
†Data from Jacobasch et al.[74]
‡Data from Benöhr and Waller.[13]

Table 12-5. Concentration of glycolytic intermediates and adenine nucleotides of human erythrocytes

Intermediate	μmoles/liter RBCs
Glucose	5.0
G-6-P	38.5
F-6-P	15.7
FDP	7.0
DHAP	17.0
Ga-3-P	5.7
1,3-DPG	0.4
2,3-DPG	5,100
3-PG	68.5
2-PG	10.0
PEP	17.0
Pyruvate	85.0
Lactate	1,430
ATP	1,500
ADP	150
AMP	50
NAD/NADH	985
Pi	1,000

Yoshikawa and Minakami[165] have provided a useful model illustrating free energy changes in the glycolytic pathway (Fig. 12-3). The model is made of two water reservoirs representing glucose and ATP at one end and lactate and NAD at the other. A connecting pipe and stopcocks and manometers represent the glycolytic enzymes and their substrates and products, respectively. The differences in the water levels in the manometers correspond to the driving forces necessary for the reaction to proceed. Enzyme reactions that are at or near equilibrium (GPI, aldolase, TPI, GAPD, PGK, PGM, enolase, and LDH) show little change in free energy when the activity at that particular step is reduced. However, large pressure differences (large changes in free energy) are observed when the activities of HK, PFK, and PK are reduced (stopcock partially closed). These three enzymes catalyze irreversible reactions of glycolysis and are the control points or regulators of the overall flux of glycolysis.

By measuring changes in the concentrations of specific glycolytic intermediates in various steady state conditions, the so-called crossover plot (Fig. 12-4), and determining the responses of the regulatory enzymes to certain external effectors such as pH, temperature, inorganic phosphate (Pi), and allosteric effectors (2,3-DPG and adenine nucleotides), one can divide glycolysis into two main

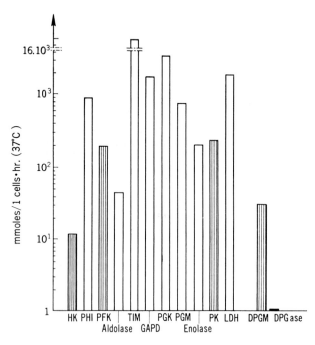

Fig. 12-2. Capacities of the glycolytic enzymes of the human erythrocyte. The shaded columns indicate enzymes that are not in thermodynamic equilibrium. (From Rapoport, S.: In Greenwalt, T. J., and Jamieson, G. A., eds.: The human red cell in vitro, New York, 1974, Grune & Stratton, Inc. Used by permission.)

units, the HK-PFK system and the PK-GAPD system.[121] The overall flux of glycolysis is determined by HK and PFK; the PK-GAPD system provides a coordinated control of the upper and lower sections of the glycolytic pathway. Thus rather than a multienzyme string proceeding inexorably from glucose to lactate, the Embden-Meyerhof pathway should be considered in terms of the key enzyme units that govern the activity of glycolysis, operate as functional units, and have similar actions, inhibitors, and effectors (Fig. 12-5).

HK-PFK system.[121] The control strength of HK is twice that of PFK at intracellular pH 7.2, most likely related to its initial position in the glycolytic chain and its low capacity. However, because of the greater sensitivity of PFK to a variety of activators and inhibitors, and the allosteric nature of these effectors, PFK exerts the greatest control over glycolytic flux. Positive effectors (activators) of PFK include the substrate F-6-P, the product FDP, the cofactor ADP, and the allosteric effectors K^+, NH_4^+, Pi, G-1,6-P, and

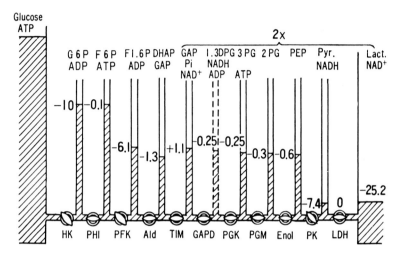

Fig. 12-3. Free energy changes in erythrocyte glycolysis. The values at the right side of columns are the free energy changes expressed as kcal/mole glucose. (From Yoshikawa, H., and Minakami, S.: Folia Haematol. **89:**357, 1968.)

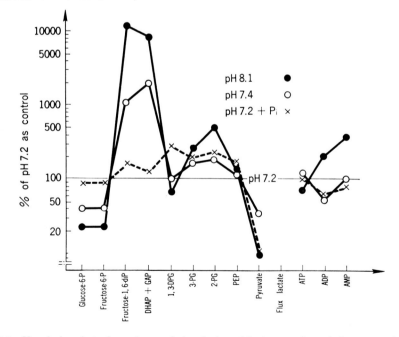

Fig. 12-4. pH and phosphate dependence of glycolysis and its intermediates in human erythrocytes at 37° C. The crossover at PFK and PK are shown. (From Jacobasch, G., et al.: In Yoshikawa, H., and Rapaport, S. M., eds.: Cellular and molecular biology of erythrocytes, Baltimore/Tokyo, 1974, University Park Press/University of Tokyo Press.)

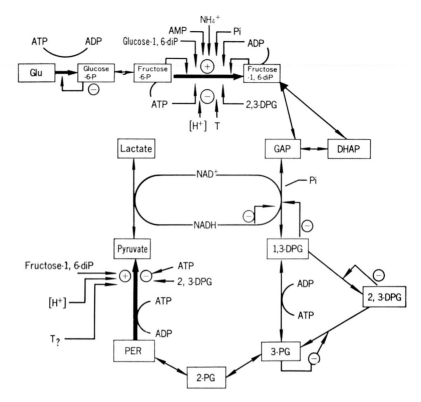

Fig. 12-5. Overall scheme of control of glycolysis. The influence of activators (+) and inhibitors (−) is shown. (From Jacobasch, G., et al.: In Yoshikawa, H., and Rapoport, S. M., eds.: Cellular and molecular biology of erythrocytes, Baltimore/Tokyo, 1974, University Park Press/University of Tokyo Press.)

AMP. Inhibitors or negative effectors include H[+], increasing temperature, ATP-Mg complex, 2,3-DPG, PEP, and citrate. When HK is activated G-6-P and F-6-P increase, and when PFK is activated these metabolites decrease.

The reciprocal relationship of substrates and products as activators and inhibitors of glycolysis is best exemplified in the HK-PFK system. G-6-P inhibits HK in a competitive manner to ATP; F-6-P, the product of HK, increases the activity of PFK competitively to ATP. A decline in the concentrations of F-6-P and G-6-P relieves the product inhibition on HK. Whereas ATP (as a complex of Mg-ATP) increases the activity of HK, it inhibits PFK.

Glycolysis is initially affected by changes in intracellular pH and Pi.[102,133] Increasing the pH increases glycolysis, and a decrease of pH lowers the rate of glycolysis. PFK is most sensitive to changes in the concentration of hydrogen ions and is markedly inhibited below pH 7.40.[111] A raised level of Pi also stimulates the PFK reaction by overcoming the inhibitory effects of ATP. Temperature also affects the activity of PFK.[65]

Two final external signals of glycolysis exerting their effects in the HK-PFK system are magnesium and 2,3-DPG. Magnesium deficiency results in a lowered glycolytic rate by decreasing the availability of the Mg-ATP complex required at the HK step.[73] A direct inhibitory effect of 2,3-DPG is exerted on both HK and PFK. This intermediate also regulates glycolysis by decreasing intracellular pH and inhibiting the PFK reaction.

PK-GAPD system.[121] The PK-GAPD system appears to regulate the middle and lower portions of glycolysis and the flux of glycolysis between the Embden-Meyerhof pathway and the Rapoport-Luebering cycle. It is most dependent on changes in intracellular pH. PK shares many of the kinetic properties of PFK. It is competitively inhibited by ATP and by 2,3-DPG. Unlike PFK, PK is inhibited by increased pH and Pi. Normally the PFK:PK ratio is 1; the higher the ratio, as in hereditary hemolytic anemia with PK deficiency, the higher the level of 2,3-DPG.

The allosteric effector FDP increases the activity of PK by increasing the affinity of the enzyme for its substrates PEP and Mg-ADP. The product of the PK reaction, pyruvate, is converted to lactate by LDH, a step requiring NADH as cofactor. The NAD generated in this step is a cofactor in the GADP reaction. The NAD:NADH ratio in the red blood cell is about 1,000. Decreased availability of NAD inhibits the GAPD

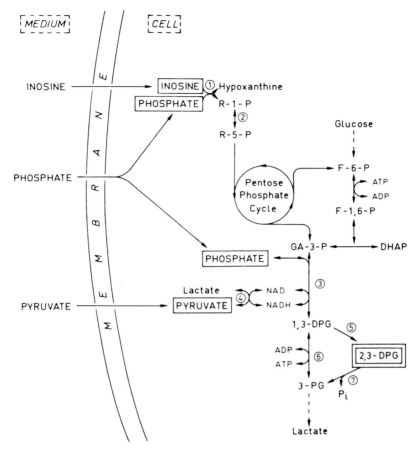

Fig. 12-6. Sequence of reactions involved in the formation of 2,3-DPG from inosine, pyruvate, and phosphate: ① purine nucleoside phosphorylase, ② phosphoribomutase, ③ Ga-3-P dehydrogenase, ④ LDH, ⑤ DPGM, ⑥ PGM, ⑦ 2,3-DPGP. (From Duhm, J., and Gerlach, E.: In Greenwalt, T. J., and Jamieson, G. A., eds.: The human red cell in vitro, New York, 1974, Grune & Stratton, Inc. Used by permission.)

reaction, resulting in an accumulation of FDP and triose phosphates (Ga-3-P and DHAP).

Rapoport-Luebering (2,3-DPG) shunt.[46,125] An important alternate pathway of glycolysis is the Rapoport-Luebering shunt, in which 2,3-DPG is synthesized from 1,3-DPG by the enzyme 2,3-DPGM and catabolized to 3-PG by 2,3-DPGP. Approximately one tenth to one quarter of glycolysis flows through the 2,3-DPG shunt.[45,139] If the flow of glycolysis is through the 2,3-DPG shunt, the production of ATP at the PGK step would be bypassed and no net synthesis of ATP would occur. The regulation of the 2,3-DPG shunt is determined by the ratio of activity of PFK:PK. The higher the PFK:PK ratio, the more 2,3-DPG formed.[145] Increased intracellular pH and increased concentrations of 1,3-DPG favor the production of 2,3-DPG.

The concentration of 1,3-DPG, in turn, is governed by the concerted actions of PFK, GAPD, PGK, and PK, but the exact kinetics and control mechanisms of the 2,3-DPG mutase reaction have

not been worked out.[134] The concentration of 2,3-DPG controls its own synthesis by exerting feedback inhibition on 2,3-DPGM. However, extremely high concentrations of 2,3-DPG are required to inhibit the mutase step. If an increasing concentration of 1,3-DPG parallels the increase in 2,3-DPG, 2,3-DPGM is not inhibited. In the presence of inosine, pyruvate, and phosphate (Fig. 12-6) large amounts of 2,3-DPG can be synthesized in normal cells or in cells depleted of 2,3-DPG by in vitro storage.[39,91] Inosine is converted to R-5-P in the hexose monophosphate shunt and enters the Embden-Meyerhof pathway at Ga-3-P and F-6-P. Phosphate stimulates the formation of R-5-P and and the conversion of triose phosphate to 1,3-DPG. Pyruvate mediates the oxidation of NADH to NAD, providing pyridine cofactor for the GADP reaction and the generation of substrate for 2,3-DPGM.

The binding of free 2,3-DPG to deoxyhemoglobin, thus relieving the feedback inhibition on 2,3-DPGM, particularly in hypoxia, appears to play a relatively minor role in controlling the production of 2,3-DPG.[5,46] At physiologic levels of 2,3-DPG the inhibition of 2,3-DPGM is 99%; thus the enzyme is working at only 1% of its potential capacity.

The intracellular concentration of 2,3-DPG exerts a control over glycolysis in general. An increased concentration of 2,3-DPG results in decreased intracellular pH.[38] This occurs because an increase in 2,3-DPG results in an intracellular increase in negative charge. The 2,3-DPG molecule, which carries at least four negative charges under physiologic conditions, cannot penetrate the red cell membrane. The Donnan equilibrium of penetrating anions and hydrogen ions is upset, choride ions exit, hydrogen ions from the plasma enter, and intracellular pH declines. The decrease of intracellular pH amounts to 0.017 pH units/μmole 2,3-DPG. Similarly each 400-μmole increase in 2,3-DPG increases the P_{50} of hemoglobin by 1 mm Hg, shifting the oxygen dissociation curve to the right and decreasing the oxygen affinity of hemoglobin.[28] Erythrocyte enzymes inhibited by 2,3-DPG are listed here:

A. Embden-Meyerhof pathway
   1. HK[16,23]
   2. GPI[4]
   3. PFK[19,148]
4. DPGM[134]
5. PGK[113]
6. PK[113]
B. Hexose monophosphate pathway: transaldolase-transketolase[41]
C. Purine nucleotide pathway
   1. RPK[67]
   2. HGPRT[163]
   3. APRT[163]
   4. Adenylate deaminase[6]

In addition to modulating intracellular pH and glycolysis, the major function of 2,3-DPG is to reduce the oxygen affinity of hemoglobin (Fig. 12-7). This is accomplished by three distinct mechanisms: (1) a direct effect of 2,3-DPG on combining with and stabilizing the deoxy conformation of hemoglobin[55,112]; (2) the effect of 2,3-DPG on the Bohr coefficient ($\Delta \log P_{50}/\Delta pH$) operating independent of its effect on lowering intracellular pH; and (3) the 2,3-DPG-induced decrease of intracellular pH, which in turn decreases the oxygen affinity of hemoglobin because of the Bohr effect.

The activity of the enzyme that degrades 2,3-DPG, 2,3-DPGP, has the lowest measurable activity of any glycolytic enzyme; it is 300 to 500 times less active than 2,3-DPGM.[63,64,135] Intracellular acidosis and phosphate ions stimulate the enzyme. Various inorganic sulfur compounds

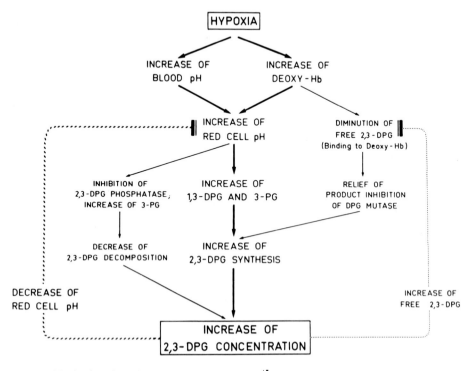

Fig. 12-7. Mechanism inducing ($\rightarrow$) and limiting ($-\,\|$) changes of 2,3-DPG concentration in red blood cells in hypoxia and alkalosis. (From Duhm, J., and Gerlach, E.: In Greenwalt, T. J., and Jamieson, G. A., eds.: The human red cell in vitro, New York, 1974, Grune & Stratton, Inc. Used by permission.)

either inhibit[88] (sulfate and thiosulfate) or activate[66] (disulfate) the enzyme but may not be of physiologic significance in normal circumstances. It appears that the levels of 2,3-DPG are controlled by synthetic rather than by degradative steps and that the rate of degradation of 2,3-DPG assumes greater importance only when the phosphatase is strongly activated or when the synthetic rate is reduced.

ATP and the adenine nucleotides. Assuming a glycolytic rate of 1.5 μmoles of glucose/liter of cells/hour, 3 μmoles of ATP are produced in steady state conditions. About 90% of the adenine nucleotides in the red cell are in the form of ATP, with 8% and 2% as ADP and AMP, respectively. The free energy change associated with the formation of two moles of ATP from the metabolism of one mole of glucose amounts to 50% of the total change in free energy for glycolysis. About one third of the ATP formed is utilized in active cation transport; part of the remaining two thirds is dissipated in the 2,3-DPG shunt, but the fate of the remainder is uncertain.

In addition to its participation in the transport of Na[+] and K[+],[56] ATP has several other important roles.[107] These include (1) functioning as a substrate and effector of the three regulatory reactions of glycolysis—HK, PFK, and PK; (2) par-

ticipating in the initial phosphorylation of glucose; (3) involvement in the maintenance of the normal biconcave shape of the red cell; (4) preservation of the deformability of the red cell through the ability to chelate calcium and serve as the energy source for calcium-ATPase, which actively extrudes calcium from the cell; (5) serving as a cofactor in the synthesis of GSH; (6) binding to deoxyhemoglobin, thus reducing the oxygen affinity of hemoglobin; (7) participation in the synthesis of purine and pyridine nucleotides; and (8) participation in lipid transport.

Metabolic defects associated with perturbations of glycolysis caused by inherited deficiencies of glycolytic enzymes often result in decreased ATP synthesis or increased ATP utilization. The common final pathway of erythrocyte destruction in these deficiency diseases may be related to a deficiency of ATP and concomitant alterations in membrane, hemoglobin, or metabolic function. The final result—a rigid, nondeformable erythrocyte—would be trapped in the microcirculation of the reticuloendothelial system, particularly the spleen, liver, and bone marrow. Stasis, acidosis, and hypoxia with inhibition of glycolytic activity and oxidative phosphorylation in reticulocytes and progression of membrane dysfunction would enhance the premature destruction of intrinsically

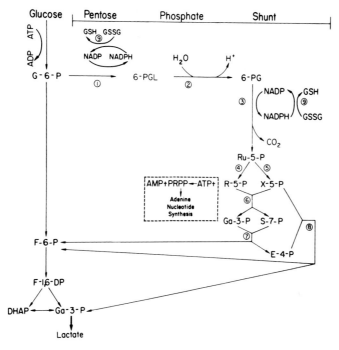

Fig. 12-8. The pentose shunt. Reactions are drawn unidirectionally although many are reversible. Circled numbers refer to the following enzymes: ① G-6-PD, ② 6-phosphogluconolactonase (or lactonase), ③ 6-phosphogluconate dehydrogenase, ④ X-5-P epimerase, ⑤ R-5-P isomerase, ⑥ transketolase, ⑦ transaldolase, ⑧ transketolase (same as ⑥), ⑨ GSSG-R. (From Eaton, J. W., and Brewer, G. J.: In Surgenor, D. M., ed.: The red cell, vol. 1, ed. 2, New York, 1974, Academic Press, Inc.)

abnormal cells whose metabolic handicaps are incapable of tolerating further stress.

Hexose monophosphate shunt[48,83]

The primary functions of the hexose monophosphate shunt are the generation of NADPH, the reduction of GSSG, and the formation of building blocks required for the synthesis of adenine nucleotides. Although the hexose monophosphate pathway accounts for less than 10% of glycolytic flux under physiologic conditions, it protects the sulfhydryl-containing proteins of the red cell (hemoglobin, enzymes, and membrane) against oxidative denaturation. The key enzyme reactions of the hexose monophosphate shunt are presented in Fig. 12-8. The reduction of NADP occurs at the initial and most important step of the hexose monophosphate shunt, G-6-PD, and again at the 6-PGD step in which 6-PG is converted to Ru-5-P, the only reaction occurring within the mature red blood cell in which oxygen is required and carbon dioxide is generated. Through a series of reactions involving pentose isomerase, epimerase, transaldolase, and transketolase, pentose phosphates are converted into F-6-P and Ga-3-P, which reenter the Embden-Meyerhof pathway and then are metabolized to lactate. For every 3 moles of pentose sugar metabolized through the hexose monophosphate shunt via the transketolase and transaldolase reactions, 2 moles of F-6-P and 1 mole of Ga-3-P and a net yield of 5 moles of ATP will be produced. Quantitative aspects of the hexose monophosphate shunt are presented in Table 12-6.

Table 12-6. Quantitative aspects of hexose monophosphate shunt

	Values
Total glucose consumption	2 μmoles/ml cells/hr
Hexose monophosphate glycolysis	0.2 μmoles/ml cells/hr
O_2 consumption	0.3-0.4 μmoles/ml cells/hr
H_2O_2 formation	0.4 moles/ml cells/hr
H_2O_2 concentration	0.1 μM
GSH concentration	2-3 mM
Enzymes	
G-6-PD	90-150 μmoles/ml cells/hr
6-PGD	45-90 μmoles/ml cells/hr
Transaldolase	40 μmoles/gm Hb/hr
Transketolase	2.7-6.9 μmoles/ml cells/hr
GSSG-R	60-175 μmoles/ml cells/hr
GSH-P	60-146 μmoles/ml cells/hr*
Catalase	3,200-7,500 $\times 10^3$ μmoles/ml cells/hr
γ-GC synthetase	8.1 μmoles/ml cells/hr
GSH synthetase	2.4 μmoles/ml cells/hr

*Decreased in premature and newborn infants.

Alternatively F-6-P can be converted to G-6-P by GPI and be recycled through the hexose monophosphate shunt. Using ^{14}C-glucose, it has been clearly demonstrated that the $^{14}CO_2$ generated in glycolytic flux through the hexose monophosphate shunt arose from the C-1 or C-2 position of glucose, with the recovery of C2 as $^{14}CO_2$ amounting to about half that from C-1-labeled glucose. Normally $^{14}CO_2$ evolution from ^{14}C-1 amounts to 0.044 to 0.062 μmoles/ml cells/hr. Following stimulation with agents such as methylene blue and other oxidant stresses, a twenty-five-fold increase in $^{14}CO_2$ evolution occurs.[106] Thus glucose-carbon labeled in several positions provides information about total hexose monophosphate shunt activity, (^{14}C-1), recycling activity (^{14}C-2), and Krebs cycle or mitochondrial activity in reticulocytes (^{14}C-6).

The NADPH generated in the hexose monophosphate shunt is utilized by the erythrocyte to reduce GSSG at the GSSG-R step. Hydrogen peroxide, the product of metabolic oxidant stress, is reduced to water by GSH, a reaction catalyzed by GSH-P, GSH itself being oxidized to GSSG. The NADPH generated in the reactions of G-6-PD and 6-PGD is utilized by the red cell to reduce GSSG at the GSSG-R step; NADP, the product of this reaction, in turn stimulates the activity of the hexose monophosphate shunt. Although catalase is also capable of detoxifying hydrogen peroxide, the contribution of GSH-P predominates at the low concentrations of hydrogen peroxide (0.1 μM) found within the red blood cell.* Unlike catalase, GSH-P reacts not only with hydrogen peroxide but also with lipid peroxide, another product of auto-oxidation that may be deleterious to cell survival. The relatively minor protective role of catalase is exemplified in patients with acatalasia who have neither hemolytic anemia nor increased sensitivity to peroxides.[144] Increased activity of the hexose monophosphate shunt in these patients may be the result of the increased activity of the GSH-P–GSSG-R systems, which result in increased amounts of NADP and GSSG, both of which stimulate the hexose monophosphate shunt.[96] Furthermore, NADPH is required to reactivate catalase after it complexes with and reduces hydrogen peroxide. Inactivation of catalase secondary to depletion of NADPH, related to decreased activity of G-6-PD, will shunt removal of peroxides through GSH-P.[47] This accounts for double jeopardy of the G-6-PD-deficient red blood cell—decreased NADPH available for the regeneration of GSH *and* for the reactivation of catalase.

Other factors that regulate the activity of the hexose monophosphate shunt are listed in Table

*References 99, 100, 108, 126.

12-7. Conditions that inhibit HK (decreased ATP and increased G-6-P) are stimulatory. The pH optimum of the HMP shunt is lower than that of the Embden-Meyerhof pathway, the latter being much more severely inhibited at pH 7.4 or less. There are further links between the two pathways. DPG inhibits not only HK but also transaldolase and transketolase. The hexose monophosphate shunt bypasses the upper half of the Embden-Meyerhof pathway, particularly the control point, PFK, and supplies substrate for the synthesis of 2,3-DPG. Decreased hexose monophosphate shunt activity is associated with increased methemoglobin formation, increased utilization of NADH through NADH-methemoglobin reductase, an increased ratio of NAD:NADH, increased activity of GAPD, increased 1,3-DPG, and ultimately increased synthesis of 2,3-DPG.

Glutathione (GSH) metabolism[17,94]

GSH is a tripeptide composed of γ-glutamic acid, cysteine, and glycine. Its concentration in the mature red cell is about 3 mM (60 to 90 mg/dl red blood cells). GSH is actively synthesized by the mature red cell in a two-step, ATP- and Mg^{++}-dependent process: The first enzyme is γ-glutamyl-cysteine synthetase, and the second is glutathione synthetase.[71,87,104] GSH has a number of critical functions within the red cell.[40] Under conditions of severe oxidative challenge, reactions occur involving hemoglobin, membrane proteins, and enzymes with highly sensitive sulfhydryl groups such as HK, GAPD, and PK. Glutathione disulfide itself inhibits the activities of HK, PFK,

Table 12-7. Regulatory factors of the hexose monophosphate shunt*

	Activators	Inhibitors
NADP	↑	↓
NADPH	↓	↑
GSSG	↑	↓
Catalase	↓	↑
Oxygen	↑	↓
ATP	↓	↑
G-6-P	↑	↓
Ascorbic acid	↑	↓
Mg^{++}	↑	↓
2,3-DPG	↓	↑
FAD	↑	↓
Thiamine	↑	↓

*Modified from Davidson, W. D., and Tanaka, K. R.: Br. J. Haemotol. 23:271, 1972.

G-6-PD, and 6-PGD in hemolysates of red cells from newborns and adults.[162] The depletion of intracellular GSH results in irreversible mixed disulfide formation between hemoglobin and GSH and the accumulation of insoluble denatured hemoglobin.[149,161] Other pathophysiologic effects include increased formation of lipid peroxides,[42] increased membrane permeability,[71] accelerated utilization of ATP, decreased deformability secondary to ATP depletion and Heinz body formation,[2] and splenic sequestration.[58,72]

Of less importance in the red cell, GSH functions as a coenzyme in the glyoxalase reactions that convert methylglyoxal to lactic acid. The biologic significance of these reactions is uncertain, although there is evidence suggesting that methylglyoxal is toxic and inhibits cell growth by interfering with protein synthesis. An inherited deficiency of glyoxalase II with coincidental hereditary elliptocytosis has been reported, but the isolated defect itself is not associated with hemolytic anemia.[154]

The rapid turnover time of GSH (half-life of 4 days) and the fact that the red cell contains only half as many molecules of GSH as of hemoglobin require that the red cell be capable of de novo synthesis of GSH and rapidly converting glutathione disulfide (GSSG) to GSH. GSSG not reduced to GSH by GSSG-R is either actively transported out of the erythrocyte in pathologic states[79] or is broken down by γ-glutamyl transpeptidase cyclotransferase of the γ-glutamyl cycle into 5-oxoproline under normal conditions.[93,110] Lacking oxoprolinase, however, the human red cell is incapable of reutilizing catabolized GSH for its own de novo synthesis.

Metabolism of adenine and pyridine nucleotides

A characteristic feature of the human red cell is the constant degradation and formation of adenine and pyridine nucleotides.[21,85] Lacking de novo synthesis of purines,[20,86] the mature erythrocyte utilizes the salvage pathway (Fig. 12-9) to synthesize AMP from either adenine or adenosine (reactions 2 and 10, respectively). A pentose phosphate of great biologic significance and of particular importance in the metabolism of purines is PRPP, formed from R-5-P generated by the hexose monophosphate shunt, and ATP, arising from the glycolytic activity of the Embden-Meyerhof pathway. This step (reaction 1, Fig. 12-7) is catalyzed by RPK. The ubiquitous 2,3-DPG inhibits four enzymes involved in purine nucleotide metabolism: RPK,[67] APRT,[66,81] HGPRT, and ADA[98] (reactions 1, 2, 5, and 9, respectively, in Fig. 12-9). The enzyme HGPRT is deficient in the Lesch-Nyhan syndrome and its assay in the readily

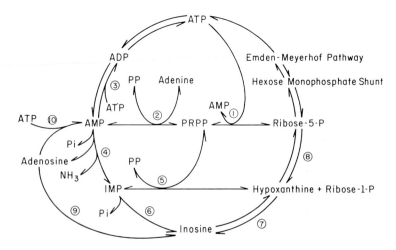

Fig. 12-9. Purine and adenine nucleotide metabolism in the red blood cell. Numbered reactions are as follows: ① RPK, ② APRT, ③ AK, ④ adenylate deaminase, ⑤ HGPRT, ⑥ nucleotidase, ⑦ nucleoside phosphorylase, ⑧ phosphoribomutase, ⑨ ADA, ⑩ AK.

accessible erythrocyte is an excellent diagnostic tool. A second key function of PRPP is as a cofactor in the synthesis of NAD.[119]

In addition to its formation in the Embden-Meyerhof pathway, ADP is generated by the action of AK (reaction 3, Fig. 12-9) in which AMP and ATP are converted to 2 moles of ADP.

Other enzymes and enzyme pathways

A number of other minor metabolic pathways will be mentioned only briefly.

Galactose pathway. The red cell is able to utilize galactose through the galactose pathway.[70] G-1-P formed from galactose-1-phosphate can be converted to G-6-P, which then enters the Embden-Meyerhof pathway or the hexose monophosphate shunt. An alternate pathway of metabolism for galactose-1-phosphate or G-1-P is the penitol pathway in which nonphosphorylated intermediates (glucuronate, gulonate, and xylitol) are formed, followed by final phosphorylation of D-xylulose to D-xylulose-5-phosphate and reentry into the hexose monophosphate shunt. The penitol pathway[69] functions as a source of NADH and NADP, the former available for the reduction of methemoglobin and the latter to stimulate the hexose monophosphate shunt.

Polyol (sorbitol) pathway. The polyol (sorbitol) pathway[152] of the red cell is activated in the presence of large amounts of glucose. The reactions of this system involve an NADPH-dependent aldose reductase that reduces glucose to sorbitol and the subsequent oxidation of sorbitol to D-fructose. Increased activity of the polyol pathway, a result of hyperglycemia, produces increased ratios of NADP:NADPH and NADH:NAD. Normally about 3% of glucose uptake is utilized for

the synthesis of sorbitol and fructose. With a tenfold increase in the concentration of glucose, the polyol pathway can account for 11% of glucose metabolism.

ATPase.[114,115,166] The ATPase system is tightly bound to the red cell membrane and is discussed in greater detail in Chapter 11. In these reactions ATP serves as the energy source for cation transport and for the maintenance of the biconcave disc shape and membrane deformability. Against gradients, sodium is extruded and potassium is pumped into erythrocytes, maintaining the intracellular conditions high in potassium and low in sodium.

The major ATPase (S-ATPase) is inhibited by cardiac glycosides such as ouabain, is stimulated by sodium and potassium, and is dependent on Mg^{++}. Of the total ATPase in the red cell, about 45% is sensitive to ouabain. The ouabain-insensitive ATPase (I-ATPase) is stimulated by Ca^{++} and Mg^{++} and is responsible for the maintenance of cell shape and membrane deformability.

Carbonic anhydrase. Carbonic anhydrase is a zinc metalloenzyme that is important in the physiologic transport of carbon dioxide. In the tissues the enzyme catalyzes the hydration of CO_2 to H_2CO_3, which then dissociates to HCO_3^-; the reverse reaction occurs in the lungs. Two carbonic anhydrase fractions designated B and C (I and II) can be readily seen in starch gel electrophoretic patterns of human red cell lysates stained for proteins.

Both isoenzymes are lower in infancy and reach their adult intensity at the second to third year of life. Even lower enzyme activity has been found in blood from premature infants.[109] Results of assay showed that normal full-term newborn infants had

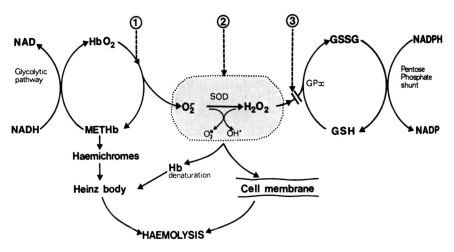

Fig. 12-10. Interrelationship of metabolism of activated oxygen and hemolysis. The production and reduction of activated oxygen (stippled area) is linked to the glycolytic and pentose phosphate pathways. The numbers indicate the mode of action of the hemolytic factors listed in Table 12-9. The processes on the left, as well as giving rise to activated oxygen, will also cause formation of hemichromes and Heinz bodies. The accumulation of activated oxygen can cause hemolysis in two ways: (1) direct oxidation of cell membrane and (2) hemoglobin denaturation and Heinz body formation. (From Carrell, R. W., Winterbourn, C. C., and Rachmilewitz, E. A.: Br. J. Haematol. **30**:259, 1975.)

approximately 25% of the enzymatic activity of adults. Premature infants without and with the respiratory distress syndrome had 12% and 5% of adult activity, respectively.[77] The reasons for the decreased activity of carbonic anhydrase in infants with respiratory distress are not clear. Zinc deficiency itself cannot explain the low enzyme activity in infants with the syndrome. Carbonic anhydrase is markedly elevated in red cells from patients with megaloblastic anemia secondary to vitamin B_{12} deficiency and is probably elevated in patients with folic acid deficiency.[156] The activity is reduced in patients with juvenile chronic granulocytic leukemia and thyrotoxicosis and is elevated in hypothyroidism, returning to normal after treatment.

Acetylcholinesterase. The presence or absence of acelytcholinesterase, a membrane-bound enzyme, serves more as a marker for pathologic states of erythropoiesis than it does for any known function. Decreased amounts of acetylcholinesterase have been found in fetal and newborn erythrocytes, in hemolytic disease of the newborn caused by ABO incompatibility, in paroxysmal nocturnal hemoglobinuria,[7] and as an inherited deficiency without apparent adverse effect on red blood cell function and metabolism.[75]

Superoxide dismutase. Superoxide dismutase (SOD), or *erythrocuprein,* is a zinc- and copper-containing metalloenzyme first discovered in bovine erythrocytes. It converts two molecules of superoxide anion, O_2^- to hydrogen peroxide and

Table 12-8. Potential causes of oxidative hemolysis by activated oxygen

Increased formation	*Decreased protection*
1. Via hemoglobin	3. Deficiencies of
Thalassemia syndromes	G-6-PD
	6-PGD
Unstable hemoglobins	GSH-P[54]
Oxidant drugs	GSSG-R
Heat	γ-Glutamyl cysteine synthetase
Metal ions (Fe^{++}, Ca^{++})	GSH synthetase
2. Direct	Catalase
Radiation	Superoxide dismutase
Oxygen exposure	
Free porphyrin	Vitamin E[147]

*From Carrell, R. W., Winterboun, C. C., and Rachmilewitz, E. A.: Br. J. Haematol. **30**:259, 1975.

oxygen.[91] (Free radicals possess a highly reactive unpaired electron, which is represented by the symbol ·, as in O_2^- superoxide radical.)

$$O_2^- + O_2^- + 2H^+ \xrightarrow{\text{SOD}} H_2O_2 + O_2$$

The superoxide radical, a highly reactive species of activated oxygen, is a toxic agent that is capable of initiating chain reactions that induce denaturation of hemoglobin,[53,58] peroxidation of membrane lipids, and eventual hemolysis. In the absence of SOD-induced conversion to H_2O_2 and eventual removal of H_2O_2 by the GSH-P and catalase systems, superoxide radicals can undergo two spontaneous reactions with the formation of two other potentially destructive forms of activated oxygen, singlet oxygen $(O_2*)*$ and hydroxyl radical $(OH^·)$:

$$O_2^- + O_2^- + 2H^+ \rightleftharpoons H_2O_2 + O_2*$$

$$O_2^- + H_2O_2 \rightleftharpoons OH^· + OH^- + O_2$$

Under physiologic conditions small amounts of activated oxygen in the form of superoxide radical are formed spontaneously by the red cell in the conversion of hemoglobin to methemoglobin.[105,158] Other sources are the exposure of hemoglobin to heavy metals such as iron and copper, heat, ultraviolet and ionizing radiation, hyperbaric oxygen, and oxidant drugs.[29] Inherited hematologic conditions may be associated with either increased production of activated oxygen (thalassemia syndromes, unstable hemoglobin, and hemolytic anemias) or decreased ability to remove activated oxygen and H_2O_2 (deficiencies of the enzymes of the hexose monophosphate shunt, catalase, and vitamin E) (Fig. 12-10 and Table 12-8).

LABORATORY EVALUATION OF INHERITED METABOLIC DISORDERS OF RED CELLS

The general laboratory features of hemolytic anemia are discussed in Chapter 9. A comprehensive approach to the laboratory evaluation of hereditary hemolytic anemias caused by deficiencies of red cell enzymes requires the performance of general, nonspecific tests including measurements of red cell indices, reticulocyte count, careful examination of the peripheral blood smear and bone marrow, and determination of bilirubin and haptoglobin levels.[174,176,179] The Coombs test, hemoglobin electrophoresis, and osmotic fragility curves are usually normal in patients with uncomplicated enzymopathies, although cases of autoimmune hemolytic anemia, hemoglobinopathies, or membrane defects in association with enzymopathies have been reported.

In 1954 Selwyn and Dacie described the autohemolysis test, which helped to classify further a group of atypical congenital hemolytic anemias.[172,184] When defibrinated blood is incubated under aseptic conditions for 48 hours at 37° C, with or without nutrient additives (saline, glucose, or neutralized ATP), the degree and correction of hemolysis follow patterns that aid in differentiating some of the hereditary hemolytic anemias. With normal blood autohemolysis in saline is less than 3.5%; with additives hemolysis is usually less than 1.0%. Whereas the addition of glucose corrected the increased autohemolysis in some patients with congenital hemolytic anemia (type I), glucose had no effect or even increased the autohemolysis in other patients, in whom neutralized ATP corrected the autohemolysis (type II). Subsequently patients with the type II pattern were found to have PK deficiency. Severe autoimmune hemolytic anemia associated with spherocytosis also shows a type II pattern. Type I patterns of autohemolysis have been observed in most other enzyme disorders including deficiencies of G-6-PD, HK, GPI, TPI, and PGK. A type I pattern has been observed in hereditary spherocytosis, hereditary stomatocytosis, the unstable hemoglobin hemolytic anemias, and paroxysmal nocturnal hemoglobinuria (Table 12-9). This test must be performed meticulously and with normal controls. It must be cautioned that the test is nonspecific and that exceptions to these patterns have been reported in individual cases. As a general screening test of enzymopathies, it has been replaced by more specific determinations of enzymes and intermediates in most laboratories. Generally, however, a type II pattern is fairly specific for PK deficiency; a type I pattern merely indicates the presence of some metabolic abnormality, whether of enzyme, membrane, or hemoglobin.

A number of simple, reliable, and inexpensive screening tests for G-6-PD deficiency are available.* The principle of most of the tests depends on the failure of the G-6-PD-deficient erythrocytes to generate NADPH. In normal red cells, the NADPH would (1) reduce dyes such as brilliant cresyl blue to a colorless state or tetrazolium to a purple formazan,[175] (2) reduce methemoglobin,[171] or (3) produce fluorescence.[170] The ascorbate-cyanide test of Jacob and Jandl,[177] originally designed to detect G-6-PD deficiency, is not specific and may be abnormal in deficiencies of GSH-P, GSSG-R, and PK and in Hb Köln disease.[174] In addition to their usefulness in G-6-PD deficiency, fluorescent screening procedures have been developed for PK and GSSG-R deficiencies.[168]

Excellent and simplified spectrophotometric methods are now available for the specific assay of the enzymes of the Embden-Meyerhof pathway and the hexose monophosphate shunt.[169,190] The glycolytic enzymes in red cells anticoagulated with heparin are fairly stable for 3 weeks when stored at 4° C. Their assay requires carefully prepared, leukocyte-free hemolysates and an accurate and preferably automated instrument. The principle of the assays is based on the linked reduction or oxidation of pyridine nucleotides and the resultant in-

---

*Asterisk represents the excited reactive state of a molecule, e.g., O_2* for singlet oxygen.

*References 167, 168, 170, 173, 177, 182, 185, 187.

Table 12-9. Autohemolysis patterns in various hemolytic disorders

Diagnosis	Degree of hemolysis*			Pattern
	Saline	Glucose	ATP	
Normal red blood cells	3.5%	1.0%	1.0%	Normal
Hereditary spherocytosis	↑	Marked ↓	Marked ↓	I
G-6-PD deficiency	Normal or slight ↑	Slight to moderate ↓	Slight to moderate ↓	I
HK deficiency†	Slight ↑	Marked ↓	Marked ↓	I
PK deficiency	Moderate ↑	Moderate ↑	Marked ↓	II
Autoimmune hemolytic anemia	↑	Variable	Marked ↓	II

*↑, Increased above normal; ↓, correction to normal.

†Also GPI and PGK deficiencies, unstable hemoglobinopathies, and paroxysmal nocturnal hemoglobinuria; TPI is completely corrected with glucose and ATP.

crease or decrease in absorbency, respectively. Controlled assay conditions—constant pH, temperature, and concentrations of substrates and cofactors—are essential for meaningful and reproducible results. Because of the heterogeneity of many enzymopathies, particularly those caused by deficiencies of G-6-PD and PK,[183] partial purification and determination of maximal activity, Michaelis constants (K_m), inhibitor constants, (K_i), utilization of substrate analogs, pH optima, thermal stability, and electrophoretic migration may be required to distinguish one mutant from another.

The measurement of glycolytic intermediates[180,181,186] and of adenine nucleotides[188,190] provides a dynamic approach to the evaluation of erythrocyte metabolism and glycolytic flux. In steady state conditions a more meaningful simulation of in vivo events can be obtained by evaluating crossover points (p. 318). Intermediates proximal to the enzymatic block are increased above the normal equilibrium concentration and those distal to the defective step are decreased below the normal equilibrium concentration. It must be emphasized that in vitro assays of glycolytic enzymes prepared from erythrocyte lysates are performed under idealized conditions that may bear little resemblance to the actual intracellular concentrations of substrates, products, activators, and inhibitors of other enzymes in the pathway under investigation.[178] Quantification of glycolytic intermediates circumvents the relative artificiality of static enzyme assays.

There are other drawbacks of the in vitro evaluation of erythrocyte metabolism in hereditary hemolytic anemias. First, only the most viable cells are available for assay, since the most deranged are rapidly removed from the circulation. Despite measurements of enzyme activity in this "fittest" population, it is still possible to detect abnormalities. Second, since enzyme activity is often increased in younger cells, particularly in reticulocytes, levels of a "deficient" glycolytic enzyme may fall in the low normal or heterozygote range. Presumptive evidence for a true deficiency may be gained if the enzyme activity is not commensurate with the youth of the cell population. The simultaneous assay of enzyme activity in red cells of control patients with reticulocytosis or the quantitative assay of enzyme activity in young and old cells obtained by density sedimentation or centrifugation helps to circumvent this dilemma. Third, patients with severe hemolytic anemia may require transfusion therapy before diagnostic tests can be performed. If this occurs, definitive studies should be delayed until the transfused cells have left the circulation (2 to 3 months). Fourth, certain mutant enzymes may show nearly normal activity under optimal conditions of substrate concentration. Kinetic studies are often required to detect the presence of aberrant enzymes. Last, the deficiency of a specific enzyme may not in itself be the cause of a particular hemolytic anemia but merely an epiphenomenon related to feedback inhibition of synthesis or activity caused by the metabolites of another enzymatic block.

Overall hexose monophosphate shunt activity can be evaluated by measuring the evolution of $^{14}CO_2$ from glucose-^{14}C (p. 324), especially when glycolytic flux through the shunt is stimulated by oxidative agents such as methylene blue and ascorbate. Functional integrity of the Embden-Meyerhof pathway can be evaluated by determining overall glucose utilization and lactate production, measuring the concentration and stability of ATP, and determining the oxygen affinity of hemoglobin. As corollaries of ATP metabolism, measurements of cation content, cation transport, and red cell deformability provide useful information relating cell metabolism and membrane function.

Enzymatic deficiencies of erythrocyte glycolysis associated with high or low concentrations of 2,3-DPG can influence the affinity of hemoglobin for oxygen. In PK deficiency the level of 2,3-DPG is markedly raised and in HK deficiency it is markedly decreased because of the location of the respective deficiencies. The oxygen dissociation curve in PK deficiency is shifted to the right (decreased affinity), and in HK deficiency it is displaced to the left (increased affinity). In PK deficiency this shift in the oxygen dissociation curve results in a 60% increase in oxygen delivery. This allows the delivery of as much oxygen from 9 gm hemoglobin/dl of PK-deficient blood as would be delivered by normal blood containing 15 gm hemoglobin/dl.

Erythrocyte survival with ^{51}Cr-labeled autologous cells and in vivo organ sequestration studies can be combined in the patient as a single procedure. The sequestration studies may indicate the main site or sites or hemolysis, supply information about the pathogenesis of hemolysis, and help in predicting the possible benefit to be expected from splenectomy. These specific studies of erythrocyte metabolism, function, and destruction will be considered in the following discussion of the clinical syndromes associated with enzyme deficiencies.

CLASSIFICATION OF RED CELL ENZYME DEFICIENCIES

Advances in biochemical methods have resulted in the identification of sixteen types of hereditary hemolytic anemias caused by well-documented deficiencies of erythrocyte enzymes* (references cited are original reports):

A. Deficiencies of Embden-Meyerhof pathway
  1. HK†[399]
  2. GPI†[202]
  3. PFK†[390]
  4. TPI[359]
  5. PGK[398]
  6. 2,3-DPGM[362]
  7. PK†[146,402]
B. Deficiencies of hexose monophosphate shunt enzymes
  1. G-6-PD*[226]
    a. Drug-induced hemolytic anemia†
    b. Chronic hemolytic anemia†
    c. Favism†
  2. PGD
  3. γ-GC synthetase[285]
  4. Glutathione synthetase
  5. GSSG-R
  6. GSH-P
C. Deficiencies of enzymes of nucleotide metabolism

  1. AK[384]
  2. Pyrimidine,5'-nucleotidase[189] (with ribophosphokinase)
  3. ATPase[254]
D. Deficiencies of uncertain or doubtful significance
  1. GAPD[251]
  2. 2,3-DPGP[383]
  3. Enolase[381]

This includes seven glycolytic enzymes in the Embden-Meyerhof pathway,* six in the hexose monophosphate shunt,† and three involving purine nucleotide metabolism.[189,254,391] Patients with hemolytic anemia and deficiencies of other glycolytic and nonglycolytic enzymes have been reported, but the uncertain relationship between the enzyme deficiency and hemolysis necessitates placing these cases in limbo until additional details of metabolic investigations have been described.

Hemolytic anemia is not a concomitance in a final group of enzymopathies that includes deficiencies of methemoglobin reductase,[265] LDH,[310] glyoxalase II,[154] catalase,[144] and ADA[242] (references cited are original reports):

  1. LDH[310]
  2. Glyoxalase II[154]
  3. ADA[242]
  4. Catalase[144]
  5. NADH-dependent methemoglobin reductase[265]
  6. NADPH-dependent methomoglobin reductase[356]
  7. Galactokinase[274]
  8. Galactose-1-phosphate uridyl transferase[274]
  9. HGPRT[371]
  10. Phosphoribosyl pyrophosphate synthetase[409]
  11. Orotidylic pyrophosphorylase[375]
  12. Orotidylic decarboxylase[375]

Enzyme deficiencies associated with other inborn errors of metabolism, such as galactokinase and galactose-1-phosphate uridyl transferase deficiency in galactosemia and HGPRT deficiency in the Lesch-Nyhan syndrome,[371] are included in this group but will not be discussed in detail.

Hemolytic disease associated with a deficiency of an erythrocyte enzyme may be caused by the decreased production of an enzyme or the production of a functionally abnormal or unstable enzyme. During the past few years the marked heterogeneity of enzyme deficiency diseases has become apparent. This genetic polymorphism has accounted for more than 100 variants of G-6-PD,[418] eight variants of PK,[306,341,385] and a few variants of HK,[399,400] GPI,[197,340] and PFK,[268] differing from each other in kinetics, electrophoretic migration, stability, and the effects of allosteric activators.

---

*References 207, 263, 305, 396, 397.
†Associated with genetic polymorphism.

*References 204, 247, 395, 410
†References 206, 285, 294, 416, 417.

DEFECTS OF THE EMBDEN-MEYERHOF PATHWAY
Hexokinase (HK) deficiency

Clinical and hematologic features. In 1965 Lohr et al.[292,293] reported the first cases of HK deficiency in two siblings and a third patient with Fanconi's aplastic anemia (pancytopenia, multiple congenital malformations, and abnormal chromosomes). The enzyme deficiency was detected in erythrocytes, leukocytes, and platelets. No subsequent reports of combined Fanconi's aplastic anemia and HK deficiency have appeared, and the relatively few cases of the disorder associated with hemolytic anemia are limited to four families.* The severity of the hemolytic process is variable. A syndrome of neonatal hyperbilirubinemia requiring exchange transfusion, hepatosplenomegaly, and severe, transfusion-dependent anemia requiring early splenectomy comprises one end of a clinical spectrum,[245] whereas mild compensated hemolytic anemia first detected in early adulthood has also been described.

A variable clinical pattern has been seen in affected family members. Valentine, et al.[399,400] described a severely affected child whose brother with a similar degree of enzyme deficit had no evidence of hemolysis. Although the possibility exists that he is a heterozygote, this finding emphasizes the fact that there is little correlation between the measured enzyme activity and the severity of the hemolytic process in HK- and other enzyme-deficiency disorders. Values for hemoglobin have ranged from low levels of 4.5 to 7.0 gm/dl to near normal. Reticulocyte counts have ranged between 15% and 4%, the higher values observed in severely affected patients. No specific erythrocyte morphologic abnormalities have been observed, although Keitt noted macrocytosis (MCV of 120 fl.) despite a reticulocyte count of 4% to 7%. The autohemolysis pattern is either type I or normal. Osmotic fragility is either increased (presplenectomy) or normal. The half-life of ^{51}Cr-labeled cells was markedly reduced when measured after splenectomy, but reports of organ sequestration are not available. After splenectomy the requirement for transfusions ceases, although milder hemolysis persists. As in other patients with hereditary hemolytic anemia, hypoplastic crises with infection and radiographic changes have been reported.

Family studies in most reports suggest an autosomal recessive mode of inheritance; the one exception is a report of hemolytic anemia in a father and son, in whom the enzyme deficiency occurred in both erythrocytes and leukocytes.[323] Thus HK deficiency appears to be a heterogenous disorder

of variable severity associated with genetic polymorphism.

Biochemical features. The initial reaction of the Embden-Meyerhof pathway is catalyzed by HK:

$$glucose + ATP \xrightarrow[Mg^{++}]{HK} G\text{-}6\text{-}P + ADP$$

The activity of HK is the least of all the enzymes of glycolysis except 2,3-DPGP. HK, like PK and G-6-PD, is an exquisitely age-dependent enzyme, its activity declining and inversely correlating with progressive senescence of the red cell. The activity of HK in nine reported cases varied between normal and 25% of normal but was significantly reduced when related to the activity of the enzyme in populations of cells with a similar degree of reticulocytosis (Fig. 12-11). Glycolytic activity as measured by glucose consumption and relative enzyme activity as measured by HK in young and old cells or by the ratios of HK:PK and HK:G-6-PD are significantly decreased when compared to either normal or reticulocyte-rich populations of red cells.[399]

Results of kinetic and stability studies have been variable. Valentine et al.[399] found normal kinetic properties. Keitt[280] reported increased enzyme lability and a high K_m of ATP in the absence of glucose, with restoration of glycolytic activity in the presence of glucose, EDTA, and mercaptoethanol, agents that protect sulfhydryl groups. Other mutants with a high K_m for glucose and ATP have been described.[323] Electrophoretic studies[192] of HK are limited and again the results are variable.[296,357,369] Altay et al.[192] found four components or bands of HK in human red cells, two major and two minor. Type II HK, the band usually increased in young red cells, was absent in a patient with hereditary hemolytic anemia caused by HK deficiency and was decreased in presumed heterozygotes. It was proposed that the absence of type II (and perhaps types III and IV) is associated with HK-deficiency hemolytic anemia and decreased glycolysis. Normal electrophoretic patterns and a deficiency of type III HK, i.e., the isozyme with the lowest K_m for glucose, have also been recorded.[323] These findings are somewhat difficult to reconcile with the fact that type I HK accounts for more than 90% of the total activity. However, a shortage of the type II isozyme, which is the major constituent of reticulocytes, may be more crucial for cell survival.

This great variability in kinetic, stability, and electrophoretic findings may be explained by the different structural and functional properties of the different isozymes and by the relatively crude evaluation of metabolic activity in a mixture of cells of varying age, containing varying amounts of four

---

*References 280, 312, 323, 399, 400.

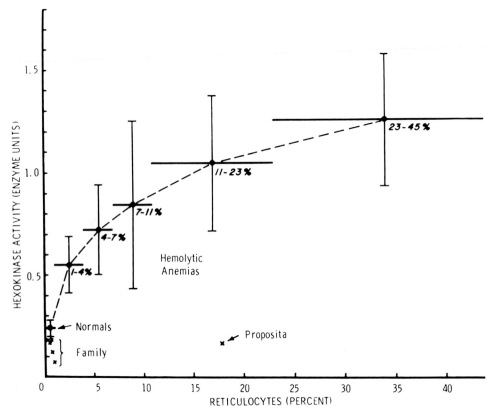

Fig. 12-11. HK activity observed in fifty-four cases of hemolytic anemia of various etiologies plotted against reticulocyte percentage in cells assayed. Cases are grouped according to reticulocyte levels. Mean HK activity for each group is plotted against mean reticulocyte percentage in cells of that group. Standard deviations are shown. Values for proposita and her family are designated separately. (From Valentine, W. N., et al.: N. Engl. J. Med. **276:**1, 1967. Reprinted by permission.)

different isozymes.[278] The combinations and permutations of clinical and biochemical syndromes are obvious. Furthermore, HK is a compartmented enzyme.[193] In the erythrocyte 85% of the HK activity is mitochondrial bound. As the erythrocyte matures and loses the subcellular organelles, the total cellular HK activity of the mature erythrocyte decreases to less than 10% of that in the reticulocyte. Cytoplasmic HK and mitochondrial bound HK have different kinetic properties.[349,354] For example, the K_m for ATP is lower and the K_i for ADP is higher for the bound form than for the soluble enzyme. The loss of a more stable or catalytically efficient HK with erythrocyte maturation may account for the inordinately low activity of HK in cells that normally have an abundance of HK. A deficiency of the enzyme would limit glycolysis and oxidative phosphorylation and result in a deranged energy supply.

As expected in erythrocytes with limited glycolysis, lowered concentrations of G-6-P, ATP, and 2,3-DPG have been reported.[280] The decreased

concentration of 2,3-DPG was associated with a leftward shift of the oxygen dissociation curve and an increased oxygen affinity (decreased P_{50} of hemoglobin).[236] The activities of other glycolytic enzymes are increased to a level expected in young red cells. The hexose monophosphate shunt functions normally, and in fact a greater percentage of glucose is metabolized through this pathway in HK-deficient than in normal erythrocytes and reticulocytes.[400] However, the ability to increase glycolytic flux through the hexose monophosphate shunt under oxidant stress is limited by the ability of HK-deficient cells to phosphorylate glucose and provide substrate for G-6-PD.

Pathogenesis of hemolysis. Although the specific mechanism of hemolysis is unknown, it can be surmised that severe impairment of glycolysis will result in critical shortages of energy in both mature and immature red cells and a deterioration of all ATP-dependent reactions that preseve normal cell function and metabolism. Furthermore, the presence of a high-K_m glucose isozyme of HK in reticulocytes makes these cells with higher energy requirements even more susceptible to glucose deprivation in the hostile environment of the spleen. In essence the HK-deficient cell suffers from early senescence. The irreversible defect may be most pronounced at the reticulocyte stage. Circulating erythrocytes and accordingly those evaluable in vitro or in vivo most likely represent a subpopulation or "survival of the fittest."

Treatment. Specific therapy for HK deficiency is not available, but the general principles of management of all cases of hemolytic anemias are applicable to this disorder. HK deficiency should be considered in the differential diagnosis of hemolysis and hyperbilirubinemia in the newborn, and exchange transfusion is indicated to prevent kernicterus. Because of the severity of hemolysis in some patients, long-term transfusion therapy may be required to maintain levels of hemoglobin above 7 to 8 gm/dl. Hypoplastic crises may be superimposed on infections. As in other hemolytic syndromes, 1 mg/day of folic acid is recommended. Splenectomy has provided a partial to marked benefit and has obviated transfusions in patients who had been transfusion dependent. Because of the associated increased risk of overwhelming infections and septicemia, prophylactic penicillin therapy is advisable. Despite splenectomy, hemolysis persists and late complications of cholelithiasis, with a need for cholecystectomy, exist in affected patients.

Depressed levels of 2,3-DPG and the resultant increased oxygen affinity and decreased delivery of oxygen to the tissues are partly responsible for the severity of clinical symptoms in these patients. Oski et al.[331] found that vigorous physical exertion in HK deficiency was associated with a prompt fall in central venous oxygen tension to levels close to those below which oxidative phosphorylation can no longer procede and with a doubling in cardiac output. Thus it is anticipated that HK-deficient patients would not be able to tolerate strenuous physical activities and that modifications in life-style would be required.

The documentation of the carrier state is difficult because many carriers posses normal or near-normal activity of HK. Complete family studies should be performed and genetic counseling should be provided with the identification of new cases of the defect.

In vitro HK-deficient cells utilize mannose more efficiently and rapidly than glucose, the phosphorylation being catalyzed by HK.[209] In turn, mannose-1-phosphate is rapidly converted to F-6-P by phosphomannose isomerase, the activity of which is increased in young cells. The product of this reaction enters the Embden-Meyerhof pathway and thus bypasses the initial metabolic block.

Attempts at biochemical reengineering have not had a clinical trial, but methods such as these, designed to alter protein function, may have applicability in the future.

Glucose phosphate isomerase (GPI) deficiency

Clinical and hematologic features. GPI deficiency, is the third most common red cell enzymopathy,[340] after G-6-PD and PK deficiency. To date twenty-nine cases in twenty-two familiies have been reported,* and fourteen different variants based on differences in electrophoretic migration,[196,217,318] stability,[197] and pH optimum[318] have been described. In two large-scale genetic studies[236,240] ten different types of electrophoretic variants were discovered in surveys of more than 5,000 individuals. The incidence of variants in both reports was 0.5%. Not all variants are associated with deficiency. Paglia et al.[334] determined that the heterozygote state occurs in approximately 0.2% of the population.[336] Most patients have been from the Western Hemisphere and northern latitudes.

The severity of anemia in GPI deficiency is variable. The clinical spectrum extends from hemolysis and hyperbilirubinemia requiring exchange transfusion to a mild well-compensated hemolytic process first detected in early adulthood. Neonatal symptoms occur in approximately one third of the reported cases. Mental retardation, perhaps related to kernicterus, has been reported in GPI Utrecht,[255,405,406] a variant associated with drug-induced hemolysis, frequent infections, and (unlike most other variants of GPI) a poor response to splenectomy. The transfusion dependency of the most severely affected patients abated after splenectomy, a procedure associated with a uniformly beneficial effect in almost all patients. Deaths in infancy and early childhood have been reported in severely affected patients who did not receive adequate transfusions or in whom splenectomy was not performed. Varying degrees of hepatosplenomegaly and a late sequela of cholelithiasis necessitating cholecystectomy have been observed. Growth and development progress normally.

Concomitant deficiencies of GPI in leukocytes and platelets have been reported in 90% and 75% of evaluated cases, respectively. Despite the enzyme defect in other cells, increased susceptibility to infection or bleeding and biochemical evidence of polymorphonuclear leukocyte or platelet dysfunction have not been observed.

---

*References 196, 197, 199, 202, 208, 217, 229, 233, 238, 255, 259, 272, 299, 308, 314, 318, 330, 334, 364, 365, 367, 405, 406.

The range and median of hemoglobin values are 4.2 to 12.3 gm/dl and 8.0 gm/dl, respectively. Similarly the reticulocyte counts ranged from 1% to 72% with a median of 20%. The age range at diagnosis of reported patients was 1 to 26 years with a median of 12 years. The morphologic changes in the peripheral blood are nonspecific; many of the described abnormalities were reported in splenectomized patients and include sporadic and slightly crenated spherocytes,[330] macrocytosis, anisopoikilocytosis, hypochromasia, polychromasia, target cells, basophilic stippling, and Howell-Jolly bodies. Oski and Fuller[330] reported the presence of prominent spherocytosis in GPI-deficiency "nonspherocytic hemolytic anemia," again emphasizing the inadequacy of a morphologic description in defining a metabolic abnormality. Hereditary elliptocytosis and heterozygosity for GPI deficiency have been reported in two siblings.

The autohemolysis test invariably reveals a type I pattern. The osmotic fragility of freshly drawn and incubated red cells is usually normal, although increased fragility has been observed in GPI Utrecht.[255] The half-life of ^{51}Cr-labeled erythrocytes is markedly reduced: The range in reported cases was 2.5 to 12 days with a median of 4.5 days. Splenic sequestration was documented in many but not all cases.

Biochemical features. GPI catalyzes the second reaction of the Embden-Myerhof pathway, converting G-6-P to F-6-P. The reaction is in equilibrium and there is virtually no change in free energy (-0.1 kcal). The molecular weight of normal GPI is 88,000 to 92,000 daltons.[393] The forward reaction is activated by G-6-P and the backward reaction by F-6-P. The backward reaction is competitively inhibited by 2,3-DPG and 6-PG. The pH optimum is 8.0 to 8.5. The activity of GPI in homozygotes or double heterozygotes (the result of the simultaneous inheritance of different mutant alleles at the locus for GPI, one from each parent) ranges from 10% to 50% of normal with a median of about 25%. Heterozygotes have about 50% of normal activity. The activity of GPI in older deficient cells is only 40% of that in a reticulocyte-rich population. There appears to be no correlation between the activity of the enzyme and the severity of the anemia. The pH optima and enzyme kinetics with regard to the K_m for G-6-P and F-6-P and K_i for 2,3-DPG and 6-PG have been normal when either hemolysates or partially purified preparations were evaluated. An exception is GPI Matsumoto with an acidic shift in the pH optimum curve.[318]

The variant enzymes in GPI deficiency have been characterized by marked to moderate thermal lability and abnormalities in electrophoretic and/or isoelectric migration.[197,318] These studies sug-

gest that the active site of the enzyme is not affected and that the deficiency is related to an amino acid substitution that critically affects the stability of the enzyme.

As a consequence of GPI deficiency the intracellular concentration of G-6-P is two to three times normal, levels that inhibit HK. The hexose monophosphate shunt functions normally and is maximally stimulated. However, because GPI in the backward reaction normally provides additional G-6-P for recycling through the shunt, $^{14}CO_2$ generation from ^{14}C-2 glucose is only 0.2% to 10% of normal in GPI deficiency.[202,334] Of interest is that the existence of double heterozygosity for G-6-PD and GPI in a male with chronic hemolytic anemia and an acute hemolytic crisis occurring after amidopyrine.[364,365] It was uncertain which defect was the key to the patient's hemolysis.

The results of other metabolic studies have been variable, but generally the concentration of 2,3-DPG is increased, and F-6-P, FDP, and other metabolites distal to the block are decreased. Glucose utilization, lactate production, and ATP concentration have been inconstant but, relative to a population of young cells, decreased.

The activity of GPI in GPI-deficient leukocytes ranged from 5% to 73% with a median of 22%;[318] in platelets GPI activity ranged between 13% and 30%.[330] Kinetic parameters were normal and the abnormalities of thermal stability and electrophoretic migration mirrored those in erythrocytes, strongly suggesting that an identical GPI, albeit a mutant or wild type, is present in all cells and tissues of the body. The one exception is GPI Valle Hermoso, in which the enzyme activity in leukocytes is normal.

Mechanism of hemolysis. Defective glycolytic activity at the GPI step and the inability of red cells to increase further any shunting of glucose through the hexose monophosphate shunt results in limited energy production of GPI-deficient cells. Decreased erythrocyte deformability,[233] particularly with acidosis, and selective phagocytosis and destruction of reticulocytes by the spleen[229] are thought to contribute to the early demise of GPI deficient cells. As in other hereditary hemolytic anemias associated with glycolytic defects, the deterioration of ATP-dependent functions results in eventual hemolysis.

Treatment. The general principles of therapy apply to GPI deficiency. Splenectomy generally results in clinical improvement and lengthening of erythrocyte survival. Transfusion therapy should not be withheld from severely affected infants who are not able to compensate adequately during the first few years of life. Arnold et al.[196] treated a mildly affected patient with intravenous Pi, which stimulates PFK, and secondarily HK. The hemoglobin level rose 14% and the reticulocyte count fell 70%. In another study these same investigators found that GPI activity and lactate formation from glucose deteriorated markedly after in vitro storage but, if mannose was used as a source of energy, the rate of glycolysis was normal after in vitro storage.[197] Mannose-6-phosphate is converted to F-6-P by phosphomannose isomerase, circumventing the block imposed by GPI. As in HK deficiency, a clinical trial using mannose has not been attempted in GPI deficiency.

Phosphofructokinase (PFK) deficiency

Clinical and hematologic features. Two major variants of PFK-deficiency hemolytic anemia have been described. The first, probably inherited as an autosomal recessive trait, was first described by Tarui et al.[390] in 1965 in patients with McArdle's syndrome or type VII glycogen storage disease and was associated with muscle fatigue, cramping pain with exercise, and intermittent myoglobinuria. The hemolytic anemia was mild with a reticulocytosis of 4% to 6% and shortened red cell survival. No PFK activity was detectable in the muscles, and the red cell activity was only 50% of normal. Immunologic studies with antihuman muscle PFK showed that, whereas the normal red cell enzyme is inhibited by about 40%, no inhibition of the enzyme occurred in affected patients, indicating that muscle and red cell PFK contain a common isoenzyme.[288]

A second variant has been reported in three other individuals; in these the deficit of PFK was restricted to the red cells.[330,412] Chronic hemolytic anemia occurred without muscle symptoms. The inheritance pattern has not been determined, although linkage to the X chromosome has been tentatively suggested. The range of red cell PFK activity was 9% to 60%. In two of the three cases in which immunologic studies were performed antimuscle PFK did not inhibit the residual red cell enzyme.[389] In a recent report by Kahn et al.[268] the activity of PFK in muscle, leukocytes, and platelets was normal but the muscle PFK was unstable and had an abnormally fast pattern on electrophoresis. The lack of deficiency of muscle PFK was attributed to the ability of this tissue to synthesize protein; in this regard the senescent red cell is important.

Biochemical features. PFK, the key rate-limiting control point of the glycolytic pathway, converts F-6-P to FDP in a one-way reaction:

$$F\text{-}6\text{-}P + ATP \xrightarrow[Mg^{++}]{PFK} FDP + ADP$$

As discussed earlier (p. 319), ATP, H^+ ions, 2, 3-DPG, and increased temperature inhibit PFK; Pi, F-6-P, AMP, ADP, NH_4^+, and FDP activate the enzyme.

Because of the paucity of cases, few detailed biochemical studies are available. Whereas the Michaelis constants are normal, pH optimum and stability with heat, dilution, and storage are altered. Lactate production appears to be normal but the ATP content is diminished.[412]

Mechanism of hemolysis. It is somewhat paradoxical that a defect at the PFK step is not characterized by more severe clinical and biochemical aberrations. Since only the muscle-type PFK is deficient in red cells, the residual isoenzymes, which are not shared by leukocytes, preserve some glycolytic function. Hemolysis is most likely related to the deficient and unstable enzyme,[267] but additional studies will be required to elucidate the pathogenic mechanisms.

Of related interest is the occurrence of relative PFK deficiency in newborns[408] and in patients with dyserythropoietic disorders, including paroxysmal nocturnal hemoglobinuria, preleukemia, and refractory anemias.[222] In all future cases it will be essential to differentiate these acquired states from PFK-deficiency hereditary hemolytic anemia.

Treatment. Hemolytic anemia of PFK deficiency is mild. Neonatal symptoms are absent, and transfusions and splenectomy have not been required. Patients with muscle symptoms require appropriate therapy for their glycogen storage disease.

Triose phosphate isomerase (TPI) deficiency[358,359]

Clinical and hematologic features. TPI deficiency is a rare multisystem disorder involving erythrocytes, skeletal and cardiac muscle, and the central nervous system. It is one of the most lethal enzyme deficiency disorders in that of the ten reported homozygotes all but three died before the age of 5 years. The longest survivor, a female patient originally described by Jaffe's group,[253] died at age 23 after lifelong confinement to a wheelchair.[266] The clinical manifestations of TPI deficiency begin in early infancy. Early deaths related to nonimmunologic hemolytic disease of the newborn have occurred in three presumably affected infants. During the first 6 to 12 months of age an atypical, severe, progressive, and debilitating neurologic deficit involving peripheral nerves and central nervous tissue occurs. Spasticity progressing to flaccidity, muscle weakness and atrophy without initial spasticity, developmental retardation, and dementia are seen. If infants survive the first few months of life, the neurologic deficit progresses. Three patients have died of sudden cardiac arrest and ventricular fibrillation.[194,358]

Frequent infections have been documented in

some patients and may be related to the concurrent deficiency of TPI in leukocytes.[359] The deficiency also occurs in skeletal muscle, serum, cerebrospinal fluid, and fibroblasts. Assays of TPI in myocardium from postmortem tissue or leukocyte function tests have yet to be performed.

Six of the ten reported cases of TPI deficiency have been in French-Negro Louisianans,[358] five of whom were members of one closely related kindred. Other single nonfamilial cases have been reported from England and the United States. The activity of TPI in the red cells of homozygotes is about 10% of normal; in heterozygotes 50% of normal TPI is present. An extensive family study by Schneider et al.[358] established an autosomal recessive mode of inheritance. Sickle cell trait and G-6-PD deficiency have been reported in the same kindred with coexisting TPI deficiency. A concurrence of all three traits was found in two members of the family.

Chromosome 5[377] is thought to be associated with the enzyme because of the demonstration of heterozygosity for TPI deficiency in a patient with cri du chat (cat cry) syndrome who had a partial deletion of the short arm of chromosome 5.

Hemolytic anemia is moderately severe. The ranges of hemoglobin values and reticulocyte counts have been 5 to 10 gm/dl and 10% to 20%, respectively. Slight macrocytosis and crenated or spiculated spherocytes have been seen in the peripheral blood. The osmotic fragility curve of fresh blood is normal, but a "tail" of cells with increased fragility has been seen after incubation. The autohemolysis pattern is type I and resembles that of hereditary spherocytosis.

Results of erythrocyte survival and organ sequestration studies have not been reported. One patient underwent splenectomy with a partial response.

Biochemical features. TPI, an enzyme in equilibrium, interconverts Ga-3-P and DHAP:

$$\text{Ga-3-P} \underset{}{\overset{\text{TPI}}{\rightleftharpoons}} \text{DHAP}$$

The mature red cell lacks α-glycerophosphate dehydrogenase and cannot convert DHAP to α-glycerophosphate, a substrate of lipid synthesis. Accordingly the major metabolite of this reaction is Ga-3-P, which is in the mainstream of glycolysis

On the basis of preliminary chromatographic and electrophoretic studies it can be said that more than one form of the enzyme exists.[276] Two enzyme peaks have been identified in normal and enzyme-deficient erythrocytes. The deficient enzyme, which has normal kinetics, was associated with the major chromatographic peak.

The glycolytic rate and stoichiometry of lactate production in TPI-deficient cells is normal.[358] The

hexose monophosphate shunt functions at a maximally stimulated rate and is not stimulated further by methylene blue. The intracellular concentration of DHAP is twenty times that found in normal erythrocytes and ten times higher than in high-reticulocyte controls. The concentrations of Ga-3-P and FDP are increased, ATP content is decreased, and 2,3-DPG is normal or increased. After incubation, with or without stimulation of the hexose monophosphate shunt, the level of DHAP rises significantly above the base line, whereas other key intermediates do not change.

Mechanism of hemolysis. Increasing glycolytic flux through the hexose monophosphate shunt theoretically could be beneficial to the TPI-deficient red cell only if more Ga-3-P than F-6-P is formed by the transketolase-transaldolase system. This would bypass the aldolase reaction, which converts F-6-P into the triose sugars DHAP and Ga-3-P. In TPI deficiency half of the trioses generated are squandered and are unavailable for ATP synthesis in the lower half of the Embden-Myerhof pathway. Paradoxically ATP is stable during incubation, and yet the morphologic abnormalities suggest ATP depletion. These inconsistencies make it difficult to relate the enzyme deficiency and an attendant deficiency of ATP to the pathogenesis of hemolysis. Although uncertain, a toxic or inhibitory effect of DHAP at an unknown site has been proposed as a possible mechanism.

Treatment. General principles of therapy apply to TPI deficiency. Multisystem involvement requires close evaluation by neurologists and cardiologists. The role of splenectomy, if any, remains to be determined.

Phosphoglycerate kinase (PGK) deficiency

Clinical and hematologic features. Since the first documentation in 1968 of PGK-deficiency hereditary hemolytic anemia in a 63-year-old woman,[398] ten other patients, seven male and three female, have been reported with the defect.*
Affected males have a moderately severe hemolytic disorder associated with mental retardation, speech impairment, emotional lability, and progressive extrapyramidal tract disease.[284] A number of male relatives of patients died in early infancy of anemia, infections, and a convulsive disorder and are presumed to have been similarly affected. The onset of symptoms in the neonatal period, varying degrees of hepatosplenomegaly, transfusion dependency until the time of splenectomy, and partial but not complete benefit from splenectomy have been recorded in some but not all patients. The affected females are most likely heterozygotes but have a mild, compensated, but nondebilitating hemolytic disorder. Heterozygous females,

---

*References 195, 227, 284, 286, 307, 418.

whether symptomatic or not, have about 40% to 80% of normal PGK activity in their erythrocytes; their affected sons' red cells contain 5% to 25% of normal PGK.

The enzyme defect has been observed in polymorphonuclear leukocytes, lymphocytes, and fibroblasts, an expected finding in view of the fact that PGK in different tissues is under the control of the same structural gene. In studies of a PGK variant from Oceania PGK in blood cells and fibroblasts was similar to that in liver, heart, kidney, and skeletal muscle. The gene frequency of one variant in New Guinea, unassociated with hereditary hemolytic anemia, was 0.014.[232] The disease has been reported in Orientals and whites.[231]

On the basis of pedigree analysis, enzyme assays in young and old erythrocytes,[398] studies of somatic cell hybridization,[281] and electrophoretic studies of enzyme activity in fibroblasts derived from a female carrier of the defect, PGK has been localized to the X chromosome.[205,238] Women heterozygous for X-linked PGK deficiency possess a mosaic of two populations of cells, one totally deficient and one totally normal. Genetic studies of PGK have established that the locus is on the long arm of the X chromosome and that the entire X chromsome, rather than random loci, is inactivated in the random inactivation of one of the two X chromosomes in females.[238]

The hemoglobin values have ranged from 5 to 10 gm/dl in hemizygotes and 10 to 11 gm/dl in symptomatic carriers. The range of reticulocyte counts has been 5% to 25%. No specific morphologic abnormalities of the red cells have been described. The autohemolysis test has not been particularly helpful. The results have been variably abnormal with patterns of both type I and type II, as well as those cases corrected by neither glucose nor ATP. When tested, osmotic fragility has been normal or increased. Red cell survival was measured in only one case, with a half-life of ^{51}Cr-labeled cells of 12 days. There are no reports of organ sequestration. The results of studies of leukocyte function are controversial. Baehner et al.[201] reported decreased bactericidal activity in an affected Chinese boy, whereas Strauss et al.[382] found normal chemotaxis, phagocytosis, ultrastructural features, and intracellular killing in the neutrophils of two boys originally described by Konrad et al.[284] The activity of PGK in the first reported patient's white cells was normal.[284]

Biochemical features. PGK catalyzes the interconversion of 1,3-PG and 3-PG and is one of the two ATP-generating steps within the mature red cell:

$$1,3\text{-PG} + \text{ADP} \xrightleftharpoons[\text{Mg}^{++}]{\text{PGK}} 3\text{-PG} + \text{ATP}$$

Purified mutant and wild-type PGK has a molecular weight of 50,000 daltons.[418,419] The func-

tional unit is a monomer. X-ray crystallography and resolution at 6Å of muscle PGK has been accomplished[212] and revealed two distinct globular subunits, one of which is involved in substrate binding. Immunologic studies with antihuman erythrocyte PGK showed that lactate formation in hemolysates was not inhibited until 30% of PGK was neutralized, confirming that PGK is in excess.[327]

Extensive biochemical characterization of PGK variants associated with hemolytic anemia has not been performed. Enzyme kinetics and stability in a probable heterozygote were normal and the activity of PGK was diminished in her older erythrocytes. Valentine et al.[398] on the other hand, found in two heterozygotes that the activity of PGK was decreased in the younger cells, which represented a mosaic of two populations of cells, one normal and the other grossly deficient. The older population of cells were all normal and had more activity than the mixed population of young cells. In homozygotes the activity of PGK is decreased in older cells.

Yoshida and Miwa[418] reported that PGK Matsue was associated with slower electrophoretic mobility, reduced affinity for 3-PG (high K_m), abnormal pH profile but normal pH optimum, increased rate of degradation in the red cells, and thermal instability. Immunologic neutralization revealed that the variant enzyme had a specific activity corresponding to 35% of normal. The erythrocytes in this patient had only 5% of normal PGK activity, a decrease related to increased degradation and decreased production of the enzyme. Because of the instability of deficient variants of PGK, purification has not been possible. Purification and structural studies of a variant with 100% catalytic activity and an abnormal electrophoretic pattern (PGK Samoa) revealed the substitution of asparagine for threonine.[420] The electrophoretic anomaly was attributed to a secondary alteration of protein charge caused by citrate in the gel rather than by the amino acid substitution itself, which was neutral.

Mechanism of hemolysis. Present work has indicated a close link between glycolysis and the activity of the ATP-dependent, sodium-potassium ion pump.[245,361] PGK and the preceding enzyme in the glycolytic chain, GAPD, are linked within the cell membrane to permit the smooth passage of intermediates from one enzyme to the next.[360] ATP generated at the PGK step is made available to the cation pump (Na,K-ATPase).[345] The ADP derived from Na,K-ATPase hydrolysis of ATP is compartmentalized in the membrane, serves as the preferred substrate in the PGK reaction, and slowly exchanges with a cytoplasmic pool of ADP.[372] This linkage is shown in Fig. 11-5.

In view of these considerations it is somewhat

surprising that cation transport is normal in PGK-deficient red cells. Glucose utilization, lactate production, and the concentration of ATP are decreased in PGK-deficient cells.[195,300] Glycolytic intermediates above the block (hexose phosphates, DHAP, 1,3-DPG, 2,3-DPG, and AMP) are increased[319]; 3-PG and 2-PG are decreased.

These alterations conceivably can be inhibitory or in some way toxic to cell metabolism and function, but the exact mechanism is once again uncertain. DHAP, which may play a role in TPI deficiency, is increased to levels four to nine times normal. Studies of red cell deformability and cation transport under the stresses of hypoxia and acidosis may elucidate possible mechanisms of hemolysis.

Treatment. Splenectomy did not mollify the hemolytic anemia in the patient reported by Kraus et al.[286] but resulted in an excellent response in two other patients. The cause of the neurologic syndrome is unknown but could be related to a deficiency of the enzyme, an effect of some glycolytic intermediate on central nervous system function, or merely an unrelated but associated inherited disorder.

2,3-Diphosphoglycerate mutase (2,3-DPGM) deficiency

Clinical and hematologic features. European investigators have described a moderately severe hemolytic anemia associated with hepatosplenomegaly, variable hyperbilirubinemia, and presumed or measured deficiency of 2,3-DPGM in fewer than 10 patients since 1963.* In some patients the evidence for the deficiency was indirect and was inferred from either the inability of 2,3-DPG-depleted cells to regenerate 2,3-DPG or a measured deficiency of 2,3-DPG-dependent PGM.[291,366] The atypical features of the cases are noteworthy. Alagille et al.[191] described two infants with transfusion-dependent hemolytic anemia hepatosplenomegaly, reticulocytosis of 11% to 50%, and decreased 2,3-DPGM activity (37% normal). The autohemolysis pattern was type I. One patient had an excellent response to splenectomy and the second improved after treatment with corticosteroids. The patients of Lohr and Waller[291] also had decreased activity of 2,3-DPG-dependent PGM but had dipyrroluria and Heinz bodies, features usually associated with unstable-hemoglobin hemolytic anemias. Both the French and German children had decreased levels of ATP and glycolytic rates. In summary, it is uncertain whether these are unequivocal cases of 2,3-DPGM deficiency in view of the nonspecificity of the methods.

*References 191, 227, 228, 287, 291, 362.

The first direct evidence of 2,3-DPGM deficiency was provided by Schröter[363]; the patient was a severely affected transfusion-dependent infant who died at 3 months of age. His parents were shown to be heterozygotes by direct assay of 2,3-DPGM. Transfused erythrocytes were rapidly destroyed, suggesting an extracorpuscular mechanism of hemolysis. An autosomal recessive pattern of inheritance was proposed in this case, but in the deficient father and son described by Labie et al.[287] an autosomal dominant characteristic was suggested. In these patients the activity of 2,3-DPGM was 50% of normal and the level of 2,3-DPG was 30% of normal. Additional studies by Cartier et al.[227,228] demonstrated increased triose phosphates and normal glycolysis and levels of ATP. As expected in the presence of decreased 2,3-DPG, oxygen affinity of hemoglobin was increased (decreased $P_{50}O_2$).

Biochemical features and mechanism of hemolysis. The enzyme 2,3-DPGM irreversibly converts 1,3-DPG to 2,3-DPG:

$$\text{1,3-DPG} + \text{3-PG} \xrightarrow{\text{2,3-DPGM}} \text{2,3-DPG} + \text{3-PG}$$

The molecular weight of purified 2,3-DPGM is 60,000 and the subunit weight is 32,000 daltons. In studies of purified enzyme from normal human erythrocytes, Rose[350] showed that 2-PG activates and 2,3-DPG potently inhibits the enzyme, with a K_i of 0.85 μM. The normal intracellular concentration of 2,3-DPG is 4 to 5 μM. Inorganic phosphate, hydrogen ions, and sulfhydryl reagents inhibit the enzyme, but other common intracellular components such as purine and pyrimidine nucleotides, GSH, and other glycolytic intermediates are neither inhibitors nor activators.[351,352] Using a different assay system, Schröter and Heyden[366] found that physiologic intracellular concentrations of ADP decreased the formation of 2,3-DPG by 70%. Electrophoretic variants have been described,[230] but these techniques have not been applied to patients with hemolytic anemia.

A deficiency of 2,3-DPG would be expected to affect hemoglobin function, but the relationship between a deficiency of 2,3-DPGM and hemolytic anemia is unclear. It is difficult to implicate a deficiency of ATP-dependent functions, since glycolysis traversing the Rapoport-Luebering cycle results in decreased synthesis of ATP. Furthermore, 2,3-DPG itself inhibits a number of rate-limiting and other important steps of the Embden-Meyerhof pathway and hexose monophosphate shunt (p. 322), and a deficiency of the metabolite would conceivably relieve the inhibition imposed on these reactions.

Treatment. Pharmacologic manipulations have been effective in raising the levels of 2,3-DPG in red cells, presumably by altering intracellular metabolism or activating 2,3-DPGM. The administration of prednisone,[374] androgens,[341] phosphate-inosine-pyruvate (in vitro),[39] and thyroid hormone[391] results in increased intracellular 2,3-DPG. It had been proposed that thyroid hormone (T_3 and T_4) directly stimulates 2,3-DPGM.[376] The results of more recent studies suggest that it is unlikely that thyroid hormones exert a direct effect on 2,3-DPG metabolism.[363] However, pharmacologic manipulations designed to increase 2,3-DPG levels may be beneficial in patients with 2,3-DPGM deficiency.

Pyruvate kinase (PK) deficiency*

Historical perspective. PK-deficiency hereditary hemolytic anemia is the first described, most common, and best-defined enzyme abnormality of the Embden-Meyerhof pathway. After Selwyn and Dacie's classification of the "congenital nonspherocytic hemolytic anemias" into two types on the basis of the autohemolysis test, De Gruchy et al.[235] noted that supplementation of whole blood with ATP would prevent autohemolysis in the type II disorder even when glucose was ineffective. A second key discovery in isolating the defect to the Embden-Meyerhof pathway was the finding of a very high content of 2,3-DPG in the erythrocytes of type II hemolytic anemia first reported by Motulsky et al.[313] in 1955 and confirmed by Robinson and her Australian associates[346] 6 years later. The raised levels of 2,3-DPG suggested that a defect in glycolysis existed between 2,3-DPG and pyruvate, and in 1961 Valentine et al. localized the predicted defect to a deficiency of PK in three patients with congenital hemolytic anemia.[387,402]

Since this classic report nearly 200 cases of PK deficiency have been described and a heterogeneous, polymorphic pattern of clinical and biochemical characteristics is now apparent. Cases have appeared worldwide, although most have been reported in the medical literature of the Western Hemisphere. The few modest population surveys suggest a gene frequency of 1%, although in Hong Kong 3% of 700 newborn Chinese infants had partial PK deficiency and 1% were suspected of being homozygotes.[242] In Germany homozygosity was calculated to occur in 0.005% of the population.[218] Despite the fact that PK deficiency is the second most common glycolytic enzyme defect of the red cell, it must be remembered that for every child with PK deficiency there are more than a half million with G-6-PD deficiency, of whom only about 100 have a chronic hemolytic disorder. Cases of PK deficiency with associated

G-6-PD deficiency or with β-thalassemia trait have been reported.[385]

Homo sapiens is not the only animal species afflicted with PK deficiency. The barkless African hunting dog, the Basenji, is also affected by a severe congenital hemolytic disorder, which usually results in death by about 3 years of age.[370]

Clinical and hematologic features. Great variation exists in the disease in homozygotes or double heterozygotes (clinically affected individuals who have inherited two different aberrant PK genes). The spectrum ranges from severe neonatal anemia and hyperbilirubinemia requiring exchange transfusions and occasionally complicated by kernicterus at one extreme[223,245] to a fully compensated mild hemolytic process first detected in senior citizens at the other.[320] Severe anemia requiring transfusions is more likely to occur in early infancy than later in childhood and adolescence, as a complication of erythroid hypoplasia secondary to infection, or during pregnancy. The requirement for transfusion is either eliminated or markedly diminished following splenectomy. Frequently a diagnosis of PK deficiency is not made until after splenectomy is performed in patients with undiagnosed or atypical hereditary hemolytic anemias not completely responsive to the surgical procedure. Dark urine, indirect hyperbilirubinemia, and slight to moderate hepatomegaly and splenomegaly are present in most patients. Growth and secondary sexual development are often delayed in more severely affected patients. Bony changes of chronic hemolytic anemias may be seen. Less common complications include severe obstructive cholelithiasis, pancreatitis,[295] and leg ulcers.[315]

Generally the range of hemoglobin values is 6 to 10 gm/dl with macrocytic normochromic indices and a normal MCHC. The reticulocyte count is 5% to 10% in unsplenectomized and 30% to 90% in splenectomized patients, the most profound reticulocytosis in any of the enzymopathies. Reticulocytopenia may be associated with infection-induced hypoplastic crises or with concomitant deficiencies of iron, folic acid, or vitamin B_{12}. Prior to splenectomy the peripheral blood smear has nonspecific abnormalities including macrocytosis, polychromatophilia, and teardrop poikilocytes (dacryocytes). Following splenectomy, crenated or spiculated spherocytes (echinocytes) and marked polychromatophilia are readily apparent.[332] The osmotic fragility curves of fresh or incubated erythrocytes are usually normal[329] but the pattern of autohemolysis is generally, but not invariably, type II; i.e., it is corrected by neutralized ATP but not glucose. Rarely the pattern may be normal or type I (correction with glucose and ATP).[249]

Erythrocyte survival measured by ^{51}Cr is vari-

---

*References 247, 263, 279, 385, 386, 395.

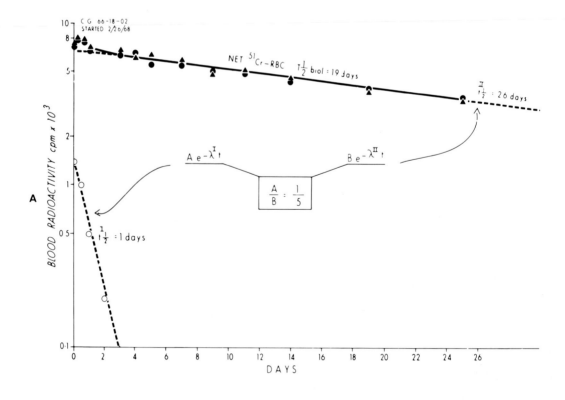

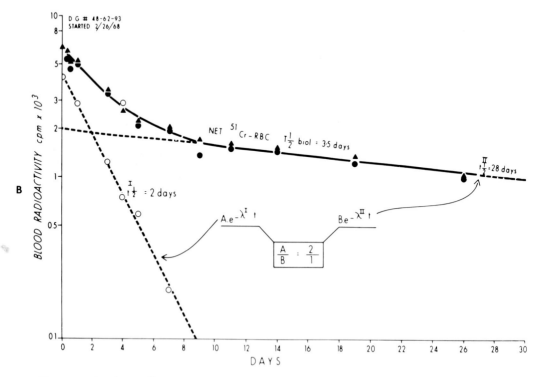

Fig. 12-12. Autologous ⁵¹Cr-labeled red cell survival in PK deficiency showing two populations of cells. **A,** Before splenectomy the larger population *(B)* has normal survival, whereas after splenectomy, **B,** more cells *(A)* have a markedly reduced survival.

ably reduced.[250,279,320] Autologous and isologous studies in splenectomized and unsplenectomized patients as well as cross-transfusion survival studies of PK-deficient cells in normal or splenectomized volunteers have demonstrated two distinct populations of PK-deficient cells and have defined the role of the spleen in premature red cell destruction. Prior to splenectomy the autologous (patient's cells in patient) and isologous (patient's cells in compatible normal or splenectomized recipients) survival curves were similar. After splenectomy two populations of PK-deficient red cells can be identified. The first, comprising 25% to 33% of the total population, has an extremely short half-life (1 day or less) when measured in an autologous or an isologous study; the second, larger population has a normal or near-normal half-life (Fig. 12-12).

Using ^{14}C-glycine as a label for reticulocytes, Nathan et al.[320] showed that PK-deficient reticulocytes have a survival that is shorter than or similar to survival of older cells, which are presumably less endowed metabolically. Autologous survival studies performed in splenectomized patients also reveal two population of cells. Unlike the pattern seen in patients with intact spleens, the larger population has the shorter survival, findings compatible with the extreme reticulocytosis present in splenectomized patients. In the splenectomized patients reticulocytes that should have been selectively destroyed still circulate.

The results of hepatic and splenic sequestration differ in splenectomized and unsplenectomized patients with PK deficiency.[146,320] In isologous studies of cells from splenectomized patients immediate splenic uptake of radioisotope was followed by a lag phase and then abrupt hepatic sequestration. In autologous and isologous studies of blood from unsplenectomized patients, hepatic and splenic uptake appeared simultaneously, decreased over the spleen after 3 to 4 days, and continued to rise over the liver. The amount of hepatic uptake far exceeds splenic uptake of ^{51}Cr and thus, by classical definition, splenic sequestration is not occurring in PK deficiency. However, splenic conditioning of reticulocytes, which are susceptible to hypoxia and dependent on oxidative phosphorylation for the production of ATP, plays a key role in the hepatic sequestration and destruction of the PK-deficient red cell.[304] For this reason splenectomy benefits the most severely affected patients and invariably decreases their transfusion requirements.

PK deficiency in other hematologic disorders. An acquired deficiency of PK has been described in patients with a wide variety of hematologic disorders[248,388] including acute myeloblastic, monomyeloblastic, and lymphoblastic leukemia; erythroleukemia; chronic granulocytic leukemia; sideroblastic anemia; chronic refractory anemia; preleukemia; congenital dyserythropoietic anemia; primary medullary insufficiency without aplasia; aplastic anemia; Diamond-Blackfan syndrome; paroxysmal nocturnal hemoglobinuria; and Chediak-Higashi syndrome.* In one large study 72 of 202 patients (36%) with leukemia and related disorders had acquired PK deficiency.[222] Nearly all of these disorders are associated with dyserythropoiesis. The PK activity is usually about 50% to 75% of normal, or within the heterozygote range, and may be associated with other abnormalities of erythrocyte metabolism including deficiencies of PFK, 2,3-DPGM, AK, and GSS6-R. The mechanism of the acquired deficiency is unknown, although a posttranslational molecular alteration leading to partial enzyme inactivation has been proposed and may be related to abnormal erythroid proliferation and differentiation.[200,269]

Genetics. An autosomal recessive inheritance has been found in all adequately studied kindreds. Heterozygous subjects are usually, but not invariably, clinically normal, and the activity of PK in their erythrocytes ranges from 50% to 70% of normal. Three examples of mild to moderate hemolytic anemia in a presumed heterozygous parent and child have been reported, and a dominant transmission has been proposed.[200,355] The PK in these patients was characterized by decreased activity, aberrant kinetics, thermal instability, or abnormal isoelectric pattern.

The marked variability of the clinical and laboratory findings in PK deficiency may be explained partially by genetic polymorphism and molecular heterogeneity. A number of variants with high, low, and normal K_m for PEP and with or without activation by the allosteric effector, FDP, have been identified (Table 12-10).

At least four isozymes or molecular forms of PK have been identified in human tissue and have been distinguished by their different electrophoretic, immunologic, and kinetic properties.[298,344]

M_1PK is present in muscle, heart, and brain. M_2 is found in spleen, lung, white blood cells, kidney, and adipose tissue and is a minor component in liver. Intermediate forms of M_1, M_3, and M_4 have been identified. L-type PK is in liver and erythrocytes. The isozyme normally present in the red cell (designated type R) is kinetically similar to the major liver isozyme (L) but can be distinguished from it by electrophoresis. Fetal tissues contain only type M_2f (or type K), considered to be the ancestral form of the enzyme. These isozymes are under control of different genes and the iso-

---

*References 198, 222, 269, 324.

Table 12-10. Summary of variants of PK-deficiency hemolytic anemia

Reference	No. of cases	PK activity (% normal)	K_m PEP (× normal)	FDP activation	pH optimum	Electrophoresis
Normal values		100	0.1-0.7	+	6.8-7.1	Normal
High K_m for PEP and decreased or "normal" activity						
Waller and Löhr[411]	2	5-7	2-4	−		
Paglia et al.[341]	4	46-115	10	+	Decreased	
Paglia et al.[335]	3	44-104	45-13	+	Decreased	
Munroe and Miller[316]	1	92	10	−	Decreased	
Boivin et al.[220]	5	88	3-10	+, −		Normal
Sachs et al.[355]	3	59-87	4-6	−		
Ohyama et al.[326]	1	137	4.5	−	Abnormal	
Mentzer and Alpers[303]	1	40-70	2-4	+		
Oski and Bowman[328]	1	79	1.8	−		
Miwa et al.[306]	2	9-50	2-3	+		Fast
Miwa and Nishina[309]	7	16-115	3-4	+	Abnormal	
Boivin et al.[220]	7	50-100	1.4-8	+		
Paglia et al.[341]	2	100-150	5-10	+	Decreased	
Kahn et al.[273]	1	28	4	+		Normal
Low K_m for PEP and decreased activity						
Rose and Warms[69]	1	10	0.2	−		
Boivin et al.[220]	5	10-60	0.2-0.3	+, −		
Oski and Bowman[328]	3	10-20	0.25-0.50	−		
Gilman[244]	1	36	0.1	−		
Miwa et al.[306]	2	27-44	0.5	+		Fast
Brandt and Hanel[224]	1	500	0.1	−	Abnormal	Fast
Normal K_m for PEP and decreased activity						
Stall et al.[379]	2	50	Normal	+	Abnormal	

zymic patterns and the rate of activity of each isoenzyme seems to depend on factors characterizing the state of differentiation of the tissue in question.[282,283]

Recent studies in erythrocyte PK deficiency have demonstrated a similar deficiency in liver PK, giving support to the idea of common genetic control of liver and red cell PK.[210,261] It is yet to be determined whether PK deficiency represents a quantitative decrease in the production of normal enzymes as a result of a defective regulating or control gene (or messenger RNA) or as a result of a mutant structural gene. That PK deficiency is caused by a structural mutation is proved by kinetic heterogeneity, electrophoretic polymorphism, modification of the isoelectric point of deficient PK variants with different electrofocusing patterns, lowered molecular specific activity, or lowered concentration of abnormal PK molecules. Other cases with decreased activity but normal kinetics suggest a "thalassemia-like" lesion, with decreased synthesis of a structurally normal molecule. However, the lowered concentration or specific activity despite normal kinetics could reflect molecular instability (an "unstable hemoglobin-like" lesion).

Biochemical features. PK catalyzes the conversion of PEP to pyruvate. The cofactor, ADP, is converted to ATP, one of the two steps in the Embden-Meyerhof pathway that generate ATP:

$$\text{PEP} + \text{ADP} \overset{\text{PK}}{\rightleftharpoons} \text{pyruvate} + \text{ATP}$$

The enzyme requires magnesium and potassium,[316] is allosterically activated by FDP,[260,339] and is inhibited by ATP.[283] The intermediate 2,3-DPG either activates or inhibits, depending on whether the concentration of magnesium is high or low, respectively.[378]

Classically assays of PK in the deficient red cells of homozygous patients yield about 10% of normal activity. In a few of the early cases, abnormal kinetics with an increased K_m for PEP were described.[411,414] Atypical cases of PK deficiency, clinically and hematologically indistinguishable from classical PK deficiency, were described with normal or slightly decreased PK activity. Paglia et al.[341] documented in two unrelated families a mutant PK characterized by a tenfold increase in the K_m for PEP, a normal K_m for ADP, decreased pH optimum, and decreased functional stability that was partially restored by mercaptoethanol, a protector of sulfhydryl groups. The mothers and maternal relatives were heterozygotes for the kinetically aberrant enzymes, and the fathers and their relatives appeared to be heterozygotes for classical PK deficiency with 50% activity and a normal K_m for PEP. The affected children inherited a variant but different PK gene from each parent.

Within a relatively short period descriptions appeared of other mutant enzymes with (1) decreased activity and a normal apparent K_m for PEP,[379] (2) decreased activity and a decreased apparent K_m for PEP,[328] and (3) slightly decreased or normal activity and an increased apparent K_m for PEP.[355] In one case hemolytic anemia was associated with markedly increased PK activity and a low K_m for PEP.[224] Further differences based on FDP activation,[216,339] ATP inhibition,[211] nucleotide specificity, thermal stability, urea inhibition, electrophoretic mobility,[317] isoelectric focusing, and reactivity to antiserum to purified PK[261] have been documented, and the molecular and biochemical heterogeneity of PK deficiency is now well established. To date no correlation between enzyme activity, kinetic aberrations, electrophoretic and immunologic differences, and clinical severity has been determined.[408]

A summary of PK variants is presented in Table 12-10. Standardization and conformity of methods will be required before the uniqueness of the individual variants is established. A useful quantitative screening test employs an in vitro assay of PK from hemolysates at high and low concentrations of the substrate PEP and has proved helpful in detecting kinetic anomalies of PK.[341] The effect of the allosteric activator, FDP, should also be determined. This activator usually converts a sigmoid kinetic curve to a hyperbolic one, thus decreasing the K_m for PEP.

Metabolism and function of the PK-deficient cell. Defective catalytic efficiency of erythrocyte PK is associated with a number of important aberrations of erythrocyte metabolism and function.[225,247] Overall glycolysis (glucose utilization and lactate production) of PK-deficient red cells is decreased as compared with youthful control cells.[289,321] The enzymatic block at the PK step results in increased concentrations of a number of glycolytic intermediates proximal to PK. Most important, the level of 2,3-DPG is two to four times normal.[346] Increased levels of 2,3-DPG decrease oxygen affinity (right-shifted oxygen dissociation curve) and increase the $P_{50}O_2$.[236] The net result is increased oxygen delivery to the tissues.[331] In-

creased 2,3-DPG decreases anaerobic glycolysis by inhibiting HK and PFK, and inhibits the activity of the pentose phosphate shunt. Glycose consumption is greater in 2,3-DPG-depleted, PK-deficient red cells than it is in 2,3-DPG-replete cells.[246]

The level of ATP within PK-deficient red cells is decreased and is unstable when cells are incubated with glucose.[321,392] The marked instability of ATP is less pronounced in PK-deficient reticulocytes, which conserve ATP more readily and make more ATP than do older cells in the absence of glucose. Oxygen consumption in deficient reticulocytes is six to seven times normal, in keeping with the absolute dependency of the PK-deficient cell on mitochondrial oxidative phosphorylation for its supply of ATP.[304] Salicylates, which uncouple oxidative phosphorylation, induce a 25% to 75% decrease in ATP, produce loss of cell potassium and water, and blunt the normal oxidant responsiveness of the hexose monophosphate shunt.[245] Even in the absence of salicylates, PK-deficient cells have a pronounced leakiness and increased cation permeability with potassium loss exceeding sodium gain, resulting in concomitant loss of water, intracellular dehydration, and the formation of crenated, rigid, viscous spherocytes (''xerocytes'' or ''desiccytes'').[211] The decreased deformability of these cells renders them susceptible to entrapment and phagocytosis by reticuloendothelial cells, shortening their survival.

The level of FDP is four to six times normal in PK-deficient erythrocytes; this activator will convert the sigmoidal kinetic pattern to a hyperbolic Michaelis-Menton curve in some but not all variants of PK deficiency.[216,378] Other phosphorylated intermediates, G-6-P, F-6-P, triose phosphates, and 2-PG, are also increased and may stimulate overall glycolytic activity.[309] Finally, the content of NAD and NADH are both decreased in PK-deficient red cells and the ratio of NADH to NAD is increased. With incubation NAD virtually vanishes.[329] The unavailability of NAD, generated at the LDH step just beyond PK, seriously impairs the activity of GAPD,[348] the step at which NAD is reduced to NADH, the substrate of NADH-dependent methemoglobin reductase.

The role of the redox state of thiol groups in the PK-deficient red cell is less certain and controversial. Some investigators have argued that PK deficiency is merely an epiphenomenon and the result of increased concentration of GSSG in the red blood cell.[403,404] Incubation with mercaptoethanol and 2-mercaptopropionyl glycine restored the kinetics of an aberrant PK isozyme to normal, but in other studies Blume et al.[213] have shown that GSSG was in the normal range and that physiologic concentrations of GSSG failed to alter the kinetics and stability of normal or abnormal enzyme. In the face of a massive body of genetic, biochemical, and immunologic data implicating a primary defect in PK, the arguments of the epiphenomenonists appear less compelling.

Mechanism of hemolysis. Premature hemolysis in PK deficiency appears to be related to the intrinsic deficiency in ATP production with resultant dysfunction of the cell membrane, the high oxygen requirements of reticulocytes for mitochondrial oxidative phosphorylation, and the hostile hypoxic, static, and acidotic environment of the spleen, which selectively affects the vulnerable reticulocyte.[304] In the spleen the low P_{O_2} diminishes or even abolishes oxidative phosphorylation. The levels of ATP decline rapidly, producing alterations in the cell membrane and allowing massive losses of potassium and water. The deformed and dehydrated product of this metabolic defect is conditioned by the spleen and eventually removed from the circulation by reticuloendothelial cells of the liver and bone marrow. A variably smaller population of certain deficient cells, more endowed with enzyme than others, survives the reticulocyte stage and has a survival that is near normal.

Treatment. Because of the right-shifted oxygen dissociation curve, decreased oxygen affinity, and increased delivery of oxygen to the tissues, patients with PK deficiency generally tolerate anemia with few symptoms.[331] Patients with ineffective erythropoiesis, relative or absolute hypoplasia, and significant growth retardation may require intermittent transfusion therapy. Splenectomy is recommended for the most severely affected, symptomatic patients who require transfusions either regularly or intermittently.[320] The response to splenectomy, unlike that in hereditary spherocytosis, is not a cessation of hemolysis, but many patients have required significantly fewer transfusions and in some this requirement has been eliminated. Increased packed cell volume, marked reticulocytosis, and improved exercise tolerance have been noted after the procedure. Because of ongoing hemolysis and impaired phagocytic function, prophylactic penicillin administration is recommended.

Gallbladder surgery for cholelithiasis is frequently necessary in teenagers and young adults, particularly those in whom gallstones were identified preceding or at the time of splenectomy.

A number of novel experimental approaches designed to alter intracellular metabolism and improve the function or increase the activity of PK have been attempted. Despite the innovative nature, the results are still unconfirmed, the benefits uncertain, and the risks considerable. In vitro incubation of red cells with inosine and adenine is known to increase the intracellular concentration

of FDP, the prime allosteric activator of PK. Intravenous infusion of these nucleosides induced a tenfold increase in the content of FDP, a prolongation of red cell survival, a decrease in reticulocytosis and hyperbilirubinemia, and a rise in the level of hemoglobin.[215] Mannose, galactose, and fructose were given to another patient in an unsuccessful effort to increase the activity of PK.[380] Finally, Zanella et al.[421] gave the sulfhydryl compound 2-mercaptopropionyl glycine intravenously to two patients with PK deficiency, claiming a correction of the qualitative and quantitative abnormalities of the enzyme in both patients. Paradoxically, they noted an *increase* in reticulocytes (from 42% to 80%), a decrease in marked hyperbilirubinemia (from 18 mg/dl to normal), and a slight increase in hemoglobin value (from 9.5 to 10.5 gm/dl). The absolute requirement for adequate base line studies and steady state conditions is emphasized by these trials.

Future perspectives. PK-deficiency hereditary hemolytic anemia represents another example of how sophisticated biochemical techniques have uncovered a vast genetic polymorphism and biochemical heterogeneity in a disorder first identified less than two decades ago. More variants will be uncovered and biochemical engineering may permit a manipulation of the intracellular environment and improvement of the stability or catalytic efficiency of the enzyme. Successful bone marrow transplantation in the Basenji, the canine model of the disease, has already been achieved,[413] but this therapeutic approach will require a tremendous improvement in the risk-benefit ratio inherent in this procedure.

Obscure Embden-Meyerhof lesions

Glyceraldehyde phosphate dehydrogenase (GAPD) deficiency. Only three cases of mild, compensated hemolytic anemia associated with GAPD deficiency have been reported.[251,333] A father and son in one family had type I autohemolysis and 30% of normal GAPD activity. The third patient, also male, had about 60% of normal enzyme activity. Hemolysis was exacerbated by infection and oxidant drugs, but defects in the hexose monophosphate shunt or in GSH stability were not observed. The enzyme catalyzes the interconversion of Ga-3-P and 1,3-DPG and requires NAD generated at the LDH step and Pi:

$$\text{Ga-3-P} + \text{NAD} \xrightleftharpoons[\text{Pi}]{\text{GAPD}} \text{1,3-DPG} + \text{NADH}$$

NADH generated in the forward reaction is the major substrate for methemoglobin reductase, but increased amounts of methemoglobin or decreased capacity for methemoglobin reduction does not occur in GAPD deficiency. The concentrations of glycolytic intermediates in GAPD deficiency were similar to those induced by iodoacetate, an inhibitor of the enzyme and of glycolysis. The presence of four free sulfhydryl groups in red cell GAPD may be related to the susceptibility of GAPD-deficient cells to oxidant drugs and sulfhydryl inhibitors.

The molecular weight of human red cell GAPD is 137,000 daltons.[325] About 20% of the enzyme is membrane bound[373] and linked to PGK and cation transport.[297] However, the membrane-associated enzyme is indistinguishable from GAPD in the cytosol on the basis of molecular weight, kinetics, and pH optima.[275,345,361] At physiologic concentrations ATP causes dissociation of tetrameric GAPD into inactive dimers and monomers and induces the release of GAPD from the membrane.[234] Interestingly, 2,3-DPG prevents the inactivation of the enzyme. The relationship between hemolysis and the deficiency of GAPD is uncertain. Future studies of cation flux, methemoglobin reduction, and oxidant hemolysis may elucidate the mechanism of hemolysis.

2,3-Diphosphoglycerate phosphatase (2,3-DPGP) deficiency. A clinical syndrome with identical features in two children with 2,3-DPGP deficiency has been described by Syllm-Rapoport et al.[262,383] These children had a mild hemolytic anemia with cerebral dysgenesis, developmental retardation, hypotonia, and light-colored hair (achromotrichia). Hematologically reticulocytosis with a count of 3%, spherocytes in the peripheral blood, increased MCHC, elevated levels of ATP and ADP, and normal levels of 2,3-DPG were observed.

No activity of 2,3-DPGP was measurable. The elevation of ATP (40% to 60% above normal) was not associated with an increase in the ATP:ADP ratio, which in normal and in 2,3-DPGP-deficient red cells is 10:1. Increased glycolytic flux through PGK was hypothesized to explain the increase in adenine nucleotides. The normal levels of 2,3-DPG in the absence of 2,3-DPGP were thought to be related to the feedback inhibition of 2,3-DPG on 2,3-DPGM.

The mechanism of hemolysis in this syndrome is unexplained and uncertain. Indeed, why hemolysis should occur at all is unclear. Obviously additional cases and more detailed metabolic studies are required. The molecular weight of 2,3-DPGP is 57,000 daltons; there are two subunits of similar mass.[347,368] Harkness and Roth[252] have purified 2,3-DPGP and separated chromatographically two enzymes of 2,3-DPGP: One, probably the more important, is bisulfite stimulated; the second is stimulated by pyrophosphate. The enzyme is also activated by glycolate-2-phosphate, a metabolite that is used in the enzymatic assay of 2,3-DPG.

Recent controversial studies have cast some doubt about the existence of 2,3-DPGP (and perforce the Rapoport-Leubering pathway) and have suggested that a single enzyme, 2,3-DPGM, has both synthetic and degradative activity for 2,3-DPG, but most of the available evidence supports the existence of a distinct 2,3-DPGP.[277]

Enolase deficiency. Two sisters with less than 10% of normal activity of enolase were reported in 1972.[381] The proposita had a hemolytic crisis following the administration of nitrofurantion for a urinary tract infection with the persistence of a mild chronic hemolytic anemia following the acute episode. Hemoglobinuria, hemoglobinemia, spherocytes, schistocytes, increased osmotic and mechanical fragility, and a type II pattern of autohemolysis were observed. All other measured glycolytic enzymes, particularly those of the hexose monophosphate shunt, were normal.

There are a number of puzzling features about this report. The positive test for Heinz bodies and a positive ascorbate-cyanide test suggest the presence of an unstable hemoglobin, but screening or specific studies for this group of disorders were not performed. It is uncertain whether the sister had chronic hemolytic anemia and whether other family members were studied, and there have been no subsequent published reports of the defect. Finally, it is unclear why an oxidant drug should precipitate a hemolytic crisis in the presence of a deficiency of enolase. Because of the paucity of information, the significance of enolase deficiency is suspect until more data is made available.

Enolase reversibly converts 2-PG to PEP; the molecular weight of the enzyme, a dimer, is 95,000 daltons.[258] The pH optimum is pH 6.5, and Mg^{++} and NH_4^+ stabilize the subunits. No differences in kinetics and pH optima were detected in enolase purified from newborn and adult erythrocytes.[415] Enolase is inhibited by calcium and fluoride. Adding fluoride to drinking water to prevent caries results in a serum concentration of fluoride that inhibits enolase by about 15%.

OTHER ENZYME DEFECTS ASSOCIATED WITH HEMOLYSIS
Pyrimidine-5'-nucleotidase deficiency

A rare hereditary hemolytic anemia with a severe deficiency of erythrocyte pyrimidine-5'-nucleotidase was first described by Valentine et al.[189] in 1974 in six members of five kindreds. Originally presumed to be caused by a deficiency of RPK,[188,645] the anemia is associated with hemoglobin values ranging from 8 to 10 gm/dl, marked to moderate reticulocytosis, persistence of hemolysis after splenectomy, indirect hyperbilirubinemia, and obstructive jaundice requiring cholecystectomy. The inheritance pattern supports an autosomal recessive mode of transmission. Further cases have been reported from Israel.[429]

Other laboratory and biochemical features of pyrimidine-5'-nucleotidase deficiency include prominent basophilic stippling in the absence of lead poisoning and greatly increased concentrations of GSH (two times normal), total nucleotides (three to six times normal), and pyrimidine nucleotides and nucleosides. Cytidine makes up about 50% and uridine 30% of the total pyrimidines with only a small contribution from inosine (10%) and adenosine (10%). In the original study the increased nucleotides were thought to represent purines or adenosine phosphates.[188] Many cases previously diagnosed as belonging to the "high-ATP syndromes" may indeed represent examples of pyrimidine-5'-nucleotidase deficiency.* The activity of pyrimidine-5'-nucleotidase in erythrocytes of affected patients was only 3% to 10% of that in normal erythrocytes, and in presumed and obligatory heterozygotes the primidine-5'-nucleotidase activity is 50% to 80% of the normal mean.

Normally ribosomal RNA is degraded intracellularly by ribonucleases to 5'-nucleotides. These nondiffusable monophosphate catabolites (cytidine [CMP] and uridine [UMP] monophosphate) are dephosphorylated by pyrimidine-5'-nucleotidase to cytidine, uridine, and Pi, which then diffuse from the cell:

$$\begin{matrix} \text{CMP} \\ \text{or} \\ \text{UMP} \end{matrix} + H_2O \xrightarrow{\substack{\text{pyrimidine-} \\ \text{5'-nucleotidase}}} \begin{matrix} \text{cytidine} \\ \text{or} \\ \text{uridine} \end{matrix} + Pi$$

In enzyme-deficient cells the concentrations of pyrimidine monophosphate is markedly increased. Basophilic stippling results from retarded degradation of ribosomal RNA. The pathogenesis of hemolysis is less certain but is considered to be related to the excess pyrimidine nucleotides, which may (1) function as competitive cofactors of ATP and ADP for HK, PFK, and PK, (2) competitively interact with ATP and ADP and alter the normal ratio of these purine nucleotides, or (3) produce deleterious feedback inhibitions at other key steps of erythrocyte metabolism.

The increased level of GSH and the deficiency of RPK are more difficult to explain. Synthesis of GSH requires ATP and alterations in the ATP:ADP ratio, or the concentration of pyrimidine nucleotides may affect the synthesis or degradation of GSH. Similarly the synthesis of RPK, rather than the enzyme itself, may be inhibited by the surfeit of pyrimidines.

An acquired defect of pyrimidine-5'-nucleotidase associated with low-level lead exposure either in vitro or in vivo has been described.[583] Unlike

---

*References 452, 458, 460, 546.

the findings in the hereditary hemolytic anemia, elevated GSH, increased intracellular pyrimidine nucleotides, basophilic stippling, and anemia were absent. However, in severe lead-induced nucleotidase deficiency, hemolytic anemia, increased basophilic stippling, and increased intracellular levels of pyrimidine nucleotides, which mimic the events in the inherited deficiency of pyrimidine-5'-nucleotidase, have been documented.[646]

The enzymatic assay for pyrimidine-5'-nucleotidase is cumbersome, but the ultraviolet spectral characteristics of deproteinized extracts provide a simple screening test based on the shift of maximal absorption from the usual 256 to 257 nm to 266 to 270 nm, which is typical of pyrimidines.

Increased adenosine deaminase (ADA)

Clinical features. In 1970 Paglia et al.[585] first described a dominantly inherited hemolytic anemia with decreased red cell ATP. Although an enzyme defect was not detected initially, subsequent studies demonstrated that the activity of ADA was markedly increased in twelve of twenty-three relatives comprising three generations.[584,647] Males and females were equally affected. Patients suffered from a mild to well-compensated hemolytic anemia. The packed cell volume ranged between 35% and 41% and the reticulocyte count between 3% and 12%. No morphologic abnormalities were noted in the peripheral blood, the Coombs test was negative, no abnormal hemoglobins were detected, and enzymes of the Embden-Meyerhof pathway and hexose monophosphate shunt were normal. The concentration of GSH and the activity of pyrimidine-5'-nucleotidase were normal. Autologous red blood cell survival was shortened, with a half-life of ^{51}Cr-labeled cells of only 5 days. Normal red cells survived normally in a proband.

The major abnormalities were (1) a decrease of ATP and total nucleotides to only 60% of normal and 50% of reticulocyte-rich cells and (2) a profound, forty-five to seventy-fold increase in erythrocyte ADA. Low levels of erythrocyte ATP are not unique to this syndrome and may be seen in patients with unstable-hemoglobin hemolytic anemias, e.g., Hb Köln disease.[560,563]

Biochemistry. Two intracellular enzymes, adenosine kinase and ADA, compete for adenosine. In the first possible reaction involving adenosine kinase, adenosine is phosphorylated and serves as a salvage pathway for replenishment of adenine nucleotides:

$$\text{adenosine} + ATP \xrightarrow{\text{adenosine kinase}} ADP + AMP$$

However, in the presence of a low ATP and markedly increased activity of ADA, as occurs in this hemolytic anemia, adenosine is deaminated rather than phosphorylated despite the low K_m for adenosine of the kinase reaction:

$$\text{adenosine} + H_2O \xrightarrow{\text{ADA}} \text{inosine} + NH_3$$

This reaction will deplete adenosine, with resultant hemolysis perhaps related to the inability to salvage the adenine nucleotides AMP, ADP, and ATP. The only other salvage pathway for adenine nucleotides in the red cell employs RPK or APRT:

$$\text{ATP} + \text{R-5-P} \xrightarrow{\text{RPK}} \text{PRPP} + \text{AMP}$$

$$\text{PRPP} + \text{adenine} \xrightarrow{\text{APRT}} \text{AMP} + \text{PP}$$

Kinetic studies of ADA revealed that the K_m for adenosine, specific activity, heat stability, inhibitory constants, and electrophoresis were all normal and suggest overproduction of a structurally normal enzyme rather than the production of a mutant protein. Other enzymes involved in nucleotide metabolism were normal: ATPase, AK, AMP deaminase, adenosine kinase, and nucleoside phosphorylase. The activity of pyrimidine-5′-nucleotidase was about twice normal, and in some patients the activities of RPK and APRT were low, conceivably related to the decreased ATP content of the cells.

Adenosine triphosphatase (ATPase) deficiency

In 1964 Harvald et al.[254] described two siblings with a mild anemia, jaundice, and splenomegaly associated with a deficiency of erythrocyte ATPase. The ATPase in question was the sodium-potassium-magnesium–stimulated, ouabian-inhibited enzyme generally considered to play a central role in the active transport of sodium and potassium across the cell membrane. Additional cases were reported by Cotte et al.[468] and by Hanel and Cohn,[514] and an autosomal dominant mode of inheritance was proposed. The evidence for hemolysis and anemia in the patients described in the latter report is sketchy. The clinical severity varied from a severe hemolytic anemia to no abnormal clinical findings. Anisopoikilocytosis was seen occasionally, the reticulocyte count ranged from normal to 4%, the lowest hemoglobin level was 10.9 gm/dl, and the haptoglobin level was decreased in only one patient. The autohemolysis pattern was type I. Bilirubin and LDH levels, Coombs test, hemoglobin electrophoresis, and the activities of ATP, PK, G-6-PD, and GSSG-R were normal. The activity of ATPase in platelets and leukocytes was normal. The total ATPase was slightly decreased but a major deficiency of glycoside-sensitive ATPase, or S-ATPase, was noted. In other reported cases ATPase activity was about 50% of normal.[515] The concentration of intracellular sodium was 2.5 times normal, but the potassium content was normal. Studies of active cation transport,

passive leak, and exchange diffusion as well as of enzyme kinetics, glycolysis, and energy metabolism have yet to be performed. The pathogenesis of this ill-defined syndrome remains uncertain. An autosomal recessive form of ATPase deficiency with increased intracellular sodium has been described in a kindred in which affected individuals did not have hemolysis.[426]

An apparent physiologic deficiency of S-ATPase exists in the red cells of full-term and premature infants.[657] Whereas ouabain produces 60% ± 5% inhibition of ATPase activity in adult red cells and a 56% ± 9% inhibition in subjects with reticulocytosis, ouabain produced an inhibition of 43% ± 6% and 39% ± 6% in the ATPase of term and premature infants' erythrocytes. This relative deficiency of ouabain-sensitive, sodium-potassium–activated ATPase may be responsible for the excessive loss of potassium that occurs with incubation of newborn erythrocytes. Newborn cells are not unique in possessing an abnormal ATPase. Red cell ghosts of patients with Duchenne or limb-girdle muscular dystrophy contain an ATPase that is stimulated rather than inhibited by ouabain.[425]

Adenylate kinase (AK) deficiency

AK catalyzes the bidirectional reaction

$$2\text{ADP} \rightleftharpoons \text{ATP} + \text{AMP}$$

Two normal isoenzymes, types 1 and 2, have been identified in normal human erythrocytes and are distinguished by electrophoretic mobility.[487] Three genetically determined wild variants have been identified: hemozygotes with only type 1 or type 2 enzymes and heterozygotes with type 2-1 enzyme. The total activity of the enzyme in type 1 individuals is higher than that found in type 2-1 individuals, suggesting differences in the amount of the two isoenzymes or differences in their catalytic properties.

The first cases of erythrocyte AK deficiency associated with hereditary hemolytic anemia were reported by Szeinberg et al.[634,635] in two siblings of an Arab family, who were identified quite accidentally during an investigation of genetic polymorphism of AK in Israel. A third case was described by Boivin et al.[221] Two of the three patients had a moderately severe congenital hemolytic anemia with mild reticulocytosis (3% to 5%), indirect hyperbilirubinemia, and hepatosplenomegaly. Concomitant G-6-PD deficiency, but not the usual Mediterranean variant, was found in one male patient. His sister had a milder anemia.

Additional laboratory studies revealed normal osmotic fragility and increased autohemolysis with variable correction by glucose (Dacie type I or II). There were increased amounts of adenine nucleotides and normal or increased activity of all measured red cell enzymes except AK, which ranged from less than 1% to 13% of the mean normal values, depending on whether the reaction was measured in the forward or backward direction. The activity of AK in the hemolysates of presumed heterozygotes was about 25% to 75% of the normal mean, and an autosomal recessive transmission has been proposed.[655] All affected patients and tested family members had type 1 AK, as determined by starch gel electrophoresis; this is not surprising since the gene frequency of AK type 1 is 0.9617.

The mechanism of hemolysis in AK deficiency is uncertain, although increased ADP content suggests a block in the forward reaction or conversion of ADP to ATP and AMP. The double enzyme defect in one patient with both AK and G-6-PD deficiency and the decreased activity of AK (25% of normal) in his mother, who was heterozygous for G-6-PD deficiency, suggests a possible interaction or potentiating effect between these enzymes.

As with PK and PFK deficiency, an acquired deficiency of AK has been reported in patients with refractory anemia, dyserythropoietic anemias, and malignant blood diseases.[447] The incidence of AK deficiency in these disorders of hematopoiesis is lower than that of PK of PFK deficiency, with which it may be associated.

DEFECTS OF THE HEXOSE MONOPHOSPHATE SHUNT
γ-Glutamyl-cysteine (γ-GC) synthetase deficiency

In the first of two steps involved in the synthesis GSH, glutamic acid and cysteine are bonded by γ-GC synthetase to form the dipeptide γ-GC. A severe deficiency of γ-GC synthetase was identified in two siblings with well-compensated hemolytic anemia, reticulocytosis (8% to 10%), type II autohemolysis, moderate anisopoikilocytosis, intermittent episodes of jaundice, splenomegaly, and gallstones requiring cholecystectomy; one patient had a progressive spinocerebellar degenerative disease and the other had dysmetria and incoordination.[285] Red cell GSH content was less than 3% of normal and the activity of γ-GC synthetase was only 8% to 13% of normal. Presumed carriers had intermediate activity of the enzyme but normal levels of GSH. The activity of the second enzyme in GSH synthesis, GSH synthetase, was normal in the affected patients and the heterozygotes. Inheritance appears to be autosomal recessive. The relationship between the neurologic disorder and the deficiency of γ-GC synthetase is uncertain.

GSH synthetase deficiency

In 1961 Dutch investigators described the first reported cases of hereditary absence of GSH in erythrocytes.[576,600] A mild compensated hemolytic anemia with normal values of hemoglobin, decreased haptoglobin, slight hyperbilirubinemia, and a virtual absence of erythrocyte GSH was detected in four siblings. Hemolysis was exacerbated by oxidant drugs and fava beans. Osmotic fragility and the activities of G-6-PD and GSSG-R were normal. Heinz bodies were present but methemoglobinemia was not. Although a defect in tripeptide synthesis was suspected, assays of GSH synthetase were not performed. In 1966 French investigators using a radioisotopic method that quantified the incorporation of ^{14}C-glycine into GSH in the presence of preformed γ-GC and ATP first pinpointed the defect at the GSH synthetase step in two other patients with hereditary hemolytic anemia associated with a marked deficiency of GSH.[446] Glycolysis, oxygen consumption during incubation with methylene blue, and the activities of other enzymes in GSH-deficient erythrocytes were normal. The autohemolysis pattern was abnormal and atypical and did not correct with either glucose or ATP. Additional cases in an American family have been reported by Mohler et al.[567] As is γ-GC synthetase deficiency, GSH synthetase deficiency is inherited as an autosomal recessive trait. The mechanism of erythrocyte destruction is most likely related to oxidant hemolysis.

An unrelated disorder has been described with a deficiency of GSH associated with stomatocytes and a severe hemolytic anemia that responded to splenectomy.[562] Stomatocytes have not been described in deficiencies of either γ-GC synthetase or GSH synthetase. Two other animal models of GSH deficiency have been described. Dwarfed Alaskan malamutes have severe hemolytic anemia, stomatocytosis, and GSH deficiency,[595] and an 80% reduction in the levels of GSH have been found in Finn sheep.[626] Decreased γ-GC synthetase is the probable cause of the deficiency in sheep.[625] A specific enzyme deficiency in the dog has not been identified. Raised erythrocyte levels of GSH and GSH synthetase have been found in acute childhood leukemia (both in remission and in relapse),[580] acute myelogenous leukemia,[442] myelofibrosis lymphoma, and iron-deficiency anemia.[551] Diminished levels of GSH have been observed in patients with G-6-PD deficiency, acute renal failure, and hepatic failure.[532] In patients with myeloproliferative disorders and acute leukemia the GSH levels correlate with the activity of GSH synthetase. The levels of GSH synthetase are significantly lower in umbilical cord blood than in maternal blood, but no relationship exists between GSH stability and GSH synthetase activity.[565]

Glutathione reductase (GSSG-R) deficiency

Biochemistry and genetics. Oxidized glutathione (GSSG) in human erythrocytes is reduced in the presence of either NADPH or NADH, the reaction catalyzed by GSSG-R:

$$2GSSG + NSDPH + H^+ \xrightarrow{\text{GSSG-R}} 2GSH + NADP^+$$

The K_m for NADH is nearly twentyfold greater than the K_m for NADPH, the preferred cofactor. The enzyme contains FAD and is activated by the riboflavin-containing coenzyme. Three phenotypes, GSSG-R A, GSSG-R AB, and GSSG-R B, have been identified by starch gel electrophoresis.[443] The gene frequencies of the three isozymes are 98.1%, 1.9%, and 0.009%, respectively.[441] An autosomal dominant mode of inheritance has been proposed.

Clinical and laboratory findings. A drug-induced, allegedly congenital hemolytic anemia with GSSG-R deficiency and normal G-6-PD activity was first reported in 1959.[473] One early patient had hemolysis during the administration of quinine and isopentaquine.[461] Another patient developed hemolysis when treated with sulfisoxazole for a urinary tract infection and had only 38% of normal GSSG-R activity.[463] In one family with GSSG-R deficiency, hemolysis occurred after ingestion of poisonous mushrooms.[461] A partial deficiency of the enzyme has been reported in association with diverse hematologic abnormalities[652] including pancytopenia,[509,510] factor IX deficiency, Hb C disease,[653] and leukemia. Nonhematologic abnormalities such as neurologic disorders and Gaucher's disease have been associated with GSSG-R deficiency.[651] An apparent deficiency has been seen in otherwise healthy individuals without disease.[490]

Recent studies have demonstrated that the great variability in the clinical and laboratory features of the deficiency are more likely related to dietary riboflavin deficiency than to a congenital deficiency of GSSG-R. A number of patients presumed to have hereditary GSSG-R deficiency were restudied after periods of adequate intake of riboflavin and were found to have normal enzyme activity. Despite the return of GSSG-R activity to normal, hematologic abnormalities such as pancytopenia and hemolytic anemia persisted.[509] The in vivo survival of deficient cells is normal and the mild deficiency has no adverse effect on the activity of the hexose monophosphate shunt. Thus in most cases GSSG-R deficiency is caused by dietary rather than genetic factors. In fact, the activation of GSSG-R by riboflavin is an excellent in vitro diagnostic test for riboflavin deficiency.[507,508]

The activity of GSSG-R is increased in patients with diabetes mellitus,[544] chronic renal failure and anemia,[484] cirrhosis, gout,[543] and G-6-PD deficiency[462] and in cord blood.[662] The cofactor, FAD, stimulates the inactive form of the enzyme, which comprises 30% of the total enzyme in normal individuals but only 21% in cord blood hemolysates, 11% in patients with uremia, 9% in patients with cirrhosis and 5% in those with G-6-PD deficiency.[663] The increased activity of GSSG-R in all of these disorders except in cord cells is related to the increased percent saturation of GSSG-R with FAD. A disproportionately large portion of the enzyme is in the active or FAD-associated form, resulting in increased GSSG-R activity. Cord cells are only partly saturated with FAD even in the presence of increased intracellular levels of FAD, suggesting that the newborn's GSSG-R is functionally and perhaps structurally different. The increased susceptibility of newborn erythrocytes to oxidant stress may be related to functional abnormalities of GSSG-R and GSH-P.[586]

Glutathione peroxidase (GSH-P) deficiency

Biochemistry. GSH-P catalyzes the oxidation of GSH by peroxides including hydrogen peroxide and hydroperoxides[493]:

$$2GSH + H_2O_2 \xrightarrow{\text{GSH-P}} GSSG + 2H_2O$$

Peroxides are highly reactive species that are constantly generated in a number of physiologic redox reactions within the red cell. Superoxide radical produced during the oxygenation of hemoglobin is converted to H_2O_2 by superoxide dismutase. Potentially destructive to sulfhydryl-containing proteins (including hemoglobin, membrane proteins, and enzymes) and unsaturated fatty acids of membrane lipoproteins, hydrogen peroxide is detoxified by GSH-P.[99,100] The enzyme is highly specific for GSH, whereas a number of peroxides are metabolized. The reaction rate of GSH-P is proportional to the concentration of GSH within a physiologic range, a key factor in explaining the similarity of the clinical symptoms resulting from a deficiency of GSH and from a genetic or physiologic deficiency of GSH-P. Kinetic studies under simulated physiologic conditions show that GSH-P rather than catalase, which has a much higher K_m for GSH than does GSH-P, is the primary enzyme responsible for the elimination of H_2O_2 in erythrocytes.[494] Cohen and Hochstein[466] showed that catalase-deficient duck or azide-treated human red cells were protected against the toxic effects of low levels of H_2O_2 by GSH-P. In fact, the property of azide inhibition of catalase is used in the spectrophotometric assay of GSH-P.[581] Controversy still exists concerning the exact K_m for GSH and for H_2O_2. The enzyme also contributes to the regulation of the hexose monophosphate shunt by influencing the NADP:NADPH ratio via the GSSG-R reaction.

Recent studies by Hockstra et al.[518] and Janther et al.[528] have shown that GSH-P is a tetrameric selenoenzyme, each molecule of the enzyme containing four tightly bound molecules of selenium, and that the activity of the enzyme is dependent on dietary intake of selenium. This situation may be analogous to the riboflavin dependence of GSSG-R, in which many cases of presumed hereditary deficiency proved to have a nutritional origin.

In a study of the red cells in mice and humans the mean activity of GSH-P was reported to be significantly higher in females than in males, suggesting some hormonal regulation of the enzyme.[445] Hopkins and Tudhope[519] were unable to confirm this sex difference in humans.

Clinical and laboratory findings. GSH-P deficiency has been reported in association with the following:

1. A physiologic deficiency in the red cells of premature and full-term newborn infants with[571] or without hemolytic anemia[658]
2. A presumed hereditary deficiency of the enzyme with hemolytic anemia[572,574]
3. Drug-induced hemolysis[449]
4. A familial deficiency in asymptomatic Ashkenazic Jews and others of Mediterranean origin[437]
5. Iron-deficiency anemia[464,552,606]

Decreased activity of GSH-P in the red cells of premature and full-term newborns has been reported by some but not all investigators.[505,649] The level in the newborn is about two thirds of that in adult red cells, and normal values are not achieved until about 6 to 12 months of age. Emerson et al.[476] found a significant relationship between serum tocopherol levels and the activity of erythrocyte GSH-P. However, despite a definite deficiency of the enzyme in newborn infants compared with older infants and adults, no evidence of hemolysis was detected. Ten percent of 120 full-term infants developed hyperbilirubinemia but none showed excessive reticulocytosis, a fall in hemoglobin level, or Heinz body formation. The degree of jaundice was not related to the level of GSH-P. The results were the same in premature infants.

In a similarly conceived study Whaun and Oski[658] explored the relationship between the activity of erythrocyte GSH-P and neonatal jaundice. Infants with a deficiency of GSH-P did not become more jaundiced than the infants with normal-for-age levels of the enzyme. However, infants with high bilirubin levels (greater than 8.6 mg/dl in term infants; greater than 11.4 mg/dl in premature infants) had lower levels of GSH-P than did infants with low bilirubin levels. However, no statistically significant correlation could be found between GSH-P and the hemoglobin level, reticulocyte count, and tocopherol level.

These findings suggest that, despite deficiencies of both tocopherol and GSH-P, adequate protective mechanisms exist and defend the newborn infant's cells against oxidative hemolysis unless further stressed by drugs or infectious agents that lead to excessive accumulation of peroxides and that over whelm the system. In fact, newborn erythrocytes responded as well as adult cells to oxidative challenges despite their decreased content of GSH-P.[505] GSH oxidation and the response of the hexose monophosphate shunt to H_2O_2 were comparable in the different cells. Necheles et al.[571] first described a partial deficiency of red cell GSH-P in four unrelated newborn infants with hyperbilirubinemia, increased formation of Heinz bodies, and a mild hemolytic anemia. Signs and symptoms of hemolysis cleared after a few months but the deficiency of GSH-P persisted. In each family tested one clinically and hematologically normal parent had slightly reduced levels of GSH-P, and it was presumed that the affected infants were heterozygotes for GSH-P deficiency and that the deficiency was inherited as an autosomal recessive trait. Additional cases of neonatal hemolysis and heterozygosity[99] or homozygosity[575] for GSH-P deficiency have been reported, but no particular ethnic grouping was apparent.

An acute hemolytic reaction has been described in a presumed homozygote after he received an autotransfusion prior to cardiac surgery.[632] Drugs and toxins that may induce hemolytic crises in patients with a partial deficiency of GSH-P include quinine, phenacetin, acetylsalicylic acid, acetanilide derivatives, sulfisoxazole, nitrofurantoin, and alcohol.

Decreased activity of GSH-P has been documented in iron-deficient red cells, whether the enzyme is expressed as activity per cell, per volume of cells, or per gram of hemoglobin.[552] A highly significant correlation exists between serum iron and red cell GSH-P, and with treatment of iron deficiency the rise in serum iron parallels the increase in enzyme activity. These findings suggest that iron or iron-containing proteins may be necessary for enzyme synthesis and/or its activity or that iron and selenium absorption, transport, or utilization may be closely linked. The decreased activity of GSH-P in iron-deficiency anemia is not related to the anemia per se or to the hypochromia since the microcytic hypochromic red cells in β-thalassemia trait have normal levels of GSH-P.

Increased GSH-P activity has been found in diverse hematologic disorders including megaloblastic anemia, acute myeloblastic leukemia, myelofibrosis, erythroleukemia, and advanced carcinomatosis.[500] This acquired abnormality may be related to nutritional factors, the dyserythropoiesis that accompanies these disorders, or the increased levels of serum iron which occur in ineffective erythropoiesis.

Mechanism of hemolysis and future research. Although it is generally accepted that GSH-P deficiency leads to oxidative hemolysis via an attack of highly reactive peroxides on hemoglobin, enzymes, membrane proteins, and lipids, causing denaturation, Heinz body formation,[451] methemoglobinemia,[643] lipid peroxidation, and eventual hemolysis, it is still uncertain whether GSH-P deficiency is a primary or secondary defect. The role of selenium deficiency[541] and the relationship of this important trace element in GSH-P synthesis and function remains to be elucidated. Unfortunately the addition of selenium in vitro will not activate the enzyme as FAD will stimulate GSH-R, the stimulation serving as a measure of riboflavin deficiency.

Glucose-6-phosphate dehydrogenase (G-6-PD) deficiency

Historical background. The investigations establishing G-6-PD deficiency as the cause of primaquine sensitivity and other drug-induced hemolytic anemias are landmarks in hematology research. Since 1926 8-aminoquinolone antimalarials were known to produce acute hemolytic anemia, primarily in blacks.[433] In a series of brilliant studies conceived and performed at the University of Chicago in the mid-1950s Dern, Beutler, Alving, Carson, and their associates established that the red cell defect in primaquine-sensitive individuals was intrinsic, that only the oldest red cells were susceptible to the drug, that other compounds such as sulfonamides, analgesics, and furantoins induced hemolysis, and that Heinz bodies were present in peripheral blood cells of patients suffering from acute hemolytic anemia and after in vitro incubation with compounds causing hemolysis or blocking sulfhydryl groups.[37] It was found that the level of the major sulfhydryl compound of the erythrocyte, GSH, was reduced

in patients with primaquine sensitivity and that the content fell precipitously after incubation with acetylphenylhydrazine — the "GSH-stability" test.[431] The next logical step in this saga of medical detective work led to the pentose phosphate shunt and established that the initial enzyme, G-6-PD, was deficient.

More than 20 years later nearly 100 variants of G-6-PD have been identified and a number of different clinical patterns have been established with a spectrum ranging from oxidative stress–induced, acute, self-limited hemolysis to a moderately severe, chronic, congenital hemolytic anemia occurring primarily in whites.[417] Now recognized as the most common inherited disorder of the red cell — or for that matter any cell — G-6-PD deficiency affects more than 125 million individuals worldwide.[206,294]

Biochemistry. G-6-PD catalyzes the first reaction of the hexose monophosphate shunt, converting G-6-P to 6-PG. In the process, NADP is reduced to NADPH:

$$G\text{-}6\text{-}P + NADP \underset{}{\overset{G\text{-}6\text{-}PD}{\rightleftharpoons}} 6\text{-}PG + NADPH$$

The active form of the normal enzyme is a dimer or tetramer with a molecular weight of approximately 200,000 daltons. The identical monomeric subunits have a molecular weight of about 50,000 daltons. The K_m for G-6-P is 40 to 60 μM and the K_m for NADP is 2 to 6 μM, depending on the method used. The pH optimum is between 8.5 and 9.0. The normal enzyme uses substrate analogs (e.g., 2-deoxyglucose-6-phosphate and deamino-NADP) much less efficiently than it does the natural substrates. Further characterization is based on electrophoretic mobility, heat stability, and inhibition by the enzyme product NADPH.[206,224]

Normal G-6-PD (B+ enzyme) has been purified and fingerprinted.[664] Single amino acid substitutions have been identified in an electrophoretically

Table 12-11. Clinical features of representative G-6-PD variants

	A−	Mediterranean	Canton	Chicago
Ethnic group	African and African descent	Greek, Sardinian, Israeli, Iraqi	Chinese	N. Europe
Prevalence	Common	Common	Common	Rare
G-6-PD activity (% normal)	10-20	0-5	4-24	0-5
Drug- and infection-induced hemolysis	+	+	+	+
Favism	0	++	+	0
Neonatal jaundice	±	++	+++	++
Increased activity in red cells after hemolysis	+	Minimal	+	+
Chronic hemolysis	0	+	0	++
Drop in hemoglobin (gm/dl) with hemolysis	2-5	4-10	4-10	Chronically <10

Table 12-12. Classification of G-6-PD variants

Class	Characteristics	No. of variants
1	Severe enzyme deficiency with chronic hemolytic anemia	23
2	Severe enzyme deficiency (<10% of normal)	15
3	Moderate to mild enzyme deficiency	20
4	Very mild to no enzyme deficiency	17
5	Increased enzyme activity	1
	TOTAL	76

fast-moving variant, A+, and a variant with a five-fold increase in enzyme activity (G-6-PD Hektoen),[470,472,665] neither of which is associated with hemolysis.

Classification. The variants of G-6-PD deficiency may be classified clinically, biochemically, and electrophoretically. Four distinct clinical syndromes have been identified: (1) oxidative stress–induced (drug, infection, and other illnesses) hemolysis,[433] (2) favism,[588] (3) neonatal jaundice,[474] and (4) chronic congenital hemolytic anemia[294] (Table 12-11). The World Health Organization has compiled a listing of these recognized variants, which now number seventy-six[417] (Table 12-12) and can be classified according to clinical severity. Certain variants have been fairly completely characterized and appear to be distinctive (group I). In group II deficiency insufficient information is available to be reasonably certain that the variant is unique. About 10% of the reported variants fall in this category. Incompletely described variants (group III) and variants that are identical to those previously reported (group IV) complete the proposed classification schema. Many of the later are similar to the class 1 Chicago variant or to the class 2 Mediterranean or Chinese variants.

Drugs and disorders inducing hemolysis. The following oxidative drugs, infections, and other disorders induce or are associated with hemolysis in G-6-PD-deficient individuals.[433]

Clinically significant hemolysis	*No significant hemolysis under normal conditions*
Antimalarials	
Pamaquine (plasmoquine)	Chloroquine
Pantaquine	Quinine*
Primaquine	Quinacrine
Quinocide	
Antipyretics and analgesics	
Acetanilid	Acetylsalicylic acid
Aminopyrine*	Acetophenetidin
Antipyrine*	p-Aminosalicylic acid

*Causes hemolysis in whites only.

Sulfonamides

Salicylazosulfapyridine	Sulfadiazine
N-Acetylsulfanilamide	Sulfamerazine
Sulfapyridine	Sulfisoxazole
Sulfamethoxypyridazine	Sulfathiazole
Thiazolsulfone	Sulfoxone

Others

Acetylphenylhydrazine	Aniline
Fava beans*	Antazolene
Nalidixic acid	Ascorbic acid
Naphthalene	Chloramphenicol
Neoarsphenamine	Dimercaprol
Phenylhydrazine	Diphenhydramine
Toluidine blue	Menadione
	Methylene blue
	p-Aminophenol
	p-Aminobenzoic acid
	Procaine amide
	Probenecid
	Pyrimethamine
	Tripelennamine

Sulfones
Diaminodiphenylsulfone (dapsone)

Certain drugs produce clinically significant hemolysis in all deficient patients, whereas only whites are affected by others. With certain drugs, hemolysis occurs only with infections or other illnesses, conditions that are themselves causative rather than the drug. Most published lists of precipitating causes of hemolysis include compounds that have no adverse effect on the G-6-PD-deficient cell. Patients with G-6-PD deficiency should avoid only those drugs associated with clinically significant hemolysis (left column, above). Acetylsalicylic acid in concentrations as high as 350 mg/dl had no inhibitory effect on the resting or stimulated rate of hexose monophosphate shunt metabolism.[504] It is unlikely that therapeutic levels of aspirin (usually below 40 mg/dl) would be toxic to G-6-PD-deficient cells. The offending compounds or conditions generate free radicals and peroxides that are not detoxified in G-6-PD-deficient cells. The attack of highly reactive peroxides on sulfhydryl groups of membrane, hemoglobin, and cytoplasmic enzymes leads to denaturation, dysfunction, and eventual hemolysis. Incubation of G-6-PD-deficient cells with many of these agents results in a fall in the level of GSH, an increase in methemoglobin, and a decrease of $^{14}CO_2$ evolved from glucose-1-^{14}C, indicating a decreased stimulation of the hexose monophosphate shunt.

Distribution and incidence. Migration has contributed to the worldwide distribution of G-6-PD deficiency, which is particularly concentrated in the Mediterranean littoral (G-6-PD Mediterranean and variants), Africa (G-6-PD A−) and the Far

*Causes hemolysis in whites only.

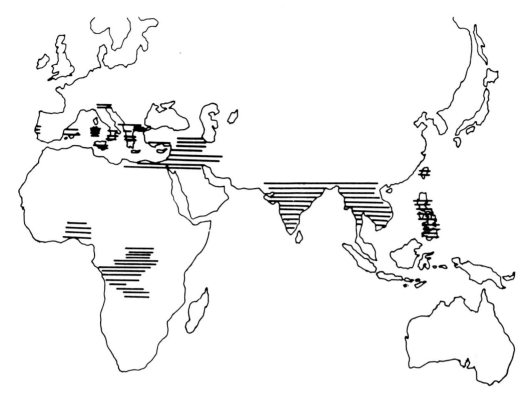

Fig. 12-13. Worldwide distribution of G-6-PD deficiency. (From Motulsky, A. G., and Campbell-Kraut, J. M.: In Blumberg, B. S., ed.: Proceedings of the conference on genetic polymorphisms and geographic variations in disease, New York, 1961, Grune & Stratton, Inc. Used by permission.)

East (Malaysia, Indochina, China, the Philippines, and Oceania).[294] Most patients with chronic congenital hemolytic anemia are from Northern Europe (Fig. 12-13).

The overlapping geographical distribution of G-6-PD deficiency (as well as sickle cell trait and thalassemia trait) and falciparum malaria has suggested a strong case for the selective advantage or balanced polymorphism of G-6-PD deficiency. Extensive investigations in Greece and in Sardinia have demonstrated a positive correlation between the incidence of G-6-PD deficiency and β-thalassemia trait and a significant relation of both to altitude and malaria parasitization.[623] Gene frequency of G-6-PD deficiency in low-lying areas (below 400 meters), previously associated with endemic malaria, was about 20%, whereas at altitudes above 400 meters the gene frequency was 3% to 8%. Confirmation of this correlation has not come from studies done in British Oceania.[549] However, other genetic and environmental factors, the heterogeneity of G-6-PD variants, and nutritional status may confer a protective effect on G-6-PD-deficient persons.

Three possible mechanisms may explain the decreased intraerythrocytic parasitization of G-6-PD-deficient erythrocytes: (1) the parasite is unable to invade the cell ("failed infection"), (2) the intra-cellular environment, with decreased levels of GSH and lowered activity of the hexose monophosphate shunt, prevents reproduction of the parasite ("abortive infection"), or (3) the parasitized red cell is destroyed by reticuloendothelial phagocytes ("suicidal infection").[549]

The incidence of G-6-PD deficiency varies in males from different ethnic groups. The gene frequency in Chinese is about 5%, in black Americans the range is from 10% to 15%, and in Kurdish Jews frequencies as high as 70% have been reported.

Genetics and X linkage. The gene for G-6-PD is located on the X chromosome. Studies of families reveal that transmission occurs from mother to son but not from father to son. Male hemizygotes ($\overline{X}Y$) and female homozygotes ($\overline{XX}$) are invariably more severely affected than female heterozygotes ($\overline{X}X$).[206] Additional evidence for the X linkage of G-6-PD deficiency has come from studies on color blindness suggesting that the gene for G-6-PD lies between the genes for color blindness.[423]

Females who are heterozygous for G-6-PD deficiency usually have levels of G-6-PD intermediate between those of fully affected males and normal subjects. Some heterozygous women, however, have normal red cell G-6-PD activity, while others have a quantitative deficiency as severe as hemizygotes. The behavior of the X-linked gene in G-6-PD deficiency bears out Lyon's hypothesis of X inactivation. The erythrocytes of female carriers of G-6-PD are either completely normal or completely abnormal. Females with two X chromosomes and individuals with more than two X chromosomes (e.g., Klinefelter's syndrome, XXY) do not have more G-6-PD activity than normal males with only one X chromosome. The variable amount of total G-6-PD activity and the double population of cells or mosaicism in heterozygous females is determined by the inactivation of the X chromosome bearing either the normal or the deficient gene for G-6-PD. Pseudomosaicism may be produced histochemically in populations of normal cells and in cells from hemizygotes, reflecting the physiologic deterioration of G-6-PD activity with normal aging of the red cell.[76] Inactivation of the abnormal gene in 90% of erythroid precursors during embryogenesis of a genotypic heterozygote could conceivably result in a phenotypically G-6-PD-deficient female. Additional evidence for Lyonization in G-6-PD deficiency has been provided by cloning studies of cultured fibroblasts and from naturally occuring clones in heterozygous patients with leiomyoma, chronic granulocytic leukemia, and lymphoma.[486] These tumors arise from a single cell bearing a single type of G-6-PD.

The levels of G-6-PD are very similar in identical twins heterozygous for G-6-PD deficiency but dissimilar in fraternal twins, suggesting either nonrandom inactivation of the X chromosome or postinactivation selection, i.e., a natural selection permitting the proliferation of a particular clone of cells over another.[453]

Electrophoretic patterns of subunits from the normal (B) and from the common A+ variant showed a single protein band indicating that the B and A enzymes each consist of different subunits and do not share subunits.[538] Since the A enzyme is a structural variant resulting from a single amino acid substitution (asparagine in B replaced by aspartic acid in A), Yoshida has proposed that human G-6-PD consists of identical subunits and that only one structural gene is involved in synthesizing the enzyme.[666]

G-6-PD in other tissues. It is generally believed that the G-6-PD in other tissues is identical to the enzyme in the red cell and that in severe deficiency states the defect is mirrored in other tissues including leukocytes, platelets, fibroblasts, liver, kidney, adrenals, saliva, and the lens of the eye.

Schlegal and Bellanti[614] proposed that there was a relationship between G-6-PD lability and/or deficiency and increased susceptibility of deficient males to infection. However, decreased bactericidal activity in G-6-PD-deficient phagocytes has

not been observed unless there is marked (<5%) or total absence of G-6-PD in the leukocytes of patients with the red cell defect. Generally the leukocyte G-6-PD activity in deficient males is about 15% of normal.[561] The metabolic and bactericidal defects in this group of severely affected individuals resemble those seen in the phagocytes of patients with chronic granulomatous disease. Alternate pathways of intracellular bacterial killing permit the partially G-6-PD-deficient phagocyte to function normally.

Approximately 10% to 15% of glucose metabolism in the resting platelet flows through the pentose shunt, a pathway coupled with lipid synthesis through the generation of NADPH. Abnormalities of platelet function have been described in some G-6-PD-deficient patients[616] but not in others.[561] Defective de novo lipid synthesis has not been reported. The citric acid cycle serves as an alternate generator of NADPH and thus protects the platelets.

The activity of G-6-PD in the lenses and cataracts of G-6-PD-deficient subjects is less than 50% of that measured in normal individuals and suggests a possible relationship.[668] Associations with other diseases, including Crohn's disease, idiopathic cardiomyopathies, hypertension, epilepsy, pernicious anemia, schizophrenia, and cancer will require confirmation.[545]

Clinical and laboratory findings

Neonatal hyperbilirubinemia. Doxiadis et al.[474] have shown that in one third of the Greek full-term infants with severe neonatal jaundice isoimmunization could be excluded. A deficiency of G-6-PD in many of these infants may have been the causative factor in jaundice and kernicterus.[587] A similar relationship has been reported from China,[529,547,624] India,[557] Italy,[556] Nigeria,[503] South Africa,[542] Thailand,[492,594] and Malaysia.[455,624] In Thai newborns G-6-PD deficiency was present in 65% of severely jaundiced (bilirubin greater than 15 mg/dl) infants. In the United States, G-6-PD deficiency in black premature infants is associated with an increased incidence of hyperbilirubinemia and a greater frequency of exchange transfusions.[478] No increased incidence of either was observed in black full-term infants with G-6-PD deficiency. The incidence of neonatal jaundice in black Africans is much higher than it is in black Americans despite the fact that both have the same A− variant, again suggesting an environmental role.

It is noteworthy that, although an increase in neonatal jaundice has been observed in Greece[475] and the Orient,[547] it could not be documented in Israel.[636] The G-6-PD variant most prevalent in these regions is the same, G-6-PD Mediterranean. The reasons for the discrepancy are unclear.

Environmental factors may play a role in neonatal hemolytic anemia associated with G-6-PD deficiency. A dye mixture used to sterilize the umbilical cord and the routine administration of vitamin K derivatives have been suggested as etiologic agents.[496] In most cases no definite exogenous agent has been determined beyond the suggestion of normal enzymatic immaturity of the newborn's red cells and liver.

The ever-present danger of kernicterus and potential death in jaundiced newborns from certain ethnic groups with a high incidence of G-6-PD deficiency should prompt the clinician to initiate appropriate diagnostic studies and therapy, including exchange transfusion. Anemia, reticulocytosis, and peripheral blood abnormalities may not be present. Clinically apparent jaundice occurs in the first 48 hours of life in three quarters of the affected infants and rapidly may reach levels of 30 to 45 mg/dl. Severe hyperbilirubinemia, kernicterus, and death have occurred in infants discharged from hospital during the first week only to return moribund a few days later.

Two preventive measures should be considered: First, administration of oxidant drugs to the mother may precipitate neonatal jaundice in the G-6-PD-deficient infant[506,592]; second, hyperbilirubinemia of G-6-PD-deficient infants may be nonhemolytic in origin, suggesting a possible hepatic defect. Phenobarbital may keep levels of bilirubin below 20 mg/dl and obviate exchange transfusion.[556] A quantitative assay for G-6-PD in the infant and the mother should be performed rather than a qualitative screening test. The indications for exchange transfusion are similar to those in infants with hemolytic disease of the newborn secondary to Rh or blood group incompatibility. A high level of suspicion and early exchange transfusion may be lifesaving.

Congenital hemolytic anemia in white newborns may commonly present as unexplained neonatal jaundice. This entity will be discussed in greater detail.

Drug-induced hemolytic anemia. Experimental studies of drug-induced hemolysis in G-6-PD-deficient persons have elucidated characteristic and reproducible clinical and laboratory manifestations, which are graphically presented in Fig. 12-14.[433] During the base line steady state period prior to drug exposure the hematocrit, reticulocyte count, and survival of ^{51}Cr-labeled autologous red cells are normal.

Acute intravascular hemolysis occurs 1 to 3 days following the daily oral administration of primaquine, 30 mg. The hematocrit drops 25% to 35%,

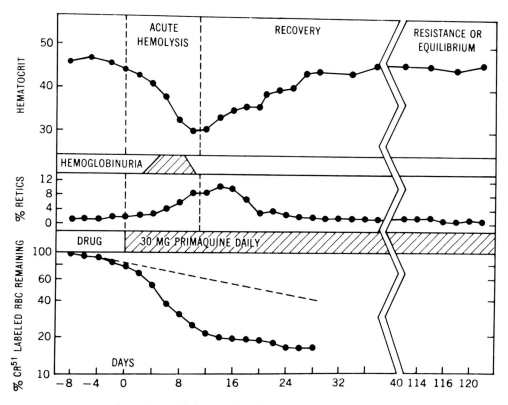

Fig. 12-14. Course of experimentally induced hemolytic anemia in primaquine-sensitive individuals. (From Alving, A. S., et al.: Bull. W.H.O. **22:**621, 1960).

reaching a nadir at 8 to 10 days, and Heinz bodies are present in peripheral blood erythrocytes stained with such supravital dyes as 1% cresyl violet. Methemalbuminemia, hemoglobinemia, hemoglobinuria, decreased haptoglobin and GSH levels, GSH instability, and bizarre red cell morphology with polychromasia, fragments, schistocytes, and cells resembling half-moons ("lunacytes") are noted. Patients may have malaise, low-grade fever, scleral icterus, abdominal or back pain, and dark urine. Hepatosplenomegaly may occur but is unusual.

The slope of the red cell survival curve plunges sharply, but 10 to 14 days after the onset of acute hemolysis a *recovery phase* begins. It is associated with a steady rise in hematocrit and hemoglobin to previous levels, reticulocytosis that reaches a peak at 14 to 16 days and decreasing thereafter. The slope of the ^{51}Cr survival curve returns to normal and clinically the patient is markedly improved despite continued administration of the offending agent. Often patients seek medical attention during the recovery phase when, because of the reticulocytosis, G-6-PD activity in the circulating red cells is normal and qualitative screening tests are negative.

In the *equilibrium phase* patients have a completely compensated hemolytic process without anemia, reticulocytosis, or jaundice. Further administration of the drug 3 to 4 months after the initial hemolysis or an increase in the amount of primaquine given will precipitate another acute hemolytice episode and a recurrence of the initial clinical and laboratory features.

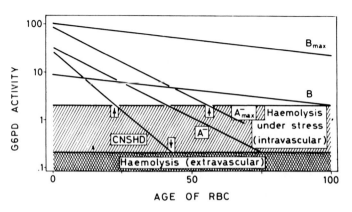

Fig. 12-15. The basis for hemolysis of red cells with different types of G-6-PD. Abscissa: red cell age as percentage of normal life span (120 days). Ordinate (log scale): G-6-PD activity as percentage of the value found in normal red cells at the time of their release into the circulation. Lines B, A−, and CNSHD represent, respectively, as a function of the age of the erythrocyte, the G-6-PD activity under basal conditions of normal cells, cells with the common African type of G-6-PD deficiency, and cells with one of the rare G-6-PD-deficient variants associated with chronic nonspherocytic haemolytic disease (CNSHD). The lines labelled B_{max} and A^-_{max} represent similarly the respective G-6-PD activities under conditions of maximal stimulation that would take place under the effect of a redox stress. The following points are illustrated. (1) Normal cells will not hemolyze through scarcity of G-6-PD activity, as sufficient activity is retained not to compromise survival to the end of normal life span. (2) Red cells with the A− type of G-6-PD deficiency can enjoy at least 75% of their normal life span under basal conditions; at that point the enzyme activity left is only about 0.2% of the original normal enzyme activity. This level seems to be the threshold below which the RE system removes erythrocytes (cross-hatched area). (3) Red cells with one of the more severe types of G-6-PD deficiency reach the same threshold long before they have completed half of their life span (downward arrow): CNSHD results. (4) A redox stress raises the level of G-6-PD activity required by the red cell for survival (the height of the new threshold depends on the severity of the stress; as an example, it is indicated by the upper hatched area at a level of about 2% of the original normal activity). As a result there will be a sudden extra-destruction, which may be largely intravascular, of the red cells, the G-6-PD activity of which falls between 0.2% and 2%. It is seen in the example shown (upward arrows) that 60% of the circulating red cells will still survive in the case of A− but less than 25% in the case of CNSHD. The degree of hemolysis, both in the absence and the presence of stress, depends primarily and critically on the slope of the fall in enzyme activity with red cell age, which is characteristic for each variant of G-6-PD. Note that the distance between the lines A^-_{max} and A− is much less than the distance between B_{max} and B, because the "reverse" capacity for NADPH production is much lower in the A− cells. (From Luzzatto, L.: Clin. Haematol. **4**:83, 1975.)

Drugs that induce hemolysis in G-6-PD-deficient individuals are presented on p. 352. Other disorders such as infectious hepatitis, infectious mononucleosis, viral respiratory infections, bacterial pneumonia and sepsis, and diabetic ketoacidosis may precipitate hemolysis as well.

Hemolysis is self-limited in patients with the G-6-PD A− variant and in patients with G-6-PD Mediterranean but is more severe in the latter group than in the former. The severity of the anemia is more likely related to the rate of decline of G-6-PD in vivo during red cell aging than it is to the activity of G-6-PD in the red cell. In normal red cells G-6-PD activity decreases as the cells age, but even at 120 days, the end of a normal lifespan, there is sufficient G-6-PD activity to ensure survival. Activity in deficient cells is lower to begin with and declines much more rapidly. Piomelli et al.[597] have shown that in the A− variant an 80-day-old erythrocyte has virtually no enzyme activity and a 15-day-old cell has only 50% of the activity present in a newborn cell. The slope of the decline is steeper in G-6-PD Mediterranean: There is no G-6-PD activity in a 10-day old cell (Fig. 12-15).

The rate of hemolysis in the unstressed state depends on the length of time red cells circulate before the activity of G-6-PD reaches a critical level. In the G-6-PD A− or Mediterranean variant the activity of enzyme falls below the critical level after 90 to 100 days, or 75% of the normal life span, when only 0.2% of the original enzyme activity remains. Deficient cells are then removed by the reticuloendothelial system. With oxidant stress the level of G-6-PD activity required to protect the cell is ten times higher than in the basal state (about 2% of original activity). Accordingly older cells are more susceptible to hemolysis. In G-6-PD A− under stress about 40% of the circulating cells will be destroyed intravascularly, but in more severe conditions progressively younger cells will be affected. In summary, the degree of hemolysis, in the absence or presence of stress, depends on the slope of the fall in enzyme activity with red cell maturity, which is characteristic for each variant.

Favism. Favism is similar to drug-induced hemolysis except that not all persons with G-6-PD deficiency are susceptible to the effects of eating broad beans *(Vicia faba)* or inhaling the pollen of the bean flower. Acute hemolytic anemia occurs almost exclusively in persons with G-6-PD Mediterranean[534] but has also been reported in Chinese patients[549] and in a German patient with chronic congenital hemolytic anemia (G-6-PD Zähringen).[659] Favism does not occur in G-6-PD A−. Sensitivity to the fava bean requires both G-6-PD deficiency and an additional factor or factors also thought to be inherited.[630] An autosomal recessive characteristic that may be age influenced has been proposed. Additional support for the genetic transmission of favism comes from the finding that the frequency of the carriers of the P^a and P^c alleles of the gene for red cell acid phosphatase was significantly higher in G-6-PD-deficient male subjects with favism than in the general population.[450] Serum from normal persons as well as serum from some patients with G-6-PD deficiency can prevent normal cells from being agglutinated by an extract of beans.[609] Serum from patients with favism does not possess this protective property, which resides in the IgA fraction of normal serum.[613] Further confirmation that enzyme deficiency is a necessary but not sufficient factor in favism comes from the experimental demonstration that enzyme-deficient siblings of patients with favism did not manifest the disease when injected with a large dose of bean extract.

It is of interest that the fava bean is a rich source of the amino acid L-dihydroxyphenylalanine, or L-dopa, the drug used to treat parkinsonism. Dopaquinone, the oxidation product of L-dopa, has the capacity to destroy GSH. However, the administration of L-dopa to G-6-PD-deficient patients failed to induce hemolysis and thus the pathogenesis of hemolysis induced by the tasty bean remains to be determined.[498]

Ingestion of small amounts of fava beans, usually in late spring when the bean first appears in the marketplace, produces in sensitive persons, especially infants and young children, a sudden acute attack of hemolysis accompanied by jaundice and often hemoglobinuria.[513] The clinical spectrum ranges from mild disease to massive and fatal hemolysis. Historically sensitivity to the bean has been held responsible for the loss of important Greek and Roman battles. Hemolysis appears from a few hours to 1 to 2 days after exposure and the episode usually lasts less than a week. Favism occurs especially in Sicily, Calabria, Sardinia, and in other countries about the Mediterranean. Sporadic cases have occurred in the United States[555] and in England.[454] When caused by inhalation of the pollen from the blossom of the bean plant, the hemolytic episode may begin within a matter of minutes. The fresh and uncooked beans are thought to be more dangerous than those that have been dried or cooked.

The precipitous drop in hemoglobin and the extreme prostration associated with hemolysis often require emergency transfusion therapy. Appropriate diagnostic studies, including a quantitative assay for G-6-PD, should be performed prior to rather than after transfusions are given.

Chronic congenital hemolytic anemia. Thirty-five variants of G-6-PD deficiency associated with chronic hemolytic anemia have been described.[417]

In general the clinical features are similar to those described in other patients with enzymopathies (Fig. 12-16). Lifelong mild to moderately severe hemolysis and exacerbations of hemolysis with infection are hallmarks of the disorder. Virtually all cases have been reported in males (99%). Sixty percent of the patients are of Northern European ancestry, 20% Mediterranean, 14% Oriental, and 6% black. Neonatal jaundice has been reported in about 75% of the cases, splenomegaly in 40%, and cholelithiasis in 20%. Anemia is usually mild — only 20% of the patients have a steady state hemoglobin level below 10 gm/dl. The range of reticulocyte counts is 2% to 35% of bilirubin, 1 to 25 mg/dl; and of ^{51}Cr survival, 3 to 20 days.

The documentation that a variant enzyme is unique requires the following biochemical studies, conventionally performed on partially purified enzyme: quantitative assay, electrophoretic mobility, K_m for G-6-P, K_m for NADP, utilization of the substrate analogs 2-deoxy-G-6-P and deamino-NADP, heat stability, pH optima, and K_i for NADPH (Tables 12-13 and 12-14). As seen in Fig. 12-16, nearly 70% of the variants associated with chronic hemolytic anemia have less than 5% of normal activity. The range is 0 to 35%. A majority (53%) have abnormal electrophoretic mobility, and most (80%) migrate slightly faster than the normal B variant. Abnormal kinetics with G-6-P, NADP, and substrate analogs have been noted in 57%, 40%, and 62%, respectively, of the reported cases. Heat stability is usually markedly diminished but the pH optima curves are variable.

The dissociation between relatively mild clinical symptoms and marked aberrations in red cell survival and in enzyme activity, kinetics, and stability is striking and emphasizes the heterogeneity of these syndromes. The physiologic activity of G-6-PD under simulated intracellular conditions may be a more important determinant of the severity of hemolysis.[666] Variants of G-6-PD associated with chronic hemolysis have a high K_m for NADP or a low apparent K_i for NADPH (e.g., G-6-PD Manchester, Alhambra, and Tripler). Variant enzymes associated with drug-induced hemolysis are characterized by a low K_m for NADP and a high K_i for NADPH (e.g., G-6-PD Mediterranean and A−). Two variants (G-6-PD Union and Markham), each with less than 10% activity, have a low K_m for G-6-P and a high K_i for NADPH, but neither is associated with hemolysis (Table 12-13).

The glycolytic rate and the levels of ATP and 2,3-DPG are elevated in patients with chronic hemolytic anemia. Both ATP and 2,3-DPG inhibit G-6-PD at physiologic concentrations. The intracellular concentration of NADPH is about 50 ± 5 μM and that of NADP about 1 to 2 μM. Even accounting for the decreased ability of the G-6-PD-deficient cell to generate NADPH, physiologic concentrations of NADPH, ATP, and 2,3-DPG suppress the activity of G-6-PD. Under simulated

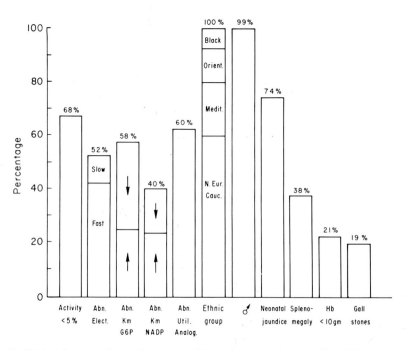

Fig. 12-16. Clinical features of chronic congenital hemolytic anemia caused by G-6-PD deficiency.

Table 12-13. Michaelis constant (K_m) for NADP and inhibition constant (K_i) for NADPH of normal and variant G-6-PD*

Enzyme	Activity (% normal)	K_m for NADP (µM)	K_i for NADPH (µM)	Hemolytic syndrome†
B+	100	12.5	9	—
A+	80	7.2	6.7	—
A−	8-20	8	13	Drug-induced hemolysis
Mediterranean	<5	3.8	9.5	Drug-induced hemolysis, favism
Union	<3	8.2	37	No hemolysis
Markham	1.5-10	6.0	16	No hemolysis
Manchester	25-30	18.5	0.8	CCHA
Alhambra	9-20	19.5	3.3	CCHA
Tripler	35	80	2.6	CCHA
Torrance	2.4	9.3	3.0	CCHA

*Modified from Yoshida, A., and Lin, M.: Blood **41**:877, 1973.
†CCHA = chronic congenital hemolytic anemia.

Table 12-14. G-6-PD deficiency associated with chronic congenital hemolytic anemia

Variant and reference	Ethnic group	G-6-PD activity (% normal)	K_m for G-6-P	K_m for NADP	Utilization of analogs
With normal electrophoretic pattern (B−)					
Aarau	Swiss	7	↓	N	Slightly abnormal
Albuquerque[436]	U.S.A. (white)	1	↑	↑	Normal
Bangkok[640]	Thai	5	N	Sl, ↑	Abnormal
Bat Yam[602]	Iraqi (Jewish)	0	↓	—	Abnormal
Boston[573]	Polish (Jewish)	5	↓	N	Abnormal
Chicago[539]	W. European	9-26	N	N	Normal
Cornell[561]	N. European	5	N	↑	Normal
Duarte[417]	U.S.A. (white)	8.5	N	N	Slightly abnormal
Englewood[604]	Italian	0.5	N	↓	Abnormal
"Hamburg"[615]	W. German	5	↑ ↑	N	—
Hayem[417]	French	0	N	N	Abnormal
Hong-Kong[661]	Chinese	0-15	↓	N	Slightly abnormal
New York[604]	Italian, black	0.6	N	N	Abnormal
Oklahoma[538]	W. European	4-10	↑ ↑	↑	Normal
Tokoshima[566]	Japanese	4.4	N	↑ ↑	Normal
"Tubingen"[430]	W. German	0.3	↓	↓	—
With fast electrophoretic pattern					
Charleston[435]	U.S.A. (black)	14	↓	↑	Abnormal
Heian[569]	Japanese	8-9	↑	N	Abnormal
Ohio[596]	Italian	2-16	Sl ↑	Sl ↑	Normal
Torrance[638]	U.S.A.	2.4	N	N	—
With slow electrophoretic pattern					
Alhambra[439]	Scandinavian	9-20	N	Sl ↓	Normal
Ashdod[602]	N. African (Jewish)	10	↑	—	Abnormal
Carswell[622]	Irish	2-6	Sl ↓	N	Abnormal
Freiburg[459]	W. German	10-20	↑	N	—
Johannesburg[427]	S. African (white)	7-35	↑	Sl ↓	Abnormal
Long Prairie[530]	U.S.A. (German)	2-8	↓	N	Abnormal
Manchester[564]	English	20-25	N	N	Slightly abnormal
Milwaukee[656]	Puerto Rican	0.5	↑ ↑	—	Normal
Ramat-Gan[602]	Iraqi (Jewish)	0	N	—	Abnormal
Rotterdam[666]	Dutch	1.9	Sl ↓	N	Abnormal
Tokyo[566]	Japanese	3	N	N	Normal
Tripler[477]	U.S.A. (white)	35	N	—	Normal
Utrecht[629]	Dutch	15	N	Sl ↑	—
Worcester[628]	U.S.A. (white)	0	↓	↑ ↑	Normal

Sl = slight; N = normal.

physiologic conditions only 0.1% to 0.2% of the maximum potential activity of G-6-PD is expressed in red blood cells. Deficient, kinetically aberrant or unstable G-6-PD associated with chronic hemolysis would be even more sensitive to the inhibitory effects of NADPH, ATP, and 2,3-DPG. The oxygen affinity is decreased and, as in other G-6-PD-deficiency states, the intracellular concentration of GSH is low and falls precipitously when cells are incubated with acetylphenylhydrazine. The autohemolysis pattern is type I with correction by glucose and ATP. Although red cell survival is shortened, splenic sequestration of ^{51}Cr-labeled cells is not seen. Infections, exposure to oxidant drugs and toxins, and occasionally fava beans exaggerate hemolysis in these patients and preventive measures should be employed.

Other disorders associated with G-6-PD deficiency

Other hereditary hemolytic anemias. A deficiency of G-6-PD has been reported in association with other enzymopathies[153] (deficiencies of GPI,[364,612] TPI, PK, and AK), membrane defects (hereditary spherocytosis),[610,629] and sickle cell anemia.[598] The presence of double heterozygosity for two distinct enzyme defects may be beneficial metabolically. For example, in combined G-6-PD-GPI deficiency, the accumulation of G-6-P may actually enhance the activity of GPI and improve the flow of energy through the Embden-Meyerhof pathway, permitting the enzyme to operate nearer to substrate saturation than do cells with isolated GPI deficiency. Catalase activity is decreased in black patients with G-6-PD deficiency and declines further when the subjects or their red cells are exposed to oxidant stress.[639]

Piomelli et al.[598] reported a significant increase of G-6-PD A− in patients with sickle cell anemia and suggested that the simultaneous inheritance of both defects may be beneficial clinically. The activity of G-6-PD is eight times greater in patients with G-6-PD A− and sickle cell anemia than in subjects with G-6-PD A− and normal hemoglobin. Similarly sickle cell patients with G-6-PD A− had higher reticulocyte counts than did sickle cell patients with normal G-6-PD. Generally cell aging in sickle cell anemia is associated with increased numbers of irreversibly sickled cells.

Lead. Significantly higher concentrations of lead in the red blood cells of G-6-PD-deficient than in G-6-PD-normal black children have been found in an urban population.[554] Although no hemolytic effects were noted, others have reported lead-induced acute hemolytic crises, decreased GSH in lead workers, and a progressive decrease in G-6-PD activity in lead-treated rats.

Endocrinopathies. In patients with either hypothyroidism or hypopituitarism, the activity of G-6-PD is below normal.[607] Following appropriate therapy with thyroid or human growth hormone, enzyme activity increases and is a sensitive index of the adequacy of hormone replacement. In hyperthyroidism the activity of G-6-PD is significantly increased and returns to normal after 1 to 2 months of euthyroidism.[648]

Myelofibrosis. Increased levels of GSH, G-6-PD and 6-PGD have been reported in patients with myelofibrosis, and assays may be helpful in distinguishing this disorder from others resembling it clinically.[512]

Other disorders. Hemolysis in *hepatitis* is four times more common in G-6-PD-deficient than in G-6-PD-normal Greek children.[535] Toxic agents that may be responsible for hepatocellular damage through the generation of activated oxygen accelerate the oxidative destruction of G-6-PD-deficient erythrocytes. *Acute renal failure* in Ghana appears to be associated with G-6-PD deficiency and may be related to acute intravascular hemolysis.[578] A higher incidence of *salmonellosis* has also been noted in Ghanians with G-6-PD deficiency.[579]

Screening tests and assays for G-6-PD. Several relatively simple rapid screening methods of detecting red cell G-6-PD are available.[432] These procedures depend on linking NADPH generation to the native fluorescence of NADPH,[170] to a visible dye (tetrazolium,[175] brilliant cresyl blue,[568,631] methylene blue,[187] or dichloroindophenol[167]), to red cell constituents (GSSG[431] or methemoglobin[173,196,559]), or to the prevention of destructive changes and the formation of denaturation products (as in the ascorbic acid–cyanide test[177]). The latter are least specific but are useful general screening tests for defects associated with oxidative hemolysis including defects of the hexose monophosphate shunt and unstable-hemoglobin hemolytic anemias. Although adequate for the detection of hemizygotes, the screening tests are less satisfactory for the detection of female heterozygotes and unsatisfactory for patients with recent hemolysis and whose older, enzyme-deficient cells have been replaced by a younger, reticulocyte-rich population with normal or near-normal activity of G-6-PD. Quantitative assays linked to the reduction of NADP and measured spectrophotometrically must be used in this situation. Quantitative assay after separation of young (top) and old (bottom) populations of cells by centrifugation and comparison of activity to that obtained in a control population of cells with an equivalent reticulocytosis should help to resolve the dilemma. Increased G-6-PD activity (1.5 to 2 times normal) in a normal subject with reticulocytosis and normal or borderline decreased activity in a patient with G-6-PD deficiency is usually found. Quantitative assays should be performed in newborns with hyperbilirubinemia and suspected hemolysis to avoid the false negative results of screening tests.

Standard methods are available for quantitative assays from hemolysates and for kinetic and electrophoretic characterization of variants from partially purified enzyme.

Treatment and prognosis. Patients with G-6-PD deficiency should avoid exposure to drugs and other toxic agents known to induce hemolysis. Bacterial and viral infections, diabetic ketoacidosis, and hepatitis should be treated appropriately and recognized as causing hemolysis. The general principles of care including transfusion for neonatal hyperbilirubinemia or hypoplastic crisis are similar to those for other hereditary hemolytic syndromes. Splenectomy in patients with chronic congenital hemolytic anemia is of dubious benefit. The lack of significant splenic sequestration must be reconciled with the commonly held concept of splenic entrapment of Heinz body–laden, rigid erythrocytes as the primary pathogenic mechanism of hemolysis. Intravascular hemolysis and sequestration in the liver, bone marrow, and other reticuloendothelial tissues occur as well. In the rare case of severe congenital hemolytic anemia, splenectomy may be indicated.

Massive screening programs are unlikely to benefit patients with the more common variants of G-6-PD deficiency (G-6-PD A− and G-6-PD Mediterranean). The self-limited nature of hemolysis in these population groups precludes a significant public health problem. Susceptible patients from racial or ethnic groups with a high gene frequency of G-6-PD deficiency should be tested prior to the administration of a potentially toxic drug. The sporadic occurrence and rarity of G-6-PD deficiency variants with chronic hemolytic anemia are too great to warrant any large-scale screening programs. A high level of suspicion and testing when indicated, particularly in neonatal jaundice, is a more realistic and practical approach.

Petrakis et al.[593] reported a decrease in the incidence of G-6-PD A− with increasing age, which suggests a higher mortality among deficient patients than among a nondeficient group. Confirmatory studies with improved methods of ascertainment of deficiency and better controls are required since old age may be associated with other disorders that mask the detection of the deficiency.

Future perspectives. The seeming heterogeneity of G-6-PD deficiency may be related to artifacts of methodology, particularly among the group associated with chronic hemolytic anemia. Studies on purification and amino acid sequencing of G-6-PD are now being reported. More exact identification of these variants will be required in the future.

Biochemical engineering exploiting the physiologic inhibition of the enzyme by NADPH, ATP, 2,3-DPG, and G-6-P may someday enhance the activity of G-6-PD. Identifying the structural abnormality in G-6-PD may permit pharmacologic or biochemical manipulations that improve the stability of the enzyme and prevent its rapid decay.

6-Phosphogluconic dehydrogenase (6-PGD) deficiency

Biochemistry. The second enzyme reaction of the hexose monophosphate shunt is catalyzed by 6-PGD, which converts 6-PG to pentose-5-phosphate. In the reaction NADP is reduced and CO_2 is generated. The activity of 6-PGD is about 75% that of G-6-PD in normal red cells. The assay system is similar to that for G-6-PD, except that 6-PG is substituted for G-6-P. Screening tests based on the fluorescence of generated NADPH are also available.

Genetics. In the few large-scale surveys performed 6-PGD polymorphism has been established by electrophoresis of hemolysates on starch gel.[488,589] About 95% of the tested subjects are 6-PGD type A; the remainder are 6-PGD type AB. Less than 1% of the population (0.3% of American blacks, 0.7% of whites) had 42% to 65% of normal red cell 6-PGD activity as determined by quantitative spectrophotometric assay. This "half-activity" phenotype did not correlate with electrophoretic phenotypes but appeared to be inherited as an autosomal dominant trait.

Clinical and laboratory findings. Heterozygotes for 6-PGD deficiency are usually free of any clinical or hematologic manifestations of hemolytic disease. ^{51}Cr-labeled red cells from a heterozygote who was also an unexpressed carrier of G-6-PD deficiency were transfused into a normal recipient; isologous survival was normal without drug challenge but was shortened when primaquine was given.[471] The shortened red cell survival was thought to be related to heterozygosity for G-6-PD deficiency. In other subjects tested the activity of G-6-PD and the reduction of methemoglobin were normal.

Partial deficiency of 6-PGD has been documented in patients with congenital hemolytic anemia, reticulocytosis, and shortened red cell survival. Primaquine sensitivity was not present.[540,617]

The cause and effect relationship has been established between 6-PGD deficiency and the extremely rare hemolytic syndrome. Dietary factors appear to regulate the synthesis of 6-PGD and conceivably could be related to decreased enzyme activity. A high-carbohydrate, fat-free diet stimulates the hepatic synthesis of 6-PGD in the rat.[601] Studies in humans are awaited.

ENZYMOPATHIES WITHOUT HEMOLYSIS

Hereditary deficiencies of a number of other erythrocyte enzymes have been described but in none is the red cell victimized. The deficiency of the red cell enzyme in certain inborn errors of metabolism is of diagnostic importance in that the red cell serves as a readily available source of biopsy material for quantitative assay and biochemical characterization.

Lactate dehydrogenase (LDH) deficiency

Five isozymes of LDH have been identified in human tissues. Each isozyme is a tetramer of A and/or B subunits. The major isozyme in red cells, which synthesizes considerably more B than A subunits, is B_4, or LDH-1. LDH-4 (B_1A_3) and LDH-5 (A_4) are primarily liver isozymes. A deficiency of LDH-1 (B subunits) in the red cells, inherited as an autosomal dominant characteristic, has been reported by Miwa et al.[310] Although the activity of red cell LDH was only 8% of normal, hemolysis was absent.

Glyoxalase II deficiency

In a two-step reaction methylglyoxal is converted to lactate by glyoxalase I and II, with GSH functioning as a cofactor. The significance of this pathway in the red cell is uncertain, but the activity of glyoxalase coincides with the concentration of GSH and is diminished in G-6-PD deficiency. Coincidental deficiency of glyoxalase II and hereditary elliptocytosis have been reported by Valentine et al.[154] but the enzyme defect does not impair cell function or metabolism, despite the presence of only 10% of normal glyoxalase activity in homozygotes and 50% in heterozygotes.

Galactosemia

Galactosemia is caused by a deficiency of one of several enzymes involved in galactose metabolism: galactose-1-phosphate uridyltransferase and its variants or galacktokinase.[621] Anemia may be a prominent feature of galactose-1-phosphate uridyltransferase–deficiency galactosemia and appears to be partly hemolytic. The hemoglobin level may drop suddenly without bleeding, followed by reticulocytosis. In one series[524] it occurred in 25% of the cases, but it is uncertain whether hemolysis is related to the accumulation of galactose-1-phosphate in red cells or to the underlying intrinsic liver disease. Oxygen uptake in red cells incubated with galactose is impaired, but decreased ATP levels have not been found. Since the liver and red cells share the same defect, assays of red cell galactose-1-phosphate uridyltransferase and galactokinase in

suspected cases confirm the diagnosis. Quantitative spectrophotometric or radioisotopic methods and a fluorescent screening test are available.

Hypoxanthine-guanine phosphoribosyl transferase (HGPRT) deficiency

HGPRT is deficient in the red cells of children with Lesch-Nyhan syndrome, a sex-linked disorder with choreoathetosis, spasticity, mental retardation, self-mutilation, and hyperuricemia.[371] A microcytic anemia and megaloblastic erythroid precursors were observed in 30% of the patients reviewed by Kelley and Wyngaarden,[537] but hemolysis was not a feature of the anemia. The high activity of HGPRT in normal red cells and the lack of interference from other related enzymes makes the erythrocyte the cell of choice for the laboratory diagnosis of the syndrome.

Acatalasemia

An autosomal recessive inherited deficiency of red cell catalase was originally reported in Japanese, Korean, and Chinese subjects by Takahara.[637] Subsequently other cases were detected in Western Europe, Israel, and the United States. The disorders in the East and the West appear to be different clinically and biochemically, with oral lesions reported in Japanese patients with acatalasemia but not in Swiss patients.[424] In the deficiency state the red cell is functionally and metabolically unperturbed by the presence of only 0.2% to 0.1% of normal catalase activity.

Acetylcholinesterase deficiency

An inherited deficiency of red cell acetylcholinesterase has no apparent adverse effect on red cell metabolism and function.[75] An acquired deficiency of acetylcholinesterase has been reported in two hemolytic disorders, paroxysmal nocturnal hemoglobinuria and ABO incompatibility, but the defect is probably an epiphenomenon of a membrane disorder.

Congenital methemoglobinemia: NADH-dependent methemoglobin reductase deficiency

An inherited deficiency of NADH-dependent methemoglobin reductase (NADH-metHb-R) has no deleterious effect on erythrocyte survival but is accompanied by severe congenital methemoglobinemia.[265] Hemolysis does not occur in either this enzymopathy or in a related disorder, NADPH-metHb-R deficiency, an oddity in which methemoglobinemia is absent as well.[358] Isologous[526] and autologous[516] survival in hereditary methemoglobinemia secondary to NADH-metHb-R deficiency is normal despite the presence of 10% to 40% methemoglobin. In fact, the presence of methemoglobin decreases sickling in vitro and prolongs the survival of sickle cells in vivo,[438] a feature that unfortunately has no useful clinical application. Methemoglobin reduction in patients with inherited deficiencies of PK, PGK, TPI, G-6-PD, and GSSG-R is normal despite the defective generation of reduced pyridine nucleotides accompanying these disorders.[265]

Definitions. Iron normally exists in the ferrous state in the heme portion of the reduced hemoglobin molecule but is in the ferric form in oxyhemoglobin (oxygenated hemoglobin). Methemoglobin is defined as an oxygenation product of hemoglobin in which the sixth coordination position of ferric heme is bound to either a water molecule or to a hydroxyl group. Congenital methemoglobinemia is caused by either a genetically determined amino acid substitution in the globin moiety of the hemoglobin molecule (see Hb M disorders, Chapter 14) or by a deficiency of NADH-metHb-R. When methemoglobin is produced in significant amounts, it reduces the oxygen-combining capacity of the blood. Methemoglobinemia is characterized by intense cyanosis and imparts a brownish color to the blood. It has a characteristic absorption spectrum at about 635 nm.

Historical background. Although congenital cyanosis was first reported in 1845,[495] it was not until 1944 that Paul and Kemp[591] showed that normal red cells produce methemoglobin. Early reports confused methemoglobinemia with sulfhemoglobinemia, which was present in patients with "enterogenous cyanosis," an ill-defined clinical syndrome characterized by attacks of cyanosis, headache, abdominal pain, and bowel dysfunction. Van den Bergh[644] identified both methemoglobin and sulfhemoglobin in this syndrome.

The abnormal pigments were attributed to the absorption of enterogenous oxidizing agents such as hydrogen sulfides. Congenital and familial sulfhemoglobinemia in the newborn was first described in 1957.[558]

In the 1940s Gibson[501] first proposed and then showed that congenital methemoglobinemia was caused by a defect in methemoglobin reduction, and in 1959 Scott and Griffith[620] proved that NADH-metHb-R was deficient in congenitally methemoglobinemic Eskimos.[619] The biochemical and genetic heterogeneity of NADH-metHb-R is now well established in that at least eight variants have been described.[264]

Biochemistry of methemoglobin reduction and pathogenesis. Methemoglobin is formed continuously in the red cell and simultaneously is reduced to hemoglobin by enzymatic (NADH-metHb-R and NADP-metHb-R) and nonenzymatic (ascorbic acid and GSH) mechanisms.[264] Hemoglobin is protected against oxidation by its innate

Table 12-15. Estimated rates of methemoglobin reduction by various systems under simulated in vivo conditions

	Percent of reducing capacity
NADH-metHb-R_I	61
Ascorbic acid	16
Glutathione	12
NADH-metHb-R_{II}	6
NADPH-metHb-R	5
TOTAL	100

*From Scott, E. M.: In Beutler, E., ed.: Hereditary disorders of erythrocyte metabolism, New York, 1968, Grune & Stratton, Inc. Used by permission.

structure, which excludes the entry of water into the heme pocket, and by other enzymes (GSH-P and catalase) and metabolites (GSH, NADPH, ergothioneine, and cysteine). The relative rates of methemoglobin reduction in vitro under simulated conditions are shown in Table 12-15.[618] In vivo, however, the varieties of NADH-metHb-R are responsible for at least 95% of methemoglobin reduction. Of the two NADH-metHb-R enzymes in the red cell, dehydrogenase I accounts for 90% of the total reductase activity, is absent in congenital methemoglobinemia, contains a flavin moiety, and is more heat stable than the minor dehydrogenase II. It is oxidized by physiologic mechanisms associated with the generation of hydrogen peroxide and superoxide radicals and by pathologic exposure to chemicals and drugs (Fig. 12-17).

Normal reduction of methemoglobin depends on the structural integrity of the red cell, is associated with carbohydrate metabolism, and requires the generation of reduced pyridine nucleotides. Thus the reduction of methemoglobin occurs only when glucose or lactate is present and is stimulated by an increase in glycolytic rate[536] or by an increase in the intracellular content of NADH.[527] Methylene blue, which stimulates the hexose monophosphate shunt and leads to the generation of NADPH, enhances methemoglobin reduction[502] through the NADPH-metHb-R system. The latter system is not of any clinical significance in that methemoglobinemia is not a feature of deficiencies of G-6-PD, GSH, catalase, and NADPH-metHb-R. Finally, although ascorbic acid can reduce methemoglobin directly, methemoglobin is absent in scurvy.

Although NADH-metHb-R has been partially purified,[517,633] uncertainties exist concerning the exact mechanism of electron transfer from NADH to methemoglobin. In this regard recent studies have suggested that cytochrome b_5 reductase may be identical to NADH-metHb-R and serve as the

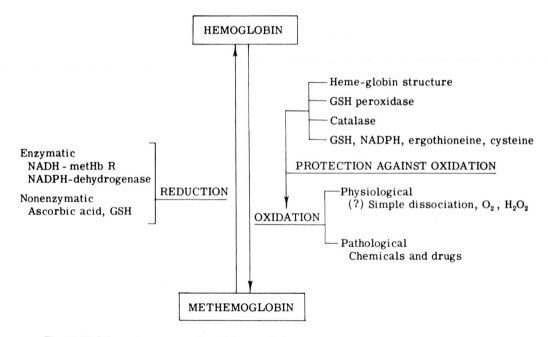

Fig. 12-17. Schematic representation of the metabolic processes presumably involved in the oxidation of hemoglobin to methemoglobin, the protection against oxidation of hemoglobin to methemoglobin, and the reduction of methemoglobin to hemoglobin in human erythrocytes. (From Hsieh, H. S., and Jaffé, E.: In Surgenor, D. M., ed.: The red blood cell, ed. 2, vol. 2, New York, 1975, Academic Press, Inc.)

naturally occurring cofactor linking NADH and methemoglobin.[525,590]

The reducing capacity of the red cell is 250 times as great as its oxidizing capacity.[618] In congenital methemoglobinemia associated with a deficiency of NADH-metHb-R, methemoglobin levels range between 10% and 40%, and the reducing capacity is only one to ten times the oxidizing capacity. Heterozygotes have intermediate levels of NADH-metHb-R, reducing capacity 126 to 130 times the oxidizing capacity, but normal levels of methemoglobin. Thus normal erythrocytes readily tolerate changes in oxidative steps; methemoglobinemia is found only in deficient erythrocytes with a severely limited reducing capacity. Furthermore, since NADH-metHb-R is an age-dependent enzyme, older red cells of deficient patients contain more methemoglobin than younger cells.[76]

The effects of the formation are twofold. First, methemoglobin is unavailable for transport of oxygen. Second, the presence of methemoglobin renders the dissociation curve more hyperbolic, shifting it to the left. The total effect is a lowered capacity for unloading oxygen to the tissues and hence a tissue susceptibility to anoxia.[444,469]

Relatively small amounts of methemoglobin, approximately 15% of the total hemoglobin, are sufficient to produce cyanosis. The relative capacities of the pigments to produce cyanosis of comparable intensity are as follows: reduced hemoglobin, 5 mg/dl; methemoglobin, 1.5 gm/dl; sulfhemoglobin, less than 0.5 gm/dl.[489]

Genetics. Congenital methemoglobinemia caused by NADH-metHb-R deficiency is familial and is transmitted as an autosomal recessive trait. Several electrophoretic variants of the enzyme have been described[522] (Table 12-16). In a large-scale survey, Hopkinson et al.[520] found six electrophoretic variants in 2,800 persons tested. As with other enzymopathies, the molecular pathology of the defect may be related to decreased synthesis or increased instability of a structurally normal enzyme or normal synthesis of a structurally abnormal enzyme with abnormal kinetics or stability. Not all of the variants are associated with decreased activity of the enzyme, and perforce methemoglobinemia, and there is no close correlation between enzyme activity, electrophoretic mobility, and clinical severity of methemoglobinemia.

A case of methemoglobinemia has been described that followed a dominant rather than the usual recessive inheritance. At first ascribed to an inability to utilize glucose for the reduction of methemoglobin,[641] the defect was later attributed to the inadequate synthesis of GSH,[642] resulting in an impairment of TPI activity, and decreased synthesis of glycolytic intermediates required for

Table 12-16. Variants of NADH-metHb-R deficiency

Variant	Electro-phoretic mobility (% normal)	NADPH-metHb-R activity (% normal)	Methemo-globinemia
Normal	100	100	0
DIA3[520]	50	?	—
DIA4[520]	60	?	—
Boston slow[522]	90	40	+
Duarte[522]	108	12	—
Princeton[522]	113	—	—
Puerto Rico[522]	117	6-23	+
Boston fast[483]	127	62	0
California[533]	133	25	+

the generation of NADH. This hypothesis is difficult to reconcile with the facts that the role of GSH in methemoglobin reduction is a minor one[618] and that methemoglobinemia does not occur in hereditary deficiency of GSH.[599]

Clinical and laboratory features. Most patients with congenital methemoglobinemia show persistent diffuse cyanosis that is generalized but particularly marked in the fingers, toes, buccal mucous membranes, legs, nose, cheeks, and conjunctivae. Clubbing of the fingers does occur. Without treatment the majority of these patients tend to reach equilibrium at about 40% methemoglobin in the blood.[489] The lethal concentration of methemoglobin in humans is estimated to be over 70% of the total,[457] a level not reached in patients with congenital methemoglobinemia. There is no anemia, but mild compensatory polycythemia may develop. Patients are usually asymptomatic except for occasional headaches, and in older patients poor exercise tolerance may be noted. Usually there is no physical disability, even with strenuous exercise. Life expectancy is unaffected.

A significant number of patients with congenital methemoglobinemia have mental retardation but there is no adequate explanation for the association.[485] Chromosomal defects, generalized enzyme deficiency, and intrauterine anoxia have been proposed without any direct supporting evidence.

The diagnosis of methemoglobinemia is supported if a sample of venous blood retains the characteristic chocolate brown color after vigorous shaking with air for 15 minutes. Methemoglobin has a well-defined absorption band spectroscopically at 630 to 635 nm, which disappears on the addition of a 5% solution of potassium cyanide. Sulfhemoglobin may accompany methemoglobin in drug-induced methemoglobinemia and can be differentiated from methemoglobin by its absorption band at 618 nm, which is unaltered by the addition of potassium cyanide. Once sulfhemoglobin is formed, it is stable and irreversible, disappearing after 3 to 4 months when the affected red cells are destroyed. Drug-induced sulfhemoglobinemia may be associated with the formation of Heinz bodies and hemolysis, events that do not occur in congenital methemoglobinemia. Hb M disorders can be differentiated on the basis of hemoglobin electrophoresis. If the amino acid substitution affects the α-chain of globin in Hb M disease, cyanosis may appear in the newborn period. Symptoms in β-chain defects occur later in life.

Newborn infants are susceptible to the development of methemoglobinemia because of a transient physiologic deficiency of NADH-metHb-R activity.[553,608,669] The deficiency is in the same range found in heterozygotes for hereditary methemoglobinemia.

Various compounds activate the oxidation of hemoglobin. These include nitrites (bismuth subnitrate), chlorates, quinones, and aniline and its derivatives sulfanilamides, acetanilid, and phenacetin. In infancy and childhood the offenders are marking ink, shoe dyes, certain red wax crayons,[605] well water containing nitrates from the soil, meat containing a high nitrate content,[577] and furniture polish containing nitrobenzene.[550] Other drugs in the pediatric armamentarium associated with toxic methemoglobinemia include the local urinary analgesic phenazopyridine hydrochloride (Azogantrisin)[465] and the antihelminthic piperazine. The following compounds and derivatives are known to produce methemoglobinemia:

Acetanilid	Nitrogen oxide
Acetophenetidin	Nitroglycerol
Alloxan	Pamaquine
p-Aminosalicylic acid	Phenetidin
Aniline derivatives	Phenazopyridine HCl
Antipyrine	Phenylenediamine
Benzene derivatives	Phenylhydroxylamine
Carrots	Phenytoin
Chlorates	Piperazine
Cyanides	Plasmaquine
Diaminodiphenyl sulfone	Prilocaine
Lidocaine	Primaquine
Methylene blue	Resorcinol
Nitrates	Sulfonamides

Nitrate from contaminated water from shallow wells used in infant feeding mixtures is converted to nitrite in the bowel and on absorption causes methemoglobinemia.[467,480,482] The absorption of aniline dyes from marking ink on diapers and other articles of infants' clothing, shoes, and blankets has been responsible for outbreaks of methemoglobinemia in premature nurseries particularly.*

---

*References 479, 521, 531, 603.

Methemoglobinemia has also resulted from application of ointments containing benzocaine.[660]

Clinically a striking feature of toxic methemoglobinemia is the intense, peculiarly grayish cyanosis that develops 1 to 2 hours after ingestion of or exposure to the toxic substance. The discoloration progresses rapidly until the skin and mucous membranes become almost black in color.[550] In mild cases the child is fully conscious and in no distress, but in severe cases the patient has considerable anoxemia and dyspnea and develops circulatory failure.

NADPH-metHb-R deficiency. One patient with NADPH-metHb-R deficiency was described by Sass et al.[356] in 1967. Methemoglobinemia was not present but methemoglobin reduction was decreased only in the presence of methylene blue. Although methylene blue–stimulated methemoglobin reduction is defective in certain unstable-hemoglobin hemolytic anemias (e.g., Hb Köln disease),[560] electrophoretic studies support the existence of this entity.[440,522]

Treatment. Patients with mild cases of acquired methemoglobinemia recover spontaneously on withdrawal of the toxic substance. In a patient with disease of any degree of severity treatment should be initiated immediately. Methylene blue acts as a specific antidote, converting methemoglobin to hemoglobin. The recommended daily dosage for infants is 2 mg/kg body weight; for older children, 1.5 mg/kg; and for adults, 1 mg/kg. It is readily available in ampules of 1% solution, which is given by slow intravenous injection. Treatment may be repeated if methemoglobinemia recurs. Ascorbic acid given orally or parenterally also reduces methemoglobin, but the conversion takes place more slowly and therefore is not practical in urgent cases.

In patients with hereditary methemoglobinemia, orally administered methylene blue or ascorbic acid may be given over prolonged periods to combat cyanosis and particularly associated symptoms such as headache. Ascorbic acid in an oral dosage of 500 mg given to a 12½-year-old boy caused a significant drop in methemoglobin concentration.[650] Intravenous methylene blue acts more promptly, but a gradual return to the original methemoglobinemia is inevitable when therapy is terminated. The drug is ineffective in the treatment of Hb M syndromes.

Toxic effects have been observed when methylene blue is given in excessive dosage.[511] These consist of a generalized bluish gray skin discoloration, which may persist for 3 to 4 days, and an acute hemolytic anemia, which may become manifest about 1 week later. The anemia may be of sufficient severity to require transfusions.

Future perspectives. Future work in this field will involve further purification of NADH-metHb-R and a better understanding of the sequence of electron transfer from enzyme to methemoglobin and the role of cytochrome b_5 in the reduction of methemoglobin. Newer, more effective agents may then be developed to treat the congenital and acquired forms of the disorder.

REFERENCES
Normal erythrocyte metabolism

1. Albson, A. C., and Burn, G. P.: Enzyme activity as a function of age in the human erythrocyte, Br. J. Haematol. **1:**291, 1955.
2. Allen, D. W., and Jandl, J. H.: Oxidative hemolysis and precipitation of hemoglobin. II. Role of thiols in oxidant drug action, J. Clin. Invest. **40:**454, 1961.
3. Altenbrunn, H. J., and Rapoport, S.: The inactivation of cytochrome oxidase by a factor in the hemolysate of rabbit reticulocytes, Acta Biol. Med. German **2:**599, 1959.
4. Arnold, H., Hoffman, A., Englehardt, R., and Löhr, G. W.: Purification and kinetic properties of glucose-phosphate isomerase from human erythrocytes. In Gerlach, E., Moser, K., and Deutsch, E., eds.: Erythrocytes, thrombocytes, leukocytes: recent advances in membrane and metabolic research, Stuttgart, 1973, Georg Thieme Verlag.
5. Asakura, T., Sato, Y., Minakami, S., and Yoshikawa, H.: Effect of deoxygenation of intracellular hemoglobin on red cell glycolysis, J. Biochem. **59:**524, 1966.
6. Askari, A., and Rao, S. N.: Regulation of AMP deaminase by 2,3-diphosphoglyceric acid: a possible mechanism for the control of adenine nucleotide metabolism in human erythrocytes, Biochim. Biophys. Acta **151:**198, 1968.
7. Auditore, J. V., and Hartmann, R. C.: Paroxysmal nocturnal hemoglobinuria. II. Erythrocyte acetylocholinesterase defect, Am. J. Med. **27:**401, 1959.
8. Bartlett, G. R.: Human red cell glycolytic intermediates, J. Biol. Chem. **234:**449, 1959.
9. Bartos, H. R., and Desforges, J. F.: Enzymes as erythrocyte age reference standards, Am. J. Med. Sci. **254:**862, 1967.
10. Bauer, C.: Antagonistic influence of CO_2 and 2,3-diphosphoglycerate on the Bohr effect of human haemoglobin, Life Sci. **8:**1041, 1969.
11. Benesch, R., and Benesch, R. E.: The effect of organic phosphates from the human erythrocyte on the allosteric properties of hemoglobin, Biochim. Biophys. Res. Commun. **26:**162, 1967.
12. Benesch, R. E., Benesch, R., and Yu, C. I.: The oxygenation of hemoglobin in the presence of 2,3-diphosphoglycerate: effect of temperature, pH, ionic strength, and hemoglobin concentration, Biochemistry **8:**2567, 1969.
13. Benohr,. H. C., and Waller, H. D.: Metabolism in haemolytic states, Clin. Haematol. **4:**45, 1975.
14. Berger, H., Zuber, C., and Miescher, P.: The reduction of methaemoglobin to haemoglobin in the aging red cell, Gerontologia **4:**220, 1960.
15. Bernstein, R. E.: Alterations in metabolic energetics and cation transport during aging of red cells, J. Clin. Invest. **38:**1572, 1959.
16. Beutler, E.: 2,3-Diphosphoglycerate affects enzymes of glucose metabolism in red blood cells, Nature (New Biol.) **232:**20, 1971.
17. Beutler, E.: Disorders of glutathione metabolism, Life Sci. **16:**1499, 1972.

18. Beutler, E., Matsumoto, F., and Quinto, E.: The effect of 2,3-DPG on red cell enzymes, Experientia **30:**190, 1974.
19. Beutler, E., and Qunito, E.: The effect of 2,3-DPG on red cell phosphofructokinase, F.E.B.S. Lett. **37:**21, 1973.
20. Bishop, C.: Purine metabolism in human blood studied in vivo by injection of C^{14}-adenine, J. Biol. Chem. **236:**1778, 1961.
21. Bishop, C., Rankine, D. M., and Talbott, J. H.: The nucleotides in normal human blood, J. Biol. Chem. **234:**1233, 1959.
22. Bishop, W. H., and VanGastel, C.: Changes in enzyme activity during reticulocyte maturation and red cell aging, Haematologica **3:**29, 1969.
23. Brewer, G. J.: Erythrocyte metabolism and function: hexokinase inhibition by 2,3-diphosphoglycerate and interaction with ATP and Mg^{2+}, Biochim. Biophys. Acta **192:**157, 1969.
24. Brewer, G. J.: General red cell metabolism. In Surgenor, D. M., ed.: The red blood cell, vol. 1, ed. 2, New York, 1974, Academic Press, Inc.
25. Brewer, G. J., Tarlov, A. R., Kellermeyer, R. W., and Alving, A. S.: Hemolytic effect of primaquine. XV. The role of methemoglobin, J. Lab. Clin. Med. **59:**905, 1962.
26. Brin, M., and Yonemoto, R. H.: Stimulation of glucose oxidative pathway in human erythrocytes by methylene blue, J. Biol. Chem. **230:**307, 1958.
27. Brok, F., Ramot, B., Zwang, E., and Danon, D.: Enzyme activities in human red blood cells of different age groups, Isr. J. Med. Sci. **2:**291, 1966.
28. Caldwell, P. R. B., Nagel, R. L., and Jaffe, E. R.: The effect of oxygen, carbon dioxide, pH, and cyanate on the binding of 2,3-diphosphoglycerate to human hemoglobin, Biochem. Biophys. Res. Commun. **44:**1504, 1971.
29. Carrell, R. W., Winterbourn, C. C., and Rachmilewitz, E. A.: Activated oxygen and haemolysis, Br. J. Haematol. **30:**259, 1975.
30. Chanutin, A., and Curnish, R. R.: Effect of organic and inorganic phosphates on the oxygen equilibrium of human erythrocytes, Arch. Biochem. **121:**96, 1967.
31. Chapman, R. G., Hennessey, M. A., Waltersdorph, A. M., et al.: Erythrocyte metabolism. V. Levels of glycolytic enzymes and regulation of glycolysis, J. Clin. Invest. **41:**1249, 1962.
32. Chapman, R. G., and Schaumberg, L.: Glycolysis and glycolytic enzyme activity of aging red cells in man: changes in hexokinase aldolase, glyceraldehyde-3-phosphate dehydrogenase, pyruvate kinase and glutamic oxalacetic transaminase, Br. J. Haematol. **13:**665, 1967.
33. Dacie, J. V., Mollison, P. L., Richardson, N., et al.: Atypical congenital haemolytic anaemia, Q. J. Med. **22:**79, 1953.
34. Danon, D., and Marikovsky, Y.: Determination of density distribution of red cell population, J. Lab. Clin. Med. **64:**668, 1964.
35. Davidson, J. N., Leslie, J., and White, J. C.: The nucleic acid content of the cell, Lancet **1:**1287, 1951.
36. Davidson, W. D., and Tanaka, K. R.: Factors affecting pentose phosphate pathway activity in human red cells, Br. J. Haematol. **23:**271, 1972.
37. Dern, R. J., Weinstein, I. M., LeRoy, G. V., et al.: The hemolytic effect of primaquine. I. The localization of the drug-induced hemolytic defect in primaquine-sensitive individuals, J. Lab. Chem. Med. **43:**303, 1954.
38. Deuticke, B., and Duhm, J.: A method of modifying the intracellular concentration of non-penetrating anions, In Rorth, M., and Astrup, P. eds.: Oxygen affinity of hemoglobin and red cell acid base status, New York, 1972, Academic Press, Inc.
39. Deuticke, B., Duhm, J., and Dierkesmann, R.: Maximal elevation of 2,3-diphosphoglycerate concentrations in human erythrocytes: influence on glycolytic metabolism and intracellular pH, Pflugers Arch. **326:**15, 1971.
40. Dimant, E., Landberg, E., and London, I. M.: The metabolic behavior of reduced glutathione in human and avian erythrocytes, J. Biol. Chem. **213:**769, 1955.
41. Dische, Z., and Igals, D.: Inhibition of transketolase and transaldolase of the human hemolyzate by multivalent anions, Arch. Biochem. Biophys. **101:**489, 1963.
42. Dormandy, T. L.: The autoxidation of red cells, Br. J. Haematol. **20:**457, 1971.
43. Duhm, J.: 2,3-Diphosphoglycerate metabolism of erythrocytes and oxygen transport function of blood. In Gerlach, E., Moser, K., and Deutsch, E., eds.: Erythrocytes, Thrombocytes, leukocytes: recent advances in membrane and metabolic research, Stuttgart, 1973, Georg Thieme Verlag.
44. Duhm, J., Deuticke, B., and Gerlach, E.: Metabolism of 2,3-diphosphoglycerate and glycolysis in human red blood cells under the influence of dipyridamole and inorganic sulfur compounds, Biochim. Biophys. Acta **170:**452, 1968.
45. Duhm, J., Deuticke, B., and Gerlach, E.: Abhängigkeit der 2,3-diphosphoglycerinsäure—synthese in Menschen —erythrocyten von der ADP-Konzentration, Pflugers Arch. **306:**329, 1969.
46. Duhm, J., and Gerlach, E.: Metabolism and function of 2,3-diphosphoglycerate in red blood cells. In Greenwalt, T. J., and Jameson, G. A., eds.: The human red cell in vitro, New York, 1974, Grune & Stratton, Inc.
47. Eaton, J. W.: Catalase activity and cancer, Lancet **2:**46, 1972.
48. Eaton, J. W., and Brewer, G. J.: Pentose phosphate metabolism. In Surgenor, D. M., ed.: The red blood cell, vol. 1, ed. 2, New York, 1974, Academic Press, Inc.
49. Edwards, M. J., Novy, M. J., Walters, C. L., and Metcalfe, J.: Improved oxygen release: an adaptation of mature cells to hypoxia, J. Clin. Invest. **47:**1851, 1968.
50. Embden, G., and Zimmerman, M.: Hoppe-Selyers Z. Physiol. Chem. **167:**114, 1927.
51. Evans, C. L.: Acid production in shed blood, J. Physiol. **56:**146, 1922.
52. Fantoni, A., De la Chapelle, A., Rifkind, R. A., and Marks, P. A.: Erythroid cell development in fetal mice: synthetic capacity for different proteins, J. Mol. Biol. **33:**79, 1968.
53. Fee, J. A., and Teitelbaum, H. D.: Evidence that superoxide dismutase plays a role in protecting red blood cells against peroxidative hemolysis, Biochem. Biophys. Res. Commun. **49:**150, 1972.
54. Flohé, L., Günzler, W. A., and Schock, H. H.: Glutathione peroxidase: a selenoenzyme, Fed. Eur. Biochem. **32:**132, 1973.
55. Garby, L., Gerber, G., and de Verdier, C. H.: Binding of 2,3-diphosphoglycerate and adenosine triphosphate to human hemoglobin A, Eur. J. Biochem. **10:**110, 1969.
56. Gardos, G., Szasz, I., and Arky, I.: Structure and function of erythrocytes. II. Relation between potassium transport and morphology, Acta Biochem. Biophys. Acad. Sci. Hung. **2:**3, 1967.
57. Gibson, Q. H.: Reduction in methemoglobin in red cells and studies on the cause of idiopathic methemoglobinemia, Biochem. J. **42:**13, 1948.
58. Gordon-Smith, E. C., and White, J. M.: Oxidative haemolysis and Heinz body haemolytic anaemia, Br. J. Haematol. **26:**513, 1974.
59. Grasso, J. A., and Woodward, J. W.: The relationship between RNA synthesis and hemoglobin synthesis in am-

phibian erythropoiesis: cytochemical evidence, J. Cell. Biol. **31:**279, 1966.

60. Greenwald, I.: A new type of phosphoric acid compound isolated from blood, with some remarks on the effect of substitution on the rotation of 1-glyceric acid, J. Biol. Chem. **63:**339, 1925.

61. Guest, G. M., and Rapoport, S. M.: Phosphorus compounds in the blood, Physiol. Rev. **21:**410, 1941.

62. Harris, J. W., and Kellermeyer, R. W.: The red cell. Production, metabolism, destruction: normal and abnormal, rev. ed., Cambridge, Mass., 1970, Harvard University Press.

63. Harkness, D. R., Ponce, J., and Grayson, V.: A comparative study on the phosphoglyceric acid cycle in mammalian erythrocytes, Comp. Biochem. Physiol. **28:**129, 1969.

64. Harkness, D. R., and Roth, S.: Purification and properties of 2,3-diphosphoglyceric acid phosphatase from human erythrocytes, Biochem. Biophys. Res. Commun. **34:**849, 1969.

65. Hasart, E., Jacobasch, G., and Rapoport, S.: Der Einfluss der Temperateur auf die Regulation der Glykolyse in Erythrocyten des Menschen und der Ratte, Acta Biol. Med. Ger. **24:**725, 1970.

66. Henderson, F. J., and LePage, G. A.: Transport of adenine-8-C^{14} among mouse tissues by blood cells, J. Biol. Chem. **234:**3219, 1959.

67. Hershko, A., Razin, A., and Mager, J.: Relation of the synthesis of 5-phospho-ribosyl-1-pyrophosphate in intact red blood cells and in cell-free preparations, Biochem. Biophys. Acta. **184:**64, 1969.

68. Hoffman, J. F.: On the relationship of certain erythrocyte characteristics to their physiological age, J. Cell. Comp. Physiol. **51:**415, 1958.

69. Horecker, B. L.: Pentoses and penitols, New York, 1969, Springer-Verlag, New York, Inc.

70. Isselbacher, K. J., Anderson, E. P., Kurahashi, K., and Kalckar, H. M.: Congenital galactosemia, a single enzymatic block in galactose metabolism, Science **123:**635, 1956.

71. Jackson, R. C.: Studies in the enzymology of glutathione metabolism in human erythrocytes, Biochem. J. **111:**309, 1969.

72. Jacob, H. S., and Jandl, J. H.: Effects of sulfhydryl inhibition on red blood cells. I. Mechanism of hemolysis, J. Clin. Invest. **38:**1555, 1959.

73. Jackobasch, G.: Einfluss des Phosphats und des Magnesiums auf die Regulation der Glykolyse, Folia Haematol. **89:**376, 1968.

74. Jacobasch, G., Minakami, S., and Rapoport, S. M.: Glycolysis of the erythrocyte, in Yoshikawa, H., and Rapoport, S. M. eds.: Cellular and molecular biology of erythrocytes. Baltimore, 1974, University Park Press.

75. Jones, R. J.: Familial reduction in red-cell cholinesterase, N. Engl. J. Med. **267:**1344, 1962.

76. Keitt, A. S., Smith, T. W., and Jandl, J. H.: Red cell "pseudomosaicism" in congenital methemoglobinemia, N. Engl. J. Med. **275:**397, 1966.

77. Kleinman, L. I., Petering, H. G., and Sutherland, J. M.: Blood carbonic anhydrase activity and zinc concentration in infants with respiratory distress syndrome, N. Engl. J. Med. **277:**1157, 1967.

78. Kosower, N. S., Song, K. R., and Kosower, E. M.: Glutathione. IV. Intracellular oxidation and membrane injury, Biochim. Biophys. Acta **192:**23, 1969.

79. Kosower, N. S., Vanderhoof, G. A., and Kosower, E. M.: Glutathione. VIII. The effects of glutathione disulfide on initiation of protein synthesis. Biochim. Biophys. Acta **272:**623, 1972.

80. LaCelle, P. L.: Alteration of deformability of the erythrocyte membrane in stored blood, Transfusion **9:**238, 1969.

81. Lajtha, L. G., and Vane, J. R.: Dependence of bone marrow on the liver for purine supply, Nature (London) **182:**191, 1958.

82. Lawaczeck, H.: Über die Dynamik der phosphorsäure des Blutes, Biochem. Z. **145:**351, 1924.

83. Lionetti, F. J.: Pentose phosphate pathway in human erythrocytes. In Yoshikawa, H., and Rapoport, S. M., eds.: Cellular and molecular biology of erythrocytes, Baltimore, 1974, University Park Press.

84. Löhr, G. W., Waller, H. D., Karges, O., et al.: Zur Biochemie der altering menschlecher Erythrozyten, Klin. Wochenschr. **36:**1008, 1958.

85. Lowy, B. A., and Williams, M. K.: Studies on the metabolism of adenosine and adenine in stored and fresh human erythrocytes, Blood **27:**623, 1966.

86. Lowy, B. A., Williams, M. K., and London, I. M.: Enzymatic deficiencies of purine nucleotide synthesis in the human erythrocyte, J. Biol. Chem. **237:**1622, 1962.

87. Majerus, P. W., Minnich, V., and Mohler, D.: De novo synthesis of glutathione in extracts from human erythrocytes, J. Clin. Invest. **49:**60a, 1970.

88. Manyai, S., and Varady, Z. S.: Elective spaltung der 2,3-Diphosphoglyzerinsäure in Erythrozyten, Biochem. Biophys. Acta **20:**594, 1956.

89. Marks, P. A., Fantoni, A., and De la Chapelle, A.: Hemoglobin synthesis and differentation of erythroid cells, Vitam. Horm. **26:**331, 1968.

90. Marks, P. A., Johnson, A. B., and Herschberg, E.: Effect of age on the enzyme activity in erythrocytes, Proc. Natl. Acad. Sci. **44:**529, 1958.

91. McCord, J. M., and Fridovich, I.: Superoxide desmutase: an enzymic function for erythrocuprein (hemocuprein), J. Biol. Chem. **244:**6049, 1969.

92. McManus, T. J., and Borgese, T. A.: Effect of pyruvate on metabolism of inosine by erythrocytes. Fed. Proc. **20:**65, 1961. (Abstract.)

93. Meister, A.: The γ-glutamyl cycle: disease associated with specific enzyme deficiencies, Ann. Intern. Med. **81:**247, 1974.

94. Meister, A.: Glutathione: metabolism and function via the γ-glutamyl cycle, Life Sci. **15:**177, 1974.

95. Meister, A.: Biochemistry of glutathione. In Metabolism of sulfur compounds, vol. 7, ed. 3, New York, 1975, Academic Press, Inc.

96. Metz, E. N., Balcerzak, S. P., and Sagone, A. L., Jr.: Regeneration of reduced glutathione in erythrocytes: stoichiometric and temporal relationship to hexose monophosphate shunt activity, Blood **44:**691, 1974.

97. Meyerhof, O.: Über die abtrennung des milchsäurebildenen Ferments aus Erythrocyten, Biochem. Z. **246:**249, 1932.

98. Meyskens, F. L., and Williams, H. E.: Adenosine metabolism in human erythrocytes, Biochim. Biophys. Acta **240:**170, 1971.

99. Mills, G. C.: Hemoglobin catabolism. I. Glutathione peroxidase, an erythrocyte enzyme which protects hemoglobin from oxidative breakdown, J. Biol. Chem. **229:**189, 1957.

100. Mills, G. C., and Randall, H. P.: Hemoglobin catabolism. II. The protection of hemoglobin from oxidative breakdown in the intact erythrocyte, J. Biol. Chem. **232:**589, 1958.

101. Minakami, S.: Regulation of glycolysis in human red cells-application of "cross over" theorem. In Deutsch, E., Gerlach, E., and Mosher, K., eds.: Metabolism and membrane permeability of erythrocytes and thrombocytes, Stuttgart, 1968, Georg Thieme Verlag.

102. Minakami, S., Saits, T., Suzuki, C., and Yoshikawa, T.: The hydrogen ion concentrations and erythrocyte glycolysis, Biochem. Biophys. Res. Commun. **17:**748, 1964.

103. Minakami, S., Suzuki, C., Takayosu, S., and Yoshikawa, H.: Studies on erythrocyte glycolysis. I. Determination of glycolytic intermediates in human erythrocytes, J. Biochem. **58:**543, 1965.

104. Minnich, V., Smith, M. D., Brauner, M. J., et al.: Glutathione biosynthesis in human erythrocytes. I. Identification of the enzymes of glutathione synthesis in hemolysates, J. Clin. Invest. **50:**507, 1971.

105. Misra, H. P., and Fridovich, I.: The generation of superoxide radical during the autioxidation of hemoglobin, J. Biol. Chem. **247:**6960, 1972.

106. Murphy, J. R.: Erythrocyte metabolism. II. Glucose metabolism and pathways, J. Lab. Clin. Med. **55:**286, 1960.

107. Nakao, M.: ATP-requiring phenomena in red-cell membranes. In Yoshikawa, H., and Rapoport, S. M., eds.: Cellular and molecular biology of erythrocytes, Baltimore, 1974, University Park Press.

108. Nicholls, P.: Contributions of catalase and glutathione peroxidase to red cell peroxide removal, Biochim. Biophys. Acta **279:**306, 1972.

109. Pablete, E., Thibeault, D. W., and Auld, P. A. M.: Carbonic anhydrase in the premature, Pediatrics **42:**429, 1968.

110. Palekar, A. G., Tate, S. S., and Meister, A.: Formation of 5-oxoproline from glutathione in erythrocytes by the γ-glutamyl-transpeptidase-cyclotransferase pathway, Proc. Natl. Acad. Sci. U.S.A. **71:**293, 1974.

111. Passaneau, J. V., and Lowry, O. H.: The role of phosphofructokinase in metabolic regulation, Adv. Enzyme Regul. **2:**265, 1964.

112. Perutz, M. F.: Stereochemistry of cooperative effects in haemoglobin, Nature **228:**726, 1970.

113. Ponce, J., Roth, S., and Harkness, D. R.: Kinetic studies on the inhibition of glycolytic kinases of human erythrocytes by 2,3-diphosphoglyceric acid, Biochim. Biophys. Acta **250:**63, 1971.

114. Post, R. L.: Relationship of an ATPase in human erythrocyte membranes to the active transport of sodium and potassium, Fed. Proc. **18:**121, 1959.

115. Post, R. L., and Jolly, P. C.: Linkage of sodium, potassium and ammonium active transport across the human erythrocyte membrane, Biochim. Biophys. Acta **25:**118, 1957.

116. Post, R. L., Merritt, C. R., Kinselving, C. R., and Albright, C. D.: Membrane adenosine triphosphatase as a participant in the active transport of sodium and potassium in the human erythrocyte, J. Biol. Chem. **235:**1796, 1960.

117. Prankerd, T. A. J.: The aging of red cells, J. Physiol. **143:**325, 1958.

118. Prankerd, T. A. J.: The red cell: an account of its chemical physiology and pathology, Oxford, 1961, Blackwell Scientific Publications.

119. Priess, J., and Handler, P.: Synthesis of diphosphopyridine nucleotide from nicotinic acid by human erythrocytes in vitro, J. Am. Chem. Soc. **79:**1514, 1957.

120. Rapoport, S.: Reifung und Alterungsvorgänge im Erythrozyten, Folia Haematol. **78:**364, 1961.

121. Rapoport, S.: Control mechanisms in red cell glycolysis, in Greenwalt, T. J. and Jameson, G. A., eds.: The human red cell in vitro, New York, 1974, Grune & Stratton, Inc.

122. Rapoport, S., and Gerishcer-Mothes, W.: Biochemische Vorgänge bci der Reticulocyten-Reifung: Auftreten und abklingen des Reticulocyten-Hemmstoffes, Hoppe Seyler Z. Physiol. Chem. **304:**213, 1956.

123. Rapoport, S., and Gerischer-Mothes, W.: Phosphatide als Inactivatoren des Reticulocyten-Hemmstoffs der Mitochondrien-Atmung, Hoppe Seyler Z. Physiol. Chem. **315:**38, 1959.

124. Rapoport, S., and Gerischer-Mothes, W.: On the knowledge of the reticulocyte supernatant inhibitor of mitochondrial flavoproteins: ferric ion and SH- as function groups, Acta Biol. Med. Ger. **3:**450, 1959.

125. Rapoport, S., and Luebering, J.: The formation of 2,3-diphosphoglycerate in rabbit erythrocytes: the existence of a diphosphoglycerate mutase, J. Biol. Chem. **183:**507, 1950.

126. Rapoport, S. M., and Müller, M.: Catalase and glutathione peroxidase. In Yoshikawa, H., and Rapoport, S. M. eds.: Cellular and molecular biology of erythrocytes, Baltimore, 1974, University Park Press.

127. Rapoport, S. M., Rosenthal, S., Schewe, T., et al.: The metabolism of the reticulocyte. In Yoshikawa, H. and Rapoport, S. M., eds.: Cellular and molecular biology of erythrocytes, Baltimore, 1974, University Park Press.

128. Rapoport, S., and Scheuch, D.: Glutathione stability and pyrophosphatase activity in reticulocytes; direct evidence for the importance of glutathione for the enzyme status in intact cells, Nature **186:**967, 1960.

129. Reed, C. F.: Studies of in vivo and in vitro exchange of erythrocyte and plasma phospholipids, J. Clin. Invest. **38:**1034, 1959.

130. Reed, C. F.: Phospholipid exchange between plasma and erythrocytes in man and dog, J. Clin. Invest. **47:**749, 1968.

131. Reed, C. F.: Incorporation of orthophosphate-^{32}P into erythrocyte phospholipids in normal subjects and in patients with hereditary spherocytosis, J. Clin. Invest. **47:**2630, 1968.

132. Rigas, D. A., and Koler, R. D.: Ultracentrifugal fractionation of human erythrocytes on the basis of cell age, J. Lab. Clin. Med. **58:**242, 1961.

133. Rose, I. A., and Warms, J. V. B.: Control of glycolysis in the human red blood cell, J. Biol. Chem. **241:**4848, 1966.

134. Rose, Z. B.: The purification and properties of diphosphoglycerate mutase from human erythrocytes, J. Biol. Chem. **243:**4810, 1968.

135. Rose, Z. B., and Liebowitz, J.: 2,3-diphosphoglycerate phosphatase from human erythrocytes, J. Biol. Chem. **245:**3232, 1970.

136. Rubinstein, D., and Denstedt, O. F.: The metabolism of the erythrocyte. III. The tricarboxylic acid cycle in the avian erythrocyte, J. Biol. Chem. **204:**623, 1953.

137. Salhany, J. M., Keitt, A. S., and Eliot, R. S.: The rate of deoxygenation of red blood cells: effect of intracellular 2,3-diphosphoglycerate and pH, F.E.B.S. Lett. **16:**257, 1971.

138. Schewe, T., Hiebsch, C., and Rapoport, S.: Biochemical events in the maturation process of the red cell: further results on the action site of the respiratory inhibitor F from reticulocytes in the respiratory chain, Acta Biol. Med. Ger. **29:**189, 1972.

139. Schröter, W.: In Deutsch, E., Gerlach, G., and Moser, K. eds.: Metabolism and membrane permeability of erythrocytes and thrombocytes, Stuttgart, 1968, Georg Thieme Verlag.

140. Segel, G. B., Feig, S. A., Baehner, R. L., and Nathan, D. G.: Fluorometric analysis of glycolytic intermediates and pyridine nucleotides in peripheral blood cells, J. Lab. Clin. Med. **78:**969, 1971.

141. Selwyn, J. G., and Dacie, J. V.: Autohemolysis and other changes resulting from patients with congenital hemolytic anemia, Blood **9:**414, 1954.

142. Siggard-Andersen, O., Salling, N., Nörgaard-Pedersen, B., et al.: Oxygen-linked hydrogen ion binding of human

hemoglobin: effects of carbon dioxide and 2,3-diphosphoglycerate, Scand. J. Clin. Lab. Invest. **29:**185, 1972.

143. Srivastava, S. K., and Beutler, E.: The transport of oxidized glutathione from human erythrocytes, J. Biol. Chem **244:**9, 1969.

144. Takahara, S.: Acatalasemia and hypocatalasemia in the Orient, Semin. Hematol. **8:**397, 1971.

145. Tanaka, K. R., and Valentine, W. N.: Pyruvate kinase deficiency. In Beutler, E., ed.: Hereditary disorders of erythrocyte metabolism, New York, 1968, Grune & Stratton, Inc.

146. Tanaka, K. R., Valentine, W. N., and Miwa, S.: Pyruvate kinase (PK) deficiency hereditary nonspherocytic hemolytic anemia, Blood **19:**267, 1962.

147. Tappel, A. L.: Selenium-glutathione peroxidase and vitamin E, Am. J. Clin. Nutr. **27:**960, 1974.

148. Tarui, N., Kono, N., and Uyeda, K.: Purification and properties of rabbit erythrocyte phosphofructokinase, J. Biol. Chem. **247:**1138, 1972.

149. Teitel, P., Marcu, I., and Xenakis, A.: Erythrocyte microrheology: its dependence on the reduced sulfhydryl groups and hemoglobin integrity, Folia Haematol. **90:**281, 1968.

150. Tomita, S., and Riggs, A.: Studies of the interaction of 2,3-diphosphoglycerate and carbon dioxide with hemoglobins from mouse, men and elephant, J. Biol. Chem. **246:**547, 1971.

151. Touster, O.: Essential pentosuria and the glucuronate-xylulose pathway, Fed. Proc. **19:**977, 1960.

152. Travis, S. F., Morrison, A. D., Clements, R. S., et al.: Metabolic alterations in the human erythrocyte produced by increases in glucose concentration: the role of the polyol pathway, J. Clin. Invest. **50:**2104, 1971.

153. Valentine, W. N.: Enzyme abnormalities in red cells, Br. J. Haematol. **31**(suppl.):11, 1975.

154. Valentine, W. N., Paglia, D. E., Neerhout, R. C., and Konrad, P. N.: Erythrocyte glyoxalase II deficiency with coincidental hereditary elliptocytosis, Blood **36:**797, 1970.

155. Warburg, O., and Christian, W.: Über activierung der Robisonchen Hexose-Mono-Phosphorsäure in roten Blutzellen und die gewinnung activierender Fermentlösungen, Biochem Z. **242:**206, 1931.

156. Weatherall, D. J., and McIntyre, P. A.: Developmental and acquired variations in erythrocyte carbonic anhydrase isozymes, Br. J. Haematol. **13:**106, 1967.

157. Weed, R. I., LaCelle, P. L., and Merrill, E. W.: Metabolic dependence of red cell deformability, J. Clin. Invest. **48:**795, 1969.

158. Wever, R., Ondega, B., and van Gelder, B. F.: Generation of superoxide radicals during the autoxidation of mammalian oxyhaemoglobin, Biochim. Biophys. Acta **302:**475, 1973.

159. Whittam, R.: The asymmetrical stimulation of a membrane adenosine triphosphatase in relation to active cation transport, Biochem. J. **84:**110, 1962.

160. Wiesner, R., and Rapoport, S.: The effect of inhibitor Rc from rabbit reticulocytes upon soluble and particulate cytochrome oxidase of beef heart mitochondria, Acta Biol. Med. Ger. **31:**289, 1973.

161. Winterbourn, C. C., and Carrell, R. W.: Studies of hemoglobin denaturation and Heinz body formation in the unstable hemoglobins, J. Clin. Invest. **54:**678, 1974.

162. Witt, I.: Influence of glutathione on enzymes from red cells of newborns and adults, Z. Kinderheilkd. **113:**71, 1972.

163. Yip, L. C., and Balis, M. E.: Inhibitory effects of 2,3-DPG on enzymes of purine nucleotide metabolism, Biochem. Biophys. Res. Commun. **63:**722, 1975.

164. Yoshikawa, H.: Introduction. In Yoshikawa, H., and Rapoport, S. M., eds.: Cellular and molecular biology of erythrocytes, Baltimore, 1974, University Park Press.

165. Yoshikawa, H., and Minakami, S.: Regulation of glycolysis in human red cells, Folia Haematol. **89:**357, 1968.

166. Yunis, A. A., and Arimura, G. K.: Sodium-potassium dependent adenoside triphosphatase of mammalian reticulocytes and mature red blood cells, Proc. Soc. Exp. Med. Biol. **121:**327, 1966.

Laboratory evaluation of inherited metabolic disorders of red cells

167. Bernstein, R. E.: A rapid screening dye test for the detection of glucose-6-phosphate dehydrogenase deficiency in red cells, Nature (London) **194:**192, 1962.

168. Beutler, E.: A series of new screening procedures for pyruvate kinase deficiency, glucose-6-phosphate dehydrogenase deficiency, and glutathione reductase deficiency, Blood **28:**553, 1966.

169. Beutler, E.: Red cell metabolism: A manual of biochemical methods, ed. 2, New York, 1973, Grune & Stratton, Inc.

170. Beutler, E., and Mitchell, M.: Special modification of the fluorescent screening method for glucose-6-phosphate dehydrogenase deficiency, Blood **32:**816, 1968.

171. Brewer, G. J., Tarlov, A. R., and Alving, A. S.: The methemoglobin reduction test for primaquine-type sensitivity of erythrocytes, J.A.M.A. **180:**386, 1962.

172. Dacie, J. V., and Lewis, S. M.: Practical Haematology ed. 5, New York, 1972, Grune & Stratton, Inc.

173. Fairbanks, V. F., and Beutler, E.: A simple method for the detection of erythrocyte glucose-6-phosphate dehydrogenase (G-6-PD spot test), Blood **20:**591, 1962.

174. Fairbanks, V. F., and Fernandez, M. N.: The identification of metabolic errors associated with hemolytic anemia, J.A.M.A. **208:**316, 1969.

175. Fairbanks, V. F., and Lampe, L. T.: A tetrazolium-linked cytochemical method for estimation of glucose-6-phosphate dehydrogenase activity in individual erythrocytes: applications in the study of heterozygotes for glucose-6-phosphate dehydrogenase deficiency, Blood **31:**589, 1968.

176. Hillman, R. S.: Hematology laboratory manual, Seattle, 1969, University of Washington Press.

177. Jacob, H. S., and Jandl, J. H.: A simple visual screening test for G-6-PD deficiency employing ascorbate and cyanide, N. Engl. J. Med. **274:**1162, 1966.

178. Jacobasch, G., Minikami, S., and Rapoport, S. M.: Glycolysis of the erythrocyte. In Yoshikawa, H., and Rapoport, S. M., eds.: Cellular and molecular biology of erythrocytes, Baltimore, 1974, University Park Press.

179. Miller, D. R.: The laboratory evaluation of hemolysis. In Weed, R. I., ed.: Hematology for internists, Boston, 1971, Little, Brown & Co.

180. Minakami, S., Suzaki, C., Sarto, T., and Yoshikawa, H.: Studies on erythrocyte glycolysis. I. Determination of the glycolytic intermediates in human erythrocytes, J. Biochem. **58:**543, 1965.

181. Niessner, H., and Beutler, E.: Fluorometric analysis of glycolytic intermediates in human red blood cells, Biochem. Med. **8:**123, 1973.

182. Oski, F. A., and Growney, P. M.: A simple micromethod for the detection of erythrocyte glucose-6-phosphate dehydrogenase deficiency, J. Pediatr. **66:**90, 1965.

183. Paglia, D. E., Valentine, W. N., Baughan, M. A., et al.: An inherited molecular lesion of erythrocyte pyruvate kinase: identification of a kinetically aberrant isozyme associated with premature hemolysis, J. Clin. Invest. **47:**1929, 1968.

184. Prager, D.: The autohemolysis test, J.A.M.A. **201:**189, 1967.

185. Sass, M. D., Caruso, C. J., and Axelrod, D. R.: Rapid screening for D-glucose-6-phosphate: NADP oxidoreductase deficiency with methylene blue, J. Lab Chem. Med. **68:**156, 1966.

186. Segel, G. B., Feig, S. A., Baehner, R. L., and Nathan, D. G.: Fluorometric analysis of glycolytic intermediates and pyridine nucleotides in peripheral blood cells, J. Lab. Clin. Med. **78:**969, 1971.

187. Tonz, O., and Betke, K.: Einfacher farbtest zur bestimmung der glucose-6-phosphat dehydrogenase in menschlichen Erythrocyten, Klin. Wochenschr. **40:**649, 1962.

188. Valentine, W. N., Anderson, H. M., and Paglia, D. E.: Studies on human erythrocyte nucleotide metabolism. II. Non-spherocytic hemolytic anemia, high red cell ATP, and ribosephosphate pyrophosphokinase (RPK, E.C. 2.7.6.1) deficiency, Blood **39:**674, 1972.

189. Valentine, W. N., Fink, K., Paglia, D. E., et al.: Hereditary hemolytic anemia with human erythrocyte pyrimidine 5'-nucleotidase deficiency, J. Clin. Invest. **54:**866, 1974.

190. Yunis, J. J., and Yasmineh, W. G.: Biochemical methods in red cell genetics, New York, 1969, Academic Press, Inc.

Classification and defects of the Embden-Meyerhof pathway

191. Alagille, D., Fleury, J., and Odièvre, M.: Déficit congénital en 2,3-diphosphoglycéromutase. Soc. Med. Hop. Paris **115:**493, 1964.

192. Altay, C., Alper, C. A., and Nathan, D. G.: Normal and variant isoenzymes of human blood cell hexokinase and the isoenzyme pattern in hemolytic anemia, Blood **36:** 219, 1970.

193. Anderson, J. W., Herman, R. H., Tyrrell, J. B., and Cohn, R. J.: Hexokinase: a compartmented enzyme, Am. J. Clin. Nutr. **24:**642, 1971.

194. Angelmann, H., Brain, M. C., and MacIver, J. E.: A case of triosephosphate isomerase deficiency with sudden death. In Abstracts of Thirteenth International Congress of Hematology, Munich, 1970.

195. Arese, P., Bozia, A., Gallo, E., et al.: Red cell glycolysis in a case of 3-phosphoglycerate kinase deficiency, Eur. J. Clin. Invest. **3:**86, 1973.

196. Arnold, H., Blume, K. G., Busch, D., et al.: Klinische und biochemische Untersuchungen zur Glucose-phosphatisomerase normaler menschlicher Erythrocyten und bei Glucose-phosphatisomerase-mangel, Klin. Wochenschr. **48:**1299, 1970.

197. Arnold, H., Blume, K. G., Engelhardt, R. and Löhr, G. W.: Glucosephosphate isomerase deficiency: evidence for in vivo instability of an enzyme variant with hemolysis, Blood **41:**691, 1973.

198. Arnold, H., Blume, K. G., Lohr, G. W., et al.: "Acquired" red cell enzyme defects in hematological diseases, Clin. Chem. Acta **57:**187, 1974.

199. Arnold, H., Blume, K. G., Löhr, G. W., et al.: Glucose phosphate isomerase deficiency with congenital non-spherocytic hemolytic anemia: a new variant (type Nordhorn). II. Purification and biochemical properties of the defective enzyme, Pediatr. Res. **8:**26, 1974.

200. Badwey, J. A., and Westhead, E. W.: Post-translational modification of human erythrocyte pyruvate kinase, Biochem. Biophys. Res. Commun. **74:**1326, 1977.

201. Baehner, R. L., Feig, S. A., Segel, G. B., et al.: Metabolic, phagocytic, and bactericidal properties of phosphoglycerate kinase deficient polymorphonuclear leukocytes, Blood **38:**833, 1971. (Abstract.)

202. Baughan, M. A., Valentine, W. N., Paglia, D. E., et al.: Hereditary hemolytic anemia associated with glucosephosphate isomerase (GPI) deficiency: a new enzyme defect of human erythrocytes, Blood **32:**236, 1968.

203. Benöhr, H. C., and Waller, H. D.: Metabolism in haemolytic states, Clin. Haematol. **4:**45, 1975.

204. Beutler, E.: Hereditary disorders of erythrocyte metabolism, New York, 1968, Grune & Stratton, Inc.

205. Beutler, E.: Electrophoresis of phosphoglycerate kinase, Biochem. Genet. **3:**189, 1969.

206. Beutler, E.: Abnormalities of the hexose monophosphate shunt, Semin. Hematol. **8:**311, 1971.

207. Beutler, E.: Genetic disorders of human red blood cells, J.A.M.A. **233:**1184, 1975.

208. Beutler, E., Sigalove, W. H., Muir, W. A., et al.: Glucose-phosphate isomerase (GPI) deficiency: GPI Elyria, Ann. Intern. Med. **80:**730, 1974.

209. Beutler, E., and Teeple, L.: Mannose metabolism in the human erythrocyte, J. Clin. Invest. **48:**461, 1909.

210. Bigley, R. H., and Koler, R. D.: Liver pyruvate kinase (PK) isoenzymes in a PK-deficient patient, Ann. Hum. Genet. **31:**383, 1968.

211. Black, J. A., and Henderson, M. H.: Activation and inhibition of human erythrocyte pyruvate kinase by organic phosphates, amino acids, dipeptides and anions, Biochem. Biophys. Acta **284:**115, 1972.

212. Blake, C. C. F., Evans, P. R., and Scopes, R. K.: Structure of horse-muscle phosphoglycerate kinase at 6Å resolution, Nature (New Biol.) **225:**195, 1972.

213. Blume, K. G., Arnold, H., Lohr, G. W., and Scholz, G.: On the molecular basis of pyruvate kinase deficiency, Biochem. Biophys. Acta **370:**601, 1974.

214. Blume, K. G., and Beutler, E.: Detection of glucose-phosphate isomerase deficiency by a screening procedure, Blood **39:**685, 1972.

215. Blume, K. G., Busch, D., et al.: The polymorphism of nucleoside effect in pyruvate kinase deficiency, Humangenetik **9:**257, 1970.

216. Blume, K. G., Hoffbauer, R. W., Busch, D., et al.: Purification and properties of erythrocyte pyruvate-kinase in normal and in pyruvate-kinase deficient human red blood cells, Biochem. Biophys. Acta **227:**364, 1971.

217. Blume, K. G., Hyrniuk, W., Powars, D., et al.: Characterization of two new variants of glucose-phosphate isomerase deficiency with hereditary non-spherocytic hemolytic anemia, J. Clin. Lab. Med. **79:**942, 1972.

218. Blume, K. G., Löhr, G. W., Praetsch, O., et al.: Beitrag zur populationsgenetik der Pyruvatkinase menschlicher Erythrocyten, Humangenetik **6:**261, 1968.

219. Boivin, P., and Galand, C.: Recherche d'une anomalie moleculaire lors des déficits en pyruvate kinase erythrocytaire, Nouv. Rev. Fr. Hématol. **8:**201, 1968.

220. Boivin, P., Galand, C., and Demartial, M. C.: Études sur la pyruvate kinase érythrocytaire II. Hétérogenéité enzymologique des déficits: Études a propos de 28 cas avec anémie hémolytique congénitale, Nouv. Rev. Fr. Hématol. **12:**569, 1972.

221. Boivin, P., Galand, C., Hakim, J., et al.: Une nouvelle érythroenzymeopathie: anémie hémolytique congénitale non-sphérocytaire et déficit héréditaire en adénylate-kinase erythrocytaire, Presse Med. **79:**215, 1971.

222. Boivin, P., Galand, C., Hakim, J., and Kahn, A.: Acquired red cell pyruvate kinase deficiency in leukemias and related disorders, Enzyme **19:**294, 1975.

223. Bowman, H. S., and Procopio, F.: Hereditary non-spherocytic hemolytic anemia of the pyruvate kinase deficient type, Ann. Intern. Med. **58:**567, 1963.

224. Brandt, N. J., and Hanel, H. K.: Atypical pyruvate kinase in a patient with haemolytic anaemia, Scand. J. Haematol. **8:**126, 1971.

225. Busch, D.: Probleme des Erythrocytenstoffwechsels bei Anämien mit Pyruvatkinase-mangel, Folia Haematol. **83:**395, 1965.

226. Carson, P. E., Flanagan, C. L., Ickes, C. E., and Alving,

A. S.: Enzymatic deficiency in primaquine-sensitive erythrocytes, Science **124:**484, 1956.

227. Cartier, P., Habibi, B., Leroux, J. P., et al.: Anemie hemolytique congenitale associe a un deficit en phosphoglycerate-kinase dans les globules rouges, les polynucleaires et les lymphocytes, Nouv. Rev. Fr. Hematol. **11:**565, 1971.

228. Cartier, P., Labie, D., Leroux, J. P., et al.: Déficit familial en diphosphoglycerate mutase: étude hématologique et biochemique, Nouv. Rev. Fr. Hematol. **12:**269, 1972.

229. Cartier, P., Temkine, H., and Griscelli, C.: Etude biochimique d'une anemie hemolytique avec deficit familial en phosphohexoisomerase, Enzym. Biol. Clin. **10:**439, 1969.

230. Chien, S.-H., Anderson, J. E., and Giblett, E. R.: 2,3-Diphosphoglycerate mutase: its demonstration by electrophoresis and the detection of a genetic variant, Biochem. Genet. **5:**481, 1971.

231. Chien, S.-H., and Giblett, E. R.: Phosphoglycerate kinase: additional variants and their geographic distribution, Am. J. Hum. Genet. **24:**229, 1972.

232. Chien, S.-H., Malcolm, L. A., Yoshida, A., and Giblett, E. R.: Phosphoglycerate kinase: an X-linked polymorphism in man, Am. J. Hum. Genet. **23:**87, 1971.

233. Chilcote, R. R., and Baehner, R. L.: Red cell (RBC) glucose phosphate isomerase deficiency (GPI): clinical and laboratory evidence of increased blood viscosity, Pediatr. Res. **8:**398, 1974.

234. Darnall, D. W., and Murray, L. V.: Effects of ATP and 2,3-diphosphoglycerate on glyceraldehyde-3-phosphate dehydrogenase activity, Biochem. Biophys. Res. Commun. **46:**1222, 1972.

235. DeGruchy, G. C., Crawford, H., and Morton, D.: Atypical (nonspherocytic) congenital haemolytic anaemia, Proc. 7th Congr. Int. Soc. Hematol., Rome, 1958. (Abstract No. 198.)

236. Delivoria-Papadopoulos, M., Oski, F. A., et al.: Oxygen-hemoglobin dissociation curves: effect of inherited enzyme defects of the red cell, Science **165:**601, 1969.

237. Detter, J. C., Ways, P. D., Giblett, E. R., et al.: Inherited variations in human phosphohexose isomerase, Ann. Hum. Genet. **31:**329, 1968.

238. Deys, B. F., Grzeschick, K. H., Grzeschick, A., et al.: Human phosphoglycerate kinase and inactivation on the X-chromosome, Science **175:**1002, 1972.

239. Dunham, P. B., and Gunn, R. B.: Adenosine triphosphatase and active cation transport in red blood cell membranes, Arch. Intern. Med. **129:**241, 1972.

240. Englehardt, R., Arnold, H., Hoffman, A., et al.: GPI-Recklinghausen: a new variant of glucosephosphate isomerase deficiency with hemolytic anemia. In Gerlach, E., Moser, K., and Deutch, E., eds.: Erythrocytes, thrombocytes, leukocytes: recent advances in membrane and metabolic research, Stuttgart, 1973, Georg Thieme Verlag.

241. Fitch, L. I., Parr, C. W., and Welch, S. G.: Phosphoglucose isomerase variation in man, Biochem. J. **110:**56P, 1968.

242. Fung, R. H., Keung, Y. K., and Chung, G. S. H.: Screening of pyruvate kinase deficiency and G-6-PD deficiency in Chinese newborns in Hong Kong, Arch. Dis. Child. **44:**373, 1969.

243. Giblett, E. R., Anderson, J. E., Cohen, F., et al.: Adenosine deaminase deficiency in two patients with severely impaired cellular immunity, Lancet **2:**1067, 1972.

244. Gilman, P. A.: An unusual form of pyruvate kinase in congenital nonspherocytic hemolytic anemia, Proc. 39th Ann. Mtg. Soc. Pediatr. Res., Atlantic City, 1969.

245. Gilman, P. A.: Hemolysis in the newborn infant resulting from deficiencies of red blood cell enzymes: diagnosis and management, J. Pediatr. **84:**625, 1974.

246. Glader, B. E.: Salicylate-induced injury of pyruvate-kinase-deficiency erythrocytes, N. Engl. J. Med. **294:**916, 1976.

247. Glader, B. E., and Nathan, D. G.: Haemolysis due to pyruvate kinase deficiency and other glycolytic enzymopathies, Clin. Haematol. **4:**123, 1975.

248. Goebel, K. M., Goebel, F. D., Janzen, R., and Kaffarnik, H.: Haemolytic anaemia with hereditary pyruvate kinase instability developing acute leukemia, Scand. J. Haematol. **14:**249, 1975.

249. Grimes, A. J., Meisler, A., and Dacie, J. V.: Hereditary non-spherocytic haemolytic anaemia: a study of red-cell carbohydrate metabolism in twelve cases of pyruvate-kinase deficiency, Br. J. Haematol. **10:**403, 1964.

250. Hanel, H. K., and Brandt, N. J.: Haemolytic anaemia due to abnormal pyruvate kinase, Lancet **2:**113, 1968.

251. Harkness, D. R.: A new erythrocytic enzyme defect with hemolytic anemia: glyceraldehyde-3-phosphate dehydrogenase deficiency, J. Lab. Clin. Med. **68:**879, 1966.

252. Harkness, D. R., and Roth, S.: Purification and properties of 2,3-diphosphoglyceric acid phosphatase from human erythrocytes, Biochem. Biophys. Res. Commun. **34:**849, 1969.

253. Harris, S. R., Paglia, D. E., Jaffé, E. R., et al.: Triose phosphate isomerase deficiency in an adult, Clin. Res. **18:**529, 1970.

254. Harvald, B., Hanel, K. H., Squires, R. and Trap-Jensen, J.: Adenosine-triphosphatase deficiency in patients with non-spherocytic haemolytic anaemia, Lancet **2:**18, 1964.

255. Helleman, P. W., and Van Biervliet, J. P.: Haematological studies in a new variant of glucosephosphate isomerase deficiency (GPI Utrecht), Helv. Paediat. Acta **30:**525, 1975.

256. Hjelm, M., and Wadman, B.: Nonspherocytic hemolytic anemia with phosphoglycerate kinase deficiency. Proc. 13th Int. Congr. Hematol., Munich, August 1970. (Abstract.)

257. Holmes, E. W., Jr., Malone, J. I., Winegrad, A. I., and Oski, F. A.: Hexokinase isoenzymes in human erythrocytes: association of type II with fetal hemoglobin, Science **156:**646, 1967.

258. Hoorn, R. K. J., Flikweert, J. P., and Staal, G. E. J.: Purification and properties of enolase of human erythrocytes, Int. J. Biochem. **5:**845, 1974.

259. Hutton, J. J., and Chilcote, R. R.: Glucose phosphate isomerase deficiency with hereditary nonspherocytic hemolytic anemia, J. Pediatr. **85:**494, 1974.

260. Ibsen, K. H., Schiller, K. W., and Hass, T. A.: Interconvertible kinetic and physical forms of human erythrocyte pyruvate-kinase, J. Biol. Chem. **246:**1233, 1971.

261. Imamura, K., Tanaka, T., Nishina, T., et al.: Studies on pyruvate kinase deficiency. II. Electrophoretic, kinetic, and immunological studies on PK of erythrocytes and other tissues. J. Biochem. **74:**1165, 1975.

262. Jacobasch, G., Syllm-Rapoport, I., Rorgas, H., and Rapoport, S.: 2,3-PGase-Mangel als mögliche Ursache erhöten ATP-gehaltes, Clin. Chem. Acta **10:**477, 1964.

263. Jaffé, E. R.: Hereditary hemolytic disorders and enzymatic deficiencies of human erythrocytes, Blood **35:**116, 1970.

264. Jaffé, E. R.: The formation and reduction of methemoglobin in human erythrocytes. In Yoshikawa, H., and Rapoport, S. M., eds.: Cellular and molecular biology of erythrocytes, Baltimore, 1974, University Park Press.

265. Jaffé, E. R. and Hsieh, H. S.: DPNH-methemoglobin reductase deficiency and hereditary methemoglobinemia, Semin. Hematol. **8:**417, 1971.

266. Jaffé, E. R., Paglia, D. E., Harris, S. R., et al.: Triosephosphate isomerase deficiency and hemolytic anemia in an adult, Proc. 13th Int. Congr. Hematol., Munich, 1970.
267. Kahn, A., Boyer, C., Cottreau, D., et al.: Immunological study of the age-related loss of six enzymes in the red cells from newborn infants and adults: evidence for a fetal type of erythrocyte phosphofructokinase, Pediatr. Res. **11:**271, 1977.
268. Kahn, A., Etiemble, J., Meienhoffer, M. C., and Boivin, P.: Erythrocyte phosphofructokinase deficiency associated with an unstable variant of muscle phosphofructokinase, Clin. Chem. Acta **61:**415, 1975.
269. Kahn, A., Marie, J., Bernard, J.-F., et al.: Mechanisms of the acquired erythrocyte enzyme deficiencies in blood diseases, Clin. Chem. Acta **71:**379, 1976.
270. Kahn, A., Marie, J., Galand, C., and Boivin, P.: Molecular mechanism of erythrocyte pyruvate kinase deficiency, Humangenetick **29:**271, 1975.
271. Kahn, A., Marie, J., Galand, C., and Boivin, P.: Chronic haemolytic anaemia in two patients heterozygous for erythrocyte pyruvate kinase deficiency, Scand. J. Haematol. **16:**250, 1976.
272. Kahn, A., Vives, J. L., Bertrand, O., et al.: Glucosephosphate isomerase deficiency due to a new variant (GPI Barcelona) and to a silent gene: biochemical, immunological and genetic studies, Clin. Chem. Acta **66:**145, 1976.
273. Kahn, A., Vives-Corron, J. L., Marie, J., et al.: A Spanish family with erythrocyte pyruvate kinase deficiency: contribution of various immunologic methods in the study of the mutant enzyme, Clin. Chem. Acta **75:**71, 1977.
274. Kalckar, H. M., Kinoshita, J. H., and Connell, G. N.: Galactosemia: biochemistry, genetics, pathophysiology and developmental aspects, Biol. Brain Dysfunction **1:**31, 1973.
275. Kant, J. A., and Steck, T. L.: Specificity in the association of glyceraldehyde-3-phosphate dehydrogenase with isolated human erythrocyte membrane, J. Biol. Chem. **248:**8457, 1973.
276. Kaplan, J. C., Teeple, J., Shore, N., and Beutler, E.: Electrophoretic abnormality in triosephosphate isomerase deficiency, Biochem. Biophys. Res. Commun. **31:**768, 1968.
277. Kappel, W. K., and Hass, L. F.: The isolation and partial characterization of diphosphoglycerate mutase from human erythrocytes, Biochemistry **15:**290, 1976.
278. Katzen, H. M., Soderman, D. D., and Cirillo, V. J.: Tissue distribution and physiological significance of multiple forms of hexokinase, Ann. N.Y. Acad. Sci. **151:**351, 1968.
279. Keitt, A. S.: Pyruvate kinase deficiency and related disorders of red cell glycolysis, Am. J. Med. **41:**762, 1966.
280. Keitt, A. S.: Hemolytic anemia with impaired hexokinase activity, J. Clin. Invest. **48:**1997, 1969.
281. Khan, P. M., Westerveld, A., Grzeschik, K. H., et al.: X-linkage of human phosphoglycerate kinase confirmed in man-mouse and man-chinese hamster somatic cell hybrids. Am. J. Hum. Genet. **23:**614, 1971.
282. Koler, R. D., Bigley, R. H., Jones, R. T., et al.: Pyruvate kinase: molecular differences between human red cell and leukocyte enzyme, Cold Spring Harbor Symp. Quant. Biol. **29:**213, 1964.
283. Koler, R. D., Bigley, R. H., and Stenzel, P.: Biochemical properties of human erythrocyte and leukocyte pyruvate kinase. In Beutler, E., ed.: Hereditary disorders of erythrocyte metabolism, New York, 1968, Grune & Stratton, Inc.
284. Konrad, P. N., McCarthy, D. J., Mauer, A. M., et al.: Erythrocyte and leukocyte phosphoglycerate kinase defi-
285. ciency with neurologic disease, J. Pediatr. **82:**456, 1973.
285. Konrad, P. N., Richards, F., Valentine, W. N., and Paglia, D. E.: γ-Glutamyl-cysteine synthetase deficiency, N. Engl. J. Med. **286:**557, 1972.
286. Kraus, A. P., Langston, M. F., and Lynch, B. L.: Red cell phosphoglycerate kinase deficiency: a new cause of non-spherocytic hemolytic anemia, Biochem. Biophys. Res. Commun. **30:**173, 1968.
287. Labie, D., Leroux, J. P., Najman, A., and Royrolle, C.: Familial diphosphoglycerate-mutase deficiency: influence on the oxygen affinity curves of hemoglobin, F.E.B.S. Lett. **9:**37, 1970.
288. Layzer, R. B., Rowland, L. P., and Ranney, H. M.: Muscle phosphofructokinase deficiency, Arch. Neurol. **17:**512, 1967.
289. Loder, P. B., and deGruchy, G. C.: Red-cell enzymes and co-enzymes in nonspherocytic congenital haemolytic anaemias, Br. J. Haematol. **11:**21, 1965.
290. Löhr, G. W., Arnold, H., Blume, K. G., et al.: Hereditary deficiency of glucosephosphate isomerase as a cause of nonspherocytic hemolytic anemia, Blut **26:**393, 1973.
291. Löhr, G. W., and Waller, H. D.: Zur biochemie einiger angeborener hämolytischer anämien, Folia Haematol. **8:**377, 1963.
292. Löhr, G. W., Waller, H. D., Anschütz, F., and Knoop, A.: Biochemische defekte in den Blutzellen bei familiärer panmyelopathie (Typ Fanconi), Humangenetik **1:**383, 1965.
293. Löhr, G. W., Waller, H. D., Anschütz, F., and Knopp, A.: Hexokinase-Mangel in Blutzellen bei einer Sippe mit familiärer panmyelopathie (Typ Fanconi), Klin. Wochenschr. **43:**870, 1965.
294. Luzzatto, L.: Inherited haemolytic states: glucose-6-phosphate dehydrogenase deficiency, Clin. Haematol. **4:**83, 1975.
295. Mahour, G. H., Lynn, H. B., and Hill, R. W.: Acute pancreatitis with biliary disease in erythrocyte pyruvate kinase deficiency, Clin. Pediatr. **8:**608, 1969.
296. Malone, J. I., Winegrad, A. I., Oski, F. A., and Holmes, E. W., Jr.: Erythrocyte hexokinase isoenzyme patterns in hereditary hemoglobinopathies, N. Engl. J. Med. **279:**1071, 1968.
297. Maretzki, D., and Rapoport, S.: Glyzeraldehyd-3-phosphat-dehydrogenase und erythrocyten des menschen, Acta Biol. Med. Germ. **29:**207, 1972.
298. Marie, J., Kahn, A., and Boivin, P.: Pyruvate kinase isozymes in man. I. M-type isozymes in adult and fetal tissues, electrofocusing and immunological studies, Hum. Genet. **31:**35, 1976.
299. Matsumota, N., Ishihara, T., Oda, E., et al.: Fine structure of the spleen and liver in glucosephosphate isomerase (GPI) deficiency hereditary nonspherocytic hemolytic anemia: selective reticulocyte destruction as a mechanism of hemolysis, Acta Haematol. Jpn. **36:**46, 1973.
300. Mazza, V., Arese, P., Bosia, A., et al.: Red cell metabolism in a case of 3-phosphoglycerate kinase deficiency. Proc. 13th Int. Congr. Hematol., Munich, August 1970, (Abstract.)
301. McDaniel, C. F., Kirtley, M. E., and Tanner, M. J. A.: The interaction of glyceraldehyde-3-phosphate dehydrogenase with human erythrocyte membranes, J. Biol. Chem. **249:**6478, 1974.
302. Meister, A.: The γ-glutamyl cycle: diseases associated with specific enzyme deficiencies, Ann. Intern. Med. **81:**247, 1974.
303. Mentzer, W., and Alpers, J.: Mild anemia with abnormal RBC pyruvate kinase, Clin. Res. **29:**209, 1971.
304. Mentzer, W. C., Jr., Baehner, R. L., Schmidt-Schoenbein, H., et al.: Selective reticulocyte destruction in

erythrocyte pyruvate kinase deficiency, J. Clin. Invest. **50:**688, 1971.

305. Miller, D. R.: The hereditary hemolytic anemias: membrane and enzyme defects, Pediatr. Clin. North Am. **19:**865, 1972.

306. Miwa, S., Nakashima, K., Ariyoshi, K., et al.: Four new pyruvate kinase (PK) variants and a classical PK deficiency, Br. J. Haematol. **29:**157, 1975.

307. Miwa, S., Nakashima, K., Oda, S., et al.: Phosphoglycerate kinase deficiency hereditary nonspherocytic hemolytic anemia: report of a case found in a Japanese family, Acta Haematol. Jpn. **35:**57, 1972.

308. Miwa, S., Nakashima, K., Oda, S., et al.: Glucosephosphate isomerase (GPI) deficiency hereditary nonspherocytic hemolytic anemia: report of the first case found in Japanese, Acta Haematol. Jpn. **36:**65, 1973.

309. Miwa, S., and Nishina, T.: Studies on pyruvate kinase (PK) deficiency. I. Clinical, hematological and erythrocyte enzyme studies, Acta Haematol. Jpn. **37:**1, 1974.

310. Miwa, S., Nishina, T., Kakahashi, Y., et al.: Studies on erythrocyte metabolism in a case with hereditary deficiency of H-subunit of lactate dehydrogenase, Acta Haematol. Jpn. **34:**228, 1971.

311. Miwa, S., Sato, T., Murao, H., et al.: A new type of phosphofructokinase deficiency hereditary nonspherocytic hemolytic anemia, Acta Haematol. Jpn. **35:**113, 1972.

312. Moser, K., Ciresa, M., and Schwarzmeier, J.: Hexokinasemangel bei hämolytischer Anämie, Med. Welt **21:**1977, 1970.

313. Motulsky, A. G., Gabrio, B. W., Burkhardt, J., and Finch, C. A.: Erythrocyte carbohydrate metabolism in hereditary hemolytic anemias, Am. J. Med. **19:**291, 1955.

314. Müller, E., Marti, H. R., Bach, J. L., et al.: Hereditäre nichtsphärozytäre hämolytische Anämie durch Glukosephosphatisomerase-Mängel: der erste in der Schweiz beobachte Fall, Schweiz. Med. Wochenschr. **104:**1379, 1974.

315. Muller-Soyano, A., deRoura, E. T., Duke, P.-R., et al.: Pyruvate kinase deficiency and leg ulcers, Blood **47:**807, 1976.

316. Munro, G. F., and Miller, D. R.: Mechanism of fructose diphosphate activation of a mutant pyruvate kinase from human red cells, Biochem. Biophys. Acta **206:**87, 1970.

317. Nakashima, K., Miwa, S., and Oda, S.: Electrophoretic and kinetic studies of mutant erythrocyte pyruvate kinases, Blood **43:**537, 1974.

318. Nakashima, K., Miwa, S., Oda, S., et al.: Electrophoretic and kinetic studies of glucosephosphate isomerase (GPI) in two different Japanese families with GPI deficiency, Am. J. Haematol. Genet. **25:**294, 1973.

319. Nakashima, K., Ogawa, H., Oda, S., and Miwa, S.: 1,3-Diphosphoglycerate in phosphoglycerate kinase deficiency, Clin. Chem. Acta. **49:**455, 1973.

320. Nathan, D. G., Oski, F. A., Miller, D. R., and Gardner, F. H.: Life-span and organ sequestration of the red cells in pyruvate kinase deficiency, N. Engl. J. Med. **278:**73, 1968.

321. Nathan, D. G., Oski, F. A., Sidel, V. W., and Diamond, L. K.: Extreme hemolysis and red cell distortion in erythrocyte pyruvate kinase deficiency. II. Measurements of erythrocyte glucose consumption, potassium flux, and adenosine triphosphate stability, N. Engl. J. Med. **272:**118, 1965.

322. Nathan, D. G., and Shohet, S. B.: Erythrocyte ion transport defects and hemolytic anemia: "hydrocytosis" and "desiccytosis," Semin. Hematol. **7:**381, 1970.

323. Necheles, T. F., Rai, U. S. and Cameron, D.: Congenital nonspherocytic hemolytic anemia associated with an unusual hexokinase abnormality, J. Lab. Clin. Med. **76:**539, 1970.

324. Nowicki, L., Behnken, L., and Biskamp, K.: Pancytopenien mit erythrocytarem Pyruvatkinase-und Glutathionoreductasedefekt, Klin. Wochenschr. **50:**566, 1972.

325. Oguchi, M.: Glyceraldehyde-3-phosphate dehydrogenase from human erythrocytes, J. Biochem. **68:**427, 1970.

326. Ohyama, H., Kumatori, T., Nishina, T., and Miwa, S.: Functionally abnormal pyruvate kinase in congenital hemolytic anemia, Acta Haematol. Jpn. **32:**330, 1969.

327. Okonkwo, P. O., Askari, A., and Korngold, L.: Human erythrocyte phosphoglycerate kinase: purification, properties and interaction with its antibody, Biochim. Biophys. Acta **321:**503, 1973.

328. Oski, F. A., and Bowman, H.: A low Km phosphoenolpyruvate mutant in the Amish with red cell pyruvate-kinase deficiency, Br. J. Haematol. **17:**289, 1969.

329. Oski, F. A., and Diamond, L. K.: Erythrocyte pyruvate kinase deficiency resulting in congenital nonspherocytic hemolytic anemia, N. Engl. J. Med. **269:**763, 1963.

330. Oski, F., and Fuller, E.: Glucose-phosphate isomerase (GPI) deficiency associated with abnormal osmotic fragility and spherocytes, Clin. Res. **19:**427, 1971.

331. Oski, F. A., Marshall, B. E., Delivoria-Papadopoulos, M., et al.: Exercise with anemia: the role of the left-shifted or right-shifted oxygen hemoglobin equilibrium curve, Ann. Intern. Med. **74:**44, 1971.

332. Oski, F. A., Nathan, D. G., Sidel, V. W., and Diamond, L. K.: Extreme hemolysis and red cell distortion in erythrocyte pyruvate kinase deficiency. I. Morphology, erythrokinetics, and family enzyme studies, N. Engl. J. Med. **270:**1023, 1964.

333. Oski, F., and Whaun, J.: Hemolytic anemia and red cell glyceraldehyde-3-phosphate dehydrogenase (G-3-PD) deficiency, Clin. Res. **17:**601, 1969. (Abstract.)

334. Paglia, D. E., Holland, P., Baughan, M. A., et al.: Occurrence of defective hexosephosphate isomerization in human erythrocytes and leukocytes, N. Engl. J. Med. **280:**66, 1969.

335. Paglia, D. E., Gray, G. R., Growe, G. J., and Valentine, W. N.: Simultaneous inheritance of mutant isoenzymes of erythrocyte pyruvate kinase associated with chronic haemolytic anaemia. Br. J. Haematol. **34:**61, 1976.

336. Paglia, D. E., Konrad, P. N., Wolff, J. A., and Valentine, W. N.: Biphasic kinetics in an anomalous isozyme of erythrocyte pyruvate kinase, Clin. Chem. Acta **73:**395, 1976.

337. Paglia, D. E., Paredis, R., Valentine, W. N., et al.: Unique phenotype expression of glucosephosphate isomerase deficiency, Am. J. Hum. Genet. **27:**62, 1975.

338. Paglia, D. E., and Valentine, W. N.: Evidence for molecular alteration of pyruvate kinase as a consequence of erythrocyte aging, J. Lab. Clin. Med. **76:**202, 1970.

339. Paglia, D. E., and Valentine, W. N.: Additional kinetic distinctions between normal pyruvate-kinase and a mutant isoenzyme from human erythrocytes: correction of the kinetic anomaly by fructose 1,6-diphosphate, Blood **37:**311, 1971.

340. Paglia, D. E., and Valentine, W. N.: Hereditary glucosephosphate isomerase deficiency, a review, Am. J. Clin. Pathol. **62:**740, 1974.

341. Paglia, D. E., Valentine, W. N., Baughan, M. A., et al.: An inherited molecular lesion of erythrocyte pyruvate kinase. Identification of a kinetically aberrant isoenzyme associated with premature hemolysis, J. Clin. Invest. **47:**1929, 1968.

342. Parker, J. P., Beirne, G. J., Desai, J. N., et al.: Androgen-induced increase in red-cell 2,3-diphosphoglycerate, N. Engl. J. Med. **287:**381, 1972.

343. Parker, J. C., and Hoffman, J. F.: The role of membrane phosphoglycerate kinase in the control of glycolytic rate by cation transport in human red blood cells, J. Gen. Physiol. **50:**893, 1967.

344. Peterson, J. S., Chern, C. J., Harkins, R. N., and Black, J. A.: The subunit structure of human muscles and human erythrocyte pyruvate kinase isozymes, F.E.B.S. Lett. **49:**73, 1974.

345. Proverbio, F., and Hoffman, J. F.: Differential behavior of the Mg-ATPase and the Na,Mg-ATPase of human red cell ghosts, Fed. Proc. **31:**215, 1972.

346. Robinson, M. A., Loder, P. B., and deGruchy, G. C.: Red cell metabolism in nonspherocytic congenital haemolytic anaemia, Br. J. Haematol. **7:**327, 1961.

347. Rosa, R., Gailbardon, J., and Rosa, J.: Characterization of 2,3-diphosphoglycerate phosphatase activity: electrophoretic study, Biochim. Biophys. Acta **293:**285, 1973.

348. Rose, I. A., and Warms, J. V. B.: Control of glycolysis in the human red blood cell, J. Biol. Chem. **241:**4848, 1966.

349. Rose, I. A., and Warms, J. V. B.: Mitrochondrial hexokinase: release, rebinding, and location, J. Biol. Chem. **242:**1635, 1967.

350. Rose, Z. B.: The purification and properties of diphosphoglycerate mutase from human erythrocytes, J. Biol. Chem. **243:**4819, 1968.

351. Rose, Z. B.: Effects of salts and pH on the rate of erythrocyte diphosphoglycerate mutase, Arch. Biochem. Biophys. **158:**903, 1973.

352. Rose Z. B., and Liebowitz, J.: 2,3-Diphosphoglycerate phosphatase from human erythrocytes, J. Biol. Chem. **245:**3232, 1970.

353. Rose, Z. B., and Whalen, R. G.: The phosphorylation of diphosphoglycerate mutase, J. Biol. Chem. **248:**1513, 1973.

354. Rubinstein, D., Ottolenghi, P., and Denstedt, D. F.: The metabolism of the erythrocyte. XIII. Enzyme activity in the reticulocyte, Can. J. Biochem. Physiol. **34:**222, 1956.

355. Sachs, J. R., Wicker, D. J., Gilcher, R. O., et al.: Familial hemolytic anemia resulting from an abnormal red blood cell pyruvate kinase, J. Lab. Clin. Med. **72:**359, 1968.

356. Sass, M. D., Caruso, C. J., and Farhangi, M.: TPNH-methemoglobin reductase deficiency: a new red-cell enzyme defect, J. Lab. Clin. Med. **70:**760, 1967.

357. Schimke, R. T., and Grossbard, L.: Studies on isozymes of hexokinase in animal tissues, Ann. N. Y. Acad. Sci. **151:**332, 1968.

358. Schneider, A. S., Dunn, I., Ibsen, K. H., and Weinstein, I. M.: Triosephosphate isomerase deficiency. In Beutler, E., ed.: Hereditary disorders of erythrocyte metabolism, New York, 1968, Grune & Stratton, Inc.

359. Schneider, A. S., Valentine, W. N., Hattori, M., and Heins, H. L., Jr.: Hereditary hemolytic anemia with triosephosphate isomerase deficiency, N. Engl. J. Med. **272:**229, 1965.

360. Schreir, S. L.: ATP synthesis in human erythrocyte membranes, Biochim. Biophys. Acta **135:**591, 1967.

361. Schrier, S. L., Ben-Bassat, I., Junga, I., et al.: Characterization of erythrocyte membrane-associated enzymes (glyceraldehyde-3-phosphate dehydrogenase and phosphoglycerate kinase), J. Lab. Clin. Med. **85:**797, 1975.

362. Schröter, W.: Kongenitale nichtophärocytäre hämolytische Anamie bei 2,3-Di-phosphoglyceratmutase-Mangel der Erythrocyten im frühen sauglinsalter, Klin. Wochenschr. **43:**1147, 1965.

363. Schröter, W.: 2,3-Diphosphoglyceratstoffwechsel und 2,3-Diphosphoglyceratmutase-Mangel in Erythrocyten, Blut **20:**1, 1970.

364. Schröter, W., Brittinger, G., Zimmerschmitt, E., et al.: A new haemolytic syndrome with glucosephosphate isomerase (GPI) and glucose-6-phosphate dehydrogenase (G6PD) deficiency of the erythrocytes: biochemical studies, Eur. J. Clin. Invest. **1:**145, 1970.

365. Schröter, W., Brittinger, G., Zimmerschmitt, E., et al.: Combined glucose-phosphate isomerase and glucose-6-phosphate dehydrogenase deficiency of the erythrocytes: a new haemolytic syndrome, Br. J. Haemat. **20:**249, 1971.

366. Schröter, W., and Heyden, H. V.: Kinetik des 2,3-diphosphoglyceratdemsatzes in menschlichen Erythrocyten, Biochem. Z. **341:**387, 1965.

367. Schröter, W., Koch, H. H., Wonneberger, B., et al: Glucose phosphate isomerase deficiency with congenital nonspherocytic hemolytic anemia: a new variant (type Nordhorn) I. Clinical and genetic studies, Pediatr. Res. **8:**18, 1974.

368. Schröter, W., and Neuvians, M.: Membrane-bound 2,3-diphosphoglycerate phosphatase of human erythrocytes, J. Membr. Biol. **2:**31, 1970.

369. Schröter, W., and Tillmann, W.: Hexokinase isoenzymes in human erythrocytes of adults and newborns, Biochem. Biophys. Res. Commun. **31:**92, 1968.

370. Searcy, G. P., Miller, D. R., and Tasker, J. B.: Congenital hemolytic anemia in the Basenji dog due to erythrocyte pyruvate kinase deficiency, Can. J. Comp. Med. **35:**67, 1971.

371. Seegmiller, J. E., Rosenbloom, F. M., and Kelley, W. N.: Enzyme defect associated with a sex-linked human neurological disorder and excessive purine synthesis, Science **155:**1682, 1967.

372. Segel, G. B., Feig, S. A., Glader, B. E., et al.: An essential role for phosphoglycerate kinase-dependent red cell cation transport, Blood **42:**982, 1973.

373. Shin, B. C., and Carraway, K. L.: Association of glyceraldehyde-3-phosphate dehydrogenase with the human erythrocyte membrane, J. Biol. Chem. **248:**1436, 1973.

374. Silken, A. B.: Pharmacologic manipulation of human erythrocyte 2,3-diphosphoglycerate levels by prednisone administration, Pediatr. Res. **9:**61, 1975.

375. Smith, L. H., Huguley, C. M., Jr., and Bain, J. A.: Hereditary orotic aciduria. In Stanbury, J. B., Wyngaarden, J. B., and Fredrickson, D. S., ed.: The metabolic basis of inherited disease, ed. 3, New York, 1972, McGraw-Hill Book Co.

376. Snyder, L. M., and Reddy, W. J.: Mechanism of action of thyroid hormones on erythrocyte 2,3-diphosphoglyceric acid synthesis, J. Clin. Invest. **49:**1993, 1970.

377. Sparkes, R. S., Carrel, R. E., and Paglia, D. E.: Probable localization of a triosephosphate isomerase gene to the short arm of the number 5 human chromosome, Nature **224:**367, 1969.

378. Staal, G. E. J., Koster, J. F., and Kamp, H., et al.: Human erythrocyte pyruvate kinase: its purification and some properties, Biochim. Biophys. Acta **227:**86, 1971.

379. Staal, G. E. J., Koster, J. F. and Nijessen, J. G.: A new variant of red blood cell pyruvate kinase deficiency, Biochim. Biophys. Acta **258:**685, 1972.

380. Staal, G. E., Sybesma, H. B., et al.: Familial haemolytic anaemia due to pyruvate kinase deficiency, Folia Med. Neerl. **14:**72, 1971.

381. Stefanini, M.: Chronic hemolytic anemia associated with erythrocyte enolase deficiency exacerbated by ingestion of nitrofurantoin, Am. J. Clin. Pathol. **58:**408, 1972.

382. Strauss, R. G., McCarthy, D. J., and Mauer, A. M.: Neutrophil function in congenital phosphoglycerate kinase deficiency, J. Pediatr. **85:**341, 1974.

383. Syllm-Rapoport, I., Jacobasch, G., Roigas, H., and Rapoport, S.: 2,3-PGase-Mangel als Ursache erhohten ATP-Gehalts, Folia Haematol. **83:**363, 1965.

384. Szeinberg, A., Kahana, D., Gavendo, S., et al.: Hereditary deficiency of adenylate kinase in red blood cells, Acta Haematol. **42:**111, 1969.

385. Tanaka, K. R., and Paglia, D. E.: Pyruvate kinase deficiency, Semin. Hematol. **8:**367, 1971.

386. Tanaka, K. R., and Valentine, W. N.: Pyruvate kinase

deficiency. In Beutler, E., ed.: Hereditary disorders of erythrocyte metabolism, New York, 1968, Grune & Stratton, Inc.

387. Tanaka, K. R., Valentine, W. N., and Miwa, S.: Pyruvate kinase (PK) deficiency hereditary non-spherocytic hemolytic anemia, Blood **19:**267, 1962.

388. Tanphaichats, V. S., and van Eys, J.: Erythrocyte pyruvate kinase activity in patients with haematological malignancies, Scand. J. Haematol. **15:**10, 1975.

389. Tarui, S., Kono, N., Nasu, T., and Nishikawa, M.: Enzymatic basis for the coexistance of myopathy and hemolytic disease in inherited muscle phosphofructo-kinase deficiency, Biochem. Biophys. Res. Commun. **34:**77, 1969.

390. Tarui, S., Okuno, G., and Ikura, Y.: Phosphofructokinase deficiency in skeletal muscle: a new type of glycogenosis, Biochem. Biophys. Res. Commun. **19:**517, 1965.

391. Torrance, J. D.: Diphosphoglycerate mutase assay: the effect of pyruvate, lactate dehydrogenase and thyroid hormone on the assay, Clin. Chem. Acta **50:**103, 1974.

392. Tsuboi, K. K., Fukunaga, K., and Chervenka, C. H.: Phosphoglucose isomerase from human erythrocyte: preparation and properties, J. Biol. Chem. **246:**7586, 1971.

393. Twomey, J. J., O'Neal, F. B., Alfrey, C. P., and Mosers, R. H.: ATP metabolism in pyruvate-kinase deficient erythrocytes, Blood **30:**376, 1967.

394. Valentine, W. N.: Hereditary hemolytic anemias associated with specific erythrocyte enzymopathies, Calif. Med. **108:**280, 1968.

395. Valentine, W. N.: Deficiencies associated with Embden-Meyerhof pathway and other metabolic pathways, Semin. Hematol. **8:**348, 1971.

396. Valentine, W. N.: Enzyme abnormalities in red cells, Br. J. Haematol. **31**(suppl.):11, 1975.

397. Valentine, W. N.: Metabolism of human erythrocytes, Arch. Intern. Med. **135:**1307, 1975.

398. Valentine, W. N., Hseih, H., Paglia, D. E., et al.: Hereditary hemolytic anemia associated with phosphoglycerate kinase deficiency in erythrocytes and leukocytes: a probable X-chromosome-linked syndrome, N. Engl. J. Med. **280:**528, 1969.

399. Valentine, W. N., Oski, F. A., Paglia, D. E., et al.: Hereditary hemolytic anemia with hexokinase deficiency. Role of hexokinase in erythrocyte aging, N. Engl. J. Med. **276:**1, 1967.

400. Valentine, W. N., Oski, F. A., Paglia, D. E., et al.: Erythrocyte hexokinase and hereditary hemolytic anemia. In Beutler, E., ed.: Hereditary disorders of erythrocyte metabolism, New York, 1968, Grune & Stratton, Inc.

401. Valentine, W. N., Schneider, A. S., Baughan, M. A., et al.: Hereditary hemolytic anemia with triosephosphate isomerase deficiency: studies in kindreds with co-existent sickle cell trait and erythrocyte glucose-6-phosphate dehydrogenase deficiency, Am. J. Med. **41:**27, 1966.

402. Valentine, W. N., Tanaka, K. R., and Miwa, S.: A specific erythrocyte glycolytic enzyme defect (pyruvate kinase) in three subjects with congenital non-spherocytic hemolytic anemia, Trans. Assoc. Am. Physicians **74:**100, 1961.

403. Van Berkel, J. C., Koster, J. F., and Staal, G. E. J.: On the molecular basis of pyruvate kinase deficiency. I. Primary defect or consequence of increased glutathione disulfide concentration, Biochim. Biophys. Acta **321:**496, 1973.

404. Van Berkel, J. D., Staal, G. E. J., Koster, J. F., and Nyessen, J. G.: On the molecular basis of pyruvate kinase deficiency. II. Role of thiol groups in pyruvate kinase from pyruvate kinase-deficient patients, Biochim. Biophys. Acta. **334:**361, 1974.

405. Van Biervliet, J. P., Van Milligen-Boersma, L., and Staal, G. E. J.: A new variant of glucosephosphate isomerase deficiency. (GPI-Utrecht), Clin. Chem. Acta **65:**157, 1975.

406. Van Biervliet, J. P., Vlug, A., Bartstra, H., et al.: A new variant of glucosephosphate isomerase deficiency, Humangenetik **30:**35, 1975.

407. Van Eys, J., and Garms, P.: Pyruvate kinase deficiency hemolytic anemia: a model for correlation of clinical syndrome and biochemical anomalies, Adv. Pediatr. **18:**203, 1971.

408. Vora, S., and Piomelli, S.: A fetal isozyme of phosphofructokinase in newborn erythrocytes, Pediatr. Res. **11:**483, 1977. (Abstract 668.)

409. Wada, Y., Nishimura, Y., Tanabu, M. et al.: Hypouricemic, mentally retarded infant with a defect of 5-phosphoribosyl-1-pyrophosphate synthetase of erythrocytes, Tohoku J. Exp. Med. **113:**149, 1974.

410. Waller, H. D., and Benöhr, H. C.: Metabolic disorders in red blood cells. In Yoshikawa, H., and Rapoport, S. M., eds.: Cellular and molecular biology of erythrocytes, Baltimore, 1974, University Park Press.

411. Waller, H. O., and Löhr, G. W.: Hereditary non-spherocytic enzymspenic hemolytic anemia with pyruvate kinase deficiency, Proc. 9th Congr. Int. Soc. Hematol., Mexico City, 1962.

412. Waterbury, L., and Frenkel, E. P.: Phosphofructokinase deficiency in congenital nonspherocytic hemolytic anemia, Clin. Res. **17:**347, 1969.

413. Weiden, P., Storb, R., Graham, T. C., and Schroeder, M.-L.: Severe hereditary haemolytic anaemia in dogs treated by marrow transplantation), Br. J. Haematol. **33:**357, 1976.

414. Weismann, V., and Tönz, O.: Investigations of the kinetics of red cell pyruvate kinase in normal individuals and in a patient with pyruvate kinase deficiency, Nature **209:**612, 1966.

415. Wilt, J., and Witz, A.: Reinigung and Charakterizierung von Phosphopyruvat-Hydratase (=Enolase; EC4.2.1.11) aus Neugeborenen und Erwachsenen-Erythrocyten, Hoppe-Seylers Z. Physiol. Chem. **351:**1232, 1970.

416. Yoshida, A.: Hemolytic anemia and G6PD deficiency, Science **179:**532, 1973.

417. Yoshida, A., Beutler, E., and Motulsky, A. G.: Human glucose-6-phosphate dehydrogenase variants, Bull. W.H.O. **45:**243, 1971.

418. Yoshida, A., and Miwa, S.: Characterization of a phosphoglycerate kinase variant associated with hemolytic anemia, Am. J. Hum. Genet. **26:**378, 1974.

419. Yoshida, A., and Watanabe, S.: Human phosphoglycerate kinase, I. Crystallization and characterization of normal enzyme, J. Biol. Chem. **247:**446, 1972.

420. Yoshida, A., Watanabe, S., Chien, S.-H., et al.: Human phosphoglycerate kinase II. Structure of a variant enzyme, J. Biol. Chem. **247:**446, 1972.

421. Zanella, A., Rebulla, P., Giovanetti, A. M., et al.: Effects of sulphydryl compounds on abnormal red cell pyruvate kinase, Br. J. Haematol. **32:**373, 1976.

422. Zuelzer, W. W., Robinson, A. R., and Hsu, T. H. J.: Erythrocyte pyruvate kinase deficiency in non-spherocytic hemolytic anemia: a system of multiple genetic markers, Blood **32:**33, 1968.

Defects of the hexose monophosphate shunt and other enzyme defects

423. Adam, A.: Linkage between deficiency of glucose-6-phosphate dehydrogenase and colour-blindness, Nature **189:**686, 1961.

424. Aebi, H., Bossi, E., Cantz, M., et al.: Acatalas(em)ia in Switzerland. In Beutler, E., ed.: Hereditary disorders

of erythrocyte metabolism, New York, 1968, Grune & Stratton, Inc.

425. Araki, S., and Mawatari, S.: Ouabain and erythrocyte ghost adenosine triphosphatase, Arch. Neurol. **24:**187, 1971.
426. Balfe, J. W., Cole, C., Smith, E. K. M., et al.: A hereditary sodium transport defect in the human red blood cell, J. Clin. Invest. **47:**4a, 1968.
427. Balinsky, D., Gomperts, E., Cayanis, E., et al.: Glucose-6-phosphate dehydrogenase Johannesburg: a new variant with reduced activity in a patient with congenital nonspherocytic haemolytic anaemia, Br. J. Haematol. **25:**385, 1973.
428. Bamji, M. S.: Glutathione reductase activity in red blood cells and riboflavin nutritional status in humans, Clin. Chem. Acta **26:**263, 1969.
429. Ben-Bassat, I., Brok-Simoni, F., Kende, G., et al.: A family with red cell pyrimidine 5'-nucleotidase deficiency, Blood **47:**919, 1976.
430. Benöhr, H. C., and Waller, H. D.: Eigenshaften der Glucose-6-P-Dehydrogenase Typ "Tubingen," Klin. Wochensch. **48:**71, 1970.
431. Beutler, E.: The glutathione instability of drug-sensitive red cells: a new method for the in vitro detection of drug sensitivity, J. Lab. Clin. Med. **49:**84, 1957.
432. Beutler, E.: Glucose-6-phosphate dehydrogenase deficiency: diagnosis, clinical and genetic implications, Am. J. Clin. Pathol. **47:**303, 1967.
433. Beutler, E.: Drug-induced hemolytic anemia, Pharmacol. Rev. **21:**73, 1969.
434. Beutler, E.: Glutathione reductase: stimulation in normal subjects by riboflavin supplementation, Science **165:**613, 1969.
435. Beutler, E., Grooms, A. M., Morgan, S. K., and Trinidad, F.: Chronic severe hemolytic disease due to G-6-PD Charleston: a new deficient variant, J. Pediatr. **80:**1005, 1972.
436. Beutler, E., Mathai, C. K., and Smith, J. E.: Biochemical variants of glucose-6-phosphate dehydrogenase giving rise to congenital nonspherocytic hemolytic disease, Blood **31:**131, 1968.
437. Beutler, E., and Matsumoto, F.: Ethnic variation in red cell glutathione peroxidase activity, Blood **46:**103, 1975.
438. Beutler, E., and Mikus, B. J.: The effect of methemoglobin formation in sickle cell disease, J. Clin. Invest. **40:**1856, 1961.
439. Beutler, E., and Rosen, R.: Nonspherocytic congenital hemolytic anemia due to a new G-6-PD variant: G-6-PD, Alhambra, Pediatrics **45:**230, 1970.
440. Bloom, G. E., and Zarkowsky, H. S.: Heterogeneity of the enzymatic defect in congenital methemoglobinemia, N. Engl. J. Med. **281:**919, 1969.
441. Blume, K. G., Gottwik, M., Lohr, G. W., and Rudiger, H. W.: Familienuntersuchungen zum Glutathionreduktasemangel menschlicher Erythrocyten, Humangenetik **6:**163, 1970.
442. Blume, K. G., Paniker, N. V., and Beutler, E.: Enzymes of glutathione synthesis in patients with myeloproliferative disorders, Clin. Chem. Acta **45:**281, 1973.
443. Blume, K. G., Von Lengen, A., Löhr, G. W., and Rüdiger, H. W.: Beitrag zur populations genetik der glutathionreduktase menschlicher erythrocyten, Humangenetik **6:**266, 1968.
444. Bodansky, O.: Methemoglobinemia and methemoglobin producing compounds, Pharmacol. Rev. **3:**144, 1951.
445. Boivin, P., Demartial, M. C., Galand, C., and Faradji, M.: Sex differences in the red blood cells glutathione peroxidase activity in the mouse and man, Nouv. Rev. Fr. Hematol. **11:**167, 1971.
446. Boivin, P., Galand, C., André, R., and Debray, J.:

Anémies hémolytiques congénitales avec déficit isolé en glutathion réduit par déficit en glutathion synthétase, Nouv. Rev. Fr. Hematol. **6:**859, 1966.
447. Boivin, P., Galand, C., and Demartial, M. C.: Acquired erythro-enzymopathies. II. Adenylate kinase deficiency in blood disorders, Pathol. Biol. **20:**781, 1972.
448. Boivin, P., Galand, G., Hakim, J., et al.: Anémie hémolytique avec déficit en glutathion-peroxydase chez un adulte, Enzymol. Bio. Clin. **10:**68, 1969.
449. Boivin, P., Galand, G., Hakin, J., and Blery, M.: Déficit en glutathion-peroxydase érythrocytaire et anémie hémolytique médicamenteuse, Press. Med. **78:**171, 1970.
450. Bottini, E., Lucarelli, P., Agostino, R. et al.: Favism: association with erythrocyte adic phosphatase, Science **171:**409, 1971.
451. Bracci, R., Corvaglia, E., Princi, P., et al.: The role of GSH-peroxidase deficiency in the increased susceptibility to Heinz body formation in the erythrocytes of newborn infants, Ital. J. Biochem. **18:**100, 1969.
452. Brewer, G. J.: A new inherited metabolic abnormality of human erythrocytes characterized by elevated levels of adenosine triphosphate (ATP), J. Clin. Invest. **43:**1287, 1964.
453. Brewer, G. J., Gall, J. C., Honeyman, M., et al.: Inheritance of quantitative expression of erythrocyte glucose-6-phosphate dehydrogenase activity in the Negro: a twin study, Biochem. Genet. **1:**41, 1967.
454. Brodribb, H. S., and Woprssam, A. R. H.: Favism in an Englishwoman, Br. Med. J. **1:**1367, 1961.
455. Brown, W. R., and Obon, W. H.: Hyperbilirubinemia and kernicterus in glucose-6-phosphate dehydrogenase deficient infants in Singapore, Pediatrics **41:**1055, 1968.
456. Brownson, C., and Spencer, N.: Partial purification and properties of the two common inherited forms of human erythrocyte adenylate kinase, Biochem. J. **130:**797, 1972.
457. Bucklin, R., and Myint, M. K.: Fatal methemoglobinemia due to well water nitrates, Ann. Intern. Med. **52:**703, 1960.
458. Busch, D.: Überhöhter Erythrocyten-ATP-Spiegel-Merkmal einer hereditären nichtsphärocytären hämolytischen anämie bei gestörter ATP-utilisation und einer Stoffwechselanomalie roter Zellen ohne Krankheitswert, Klin. Wochenschr. **48:**543, 1970.
459. Busch, D., and Boie, K.: Glucose-6-phosphat-Dehydrogenase—Defekt in Deutschland. II. Eigenshaften des Enzyms (Typ "Freiburg"), Klin. Wochenschr. **48:**74, 1970.
460. Busch, D., and Heimpel, H.: Hereditäre nichtsphärozytäre hämolytische Anämie mit hohem Erythrocyten-ATP, Blut **19:**293, 1969.
461. Carson, P. E., Brewer, G. J., and Ickes, C. E.: Decreased glutathione reductase with susceptibility to hemolysis, J. Lab. Clin. Med. **58:**840, 1961.
462. Carson, P. E., and Frischer, H.: Glucose-6-phosphate dehydrogenase deficiency and related disorders of the pentose phosphate pathway, Am. J. Med. **41:**744, 1966.
463. Carson, P. E., Okita, G. T., Frischer, H., et al.: Patterns of hemolytic susceptibility and metabolism, Proc. 9th Congr. Eur. Soc. Haematol., Lisbon, 1963.
464. Cellerino, R., Guidi, G., and Perona, G.: Plasma iron and erythrocyte glutathione peroxidase activity, Scand. J. Haematol. **17:**111, 1976.
465. Cohen, B. L., and Bovasso, G. J.: Acquired methemoglobinemia and hemolytic anemia following excessive pyridium (phenazopyridine hydrochloride) ingestion, Clin. Pediatr. **10:**537, 1971.
466. Cohen, J., and Hochstein, P.: Glutathione peroxidase: the primary agent for the elimination of hydrogen peroxide in erythrocytes, Biochemistry **2:**1420, 1963.

467. Cornblath, M., and Hartmann, A. F.: Methemoglobinemia in young infants, J. Pediatr. **33:**421, 1948.

468. Cotte, J., Kissin, C., Mathieu, M., et al.: Observation d'un cas de déficit partiel en ATPase intraerythrocytaire, Rev. Fr. Etud. Clin. Biol. **13:**284, 1968.

469. Darling, R. C., and Roughton, F. J. W.: The effect of methemoglobin on the equilibrium between oxygen and hemoglobin, Am. J. Physiol. **137:**56, 1942.

470. Dern, R. J.: A new hereditary quantitative variant of glucose-6-phosphate dehydrogenase characterized by a marked increase in enzyme activity, J. Lab. Clin. Med. **68:**560, 1966.

471. Dern, R. J., Brewer, G. J., Tashian, R. E., and Shows, T. B.: Hereditary variation of erythrocytic 6-phosphogluconic dehydrogenase, J. Lab. Clin. Med. **67:**255, 1966.

472. Dern, R. J., McCurdy, P. R., and Yoshida, A.: A new structural variant of glucose-6-phosphate dehydrogenase with a high production rate (G6PD Hektoen), J. Lab. Clin. Med. **73:**283, 1969.

473. Desforges, J. F., Thayer, W. W., and Dawson, J. P.: Hemolytic anemia induced by sulfoxone therapy, with investigations into the mechanisms of its action, Am. J. Med. **27:**132, 1959.

474. Doxiadis, S. A., Fessas, P. H., and Valoes, T.: Glucose-6-phosphate dehydrogenase deficiency: a new aetiological factor of severe neonatal jaundice, Lancet **1:**297, 1961.

475. Doxiadis, S. A., Valoes, T., Karaklis, A., and Stavrakakis, D.: Risk of severe jaundice in glucose-6-phosphate dehydrogenase deficiency of the newborn; differences in population groups, Lancet **2:**1210, 1964.

476. Emerson, P. M., Mason, D. Y., and Cuthbert, J. E.: Erythrocyte glutathione peroxidase content and serum tocopherol levels in newborn infants, Br. J. Haematol. **22:**667, 1972.

477. Engstrom, P. F., and Beutler, E.: G-6-PD Tripler: a unique variant associated with chronic hemolytic disease, Blood **36:**10, 1970.

478. Eshaghpour, E., Oski, F. A., and Williams, M.: The relationship of erythrocyte glucose-6-phosphate dehydrogenase deficiency to hyperbilirubinemia in Negro premature infants, J. Pediatr. **70:**595, 1967.

479. Etteldorf, J. N.: Methylene blue in the treatment of methemoglobinemia in premature infants caused by marking ink, J. Pediatr. **38:**24, 1951.

480. Ewing, M. C., and Mayon-White, R. M.: Cyanosis in infancy from nitrates in drinking water, Lancet **1:**931, 1951.

481. Fairbanks, V. F., and Lampe, L. T.: A tetrazolium linked cytochemical method for estimation of glucose-6-phosphate dehydrogenase activity in individual erythrocytes: applications in the study of heterozygotes for glucose-6-phosphate dehydrogenase deficiency, Blood **31:**589, 1968.

482. Faucett, R. L., and Miller, H. C.: Methemoglobinemia occuring in infants fed milk diluted with well water of high nitrate content, J. Pediatr. **29:**593, 1946.

483. Feig, S. A., Nathan, D. G., Gerald, P. S., et al.: Congenital methemoglobinemia: the result of age-dependent decay of methemoglobin reductase, Blood **39:**407, 1972.

484. Ferrone, S., Zanella, A., and Sirchia, G.: Erythrocyte glutathione reductase activity in chronic renal disease, Scand. J. Haematol. **7:**409, 1970.

485. Fialkow, R. J., Browder, J. A., Sparkes, R. S., et al.: Mental retardation in methemoglobinemia due to diaphorase deficiency, N. Engl. J. Med. **273:**840, 1965.

486. Fialkow, P. J., Gartler, S. M., and Yoshida, A.: Clonal origin of chronic myelocytic leukemia in man, Proc. Natl. Acad. Sci. **58:**1468, 1967.

487. Fildes, R. A., and Harris, H.: Genetically determined

488. Fildes, R. A., and Parr, C. W.: Human red cell phosphogluconate dehydrogenase, Nature **200:**890, 1963.

489. Finch, C. A.: Methemoglobinemia and sulfhemoglobinemia, N. Engl. J. Med. **239:**470, 1948.

490. Flatz, J.: Population study of erythrocyte glutathione reductase activity. I. Stimulation of the enzyme by flavin adenine denucleotide and by riboflavin supplementation, Humangenetik **11:**269, 1971.

491. Flatz, J.: Population study of erythrocyte glutathione reductase activity. II. Hematological data of subjects with low enzyme activity and stimulation characteristics in their families, Humangenetik **11:**278, 1971.

492. Flatz, J., Sringam, S., and Kokris, V.: Neonatal jaundice in glucose-6-phosphate dehydrogenase deficiency, Lancet **1:**1382, 1962.

493. Flohé, L.: Glutathione peroxidase: enzymology and biologic aspects, Klin. Wochenschr. **49:**669, 1971.

494. Flohé, L., and Brand, I.: Kinetics of glutathione peroxidase, Biochim. Biophys. Acta **191:**541, 1969.

495. François, D.: Cas de cyanose congéniale sans cause apparente, Bull. Acad. R. Med. Belg. **4:**698, 1845.

496. Freier, S., Mayer, K., Abrahamov, A., and Leven, C.: Neonatal jaundice in infants with enzymatic defect of the red cell, Is. J. Med. Sci. **1:**844, 1965.

497. Frischer, H., Carson, P. E., Bowman, G. E., and Ruckmann, K. H.: Visual test for erythrocytic glucose-6-phosphate dehydrogenase, 6-phosphogluconic dehydrogenase, and glutathione reductase deficiencies, J. Lab. Clin. Med. **81:**613, 1973.

498. Gaetani, G., Salvidio, E., Panacciulli, I., et al.: Absence of haemolytic effects on transfused G6PD-deficient erythrocytes, Experientia **26:**785, 1970.

499. Gahr, M., Schröter, W., Sturzenegger, M., et al.: Glucose-6-phosphate dehydrogenase (G-6-PD) deficiency in Switzerland: demonstration of a new variant (G-6-PD Aarau) with chronic nonsphaerocytic haemolytic anaemia, Helv. Pediatr. Acta **31:**159, 1976.

500. Gharib, H., Fairbanks, V. F., and Bartholomew, L. G.: Hepatic failure with acanthocytosis associated with hemolytic anemia and deficiency of glutathione peroxidase, Proc. Staff Meet. Mayo Clin. **44:**96, 1969.

501. Gibson, Q. H.: The reduction of methemoglobin by ascorbic acid, Biochem. J. **37:**615, 1943.

502. Gibson, Q. H.: The reduction of methaemoglobin in red blood cells and studies on the cause of idiopathic methaemoglobinaemia, Biochem. J. **42:**13, 1948.

503. Gilles, H. M., and Taylor, B. G.: The existance of the glucose-6-phosphate dehydrogenase deficiency trait in Nigeria and its clinical implications, Ann. Trop. Med. Parasitol. **55:**64, 1961.

504. Glader, B. E.: Evaluation of the hemolytic role of aspirin in glucose-6-phosphate dehydrogenase deficiency, J. Pediatr. **89:**1027, 1976.

505. Glader, B. E., and Conrad, M. E.: Decreased glutathione peroxidase in neonatal erythrocytes: lack of relation to hydrogen peroxide metabolism, Pediatr. Res. **6:**900, 1972.

506. Glass, L., Rajegowda, B. K., Bowen, E., and Evans, H. E.: Exposure to quinine and jaundice in a glucose-6-phosphate dehydrogenase-deficient newborn infant, J. Pediatr. **82:**734, 1973.

507. Glatzle, D., Körner, W. F., Christellu, S., and Wiss, O.: Method for the detection of a biochemical riboflavin deficiency stimulation of NADPH$_2$-dependent glutathione reductase from human erythrocytes by FAD in vitro: investigations on the vitamin B$_2$ status in healthy people and geriatric patients, Int. J. Vit. Res. **40:**166, 1970.

508. Glatzle, D., Weber, F., and Wiss, O.: Enzymatic test for the detection of a riboflavin deficiency: NADPH-de-

variation of adenylate kinase in man, Nature **209:**261, 1966.

pendent glutathione reductase of red blood cells and its activation by FAD in vitro, Experientia **24:**1122, 1968.

509. Goebel, K. M., and Goebel, F. D.: Hemolytic anemia and pancytopenia in glutathione reductase deficiency: further experience with riboflavin, Acta Haematol. **47:** 292, 1972.

510. Goebel, K. M., Hausmann, L., and Kaffarnik, H.: Pancytopenia with hemolytic anemia in glutathione deficiency: In vivo and in vitro studies with riboflavin/FAD, Enzyme **12:**375, 1971.

511. Goluboff, N., and Wheaton, R.: Methylene blue induced cyanosis and acute hemolytic anemia complicating the treatment of methemoglobinemia, J. Pediatr. **58:**86, 1961.

512. Goswitz, F., Lee, G. R., Cartwright, G. E., and Wintrobe, M. M.: Erythrocyte reduced glutathione, glucose-6-phosphate dehydrogenase, and 6-phosphogluconic dehydrogenase in patients with myelofibrosis, J. Lab. Clin. Med. **67:**615, 1966.

513. Greenberg, M. S., and Wong, H.: Studies on the destruction of glutathione unstable red blood cells: the influence of fava beans and primaquine upon such cells in vivo, J. Lab. Clin. Med. **57:**733, 1961.

514. Hanel, H. K., and Cohn, J.: Adenosine triphosphatase deficiency in a family with non-spherocytic haemolytic anaemia, Scand. J. Haematol. **9:**28, 1972.

515. Hanel, H. K., Cohn, J., and Harvald, B.: Adenosine-triphosphatase deficiency in a family with non-spherocytic haemolytic anaemia, Hum. Hered. **21:**313, 1971.

516. Harris, J. W., and Kellermeyer, R. W.: In The red cell: production, metabolism, destruction: normal and abnormal, rev. ed., Cambridge, Mass., 1970, Harvard University Press.

517. Hegesh, E., and Avron, M.: The enzymatic reduction of ferrihemoglobin. II. Purification of a ferrihemoglobin reductase from human erythrocytes, Biochim. Biophys. Acta **146:**397, 1967.

518. Hockstra, W. G., Hofeman, O., Oh, S. H., et al.: Effect of dietary selenium on liver and erythrocyte glutathione peroxidase in the rat, Fed. Proc. **32:**885, 1973.

519. Hopkins, J., and Tudhope, G. R.: Glutathione peroxidase in human red cells in health and disease, Br. J. Haematol. **25:**563, 1973.

520. Hopkinson, D. A., Corney, G., Cook, P. J. L., et al.: Genetically determined electrophoretic variants of human red-cell NADH diaphorase, Ann. Hum. Genet. **34:**1, 1970.

521. Howarth, B. E.: Epidemic of aniline methaemoglobinaemia in newborn babies, Lancet **1:**934, 1951.

522. Hseih, H.-S., and Jaffé, E. R.: Electrophoretic and functional variants of NADH-methemoglobin reductase in hereditary methemoglobinemia, J. Clin. Invest. **50:**196, 1971.

523. Hseih, H.-S., and Jaffé, E. R.: The metabolism of methemoglobin in human erythrocytes. In Surgenor, D. MacN., ed.: The red cell, vol. 2, New York, 1974, Academic Press, Inc.

524. Hsia, D. Y.-Y., and Walker, F. A.: Variability in the clinical manifestations of galactosemia, J. Pediatr. **59:** 872, 1961.

525. Hultquist, D. E., and Passon, P. G.: Catalysis of methemoglobin reduction by erythrocyte cytochrome b_5 and cytochrome b_5 reductase, Nature (New Biol.) **229:**252, 1971.

526. Hurley, T. H., Weisman, R., Jr., and Pasquariello, A. E.: The determination of the survival of transfused red cells by a method of differential hemolysis, J. Clin. Invest. **33:**385, 1954.

527. Jaffé, E. R., and Neumann, G.: Hereditary methemoglobinemia and the reduction of methemoglobin, Ann. N.Y. Acad. Sci. **151:**795, 1968.

528. Janther, H. E., Hafeman, D. G., Hockstra, W. G., et al.: Selenium and glutathione peroxidase in health and disease: a review. In Prosad, A. S., ed.: Trace elements in human health and disease, vol. 2, New York, 1976, Academic Press, Inc.

529. Jim, R. T. S., and Chu, F. K.: Hyperbilirubinemia due to glucose-6-phosphate dehydrogenase in a newborn Chinese infant, Pediatrics **31:**1046, 1963.

530. Johnson, G. J., Kaplan, M. E., and Beutler, E.: G-6-PD Long Prairie: a new glucose-6-phosphate dehydrogenase mutant exhibiting normal sensitivity to inhibition by NADPH and accompanied by nonspherocytic hemolytic anemia, Blood **49:**247, 1977.

531. Kagan, B. M., Mirman, B., Calvin, J., et al.: Cyanosis in premature infants due to aniline dye intoxication, J. Pediatr. **34:**574, 1949.

532. Kaplan, J.-C.: Defects of glutathione reducing and synthesizing reactions in the red cells, Rev. Eur. Étud. Clin. Biol. **16:**523, 1971.

533. Kaplan, J.-C., and Beutler, E.: Electrophoresis of red cell NADH- and NADPH-diaphorases in normal subjects and patients with congenital methemoglobinemia, Biochem. Biophys. Res. Commun. **29:**605, 1967.

534. Kattamis, C. A., Chaidas, A., and Chaidas, S.: G6PD deficiency and favism in the island of Rhodes (Greece), J. Med. Genet. **6:**286, 1969.

535. Kattamis, C. A., and Tjortjatou, F.: The hemolytic process of viral hepatitis in children with normal or deficient glucose-6-phosphate dehydrogenase activity, J. Pediatr. **77:**422, 1970.

536. Keitt, A. S.: Hereditary methemoglobinemia with deficiency of NADH methemoglobin reductase. In Stanbury, J. B., Wyngaarden, J. B., and Fredrickson, D. S., eds.: The metabolic basis of inherited disease, ed. 3, New York, 1972, McGraw-Hill Book Co.

537. Kelley, W. N., and Wyngaarden, J. B.: The Lesch-Nyhan syndrome. In Standury, J. B., Wyngaarden, J. B., and Fredrickson, D. S., eds.: The metabolic basis of inherited disease, ed. 3, New York, 1972, McGraw-Hill Book Co.

538. Kirkman, H. N., McCurdy, P. R., and Naiman, J. L.: Functionally abnormal glucose-6-phosphate dehydrogenase, Cold Spring Harbor Symp. Quant. Biol. **29:**391, 1964.

539. Kirkman, H. N., Rosenthal, I. M., Simon, E. R., et al.: ''Chicago 1'' variant of glucose-6-phosphate dehydrogenase in congenital hemolytic disease, J. Lab. Clin. Med. **63:**715, 1964.

540. Lausecker, C., Heidt, P., Fischer, D., et al.: Anémie hémolytique constitutionnelle avec déficit en 6-phosphogluconate-dehydrogenase, Arch. Fr. Pediatr. **22:**789, 1965.

541. Lawrence, R. A., and Burk, R. F.: Glutathione peroxidase activity in selenium-deficient rat liver, Biochem. Biophys. Res. Commun. **71:**952, 1976.

542. Levin, S. E., Charlton, R. W., and Freeman, I.: Glucose-6-phosphate dehydrogenase deficiency and neonatal jaundice in South African Bantu infants, J. Pediatr. **65:** 757, 1964.

543. Long, W. K.: Glutathione reductase in red blood cells: variant associated with gout, Science **155:**712, 1967.

544. Long, W. K., and Carson, P. E.: Increased erythrocyte glutathione reductase activity in diabetes mellitus, Biochem. Biophys. Res. Comm. **5:**394, 1961.

545. Long, W. K., Wilson, S. W., and Frenkel, E. P.: Associations between red cell glucose-6-phosphate dehydrogenase variants and vascular diseases, Am. J. Hum. Genet. **19:**35, 1967.

546. Loos, J. A., Prins, H. K., and Zurcher, C.: Elevated ATP levels in human erythrocytes. In Beutler, E., ed.: Hereditary disorders of erythrocyte metabolism, New York, 1968, Grune & Stratton, Inc.

547. Lu, T. C., Wei, H., and Blackwell, R. Q.: Increased incidence of severe hyperbilirubinemia among newborn Chinese infants with G6PD deficiency, Pediatrics **37:**994, 1966.
548. Luisada, L.: Favism: singular disease affecting chiefly red blood cells, Medicine **20:**229, 1941.
549. Luzzatto, L.: Interactions between gentic red-cell defects and the environment, Br. J. Haemat. **31**(suppl.):21, 1975.
550. MacDonald, W. P.: Methaemoglobinaemia resulting from poisoning in children, Med. J. Aust. **1:**145, 1951.
551. MacDougall, L. G.: Red cell metabolism in iron-deficiency anemia, J. Pediatr. **72:**303, 1968.
552. MacDougall, L. G.: Red cell metabolism in iron deficiency anemia: the relationship between glutathione peroxidase, catalase, serum vitamin E and susceptibility of iron-deficient red cells to oxidative hemolysis, J. Pediatr. **80:**775, 1972.
553. McDonald, C. D., Jr., and Huisman, T. H. J.: A comparative study of enzyme activities in normal adult and cord blood erythrocytes as related to the reduction of methemoglobin, Clin. Chim. Acta **7:**555, 1962.
554. McIntire, M. S., and Angle, C. R.: Air lead: Relation to lead in blood of black school children deficient in glucose-6-phosphate dehydrogenase, Science **177:**520, 1972.
555. McPhee, W. R.: Acquired hemolytic anemia caused by ingestion of fava beans, Am. J. Clin. Pathol. **26:**1287, 1956.
556. Meloni, T., Cagnazzo, G., Dore, A., and Cutillo, S.: Phenobarbital for prevention of hyperbilirubinemia in glucose-6-phosphate dehydrogenase-deficient newborn infants, J. Pediatr. **82:**1048, 1973.
557. Mijia, J. D., and Hasan, M. I.: Neonatal jaundice due to glucose-6-phosphate dehydrogenase deficiency, J. Indian Med. Assoc. **44:**143, 1965.
558. Miller, A. A.: Congenital sulfhemoglobinemia, J. Pediatr. **51:**223, 1957.
559. Miller, D. R., and Kotok, D.: The micro-methemoglobin reduction screening test for G6PD deficiency in childhood, Pediatrics **41:**528, 1968.
560. Miller, D. R., Weed, R. I., Stamatoyannopolous, G., and Yoshida, A.: Hemoglobin Köln disease occurring as a fresh mutation: erythrocyte metabolism and survival, Blood **38:**715, 1971.
561. Miller, D. R., and Wollman, M. R.: A new variant of glucose-6-phosphate dehydrogenase deficiency hereditary hemolytic anemia, G6PD Cornell: erythrocyte, leukocyte, and platelet studies, Blood **44:**323, 1974.
562. Miller, J., Townes, P. L., and MacWhinney, J. B.: A new congenital hemolytic anemia with deformed erythrocytes (?"stomatocytes") and remarkable susceptibility of erythrocytes to cold hemolysis in vitro. I. Clinical and hematologic studies, Pediatrics **35:**906, 1965.
563. Mills, G. C., Levin, W. C., and Alperin, J. B.: Hemolytic anemia associated with low erythrocyte ATP, Blood **32:**15, 1968.
564. Milner, J., Delamore, I. W., and Yoshida, A.: G6PD Manchester: a new variant associated with chronic nonspherocytic hemolytic anemia, Blood **43:**271, 1974.
565. Minnick, F., Smith, E., Rajanasatkit, C., and Majerus, P. W.: Erythrocyte glutathione synthesis in the neonate, Biol. Neonate **24:**128, 1974.
566. Miwa, S., Ons, J., Nakashima, K., et al.: Two new glucose-6-phosphate dehydrogenase variants associated with congenital nonspherocytic hemolytic anemia found in Japan: Gd(-) Tokoshima and Gd(-) Tokyo, Am. J. Hematol. **1:**433, 1976.
567. Mohler, D. N., Majerus, P. W., Minnick, V., et al.: Glutathione synthetase deficiency as a cause of hereditary hemolytic disease, N. Engl. J. Med. **283:**1253, 1970.
568. Motulsky, A. G., and Campbell-Kraut, J. M.: Population genetics of glucose-6-phosphate dehydrogenase deficiency of the red cell. In Blumberg, B. S., ed.: Proceedings of the conference on genetric polymorphisms and geographic variations in diseases, New York, 1961, Grune & Stratton, Inc.
569. Nakai, T., and Yoshida, A.: G6PD Heian, a glucose-6-phosphate dehydrogenase variant associated with hemolytic anemia found in Japan, Clin. Chem. Acta **51:**199, 1974.
570. Nathan, R. D., Pachtman, E. A., Fiorelli, G., and Frumen, A. M.: A serum defect in favism, Am. J. Clin. Pathol. **61:**462, 1974.
571. Necheles, T. F., Boles, T. A., and Allen, D. M.: Erythrocyte glutathione peroxidase deficiency and hemolytic disease of the newborn infant, J. Pediatr. **72:**319, 1968.
572. Necheles, T. F., Maldonado, N., Barquet-Chediak, A., and Allen, D. M.: Homozygous erythrocyte glutathione peroxidase deficiency: clinical and biochemical studies, Blood **33:**164, 1969.
573. Necheles, T. F., Snyder, L. M., and Strauss, W.: Glucose-6-phosphate dehydrogenase Boston, Humangenetik **13:**218, 1971.
574. Necheles, T. F., Steinberg, M. H., and Cameron, D.: Erythrocyte glutathione peroxidase deficiency, Br. J. Haematol. **19:**605, 1970.
575. Nishimura, Y., Chida, N., Hayashi, T., and Arakawa, T.: Homozygous glutathione-peroxidase deficiency of erythrocytes and leukocytes, Tohoku J. Exp. Med. **108:**207, 1972.
576. Oort, M., Loos, J. A., and Prins, H. K.: Hereditary absence of reduced glutathione in the erythrocytes: a new clinical and biochemical entity? Vox Sang. **6:**370, 1961.
577. Orgeron, J. D., Martin, J. D., Caraway, C. T., et al.: Methemoglobinemia from eating meat with high nitrite content, Pub. Health Rep. **72:**189, 1957.
578. Owusu, S. K., Addy, J. H., Foli, A. K. et al.: Acute reversible renal failure associated with glucose-6-phosphate dehydrogenase deficiency, Lancet **1:**1255, 1972.
579. Owusu, S. K., Goli, A. K., Konotey-Ahulu, F. I. D., et al.: Frequency of glucose-6-phosphate dehydrogenase deficiency in typhoid fever in Ghana, Lancet **1:**320, 1972.
580. Ozsoylu, S.: Glutathione concentration and stability of the red blood cells in acute childhood leukemia, Acta Haematol. **44:**233, 1970.
581. Paglia, D. E., and Valentine, W. N.: Studies on the quantitative and qualitative characterization of erythrocyte glutathione peroxidase, J. Lab. Clin. Med. **70:**158, 1967.
582. Paglia, D. E., and Valentine, W. N.: Characteristics of a pyrimidine specific 5'-nucleotidase in human erythrocytes, J. Biol. Chem. **250:**7973, 1975.
583. Paglia, D. E., Valentine, W. N., and Dahlgren, J. G.: Effects of low-level lead exposure on pyrimidine 5'-nucleotidase and other erythrocyte enzymes. Possible role of pyrimidine 5'-nucleotidase in the pathogenesis of lead-induced anemia, J. Clin. Invest. **56:**1164, 1975.
584. Paglia, D. E., Valentine, W. N., Tartaglia, A. P., and Gilsanz, F.: Perturbations in erythrocyte adenine nucleotide metabolism: A dominantly inherited hemolytic anemia with implications regarding normal mechanisms of adenine nucleotide preservation, Blood **48:**959, 1976. (Abstract.)
585. Paglia, D. E., Valentine, W. N., Tartaglia, A. P., and Konrad, P. N.: Adenine nucleotide reductions associated with a dominantly transmitted form of nonspherocytic hemolytic anemia, Blood **36:**837, 1970.
586. Paniker, N. V., Srivastava, S. K., and Beutler, E.: Glutathione metabolism of the red cells: effect of glutathione reductase deficiency on the stimulation of hexose mono-

phosphate shunt under oxidative stress, Biochim. Biophys. Acta **215:**456, 1970.
587. Panizon, F.: Erythrocyte enzyme deficiency in unexplained kernicterus, Lancet **2:**1093, 1960.
588. Panizon, F., and Vulls, C.: The mechanism of haemolysis in favism, Acta Haematol. **26:**337, 1961.
589. Parr, C. W.: Erythrocyte phosphogluconate dehydrogenase polymorphism, Nature **210:**487, 1966.
590. Passon, P. G., and Hultquist, D. E.: Soluble cytochrome b_5, reductase from human erythrocytes, Biochim. Biophys. Acta. **275:**62, 1972.
591. Paul, W. D., and Kemp, C. G.: Methemoglobin: a normal constituent of blood, Proc. Soc. Exp. Biol. Med. **56:**55, 1944.
592. Perkins, R. P.: Hydrops fetalis and stillbirth in a male glucose-6-phosphate dehydrogenase-deficient fetus possibly due to maternal ingestion of sulfisoxazole, Am. J. Obstet. Gynecol. **111:**379, 1971.
593. Petrakis, N. L., Wiesenfeld, S. L., Sams, B. J., et al.: Prevalence of sickle cell trait and glucose-6-phosphate dehydrogenase deficiency: decline with age in the frequency of G6PD deficient males — a preliminary report, N. Engl. J. Med. **282:**767, 1970.
594. Phornphutkul, C., Whitaker, J. A., and Worathumrong, N.: Severe hyperbilirubinemia in Thai newborns in association with erythrocyte G6PD deficiency, Clin. Pediatr. **8:**275, 1969.
595. Pinkerton, P. H., Fletch, S. M., Brueckner, P. J., and Miller, D. R.: Hereditary stomatocytosis with hemolytic anemia in the dog, Blood **44:**557, 1974.
596. Pinto, P. V. C., Newton, W. A., Jr., and Richardson, K. E.: Evidence for four types of erythrocyte glucose-6-phosphate dehydrogenase from G-6-PD deficient human subjects, J. Clin. Invest. **45:**823, 1966.
597. Piomelli, S., Corash, L. M., Davenport, D. D., et al.: In vivo lability of glucose-6-phosphate dehydrogenase in Gd^A and Gd mediterranean deficiency, J. Clin. Invest. **47:**940, 1968.
598. Piomelli, S., Reindorf, C. A., Arzanian, M. T., and Corash, L. M.: Clinical and biochemical interactions of glucose-6-phosphate dehydrogenase deficiency and sickle-cell anemia, N. Engl. J. Med. **287:**213, 1972.
599. Prins, H. K., Loos, J. A., and Zurcher, C.: Glutathione deficiency. In Beutler, E., ed.: Hereditary disorders of erythrocyte metabolism, New York, 1968, Grune & Stratton, Inc.
600. Prins, H. K., Oort, M., Loos, J. A., et al.: Congenital nonspherocytic hemolytic anemia, associated with glutathione deficiency of the erythrocytes, Blood **27:**145, 1966.
601. Procsal, D., Winberry, L., and Holten, D.: Dietary regulation of 6-phosphogluconate dehydrogenase, J. Biol. Chem. **251:**2539, 1976.
602. Ramot, B., Ben-Bassat, I., and Shchory, M.: New glucose-6-phosphate dehydrogenase variants observed in Israel: association with congenital nonspherocytic hemolytic disease, J. Lab. Clin. Med. **74:**895, 1969.
603. Ramsay, D. H. E., and Harvey, C. C.: Marking-ink poisoning: an outbreak of methemoglobin cyanosis in newborn infants, Lancet **1:**910, 1959.
604. Rattazzi, M. C., Corash, L. M., van Zanen, G. E., et al.: G-6-PD deficiency and chronic hemolysis: four new mutants: relationships between clinical syndrome and enzyme kinetics, Blood **38:**205, 1971.
605. Rieders, F., and Brieger, H.: Mechanism of poisoning from wax crayons, J.A.M.A. **151:**1490, 1953.
606. Rodveim, R., Gellum, A., and Weintraub, L. R.: Decreased glutathione peroxidase activity secondary to severe iron deficiency: a possible mechanism responsible for the shortened life span of the iron-deficient red cell, Blood **43:**281, 1974.
607. Root, A. W., Oski, F. A., Bongiovanni, A. M., and Eberlein, W. R.: Erythrocyte glucose-6-phosphate dehydrogenase activity in children with hypothroidism and hypopituitarism, J. Pediatr. **70:**369, 1967.
608. Ross, J. D.: Deficient activity of DPNH-dependent methemoglobin diaphorase in cord blood erythrocytes, Blood **21:**51, 1963.
609. Roth, K. L., and Frumen, A. M.: Studies on the hemolytic principle of the fava bean, J. Lab. Clin. Med. **56:**695, 1960.
610. Rubins, J., and Young, L. E.: Hereditary sperhocytosis and glucose-6-phosphate dehydrogenase deficiency, J.A.M.A. **237:**797, 1977.
611. Russo, G., Mollica, F., Pavone, L., and Schaliro, G.: Hemolytic crises of favism in Sicilian females heterozygous for G-6-PD deficiency, Pediatrics **49:**854, 1972.
612. Sanpitak, N., Supalert, Y., Chayutimonkul, L., and Glatz, G.: Combined erythrocyte phosphohexose isomerase and glucose-6-phosphate dehydrogenase deficiency, Hum. Hered. **23:**83, 1973.
613. Sartori, E.: On the pathogenesis of favism, J. Med. Genet. **8:**462, 1971.
614. Schlegal, R. S., and Bellanti, J. A.: Increased susceptibility of males to infection, Lancet **2:**826, 1969.
615. Schröter, W., Drescher, J., and Fischer, K.: Über eine seltene form des glucose-6-phosphatedehydrogenase-Mangels mit kongenitaler nichtsphärocytärer hämolytischen Anämie, Klin. Wochenschr. **45:**355, 1967.
616. Schwartz, J. P., Cooperberg, A. A., and Rosenberg, A.: Platelet function studies in patients with glucose-6-phosphate dehydrogenase deficiency, Br. J. Haematol. **27:**273, 1974.
617. Scialom, C., and Bernard, J.: Anémie hémolytique congénital non sphérocytaire avec déficit incomplet en 6-phosphogluconate deshydrogenase, Nouv. Rev. Fr. Hematol. **6:**452, 1966.
618. Scott, E. M.: Congenital methemoglobinemia due to DPNH-diaphorase deficiency. In Beutler, E., ed.: Hereditary disorders of erythrocyte metabolism, New York, 1968, Grune & Stratton, Inc.
619. Scott, E. M., and Hoskins, D. D.: Hereditary methemoglobinemia in Alaskan Eskimos and Indians, Blood **13:**795, 1958.
620. Scott, E. M., and Griffith, I. V.: The enzymic defect of hereditary methemoglobinemia: diaphorase, Biochim. Biophys. Acta **34:**584, 1959.
621. Segal, S.: Disorders of galactose metabolism. In Stanbury, J. B., Wyngaarden, J. B., and Fredrickson, D. S., eds.: The metabolic basis of inherited disease, ed. 3, New York, 1972, McGraw-Hill Book Co.
622. Siegel, N. H., and Beutler, E.: Hemolytic anemia caused by G6PD Carswell, a new variant, Ann. Intern Med. **75:**437, 1971.
623. Sinisalco, M., Bernini, L., Filippi, G., et al.: Population genetics of haemoglobin variants, thalassemia and G-6-PD deficiency, with particular reference to the malaria hypothesis, Bull. W.H.O. **34:**379, 1966.
624. Smith, G. D., and Vella, F.: Erythrocyte enzyme deficiency in unexplained kernicterus, Lancet **1:**1133, 1960.
625. Smith, J. E., Lee, M. S., and Mia, A. S.: Decreased γ-glutamylcysteine synthetase: the probable cause of glutathione deficiency in sheep erythrocytes, J. Lab. Clin. Med. **82:**713, 1973.
626. Smith, J. E., and Osburn, B. I.: Glutathione deficiency in sheep erythrocytes, Science, **158:**374, 1967.
627. Smith, J. E., Ryer, K., and Wallace, L.: Glucose-6-phosphate dehydrogenase deficiency in a dog, Enzyme **21:**379, 1976.
628. Snyder, L. M., Necheles, T. F., Reddy, W. J., et al.: G6PD Worcester; a new variant associated with X-linked optic atrophy, Am. J. Med. **49:**125, 1970.

629. Staal, G. E. J., Punt, K., Geerdink, R. A., et al.: A possible new variant of G6PD with decreased activity (G6PD Utrecht) in a Dutch family with hereditary spherocytosis, Scand. J. Haematol. 7:401, 1970.

630. Stamatoyannopoulos, G., Fraser, G., Motulsky, A. G., et al.: On the familial predisposition to favism, Am. J. Hum. Genet. 18:253, 1966.

631. Stamatoyannopoulos, G., Papayannopoulou, T., Bakopoulos, C., and Motulsky, A. G.: Detection of glucose-6-phosphate dehydrogenase deficient heterozygotes, Blood 29:87, 1967.

632. Steinberg, M., Brauer, M. J., and Necheles, T. F.: Acute hemolytic anemia associated with erythrocyte glutathione-peroxidase deficiency, Arch. Intern. Med. 125:302, 1970.

633. Sugita, Y., Nomura, S., and Yoneyama, Y.: Purification of reduced pyridine nucleotide dehydrogenase from human erythrocytes and methemoglobin reduction by the enzyme, J. Biol. Chem. 246:6072, 1971.

634. Szeinberg, A., Gavendo, S., and Cahane, D.: Erythrocyte adenylate kinase deficiency, Lancet 1:315, 1969.

635. Szeinberg, A., Kahana, D., Gavendo, S. et al.: Hereditary deficiency of adenylate kinase in red blood cells, Acta Haematol. 42:111, 1969.

636. Szeinberg, A., Oliver, M., Schmidt, R., et al.: Glucose-6-phosphate dehydrogenase deficiency and haemolytic disease of the newborn in Israel, Arch. Dis. Child. 38:23, 1963.

637. Takahara, S.: Actalasemia and hypocatalasemia in the Orient, Semin. Hematol. 8:397, 1971.

638. Tanaka, K., and Beutler, E.: Hereditary hemolytic anemia due to glucose-6-phosphate dehydrogenase Torrance, a new variant, J. Lab. Clin. Med. 73:657, 1969.

639. Tarlov, A. R., and Kellermeyer, R. W.: Hemolytic effect of primaquine. XI Decreased catalase activity in primaquine-sensitive erythrocytes, J. Lab. Clin. Med. 58:204, 1961.

640. Tololak, P., and Beutler, E.: G-6-PD Bangkok: a new variant found in congenital nonspherocytic hemolytic disease (CNHD), Blood 39:772, 1969.

641. Townes, P. L., and Lovell, G. R.: Hereditary methemoglobinemia: a new variant exhibiting dominant inheritance of methemoglobin A, Blood 18:18, 1961.

642. Townes, P. L., and Morrison, M.: Investigation of the defect of a variant of hereditary methemoglobinemia, Blood 19:60, 1962.

643. Tudhope, G. R., and Leece, S. P.: Red-cell catalase and the production of methemoglobin, Heinz bodies, and changes in osmotic fragility due to drugs, Acta Haematol. 45:290, 1971.

644. Van den Burgh, A. A. H.: Enterogene cyanose, Deutsch. Arch. Klin. Med. 83:86, 1905.

645. Valentine, W. N., Bennett, J. M., Krivit, W., et al.: Nonspherocytic hemolytic anaemia with increased red cell adenine nucleotides, glutathione and basophilic stippling and ribosephosphate pyrophosphokinase (RPK) deficiency: studies on two new kindreds, Br. J. Haematol. 24:157, 1973.

646. Valentine, W. N., Paglia, D. E., Fink, K., and Madokoro, G.: Lead poisoning association with hemolytic anemia, basophilic stippling, erythrocyte pyrimidine 5'nucleotidase deficiency, and intraerythrocytic accumulation of pyrimidines, J. Clin Invest. 58:926, 1976.

647. Valentine, W. N., Paglia, D. E., Tartaglia, A. P., and Gilsanz, F.: Hereditary hemolytic anemia with increased red cell adenosine deaminase (45- to 70-fold) and decreased adenosine triphosphate, Science 195:783, 1977.

648. Veherkoski, M., and Lamberg, B. A.: The glucose-6-phosphate dehydrogenase activity (G6PD) of the red blood cell in hyperthyroidism and hypothyroidism, Scand. J. Clin. Lab. Invest. 25:137, 1970.

649. Vetrella, M., Barthelmai, W., and Rietkotter, J.: Activity of glutathione peroxidase in erythrocytes from fetal life to adulthood, Klin. Wochenschr. 48:85, 1970.

650. Waisman, H. A., Bain, J. A., Richmond, J. B., et al.: Laboratory and clinical studies in congenital methemoglobinemia, Pediatrics 10:293, 1952.

651. Waller, H. D.: Glutathione reductase deficiency. In Beutler, E., ed.: Hereditary disorders of erythrocyte metabolism, New York, 1968, Grune & Stratton, Inc.

652. Waller, H. D., Benöhr, H. C., Hener, B., and Nerke, O.: Die glutathionreduktion in erythrocyten von gesunden und enzymedifekttragern, Klin. Wochenschr. 48:79, 1970.

653. Waller, H. D., Bremer, J., Schonthal, H., and Dorow, W.: Hb C-Homozygotic mit glutathion-reduktase-mangel in den blutzellen, Klin. Wochenschr. 45:824, 1967.

654. Waller, H. D., Löhr, G. W., and Gayer, J.: Hereditäre nichsphärocytäre hämolitische Anämie durch glucose-6-phosphatedehydrogenase-Mangel, Klin. Wochenschr. 44:122, 1966.

655. Wendt, G. G., Ritter, H., Zilch, I., et al.: Genetics and linkage analysis on adenylate kinase, Humangenetik 13:347, 1971.

656. Westring, D. W., and Pisciotta, A. V.: Anemia, cataracts, and seizures in a patient with glucose-6-phosphate dehydrogenase deficiency, Arch. Intern. Med. 118:385, 1966.

657. Whaun, J. M., and Oski, F. A.: Red cell stromal adenosine triphosphatase (ATPase) of newborn infants, Pediatr. Res. 3:105, 1969.

658. Whaun, J. M., and Oski, F. A.: Relation of red blood cell glutathione peroxidase to neonatal jaundice, J. Pediatr. 76:555, 1970.

659. Witt, I., and Yoshioka, S.: Biochemical characterization of a glucose-6-phosphate dehydrogenase variant with favism: G-6-PD Zähringen, Klin. Wochenschr. 50:205, 1972.

660. Wolff, J. A.: Methemoglobinemia due to benzocaine, Pediatrics 20:915, 1957.

661. Wong, P. W. K., Shih, L.-Y., and Hsia, D. Y.-Y.: Characterization of glucose-6-phosphate dehydrogenase among Chinese, Nature 208:1323, 1965.

662. Yawata, Y., and Tanaka, K. R.: Studies on glutathione reductase and regeneration of reduced glutathione in normal human adult and cord red cells, Clin. Chem. Acta 46:267, 1973.

663. Yawata, Y., and Tanaka, K. R.: Regulatory mechanism of glutathione reductase activity in human red cells, Blood 43:99, 1974.

664. Yoshida, A.: A single amino acid substitution (asparagine to aspartic acid) between normal (B+) and the common Negro variant (A+) of human glucose-6-phosphate dehydrogenase, Proc. Natl. Acad. Sci. 57:835, 1967.

665. Yoshida, A., and Lin, M.: Amino acid substitution (histidine to tyrosine) in a glucose-6-phosphate dehydrogenase variant (G6PD Hektoen) associated with over production, J. Mol. Biol. 52:483, 1970.

666. Yoshida, A.: Regulation of glucose-6-phosphate dehydrogenase activity in red blood cells from hemolytic and nonhemolytic variant subjects, Blood 41:877, 1973.

667. Yue, P. C. K., and Strickland, M.: Glucose-6-phosphate dehydrogenase deficiency and neonatal jaundice in Chinese male infants in Hong Kong, Lancet 1:350, 1965.

668. Zinkham, W. H.: A deficiency of glucose-6-phosphate dehydrogenase activity in lens from individuals with primaquine-sensitive erythrocytes, Bull. Johns Hopkins Hosp. 109:206, 1961.

669. Zipursky, A.: The erythrocytes of the newborn infant, Semin. Hematol. 2:167, 1965.

13 □ The human hemoglobins

Normal hemoglobins and methods for characterization

HOWARD A. PEARSON

The seminal observations by Pauling et al.[36] demonstrating that sickle cell anemia and the sickling phenomenon are associated with an abnormal hemoglobin stimulated an enormous surge of interest in human hemoglobin and its perturbations. This interest, combined with improved methods for detection and characterization, has resulted in identification of a large number of hemoglobins— nearly 300 variants at the latest tabulation.

The hereditary hemoglobinopathies comprise a diverse clinical group varying from clinical and hematologic normalcy to severe and life-threatening disease. In these disorders, a portion or virtually all of the hemoglobin within the red cells of the affected individual is replaced by a species that chemically differs from normal hemoglobin.

HEMOGLOBIN STRUCTURE

The human hemoglobin molecule is approximately spherical and has a molecular weight of 64,400 daltons. The protein or globin portion of most human hemoglobins is made up of two unlike polypeptide chains composed of sequences of about 140 amino acid residues. A number of polypeptide chains differ in their amino acid sequences and are designated by sequential Greek letters (α, β, γ, δ, ϵ, etc.). A heme group is covalently linked to each of the polypeptide chains, and the iron within the heme portion is normally in the divalent or ferrous form. The hemes of most mammalian species are invariant; however, the globin portion shows considerable intra- and interspecies variations.

The primary structure (i.e., the exact amino acid composition and sequence of each of the human polypeptide chains) has been described. It is thought that the primary structure in turn determines the three-dimensional helical form of the chains (secondary and tertiary structures) and the interaction of the four chains together (quaternary structure). Tertiary and quaternary configurations are crucial for physiologic function.

The normal human hemoglobins are designated by capital letters. Hb A (or A_1) refers to the predominant ($> 95\%$) hemoglobin found in normal adults. Hb A_2 refers to the normal adult minor component that constitutes 2.5% to 3.5% of the total hemoglobin. Hb F, or fetal hemoglobin, is the predominant hemoglobin of the fetus and young infant but is present only in trace amounts ($< 2.0\%$) in the adult. These normal human hemoglobins have specific polypeptide chain constituents:

Name	Structure
Embryonic hemoglobins	
Hb Gower 1	$\zeta_2\epsilon_2$
Hb Gower 2	$\alpha_2\epsilon_2$
Hb Portland	$\zeta_2\gamma_2$
Fetal hemoglobins (Hb F)	$\alpha_2\gamma_2{}^{136\ ala}$
	$\alpha_2\gamma_2{}^{136\ gly}$
Adult hemoglobins	
Hb A	$\alpha_2\beta_2$
Hb A_2	$\alpha_2\delta_2$

Hgb A is comprised of two different chains. One set, designated the α-chain, is composed of 141 amino acid residues, and the other set, designated β-chain, has 146 amino acids. The structure of Hgb A can therefore be presented schematically as $\alpha_2\beta_2$. Hemoglobin A_2 has the structure $\alpha_2\delta_2$. δ-Chains are similar to β-chains, differing in only ten amino acid residues; however, these differences produce a distinct change in molecular charge, conferring a slow electrophoretic mobility to Hb A_2. Hb F, the other normal minor component, contains yet another polypeptide chain, designated the γ-chain. The structure of Hb F can be represented as $\alpha_2\gamma_2$. γ-Chains differ from β-chains in thirty nine amino acid residues and are characterized by the presence of isoleucine, an amino acid not found in other polypeptide chains. The γ-chains are heterogenous, for there are two types of γ-chains differing in the number 136 position, where either a glycine or alanine residue is found.[42]

Other minor components can be identified in hemoglobin solutions of normal adults (Hb A_3, A_{IC}, etc.). However, these fractions are thought to result from spontaneous chemical changes rather than being genetically determined. For example, the level of Hb A_{IC}, a glycosylated hemoglobin, increases in hyperglycemic states such as diabetes mellitus.[30]

In addition to the various hemoglobins characteristic of fetal and postnatal life, embryonic or primitive hemoglobins are also found early in intrauterine life. For a long time the existence of embryonic hemoglobins was controversial because it was difficult to obtain adequate blood samples early in gestation. Drescher and Kunzer[13] in 1954 and, more definitively, Huehns et al.[19] convincingly demonstrated unique hemoglobins, which have been designated the Gower hemoglobins, in embryos of less than 12 weeks gestation. The embryonic hemoglobins contain unique types of polypeptide chains, designated epsilon (ϵ) and zeta (ζ). Hb Gower 1 has the structure $\zeta_2\epsilon_2$, whereas the structure of Hb Gower 2 is $\alpha_2\epsilon_2$. Another embryonic hemoglobin with Hb A–like electrophoretic mobility has been designated Hb Portland 1; it has the structure $\zeta_2\gamma_2$.[6,18]

Because α, β, γ, δ, ϵ, and ζ chains are chemically different, the modern genetic tenet of one gene, one polypeptide chain dictates that their synthesis must be governed by different genes. There is convincing data that a number of genes direct hemoglobin synthesis. Biochemical and genetic evidence indicates that there are at least two α genes in many ethnic groups, one β gene, two γ genes, one δ gene, and one ϵ gene. Each individual, being diploid, possesses sets of these (four α, two β, four γ, and two δ genes). γ^G, γ^A, δ, and β genes are closely linked on the same autosomal chromosome in that order. The α genes are located at considerable distance from the $\gamma\delta\beta$ complex, perhaps on a different chromosome.[3,44,46]

DEVELOPMENTAL ASPECTS OF HUMAN HEMOGLOBINS

The hemoglobin of the human embryo and fetus demonstrates remarkable developmental changes, with several varieties detectable within human red cells at successive developmental stages. Fig. 13-1 depicts the changing relationships between these chains during development.

In embryos of less than 8 weeks of gestational age, the two Gower hemoglobins and Hb Portland account for almost one half of the total circulating hemoglobin. Synthesis of these components rapidly diminishes with advancing fetal age; therefore by 90 days embryonic hemoglobins can no longer be detected in the circulation. Although Gower hemoglobins normally disappear after the third fetal month, Huehns and associates detected their presence in a few newborns with D-1 trisomy, suggesting an alteration of genetic control mechanisms in this condition.[20]

Hb F ($\alpha_2\gamma_2$) constitutes the predominant hemoglobin during most of fetal life, and there is a general correlation between gestational age and the proportions of Hb F. Before 35 weeks of gestation more than 90% of the hemoglobin of the blood is Hb F, but its proportion decreases at a rate of about 3% to 4%/week.[9] Thus the blood of full-term infants has a lower proportion of Hb F than that of premature infants.[2] During prolonged gestation the level of Hb F continues to decrease steadily, so

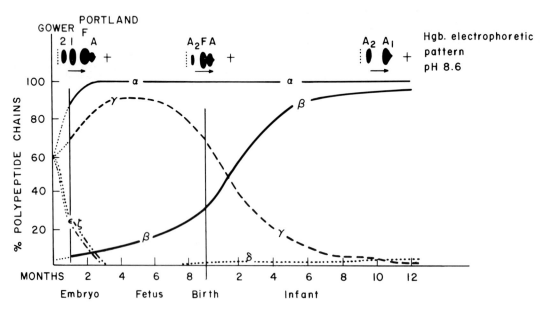

Fig. 13-1. Changes in hemoglobin polypeptide chains and electrophoretic patterns during human development.

that postmature infants characteristically have even lower proportions of Hb F in their blood.[10] Although the inverse relationship between maturity and Hb F is valid for groups of infants, gestational age cannot be precisely predicted by Hb F levels alone because of considerable individual variation. In addition, conditions that cause fetal anemia, such as fetal-maternal transfusion and erythroblastosis fetalis, have generally found to be associated with a decrease in the expected level of Hb F at birth.[15] Because actual synthesis rates of Hb A and Hb F are not affected in these instances, preferential destruction of older fetal cells containing larger amounts of Hb F is probably responsible for this difference.[15]

At the time of birth an abrupt decrease in the rate of synthesis of Hb F occurs whether the infant is premature or full term. During and after the neonatal period, levels of Hb F decrease rapidly, so that by 9 to 12 months of age the usual adult concentration of about 2% Hb F is attained by the majority of infants.

When the blood of fetuses less than 35 weeks of gestational age is examined by the acid elution technique (Kleihauer-Betke), all of the red cells contain a large proportion of Hb F ("fetal cells"). At 35 weeks of gestation small numbers of red cells containing Hb A begin to be seen, and in the cord blood of term infants about 5% of the circulating red cells contain predominantly Hb A ("adult cells").[16] After birth the percentage of fetal cells decreases rapidly. Small numbers of cells containing small amounts of Hb F ("intermediate cells") may persist after infancy, but in absolute numbers are less than 0.1% of the total.[17] Serial studies with the acid elution test thus generally parallel the pattern obtained with alkali denaturation techniques, but they also indicate that both Hb A and Hb F are synthesized within a single cell.

Although small amounts of normal Hb A ($\alpha_2\beta_2$) can be detected in the blood of very small embryos and fetuses, this component accounts for only a small proportion of the total hemoglobin until about 35 weeks of gestation.[24] Thereafter Hb A increases in a reciprocal fashion to the decreasing amount of Hb F. This appearance of Hb A synthesis within individual red cells is nicely demonstrated by the acid elution test. Minute quantities of normal adult hemoglobin Hb A_2 ($\alpha_2\delta_2$) are also present in late gestation; production of Hb A_2 parallels that of Hb A_1 although in only about $\frac{1}{30}$ the quantity.

Regulation of the reciprocal relationshhip between Hb F and Hb A throughout fetal life and infancy has been attributed to a "switch mechanism." This mechanism facilitates γ-chain synthesis while inhibiting β- and δ- chain synthesis

during most of fetal life and has the opposite effect later. A similar regulation may occur in early gestation between ϵ- and γ-chains. The exact mechanisms and factors that constitute and regulate such switches are for the most part undefined. Although birth has an obvious influence, it is not the sole one. As indicated by the continuing prenatal drop of Hb F in postmature infants and indirectly by the observation that in some mammals, fetal hemoglobins disappear before birth.[24] Erythropoietin does not appear to have a crucial role in the switch. Blood oxygenation also does not appear to be crucial, for the switchover occurs normally in infants with congenital cardiac defects associated with profound cyanosis.[40] In early pregnancy Hb F synthesis is reactivated under the stress of chorionic gonadotropin.[38] Finally in a variety of hematologic diseases associated with severe, chronic erythropoietic stress, including genetically determined defects of hemoglobin, Hb F levels of the blood may persist in later life, although such synthesis appears confined to a small clone of red cells. Levels of Hb F may be elevated in leukemia, and extraordinary levels of Hb F are found in the juvenile form of chronic myelogenous leukemia.[32]

Genetic regulatory mechanisms controlling the relative proportions of proteins (elegantly described in bacterial systems) have led to a theory of regulation of protein synthesis by a hierarchy of regulatory genes,[23] a model with many attractive features that might be relevant to the switch mechanism for reciprocal γ- and β-chain synthesis. Much still remains to be learned, however, about the regulation of hemoglobin synthesis and the effect of environmental and physiologic factors in its control.

Synthesis of the embryonic (Gower) hemoglobins and Hb Portland predominates during the mesoblastic phase of hematopoiesis; presumably these hemoglobins are synthesized in hematopoietic centers of the yolk stalk. Hb F is the major hemoglobin during the time when hematopoiesis is centered in the liver, and Hb A appears in increasing amounts as the bone marrow becomes progressively more active in the blood formation. Despite the coincidence, there appear to be no specific anatomic localizations for synthesis of the various types of hemoglobin. Thomas et al.[45] showed that erythroblasts obtained from the liver of human fetuses formed Hb F and Hb A in proportions equivalent to those of erythroblasts obtained from the bone marrow; Wood and Weatherall[47] also noted identical ratios of Hb A and Hb F synthesis in erythroblasts derived from the bone marrow or viscera. Thus the anatomic sources of erythropoietic tissue do not appear to be specific for the type of hemoglobin fabricated.

Since multiple hemoglobins have been found in

many species during embryonic and fetal development, it would be logical to assume that this variability has physiologic importance. No physiologic studies of the Gower or Portland hemoglobins have been performed, so it is not possible to state whether they have a unique function during embryonic life. On the other hand, the possible physiologic advantages conferred by Hb F have been much discussed. Although fetal blood shows a shifted oxygen dissociation curve when compared to maternal blood, Allen et al.[1] demonstrated that the oxygen dissociation curves of *pure* solutions of Hb F and Hb A were identical. This apparent contradiction has been resolved by the demonstration that Hb F binds 2,3-DPG in the red cell only about 20% as effectively as does Hb A. This difference causes the oxygen-hemoglobin equilibrium curve of fetal red cells to be shifted to the left of the adult position.

The observation of a physiologic difference in Hb F function also necessitates reconsideration of older concepts that the complex sequential changes in hemoglobin types occurring during development merely represent "ontogeny recapitulating phylogeny." It seems likely that the system of embryonic, fetal, and adult hemoglobins occurring extensively throughout the evolutionary ladder might be of importance to survival.

HEMOGLOBIN-OXYGEN INTERACTIONS

The hemoglobin molecule is uniquely structured to perform its vital role of oxygen transport from the lungs to the tissues without expending energy. The interactions between hemoglobin and oxygen are characterized by the oxygen dissociation curve obtained when the percentage of hemoglobin saturated with oxygen is plotted against the partial pressure of oxygen at standardized temperature and pH and atmospheric pressure; the resultant curve is sigmoidal. Oxygenation of one heme group induces an intermolecular spatial change that facilitates oxygenation of the remaining heme groups at a lower increment of partial pressure of oxygen—a process called heme-heme interaction.

The position and configuration of the oxygen dissociation curve is also influenced by changes in pH. Lowering of pH reduces oxygen affinity, the so-called Bohr effect. These phenomena (heme-heme interaction and the Bohr effect) combine to increase the efficiency of oxygen uptake in the lungs and promote oxygen release at the tissues.

A final reaction of hemoglobin that further enhances the physiologic function of this remarkable molecule is its capacity to combine with phosphorylated glycolytic intermediates, especially 2,3-DPG. 2,3-DPG has a preferential affinity for reduced (as opposed to oxy-) hemoglobin and so facilitates the dissociation of oxygen. 2,3-DPG has a higher binding affinity for deoxy- than oxyhemoglobin and does not bind to methemoglobin or cyanmethemoglobin. These properties indicate that 2,3-DPG binds selectively with the deoxyhemoglobin configuration. Isolated α- or β-polypeptide chains do not bind 2-3 DPG, implying that binding requires complete tetramers. 2,3-DPG binds β-4 tetramers, but not α-4 tetramers, suggesting that the site of attachment is on the β-chains of hemoglobin. The 2,3-DPG mechanism provides considerable adaptive flexibility of oxygen transport in a variety of clinical situations.

2,3-DPG, an intermediate of the glycolytic pathway, reaches a higher concentration within the red cell than any other tissue. The level of 2,3-DPG shows marked variability in response to a number of factors. For example, an elevation in the level of red cell 2,3-DPG occurs within 24 to 48 hours after the exposure of humans to high altitudes. In hypoxic states secondary to pulmonary or congenital heart disease, increased levels of 2,3-DPG are also noted. Most anemias of diverse etiologies (hemolytic, aregenerative, iron deficiency) are also characterized by high levels of red cell 2,3-DPG. This probably indicates that tissue hypoxia is a potent stimulator of 2,3-DPG synthesis. Other contributing factors to increased levels of 2,3-DPG include acidosis, hyperphosphotemia, androgens, and other hormones.[4,14,35] (See Chapter 12.)

The major reason for the left shift of the oxygen-hemoglobin equilibrium curve of neonatal blood is the relatively poor binding of 2,3-DPG by Hb F. As the level of Hb F declines postnatally, the curve gradually changes and attains the adult pattern by 4 to 6 months of age.[34] However, the position of the curve is not only determined by Hb F; it may differ considerably in infants with the same level of Hgb F. This is because *both* the level of Hb F and the level of 2,3-DPG affect the oxygen-hemoglobin equilibrium curve. Delivoria-Papadopoulous and Oski et al. have used the term "functioning 2,3-DPG fraction" to describe the interaction of both these variables.[11,12] The equilibrium curves of premature infants are in general shifted more to the left than those of term infants because of higher levels of Hb F. In addition, in premature infants with the respiratory distress syndrome the shift is even more extreme because a marked reduction of 2,3-DPG accompanies acidosis.

The left-shifted oxygen-hemoglobin equilibrium, which is physiologically advantageous in utero, may impose a handicap after birth by inhibiting the release of oxygen to the tissues. Transfusion of fresh adult blood to newborns results in a prompt shift to the right of the equilibrium, permitting the infant's blood to deliver more oxygen to the tissues at higher partial pressures. This observation has prompted the suggestion that exchange transfusions with normal adult blood might be beneficial for hypoxemic infants.[12] Whether the degree of improvement to be gained in oxygen transport by the replacement of Hb F by Hb A will have clinical significance has not been determined.

LABORATORY TECHNIQUES FOR DIAGNOSIS

Hemoglobinopathies are defined as disorders in which the production of a normal polypeptide chain is partially or completely replaced by production of a chemically different polypeptide chain. However, before consideration of specific chemical entities and syndromes, some of the techniques that are utilized for diagnosis of hemoglobin abnormalities will be presented.

Alkali denaturation methods

The first chemical difference in human hemoglobins was demonstrated by Korber more than a century ago. He noted that the hemoglobin from fetuses and young infants was not affected by strong alkali solutions, whereas that of older children and adults was rapidly denatured. The property of alkali resistance is still used in most techniques for the quantitation of Hb F. Singer et al.[43] described the 1-minute alkali denaturation test, the most widely used method for measuring levels of Hb F. However, this method is relatively inaccurate for Hb F concentrations in excess of 50%, such as obtain in early life. Jonxis and Huisman[25] devised a modification of the alkali denaturation method which is accurate and reproducible at high levels of Hgb F. Betke et al.[5] modified the Singer technique to provide greater accuracy at low levels (<2.0%) of Hb F. A reliable and reproducible column chromatographic technique has been described; the results, however, are 10% to 15% higher than those of the alkali denaturation method.[27]

In the individual red cell Hb F can be identified and its concentration roughly estimated by the practical and useful acid elution slide test of Kleihauer and Betke,[28] which is based on the fact that, in addition to being resistant to denaturation by strong alkalis, Hb F is also resistant at acid pH. In the Kleihauer technique blood smears are exposed to a citrate-phosphate buffer of pH 3.2. When the concentration of Hb F in a red cell exceeds about 20%, the intracellular hemoglobin is

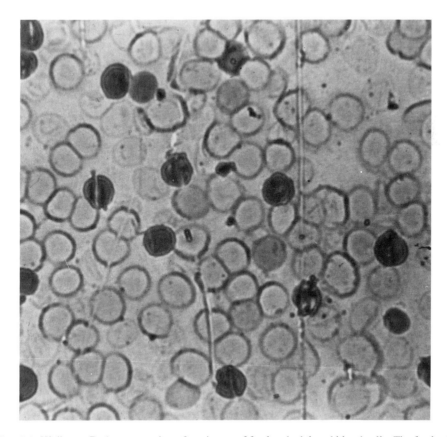

Fig. 13-2. Kleihauer-Betke preparation of a mixture of fetal and adult red blood cells. The fetal cells are normally stained; the adult cells appear as ''ghosts.''

not denatured and the red cell maintains its usual tinctorial properties when stained with hematoxylin-eosin or Giemsa stain. These darkly stained erythrocytes are designated fetal cells. In red cells that contain a predominance of Hb A (as well as most other hemoglobins), the intracellular hemoglobin is denatured and eluted. The red cells devoid of hemoglobin are not stained and appear as empty membrane ghosts designated adult cells (Fig. 13-2). Cells that contain approximately 5% to 20% of Hb F appear partially stained and are designated intermediate cells. The Kleihauer technique has also been used to demonstrate Gower hemoglobins in red cells of young fetuses because the embryonic Gower hemoglobins have an elution pattern intermediate between those of Hb A and Hb F.[39]

Hemoglobin electrophoresis

The most utilitarian and widely employed method for detection of hemoglobin variants involves electrophoresis, the migration induced by an electric current of charged particles suspended in an electrolyte solution. Particles that have positive charges migrate to the cathode, while negatively charged particles move anodally. Changes in the amino acid composition of a hemoglobin polypeptide chain often alter the charge of the whole molecule and so influence its electrophoretic mobility.

The first electrophoretic technique, the so-called moving boundary method of Tiselius, was used by Pauling et al.[36] in their epochal discovery of Hb S. This rather cumbersome technique has been supplanted by methods using a variety of supporting media and electrolyte solutions. Most methods for studying hemoglobin utilize a buffer solution (usu-

ally sodium barbital) with alkaline pH (8.2 to 8.6). In those solutions, negatively charged protein molecules migrate to the anode. Diverse supporting media have been used, including filter paper, starch gel or starch granules, cellulose acetate, acrylamide, agar gels, and others. The cellulose acetate technique using a discontinuous borate-barbital buffer has proved eminently practical and satisfactory for diagnosis. Fig. 13-3 depicts the electrophoretic mobility of some of the more common variants.

Electrophoretic systems only permit definition of those hemoglobin variants with changes in total molecular charge. Variants in which the amino acid substitution does not result in a net charge difference cannot be separated. For example, a variant in which one neutral amino acid was substituted for a different neutral amino acid could not be demonstrated electrophoretically (electrophoretically silent). It is also apparent that substitution of any one of several like-charged amino acids would produce a number of variants with identical electrophoretic mobilities—a situation seen in the several variants designated as Hb D.

Agar gel electrophoresis at acid pH 6.2 has provided a useful supplemental adjunct to alkaline electrophoresis. All hemoglobins move cathodally in this system, but there are important differences in relative mobilities of a number of important hemoglobins, permitting more exact definition.[29] Agar gel is especially useful in the newborn period because of the very rapid mobility of Hb F.[37] Fig. 13-4 compares mobilities at pH 6.2 and 8.6.

Accurate quantitation of minor hemoglobin components such as Hb A_2 requires spectophotometric determination after separation and elution. Starch block electrophoresis and column chroma-

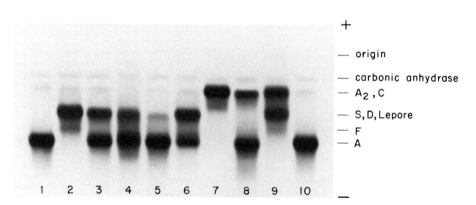

Fig. 13-3. Electrophoretic patterns of some common hemoglobins at pH 8.6. The origin is at the top, and migration is downward toward the anode. The patterns represent, *1,* normal, AA; *2,* homozygous sickle, SS; *3,* heterozygous sickle, AS (more A than S); *4,* AD; *5,* A-Lepore; *6,* sickle-thalassemia (more S than A); *7,* CC; *8,* AC; *9,* SC; and *10,* AA. (From McPhedran, P., and Weissman, S. M.: In Conn, H. F.: Current diagnosis, Philadelphia, 1974, W. B. Saunders Co.)

tography have been used extensively for this purpose.[7,31] Attempts have been made to develop immunologic systems for identification and quantitation of various hemoglobins. Antibodies have been prepared that are specific for different polypeptide chains and even for specific hemoglobin types. These have been used to identify the kind of hemoglobin within individual red cells. The antisera may ultimately permit development of automated techniques for quantitation of Hb A_2.[41]

Hemoglobin hybridization and polypeptide chain separation

More precise identification of hemoglobin variants and delineation of their characteristic primary sequence requires more sophisticated techniques than those discussed so far. One such specialized method is designated hemoglobin hybridization. When a solution of hemoglobin is subjected to low pH, it dissociates into two identical fragments approximately one-half the size of the intact molecule. When the pH is restored to neutral, recombination of these fragments occurs in a random fashion.[22] The dissociation-reassociation technique can be applied to mixtures of an unknown hemoglobin variant with a variant with a known chain abnormality to localize which polypeptide chain of

the unknown variant is affected. When the abnormality of the unknown variant is on a different polypeptide chain from the known one, a hybrid molecule is formed.

It is also possible to separate hemoglobin (or globin) into its constituent chains chromatographically using a carboxymethyl cellulose column in the presence of 8M urea.[9] Clean separations of α- and β-chains can be readily accomplished. The component chains of hemoglobins can also be separated electrophoretically using a starch gel–urea medium.[33] All of these techniques permit localization of an electrophoretic abnormality to a specific polypeptide chain.

Fingerprinting

The exact amino acid substitution characterizing a hemoglobin variant can be precisely identified by a technique called fingerprinting.[21] Purified globin is reacted with the proteolytic enzyme trypsin under stringent conditions of pH, temperature, and ionic concentration. Trypsin cleaves proteins only where arginine or lysine participate in a peptide linkage. Trypsin digestion breaks intact globin into about thirty smaller fragments containing five to ten amino acids each, and this cleavage is predictable and reproducible. The mixture of trypsin-

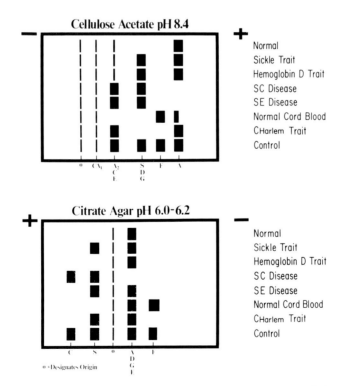

Fig. 13-4. Comparison of various hemoglobin samples on cellulose acetate and citrate agar. (From Schmidt, R. M., and Brosious, E. M.: Basic laboratory methods of hemoglobinopathy detection, DHEW Pub. No. (CDC) 76-8266.

digested peptides can then be subjected to high-voltage electrophoresis followed by cross-dimension chromatography, resulting in a pattern of peptide spots that is as characteristic of a hemoglobin species as the fingerprint is for an individual human. In most hemoglobin variants only one aberrant trypsin-digested peptide is observed. Amino acid analysis and sequencing can be performed on the aberrant peptide to determine how it differs from the normal. Because of the complexity of this analytic technique, not all hemoglobin variants have had their amino acid substitution located and specified, but in most reported instances the aberrant chain has been identified.

NOMENCLATURE

In the early days of hemoglobin nomenclature, variants were designated by sequential capital letters (C, D, E, etc.) in the order of their discovery. This system soon proved too cumbersome. A proliferation of species, some of which were indistinguishable electrophoretically, posed difficulty in deciding on priorities. It then became common practice to specify a hemoglobin variant on the basis of the city or geographical area of discovery. Currently a geographical designation is given until the substitution is determined.

Abnormal hemoglobins
RUTH N. WRIGHTSTONE

Abnormal human hemoglobin variants may result from a variety of mechanisms. Most hemoglobin variants result from substitution of a single amino acid (point mutation) in one or another of the polypeptide chains. This results from a change in the DNA code triplet that is responsible for insertion of a specific amino acid into the chain. Other genetic mechanisms have been described as the basis for chemically altered polypeptide chains. These mechanisms include (1) a deletion of a segment of DNA, resulting in a foreshortened polypeptide chain, (2) the occurrence of two or even more separate amino acid substitutions in a polypeptide chain, (3) fusion hemoglobins resulting from nonhomologous crossing over between chains, and (4) substitutions that result in failure to terminate polypeptide chain propogation.

It is also possible to categorize the hemoglobinopathies functionally: (1) hemoglobin variants with no abnormal physical or physiologic properties, (2) hemoglobin variants with altered solubilities or abnormal properties of aggregation or molecular stability (this often results in hemolysis as exemplified by Hb S and Hb C), (3) hemoglobin

Text continued on p. 395.

Table 13-1. Variants of the α-chain

Residue	Substitution	Name	Major abnormal property	Reference No.
5 (A3)	Ala → Asp	Hb J Toronto		133
6 (A4)	Asp → Ala	Hb Sawara		312
11 (A9)	Lys → Glu	Hb Anantharaj		264
12 (A10)	Ala → Asp	Hb J Paris I		286
15 (A13)	Gly → Asp	Hb I Interlaken		232
	Gly → Arg	Hb Ottawa		325
16 (A14)	Lys → Glu	Hb I Philadelphia		74
19 (AB1)	Ala → Asp	Hb J Kurosh		268
21 (B2)	Ala → Asp	Hb J Nyanza		194
22 (B3)	Gly → Asp	Hb J Medellin		159
23 (B4)	Glu → Gln	Hb Memphis		206
	Glu → Lys	Hb Chad		99
	Glu → Val	Hb G Audhali		230
27 (B8)	Glu → Gly	Hb Ft. Worth		295
	Glu → Val	Hb Spanish Town		53
30 (B11)	Glu → Lys	Hb O Padova		330
	Glu → Gln	Hb G Honolulu		313
43 (CE1)	Phe → Val	Hb Torino	Unstable, decreased O_2 affinity	76
	Phe → Leu	Hb Hirosaki		255
47 (CE5)	Asp → Gly	Hb Umi (Mugino)		311
	Asp → His	Hb Hasharon	Unstable	161
	Asp → Asn	Hb Arya	Slightly unstable	271
48 (CE6)	Leu → Arg	Hb Montgomery		105
50 (CE8)	His → Asp	Hb J Sardegna		316
51 (CE9)	Gly → Asp	Hb J Abidjan		111
	Gly → Arg	Hb Russ		279

Table 13-1. Variants of the α-chain—cont'd

Residue	Substitution	Name	Major abnormal property	Reference No.
53 (E2)	Ala → Asp	Hb J_{Rovigo}	Unstable	58
54 (E3)	Gln → Arg	Hb Shimonoseki		236
	Gln → Glu	Hb J_{Mexico}		188
57 (E6)	Gly → Arg	Hb L_{Persian Gulf}		270
	Gly → Asp	Hb J_{Norfolk}		63
58 (E7)	His → Tyr	Hb M_{Boston}	Decreased O_2 affinity	155
60 (E9)	Lys → Asn	Hb Zambia		71
61 (E10)	Lys → Asn	Hb J_{Buda}		103
64 (E13)	Asp → Asn	Hb G_{Waimanalo}		79
	Asp → His	Hb Q_{India}		310
	Asp → Tyr	Hb Perspolis		268
68 (E17)	Asn → Asp	Hb Ube 2		237
	Asn → Lys	Hb G_{Philadelphia}		66
71 (E20)	Ala → Glu	Hb J_{Habana}		132
72 (EF1)	His → Arg	Hb Daneskgah-Tehran		272
74 (EF3)	Asp → His	Hb Mahidol		263
	Asp → Asn	Hb G_{Pest}		103
	Asp → Gly	Hb Chapel Hill		257
75 (EF4)	Asp → His	Hb Q_{Iran}		219
	Asp → Tyr	Hb Winnipeg		329
	Asp → Asn	Hb Matsue-Oki		254
78 (EF7)	Asn → Lys	Hb Stanleyville II		324
80 (F1)	Leu → Arg	Hb Ann Arbor	Unstable	50,288
82 (F3)	Ala → Asp	Hb Garden State		287
84 (F5)	Ser → Arg	Hb Etobicoke	Increased O_2 affinity	134
85 (F6)	Asp → Asn	Hb G_{Norfolk}	Increased (?) O_2 affinity	130,220
	Asp → Tyr	Hb Atago		148
	Asp → Val	Hb Inkster		278
87 (F8)	His → Tyr	Hb M_{Iwate}	Ferrihemoglobin, decreased O_2 affinity	241
90 (FG2)	Lys → Asn	Hb J_{Broussais}		141
	Lys → Thr	Hb J_{Rajappen}		173
92 (FG4)	Arg → Gln	Hb J_{Cape Town}	Increased O_2 affinity	96, 217
	Arg → Leu	Hb Chesapeake	Increased O_2 affinity	122, 123
94 (G1)	Asp → Tyr	Hb Setif	Unstable	334
	Asp → Asn	Hb Titusville	Decreased O_2 affinity, increased dissociation	293
95 (G2)	Pro → Leu	Hb G_{Georgia}	Increased dissociation	167, 307
	Pro → Ser	Hb Rampa	Increased dissociation	138
	Pro → Ala	Hb Denmark Hill	Increased O_2 affinity	342
	Pro → Arg	Hb St. Lukes	Increased dissociation	70
102 (G9)	Ser → Arg	Hb Manitoba		135
112 (G19)	His → Asp	Hb Hopkins 2	Unstable, increased O_2 affinity	121
	His → Arg	Hb Strumica		251
114 (GH2)	Pro → Arg	Hb Chiapas		188
115 (GH3)	Ala → Asp	Hb J_{Tongariki}		151
116 (GH4)	Glu → Lys	Hb O_{Indonesia}		67
118 (H1)	Thr → Gly	Hb Hopkins 2-II		259
120 (H3)	Ala → Glu	Hb J_{Meerut} (J_{Birmingham})		87
126 (H9)	Asp → Asn	Hb Tarrant		248
127 (H10)	Lys → Thr	Hb St. Claude		326
	Lys → Asn	Hb Jackson		244
136 (H19)	Leu → Pro	Hb Bibba	Unstable, increased dissociation	200
141 (HC3)	Arg → Pro	Hb Singapore		127
	Arg → His	Hb Suresnes	Increased O_2 affinity	265

Table 13-2. Variants of the β-chain

Residue	Substitution	Name	Major abnormal property	Reference No.
1 (NA1)	Val → Ala(NAc)	Hb Raleigh		243
2 (NA2)	His → Arg	Hb Deer Lodge		209
6 (A3)	Glu → Val	Hb S	Sickling	179
	Glu → Lys	Hb C		172
	Glu → Ala	Hb G$_{Makassar}$		84
7 (A4)	Glu → Gly	Hb G$_{San Jose}$		164
	Glu → Lys	Hb C$_{Siriraj}$		323
9 (A6)	Ser → Cys	Hb Pôrto Alegre	Polymerization	94
10 (A7)	Ala → Asp	Hb Ankara		61
14 (A11)	Leu → Arg	Hb Sögn		242
	Leu → Pro	Hb Saki	Unstable	78, 234
15 (A12)	Trp → Arg	Hb Belfast	Unstable, increased O$_2$ affinity	150, 196
16 (A13)	Gly → Asp	Hb J$_{Baltimore}$		68
	Gly → Arg	Hb D$_{Bushman}$		332
17 (A14)	Lys → Glu	Hb Nagasaki		228
19 (B1)	Asn → Lys	Hb D$_{Ouled Rabah}$		145
20 (B2)	Val → Met	Hb Olympia	Increased O$_2$ affinity	308
	Val → Asp	Hb Strasbourg	Unstable (slightly)	152
22 (B4)	Glu → Lys	Hb E$_{Saskatoon}$		328
	Glu → Gly	Hb G$_{Taipei}$		89
	Glu → Ala	Hb G$_{Saskatoon}$		327
	Glu → Gln	Hb D$_{Iran}$		267
24 (B6)	Gly → Arg	Hb Riverdale-Bronx	Unstable	276
	Gly → Val	Hb Savannah	Unstable	168
	Gly → Asp	Hb Moscva	Unstable, decreased O$_2$ affinity	174
25 (B7)	Gly → Arg	Hb G$_{Taiwan Ami}$		80
26 (B8)	Glu → Lys	Hb E		171
	Glu → Val	Hb Henri Mondor	Unstable (slightly)	91
27 (B9)	Ala → Asp	Hb Volga	Unstable	175
28 (B10)	Leu → Gln	Hb St. Louis	Unstable, ferrihemoglobin, increased O$_2$ affinity	131
	Leu → Pro	Hb Genova	Unstable, increased O$_2$ affinity	291
29 (B11)	Gly → Asp	Hb Lufkin		243
30 (B12)	Arg → Ser	Hb Tacoma	Unstable, decreased Bohr effect, decreased heme-heme, normal O$_2$ affinity	104
32 (B14)	Leu → Pro	Hb Perth	Unstable	180
	Leu → Arg	Hb Castilla	Unstable	153
35 (C1)	Tyr → Phe	Hb Philly	Unstable, increased O$_2$ affinity	282
37 (C3)	Trp → Ser	Hb Hirose	Increased O$_2$ affinity	345
39 (C5)	Gln → Lys	Hb Alabama		105
	Gln → Glu	Hb Vaasa		195
40 (C6)	Arg → Lys	Hb Athens, Ga.	Increased O$_2$ affinity	108
	Arg → Ser	Hb Austin		246
41 (C7)	Phe → Tyr	Hb Mequon		109
42 (CD1)	Phe → Ser	Hb Hammersmith	Unstable, decreased O$_2$ affinity	136
	Phe → Leu	Hb Louisville	Unstable, decreased O$_2$ affinity	193
43 (CD2)	Glu → Ala	Hb G$_{Galveston}$		98
46 (CD5)	Gly → Glu	Hb K$_{Ibadan}$		59
47 (CD6)	Asp → Asn	Hb G$_{Copenhagen}$		306

Table 13-2. Variants of the β-chain—cont'd

Residue	Substitution	Name	Major abnormal property	Reference No.
48 (CD7)	Leu → Arg	Hb Okaloosa	Unstable, decreased O₂ affinity	118
50 (D1)	Thr → Lys	Hb Edmonton		208
51 (D2)	Pro → Arg	Hb Willamette		191
52 (D3)	Asp → Asn	Hb Osu Christiansborg		205
	Asp → Ala	Hb Ocho Rios		75
56 (D7)	Gly → Asp	Hb J$_{Bangkok}$		81, 123
	Gly → Arg	Hb Hamadan		273
57 (E1)	Asn → Lys	Hb G$_{Ferrara}$		331
58 (E2)	Pro → Arg	Hb Dhofar		231
59 (E3)	Lys → Glu	Hb I$_{High\ Wycombe}$		97
	Lys → Thr	Hb J$_{Kaohsiung}$		83
61 (E5)	Lys → Glu	Hb N$_{Seattle}$		186
	Lys → Asn	Hb Hikari		303
62 (E6)	Ala → Pro	Hb Duarte	Unstable, increased O₂ affinity	77
63 (E7)	His → Arg	Hb Zürich	Unstable, increased O₂ affinity	249
	His → Tyr	Hb M$_{Saskatoon}$	Ferrihemoglobin, increased O₂ affinity	155
	His → Pro	Hb Bicêtre		335
64 (E8)	Gly → Asp	Hb J$_{Calabria}$	Unstable	320
65 (E9)	Lys → Asn	Hb Sicilia		280
	Lys → Gln	Hb J$_{Cairo}$		154
66 (E10)	Lys → Glu	Hb I$_{Toulouse}$	Unstable, ferri-hemoglobin	285
67 (E11)	Val → Asp	Hb Bristol	Unstable	309
	Val → Glu	Hb M$_{Milwaukee\ I}$	Ferrihemoglobin, decreased O₂ affinity	155
	Val → Ala	Hb Sydney	Unstable	113
68 (E12)	Leu → Pro	Hb Mizuho		253
69 (E13)	Gly → Asp	Hb J$_{Cambridge}$		306
70 (E14)	Ala → Asp	Hb Seattle	Decreased O₂ affinity	207
71 (E15)	Phe → Ser	Hb Christchurch	Unstable	114
73 (E17)	Asp → Tyr	Hb Vancouver		189
	Asp → Asn	Hb Korle Bu		204
	Asp → Val	Hb Mobile		298
74 (E18)	Gly → Val	Hb Bushwick		283
	Gly → Asp	Hb Shepherds Bush	Unstable, increased O₂ affinity	339
75 (E19)	Leu → Pro	Hb Atlanta	Unstable	166
76 (E20)	Ala → Asp	Hb J$_{Chicago}$		284
77 (EF1)	His → Asp	Hb J$_{Iran}$		269
79 (EF3)	Asp → Gly	Hb G$_{Hsi-Tsou}$	Increased O₂ affinity	85
80 (EF4)	Asn → Lys	Hb G$_{Szuhu}$		88
81 (EF5)	Leu → Arg	Hb Baylor	Increased O₂ affinity	297
82 (EF6)	Lys → Asn → Asp	Hb Providence	Decreased O₂ affinity	92, 120, 227, 247
	Lys → Thr	Hb Rahere	Increased O₂ affinity	223
	Lys → Met	Hb Helsinki	Increased O₂ affinity	176
83 (EF7)	Gly → Cys	Hb Ta-li		82
	Gly → Asp	Hb Pyrgos		317, 318
85 (F1)	Phe → Ser	Hb Bryn Mawr	Unstable, increased O₂ affinity	100
87 (F3)	Thr → Lys	Hb D$_{Ibadan}$		337
88 (F4)	Leu → Arg	Hb Borås	Unstable	165
	Leu → Pro	Hb Santa Ana	Unstable	256
89 (F5)	Ser → Asn	Hb Creteil	Increased O₂ affinity	128
	Ser → Arg	Hb Vanderbilt		261
90 (F6)	Glu → Lys	Hb Agenogi	Decreased O₂ affinity	240

Continued.

Table 13-2. Variants of the β-chain—cont'd

Residue	Substitution	Name	Major abnormal property	Reference No.
91 (F7)	Leu → Pro	Hb Sabine	Unstable	299
	Leu → Arg	Hb Caribbean	Unstable, decreased O₂ affinity	52
92 (F8)	His → Tyr	Hb M_Hyde Park	Normal O₂, ferri-hemoglobin	163, 305
	His → Gln	Hb Istanbul	Unstable, increased O₂ affinity, decreased dissociation	57
	His → Asp	Hb J_Altgeld Gardens	Normal O₂ affinity	49
	His → Pro	Hb Newcastle		146
95 (FG2)	Lys → Glu	Hb N_Baltimore		124
97 (FG4)	His → Gln	Hb Malmö	Increased O₂ affinity	221
	His → Leu	Hb Wood	Increased O₂ affinity	314, 315
98 (FG5)	Val → Met	Hb Köln	Unstable, increased O₂ affinity	112
	Val → Gly	Hb Nottingham	Unstable, increased O₂ affinity	158
	Val → Ala	Hb Djelfa	Unstable, increased O₂ affinity	149
99 (G1)	Asp → Asn	Hb Kempsey	Increased O₂ affinity	277
	Asp → Ala	Hb Radcliffe	Increased O₂ affinity	338
	Asp → His	Hb Yakima	Increased O₂ affinity	192
	Asp → Tyr	Hb Ypsilanti	Increased O₂ affinity	156, 289
100 (G2)	Pro → Leu	Hb Brigham	Increased O₂ affinity	218
101 (G3)	Glu → Lys	Hb British Columbia	Increased O₂ affinity	184
	Glu → Gln	Hb Rush	Unstable	51
	Glu → Gly	Hb Alberta		229
	Glu → Asp	Hb Potomac	Increased O₂ affinity	119
102 (G4)	Asn → Lys	Hb Richmond	Asymmetric hybrids	143
	Asn → Thr	Hb Kansas	Decreased O₂ affinity, increased dissociation	93
	Asn → Ser	Hb Beth Israel	Decreased O₂ affinity	250
103 (G5)	Phe → Leu	Hb Heathrow	Increased O₂ affinity	340
104 (G6)	Arg → Ser	Hb Camperdown	Unstable (slightly)	341
106 (G8)	Leu → Pro	Hb Casper	Increased O₂ affinity	203
	Leu → Gln	Hb Tübingen	Unstable, increased O₂ affinity	201, 202
107 (G9)	Gly → Arg	Hb Burke		190
108 (G10)	Asn → Asp	Hb Yoshizuka	Decreased O₂ affinity	178
109 (G11)	Val → Met	Hb San Diego	Increased O₂ affinity	252
111 (G13)	Val → Phe	Hb Peterborough	Unstable, decreased O₂ affinity	198
113 (G15)	Val → Glu	Hb New York		274
115 (G17)	Ala → Pro	Hb Madrid	Unstable	260
117 (G19)	His → Arg	Hb P_Galveston		292
119 (GH2)	Gly → Asp	Hb Fannin-Lubbock	Unstable (slightly)	245, 294
120 (GH3)	Lys → Glu	Hb Hijiyama		238
	Lys → Asn	Hb Riyadh		144
121 (GH4)	Glu → Gln	Hb D	Increased O₂ affinity	64
	Glu → Lys	Hb O_Arab		67
	Glu → Val	Hb Beograd		142
124 (H2)	Pro → Arg	Hb Khartoum	Unstable	127
126 (H4)	Val → Glu	Hb Hofu		239
127 (H5)	Gln → Glu	Hb Hacettepe		60
129 (H7)	Ala → Asp	Hb J_Taichung		90
	Ala → Glu or Asp	Hb K_Cameroon		59
130 (H8)	Tyr → Asp	Hb Wien	Unstable	222

Table 13-2. Variants of the β-chain—cont'd

Residue	Substitution	Name	Major abnormal property	Reference No.
131 (H9)	Gln → Glu	Hb Camden		333
132 (H10)	Lys → Gln	Hb K Woolwich		59
135 (H13)	Ala → Pro	Hb Altdorf	Unstable, increased O₂ affinity	233
136 (H14)	Gly → Asp	Hb Hope	Unstable	235
141 (H19)	Leu → Arg	Hb Olmsted		221
143 (H21)	His → Arg	Hb Abruzzo	Increased O₂ affinity	321
	His → Gln	Hb Little Rock	Increased O₂ affinity	107
	His → Pro	Hb Syracuse	Increased O₂ affinity	182
144 (HC1)	Lys → Asn	Hb Andrew-Minneapolis	Increased O₂ affinity	347
145 (HC2)	Tyr → His	Hb Bethesda	Increased O₂ affinity	162
	Tyr → Cys	Hb Rainier	Increased O₂ affinity, alkali resistant	162
	Tyr → Asp	Hb Ft. Gordon	Increased O₂ affinity	199
	Tyr → Term	Hb McKees Rocks	Increased O₂ affinity	343
146 (HC3)	His → Asp	Hb Hiroshima	Increased O₂ affinity	262
	His → Pro	Hb York	Increased O₂ affinity	72
	His → Arg	Hb Cochin-Port Royal		197

variants with altered oxygen affinity or heme function as in the Hb M and heat-unstable hemoglobins, and (4) thalassemias and hereditary persistence of Hb F, syndrome states associated with abnormal and unbalanced rates of production of normal polypeptide chains.

In Tables 13-1 to 13-8 the human hemoglobin variants are categorized on the basis of the chain and position of the amino acid substitution. Fusion hemoglobins, variants with extended chains, deletions, and double substitution variants are also indicated. For each variant the major abnormal property, if any, and a representative reference have been cited.

Table 13-3. Variants of the δ-chain

Residue	Substitution	Name	Reference No.
2 (NA2)	His → Arg	Hb A₂ Sphakia	185
12 (A9)	Asn → Lys	Hb A₂ NYU	275
16 (A13)	Gly → Arg	Hb A₂ (B₂)	69
20 (B2)	Val → Glu	Hb A₂ Roosevelt	281
22 (B4)	Ala → Glu	Hb A₂ Flatbush	183
43 (CD2)	Glu → Lys	Hb A₂ Melbourne	301
69 (E13)	Gly → Arg	Hb A₂ Indonesia	215
116 (G18)	Arg → His	Hb A₂ Coburg	302
136 (H14)	Gly → Asp	Hb A₂ Babinga	137

Table 13-4. Variants of the γ-chain

Residue	Substitution	Name	Reference No.
1 (NA1)	Gly → Cys (136 gly)	Hb F Malaysia	214
5 (A2)	Glu → Lys (136 ala)	Hb F Texas I	56, 181
6 (A3)	Glu → Lys	Hb F Texas II	210
7 (A4)	Asp → Asn (136 gly)	Hb F Auckland	115
12 (A9)	Thr → Lys	Hb Alexandra	224
16 (A13)	Gly → Arg (136 gly)	Hb F Melbourne	102
22 (B4)	Asp → Gly (136 ala)	Hb F Kuala Lumpur	216
61 (E5)	Lys → Glu (136 ala)	Hb F Jamaica	55
75 (E19)	Ile → Thr (136 gly [?])	Hb F Sardinia	160
80 (EF4)	Asp → Tyr (136 ala)	Hb F Victoria Jubilee	54
97 (FG4)	His → Arg (136 ala)	Hb F Dickinson	296
117 (G19)	His → Arg (136 gly)	Hb F Malta I	117
121 (GH4)	Glu → Lys (136 ala)	Hb F Hull	290
121 (GH4)	Glu → Lys (136 gly)	Hb F Carlton	102
125 (H3)	Glu → Ala (136 gly)	Hb F Port Royal	106
130 (H8)	Trp → Gly (136 gly)	Hb F Poole	211

Table 13-5. Fusion hemoglobins

RESIDUE: δ-CHAIN: β-CHAIN:	9 (A6) Thr Ser	12 (A9) Asn Thr	22 (B4) Ala Glu	50 (D1) Ser Thr	86 (F2) Ser Ala	87 (F3) Gln Thr	116 (G18) Arg His	117 (G19) Asn His	124 (H2) Gln Pro	126 (H4) Met Val	Reference No.
Hb Lepore Hollandia	δ———————————————δ – – – β————————————————————————										73
Hb Lepore Baltimore	δ———————————————————δ – – – β————————————————————										258
Hb Lepore Washington-Boston	δ——————————————————————————δ – – – β——————————————										65
Hb Miyada	δ—————β – – – δ——————————————————————————————————										346
Hb P Congo	δ—————β – – – – – – – – – – – – – – – – – δ————————										213
Hb P Nilotic	δ—————β – – – δ——————————————————————————————————										62

RESIDUE: γ-CHAIN: β-CHAIN:	1 (NA1) Gly Val		80 (EF4) Asp Asn	81 (EF5) Leu Leu	86 (F2) Ala Ala	87 (F3) Gln Thr				146 (HC3) His His	Reference No.
Hb Kenya	γ—————————————————————γ – – – β———————————————————										170

Table 13-6. Variants with extended chains

	Residue	Name	Major abnormal property	Reference No.
α141	31 additional residues: tyr-arg-gln-ala-gly- ala-ser-val-ala-val-pro-pro-ala-arg-trp- ala-ser-gln-arg-ala-leu-leu-pro-ser-leu- his-arg-pro-phe-leu-val-phe-glu (residues numbered 140, 150, 160, 170)	Hb Constant Spring		126
α141	31 additional residues: identical to Hb Constant Spring except for residue 142, which is lysine instead of glutamine	Hb Icaria		125
α141	16 or 17 additional residues: tyr-arg-(ser, ala,gly,ala,ser,val,ala,val,pro,pro, ala)-arg(?,ala,ser,gln)-arg-COOH (residues numbered 140, 160)	Hb Koya Dora		139
β146	10 additional residues: thr-lys-leu-leu- ala-ser,leu,asn,phe-tyr	Hb Tak	Increased O$_2$ affinity	147, 177, 212
α139-141	thr-ser-asn-thr-val-lys-leu-glu-pro-arg (Frameshift) (residue numbered 140)	Hb Wayne		300
β145	lys-ser-ile-thr-lys-(leu-asn-ala-ser)- leu-phe-tyr-COOH (residue numbered 144)	Hb Cranston	Unstable	110
α115-118	ala-glu-phe-thr-*glu-phe-thr*-pro (Insertion) (residues numbered 115 116 117 118 119)	Hb Grady (Dakar)		169, 319

Table 13-7. Variants with deleted residues

Residue	Substitution	Name	Major abnormal property	Reference No.
$\beta 6$ or 7	Glu → O	Hb Leiden	Unstable, slightly increased O_2 affinity	140
$\beta 17$-18	(Lys-Val) → O	Hb Lyon	Increased O_2 affinity	129
$\beta 23$	Val → O	Hb Freiburg	Increased O_2 affinity	187
$\beta 42$-44 or 43-45	(Phe-Glu-Ser) → O or (Glu-Ser-Phe) → O	Hb Niteroi	Decreased O_2 affinity, unstable	266
$\beta 56$-59	(Gly-Asn-Pro-Lys) → O	Hb Tochigi	Unstable, O_2 affinity not known	304
$\beta 74$-75	(Gly-Leu) → O	Hb St. Antoine	Unstable, normal O_2 affinity	336
$\beta 87$	Thr → O	Hb Tours	Increased O_2 affinity, unstable	336
$\beta 91$-95	(Leu-His-Cys-Asp-Lys) → O	Hb Gun Hill	Unstable, increased O_2 affinity	101
$\beta 131$	Gln → O	Hb Leslie	Unstable, normal O_2 affinity	225, 226
$\beta 141$	Leu → O	Hb Coventry		116

Table 13-8. Variants with more than one point mutation in the same polypeptide chain

Residue	Substitution	Name	Major abnormal property	Reference No.
$\beta 6$ (A3)	Glu → Val, 73 Asp → Asn	Hb C$_{Harlem}$	Normal O_2 affinity	95
	Glu → Lys, 95 Lys → Glu	Hb Arlington Park		48
$\alpha 78$-79	Asn → Asp, Ala → Gly	Hb J$_{Singapore}$		86
$\beta 6$ (A3)	Glu → Val, 58 Pro → Arg	Hb C$_{Ziguinchor}$		157
$\beta 6$ (A3)	Glu → Val, 142 Ala → Val	Hb Travis	Increased O_2 affinity	243

REFERENCES
Normal hemoglobins

1. Allen, D. N., Wyman, J., and Smith, C. I.: The oxygen equilibrium of fetal and adult hemoglobin, J. Biol. Chem. **203**:81, 1953.
2. Andrews, B. F., and Willet, G. P.: Fetal hemoglobin concentration in the newborn: index of maturity as supportive evidence for maternal fetal transfusion, Am. J. Obstet. Gynecol. **91**:85, 1965.
3. Baglioni, C.: The fusion of two peptide chains in hemoglobin Lepore and its interpretation as a genetic deletion, Proc. Natl. Acad. Sci. **48**:1880, 1962.
4. Benesch, R., and Benesch, R. E.: Intracellular organic phosphates as regulators of oxygen release by haemoglobin, Nature **221**:618, 1969.
5. Betke, K., Marti, H. R., and Schlicht, I.: Estimation of small percentages of foetal haemoglobin, Nature **184**:1877, 1959.
6. Capp, G. L., Rigas, D. A., and Jones, R. T.: Hemoglobin Portland 1: a new human hemoglobin unique in structure, Science **157**:65, 1967.
7. Chemoff, A. I.: A method for the quantitative determination of H_bA_2, Ann. N.Y. Acad. Sci. **119**:557, 1964.
8. Clegg, J. B., Naughton, M. A., and Weatherall, D. J.: An improved method for the characterization of human haemoglobin mutants: identification of a_2b_2 95 glu haemoglobin N (Baltimore), Nature **207**:945, 1965.
9. Cook, C. D., Brodie, H. R., and Allen, D. W.: Measurement of fetal hemoglobin in premature infants: correlation with gestational age and intrauterine hypoxia, Pediatrics **20**:272, 1959.

10. Cotter, J., and Prystowsky, H.: Fetal blood studies. XIX. Adult and fetal hemoglobin levels of human fetal blood in term pregnancy and in prolonged pregnancy, Am. J. Obstet. Gynecol. **22**:745, 1963.
11. Delivoria-Papadopoulos, M., Miller, L. D., Forster, R. E., II, and Oski, F. A.: The role of exchange transfusion in the management of low-birth weight infants with and without severe respiratory distress syndrome, J. Pediatr. **89**:273, 1976.
12. Delivoria-Papadopoulos, M., Oski, F. A., and Gottlieb, A. J.: Oxygen-hemoglobin dissociation curves: effects of inherited enzyme defects of the red cell, Science **165**:601, 1969.
13. Drescher, H., and Kunzer, W.: Der Blutfarbstoff des menschlichen feten, Klin. Wochenschr. **32**:92, 1954.
14. Finch, C. A., and Lenfant, C.: Oxygen transport in man, N. Engl. J. Med. **286**:407, 1972.
15. Fraser, I. D.: Adult and foetal haemoglobin in Rh haemolytic disease, Br. J. Haematol. **23**:269, 1972.
16. Fraser, I. D., and Raper, A. B.: Observations on the change from foetal to adult erythropoiesis, Arch. Dis. Child. **37**:289, 1962.
17. Hollenberg, M. D., Kaback, M. M., and Kazazian, H. H. Jr.: Adult hemoglobin synthesis by reticulocytes from the human fetus at midtrimester, Science **174**:698, 1971.
18. Huehns, E. R., and Farooqui, A. M.: Oxygen dissociation properties of human embryonic red cells, Nature **254**:335, 1975.
19. Huehns, E. R., Flynn, F. V., Butler, E. A., and Beaven,

G. H.: Two new haemoglobin variants in a very young human embryo, Nature **189:**496, 1961.

20. Huehns, E. R., Hecht, F., Keil, J. V., and Motulsky, A. G.: Developmental hemoglobin anomalies in a chromosomal triplication: D trisomy syndrome, Proc. Natl. Acad. Sci. **51:**89, 1964.

21. Ingram, V. M.: Abnormal human haemoglobin. I. The comparison of normal human and sickle cell haemoglobins by fingerprinting, Biochem. Biophys. Acta **28:** 539, 1958.

22. Itano, H. A., and Singer, S. J.: On dissociation and recombination of human adult hemoglobins: A, S, and C, Proc. Natl. Acad. Sci. **44:**522, 1958.

23. Jacob, F., and Monad, J.: Genetic regulatory mechanisms in the synthesis of proteins, J. Mol. Biol. **3:**318, 1961.

24. Jonxis, J. H. P.: The development of hemoglobin, Pediatr. Clin. N. Am. **12:**535, 1965.

25. Jonxis, J. H. P., and Huisman, T. H. J.: The detection and estimation of fetal hemoglobin by means of the alkali denaturation test, Blood **11:**1009, 1956.

26. Kan, Y. W., Forget, B. G., and Nathan, D. G.: Gamabeta thalassemia: a cause of hemolytic disease of newborns, N. Engl. J. Med. **286:**129, 1972.

27. Kirschbaum, T. H.: Fetal hemoglobin content of cord blood determined by column chromatography, Am. J. Obstet. Gynecol. **84:**1375, 1962.

28. Kleihauer, E., Braun, H., and Betke, K.: Demonstration von fetalin Hämoglobin in den erythrocyten eines Blutausstrichs, Klin. Wochenschr. **35:**637, 1957.

29. Kleihauer, E. F., Tang, T. E., and Betke, K.: Die intrazellulare verteilung von embryonalem haemoglobin in roten blutzellen menschlicher embryonen, Acta Haematol. **38:**264, 1967.

30. Koenig, R. J., Peterson, C. M., Jones, R. L., Sandek, C., Lehrman, M., and Cerami, A.: Correlation of glucose regulation on hemoglobin AIC in diabetes mellitus, N. Engl. J. Med. **295:**417, 1976.

31. Kunkel, H. G., and Wallenius, G.: New hemoglobin in normal adult blood, Science **122:**228, 1955.

32. Maurer, H. S., Veda, L. N., and Honig, G. R.: Similarities of the erythrocytes in juvenile chronic myelogenic leukemia to fetal erythrocytes, Blood **39:**778, 1972.

33. Muller, C. J.: Separation of the α and β chains of globins by means of starch gel electrophoresis, Nature **186:**643, 1960.

34. Oski, F. A., and Delivoria-Papadopoulos, M.: The red cell, 2,3 diphosphoglycerate (DPG), and tissue oxygen release, J. Pediatr. **77:**941, 1970.

35. Oski, F. A., and Gottlieb, A. J.: The interrelationships between red blood cell metabolites, hemoglobin, and the oxygen-equilibrium curve, Prog. Hematol. **7:**33, 1971.

36. Pauling, L., Itano, H. A., Singers, S. J., and Wells, I. C.: Sickle cell anemia: a molecular disease, Science **110:**543, 1949.

37. Pearson, H. A., et al.: Routine screening of umbilical cord blood for sickle cell diseases, J.A.M.A. **227:**420, 1974.

38. Pembrey, M. E., Weatherall, D. J., and Clegg, J. B.: Maternal synthesis of haemoglobin F in pregnancy, Lancet **1:**1350, 1973.

39. Robinson, A. R., Robson, M., Harrison, A. P., and Zuelzer, W. W.: A new technique for differentiation of hemoglobin, J. Lab. Clin. Med. **50:**745, 1957.

40. Rudolph, A. M., Nadas, A. S., and Borges, W. H.: Hematological adjustments and cyanotic congenital heart disease, Pediatrics **11:**454, 1953.

41. Schmidt, R. M., Rucknagel, D. L., and Nechiles, T. F.: Comparison of methodologies for thalassemia screening by Hgb A₂ quantitation, J. Lab. Clin. Med. **86:**873, 1975.

42. Schroeder, W. A., Huisman, T. J. H., Shelton, J. B., et al.: Evidence for multiple structural genes for the γ chain of human fetal hemoglobin, Proc. Nat. Acad. Sci. **60:**537, 1968.

43. Singer, K., Chemoff, A. J., and Singer, L.: Studies on abnormal hemoglobin. I. Their demonstration in sickle cell anemia and other hematologic disorders by means of alkali denaturation, Blood **11:**1009, 1956.

44. Smith, E. W., and Torbert, J. V.: Two abnormal hemoglobins with evidence for a new genetic locus for hemoglobin formation, Bull. Johns Hopkins Hosp. **102:**38, 1958.

45. Thomas, E. D., Lochte, H. L., Jr., Greenough, W. B., III, and Wales, M.: In vitro synthesis of foetal and adult haemoglobin by foetal haematopoietic tissues, Nature **185:**396, 1960.

46. Weatherall, D. V., and Clegg, J. B.: The thalassemia syndrome, ed. 2, Oxford, 1972, Blackwell Scientific Publications.

47. Wood, W. G., and Weatherall, D. J.: Haemoglobin synthesis during foetal development, Nature **244:**162, 1973.

Abnormal hemoglobins

48. Adams, J. G., and Heller, P.: Hemoglobin Arlington Park (β6 Glu → Lys 95 Lys → Glu): electrophoretically "silent" hemoglobin variant with two amino acid substitutions in the same polypeptide chain, Blood **42:**990, 1973.

49. Adams III, J. G., Przywara, K. P., Shamsuddin, M., and Heller, P.: Hemoglobin J Altgeld Gardens (β92 (F8) His → Asp): a new hemoglobin variant involving a substitution of the proximal histidine, Am. Soc. Hematol. 18th Ann. Meet., Dallas, December 1975.

50. Adams III, J. G., Winter, W. P., Rucknagel, D. L., and Spencer, H. H.: Biosynthesis of hemoglobin Ann Arbor: evidence for catabolic and feedback regulation, Science **176:**1427, 1972.

51. Adams, J. G., Winter, W. P., Tausk, K., and Heller P.: Hemoglobin Rush [β101 (G3) Glutamine]: a new unstable hemoglobin causing mild hemolytic anemia, Blood **43:**261, 1974.

52. Ahern, E., Ahern, V., Hilton, T., Serjeant, G. R., Serjeant, B. E., Seakins, M., Lang, A., Middleton, A. and Lehmann, H.: Haemoglobin Caribbean β 91 (F7) Leu → Arg: a mildly unstable haemoglobin with a low oxygen affinity, F.E.B.S. Lett. **69:**99, 1976.

53. Ahern, E., Ahern, V., Holder, W., Palomino, E., Serjeant, G. R., Serjeant, B. E., Forbes, M., Brimhall, B., and Jones, R. T.: Haemoglobin Spanish Town α27 Glu → Val (B8), Biochim. Biophys. Acta **427:**530, 1976.

54. Ahern, E., Holder, W., Ahern, V., Serjeant, G. R., Serjeant, B. E., Forbes, M., Brimhall, B., and Jones, R. T.: Haemoglobin F Victoria Jubilee (α2Aγ2 80 Asp → Tyr), Biochim. Biophys. Acta **393:**188, 1975.

55. Ahern, E. J., Jones, R. T., Brimhall, B., and Gray, R. H.: Haemoglobin F Jamaica (α2γ2 61 Lys → Glu; 136 Ala), Br. J. Haematol. **18:**369, 1970.

56. Ahern, E. J., Wiltshire, B. G., and Lehmann, H.: Further characterization of haemoglobin F Texas-I γ5 Glutamic acid → Lysine: γ136 Alanine, Biochim. Biophys. Acta **271:**61, 1972.

57. Aksoy, M., Erden, S., Efremov, G. D., Wilson, J. B., Huisman, T. H. J., Schroeder, W. A., Shelton, J. R., Shelton, J. B., Ulitin, O. N., and Müftüglu, A.: Hemoglobin Istanbul: substitution of glutamine for histidine in a proximal histidine (F8(92)β), J. Clin. Invest. **51:**2380, 1972.

58. Alberti, R., Mariuzzi, G. M., Artibani, L., Bruni, E., and Tentori, L.: A new haemoglobin variant: J-Rovigo

alpha 53 (E-2) alanine → aspartic acid, Biochim. Biophys. Acta **342**:1, 1974.

59. Allan, N., Beale, D., Irvine, D., and Lehmann, H.: Three haemoglobins K: Woolwich, an abnormal, Cameroon, and Ibadan, two unusual variants of human haemoglobin A, Nature **208**:658, 1965.
60. Altay, C., Altinöz, N., Wilson, J. B., Bolch, K. C., and Huisman, T. H. J.: Hemoglobin Hacettepe or α2β2 127(H5)Gln → Glu, Biochim. Biophys. Acta **434**:1, 1976.
61. Arcasoy, A., Casey, R., Lehmann, H., Cavdar, A. O., and Berki, A.: A new haemoglobin J from Turkey: Hb Ankara (β10 (A7)Ala → Asp), F.E.B.S. Lett. **42**:121, 1974.
62. Badr, F. M., Lorkin, P. A., and Lehmann, H.: Haemoglobin P-Nilotic: containing a β-δ chain, Nature (New Biol.) **242**:107, 1973.
63. Baglioni, C.: A chemical study of Hemoglobin Norfolk, J. Biol. Chem. **237**:69, 1962.
64. Baglioni, C.: Abnormal human haemoglobins. VIII. Chemical studies on Haemoglobin D, Biochim. Biophys. Acta **59**:437, 1962.
65. Baglioni, C.: The fusion of two peptide chains in hemoglobin Lepore and its interpretation as a genetic deletion, Proc. Natl. Acad. Sci. **48**:1880, 1962.
66. Baglioni, C., and Ingram, V. M.: Abnormal human haemoglobins. V. Chemical investigation of haemoglobins A, G, C, X from one individual, Biochim. Biophys. Acta **48**:253, 1961.
67. Baglioni, C., and Lehmann, H.: Chemical heterogeneity of haemoglobin O, Nature **196**:229, 1962.
68. Baglioni, C., and Weatherall, D. J.: Abnormal human hemoglobins. IX. Chemistry of Hemoglobin J Baltimore, Biochim. Biophys. Acta **78**:637, 1963.
69. Ball, E. W., Meynell, M. J., Beale, D., Kynoch, P., Lehmann, H., and Stretton, A. O. W.: Haemoglobin A₂': α2δ2 16 Glycine → Arginine, Nature **209**:1217, 1968.
70. Bannister, W. H., Grech, J. L., Plese, C. F., Smith, L. L., Barton, B. P., Wilson, J. B., Reynolds, C. A., and Huisman, T. H. J.: Hemoglobin St. Luke's or α2 95 Arg (G2) β2, Eur. J. Biochem. **29**:301, 1972.
71. Barclay, G. P. T., Charlesworth, D., and Lehmann, H.: Abnormal haemoglobins in Zambia: a new haemoglobin Zambia α60 (E9) Lysine → Asparagine, Br. Med. J. **4**:595, 1969.
72. Bare, G. H., Bromberg, P. A., Alben, J. O., Brimhall, B., Jones, R. T., Mintz, S., and Rother, I.: Altered C-terminal salt bridges in haemoglobin York cause high oxygen affinity, Nature **259**:155, 1976.
73. Barnabas, J., and Muller, C. J.: Haemoglobin Lepore Hollandia, Nature **194**:931, 1962.
74. Beale, D., and Lehmann, H.: Abnormal haemoglobins and the genetic code, Nature **207**:259, 1965.
75. Beresford, C. H., Clegg, J. B., and Weatherall, D. J.: Haemoglobin Ocho Rios (β52(D3) Aspartic acid → Alanine): a new β-chain variant of haemoglobin A found in combination with haemoglobin S, J. Med. Genet. **9**:151, 1972.
76. Beretta, A., Prato, V., Gallo, E., and Lehmann, H.: Haemoglobin Torino — α43 (CD1) Phenylalanine → Valine, Nature **217**:1016, 1968.
77. Beutler, E., Lang, A., and Lehmann, H.: Hemoglobin Duarte: α2β2 62(E6)Ala → Pro: a new unstable hemoglobin with increased oxygen affinity, Blood **43**:527, 1974.
78. Beuzard, Y., Basset, P., Braconnier, F., El Gammal, H., Martin, L., Oudard, J. L., and Thillet, J.: Haemoglobin Saki α2β2 14 Leu → Pro (A11) structure and function, Biochim. Biophys. Acta **393**:182, 1975.

79. Blackwell, R. Q., Jim, R. T. S., Tan, T. G. H., Weng, M. I., Liu, C. S., and Wang, C. L.: Hemoglobin G Waimanalo: α64 Asp → Asn, Biochim. Biophys. Acta **322**:27, 1973.
80. Blackwell, R. Q., and Liu, C.-S.: Hemoglobin G Taiwan-Ami α2β2 25 Gly → Arg, Biochem. Biophys. Res. Comm. **30**:690, 1968.
81. Blackwell, R. Q., and Liu, C.-S.: The identical structural anomalies of hemoglobins J Meinung and J Korat, Biochem. Biophys. Res. Comm. **24**:732, 1966.
82. Blackwell, R. Q., Liu, C.-S., and Wang, C.-L.: Hemoglobin Ta-Li: β83 Gly → Cys. Biochim. Biophys. Acta **243**:467, 1971.
83. Blackwell, R. Q., Liu, C.-S., and Shih, T.-B.: Hemoglobin J Kaohsiung: β59 Lys → Thr, Biochim. Biophys. Acta **229**:343, 1971.
84. Blackwell, R. Q., Oemijati, S., Pribadi, W., Weng, M.-I., and Liu, C.-S. Hemoglobin G Makassar: β6 Glu → Ala, Biochim. Biophys. Acta **214**:396, 1970.
85. Blackwell, R. Q., Shih, T.-B., Wang, C.-L., and Liu, C. S.: Hemoglobin G-Hsi-Tsou: β79 Asp → Gly, Biochim. Biophys. Acta **257**:49, 1972.
86. Blackwell, R. Q., Wong Hock Boon, Liu, C. S., and Weng, M. I.: Hemoglobin J Singapore: α78 Asn → Asp; α79 Ala → Gly, Biochim. Biophys. Acta **278**:482, 1972.
87. Blackwell, R. Q., Wong, H. B., Wand, C. L., Weng, M. L., and Liu, C. S.: Hemoglobin J Meerut: α120 Ala → Glu, Biochim. Biophys. Acta **351**:7, 1974.
88. Blackwell, R. Q., Yang, H. T., and Wang, C. C.: Hemoglobin G Szuhu: β80 Asn → Lys, Biochim. Biophys. Acta **188**:59, 1969.
89. Blackwell, R. Q., Yang, H. J., and Wang, C. C.: Hemoglobin G Taipei: α2β2 22 Glu → Gly, Biochim. Biophys. Acta **175**:237, 1969.
90. Blackwell, R. Q., Yang, Y.-J., and Wang, C.-C.: Hemoglobin J Taichung: β129 Ala → Asp, Biochim. Biophys. Acta **194**:1, 1969.
91. Blouquit, Y., Arous, N., Machado, P. E. A., Garel, M. C., and Perrone, F.: Hb Henri Mondor: β26 (B8) Glu → Val: a variant with a substitution localized at the same position as that of Hb E β26 Glu → Lys, F.E.B.S. Lett. **72**:5, 1976.
92. Bonaventura, J., Bonaventura, C., Sullivan, B., Ferruzzi, G., McCurdy, P. R., Fox, J., and Moo-Penn, W. F.: Hemoglobin Providence: functional consequences of two alterations of the 2,3-diphosphoglycerate binding site at position β82, J. Biol. Chem. **251**:7563, 1976.
93. Bonaventura, J., and Riggs, A.: Hemoglobin Kansas, a human hemoglobin with a neutral amino acid substitution and an abnormal oxygen equilibrium, J. Biol. Chem. **243**:980, 1968.
94. Bonaventura, J., and Riggs, A.: Polymerization of hemoglobins of mouse and man: structural basis, Science **158**:800, 1967.
95. Bookchin, R. M., Nagel, R. L., and Ranney, H. M.: Structure and properties of hemoglobin C Harlem, a human hemoglobin variant with amino acid substitutions in 2 residues of the β-polypeptide chain, J. Biol. Chem. **242**:248, 1967.
96. Botha, M. C., Beale, D., Isaacs, W. A., and Lehmann, H.: Haemoglobin J Cape Town α2 92 Arginine → Glutamine β2, Nature. **212**:792, 1966.
97. Boulton, F. E., Huntsman, R. G., Lehmann, H., Lorkin, P., and Romero Herrera, A.: Hb I High Wycombe β59 Lys → Glu, Proc. Br. Soc. Haematol. April 1970.
98. Bowman, B. H., Oliver, C. P., Barnett, D. R., Cunningham, J. R., and Schneider, R. G.: Chemical characterization of three hemoglobins G, Blood **23**:193, 1964.
99. Boyer, S. H., Crosby, E. F., Fuller, G. F., Ulenurm, L.,

and Buck, A. A.: A survey of hemoglobins in the Republic of Chad and characterization of hemoglobin Chad: $\alpha2$ 23Glu → Lys $\beta2$, Am. J. Human Genet. **20:**570, 1968.

100. Bradley, T. B., Wohl, R. C., Murphy, S. B., Oski, F. A., and Bunn, H. F.: Properties of hemoglobin Bryn Mawr, β85Phe → Ser: a new spontaneous mutation producing an unstable hemoglobin with high oxygen affinity, Proc. Ann. Meet. Am. Soc. Hematol., 1972. (Abstract No. 67.)

101. Bradley, T. B., Wohl, R. C., and Rieder, R. F.: Hemoglobin Gun Hill: deletion of five amino acid residues and impaired heme-globin binding, Science **157:**1581, 1967.

102. Brennan, S. O., Smith, M. B., and Carrell, R. W.: Haemoglobin F Melbourne Gγ16 Gly → Arg and Haemoglobin F Carlton Gγ121 Glu → Lys, Biochim. Biophys. Acta **490:**452, 1977.

103. Brimhall, B., Duerst, M., Hollán, S. R., Stenzel, P., Szelenyi, I., and Jones, R. T.: Structural characterizations of hemoglobins J Buda (α61 (E10) Lys → Asn) and G Pest (α74 (EF3) Asp → Asn), Biochim. Biophys. Acta **336:**344, 1974.

104. Brimhall, B., Jones, R. T., Baur, E. W., and Motulsky, A. G.: Structural characterization of hemoglobin Tacoma, Biochem. **8:**2125, 1969.

105. Brimhall, B., Jones, R. T., Schneider, R. G., Hosty, T. S., Tomlin, G., and Atkins, R.: Two new hemoglobins: Hemoglobin Alabama (β39(C5)Gln → Lys) and Hemoglobin Montgomery (α48(CD6)Leu → Arg), Biochim. Biophys. Acta **379:**28, 1975.

106. Brimhall, B., Vedvick, T. S., Jones, R. T., Ahern, E., Palomino, E., and Ahern, V.: Haemoglobin F Port Royal (α2Gγ 125 Glu → Ala), Br. J. Haematol. **27:**313, 1974.

107. Bromberg, P. A., Alben, J. O., Bare, G. H., Balcerzak, S. P., Jones, R. T., Brimhall, B., and Padilla, F.: Haemoglobin Little Rock (β143 His → Gln; H21): a high oxygen affinity haemoglobin variant with unique properties. Nature (New Biol.) **243:**177, 1973.

108. Brown, W. J., Niazi, G. A., Jayalakshmi, M., Abraham, E. C., and Huisman, T. H. J.: Hemoglobin Athens-Georgia, or $\alpha2\beta2$ 40(C6)Arg → Lys, a hemoglobin variant with an increased oxygen affinity, Biochim. Biophys. Acta **439:**70, 1976.

109. Buckett, L. B., Sharma, V. S., Piscotta, A. V., Ranney, H., and Bruckheimer, P.: Hemoglobin Mequon β41 (C7) Phenylalanine → Tyrosine, Clin. Res. **22:**176A, 1974.

110. Bunn, H. F., Schmidt, G. J., Haney, D. N., and Dluhy, R. G.: Hemoglobin Cranston: an unstable variant having an elongated β chain due to nonhomologous crossover between two normal β chain genes, Proc. Natl. Acad. Sci. **72:**3609, 1975.

111. Cabannes, R., Renaud, R., Mauran, A., Pennors, H., Charlesworth, D., Price, B. G., and Lehmann, H.: Deux hémoglobines rapides an Côte-D'Ivoire: l'Hb K Woolwich et une nouvelle hémoglobine, l'Hb J Abidjan (α51 Gly → Asp), Nouv. Rev. Fr. Hematol. **12:**289, 1972.

112. Carrell, R. W., Lehmann, H., and Hutchison, H. E.: Haemoglobin Köln (β-98 Valine → Methionine): an unstable protein causing inclusion-body anaemia, Nature (London) **210:**915, 1966.

113. Carrell, R. W., Lehmann, H., Lorkin, P. A., Raik, E., and Hunter, E.: Haemoglobin Sydney: β67(E11)Valine → Alanine: an emerging pattern of unstable haemoglobins, Nature **215:**626, 1967.

114. Carrell, R. W., and Owen, M. C.: A new approach to haemoglobin variant identification: Haemoglobin Christchurch β71(E15)Phenylalanine → Serine, Biochim. Biophys. Acta **236:**507, 1971.

115. Carrell, R. W., Owen, M. C., Anderson, R., and Berry, E.: Haemoglobin F Auckland Gγ7 Asp → Asn: further

evidence for multiple genes for the gamma chain, Biochim. Biophys. Acta **365:**323, 1974.

116. Casey, R., Lang, A., Lehmann, H., and Shinton, N. K.: Double heterozygosity for two unstable haemoglobins: Hb Sydney (β67 E11) (Val → Ala) and Hb Coventry (β141 (H19) Leu deleted), Br. J. Haematol. **33:**143, 1976.

117. Cauchi, M. N., Clegg, J. B., and Weatherall, D. J.: Haemoglobin F (Malta): a new foetal haemoglobin variant with a high incidence in Maltese infants, Nature **223:**311, 1969.

118. Charache, S., Brimhall, B., Milner, P., and Cobb, L.: Hemoglobin Okaloosa β48(CD7)Leu → Arg): an unstable hemoglobin with decreased oxygen affinity, J. Clin. Invest. **52:**2858, 1973.

119. Charache, S., Jacobson, R., Brimhall, B., Winslow, R., Murphy, E. A., Rath, C., and Jones, R. T.: Hemoglobin Potomac (β101Glu → Asp): speculations on fetal oxygenation, Clin. Res. **25:**517A, 1977.

120. Charache, S., McCurdy, P., and Fox, J.: Hemoglobin Providence (Hb Prov.), a fetal-like hemoglobin, Paper presented at American Society of Hematology, eighteenth annual meeting, Dallas, December, 1975.

121. Charache, S., and Ostertag, W.: Hemoglobin Hopkins-2 (α112 Asp)2β2): "low output" protects from potentially harmful effects, Blood **36:**852, 1970.

122. Charache, S., Weatherall, D. J., and Clegg, J. B.: Polycythemia associated with a hemoglobinopathy, J. Clin. Invest. **45:**813, 1966.

123. Clegg, J. B., Naughton, M. A., and Weatherall, D. J.: Abnormal human haemoglobins: separation and characterization of the α and β chains by chromatography, and the determination of two new variants, Hb Chesapeake and Hb J (Bangkok), J. Mol. Biol. **19:**91, 1966.

124. Clegg, J. B., Naughton, M. A., and Weatherall, D. J.: An improved method for the characterization of human haemoglobin mutants: identification of $\alpha2\beta2$ 95Glu, Haemoglobin N (Baltimore), Nature **207:**945, 1965.

125. Clegg, J. B., Weatherall, D. J., Contopolou-Griva, I., Caroutsos, K., Poungouras, P., and Tsevrenis, H.: Haemoglobin Icaria, a new chain-termination mutant which causes α thalassaemia, Nature **251:**245, 1974.

126. Clegg, J. B., Weatherall, D. J., and Milner, P. F.: Haemoglobin Constant Spring: a chain termination mutant, Nature **234:**337, 1971.

127. Clegg, J. B., Weatherall, D. J., Wong Hock Boon, and Mustafa, D.: Two new haemoglobin variants involving proline substitutions, Nature **222:**379, 1969.

128. Cohen-Solal, M., Blouquit, Y., Carel, M. C., Reyes, F., Thillet, J., Caburi, J., Beuzard, Y., and Rosa, J.: Hemoglobin Creteil (β89Ser → Asn): a new hemoglobin variant present in a frozen state, associated with familial erythrocytosis. In International symposium on abnormal hemoglobins and thalassemia, Istanbul, 1974. (Abstract No. 5.)

129. Cohen-Solal, M., Blouquit, Y., Garel, M. C., Thillet, J., Gaillard, L., Creyssel, R., Gibaud, A., and Rosa, J.: Haemoglobin Lyon (β17-18(A14-15) Lys-Val → O) determination by sequenator analysis, Biochim. Biophys. Acta **351:**306, 1974.

130. Cohen-Solal, M., Manesse, B., Thillet, J., and Rosa, J.: Haemoglobin G Norfolk α85 (F6) Asp → Asn: structural characterization by sequenator analysis and functional properties of a new variant with high oxygen affinity, F.E.B.S. Lett. **50:**163, 1975.

131. Cohen-Solal, M., Seligmann, M., Thillet, J., and Rosa, J.: Haemoglobin St. Louis β28(B10)Leucine → Glutamine: a new unstable haemoglobin only present in a ferri form (Abstract 408, XIV International Congress of Hematology, Sao Paulo, 1972), F.E.B.S. Lett. **33:**37, 1973.

132. Colombo, B., Vidal, H., Kamuzora, H., and Lehmann, H.: A new haemoglobin J-Habana α71 (E20) Alanine → Glutamic acid, Biochim. Biophys. Acta **351**:1, 1974.

133. Crookston, J. H., Beale, D., Irvine, D., and Lehmann, H. A new haemoglobin, J Toronto (α5 Alanine → Aspartic acid), Nature **208**:1059, 1965.

134. Crookston, J. H., Farquharson, H. A., Beale, D., and Lehmann, H.: Hemoglobin Etobicoke: α84 (F5) Serine replaced by Arginine, Can. J. Biochem. **47**:143, 1969.

135. Crookston, J. H., Farquharson, H., Kinderlerer, J., and Lehmann, H.: Hemoglobin Manitoba: α102 (G9) Serine replaced by arginine, Can. J. Biochem. **48**:911, 1970.

136. Dacie, J. V., Shinton, N. K. Gaffney, P. J., Jr., Carrell, R. W., and Lehmann, H.: Haemoglobin Hammersmith (β42(CD1)Phe → Ser), Nature **216**:663, 1967.

137. DeJong, W. W. W., and Bernini, L. F.: Haemoglobin Babinga (δ136 Glycine → Aspartic acid): a new delta chain variant, Nature **219**:1360, 1968.

138. DeJong, W. W. W., Bernini, L. F. and Khan, P. M.: Haemoglobin Rampa: α95 Pro → Ser, Biochim. Biophys. Acta **236**:197, 1971.

139. DeJong, W. W. W., Meera Khan, P., and Bernini, L. F.: Hemoglobin Koya Dora: high frequency of a chain termination mutant, Am. J. Hum. Genet. **27**:81, 1975.

140. DeJong, W. W. W., Went, L. N., and Bernini, L. F.: Haemoglobin Leiden: deletion of β6 or 7 glutamic acid, Nature **220**:788, 1968.

141. DeTraverse, P. M., Lehmann, H., Coquelet, M. L., Beale, D., Isaacs, W. A.: Etude d'une hemoglobine Jα non encore décrite, Dans une famille française, Compt. R. Scéance. Soc. Biol. **160**:2270, 1966.

142. Efremov, G. D., Duma, H., Ruvidic, R., Rolovic, Z., Wilson, J. B., and Huisman, T. H. J.: Hemoglobin Beograd or α2β2 121Glu → Val(GH4), Biochim. Biophys. Acta **328**:81, 1973.

143. Efremov, G. D., Huisman, T. H. J., Smith, L. L., Wilson, J. B., Kitchens, J. L., Wrightstone, R. N., and Adams, H. R.: Hemoglobin Richmond, a human hemoglobin which forms asymmetric hybrids with other hemoglobins, J. Biol. Chem. **244**:6105, 1969.

144. El-Hazmi, M. A. F., and Lehmann, H.: Hemoglobin Riyadh [α2β2 120(GH3) Lys → Asn]: a new variant found in association with α-thalassemia and iron deficiency, Hemoglobin **1**:59, 1976.

145. Elion, J., Belkhodja, O., Wajcman, H., and Labie, D.: Two variants of hemoglobin D in the Algerian population: Hemoglobin D Ouled Rabah β19(B1)Asn → Lys and Hemoglobin D Iran β22(B4) Glu → Gln, Biochim. Biophys. Acta **310**:360, 1973.

146. Finney, R., Casey, R., Lehmann, H., and Walder, W.: Hb Newcastle: β92 (F8) His → Pro, F.E.B.S. Lett. **60**:435, 1975.

147. Flatz, G., Kinderlerer, J. L., Kilmartin, J. V., and Lehmann, H.: Haemoglobin Tak: a variant with additional residues at the end of the β-chains, Lancet **10**:732, 1971.

148. Fujiwara, N., Maekawa, T., and Matsuda, G.: Hemoglobin Atago (α2 85 Tyr β2): a new abnormal human hemoglobin found in Nagasaki, Int. J. Protein Res. **3**:35, 1971.

149. Gacon, G., Wajcman, H., and Labie, D.: A new unstable hemoglobin mutated in β98(FG5)Val → Ala: Hb Djelfa, F.E.B.S. Lett. **58**:238, 1975.

150. Gacon, G., Wajcman, H., Labie, D., Varet, B., and Christoforov, B.: A second case of haemoglobin Belfast (β15[A12]Trp → Arg) observed in a French patient, Acta Haematol. **55**:319, 1976.

151. Gajdusek, D. C., Guiart, J., Kirk, R. L., Carrell, R. W., Irvine, D., Kynoch, P. A. M., and Lehmann, H.: Haemoglobin J Tongariki (α115 Alanine → Aspartic acid): the first new haemoglobin variant found in a Pacific (Melanesian) population, J. Med. Genet. **4**:1, 1967.

152. Garel, M. C., Blouquit, Y., Arous, N., Rosa, J., and North, M. L.: Hb Strasbourg α2β2 20(B2) Val → Asp: a variant at the same locus as Hb Olympia β20 Val → Met. F.E.B.S. Lett. **72**:1, 1976.

153. Garel, M. C., Blouquit, Y., and Rosa, J.: Hemoglobin Castilla β32 (B14) Leu → Arg: a new unstable variant producing severe hemolytic disease, F.E.B.S. Lett. **58**:145, 1975.

154. Garel, M. C., Hassan, W., Coquelet, M. T., Goossens, M., and Rosa, J.: Hemoglobin J Cairo: β 65 (E9) Lys → Gln, a new hemoglobin variant discovered in an Egyptian family, Biochim. Biophys. Acta **420**:97, 1976.

155. Gerald, P. S., and Efron, M. L.: Chemical studies of several varieties of Hb M, Proc. Nat. Acad. Sci. (Wash.) **47**:1758, 1961.

156. Glynn, K. P., Penner, J. A., Smith, J. R., Rucknagel, D. L.: Familial erythrocytosis: a description of three families, one with Hemoglobin Ypsilanti, Ann. Intern. Med. **69**:769, 1968.

157. Goossens, M., Garel, M. C., Auvinet, J., Basset, P., Gomes, P. F., and Rosa, J.: Hemoglobin C Ziguinchor $\alpha_2^A \beta_2^6$ (A3) Glu → Val β58 (E2) Pro → Arg: the second sickling variant with amino acid substitutions in 2 residues of the β polypeptide chain, F.E.B.S. Lett. **58**:149, 1975.

158. Gordon-Smith, E. C., Dacie, J. V., Blecher, T. E., French, E. A., Wiltshire, B. G., and Lehmann, H.: Haemoglobin Nottingham, β98(FG5)Val → Gly: a new unstable haemoglobin producing severe haemolysis, Proc. R. Soc. Med. **66**:507, 1973.

159. Gottlieb, A. J., Restrepo, A., and Itano, H. A.: Hemoglobin J Medellin: chemical and genetic study, Fed. Proc. **23**:172, 1964.

160. Grifoni, V., Kamuzora, H., Lehmann, H., and Charlesworth, D.: A new Hb variant: Hb-F Sardinia γ75 (E19) Isoleucine → Threonine found in a family with Hb G Philadelphia, β-chain deficiency and a Lepore-like haemoglobin indistinguishable from Hb A₂, Acta Haematol. **53**:347, 1975.

161. Halbrecht, I., Isaacs, W. A., Lehmann, H., and Ben-Porat, F.: Hemoglobin Hasharon (α47 Aspartic acid → Histidine), Isr. J. Med. Sci. **3**:827, 1967.

162. Hayashi, A., Stamatoyannopoulos, G., Yoshida, A., and Adamson, J.: Haemoglobin Rainier: β145(HC2) Tyrosine → Cysteine and Haemoglobin Bethesda: β145 (HC2)Tyrosine → Histidine, Nature (New Biol.) **230**:264, 1971.

163. Heller, P., Coleman, R. D., and Yakulis, V.: Hemoglobin M Hyde Park: A new variant of abnormal methemoglobin, J. Clin. Invest. **45**:1021, 1966.

164. Hill, R. I., Swenson, R. T., and Schwartz, H. C.: Characterization of a chemical abnormality in hemoglobin G, J. Biol. Chem. **235**:3182, 1960.

165. Hollender, A., Lorkin, P. A., Lehmann, H., and Svensson, B.: New unstable Haemoglobin Böras: β88(F4) Leucine → Arginine, Nature **222**:953, 1969.

166. Hubbard, M., Winton, E., Lindeman, J. G., Dessauer, P. L., Wilson, J. B., Wrightstone, R. N., and Huisman, T. H. J. Hemoglobin Atlanta or α2β2 75 Leu → Pro (E19): an unstable variant found in several members of a Caucasian family, Biochim. Biophys. Acta **386**:538, 1975.

167. Huisman, T. H. J., Adams, H. R., Wilson, J. B., Efremov, G. D., Reynolds, C. A., and Wrightstone, R. N.: Hemoglobin G Georgia or α2 95Leu (G2) β2, Biochim. Biophys. Acta **200**:578, 1970.

168. Huisman, T. H. J., Brown, A. K., Efremov, G. D., Wilson, J. B., Reynolds, C. A., Uy, R., and Smith, L. L.: Hemoglobin Savannah (B6(24)β-glycine → Valine): an

unstable variant causing anemia with inclusion bodies, J. Clin. Invest. **50:**650, 1971.

169. Huisman, T. H. J., Wilson, J. B., Gravely, M., and Hubbard, M.: Hemoglobin Grady: the first example of a variant with elongated chains due to an insertion of residues, Proc. Natl. Acad. Sci. **71:**3270, 1974.

170. Huisman, T. H. J., Wrightstone, R. N., Wilson, J. B., Schroeder, W. A., and Kendall, A. G.: Hemoglobin Kenya, the product of fusion of γ and β polypeptide chains, Arch. Biochem. Biophys. **153:**850, 1972.

171. Hunt, J. A., and Ingram, V. M.: Abnormal Human Haemoglobins. VI. The chemical difference between haemoglobins A and E, Biochim. Biophys. Acta **49:**520, 1961.

172. Hunt, J. A., and Ingram, V. M.: Abnormal Human Haemoglobins. IV. The chemical difference between normal human haemoglobin and haemoglobin C, Biochim. Biophys. Acta **42:**409, 1960.

173. Hyde, R. D., Kinderlerer, J. L., Lehmann, H., and Hall, M. D.: Haemoglobin J Rajappen: α90 (FG2) Lys → Thr, Biochim. Biophys. Acta **243:**515, 1971.

174. Idelson, L. I., Didkowsky, N. A., Casey, R., Lorkin, P. A., and Lehmann, H.: New unstable haemoglobin (Hb Moscva, β24(B6)Gly → Asp) found in the U.S.S.R., Nature **249:**768, 1974.

175. Idelson, L. I., Didkovsky, N. A., Filippova, A. V., Casey, R., Kynoch, P. A. M., and Lehmann, H.: Haemoglobin Volga, β27, (B9)Ala → Asp: a new highly unstable haemoglobin with a suppressed charge. F.E.B.S. Lett. **58:**122, 1975.

176. Ikkala, E., Koskela, J., Pikkarainen, P., and Rahiala, E.: Hb Helsinki: a variant with a high oxygen affinity and a substitution at a 2,3-DPG binding site (β^{82} [EF6]Lys → Met), Acta Haematol. **56:**257, 1976.

177. Imai, K., and Lehmann, H.: The oxygen affinity of haemoglobin Tak: a variant with an elongated β chain, Biochim. Biophys. Acta **412:**288, 1975.

178. Imamura, T., Fujita, S., Ohta, Y., Hanada, M., and Yanase, T.: Hemoglobin Yoshizuka (G10(108)βAsparagine → Aspartic acid): a new variant with a reduced oxygen affinity from a Japanese family, J. Clin. Invest. **48:**2341, 1969.

179. Ingram, V. M.: Abnormal human Haemoglobins. III. The chemical difference between normal and sickle cell hemoglobins, Biochim. Biophys. Acta **36:**402, 1959.

180. Jackson, J. M., Yates, A., and Huehns, E. R.: Haemoglobin Perth: β32(B14) Leu → Pro: an unstable haemoglobin causing haemolysis, Br. J. Haematol. **25:**607, 1973.

181. Jenkins, G. C., Beale, D., Black, A. J., Huntsman, G. R., and Lehmann, H.: Haemoglobin F Texas-I (α2γ2 5 Glu → Lys): a variant of haemoglobin F, Br. J. Haematol. **13:**252, 1967.

182. Jensen, M., Oski, F. A., Nathan, D. G., and Bunn, H. F.: Hemoglobin Syracuse (α2β2 143(H21)His → Pro): a new high-affinity variant detected by special electrophoretic methods, J. Clin. Invest. **55:**469, 1975.

183. Jones, R. T., and Brimhall, B.: Structural characterization of two δ chain variants, J. Biol. Chem. **242:**5141, 1967.

184. Jones, R. T., Brimhall, B., and Gray, G.: Hemoglobin British Columbia [α2β2 101(G3)Glu → Lys]: a new variant with high oxygen affinity, Hemoglobin **1:**171, 1976.

185. Jones, R. T., Brimhall, B., Huehns, E. R., and Barnicot, N. A.: Hemoglobin Sphakiá: a delta chain variant of hemoglobin A$_2$ from Crete, Science **151:**1406, 1966.

186. Jones, R. T., Brimhall, B., Huehns, E. R., and Motulsky, A. G.: Structural characterization of hemoglobin N Seattle: α2Aβ2 61 Lys → Glu, Biochim. Biophys. Acta **154:**278, 1968.

187. Jones, R. T., Brimhall, B., Huisman, T. H. J., Klei-

hauer, E., and Betke, K.: Hemoglobin Freiburg: abnormal hemoglobin due to deletion of a single amino acid residue, Science **154:**1024, 1966.

188. Jones, R. T., Brimhall, B., and Lisker, R.: Chemical characterization of hemoglobin Mexico and hemoglobin Chiapas, Biochim. Biophys. Acta **154:**488, 1968.

189. Jones, R. T., Brimhall, B., Pootrakul, S., and Gray, G.: Hemoglobin Vancouver [α$_2$β$_2$73(E17)Asp → Tyr]: its structure and function, J. Mol. Evol. **9:**37, 1976.

190. Jones, R. T., and Koler, R. D.: Functional studies of seven new abnormal hemoglobins. In sixteenth International Congress of Hematology, September 1976. (Abstract Nos. 1 to 21, p. 48)

191. Jones, R. T., Koler, R. D., Duerst, M. L., and Dhindsa, S.: Hemoglobin Willamette [α2β2 51Pro → Arg (D2)]: a new abnormal human hemoglobin, Hemoglobin **1:**45, 1976.

192. Jones, R. T., Osgood, E. E., Brimhall, B., and Koler, R. D.: Hemoglobin Yakima: 1. clinical and biochemical studies, J. Clin. Invest. **46:**1840, 1967.

193. Keeling, M. M., Ogden, L. L., Wrightstone, R. N., Wilson, J. B., Reynolds, C. A., Kitchens, J. L., and Huisman, T. H. J.: Hemoglobin Louisville (β42 (CD1) Phe → Leu): an unstable variant causing mild hemolytic anemia, J. Clin. Invest. **50:**2395, 1971.

194. Kendall, A. G., Lang, A., and Lehmann, H.: Haemoglobin J Nyanza: α21 (B2) Ala → Asp, Biochim. Biophys. Acta **310:**357, 1973.

195. Kendall, A. G., Wilson, J. B., Cope, N., Bolch, K., and Huisman, T. H. J.: Hb Vaasa or α2β2 (39(C5) Gln → Glu): a mildly unstable variant found in a Finnish family, Hemoglobin **1:**292, 1977.

196. Kennedy, C. C., Blundell, G., Lorkin, P. A., Lang, A., and Lehmann, H.: Haemoglobin Belfast 15(A12) Tryptophan → Arginine: a new unstable haemoglobin variant, Br. Med. J. **4:**324, 1974.

197. Kilmartin, J. V., Najman, A., and Labie, D.: Hemoglobin Cochin Port-Royal consequences of the replacement of the β chain C-terminal by an arginine, Biochim. Biophys. Acta **400:**354, 1975.

198. King, M. A. R., Wiltshire, B. G., Lehmann, H., and Morimoto, H.: An unstable haemoglobin with reduced oxygen affinity: Haemoglobin Peterborough, β111(G13) Valine → Phenylalanine, its interaction with normal haemoglobin and with haemoglobin Lepore, Br. J. Haematol. **22:**125, 1972.

199. Kleckner, H. B., Wilson, J. B., Lindeman, J. G., Stevens, P. D., Niazi, G., Hunter, E., Chen, C. J., and Huisman, T. H. J.: Hemoglobin Fort Gordon or α2β2 145 Tyr → Asp: a new high-oxygen-affinity-hemoglobin variant, Biochim. Biophys. Acta **400:**343, 1975.

200. Kleihauer, E. F., Reynolds, C. A., Dozy, A. M., Wilson, J. B., Moores, R. R., Berenson, M. P., Wright, C.-S., and Huisman, T. H. J.: Hemoglobin Bibba Biochim. Biophys. Acta **154:**220, 1968.

201. Kleihauer, E., Waller, H. D., Benöhr, H. C., Kohne, E., and Gelinsky, P.: Hb Tübingen eine neue β-Kettenvariante (βTp 10-12) mit erhöhter Spontanoxydation, Klin. Wochenschr. **48:**651, 1971.

202. Kohne, E., Kley, H. P., and Kleihauer, E.: Structural and functional characteristics of Hb Tübingen: β^{106} (G8) Leu → Gln, F.E.B.S. Lett. **64:**443, 1976.

203. Koler, R. D., Jones, R. T., Bigley, R. H., Litt, M., Lovrien, E., Brooks, R., Lahey, M. E., and Fowler, R.: Hemoglobin Casper: β106(G8)Leu → Pro, a contemporary mutation, Am. J. Med. **55:**549, 1973.

204. Konotey-Ahulu, F. I. D., Gallo, E., Lehmann, H., and Ringelhann, B.: Haemoglobin Korle-Bu (β73 Aspartic acid → Asparagine) showing one of the two amino acid substitutions of haemoglobin C Harlem, J. Med. Genet. **5:**107, 1968.

205. Konotey-Ahulu, F. I. D., Kinderlerer, J. L., Lehmann, H., and Ringelhann, B.: Haemoglobin Osu-Christiansborg: a new β-chain variant of haemoglobin A (β52(D3) Aspartic acid → Asparagine) in combination with haemoglobin S, J. Med. Genet. **8**:302, 1971.

206. Kraus, A. P., Miyaji, T., Iuchi, I., and Kraus, L. M.: Memphis: a new variety of sickle cell anemia with clinically mild symptoms due to an α-chain variant of hemoglobin (α23Glu NH2), J. Lab. Clin. Med. **66**:886, 1965.

207. Kurachi, S., Hermodson, M., Hornung, S., and Stamatoyannopoulos, G.: Structure of Haemoglobin Seattle, Nature (New Biol.) **243**:275, 1973.

208. Labossiere, A., Hill, J. R., and Vella, F.: A new βTp V Hemoglobin variant: Hb Edmonton, Clin. Biochem. **4**:114, 1971.

209. Labossiere, A., Vella, F., Hiebert, J., and Galbraith, P.: Hemoglobin Deer Lodge: α2β2 2 His → Arg, Clin. Biochem. **5**:46, 1972.

210. Larkin, I. L. M., Baker, T., Lorkin, P. A., Lehmann, H., Black, A. J., and Huntsman, R. G.: Haemoglobin F Texas-II (α2γ2 6 Glu → Lys): the second of the haemoglobin F Texas variants, Br. J. Haematol. **14**:233, 1968.

211. Lee-Potter, J. P., Deacon-Smith, R. A., Simpkiss, M. J., Kamuzora, H., and Lehmann, H.: A new cause of haemolytic anaemia in the newborn: a description of an unstable fetal haemoglobin: F Poole, α2Gγ2 130 Tryptophan → Glycine, J. Clin. Pathol. **28**:317, 1975.

212. Lehmann, H., Casey, R., Lang, A., Stathopoulou, R., Imai, K., Tuchinda, S., Vinai, P., and Flatz, G.: Haemoglobin Tak: a β-chain elongation, Br. J. Haematol. **31**(suppl.):119, 1975.

213. Lehmann, H., and Charlesworth, D.: Observations on haemoglobin P (Congo type), Biochem. J. **119**:43, 1970.

214. Lie Injo, L. E., Kamuzora, H., and Lehmann, H.: Haemoglobin F Malaysia: α2γ2 1(NA1) Glycine → Cysteine: 136 Glycine, J. Med. Genet. **11**:25, 1974.

215. Lie Injo, Luan Eng, Pribada, W., Boerma, F. W., Efremov, G. D., Wilson, J. B., Reynolds, C. A., and Huisman, T. H. J.: Hemoglobin A2: Indonesia or α2δ2 69(E13) Gly → Arg, Biochim. Biophys. Acta **229**:335, 1971.

216. Lie Injo, Luan Eng, Wiltshire, B. G., and Lehmann, H.: Structural identification of haemoglobin F Kuala Lumpur (α2γ2 22(B4)Asp → Gly: 136 Ala). Biochim. Biophys. Acta **322**:224, 1973.

217. Lines, J. G., and McIntosh, R.: Oxygen binding by Haemoglobin J Cape Town (α2 92 Arg → Gln), Nature **215**:297, 1967.

218. Lokich, J. J., Mahoney, C., Bunn, H. F., Bruckheimer, S. M., and Ranney, H.: Hemoglobin Brigham (α2Aβ2 100 Pro → Leu): hemoglobin variant associated with familial erythrocytosis, J. Clin. Invest. **52**:2060, 1973.

219. Lorkin, P. A., Charlesworth, D., Lehmann, H., Rahbar, S., Tuchinda, S., and Lie Injo Luan Eng.: two haemoglobins Q, α74(EF3) and α75(EF4) Aspartic acid → Histidine, Br. J. Haematol. **19**:117, 1970.

220. Lorkin, P. A., Huntsman, R. G., Ager, J. A. M., Lehmann, H., Vella, F., and Darbre, P. D.: Haemoglobin G Norfolk: α85 (F6) Asp → Asn, Biochim. Biophys. Acta **379**:22, 1975.

221. Lorkin, P. A., Lehmann, H., Fairbanks, V. F., Berglund, G., and Leonhardt, T.: Two new pathological haemoglobins: Olmsted β141(H19) Leu → Arg and Malmö: β97(FG4) His → Gln, Biochem. J. **119**:68, 1970.

222. Lorkin, P. A., Pietschmann, H., Braunsteiner, H., and Lehmann, H.: Structure of Haemoglobin Wien β130 (H8)Tyrosine → Aspartic acid: an unstable haemoglobin variant, Acta Haematol. **51**:351, 1974.

223. Lorkin, P. A., Stephens, A. D., Beard, M. E. J., Wrigley, P. F. M., Adams, L., and Lehmann, H.: Haemoglobin Rahere (β82 Lys → Thr): a new high affinity haemoglobin associated with decreased 2,3-diphosphoglycerate binding and relative polycythaemia, Br. Med. J. **4**:200, 1975.

224. Loukopoulos, D., Kaltsoya, A., and Fessas, Ph.: On the chemical abnormality of Hb "Alexandra" a fetal hemoglobin variant, Blood **33**:114, 1969.

225. Lutcher, C. L., and Huisman, T. H. J.: Hb-Leslie, an unstable variant due to deletion of Gln β131, occurring in combination with β⁰-thalassemia, Hb-S, and Hb-C, Clin. Res. **23**:278A, 1975.

226. Lutcher, C. L., Wilson, J. B., Gravely, M. E., Stevens, P. D., Chen, C. J., Lindeman, J. G., Wong, S. C., Miller, A., Gottlieb, M., and Huisman, T. H. J.: Hb Leslie: an unstable hemoglobin due to deletion of Glutaminyl residue β131 (H9) occurring in association with β⁰-thalassemia, Hb C, and Hb S, Blood **47**:99, 1976.

227. McCurdy, P. R., Fox, J., and Moo-Penn, W.: Apparent duplication of the β-chain gene in man, Am. J. Hum. Genet. **27**:62A, 1975.

228. Maekawa, M., Maekawa, T., Fujiwara, N., Tabara, K., and Matsuda, G.: Hemoglobin Nagasaki: α2β2 17 Glu: a new abnormal human hemoglobin found in one family in Nagasaki, Int. J. Protein Res. **2**:147, 1970.

229. Mant, M. J., and Salkie, M. L., Cope, N., Appling, F., Bolch, K., Jayalakshmi, M., Gravely, M., Wilson, J. B., and Huisman, T. H. J.: Hb Alberta or α2β2 (101(G3) Glu → Gly): a new high-oxygen-affinity variant causing erythrocytosis, Hemoglobin **1**:183, 1976.

230. Marengo-Rowe, A. J., Beale, D., and Lehmann, H.: New human haemoglobin variant from Southern Arabia: G-Audhali (α23 (B4) Glutamic acid → Valine) and the variability of B4 in human haemoglobin, Nature **219**:1164, 1968.

231. Marengo-Rowe, A. J., Lorkin, P. A., Gallo, E., and Lehmann, H.: Haemoglobin Dhofar: a new variant from Southern Arabia, Biochim. Biophys. Acta **168**:58, 1968.

232. Marti, H. R., Pik, C., and Mosimann, P.: Eine neue Hämoglobin I-variante: Hb I Interlaken, Acta Haematol. **32**:9, 1964.

233. Marti, H. R., Winterhalter, K. H., Di Iorio, E. E., Lorkin, P. A., and Lehmann, H.: Hb Altdorf α2β2(H13) Ala → Pro: a new electrophoretically silent unstable haemoglobin variant from Switzerland, F.E.B.S. Lett. **63**:193, 1976.

234. Milner, P. F., Corley, C. C., Pomeroy, W. L., Wilson, J. B., Gravely, M., and Huisman, T. H. J.: Thalassemia intermedia caused by heterozygosity for both β-thalassemia and hemoglobin Saki (β14 (A11)Leu → Pro), Am. J. Hematol. **1**:283, 1976.

235. Minnich, V., Hill, R. J., Khuri, P. D., and Anderson, M. E.: Hemoglobin Hope: a beta chain variant, Blood **25**:830, 1965.

236. Miyaji, T., Iuchi, I., Takeda, I., and Shibata, S.: Hemoglobin Shimonoseki (α2 54Arg β2A): a slow-moving hemoglobin found in a Japanese family, with special reference to its chemistry, Acta Haematol. Jpn. **26**:531, 1963.

237. Miyaji, T., Iuchi, I., Yamamoto, K., Ohba, Y., and Shibata, S.: Amino acid substitution of hemoglobin Ube 2 (α2 68Asp β2): an example of successful application of partial hydrolysis of peptide with 5% acetic acid, Clin. Chim. Acta **16**:347, 1967.

238. Miyaji, T., Oba, Y., Yamamoto, K., Shibata, S., Iuchi, I., and Hamilton, H. B.: Hemoglobin Hijiyama: a new fast-moving hemoglobin in a Japanese family, Science **159**:204, 1968.

239. Miyaji, T., Ohba, Y., Yamamoto, K., Shibata, S., Iuchi, I., and Takenaka, H.: Japanese haemoglobin variant, Nature **217**:89, 1968.

240. Miyaji, T., Suzuki, H., Ohba, Y., and Shibata, S.: Hemoglobin Agenogi (α2β2 90 Lys): a slow-moving hemo-

globin of a Japanese family resembling Hb-E, Clin. Chim. Acta **14**:624, 1966.

241. Miyaji, T., Iuchi, I., Shibata, S., Takeda, I., and Tamura, A.: Possible amino acid substitution in the α-chain (α87 Tyr) of Hb M Iwate, Acta Haematol. Jpn. **26**:538, 1963.

242. Monn, E., Gaffney, P. J., and Lehmann, H.: Hemoglobin Sögn (β14 Arginine): a new haemoglobin variant, Scand. J. Haematol. **5**:353, 1968.

243. Moo-Penn, W. F.: Personal communication, 1977.

244. Moo-Penn, W. F., Bechtel, K. C., Johnson, M. H., Jue, D. L., Holland, S., Huff, C., and Schmidt, R. M.: Hemoglobin Jackson, α127 (H10) Lys → Asn, Am. J. Clin. Pathol. **66**:453, 1976.

245. Moo-Penn, W. F., Bechtel, K. C., Johnson, M. H., Jue, D. L., Therrell, B. L., Jr., Morrison, B. Y., and Schmidt, R. M.: Hemoglobin Fannin-Lubbock [α2β2¹¹⁹ (GH2) Gly → Asp]: a new hemoglobin variant at the α₁β₁ contact, Biochim. Biophys. Acta **453**:472, 1976.

246. Moo-Penn, W. F., Johnson, M. H., Bechtel, K. C., Jue, D. L., Therrell, Jr., B. L., and Schmidt, R. M.: Hemoglobins Austin and Waco: two hemoglobins with substitutions in the α₁β₂ contact region, Arch. Biochem. Biophys. **179**:86, 1977.

247. Moo-Penn, W. F., Jue, D. L., Bechtel, K. C., Johnson, M. H., and Schmidt, R. M.: Hemoglobin Providence: a human hemoglobin variant occurring in two forms *in vivo*, J. Biol. Chem. **251**:7557, 1976.

248. Moo-Penn, W. F., Jue, D. L., Johnson, M. H., Wilson, S. M., Therrell, Jr., B., and Schmidt, R. M.: Hemoglobin Tarrant: α126(H9)Asp → Asn: a new hemoglobin variant in the α₁β₁ contact region showing high oxygen affinity and reduced cooperativity, Biochim. Biophys. Acta **490**:443, 1977.

249. Muller, C. J., and Kingma, S.: Haemoglobin Zürich α2β2 63 Arg, Biochim. Biophys. Acta **50**:595, 1961.

250. Nagel, R. L., Joshua, L., Johnson, J., Landau, L., Bookchin, R. M., and Harris, M. B.: Hemoglobin Beth Israel: a mutant causing clinically apparent cyanosis, N. Engl. J. Med. **295**:125, 1976.

251. Niazi, G. A., Efremov, G. D., Nikolov, N., Hunter, E., Jr., and Huisman, T. H. J.: Hemoglobin Strumica or α₂¹¹²(G19)His → Argβ₂. (With an addendum: Hemoglobin J Paris-I, α₂¹²(A10)Ala → Asp β₂ in the same population), Biochim. Biophys. Acta **412**:181, 1975.

252. Nute, P. E., Stamatoyannopoulos, G., Hermodson, M. A., Roth, D., and Hornung, S.: Hemoglobinopathic erythrocytosis due to a new electrophoretically silent variant, Hemoglobin San Diego (β109(G11)Val → Met), J. Clin. Invest. **53**:320, 1974.

253. Ohba, Y., Miyaji, T., Matsuoka, M., Sugiyama, K., Suzuki, T., and Sugiura, T.: Hemoglobin Mizuho or beta 68 (E 12) Leucine → Proline: a new unstable variant associated with severe hemolytic anemia, Hemoglobin **1**:467, 1977.

254. Ohba, Y., Miyaji, T., Matsuoka, M., Takeda, I., Fukuba, Y., Shibata, S., and Ohkura, K.: Hemoglobin Matsue-Oki: Alpha 75 (EF4) Aspartic acid → Asparagine, Hemoglobin **1**:383, 1977.

255. Ohba, Y., Miyaji, T., Matsuoka, M., Yokoyama, M., Numakura, H., Nagata, K., Takebe, Y., Izumi, Y., and Shibata, S.: Hemoglobin Hirosaki (α43[CE 1]Phe → Leu): a new unstable variant, Biochim. Biophys. Acta **405**:155, 1975.

256. Opfell, R. W., Lorkin, P. A., and Lehmann, H.: Hereditary nonspherocytic haemolytic anaemia with postsplenectomy inclusion bodies and pigmenturia caused by an unstable haemoglobin Santa Ana: β88(F4)Leucine → Proline, J. Med. Genet. **5**:292, 1968.

257. Orringer, E. P., Wilson, J. B., Huisman, T. H. J.: Hemoglobin Chapel Hill or α₂ 74 (Asp → Gly) β₂, F.E.B.S. Lett. **65**:297, 1976.

258. Ostertag, W., and Smith, E. W.: Hemoglobin-Lepore Baltimore: a third type of a δβ crossover (δ50, β86), European J. Biochem. **10**:371, 1969.

259. Ostertag, W., von Ehrenstein, G., and Charache, S.: Duplicated α-chain genes in Hopkins-2 haemoglobin from man and evidence for unequal crossing over between them, Nature (New Biology) **237**:90, 1972.

260. Outeirino, J., Casey, R., White, J. M., and Lehmann, H.: Haemoglobin Madrid, β115(G17)Alanine → Proline: an unstable variant associated with haemolytic anaemia, Acta Haematol. **52**:53, 1974.

261. Paniker, N. V., Lin, K. D., Krantz, S. B., Flexner, J. M., Wasserman, B. K., and Puett, D.: Hemoglobin Vanderbilt (α2β2 89(F5)Ser → Arg): a new mutant with decreased response to 2,3-diphosphoglycerate, Hemoglobin **1**:302, 1977.

262. Perutz, M. F., del Pulsinelli, P., Ten Eyck, L., Kilmartin, J. V., Shibata, S., Iuchi, I., Miyaji, T., and Hamilton, H.: Haemoglobin Hiroshima and the mechanism of the alkaline Bohr effect, Nature (New Biol.) **232**:147, 1971.

263. Pootrakul, S., and Dixon, G. H.: Hemoglobin Mahidol: a new hemoglobin α-chain mutant, Canad. J. Biochem. **48**:1066, 1970.

264. Pootrakul, S., Kematorn, B., Na-Nakorn, S., and Suanpan, S.: A new haemoglobin variant: Haemoglobin Anantharaj alpha 11 (A9) Lysine → Glutamic acid, Biochim. Biophys. Acta **405**:161, 1975.

265. Poyart, C., Krishnamoorth, R., Bursaux, E., Gacon, G., and Labie, D.: Structural and functional studies of haemoglobin Suresnes or α2 141 (HC3) Arg → His β2: a new high oxygen affinity mutant, F.E.B.S. Lett. **69**:103, 1976.

266. Praxedes, H., and Lehmann, H.: Haemoglobin Niteroi: a new unstable variant, Paper presented at fourteenth international congress of hematology, Sao Paulo, 1972.

267. Rahbar, S.: Haemoglobin D Iran: β2 22 Glutamic acid → Glutamine (B4), Br. J. Haematol. **24**:31, 1973.

268. Rahbar, S., Ala, F., Akhavan, E., Nowzari, G., Shoa'I, I., and Zamanianpoor, H.: Two new haemoglobins: Haemoglobin Perspolis [α64 (E13) Asp → Tyr] and Haemoglobin J-Kurosh [α19 (AB) Ala → Asp], Biochim. Biophys. Acta **427**:119, 1976.

269. Rahbar, S., Beale, D., Isaacs, W. A., and Lehmann, H.: Abnormal haemoglobins in Iran: observations of a new variant, haemoglobin J Iran (α2β2 77His → Arg), Br. Med. J. **1**:674, 1967.

270. Rahbar, S., Kinderlerer, J. L., and Lehmann, H.: Haemoglobin L Persian Gulf: α57 (E6) Glycine → Arginine, Acta Haematol. **42**:169, 1969.

271. Rahbar, S., Mahdavi, N., Nowzari, G., and Mostafavi, I.: Hemoglobin Arya: α₂47(CD5) Aspartic acid → Asparagine, Biochim. Biophys. Acta **386**:525, 1975.

272. Rahbar, S., Nowzari, G., and Daneshmand, P.: Haemoglobin Daneshgah-Tehran α2 72(EF1) Histidine → Arginine β2A, Nature (New Biol.) **245**:268, 1973.

273. Rahbar, S., Nowzari, G., Haydari, H. and Daneshmand, P.: Haemoglobin Hamadan αA2β2 56 Glycine → Arginine(D7), Biochim. Biophys. Acta **379**:645, 1975.

274. Ranney, H. M., Jacobs, A. S., and Nagel, R. L.: Haemoglobin New York, Nature **213**:876, 1967.

275. Ranney, H. M., Jacobs, A. S., Ramot, B., and Bradley, Jr., T. B.: Hemoglobin NYU: a delta chain variant, α2δ2 12Lys, J. Clin. Invest. **48**:2057, 1969.

276. Ranney, H. M., Jacobs, A. S., Udem, L., and Zalusky, R.: Hemoglobin Riverdale-Bronx: an unstable hemoglobin resulting from the substitution of arginine for glycine at helical residue B6 of the β polypeptide chain, Biochim. Biophys. Acta **33**:1004, 1968.

277. Reed, C. S., Hampson, R., Gordon, S., Jones, R. T., Novy, M. J., Brimhall, B., Edwards, M. J., and Koler, R. D.: Erythrocytosis secondary to increased oxygen af-

finity of a mutant hemoglobin, hemoglobin Kempsey, Blood **31**:623, 1968.

278. Reed, R. E., Winter, W. P., and Rucknagel, D. L.: Haemoglobin Inkster (α2 85 Aspartic acid → Valine β2) coexisting with β-thalassemia in a Caucasian family, Br. J. Haematol. **26**:475, 1974.

279. Reynolds, C. A., and Huisman, T. H. J.: Hemoglobin Russ or α2 51Arg β2, Biochim. Biophys. Acta **130**:541, 1966.

280. Ricco, G., Pich, P. G., Mazza, U., Rossi, G., Ajmar, F., Arese, P., and Gallo, E.: Hb J Sicilia: β65 (E9)Lys → Asn, a beta homologue of Hb Zambia, F.E.B.S. Lett. **39**:200, 1974.

281. Rieder, R. F., Clegg, J. B., Weiss, H. J., Christy, N. P., and Rabinowitz, R.: Hemoglobin A₂-Roosevelt: α2δ2 20 Val → Glu, Biochim. Biophys. Acta **439**:501, 1976.

282. Rieder, R. F., Oski, F. A., and Clegg, J. B.: Hemoglobin Philly (β35 Tyrosine → Phenylalanine): studies in the molecular pathology of hemoglobin, J. Clin. Invest. **48**:1627, 1969.

283. Rieder, R. F., Wolf, D. J., Clegg, J. B. and Lee, S. L.: Rapid postsynthetic destruction of unstable haemoglobin Bushwick, Nature **254**:725, 1975.

234. Romain, P. L., Schwartz, A. D., Shamsuddin, M., Adams III, J. G., Mason, R. G., Vida, L. N., and Honig, G. R.: Hemoglobin J Chicago (β76(E20)Ala → Asp): a new hemoglobin variant resulting from substitution of an external residue, Blood **45**:387, 1975.

285. Rosa, J., Labie, D., Wajcman, H., Boigne, J. M., Cabannes, R., Bierme, R., and Ruffie, J.: Haemoglobin I Toulouse: β66(E10)Lys → Glu: a new abnormal hemoglobin with a mutation localized on the E10 porphyrin surrounding zone, Nature **223**:190, 1969.

286. Rosa, J., Maleknia, N., Vergoz, D., and Dunet, R.: Une nouvelle hémoglobine anormale: l'hémoglobin Jα Paris 12 Ala → Asp. Nov, Rev. Fr. Hematol. **6**:423, 1965.

287. Rucknagel, D. L., et al.: Clin. Res. **26**:22A, 1978.

288. Rucknagel, D. L., Brandt, N. J., and Spencer, H. H.: α-chain mutants of human hemoglobin contributing to the genetics of the α-chain locus. In Proceedings of first inter-American symposium on hemoglobins, Caracus, 1969.

289. Rucknagel, D. L., Glynn, K. P., and Smith, J. R.: Hemoglobin Ypsilanti characterized by increased oxygen affinity, abnormal polymerization, and erythremia, Clin. Res. **15**:270, 1967.

290. Sacker, L. S., Beale, D., Black, A. J., Huntsman, R. G., Lehmann, H., and Lorkin, P. A.: Haemoglobin F Hull (γ121 Glutamic acid → Lysine), homologous with Haemoglobins O and O Indonesia, Br. Med. J. **3**:531, 1967.

291. Sansone, G., Carrell, R. W., and Lehmann, H.: Haemoglobin Genova: β28(B10) Leucine → Proline, Nature **214**:877, 1967.

292. Schneider, R. G., Alperin, J. B., Brimhall, B., and Jones, R. T.: Hemoglobin P (α2β2 117 Arg): structure and properties, J. Lab. Clin. Med. **73**:616, 1969.

293. Schneider, R. G., Atkins, R. J., Hosty, T. S., Tomlin, G., Casey, R., Lehmann, H., Lorkin, P. A., and Nagai, K.: Haemoglobin Titusville: α94 Asp → Asn, a new haemoglobin with a lowered affinity for oxygen, Biochim. Biophys. Acta **400**:365, 1975.

294. Schneider, R. G., Berkman, N. L., Brimhall, B., and Jones, R. T.: Hemoglobin Fannin-Lubbock [α₂β₂¹¹⁹ (GH2)Gly → Asp]: a slightly unstable mutant, Biochim. Biophys. Acta **453**:478, 1976.

295. Schneider, R. G., Brimhall, B., Jones, R. T., Bryant, R., Mitzhell, C. B., and Goldberg, A. I.: Hb Fort Worth: α27Glu → Gly (B8) a variant present in unusually low concentration, Biochim. Biophys. Acta **243**:164, 1971.

296. Schneider, R. G., Haggard, M. E., Gustavson, L. P., Brimhall, B., and Jones, R. T.: Genetic haemoglobin abnormalities in about 9,000 Black and 7,000 White newborns: Haemoglobin F Dickinson (Aγ97 His → Arg), a new variant, Br. J. Haematol. **28**:515, 1974.

297. Schneider, R. G., Hettig, R. A., Bilunos, M., and Brimhall, B.: Hemoglobin Baylor [α2β2 81(EF5) Leu → Arg]: an unstable mutant with high oxygen affinity, Hemoglobin **1**:85, 1976.

298. Schneider, R. G., Hosty, T. S., Tomlin, G., Atkins, R., Brimhall, B., and Jones, R. T.: Hb Mobile [α2β2 73(E17)Asp → Val]: a new variant, Biochem. Genet. **13**:411, 1975.

299. Schneider, R. G., Satoshi, U., Alperin, J. B., Brimhall, B., and Jones, R. T.: Hemoglobin Sabine, Beta 91(F7) Leu → Pro: an unstable variant causing severe anemia with inclusion bodies, N. Engl. J. Med. **280**:739, 1969.

300. Seid-Akhaven, M., Winter, W. P., Abramson, R. K., and Rucknagel, D. L.: Hemoglobin Wayne: a frameshift variant occurring in two distinct forms, Ann. Meeting Am. Soc. Hemat. Miami (Abstract No. 9), 1972.

301. Sharma, R. S., Harding, D. L., Wong, S. C., Wilson, J. B., Gravely, M. E., and Huisman, T. H. J.: A new δ chain variant: haemoglobin-A₂-Melbourne or α2δ2 43Glu → Lys(CD2), Biochim. Biophys. Acta **359**:233, 1974.

302. Sharma, R. S., Williams, L., Wilson, J. B., and Huisman, T. H. J.: Hemoglobin-A₂-Coburg or α2δ2 116 Arg → His (G18), Biochim. Biophys. Acta **393**:379, 1975.

303. Shibata, S., Miyaji, T., Iuchi, I., Ueda, S., and Takeda, I.: Hemoglobin Hikari (α2Aβ2 61Asp NH2): a fast moving hemoglobin found in two unrelated Japanese families, Clin. Chim. Acta **10**:101, 1964.

304. Shibata, S., Miyaji, T., Ueda, S., Matsuoka, M., Iuchi, I., Yamada, K., and Shinkai, N.: Hemoglobin Tochigi (Beta 56-59 deleted): a new unstable hemoglobin discovered in a Japanese family, Proc. Jpn. Acad. **46**:440, 1970.

305. Shibata, S., Yawata, Y., Yamada, O., Koresawa, S., and Ueda, S.: Altered erythropoiesis and increased hemolysis in hemoglobin M Akita (M Hyde Park β92 His → Tyr) disease, Hemoglobin **1**:111, 1976.

306. Sick, K., Beale, D., Irvine, D., Lehmann, H., Goodall, P. T., and MacDougall, S.: Haemoglobin G Copenhagen and haemoglobin J Cambridge: two new β-chain variants of haemoglobin A, Biochim. Biophys. Acta **140**:231, 1967.

307. Smith, L. L., Plese, C. L., Barton, B. P., Charache, S., Wilson, J. B., and Huisman, T. H. J.: Subunit dissociation of the abnormal hemoglobins G Georgia (α2 95 Leu (G2)β2) and Rampa (α2 95 Ser (G2)β2), J. Biol. Chem. **247**:1433, 1972.

308. Stamatoyannopoulos, G., Nute, P. E., Adamson, J. W., Bellingham, A. J., Funk, D., and Hornung, S.: Hemoglobin Olympia (β20 Valine → Methionine): an electrophoretically silent variant associated with high oxygen affinity and erythrocytosis, J. Clin. Invest. **52**:342, 1973.

309. Steadman, J. H., Yates, A., and Huehns, E. R.: Idiopathic Heinz body anaemia: Hb-Bristol (β67(E11)Val → Asp), Br. J. Haematol. **18**:435, 1970.

310. Sukumaran, P. K., Merchant, S. M., Desai, M. P., Wiltshire, B. G., and Lehmann, H.: Haemoglobin Q (α64 (E 13) Aspartic acid → Histidine) associated with β-thalassemia in three Sindhi families, J. Med. Genet. **9**:436, 1972.

311. Sumida, I.: Studies of abnormal hemoglobins in western Japan, Frequency of visible hemoglobin variants, and chemical characterization of hemoglobin Sawara (α₂⁶ᴬˡᵃβ₂) and hemoglobin Mugino (Hb L Ferrara: α₂⁴⁷ᴳˡʸβ₂). Jap. J. Human Genet. **19**:343, 1975.

312. Sumida, I., Ohta, Y., Imamura, T., and Yanase, T.: Hemoglobin Sawara: α6 (A4) Aspartic acid → Alanine, Biochim. Biophys. Acta **322**:23, 1973.

313. Swenson, R. T., Hill, R. L., Lehmann, H., and Jim, R. T. S.: A chemical abnormality in hemoglobin G from Chinese individuals, J. Biol. Chem. **237:**1517, 1962.

314. Taketa, F., Antholine, W. E., Mauk, A. G., and Libnoch, J. A.: Nitrosyl-hemoglobin Wood: effects of inositol hexaphosphate on thiol reactivity and electron paramagnetic resonance spectrum, Biochemistry **14:**3229, 1975.

315. Taketa, F., Huang, Y. P., Libnoch, J. A., and Dessel, B. H.: Hemoglobin Wood β97(FG4) His → Leu: a new high-oxygen-affinity hemoglobin associated with familial erythrocytosis, Biochim. Biophys. Acta **400:**348, 1975.

316. Tangheroni, W., Zorcolo, G., Gallo, E., and Lehmann, H.: Haemoglobin J Sardegna: α50 (CD8) Histidine → Aspartic acid, Nature (London) **218:**470, 1968.

317. Tatsis, B., Sofroniadou, K., and Stergiopoulos, C. I.: Hemoglobin Pyrgos α2β2 83(EF7)Gly → Asp: a new hemoglobin variant in double heterozygosity with hemoglobin S, Blood **47:**827, 1976.

318. Tatsis, B., Sofroniadou, K., and Stergiopoulos, K.: Hemoglobin Pyrgos (α2β2 83Gly → Asp): a new hemoglobin (Hb) variant, In Annual meeting of American Society of Hematology, Miami, 1972. (Abstract No. 168.)

319. Tentori, L.: Personal Communication, International Committee for Standardization in Hematology, Kyoto, Japan, 1976.

320. Tentori, L.: Three examples of double heterozygosis beta-thalassemia and rare hemoglobin variant. In International symposium on abnormal hemoglobins and thalassemia, Istanbul, 1974. (Abstract 68.)

321. Tentori, L., Carta Sorcini, M., and Buccella, C.: Hemoglobin Abruzzo: beta 143 (H21)His → Arg, Clin. Chim. Acta **38:**258, 1972.

322. Thillet, J., Cohen-Solal, M., Seligmann, M., and Rosa, J.: Functional and physicochemical studies of Hemoglobin St. Louis β^{28} (B10) Leu → Gln, J. Clin. Invest. **58:**1098, 1976.

323. Tuchinda, S., Beale, D., and Lehmann, H.: A new haemoglobin in a Thai family: a case of haemoglobin Siriraj-β thalassemia, Br. Med. J. **1:**1583, 1965.

324. Van Ros, G., Beale, D., and Lehmann, H.: Haemoglobin Stanleyville II (α78 Asparagine → Lysine), Br. Med. J. **4:**92, 1968.

325. Vella, F., Casey, R., Lehmann, H., Labossiere, A., and Jones, T. G.: Haemoglobin Ottawa: α2 15(A13) Gly → Arg β2, Biochim. Biophys. Acta **336:**25, 1974.

326. Vella, F., Galbraith, P., Wilson, J. B., Wong, S. C., Folger, G. C., and Huisman, T. H. J.: Hemoglobin St. Claude or α2 127 (H10)Lys → Thr β2, Biochim. Biophys. Acta **365:**318, 1974.

327. Vella, F., Isaacs, W. A., and Lehmann, H.: Hemoglobin G Saskatoon: β22 Glu → Ala, Canad. J. Biochem. **45:**351, 1967.

328. Vella, F., Lorkin, P. A., Carrell, R. W., and Lehmann, H.: A new hemoglobin variant resembling hemoglobin E. Hemoglobin E Saskatoon: β22 Glu → Lys, Canad. J. Biochem. **45:**1385, 1967.

329. Vella, F., Wiltshire, B. G., Lehmann, H., and Galbraith, P.: Hemoglobin Winnipeg: α2 75 Asp → Tyr β2, Clin. Biochem. **6:**66, 1973.

330. Vettore, L., DeSandre, G., Dilorio, E. E., Winterhalter, K. H., Lang, A., and Lehmann, H.: A new abnormal hemoglobin O Padova, α30 (B11) Glu → Lys and a dyserythropoietic anemia with erythroblastic multinuclearity coexisting in the same patient, Blood **44:**869, 1974.

331. Vullo, C., Christofori, G., Salsini, G., Tentori, L., Marinucci, M., and Bruni, E.: Haemoglobin G Ferrara: β2 57(E1)Asn → Lys, Int. Res. Comm. System.

332. Wade, P. T., Jenkins, T., and Huehns, E. R.: Haemoglobin variant in a Bushman: Haemoglobin D β Bushman α2β2 16 Gly → Arg, Nature **216:**688, 1967.

333. Wade Cohen, P. T., Yates, A., Bellingham, A. J., and Huehns, E. R.: Amino-acid substitution on the α1β1 intersubunit contact of haemoglobin Camden β131(H9) Gln → Glu, Nature (New Biol.) **243:**467, 1973.

334. Wajcman, H., Belkhodja, O., and Labie, D.: Hb Setif: G1(94) αAsp → Tyr: a new α chain hemoglobin variant with substitution of the residue involved in a hydrogen bond between unlike subunits, F.E.B.S. Lett. **27:**298, 1972.

335. Wajcman, H., Krishnamoorthy, R., Gacon, G., Elion, J., Allard, C., and Labie, D.: A new hemoglobin variant involving the distal histidine: Hb Bicêtre (β 63 (E7) His → Pro), J. Mole. Med. **1:**187, 1976.

336. Wajcman, H., Labie, D., and Schapira, G.: Two new hemoglobin variants with deletion. Hemoglobin Tours: Thr β87 (F3) deleted and hemoglobin St. Antoine: Gly → Leu β74-75 (E18-19) deleted. Consequences for oxygen affinity and protein stability, Biochim. Biophys. Acta **295:**495, 1973.

337. Watson-Williams, E. J., Beale, D., Irvine, D., and Lehmann, H.: A new haemoglobin, D Ibadan (β87Threonine → Lysine), producing no sickle cell haemoglobin D disease with haemoglobin S, Nature **205:**1273, 1965.

338. Weatherall, D. J., Clegg, J. B., Callender, S. T., Wells, R. M. G., Gale, R. E., Huehns, E. R., Perutz, M. F., Viggiano, G., and Ho, C.: Haemoglobin Radcliffe (α2β2 99(GI)Ala): a high oxygen-affinity variant causing familial polycythaemia, Br. J. Haematol. **35:**177, 1977.

339. White, J. M., Brain, M. C., Lorkin, P. A., Lehmann, H., and Smith, M.: Mild "unstable haemoglobin haemolytic anaemia" caused by haemoglobin Shepherds Bush (β74(E18) Gly → Asp), Nature (London) **225:**939, 1970.

340. White, J. M., Szur, L., Gillies, I. D. S., Lorkin, P. A., and Lehmann, H.: Familial polycythaemia caused by a new haemoglobin variant: Hb Heathrow β103(G5)Phe → Leu, Br. Med. J. **3:**665, 1973.

341. Wilkinson, T., Ching Geh Chua, Carrell, R. W., Robin, H., Exner, T., Kit Ming Lee, and Kronenberg, H.: A new haemoglobin variant, Haemoglobin Camperdown β104(G6) Arginine → Serine, which has normal physiological function, Biochim. Biophys. Acta **393:**195, 1975.

342. Wiltshire, B. G., Clark, K. G. A., Lorkin, P. A., and Lehmann, H.: Haemoglobin Denmark Hill α95 (G2) Pro → Ala: a variant with unusual electrophoretic and oxygen binding properties, Biochim. Biophys. Acta **278:**459, 1972.

343. Winslow, R. M., Swenberg, M.-L., Gross, E., Chervenick, P. A., Buchman, R. R., and Anderson, W. F.: Hemoglobin McKees Rocks (α2β2 145Tyr → Term): a human "nonsense" mutation leading to a shortened β-chain, J. Clin. Invest. **57:**772, 1976.

344. Winter, W. P., Rucknagel, D. L., and Fielding, J.: Identification of several rare hemoglobin variants discovered in a population survey including a new variant Hb Garden State α82 Ala → Asp, Clin. Res. **26**(1):22A, 1978.

345. Yamaoka, K.: Hemoglobin Hirose: α2β2 37(C3)Tryptophan yielding Serine, Blood **38:**730, 1971.

346. Yanase, T., Hanada, M., Seita, M., Obya, I., Ohta, Y., Imamura, T., Fijimura, T., Kawasaki, K., and Yamaoka, K.: Molecular basis of morbidity: from a series of studies of hemoglobinopathies in Western Japan, Jpn. J. Human Genet. **13:**40, 1968.

347. Zak, S. J., Brimhall, B., Jones, R. T., and Kaplan, M. E.: Hemoglobin Andrew-Minneapolis α2Aβ2 144 Lys → Asn: a new high-oxygen-affinity mutant human hemoglobin, Blood **44:**543, 1974.

14 □ Sickle cell syndromes and other hemoglobinopathies

Howard A. Pearson

The sickle cell syndromes constitute a most important and clinically varied group of diseases.[151] Because the mutant autosomal gene responsible for the synthesis of Hb S reaches a high prevalence in certain geographic areas and ethnic groups, it has enormous clinical significance. In addition, the study of sickle cell conditions has led to monumental advances in the understanding of biochemical and population genetics.

The symptomatic disorder now designated as sickle cell anemia (Hb SS disease) was first described by Herrick in 1910 in a 20-year-old West Indian student who had recurrent jaundice, fever, and chronic ulceration of his lower extremities. The patient was anemic and striking morphologic abnormalities were present. His circulating blood contained bizarre, elongated, crescent-shaped red cells, which were fancifully compared to the blade of a sickle.[70] In subsequent years a series of reports described the induction of sickling by deoxygenation of red cells of clinically affected persons as well as asymptomatic ones. The disease and sickling phenomenon were shown to be familial, and by 1933 Diggs et al.[47] pointed out the clinical differences between the asymptomatic state now designated as sickle cell trait and the overt disease. Neel[115] clearly showed that both parents of children with sickle cell anemia had the trait. The sickling defect was shown to be caused by an abnormality of the red cells rather than the plasma.[64]

It was at the suggestion of William Castle that Pauling and his associates initiated their studies, launching the modern era of understanding about the hemoglobinopathies. When hemoglobin solutions from a patient with sickle cell anemia were subjected to electrophoresis, virtually all of the hemoglobin was electrophoretically abnormal, migrating considerably more slowly than Hb A. This abnormal protein was designated Hb S, or sickle hemoglobin. Studies of hemolysates from the parents of a patient with sickle cell anemia (obligate heterozygotes) revealed that approximately 40% of their hemoglobin was abnormal, the rest being normal Hb A.[122] The parents thus possess one normal Hb A gene and one responsible for the synthesis of Hb S. This gene is autosomal and the inheritance follows a standard Mendelian pattern (Fig. 14-1).

As hemoglobin biochemical methodology became more refined, it was demonstrated that the chemical abnormality characteristic of Hb S resides in the β-polypeptide chains. Hb S can therefore be designated as $\alpha_2\beta_2^S$. By means of the fingerprinting technique Ingram was able to show that the abnormality of Hb S is located in the number 26 tryptic digest peptide. Amino acid analysis revealed that in the number 6 amino acid position of that peptide, the normal negatively charged glutamic acid had been replaced by a neutral valine ($\beta6$ glu $\rightarrow$ val).[73] This change in molecular charge from -1 to 0 induces the different electrophoretic mobility. Finally, it has been determined that the number 6 tryptic digest peptide constitutes the *N*-

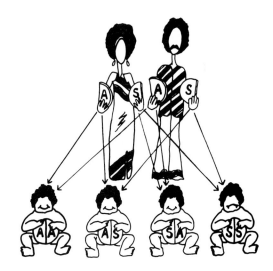

Fig. 14-1. Genetics of sickle cell anemia. Both parents possess one gene for normal hemoglobin (A) and one for sickle hemoglobin (S). With each pregnancy there is a 25% statistical chance that the child will have normal hemoglobin (AA) and a 25% chance of sickle cell anemia (SS). Fifty percent will have sickle cell trait (AS).

Table 14-1. Minimal gelling concentration and clinical severity in various sickle cell syndromes*

Disease	Degree of clinical severity	Hb S (%)	Other hemo-globins (%)	Minimum gelling concentration (gm/dl)
Hb SS	4+	≈90%	≈10 (F, A₂)	24
Hb S-β-thalassemia	2+, 3+	60-90	10-40 F (±A)	Variable
Hb SD	3+	45	55 (D)	20
Hb SO$_{Arab}$	3+	50	50 (O$_{Arab}$)	22
Hb SC	2+	50	50 (C)	27
Hb AS	0	40	60 (A)	30
Hb S–HPFH	0	70	30 (F)	37

*From Nathan, D. G., and Pearson, H. A.: In Nathan, D. G., and Oski, F. A., eds.: Hematology of infancy and childhood, Philadephia, 1974, W. B. Saunders Co.

terminal sequence of the polypeptide chain, thus precisely pinpointing the molecular pathology of sickle cell anemia.

PATHOPHYSIOLOGIC MECHANISM OF THE SICKLING PHENOMENA

The substitution of valine for glutamic acid in the number 6 position of the β-chain, the ultimate basis of sickling, produces its effect through profound changes in molecular stability and solubility. Solutions of Hb S, when fully oxygenated, are indistinguishable from normal. However, when these solutions are deoxygenated, a marked increase in viscosity and decrease in solubility occurs, indicating hemoglobin polymerization. When a solution containing 30% Hb S (approximately the concentration of Hb S within an intact red cell) is deoxygenated, the solution forms a semisolid gel. This physical change results from formation of light-polarizing tactoids or nematic liquid crystals.[67] The structure of these tactoids has been investigated in solutions of hemoglobin as well as in intact red cells. Tactoids are long rodlike structures formed from six or eight monomolecular filaments of deoxygenated Hb S molecules twisted around each other.[79,111] Multiple rods are organized in bundles arranged parallel to the long axis of the sickled red cells. At the present time the precise intermolecular and intramolecular interactions that produce sickling are not completely defined, but they clearly involve both hydrophobic and electrostatic bonds.[20,111]

Polymer formation occurs most effectively between molecules of Hb S, but some degree of copolymerization may be seen with other types of hemoglobin variants that have different capacities to participate in tactoid formation. This property can be quantitatively assessed by techniques measuring the minimal concentration at which various proportions of hemoglobins form gels after complete deoxygenation. The minimal gelling concentrations of hemolysates prepared from red cells of patients with several Hb S syndromes containing different hemoglobins are listed in Table 14-1. A progressively reduced degree of interaction with Hb S is noted, with a sequence of Hb S > D > O$_{Arab}$ > A > F. There is a good correlation between lower minimum gelling concentrations and clinical severity of syndromes involving these variants.[29]

TESTS FOR SICKLING

Hb S may be detected within red cells or hemoglobin solutions by a variety of simple tests. When red cells containing at least 20% Hb S are deoxygenated, they assume a crescent shape, whereas red cells lacking Hb S maintain a normal configuration. The rate of sickling as well as the degree of morphologic abnormality reflect both the proportion of Hb S and which other hemoglobins that are present in the red cells. In early studies of the sickling phenomenon, when deoxygenation was accomplished by merely sealing blood between glass slides, sickling often took 24 hours or more. Greater reliability and speed were obtained by the classic sickle cell preparation of Daland and Castle.[41] The blood to be tested is mixed with a freshly prepared solution of 2% sodium metabisulfite ($Na_2S_2O_2$) and sealed under a glass coverslip. Sickling ensues within a few minutes to several hours. Individual red cells containing less than 40% Hb S (as in sickle cell trait) sickle relatively slowly and assume a "holly" or "mulberry leaf" configuration. Cells that contain 50% or more of Hb S sickle much more rapidly, usually in a matter of minutes, and take on a filamentous shape (Fig. 14-2). Except in the early months of life when large amounts of Hb F are present, virtually all of the red cells of a person who possesses at least one Hb S gene can be induced to sickle, clearly indicating that Hb S is synthesized in every red cell. After infancy transfusions are the usual explanation for less than complete sickling, and a quantitative preparation offers a practical way to assess the adequacy of transfusion therapy in sickle cell anemia.[126]

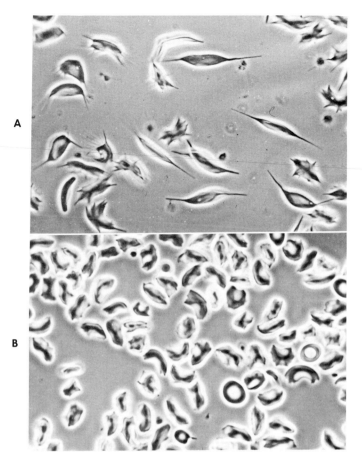

Fig. 14-2. Phase contrast microscopy of sickle cells in homozygous SS disease, **A**, and heterozygous AS trait, **B**. (Courtesy Dr. Julius Rutzky, Pontiac, Mich.)

The unique property of the markedly decreased solubility of solutions of deoxygenated Hb S may be used to identify Hb S. Solubility tests employ a buffered solution of a reducing agent such as sodium dithionate ($Na_2S_2O_4$) to which a small amount of blood or hemoglobin solution is added. If Hb S is present, it becomes deoxygenated and precipitates, making the solution turbid. Other hemoglobins stay in solution and the solution remains clear.[74]

Homemade solutions can be formulated for performance of solubility tests, and commercial reagents are also available. Solubility tests for the detection of Hb S can be performed by automated techniques, which are advantageous if mass screening is to be considered.[114] As ordinarily performed and interpreted, neither sickle cell preparation nor solubility tests provide definitive genotypic information. They do not reliably distinguish between persons who are heterozygous or homozygous for the Hb S gene. Furthermore, they do not detect other hemoglobin variants, such as Hb C or Hb D, that may interact with Hb S and have

genetic importance. Definitive diagnosis must be based on reliable electrophoretic or chromatographic techniques supplemented by family studies when possible.

GEOGRAPHIC DISTRIBUTION AND FREQUENCY OF THE SICKLE GENE

The sickle gene reaches a high prevalence in some ethnic groups and geographic areas (Fig. 14-3). The highest gene concentration occurs in equatorial Africa, where up to 40% of certain West African peoples possess the Hb S gene. The prevalence in regions of Africa away from the Equator both north and south, is considerably lower. The seventeenth and eighteenth century slave trade, exploiting predominantly West African peoples, resulted in the spread of the sickle gene into the New World. It occurs in about 8% of blacks in the United States and is relatively common in those regions in Latin America directly linked to the Spanish empire by the sea (Cuba, Puerto Rico, Panama, and Brazil), but not in others such as Mexico, Chile, and Peru.[151]

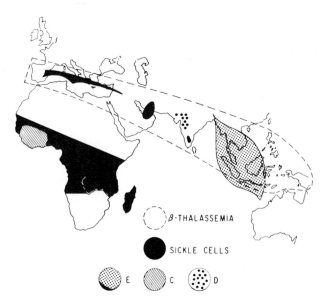

Fig. 14-3. World distribution of major hemoglobin abnormalities and thalassemias. (From Lehmann, H., Huntsman, R. G., and Ager, J. A. M.: In Stanbury, J. B., Wyngaarden, J. B., and Frederickson, D. S., eds.: The metabolic basis of inherited disease, ed. 2, New York, 1966, McGraw-Hill Book Co. Copyright 1966 by McGraw-Hill Book Co. Used by permission of McGraw-Hill Book Co.)

In addition to these areas in which the prevalence of the gene can be explained by links to Africa, the gene is also found elsewhere. In the Mediterranean area it is present in southern Italy and Sicily. In central regions of Greece there are foci where the Hb S gene frequency is 20%.[167] Certain Veddoid tribes in India also have a high prevalence of the sickle gene.

Population surveys of those areas in Africa where the sickle gene is extraordinarily prevalent revealed relatively few persons with the homozygous state, indicating that the disease is usually fatal in childhood. In areas of equatorial Africa where 40% of the persons are heterozygous for the sickle cell gene, 4% of all births result in homozygotes. Since most homozygotes in equatorial Africa die before the age of reproduction, it is evident that some potent factor must operate to maintain the gene frequency at such a high and stable level. The most widely held theory to explain this phenomenon invokes balanced polymorphism. This theory postulates that possession of a single sickle gene confers some degree of protection against falciparum malaria, particularly in young children susceptible to the lethal cerebral form of that disease.[6,7] This heterozygous advantage more than compensates for the loss of homozygotes. The mechanism for enhanced resistance to malaria conferred by sickle trait is not absolutely clear; however, it appears that when red cells containing Hb S are parasitized they become sickled and are removed from the circulation before parasite mul-

tiplication has occurred. Thus the degree of parasitemia is substantially reduced and the overwhelming, frequently lethal disease is aborted.[108]

DEFINITIONS

There are a number of syndromes characterized by the presence of Hb S in the red cells. In this chapter the term "Hb S diseases" refers to major, symptomatic sickle hemoglobinopathies. In the Hb S diseases quantitatively more than one half of the intraerythrocytic hemoglobin is Hb S. Spontaneous in vivo sickling occurs under physiologic conditions and results in hemolysis and vaso-occlusive phenomena. Specifically, homozygous Hb SS disease (sickle cell anemia), Hb SC, Hb SD, Hb SO$_{Arab}$, and Hb S — β-thalassemia are considered to be major Hb S diseases. Heterozygosity for Hb S (sickle cell trait) and the Hb S — HPFH (hereditary persistence of fetal hemoglobin) syndrome are not considered Hb S diseases by this definition.

SICKLE CELL TRAIT

Sickle cell trait, resulting from heterozygosity for the sickle hemoglobin gene, is associated with red cells that contain less than 50% Hb S. As previously noted, solutions of Hb A and S in the concentration and proportions found in the red cells of persons with the trait do not undergo gelation or change in viscosity under physiologic conditions. The proportion of Hb S usually varies between 34% to 45% and is relatively constant within families. There appear to be no consequences of these varying amounts of Hb S. Hb S proportions of less than 30% or greater than 50% indicate modifying environmental factors such as iron-deficiency anemia, which decreases the amount of Hb S,[93] or the concomitant presence of β- or α-thalassemia genes that increase or decrease the proportion, respectively. Hb S trait is diagnosed by electrophoretic studies showing an Hb AS pattern, the S component comprising less than half of the total. The sickle cell preparation with metabisulfite is positive and usually all cells can be induced to assume a sickled shape resembling holly or ivy leaves (Fig. 14-2, *B*). Solubility studies are positive.

COMPLICATIONS

Under usual physiologic conditions sickle cell trait has few, if any, physiologic or hematologic consequences. Population studies have generally revealed no effects on longevity or morbidity.[21] Red cell morphology, hematologic parameters, red cell survival, and bone marrow findings do not deviate from normal values. A case of concomitant cyanotic congenital heart defect and sickle cell trait has been described in which an obvious hemolytic process disappeared after an effective shunting procedure was performed.[161] A report describing apparent impairment of growth in children with sickle cell trait clearly requires confirmation before it can be accepted.[103] In fact, we have recently demonstrated no differences between 3- to 5-year-old children with Hg AA and AS genotypes in a variety of measures of growth and development.[89a]

Intrarenal sickling may be promoted by changes in pH, oxygenation, and ionic concentration in the region of the loop of Henle. Most persons with sickle cell trait have a somewhat impaired ability to concentrate urine, but hyposthenuria is not as common nor as extreme as that encountered in the major sickle hemoglobinopathies and causes no recognizable symptoms.[144] Spontaneous hematuria, usually from the left kidney, occurs with an increased frequency in individuals with sickle cell trait; it is caused by infarction of the renal pelvis.[10] In some instances renal papillary necrosis has been demonstrated.[95] Consistently effective therapy for hematuria has not been described. Bed rest is commonly of value. The use of diuretics, cautious administration of ε-amino caproic acid, and infusion of distilled water have also been advocated.[19,87] Replacement transfusions should be considered in severe refractory cases. Nephrectomy is rarely necessary. Instances of priapism in persons with sickle cell trait have also been described, but it is unclear whether the frequency of this is increased.[50]

A panoply of serious and occasionally life-threatening complications has been reported in relatively small numbers of persons with sickle cell trait; most have occurred under rather unphysiologic circumstances. It should be remembered that since 8% of black Americans have sickle cell trait, a coincidental association of the trait and other disease states often occurs. Mere coincidence must always be excluded before a causal relationship is assumed.

Splenic infarction in persons with sickle cell trait was first recognized during flying at high altitudes in aircraft with unpressurized cabins.[162] Since modern aircraft maintain altitudes of about 7,000 feet within their pressurized cabins and provide supplemental oxygen if there is a failure of cabin pressure, there is no contraindication to the usual forms of air travel. However, testing for sickle cell trait is logical before advice can be given about occupational or recreational activities that might involve extreme ranges of altitudes or oxygenation.

Isolated descriptions of unexpected death have been reported in persons who were subsequently found to have sickle cell trait. At autopsy in some of these cases large numbers of sickled cells have been found in the viscera, and death has been attributed to in vivo sickling.[78] In evaluating such cases it should be remembered that the sickling observed at autopsy may represent a phenomenon induced by the acidosis, hypoxia, and reduced circulation that occur agonally.

Cases of anesthesia or postoperative deaths associated with sickle cell trait have been reported.[106] Again, it is unclear whether sickling occurred antemortem and whether the incidence is really greater than in the nonsickling population. If a life-threatening effect of sickle cell trait exists, it is not sufficient to significantly affect life expectancy, for there are no age-related differences in the prevalence of the trait in prospectively studied populations.[21]

At the present time there is no concensus that the person with sickle cell trait needs to take special precautions other than avoiding extremes of altitude or other situations that might result in hypoxia. Clearly, hypoxia and shock should be avoided during anesthesia and surgery in all patients when possible! No specific restrictions in physical activity are necessary. It is reassuring to note that the proportion of professional football players (including the Denver Broncos, whose home playing field is at 6,000 feet elevation) with sickle cell trait is similar to that of the national population.[112]

Perhaps the most important implication of sickle cell trait is a genetic one. Persons with sickle cell trait may pass the gene on to their offspring. Should they mate with another person who has the trait, there is one chance in four that any child will have sickle cell anemia. The major aim of mass testing procedures after the first few years of life should be to detect persons with sickle cell trait to give them the information necessary for marital and family planning. To be effective such information must be combined with meaningful educational and counseling programs. The prenatal diagnosis of sickle cell anemia is becoming more feasible and is discussed in Chapter 15.

SICKLE CELL ANEMIA

Sickle cell anemia (Hb SS disease) results from homozygosity for the Hb S gene. As previously mentioned, the disease was first specifically reported in 1910 by Herrick.[70] However, a much earlier report published in the American literature in 1846 by Lebby[91] described a man who had splenic atrophy and a suggestive clinical course. The disease has also long been recognized in West Africa. Konotey-Ahulu has listed various tribal terms for the disease. These names have in common a long repetitive, onomatopoeic quality suggesting the bone-crushing, chronic, and relapsing nature of this disease or perhaps the persistent, protracted moaning of afflicted children.[89]

The red cells in sickle cell anemia contain large amounts of Hb S, variable amounts of Hb F (usually less than 10% after childhood), and normal levels of Hb A_2. Because these high concentrations of Hb S produce a low minimal gelling concentration, spontaneous sickling occurs at the physiologic conditions of oxygenation that occur in vivo. Circulating sickled cells, usually designated irreversibly sickled cells (ISC), are fragile, nondeformable, and rapidly destroyed. The clinical features of sickle cell anemia therefore include symptoms such as pallor, weakness, and fatigability.

In addition to the features found in any chronic and severe hemolytic state, unique clinical aspects of sickle cell anemia result from occlusion of small blood vessels by entangled masses of sickled cells. The consequence of this vaso-occlusion is infarction of the tissues. The clinical and hematologic manifestations of sickle cell anemia thus reflect these two processes: (1) severe hemolysis and the compensatory mechanisms evoked by hemolytic anemia and (2) widespread vaso-occlusion and infarction involving many tissues and organs.

The natural history of Hb SS disease during infancy has been described by O'Brien et al.[117] and Powars.[132] Affected infants can be diagnosed at birth with acid agar gel electrophoresis or microcolumn chromatography, techniques that permit detection of small hemoglobin components despite the predominating presence of Hb F (Fig. 14-4).[133] In addition, certain cellulose acetate methods also permit good separation.[155]

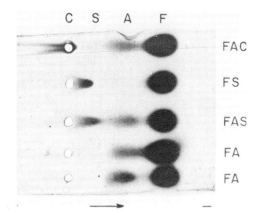

Fig. 14-4. Acid agar gel electrophoresis of cord blood hemoglobin from newborn infants. Under these conditions Hb F has a rapid cathodal mobility. Small amounts of the adult hemoglobins A, S, and C can be readily recognized. The second pattern from the top is from a newborn with homozygous Hb SS disease (sickle cell anemia). The pattern of Hb S—β-thalassemia and Hb S–HPFH would be similar.

Infants with Hb SS disease are not anemic at birth. The development of a hemolytic anemia parallels the declining level of Hb F postnatally and becomes obvious by 4 months of age (Figs. 14-5 and 14-6). The onset of clinical symptoms attributable to intravascular sickling shows considerable variability. Symptoms may occur as early as 3 months of age, are noted in half the cases by the age of 1 year, and appear in virtually all cases by 5 to 6 years of age.[132]

Sickle cell anemia has significant effects on growth. During childhood both height and weight are below average.[180] Delayed adolescence is usual and an elongated eunuchoid habitus is characteristic in adult life.[76,156] Chronic refractory ulceration about the ankles is probably a consequence of the anemia. Leg ulcers do not usually occur until later childhood and are more common in tropical than temperate areas.[150]

Effects of sickling on organs and tissues

Chronic vaso-occlusive phenomena, as well as acute and sometimes catastrophic events, produce progressive abnormalities and dysfunction of many organs and tissues. Distorted sickled cells that have the capacity to obstruct small blood vessels occur in the circulation of these patients. This phenomenon can be directly demonstrated by slit lamp ophthalmologic examination of the bulbar conjunctiva. Small areas of precapillary arterioles contain entrapped sickled cells imparting a beaded, sacculated appearance.[120]

Heart. The heart is usually enlarged in patients with Hb SS disease even in early childhood, reflecting the increased cardiac output necessary to

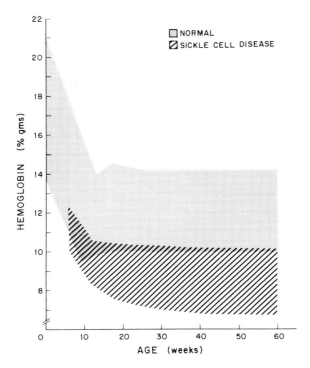

Fig. 14-5. Hemoglobin levels in young infants with Hb SS disease followed serially from birth. Significant anemia is noted by 15 to 20 weeks. Elevated reticulocyte counts are also noted, indicating onset of hemolytic process. (From O'Brien, R. T., et al.: J. Pediatr. **89:**205, 1976.)

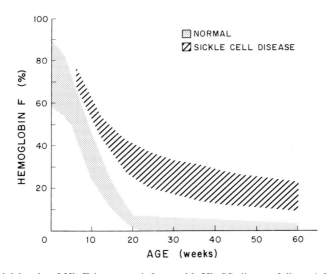

Fig. 14-6. Serial levels of Hb F in young infants with Hb SS disease followed from birth. Hb F fall-off is considerably slower than normal. (From O'Brien, R. T., et al.: J. Pediatr. **89:**205, 1976.)

compensate for chronic severe anemia.[98] By adolescence cardiomegaly and a left parasternal heave are evident. An assortment of systolic murmurs may be heard. The most prominent in childhood is a left parasternal "flow-type" systolic murmur, but an ejection murmur suggesting relative mitral insufficiency may also be noted. These auscultatory findings may suggest rheumatic fever, and in some series this was the initially suspected diagnosis in one third of the cases.[1] The absence of true arthritis (as opposed to pain in an extremity), lack of high fever, and failure to respond to aspirin are key differential features.[85] Concurrence of rheumatic heart disease and sickle cell anemia is occasionally seen but is probably rare.[176] Coincidental occurrence of sickle cell anemia and congenital heart disease is occasionally noted. Incredibly, even cyanotic tetralogy of Fallot has been described.[127]

Radiologic examination reveals cardiac enlargement involving all chambers. The pulmonary artery segment of the left heart border is frequently prominent. Electrocardiograms show left ventricular hypertrophy in about one half of the cases. Prolongation of the P-R interval may be present.[97,175] Myocardial infarction caused by coronary artery occlusion is unusual.[182]

Ultrasound examination of the heart in sickle cell anemia has been reported to show both left and right ventricular dilatation and increased stroke volume and abnormal septal motion.[98]

Lungs. Pulmonary function is significantly altered in sickle cell anemia.[26,110] Although few systematic studies have been reported in children, reductions of vital and total lung capacities have been described in older patients.[107,166] A consistent finding is reduction of Pao_2 and arterial oxygen saturation, even in young children, probably reflecting shunting rather than intrinsic anatomic pulmonary pathology.[54] A marked right shift of the oxygen dissociation curve is also noted.

The patient with sickle cell anemia is susceptible to acute pneumonic processes.[14] Some of these are clearly infectious in etiology, often pneumococcal, whereas others may result primarily from vaso-occlusion. It may be impossible to differentiate between the two processes and in fact they may merge imperceptibly. A double etiology for pulmonary infiltrative processes may account for the unusual severity and slow resolution when compared with hematologically normal persons.[130] Red cell morphology, including ''blister cells,'' and microangiopathic changes have been described in pulmonary infarctive episodes and may be of diagnostic importance.[12] Unusually severe mycoplasmal infections have also been reported.[158]

Kidney. Renal dysfunction is nearly always present.[5,28] In childhood increased renal blood flow and glomerular filtration rate, at least in part reflecting anemia, are present.[69] This is followed by an inexorably decreasing renal circulation with advancing age.[94] The biochemical milieu of the renal medulla enhances sickling, leading to progressive obliteration of the vasa rectae, parenchymal infarction, and papillary necrosis.[129,170]

Intravenous pyelography reveals enlargement of the kidneys and distortion of the collection system.[83] Frank papillary necrosis may be noted. Urine specific gravity is decreased to about 1.010 after 6 months of age (maximum urine osmolarity 360 to 760 mOsm/kg). Hyposthenuria can be temporarily reversed by transfusions of normal red blood cells in children younger than 4 or 5 years

of age but not thereafter.[82] A number of possible mechanisms for hyposthenuria have been suggested. Obstruction of blood flow through the vasa rectae, at first caused by stasis and later by vaso-occlusion, would disrupt the countercurrent multiplication system and the normal solute gradient within the renal medullae.[82] This proposed mechanism has been challenged. An alternative mechanism involving decreased perfusion and progressive destruction of the renal papilla has been suggested.[28] A clinical consequence of hyposthenuria, as well as the high fluid intake common in these children, is enuresis and nocturia that occur in more than 50% of children with Hb SS disease.[173]

Frank nephrotic syndrome is also seen from time to time, and electron microscopic examination of splitting of the basement membrane and fused foot processes.[104,174] The predominant lesion is a mesangial capillary nephritis. The nephrotic syndrome responds unpredictably, often not at all, to corticosteroid or immunosuppressive therapy and may progress to renal failure and uremia requiring dialysis.[57]

Recently interest has been focused on the development of an immune complex glomerulonephritis in patients with sickle cell anemia. This glomerulonephropathy is associated with normal levels of complement and deposits of immune complex of antigen and antibody derived from damaged renal cells on the glomerulus. The nephritis is hypothesized to result from deposition of immune complexes of renal tubular epithelial antigen, possibly released after tubular damage, and antibody directed against this antigen.[119]

Priapism is an infrequent but distressing complication in boys and men with sickle cell anemia.[68] Various forms of treatment have been suggested. A conservative approach, including analgesia, hydration, and transfusions to reduce the number of circulating sickled red cells, is probably indicated.[148] Surgical approaches include aspiration of the corpora cavernosa and venous shunts, but these have been of uncertain value and may cause subsequent impotence.[81,102,164]

Liver and biliary system. Hepatomegaly is regularly observed by 1 year of age and persists to a moderate degree throughout childhood and early adult life. Histologic examination of the liver reveals distension of sinusoids by sickled cells with variable degrees of focal necrosis and fibrosis.[165] These histologic abnormalities are accompanied by changes in liver function tests, including elevations of levels serum bilirubin (averaging 3.0 mg/dl), alkaline phosphatase, SGOT, SPT and LDH and increased BSP (Bromsulphalein) retention.[71] Elevated levels of γ-globulin are also noted. These abnormalities tend to progress with age.[45]

Fatal episodes of severe obstructive jaundice with extremely high levels of conjugated bilirubin and hepatic dysfunction have been described.[86] Histologic examination in some of these cases has revealed intrahepatic cholestasis caused by Kupfer cells engorged with sickle cells, resulting in sinusoidal obstruction and hepatocellular necrosis. Death from hepatic coma may occur.[118] Less severe episodes may be difficult to distinguish from extrahepatic obstruction by gallstones. Posttransfusional hepatitis may also occur.

The extreme hemolytic anemia results in a high frequency of pigmentary gallstones. These bilirubin stones may be either radiolucent or radiopaque. They have been seen even in the first 5 years of life and ultimately reach a rate of 5% to 30%, being most common in patients older than 20 years.[16,179] There is controversy concerning the management of asymptomatic gallstones coincidentally noted in these patients.[8] Because actual obstruction of the common duct by stones is unusual, most authorities do not recommend ''prophylactic'' cholecystectomy. However, when the patient has recurrent episodes of upper abdominal pain with demonstrated gallstones, cholecystectomy may be indicated although it may not ameliorate the symptoms.[3]

Spleen. The spleen in sickle cell anemia undergoes characteristic changes during infancy and childhood. By 6 months of age significant splenomegaly is apparent and persists during childhood. By 6 months of age significant splenomegaly becomes less common.[46] In the United States persistence of splenomegaly after adolescence suggests a mixed hemoglobin variant rather than homozygous Hb SS disease. The spleen, which is enlarged and congested in early years, undergoes progressive fibrosis, usually without clearly defined episodes of abdominal pain. Perivascular hemorrhage and infarction ultimately result in a minute, siderofibrotic nubbin, a phenomenon designated as autosplenectomy.

Evidence has accumulated indicating that a functional reduction of splenic activity preceding the occurrence of autosplenectomy is nearly invariable in early life. Functional hyposplenia is defined as defective splenic reticuloendothelial activity of the anatomically enlarged spleens of young children with sickle cell anemia.[128] This appears to be a consequence of altered perfusion caused by intrasplenic sickling and can be temporarily reversed by transfusions of normal red cells.[125] Functional hyposplenia is not congenital but an acquired defect occurring between 5 to 36 months of age when the proportion of Hb F falls to less than 20%[117] (Fig. 14-7).

There are hematologic and immunologic manifestations of functional hyposplenia. The circu-

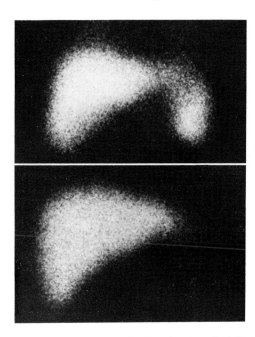

Fig. 14-7. Development of "functional asplenia" in sickle cell anemia. A ^{99m}Tc sulfur colloid scan at age 5 months shows normal splenic size and activity. Three months later there is no evidence of splenic reticuloendothelial activity. (From O'Brien, R. T., et al.: J. Pediatr. **89:**205, 1976.)

lating red blood cells contain Howell-Jolly bodies and membrane "pits" reflecting deficient splenic "pitting" function.[31,40] The spleens of these children also fail to form antibodies in response to intravenous immunization with small doses of particulate antigens.[146] Finally, these children are 300 to 600 times more likely to develop overwhelming pneumococcal and *Haemophilus influenzae* sepsis and meningitis than normal children.[15] This propensity to serious infection is similar to that seen after surgical splenectomy in young children.

Studies of sickle cell anemia in infancy indicate that the period of greatest risk for death from severe infection is during the first 5 years of life.[132] To reduce this inordinately high rate in early life, populations at risk should be screened for sickle cell anemia, ideally at birth. Careful follow-up and ready access to medical care are essential.

Several types of immunologic abnormalities have been described in these patients. A deficiency of circulating, heat-labile, pneumococcal opsonins has been described.[181] A defect in the properdin system (the alternate pathway of complement activations) has been described by some researchers but refuted by others.[77,172] Deficiency of "tuftsin," a phagocytosis-promoting peptide has also been noted.[38]

Eyes. Intravascular sickling can be directly observed in ocular blood vessels.[9] Ophthalmoscopic examination of conjunctival blood vessels shows saccular abnormalities with "multiple short comma-shaped or curlicued capillary segments often seemingly isolated from the vascular network."[121] A variety of intraocular abnormalities can be noted.

The retinal vessels are tortuous and their occlusion may lead to ischemic infarcts and retinal hemorrhage. The changes that begin at the periphery of the retina are best appreciated with indirect ophthalmoscopy. Neovascularization may be associated with abnormal arteriovenous connections causing a proliferation of new vessels that resemble "sea fans."[37] Pigmented chorioretinal lesions ("black sunbursts") and other evidence of choroidal disease may be seen. Although ocular abnormalities are common in sickle cell anemia, they are less severe and a relentless progression to retinal detachment and blindness occurs less often than in Hb SC disease.

Ulceration of the ankles. Chronic, indolent ulceration about the ankles is a regular complication of sickle cell anemia. Ulcers are unusual in the first decade of life, but in some areas as many as 75% of adults may develop them.[150] These ulcers are thought in most instances to result from poor circulation and anemia, which impede healing of minor traumatic lesions. Infarction of the skin may also occur. These ulcers are more common in the tropics because of the greater likelihood of trauma and infection where shoes are not worn and because hygiene may be less than optimal. Conservative therapy, including clean dressings and immobilization, is indicated. In refractory or progressive cases multiple transfusions with or without skin grafting and antibiotics may be necessary. Oral zinc therapy has also been described to hasten healing.[154]

Laboratory findings

Selected laboratory findings in sickle cell anemia are listed in Table 14-2. A moderately severe normochromic-normocytic, hemolytic anemia with morphologic abnormalities (including Howell-Jolly bodies, target cells, polychromatophilia, and the presence of varying numbers of irreversibly sickled cells) are characteristic. The white blood cell count is consistently elevated (15 to 20 × 10⁹/liter) with a polymorphonuclear leukocytosis. This increase probably reflects a relative shift of granulocytes from the marginated to the circulating compartment. Platelet counts are usually increased. The bone marrow shows hypercellularity and marked erythroid hyperplasia. Serum ferritin, serum iron-binding capacity, and iron stores are normal during childhood unless repeated transfusions have been given.[116]

Studies of the coagulation factors in patients

Table 14-2. Selected laboratory values in children with sickle cell anemia

	Average	Range
Hemoglobin (gm/dl)	7.5	5.5-9.5
Hematocrit (%)	22	17-29
Reticulocyte count (%)	12	5-30
Nucleated red blood cells (/100 white blood cells)	3	1-20
White blood cell count (×10⁹/liter)	15	12-30
Bilirubin (mg/dl)	2.5	1.5-4.0

with sickle cell anemia reveal elevated levels of factor VIII and fibrinogen as well as increased fibrinolytic activity. Platelet counts are usually elevated but may decrease slightly during vaso-occlusive crises. These abnormalities are believed to reflect vascular endothelial damage induced by the sickling process. However, hypercoagulability and thrombosis are not considered primary pathogenic phenomena in this disease.[140]

Sickle cell crises

The clinical courses of patients with sickle cell anemia are punctuated by episodic events that threaten their lives and comfort. These acute events have traditionally been termed crises, but in fact a number of types of crises with different pathophysiologic mechanisms and symptoms may require different types of therapy. These include (1) vaso-occlusive or symptomatic crises, (2) acute splenic sequestration crises, (3) aplastic crises, and (4) hyperhemolytic crises.

Vaso-occlusive crises. Vaso-occlusive crises are painful episodes that are the most common type of crises seen in children with sickle cell anemia. The manifestations may vary markedly, depending on the tissues or organs involved and the extent of the ischemic damage. The basic cause of such a crisis is obstruction of blood flow by tangled masses of sickled cells and some degree of vasospasm. There are few or no changes in the hematologic parameters during these episodes. The events that trigger vaso-occlusion are largely undefined, although infections often are associated with or followed by painful crises, perhaps because of accompanying fever, acidosis, and dehydration. Exposure to the cold may sometimes by implicated, but there appears to be no seasonal variability in the United States.[48] In most instances there is no discernable antecedent cause.

"Hand-foot syndrome." Dactylitis is a common initial manifestation of sickle cell anemia during infancy. This results from symmetrical infarction of the metacarpals and metatarsals, and painful swelling of the dorsa of the hands and feet occurs.

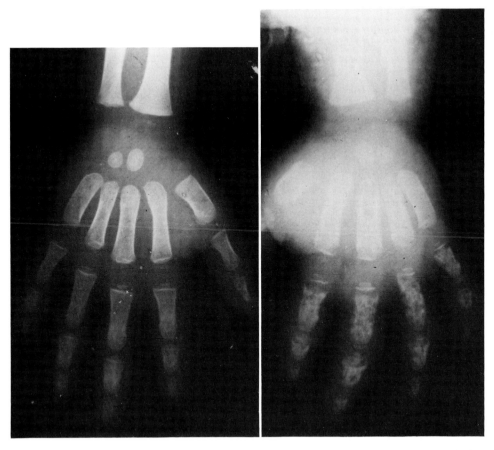

Fig. 14-8. Hand roentgenograms of a child with Hb SS disease with the ''hand-foot syndrome.'' At the onset of the event no osseous abnormalities are evident. Three weeks later almost every bone is involved by osteolytic and periosteal processes.

The hand-foot syndrome occurs in 10% to 30% of cases and is often the first clinical symptom of the disease.[89,178] Low-grade fever may accompany the hand-foot syndrome; occasionally there may be high fever. Characteristic hematologic changes are not seen. X-ray films show no abnormalities initially, but later areas of osteolysis, periostitis, and bone reabsorption may appear (Fig. 14-8). The diffuse and symmetrical pattern of involvement of multiple bones and especially the lack of systemic signs and sterile blood cultures usually permit differentiation of the hand-foot syndrome from osteomyelitis, which may be suggested by roentgenograms. There is no specific therapy. Attacks may repetitively occur for many months, but after the second or third year of life the syndrome does not usually recur. There are usually no permanent orthopedic sequelae, but premature epiphyseal fusion and bone shortening have been described.[153]

Involvement of joints and extremities. Symptomatic, painful crises involving the joints and extremities usually begin after the third or fourth year of life. Pains in the extremities result from infarction of the small areas of the long bones or bone marrow or involvement of the periosteum and periarticular tissues of the larger joints. There may be swelling and moderate limitation of motion, but redness and heat are not prominent. Episodes of joint pain may mimic acute episodes of rheumatic fever or rheumatoid arthritis. X-ray studies may ultimately show areas of bone infarction and periostitis but are usually negative at the onset of crises. Scanning techniques employing radioisotopes are being increasingly used to diagnose vasoocclusive processes involving the marrow or the bones.[4] Acute areas of decreased bone or marrow perfusion are noted using ^{99m}Tc gelatin sulfur colloid; later as healing occurs increased osteoblastic activity can be demonstrated with ^{99m}Tc diphosphonate or ^{85}Sr.[65,84] In general few hematologic changes occur during these painful crises, although the total white blood cell count may increase without a greater shift to the left. Significant fever is usually not observed.

Abdominal involvement. Episodes of abdominal involvement are thought to occur when areas of infarction or hemorrhage within abdominal structures such as the liver, spleen, or abdominal lymph nodes result in capsular stretching. Occasionally the pain may be incapacitating, severe, and episodic in character, and signs of peritoneal irritation may be present. However, peristalsis usually persists, and this finding helps to differentiate abdominal crises from inflammatory processes that require surgical intervention, such as appendicitis or peritonitis. Painful abdominal crises are often associated with low-grade fever, but severe abdominal crises may be accompanied by hyperpyrexia and incapacitation.

The duration of the painful crises averages 3 to 4 days. There may be early spontaneous termination, but protracted episodes lasting a week or more also can occur. Variability of individual crises and irregularity in their frequency even in the same patient make evaluation of any specific drug or other method of treatment difficult.

Central nervous system crises. Children with sickle cell anemia may develop hemiplegia with other neurologic findings suggestive of extensive central nervous system damage. The consequences of these "strokes" are variable. Some patients recover rapidly without residual disability, indicating that there had been a significant element of vasospasm present. Others are left with permanent neurologic deficits, showing that actual infarction has occurred. Cerebral angiographic studies are *not* indicated unless the patient has been prepared with transfusions, for hypertonic contrast media produce immediate sickling of red cells exposed to them, which could well aggravate vaso-occlusion. However, when properly performed these studies demonstrate blood vessel abnormalities involving the larger cerebral vessels that may reflect disease in the vasa vasorum.[171]

The treatment of central nervous system crises includes prompt and vigorous hydration, administration of oxygen, and multiple transfusions of packed red cells. Recent reports describe the effectiveness of a program of repeated transfusions for a year or more, resulting in marked improvement of vascular abnormalities in patients who have suffered strokes.[143] Such a program should be strongly considered because these strokes tend to be repetitive and progressive.

Pulmonary crises. Children with sickle cell anemia often have severe and protracted episodes of pulmonary disease. Although the precipitating event may be bacterial infection with pneumococcus or even mycoplasma organisms, infarction may also be a significant component. It may be difficult to separate infection from infarction, even with careful x-ray scanning studies. In fact, both processes may be operative. After appropriate cultures have been taken, antibiotic therapy, including penicillin, should be administered. Multiple transfusions of packed red cells are also indicated if the pulmonary involvement is extensive or protracted and is causing significant pulmonary insufficiency or arterial desaturation. Such transfusions appear to hasten recovery.

Treatment. There is no specific therapy for vaso-occlusive crises.[33] Many medications of possible value have been proposed at various times. These include anticoagulants, low molecular weight dextran, carbonic anhydrase inhibitors, alkalis, phenothiazides, stimulators of erythropoiesis (such as cobalt and androgens), and many others as well. Most recently urea, cyanate, and zinc have been extolled. Suitably controlled studies have not proved the efficacy of most of these. Management of the vaso-occlusive crises is for the most part symptomatic and supportive but must include therapy directed at the following conditions that are known to enhance sickling.

Hypertonicity, which enhances the sickling process in vitro, may occur in vivo by several mechanisms. The expanded plasma volume of these patients may become constricted during painful crises or infection.[13,52] As previously described, these patients have fixed hyposthenuria and polyuria and may become dehydrated easily. Optimal hydration should be ensured.

Oral fluids can be relied on in milder symptomatic episodes, but when the pain is severe and particularly when fever, vomiting, or diarrhea contributes to dehydration, parenteral hydration is indicated. A mixture of equal amounts of normal saline and 5% dextrose, infused at the rate of 2,000 to 2,500 ml/m²/day, should be given.

Acidosis aggravates sickling, and pain can be produced immediately by the intravenous infusion of acidifying compounds such as ammonium sulfate.[61] Accordingly alkali therapy is often administered to rectify potential or actual acidosis.[39,147] Although controlled studies showed little beneficial effect of such therapy, oral sodium bicarbonate or polycitrate solutions may be used in mild vaso-occlusive crises. When intravenous therapy is given, sodium bicarbonate is often added to the hydrating solution.

Reduced oxygenation and hypoxia increase sickling; therefore an atmosphere of well-humidified oxygen may be used when the child is experiencing pain. Although hyperbaric oxygen is probably effective, the modest increase in blood oxygenation accomplished with an oxygen tent or mask is of uncertain value.[139]

Infection may be a precipitating cause of vaso-occlusive crises and in the tropics it may be the most important one.[89] When evidence of bacterial infection is found, appropriate antibiotic therapy is indicated after cultures are taken.

Besides giving attention to the possible contributing factors, one should also consider the use of transfusion if the crisis is severe. Since the ordinary vaso-occlusive crisis is not associated with hematologic deterioration, blood is not given for anemia per se. In fact, the beneficial effects of a single blood transfusion in increasing oxygen transport may be counterbalanced by the increased blood viscosity resulting from an increase in hematocrit. In severe or prolonged vaso-occlusive crises, vigorous multiple transfusion therapy designed to "dilute" the patient's sickle cells may be considered. If the number of sickle cells in the circulation can be reduced effectively, vaso-occlusive manifestations of the disease can usually be ameliorated. The most effective way to accomplish such a reduction is by transfusion of normal red blood cells from non–sickle cell donors. When at least 60% of the patient's circulating red blood cells are replaced by normal cells, the progression of vaso-occlusive symptoms usually stops. Transfusions of fresh packed red blood cells, 10 to 15 ml/kg, can be given every 12 hours until the hemoglobin level has increased to 12 to 13 gm/dl. At this point simple dilution will have significantly decreased the proportion of the patient's circulating red blood cells. Limited exchange transfusions have been suggested as a more rapid way of accomplishing this.[25,33] Further erythropoiesis will be suppressed. Because of their only 10- to 20-day survival rate, the patient's own red blood cells, which predominantly contain Hb S, disappear rapidly. With small packed cell transfusions given to maintain the hemoglobin level above 12 gm/dl, the proportion of circulating cells containing Hb S will rapidly fall to low levels, thus producing the same effects as an exchange transfusion in a few days. Packed cell transfusions every 2 to 3 weeks will usually ensure that the circulating blood contains predominantly normal red blood cells. A quantitative sickle cell preparation, using sodium metabisulfite in which red cells of the patient and donor can be morphologically differentiated, is an accurate method for assessing the completeness of replacement transfusion and is more rapid than quantitative hemoglobin electrophoresis.

Although this "hypertransfusion regimen" is symptomatically effective, there are inherent risks of isoimmunization, hepatitis, and hemosiderosis. This type of program usually is advocated therefore only for specific indications such as in prolonged or severe vaso-occlusive crises, especially those involving the central nervous system; as preparation for anesthesia and surgery; as management of pregnancy; and as supportive therapy during complicating medical conditions. In critical situations exchange transfusions with fresh blood may be the most effective way to rapidly reduce the proportion of cells containing Hb S.

SEDATION AND ANALGESIA. Considerable relief of pain and discomfort may be obtained with the judicious use of sedatives and analgesics. Aspirin in large doses should be avoided so as not to aggravate a tendency to metabolic acidosis. Acetaminophen (Tylenol) in a dose of 120 to 240 mg every 4 to 6 hours may provide some relief in mild painful crises and may be further beneficial by acting as an antipyretic. When pain is more severe, codeine sulfate (30 to 60 mg) may be necessary. The use of meperidine hydrochloride or morphine sulfate may lead to addiction and should be used only when pain is extreme. Compounds such as prochlorperazine and chlorpromazine are useful adjuncts for treatment of painful crises because of their sedative and tranquilizing action; their use may reduce the need for narcotics.

UREA, CYANATE, AND ZINC THERAPIES. The history of sickle cell anemia is studded with enthusiastic preliminary reports of effective therapies. However, when these reports have been subjected to tests in larger controlled studies, no significant benefit has usually been shown.[29] The problems of evaluation are compounded by the extreme diversity and variability of the sickle cell crises. Ultimately any beneficial therapy of sickle cell anemia must be reflected in a decrease of in vivo sickling. Furthermore, careful, controlled crossover studies in which the patient serves as his own control must demonstrate a decrease in the number and frequency of vaso-occlusive episodes. Unless unequivocal proof is demonstrated, a degree of healthy skepticism must be maintained, especially if the proposed therapy has some possibility of danger. The use of urea, cyanate, and zinc merits special attention.

Considerable publicity (much of it in the lay press) extolled the possible benefit of intravenous urea in invert sugar for the painful crises of sickle cell disease. The rationale for this therapy was that high concentrations of urea disrupt molecular bonds that participate in the sickling process.[113] The therapeutic use of urea increases the patient's blood urea nitrogen level to 150 to 200 mg/dl and evokes a diuresis that must be treated vigorously if dehydration is to be avoided. Despite preliminary and uncontrolled clinical reports suggesting the efficacy of urea, the supposed therapeutic level of urea attained in patients was shown to have no effect on in vitro sickling and controlled studies of both intravenous and oral urea did not demonstrate significant benefit.[39,99] Therefore the use of urea is not indicated in the management of sickle cell disease.

The possible value of cyanate has been investigated vigorously in patients with Hb SS disease. This compound interacts with the sickle hemoglobin molecule by a process called carbamylation. Cyanate directly inhibits the sickling process probably by changing the affinity between hemoglobin, oxygen, and 2,3-DPG or by altering molecular configuration.[60] The same kind of approach had previously been attempted without clear benefit using carbon monoxide or agents that produce methemoglobin.[18,136] Although oral cyanate treatment decreases the rate of hemolysis and leads to an increased hemoglobin level, a controlled study did not demonstrate significant reduction in the number or severity of vaso-occlusive episodes. In addition, considerable drug toxicity was observed, including peripheral neuropathy, interference with nutrition, and in two patients the development of cataracts.[66] The use of oral cyanate is not currently indicated in sickle cell disease, although methods using extracorporeal carbamylation are still being actively investigated.[42] Despite formidable technical problems, some form of treatment may be evolved.

Delayed physical and sexual maturation are common in sickle cell anemia and are also features of a zinc-deficiency syndrome. Studies of zinc metabolism in sickle cell anemia revealed increased urinary zinc excretion and low plasma levels of zinc in many patients.[134] It has been postulated that zinc might replace calcium in the red cell membrane and so inhibit intravascular sickling.[23] The possible efficacy of zinc therapy is still being investigated.

A large number of compounds have the capacity to interfere with the sickling phenomenon in in vitro preparations. Some of these agents interact with the red cell membrane, whereas others interfere with hemoglobin polymerization. Careful pharmacologic and toxicologic studies are necessary. A safe and effective pharmacologic approach to sickle cell anemia remains elusive.[24] A reliable animal test system would be of great value in the testing of potential drugs for the treatment of sickle cell anemia, and an animal model for measuring in vivo survival of Hb SS red cells has been described.[32]

Splenic sequestration crises. Infants and young children with Hb SS disease whose spleens have not yet undergone multiple infarctions and subsequent fibrosis and children with other major Hb S syndromes whose spleens remain enlarged into adult life may suddenly have pooling of vast amounts of blood in the spleen. During these sequestration crises the spleen becomes enormous, fills the abdomen, and even reaches into the pelvis. The hemoglobin level may drop so precipitously that hypovolemic shock and death may occur (Fig. 14-9). This is the most acutely dangerous crisis in the life of the young child with sickle cell anemia, and it must be recognized and treated promptly.[75,123] Infants between the ages of 8 months and 5 years are particularly susceptible and may die within hours of the first signs of this disturbance.

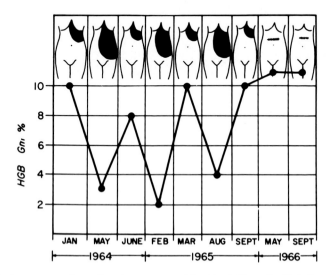

Fig. 14-9. Splenic sequestration crises in a young girl with sickle cell–β^0-thalassemia. On three occasions over 1½ years acute massive enlargement of the spleen accompanied by profound anemia occurred. Splenectomy was then performed. (From Pearson, H. A.: Ann. N.Y. Acad. Sci. **165:** 83, 1969.)

The usual clinical indications of this complication are the sudden development of weakness, pallor of the lips and mucous membranes, breathlessness, rapid pulse, faintness, and abdominal fullness. Death is not uncommon.[149]

Treatment of the sequestration crisis is directed toward the prompt correction of hypovolemia with plasma expanders and particularly with whole blood transfusions. If the shock can be reversed, much of the blood sequestered in the spleen is remobilized and dramatic regression of splenomegaly may occur in a short time. This occurrence has been called the syndrome of the "yo-yo" spleen. Because of the rapidity with which a sequestration crisis can occur and even recur and because of its potential fatality in a matter of hours, splenectomy should be strongly considered if a child has had one or more of these severe crises.

Aplastic crises. In patients with sickle cell anemia red cell survival is only between 10 and 20 days, compared with 120 in normal persons. Despite this extreme hemolysis the patient usually maintains a hemoglobin level of 5.5 to 9.5 gm/dl by increasing red cell production fivefold to eightfold. If this maximal compensatory response is compromised, profound anemia develops rapidly. The patient rapidly develops weakness, listlessness, rapid breathing, and tachycardia. Diminished red cell production superimposed on the usual rapid destruction rather than hyperhemolysis is the basis of the aplastic crisis.[160]

A number of infections, usually viral in type, may in some way damage the erythroid bone marrow and result in a cessation of red cell production that may persist for 10 to 14 days. Aplastic crises may occur in several members of a family (further evidence suggesting an infectious origin).[92] Although nutritional deficiency of folic acid has been invoked in the genesis of some of these crises,[96,131] later studies do not confirm a relationship in childhood.[124]

During aplastic episodes, reticulocytes disappear from the blood and a markedly reduced number of erythroid precursors are present in the bone marrow. However, the hematologic findings during aplastic crises differ, depending on the stage at which the patient is studied. Early the degree of anemia is more extreme than usual, but the degree of jaundice may decrease. The numbers of reticulocytes in the blood and nucleated red cells in the bone marrow are sharply decreased. Platelet and white blood cell counts are usually not affected. At the nadir of the aplastic crisis the hemoglobin level may fall as low as 1 gm/dl and death may result from severe anemia and congestive heart failure.

Erythroid aplasia usually terminates spontaneously after 5 to 10 days, and recovery is accompanied by a surge of reticulocytes and nucleated red cells in the blood. The reticulocyte count may then reach 50% to 60%, and the hemoglobin quickly returns to its precrisis level. If the patient is studied early in the recovery stage from an aplastic crisis, a mistaken diagnosis of hemolytic crisis may be reached because severe anemia and marked reticulocytosis are still present.

The treatment for an aplastic crisis is transfusion of fresh packed red cells, given slowly in a dose of not more than 2 to 3 ml/kg of body weight every 6 to 8 hours until the hemoglobin level is increased by about 5 gm/dl. For the small child a whole unit of packed cells (250 to 300 ml) can be divided and used sequentially, thereby reducing the risk of transfusion hepatitis. When profound anemia is present, fresh packed red cells, preferably collected with CPD anticoagulant, should be used to assure normal levels of 2,3-DPG so that oxygen transport by the transfused red cells is normal. Oxygen should be administered if the patient is dyspneic, but the use of digitalis is not generally indicated. If signs of congestive heart failure are present, venous pressure should be monitored by a central venous catheter during transfusion. Blood can be withdrawn from the patient as the donor blood is given, effecting a partial exchange transfusion. Parents of children with major Hb S diseases should be made aware of the manifestations of the aplastic crisis. They should seek medical attention promptly if the child becomes weak or pale, especially in the wake of infections.

Hyperhemolytic crises. The frequency and even existence of so-called hyperhemolytic crises is somewhat controversial because of the difficulty of proving a more rapid rate of hemolysis superimposed on an already severe process.[45] Nevertheless, although it is probably very unusual, hyperhemolysis may ensue in association with certain drugs or acute infections. The concomitant presence of G-6-PD deficiency has been suggested as a possible contributing cause of hyperhemolytic episodes, especially when combined with infections.[163]

During these episodes the patient begins to feel weak, look paler, and show more scleral icterus. There may be abdominal pain. The hematocrit falls from its usual 21% to 25% to 15% or less in a few days, and at the same time the reticulocyte count rises. The patient becomes more jaundiced. After several days the excessive hemolysis tends to gradually subside.

If evidence of bacterial infection is found, appropriate antibiotic therapy is indicated. Oxidant drugs that may produce hemolysis should be discontinued. At the same time dehydration and acidosis should be corrected. Transfusions of packed red cells should be given to reverse or prevent incipient heart failure from anemic hypoxia.

Miscellaneous problems

Folic acid deficiency. A deficiency of folic acid has been suggested as a frequent occurrence in sickle cell anemia. The hyperactive bone marrow is postulated to increase the requirements for this vitamin, especially when the diet is poor and in infants, pregnant women, and alcoholics.[100] Many authorities recommend daily administration of 1 to 5 mg of oral folic acid to patients with chronic hemolytic anemias, including sickle cell anemia. This has no demonstrable effect on the hemoglobin level in children despite a relatively high frequency of biochemical indicators of folic acid.[124]

Pregnancy. Pregnancy poses serious problems to the woman with sickle cell anemia, especially to the teenager. Pregnancy should be only undertaken with full understanding of the implications and with the assured availability of excellent medical supervision. Oral contraception, although probably associated with a greater thromboembolic risk than in normal women, is still much safer than an unplanned pregnancy.[33,62]

In poorly supervised pregnancies maternal mortality as high as 20% has been noted, but serious complications are much lower with good care.[51] Nevertheless, even the best series report a high rate of fetal prematurity and stillbirth.[55] Some authorities recommend a transfusion program during the last trimester of pregnancy or even earlier to reduce both placental insufficiency resulting from infarction with its effect on the fetus and the maternal risk in the perinatal period.[135]

Osteomyelitis. Osteomyelitis occurs with increased frequency in all of the major sickle cell diseases. In the non–sickle cell population staphylococci account for more than 80% of cases of hematogenous osteomyelitis, and salmonellae are decidedly uncommon pathogens. In contrast, in sickle cell states more than half the cases of osteomyelitis are caused by salmonellae of various types.[44] Osteomyelitis is most common during the first 5 years of life.[132]

It may be difficult to differentiate bone infarction from osteomyelitis. The absence of fever, leukocytosis, and a markedly elevated sedimentation rate favor the former. Diagnosis ultimately depends on isolation of the organism from the blood or bone. Scanning techniques may also be useful, for uptake of ^{99m}Tc sulfur colloid is usually decreased in vaso-occlusion whereas uptake of ^{99m}Tc diphosphonate is characteristically increased in osteomyelitis.[84,137]

The factors predisposing to salmonella osteomyelitis are doubtless multiple. Decreased and impaired reticuloendothelial activity facilitate bacteremia, but the propensity of salmonellae to grow in necrotic bone is probably the most important predisposition. Once salmonella infection is established, the immune mechanisms marshaled by the sickle cell patient are normal.[141]

Prognosis

An accurate definition of the prognosis of sickle cell anemia is difficult. There is a paucity of careful, long-term prospective studies. Prognosis is markedly affected by the kind of available medical care and supervision. In a retrospective analysis of autopsy cases Diggs[43] suggested that 20% to 30% of patients die in the first 5 years of life. The median age of death was less than two decades, and survival beyond 40 years was unusual.[43] The causes of the inordinate mortality during the first years of life are overwhelming sepsis and sequestration crises, complications that should be preventable to a great extent by good medical supervision.

Occasionally patients with sickle cell anemia have relatively benign clinical courses. The reasons for this variability are not entirely clear. The disease process in some cases is clearly modified by the presence of other genetic traits, such as α-thalassemia[177] or Hb Memphis.[90] Doubly heterozygous states—especially Hb S–β^0-thalassemia disease and Hb S–HPHF syndrome[27]—may sometimes be confused with mild sickle cell anemia.

However, when all of the usual explanations are excluded by careful biochemical and genetic studies, clinical variability remains. Occasionally very old patients have been reported, and in some populations high levels of Hb F appear to ameliorate this disease.[27]

Hb C SYNDROMES

Hb C ($\alpha_2\beta_2^{6\ glu\rightarrow lys}$) variant results from substitution of a positively charged lysine instead of the negatively charged glutamic acid residue in the number 6 position of the β-polypeptide chain. The chemical structure can be represented as $\alpha_2\beta_2^C$. Hb C has a number of physical properties differing from normal Hb A. These include a different molecular charge (-1 to $+1$) that imparts an extremely slow electrophoretic mobility at both alkali and acid pH (Fig. 13-4). The gene for Hb C appears to have originated in West Africa in the area comprising northern Ghana where its frequency approaches 50%. It is present in about 2.5% of black Americans.

Hb CC disease

Homozygosity for the Hb C gene results in red cells that contain Hb C plus a small proportion of Hb F. Hb A_2 is present in normal amounts but cannot be separated electrophoretically. Hb C has decreased solubility and may be predisposed to a "precrystallization" process in the red cell. Under conditions of dehydration and increased hemoglobin concentration, actual rectangular crystal-like structures may be found in the red cell, especially in the postsplenectomy state.[49] However, unlike Hb S, the altered solubility of Hb C is not a consequence of deoxygenation. The large amounts of intracellular Hb C impart a degree of cellular rigidity predisposing these cells to a slightly shortened rate of survival.

The disease is characterized by a mild chronic hemolytic anemia with splenomegaly, and the diagnosis may be made during the course of investigation of a patient with asymptomatic anemia or splenomegaly. The hemoglobin level ranges between 10 to 12 gm/dl and reticulocytes average 5% to 10%. A most impressive morphologic feature is the presence of large numbers (>90%) of target cells. Additionally, microspherocytosis, polychromasia, and an unusual folded cell form resembling a conch shell are present. Hb C–β-thalassemia is characterized by 70% to 95% Hb C. Clinically and hematologically it resembles Hb CC disease.

Hb C trait

Heterozygous individuals have 30% to 50% of Hb C in their red cells, the remainder being Hb A and a small amount of Hb F. Because Hb A_2 has similar electrophoretic mobility, it cannot be quantitated unless special techniques are used.[72] Hb C trait is hematologically and clinically benign. Moderate numbers (10% to 30%) of target cells are noted on peripheral blood smears.

OTHER COMMON HEMOGLOBIN VARIANTS
Hb E

Hb E ($\alpha_2\beta_2^{26\ lys\rightarrow glu}$) is a variant in which a lysine has been substituted for glutamic acid in the number 26 position of the β-chain. It is designated $\alpha_2\beta_2^E$. Hb E has slow electrophoretic mobility, only slightly more rapid than Hb C at alkaline pH, but on agar gel at acid pH it moves with Hb A. The gene occurs with high frequency in peoples from southeast Asia and has been documented in 35% of Cambodians and 15% of peoples from Thailand.[53]

Hb E trait is an entirely asymptomatic state characterized by 30% to 45% Hb E in the red cells. No significant morphologic features are seen. Homozygous Hb EE disease results in a clinical state similar to Hb CC disease, which it resembles electrophoretically. Target cells and microcytosis are prominent morphologic features. The two conditions may be distinguished by their different racial predilections. In addition, Hb E and Hb C

can be easily distinguished by their different electrophoretic mobilities in acid agar gel (Fig. 13-4).

Hb D

The letter designation "D" (sometimes also "G") is applied to a number of variants having an electrophoretic mobility similar to that of Hb S at alkaline pH. A number of these have substitutions in the β-chain such as Hb D_{Punjab} ($\alpha_2\beta_2^{121\ glu\rightarrow glu}$) and Hb D_{Ibidan} ($\alpha_2\beta_2^{87\ thr\rightarrow lys}$). There are also Hb D variants with α-chain substitutions such as Hb $D_{St.\ Louis}$ ($\alpha_2^{68\ asp\rightarrow lys}\beta_2$). The most common variant is Hb D_{Punjab}, found in about 1 in 2,000 American blacks.[101]

Although the Hb D variants may be mistaken for Hb S on ordinary alkaline electrophoresis, they have normal solubilities and do not sickle. They can be differentiated by acid agar gel electrophoresis by which technique they migrate with Hb A. (See Fig. 13-4.) Hb D trait is associated with no clinical or hematologic abnormalities. A few persons with homozygous Hgb D have been reported to have a mild anemia and splenomegaly.[35]

Hb O_{Arab} ($\alpha_2\beta^{121\ glu\rightarrow lys}$)

This β chain variant is caused by substitution of a glutamic acid for the normal position 121 lysine. It has a mobility similar to that of Hb C on alkaline electrophoresis, but electrophoretically it resembles Hb S on acid agar gel. In our laboratory about one in twenty black persons thought to have Hb C on initial electrophoretic screening are subsequently found to have Hb O_{Arab} trait.

Hb $C_{Georgetown}$ (Hb C_{Harlem})

This variant results from two separate β-chain mutations. One is the $\beta^{6\ glu\rightarrow valine}$ characteristic of sickle hemoglobin and the other is the $\beta^{73\ asp\rightarrow asn}$. The alkaline electrophoretic mobility is similar to that of Hb C. However, Hb $C_{Georgetown}$ has the solubility abnormalities of Hb S and can be induced to sickle by deoxygenation.

Hb I ($\alpha_2^{16\ lys\rightarrow glu}\beta_2$)

α-Variants are by far more uncommon than β-chain abnormal hemoglobins. Further, in α-chain heterozygotes the proportion of the abnormal hemoglobin is lower than that which generally occurs in β-chain types; 10% to 35% versus 35% to 50%. This is one of the strongest bits of evidence supporting the concept of duplication of α-genes in humans. Hb I is probably the most common α-chain abnormality. A person doubly heterozygous for Hb I and an α-thalassemia 2 gene had 70% Hb I and 30% Hb A.[11] In the heterozygous state Hb I has no hematologic manifestations.

DOUBLY HETEROZYGOUS SICKLE CELL SYNDROMES
Hb SC disease

This fairly common hemoglobinopathy results from inheritance of both a sickle gene and the Hb C gene. The red cells contain a roughly equal mixture of the two hemoglobins plus normal or slightly increased levels of Hb F. Hb A is totally absent.

Hb SC disease is characterized hematologically by a moderate, chronic hemolytic anemia. Hemoglobin levels range between 9 and 12 gm/dl. The blood smear contains about 50% target cells but few if any sickled cells are seen. Occasionally cells containing condensed Hb C crystals may be noted. Genetic studies usually reveal one parent with sickle trait and the other with Hb C trait.

Clinically the patient with Hb SC disease appears well and has a normal habitus. The spleen is palpably enlarged in about two thirds of cases. Because of the relatively high hemoglobin level in this disease and the capacity of Hb C to interact with Hb S in the sickling process, acute vaso-occlusive phenomena ("crises") occur, although they are less severe than those of sickle cell anemia. Progressive retinal thrombosis culminating in retinal detachment and necrosis of the femoral head are more common in Hb SC than in sickle cell anemia. These complications may develop in 25% to 50% of patients, although they usually do not occur until after adolescence.[17,36] Splenic sequestration crises have occurred even in later life. Pregnancy has been reported to have an inordinately high maternal risk in Africa, but less so in the United States.[55,58] Splenomegaly and intact splenic function are usually maintained at least throughout childhood and adolescence. However, a few deaths from overwhelming pneumococcal sepsis suggesting transient functional hyposplenia have been reported.[80]

Hb SO$_{Arab}$ disease

Hb O$_{Arab}$ interacts strongly with Hb S in the sickling process and the doubly heterozygous state is usually more severe than Hb SC disease, approaching sickle cell anemia in clinical and hematologic severity.[109] The alkaline electrophoretic pattern is identical to that of Hb SC disease, but on acid agar gel resembles Hb SS. Family studies are confirmatory. Functional asplenia and subsequent autosplenectomy occur in this disease as they do in sickle cell anemia.

Hb SD$_{Punjab}$ disease

At least nine hemoglobins with a D- or G-like mobility have been described as occurring with Hb S.[105] Only Hb S–D$_{Punjab}$ disease has been associated with hemolytic anemia and vaso-occlusive phenomena.

Hb S–HPHF syndrome

Those persons doubly heterozygous for Hb S and HPFH genes have no evidence of an in vivo sickling or hemolysis, despite red cells that contain 70% to 80% Hb S.[22] The 20% to 30% Hb F is uniformly distributed in the red cells as demonstrated by the Kleihauer-Betke technique. This high intracellular content of Hb F effectively prevents sickling under physiologic levels of oxygenation.[34] There is no significant anemia or evidence of hemolysis. Blood morphology is characterized by moderate targeting of the red cells.

Hb S–β-thalassemia

The doubly heterozygous occurrence of the genes for Hb S and β-thalassemia has been found in a wide geographic distribution. It was first described in Italy and designated as microdrepanocytic disease.[159] Because the clinical course more resembles the sickle than the thalassemia syndromes, it is discussed here.

Hb S–β-thalassemia disease is characterized by a moderate to moderately severe hemolytic anemia. The degree of in vivo sickling is usually considerably less than in sickle cell anemia, but hand-foot syndrome and other vaso-occlusive symptoms involving extremities, abdomen, and chest may occur. Careful biochemical and family studies in presumed cases of sickle cell anemia may reveal Hb S–β-thalassemia.[123] Some cases are diagnosed coincidentally during family studies or admission to the hospital for an unrelated condition such as pregnancy.

In contrast to sickle cell anemia, the spleen remains palpably enlarged into adult life and functional asplenia does not usually occur. Growth retardation and delayed osseous maturation are common during childhood.[123,152] The blood smear shows significant thalassemic morphologic changes—microcytosis, hypochromia, and targeting. These can be confirmed by red cell indices, which show the MCV to average 68 fl and the MCH 20 pg. Irreversibly sickled cells are infrequent.

The hemoglobin electrophoretic pattern depends on the kind of thalassemia gene that is present. If it is of the β⁺-thalassemia variety, a small amount (<30%) of Hb A will be noted. This increase in Hb S proportion greater than that noted in the simple Hb S heterozygote is described as interaction, and an Hb SA rather than AS electrophoretic pattern strongly suggests Hb S–β-thalassemia. Hb A$_2$ is also elevated. However, it may be difficult to accurately quantitate Hb A$_2$ by means of electrophoresis because of the difficulty in separating the A$_2$ and S bands.

When a β⁰-thalassemia gene is present, the hemoglobin electrophoretic pattern reveals only Hb S and Hb F, accounting for the frequent confusing of the several conditions Hb SS disease,

Hb S–β^0-thalassemia, and Hb S–HPFH. Family studies that show a microcytic anemia with elevated Hb A$_2$ levels in a parent or another first-degree relative are helpful. Hemoglobin polypeptide chain synthetic studies that show a $\beta:\alpha$ ratio below 1 establish the diagnosis.

The clinical course of Hb S–β-thalassemia is variable. Some authorities think that Hb S–β^+-thalassemia has milder clinical and hematologic manifestations than Hb S–β^0-thalassemia.[152] However, most of the vaso-occlusive complications and other crises of sickle cell anemia have been observed in these patients and they should be managed in the same way.

UNSTABLE HEMOGLOBIN VARIANTS

A group of variants, currently about fifty in number, possess molecular instability as a common property (see Tables 13-1 and 13-2). Because of their susceptibility to denaturation, precipitation of hemoglobin occurs within the red cell, forming Heinz bodies. These lead to membrane damage, premature red cell destruction, and a hemolytic process. The name "congenital Heinz body anemia" (CHBA) is frequently used for these syndromes. Unstable hemoglobins have been recognized in a significant proportion of patients with the syndrome of congenital nonspherocytic hemolytic anemia.

Both α- and β-chain substitutions may cause molecular instability, but β-chain variants are more common. Most substitutions are crucially located in the molecular regions adjacent to a heme group attachment, resulting in either enhanced methemoglobin formation or a reduced binding and subsequent loss of the heme groups from the hemoglobin molecule. Both kinds of changes result in marked molecular instability and subsequent hemoglobin precipitation. In other unstable variants amino acid substitutions or deletions in critical areas so distort secondary, tertiary, and quaternary structure that the molecule cannot hang together.

The congenital Heinz body anemias result from heterozygosity for these abnormal hemoglobin genes. Hemozygous persons have not been described and, in fact, such a condition would probably be lethal. Many patients have negative family histories and are thought to represent new mutations. The clinical and hematologic manifestations of the unstable hemoglobin syndromes vary from relatively mild anemia such as occurs in Hb Köln disease to a severe hemolytic process as is seen with Hb Bristol and Hb Hammersmith.

The red cells in these diseases are usually normocytic but may manifest hypochromia because of loss of hemoglobin through the splenic pitting action on precipitated hemoglobin. Poikilocytosis, stippling, and polychromasia are usually noted.

The reticulocyte count may be spuriously elevated.[88] Some patients excrete dark urine caused by excretion of dipyrrole pigment, and this may increase after splenectomy.[145] Heinz bodies are not usually noted in fresh blood; however, after a few hours of incubation in the presence of methylene blue, they are usually demonstrable. The abnormal hemoglobin may or may not be demonstrable by electrophoresis, but when found it occurs in relatively small proportions (5% to 20%) before splenectomy.

These variants can often be demonstrated by the heat stability test. A solution of fresh stroma-free hemolysate is heated at 50° C for 1 hour in a neutral buffer. A flocculent, brownish precipitate indicates the presence of one of these variants.[63] Alternatively a buffered solution of 17% isopropanol may be used to precipitate unstable hemoglobins.[30] Because the unstable hemoglobins often affect heme-globin interactions, oxygen affinity as indicated by the shape and position of the oxygen dissociation curve or the P$_{50}$ may be abnormally shifted either to the right or the left.

There is no specific therapy for these disorders. When the hemolytic anemia is severe and symptomatic, splenectomy may produce some benefit but is not curative.[88] Following splenectomy the proportion of unstable hemoglobin increases and large numbers of Heinz bodies may often be demonstrated in the circulating blood. In some of the variants it is advisable to avoid oxidant drugs that may aggravate hemolysis. In fact with one of these variants, Hb Zurich, hemolysis may be precipitated by administration of sulfonamides.[56]

Hb M DISORDERS

Abnormal hemoglobin variants, identified as the cause of familial cyanosis, are classified as Hb M (methemoglobin) (see Tables 13-1 and 13-2). Five such variants have been characterized. The substitutions are crucially located in the vicinity of the heme groups of either α- or β-chains. In most of the variants a histidine is replaced by a tyrosine residue. This substitution appears to stabilize heme iron in the ferric (oxidized) rather than ferrous valence as is characteristic of methemoglobin. The person with Hb M disease has visible cyanosis that cannot be corrected by oxygen administration or by administration of methylene blue.

Hb M may be detected electrophoretically on starch block or gel in phosphate buffer at pH 7.0 using potassium ferricyanide–treated hemolysate (methemoglobin).[59] In addition, the hemoglobin solutions containing the Hb M have a characteristic spectral absorption pattern differing from that of ordinary methemoglobin.[157]

In contrast to congenital enzymatic methemoglobinemias caused by diaphorase deficiency, genetic analysis of Hb M pedigrees demonstrates an autosomal dominant rather than recessive mode of transmission. Affected persons are heterozygotes. In α-chain Hb M diseases cyanosis is noted at birth, while in β-variants, it is not obvious until later in infancy. No therapy is indicated for affected persons. However, correct diagnosis is essential to avoid unnecessary diagnostic studies or restriction of activity.

HEMOGLOBINS WITH ALTERED OXYGEN AFFINITY
High-affinity hemoglobins

A group of about two dozen hemoglobin variants have been described in which amino acid substitutions drastically alter the reversible affinity between hemoglobins and oxygen[2] (see Tables 13-1 and 13-2). As previously mentioned, many of the unstable variants also have altered affinity, but the hemoglobins of this group are stable. The amino acid substitutions in many of these variants occur in portions of the molecule where α- and β-chains contact one another. This leads to alterations of the conformational relationships during oxygenation and deoxygenation. Other variants are abnormal in positions near the C-terminal position of the β-chains affecting interaction with 2,3-DPG and heme-heme interaction.

In many instances variants with increased oxygen affinity have been uncovered during the investigation of persons with familial polycythemia, or, more accurately, erythrocytosis. Hemoglobin values of affected patients range between 17.5 and 24.0 gm/dl and red blood cell volumes as measured by the ^{51}Cr technique are also elevated. Platelet and white blood cell counts are normal; this assists in differentiation of these syndromes from polycythemia vera.

The whole blood oxygen dissociation curve is shifted to the left with a P_{50} range of 12 to 18 mm Hg; the Pao_2 is normal. The patients are usually asymptomatic, longevity and fertility are not affected, and no therapy is indicated.

Low-affinity hemoglobins

About six variants have been described with decreased affinity for oxygen resulting in a right shift of the oxygen dissociation curve and low P_{50} (see Tables 13-1 and 13-2). The most remarkable of these variants is Hb Kansas, which is manifested by reduced Pao_2 and clinical cyanosis.[138] These patients may have lower than normal hemoglobin levels but have no symptoms of anemia.[168]

REFERENCES

1. Aaron, R. S.: Sickle cell anemia: a clinical study with emphasis on cardiac status, N.Y. J. Med. **51:**1511, 1951.
2. Adamson, J. W.: Familial polycythemia seminars, Hematology **12:**383, 1975.
3. Ahrens, W. E.: Gallbladder disease in children, Clin. Proc. Child. Hosp. **13:**94, 1957.
4. Alavi, A., Bond, J. P., Kuhl, D. E., and Creech, R. H.: Scan detection of bone marrow infarcts in sickle cell disorders, J. Nucl. Med. **15:**1003, 1974.
5. Alleyne, G. A., Statius Van Eps, L. W., Acedae, S. K., Nicholson, G. D., and Schrouten, H.: The kidney in sickle cell anemia, Kidney Int. **7:**371, 1975.
6. Allison, A. C.: Malaria in carriers of the sickle cell trait and in newborn children, Exp. Parasitol. **6:**418, 1957.
7. Allison, A. C.: Protection afforded by sickle cell trait against subtertian malarial infection, Br. Med. J. **1:**290, 1954.
8. Ariyan, S., Shessel, F. S., and Pickett, L. K.: Cholecystitis and cholelithiasis masking as abdominal crises in sickle cell disease, Pediatrics **58:**252, 1976.
9. Armaly, M. F.: Ocular manifestations in sickle cell disease, Arch. Intern. Med. **133:**670, 1974.
10. Atkinson, D. W.: Sickling and hematuria, Blood **34:**736, 1969. (Abstract.)
11. Atwater, J., Schwartz, I. R., Erslev, A. J., Montgomery, T. L., and Tocantins, L. M.: Sickling of erythrocytes in a patient with thalassemia-hemoglobin I disease, N. Engl. J. Med. **263:**1215, 1960.
12. Barreras, L., Diggs, L. W., and Bill, A.: Erythrocyte morphology in patients with sickle cell anemia and pulmonary emboli, J.A.M.A. **203:**569, 1968.
13. Barreras, L., Diggs, L. W., and Lipscomb, A.: Plasma volume in sickle cell disease, South. Med. J. **59:**456, 1966.
14. Barrett-Connor, E.: Pneumonia and pulmonary infarction in sickle cell anemia, J.A.M.A. **224:**997, 1973.
15. Barrett-Connor, E.: Bacterial infection and sickle cell anemia, Medicine **50:**97, 1971.
16. Barrett-Connor, E.: Cholelithiasis in sickle cell anemia, Am. J. Med. **45:**889, 1968.
17. Barton, C. J., and Cockshott, W. P.: Bone changes in hemoglobin SC disease, Am. J. Roentgenol. **88:**523, 1962.
18. Beutler, E.: The effect of methemoglobin formation in sickle cell disease, J. Clin. Invest. **40:**1856, 1961.
19. Bilinsky, R. T., Kandel, G. L., and Rabiner, S. F.: Epsilon amino caproic acid therapy of hematuria due to heterozygous sickle cell diseases, J. Urol. **102:**93, 1969.
20. Bookchin, R., and Nagel, R. L.: Molecular interactions of sickling hemoglobins. In Abramson, H., Bertles, J. F., and Wethers, D. L., eds.: Sickle cell disease; diagnosis, management, education, and research, St. Louis, 1973, The C. V. Mosby Co.
21. Boyle, E., Jr., Thompson, C., and Tyroler, H. A.: Prevalence of sickle cell trait in adults of Charleston County, Arch. Environ. Health **17:**891, 1968.
22. Bradley, T. B., Jr., Brawner, J. N., III, and Conley, C. L.: Further observations on an inherited anomaly characterized by persistence of fetal hemoglobin; Bull. Johns Hopkins Hosp. **108:**242, 1961.
23. Brewer, G. J., Oelshlegel, F. J., Jr., Prasad, A. S., Knutsen, C. A., and Meyers, N.: Antisickling effects of zinc. In Hercules, J. I., Schechter, A. N., Eaton, W. A., and Jackson, R. E., eds.: Proceedings of the first national symposium on sickle cell disease, Publication No. (NIH) 75-723, Bethesda, Md., 1974, U.S. Department of Health, Education and Welfare.
24. Brewer, G. J.: A view of the current status of antisickling therapy, Am. J. Hematol. **1:**121, 1976.
25. Brody, J. I., Goldsmith, M. H., Park, S. K., and Soltys, H. D.: Symptomatic crises of sickle cell anemia treated by limited exchange transfusion, Ann. Intern. Med. **72:**327, 1970.
26. Bromberg, P. A.: Pulmonary aspects of sickle cell disease, Arch. Intern. Med. **133:**652, 1974.

27. Brown, M. J., Weatherall, D. J., and Clegg, J. B.: Benign sickle cell anaemia, Br. J. Haematol. **22:**635, 1972.

28. Buckalew, V. M., and Someren, A.: Renal manifestations of sickle cell disease, Arch. Int. Med. **133:**660, 1974.

29. Bunn, H. F., Forget, B. G., and Ranney, H. M.: Hemoglobinopathies. In Major problems in internal medicine. XII, Philadelphia, 1977, W. B. Saunders Co.

30. Carrell, R. W., and Kay, R.: A simple method for the detection of unstable haemoglobins, Br. J. Haematol. **23:**615, 1972.

31. Caspar, J. T., Koethe, S., Rodey, G. E., and Thatcher, L. G.: A new method for studying splenic reticuloendothelial dysfunction in sickle cell disease patients and its clinical application, Blood **47:**183, 1976.

32. Castro, O., Osbaldiston, G. W., Orlin, J., Rosen, M. W., and Finch, S. F.: Oxygen dependent circulation of human sickle cells in an animal model. In Hercules, J. I., Schechter, A. N., Eaton, W. A., and Jackson, R. E., editors: Proceedings of the first national symposium on sickle cell disease, Publication No. (NIH) 75-723, Bethesda, Md., 1974, U.S. Department of Health, Education and Welfare.

33. Charache, S.: The treatment of sickle cell anemia, Arch. Int. Med. **133:**698, 1974.

34. Charache, S., and Conley, C. L.: Rate of sickling of red cells during deoxygenation of blood from persons with various sickling disorders, Blood **24:**25, 1964.

35. Chernoff, A. I.: The hemoglobin D syndromes, Blood **13:**116, 1958.

36. Condon, P. I., and Serjeant, G. R.: Ocular findings in hemoglobin SC disease in Jamaica, Am. J. Ophthalmol. **74:**921, 1972.

37. Condon, P. I., and Serjeant, G. R.: Ocular findings in homozygous sickle cell anemia in Jamaica, Am. J. Ophthalmol. **73:**533, 1972.

38. Constantopoulos, A., Najjar, V. A., and Smith, J. W.: Tuftsin deficiency: a new syndrome with defective phagocytosis, J. Pediatr. **80:**564, 1972.

39. Cooperative Urea Trials Group: Clinical trials of therapy for sickle cell vaso-occlusive cases, J.A.M.A. **228:**1120, 1974.

40. Crosby, W. H.: Normal functions of the spleen relative to red blood cells: a review, Blood **14:**399, 1959.

41. Daland, G. A., and Castle, W. B.: A simple and rapid method for demonstrating sickling of the red cells: the use of reducing agents, J. Lab. Clin. Med. **33:**1082, 1948.

42. Diederich, D., Gill, P., Trueworthy, R., and Larson, W.: In vitro carbomylation in sickle cell anemia. In Brewer, G. J., ed.: Erythrocyte structure and function, New York, 1975, Alan R. Liss Co.

43. Diggs, L. W.: Anatomic lesions in sickle cell diseases. In Abramson, H. F., Bertles, J. F., and Wethers, D. L., eds.: Sickle cell disease: diagnosis, management, education, and research, St. Louis, 1973, The C. V. Mosby Co.

44. Diggs, L. W.: Bone and joint lesions in sickle cell disease, Clin. Orthopaed. **52:**119, 1967.

45. Diggs, L. W.: Sickle cell crises, Am. J. Clin. Pathol. **44:**1, 1965.

46. Diggs, L. W.: Siderofibrosis of the spleen in sickle cell anemia, J.A.M.A. **104:**538, 1935.

47. Diggs, L. W., Ahmann, C. F., and Bibb, J.: The incidence and significance of the sickle cell trait, Ann. Intern. Med. **7:**769, 1933.

48. Diggs, L. W., and Flowers, E.: Sickle cell anemia in the home environment, Clin. Pediatr. **10:**697, 1971.

49. Diggs, L. W., Kraus, A. P., Morrison, D. B., and Rudnicki, R. P. T.: Intraerythrocytic crystals in a white

patient with hemoglobin C in the absence of other types of hemoglobin, Blood **9:**1172, 1954.

50. Duback, R. T., and Ramey, J. A.: Priapism in sickle cell trait: case report utilizing hemovac suction as an adjunct to therapy, J. Urol. **100:**175, 1968.

51. Eisenstein, M. I., Posner, A. C., and Friedman, S.: Sickle cell anemia in pregnancy, Am. J. Obstet. Gynecol. **72:**622, 1956.

52. Erlandson, M. E., Schulman, I., and Smith, C. H.: Studies on congenital hemolytic syndromes. III. Rates of destruction and production of erythrocytes in sickle cell anemia, Pediatrics **25:**629, 1960.

53. Flatz, G. Hemoglobin E: distribution and population dynamics, Humangenetik **3:**189, 1967.

54. Fowler, N. O., Smith, O., and Greenfield, J. C.: Arterial blood oxygenation in sickle cell anemia, Am. J. Med. Sci. **234:**449, 1957.

55. Freeman, M. G., and Ruth, G. J.: SS disease—SC disease—CC disease: obstetric considerations and treatment, Clin. Obstet. Gynecol. **12:**134, 1969.

56. Frick, P. G., Hitzig, W. H., and Betke, K.: Hemoglobin Zürich: a new hemoglobin anomaly associated with acute hemolytic episodes with inclusion bodies after sulfonamide therapy, Blood **20:**261, 1962.

57. Friedman, E. A., Sreepada Rao, T. K., Sprung, C. L., Smith, A., Manis, T., Bellevici, R., Britt, K. M. H., Levere, R. D., and Holden, D. M.: Uremia in sickle cell anemia treated by maintainence hemodialysis, N. Engl. J. Med. **291:**431, 1974.

58. Fullerton, W. T., Hendrickse, J. P. de V., and Watson-Williams, E. J.: Haemoglobin SC disease in pregnancy. In Jonxis, J. H. P., ed.: Abnormal haemoglobin in Africa, Oxford, 1965, Blackwell Scientific Publications, Ltd.

59. Gerald, P. S.: The electrophoretic and spectroscopic characterization of Hgb M, Blood **13:**936, 1958.

60. Gillette, P. N., Lu, Y. S., and Peterson, C. M.: The pharmacology of cyanate with a summary of its initial usage in sickle cell disease, Prog. Hematol. **8:**181, 1973.

61. Greenberg, M. S., and Kass, E. H.: Studies on the destruction of red blood cells. XIII. Observations on the role of pH in the pathogenesis and treatment of painful crises in sickle cell disease, Arch. Int. Med. **101:**355, 1958.

62. Greenwald, J. G.: Stroke, sickle cell trait, and oral contraceptives, Ann. Intern. Med. **72:**960, 1970.

63. Grimes, A. J., Meisler, A., and Dacie, J. V.: Congenital Heinz-body anaemia: further evidence on the cause of Heinz-body production in red cells, Br. J. Haematol. **10:**281, 1964.

64. Hahn, E. V., and Gillespie, E. B.: Sickle cell anemia: report of a case greatly improved by splenectomy, Arch. Intern. Med. **39:**233, 1927.

65. Hammel, C. F., DeNardo, S. J., DeNardo, G. L., and Lewis, J. P.: Bone marrow and bone mineral scintigraphic studies in sickle cell disease, Br. J. Haematol. **25:**593, 1973.

66. Harkness, D. R., and Roth, S.: Clinical evaluation of cyanate in sickle cell anemia, Prog. Hematol. **9:**157, 1975.

67. Harris, J. W., Brewster, H. H., Ham, T. H., and Castle, W. B.: Studies on the destruction of red blood cells. X. The biophysics and biology of sickle cell disease, Arch. Intern. Med. **97:**145, 1956.

68. Hasen, H. B., and Raines, S. L.: Priapism associated with sickle cell disease, J. Urol. **88:**71, 1962.

69. Hatch, F. E., Jr., Azar, S. H., Ainsworth, T. E., Nardo, J. M., and Culbertson, J. W.: Renal circulatory studies in young adults with sickle cell anemia, J. Lab. Clin. Med. **76:**632, 1970.

70. Herrick, J. B.: Peculiar elongated and sickle shaped

red blood corpuscles in a case of severe anemia, Arch. Intern. Med. **6:**517, 1910.

71. Hilkovitz, G., and Jacobson, A.: Hepatic dysfunction and abnormalities of the serum proteins and serum enzymes in sickle cell anemia, J. Lab. Clin. Med. **57:**856, 1961.

72. Huisman, T. H. J.: Chromatographic separation of Hemoglobins A$_2$ and C: The quantitation of hemoglobin A$_2$ in patients with A-C trait, C-C disease, and C-β-thalassemia, Clin. Chem. Acta **40:**159, 1972.

73. Ingram, V. M.: Abnormal human haemoglobins. I. The comparison of normal human and sickle cell haemoglobins by fingerprinting, Bio. Chem. Biophys. Acta **28:**539, 1957.

74. Itano, H. A.: Solubilities of naturally occurring mixtures of human hemoglobins, Arch. Biochem. Biophys. **47:**148, 1953.

75. Jenkins, M. E., Scott, R. B., and Baird, R. L.: Studies in sickle cell anemia. XVI. Sudden death during sickle cell anemia crisis in young children, J. Pediatr. **56:**30, 1960.

76. Jiminez, C. T., Scott, R. B., Henry, W. L., Sampson, C. C., and Ferguson, A. D.: Studies in sickle cell anemia. XXVI. The effects of homozygous sickle cell disease on the onset of menarche, pregnancy, fertility, pubescent changes, and body growth in Negro subjects, Am. J. Dis. Child. **111:**467, 1966.

77. Johnston, R. B., Jr., Newman, S. L., and Struth, A. G.: An abnormality of the alternate pathway of complement activation in sickle cell diseases, N. Engl. J. Med. **288:**803, 1973.

78. Jones, S. R., Bender, R. A., and Denowho, E. M., Jr.: Sudden death in sickle cell trait, N. Engl. J. Med. **282:**323, 1970.

79. Josephs, R., Jarosch, H. S., and Edelstein, S. J.: Polymorphism of sickle cell hemoglobin fibers, J. Mol. Biol. **102:**409, 1976.

80. Joshpe, G., Rothenberg, S. P., and Baum, S.: Transient functional asplenism in sickle cell-Hb C disease, Am. J. Med. **55:**720, 1973.

81. Karayalcino, G., Imran, M., and Rosner, F.: Priapism in sickle cell disease: report of five cases, Am. J. Med. Sci. **264:**289, 1972.

82. Keitel, H. G., Thompson, D., and Itano, H. A.: Hyposthenuria in sickle cell anemia—a reversible defect, J. Clin. Invest. **35:**998, 1956.

83. Khademi, M., and Marquis, J. R.: Renal angiography in sickle cell disease, Radiology **107:**41, 1973.

84. Kim, H. C., Alavi, A., Russell, M. O., and Schwartz, E.: Scintigraphic detection of bone and bone marrow infarcts in sickle cell disorders, Pediatr. Res. **11:**473, 1977. (Abstract.)

85. Klinefelter, H. F.: The heart in sickle cell anemia, Am. J. Med. Sci. **203:**34, 1942.

86. Klion, F. M., Weiner, M. J., and Schaffner, F.: Cholestasis in sickle cell anemia, Am. J. Med. **37:**829, 1964.

87. Knochel, J. P.: Hematuria in sickle cell trait: the effect of intravenous administration of distilled water, alkalinization, and diuresis, Arch. Intern. Med. **123:**160, 1969.

88. Koler, R. D., Jones, R. T., Begley, R. H., et al.: Hemoglobin casper β106 (G8) LewPro: a contemporary mutation, Am. J. Med. **55:**549, 1973.

89. Konatey-Ahulu, F. I. D.: The sickle cell diseases—clinical manifestations including the "sickle crisis," Arch. Intern. Med. **133:**611, 1974.

89a. Kramer, M. S., Rooks, Y. and Pearson, H. A.: Growth and development in children with sickle cell trait: a matched pair prospective study, Pediatr. Res. **12:**467, 1978.

90. Kraus, L. M., Miyaji, T., Iuchi, I., and Kraus, A. P.: Characterization of $\alpha^{23glu\ NH_2}$ in hemoglobin Memphis:

hemoglobin memphis/S, is a new variant of molecular disease. Biochemistry **5:**3701, 1966.

91. Lebby, R.: Case of absence of the spleen, South. Pharm. J. **1:**481, 1846.

92. Leikin, S. L.: The aplastic crisis of sickle cell disease: occurrence in several members of families within a short period of time, Am. J. Dis. Child. **93:**128, 1957.

93. Levere, R. D., Lichtman, H. C., and Levine, J.: Effect of iron deficiency anaemia on the metabolism of the heterogenic haemoglobins in sickle cell trait, Nature **202:**499, 1964.

94. Levitt, M. F., Hauser, A. D., Levy, M. S., and Palemeros, D.: The renal concentrating defect in sickle cell disease, Am. J. Med. **29:**611, 1960.

95. Liebman, N. C.: Renal papillary necrosis and sickle cell disease, J. Urol. **102:**294, 1969.

96. Lindenbaum, J., Klipstein, F. A.: Folic acid deficiency in sickle cell anemia, N. Engl. J. Med. **269:**875, 1963.

97. Lindo, C. L., and Doctor, L. R.: The electrocardiogram in sickle cell anemia, Am. Heart J. **50:**218, 1955.

98. Lindsay, J., Jr., Meshel, J. C., and Patterson, R. H.: The cardiovascular manifestations of sickle cell disease, Arch. Intern. Med. **133:**643, 1974.

99. Lubin, B. H., and Oski, F. A.: Oral urea therapy for sickle cell vaso-occlusive crisis, J. Pediatr. **82:**311, 1973.

100. MacIver, J. E., and Went, L. N.: Sickle cell anemia complicated by megaloblastic anaemia of infancy, Br. Med. J. **1:**775, 1960.

101. Marder, V. J., and Conley, C. L.: Frequency of Hgb D in Negro populations: electrophoresis of hemoglobin on agar gel, Bull. John Hopkins Hosp. **105:**77, 1959.

102. Martinez, M., Sharma, T. C., MacDonald, C., and Smyth, N. P. D.: Operative management of priapism secondary to sickle cell trait, Arch. Surg. **98:**81, 1969.

103. McCormack, M. K., Scarr-Salapatek, S., Polesky, H., Thompson, W., Katz, S. H., and Barker, W. B.: A comparison of physical and intellectual development of black children with and without sickle cell trait, Pediatrics **56:**1021, 1975.

104. McCoy, R. C.: Ultrastructural alterations in the kidney of patients with sickle cell disease and the nephrotic syndrome, Lab. Invest. **21:**85, 1969.

105. McCurdy, P. R., Lorkin, P. A., Casey, R., et al.: Hemoglobin S-G (S-D) syndrome, Am. J. Med. **57:**665, 1974.

106. McGarry, P. and Duncan, C.: Anesthetic risks in sickle cell trait, Pediatrics **51:**507, 1973.

107. Miller, G. J., and Serjeant, G. R.: An assessment of lung volume and gas transfer in sickle cell anaemia, Thorax **26:**309, 1971.

108. Miller, M. J., Neel, J. V., and Livingstone, F. B.: Distribution of parasites in the red cells of sickle cell trait-carriers infected with *Plasmodium falciparum*, Trans. R. Soc. Trop. Med. Hyg. **50:**294, 1956.

109. Milner, P. F., Miller, C., Grey, R., Seakins, M., DeJong, W. W., and Went, L. N.: Hemoglobin O$_{Arab}$ in four Negro families and its interaction with hemoglobin S and hemoglobin C, N. Engl. J. Med. **283:**1417, 1970.

110. Moser, K. M., Luchsinger, P. C., and Katz, S.: Pulmonary and cardiac function in sickle cell lung disease, Dis. Chest **37:**637, 1957. 1960.

111. Murayama, M.: Molecular mechanism of red cell "sickling," Science **153:**145, 1966.

112. Murphy, J. R.: Sickle cell hemoglobin (Hb AS) in black football players, J.A.M.A. **225:**981, 1973.

113. Nalbandian, R. M.: Urea for sickle cell crises, N. Engl. J. Med. **284:**1381, 1971.

114. Nalbandian, R. M., Nichols, B. M., Heustis, A. E., Prothro, W. B., and Ludwig, F. E.: An automated mass screening program for sickle cell disease, J.A.M.A. **218:**1680, 1971.

115. Neel, J. V.: The inheritance of sickle cell anemia, Science **110**:64, 1949.
116. O'Brien, R. T.: Body iron burden in sickle cell anemia, J. Pediatr. **92**:579, 1978.
117. O'Brien, R. T., McIntosh, L. S., Aspnes, G. T., and Pearson, H. A.: Prospective study of sickle cell anemia in infancy, J. Pediatr. **89**:205, 1976.
118. Owen, D. M., Aldridge, J. E., and Thompson, R. B.: An unusual hepatic sequelae of sickle cell anemia: a report of 5 cases, Am. J. Med. Sci. **249**:175, 1965.
119. Pardo, V., Strauss, J., Kramer, H., Ozawa, T., and McIntosh, R. M.: Nephropathy associated with sickle cell anemia: an autologous, immune complex nephritis, Am. J. Med. **59**:650, 1975.
120. Paton, D.: Conjunctival signs of sickle cell disease: further observations, Arch. Opthalmol. **68**:627, 1962.
121. Paton, D.: The conjunctival sign in sickle cell disease, Arch. Opthalmol. **66**:90, 1961.
122. Pauling, L., Itano, H. A., Sengers, S. J., and Wells, I. C.: Sickle cell anemia molecular disease, Science **110**:543, 1949.
123. Pearson, H. A.: Hemoglobin- S Thalassemia syndrome in Negro children, Ann. N.Y. Acad. Sci. **165**:83, 1969.
124. Pearson, H. A., and Cobb, W. T.: Folic acid studies in sickle cell anemia, J. Lab. Clin. Med. **64**:913, 1964.
125. Pearson, H. A., Cornelius, E. A., Schwartz, A. D., Zelson, J. H., Wolfson, S. L., and Spencer, R. P.: Transfusional reversible, functional asplenia in young children with sickle cell anemia, N. Engl. J. Med. **283**:334, 1970.
126. Pearson, H. A., and Diamond, L. K.: Sickle cell disease crises and their management in the critically ill child. In Smith, C. A., ed.: Diagnosis and management, ed. 2, Philadelphia, 1977, W. B. Saunders Co.
127. Pearson, H. A., Schiebler, G. L., Krovetz, L. J., Bartley, T. D., and David, J. K.: Sickle cell anemia associated with tetrology of Fallot, N. Engl. J. Med. **273**:1079, 1965.
128. Pearson, H. A., Spencer, R. P., and Corneluis, E. A.: Functional asplenia in sickle cell anemia, N. Engl. J. Med. **281**:923, 1969.
129. Perillie, P. E., and Epstein, F. H.: Sickling phenomenon produced by hypertonic solutions; a possible explanation for the hyposthenuria of sicklemia, J. Clin. Invest. **42**:570, 1963.
130. Petch, M. C., and Serjeant, G. R.: Clinical features of pulmonary lesions in sickle cell anemia, Br. Med. J. **2**:31, 1970.
131. Pierce, L. E., and Rath, C. E.: Evidence of folic acid deficiency in the genesis of anemic sickle cell crisis, Blood **20**:192, 1962.
132. Powars, D. R.: Natural history of sickle cell disease—the first ten years, Semin. Hematol. **12**:267, 1975.
133. Powars, D., Schroeder, W. A., and White, L.: Rapid diagnosis of sickle cell disease at birth by microcolumn chromatography, Pediatrics **55**:630, 1975.
134. Prasad, A. S., Schoomaker, E. B., Ortega, J., Brewer, G. J., Oberleas, D., and Oelshlegel, F.: Deficiency of zinc in Sickle cell disease patients. In Hercules, J. A., Schecter, A. N., Eaton, W. A., and Jackson, R. E., eds.: Proceedings of the first national symposium on sickle cell disease, Publication No. (NIH) 75-723, Bethesda, Md., 1974, U.S. Department of Health, Education and Welfare.
135. Pritchard, J. A., Scott, D. E., Whalley, P., et al.: The effects of maternal sickle cell hemoglobinopathea and sickle cell trait on reproductive performance, Am. J. Obstet. Gynecol. **117**:662, 1971.
136. Purugganan, H. B., and McElfresh, A. E.: Failure of carbonmonoxy sickle cell haemoglobin to alter the sickle state, Lancet **1**:79, 1964.
137. Rao, S. P., Tavormins, A., Rao, A. N., Solomon, N. A., and Brown, A. K.: The usefulness of bone scans in differentiating osteomyclite from thrombolic crisis in children with sickle cell disease, Pediatr. Res. **11**:479, 1977. (Abstract.)
138. Reissmann, K. R., Ruth, W. E., and Nomura, T.: A human hemoglobin with lowered oxygen affinity and impaired heme-heme interactions, J. Clin. Invest. **40**:1826, 1961.
139. Reynolds, J. D. H.: Painful sickle cell crisis—successful treatment with hyperbaric oxygen therapy, J.A.M.A. **216**:1977, 1971.
140. Rickles, F. R., and O'Leary, D. S.: Role of coagulation system in the pathophysiology of sickle cell disease, Arch. Int. Med. **133**:635, 1974.
141. Robbins, J. B., and Pearson, H. A.: Normal response of sickle cell anemia patients to immunization with Salmonella vaccines, J. Pediatr. **66**:877, 1965.
142. Robinson, A. R., Robson, M., Harrison, A. P., and Zuelzer, W. W.: A new technique for differentiation of hemoglobin, J. Lab. Clin. Med. **50**:745, 1957.
143. Russell, M. O., Goldberg, H. I., Reis, L., Freidman, S. H., Slater, R., Reivich, M., and Schwartz, E.: Transfusion therapy for cerebrovascular abnormalities in sickle cell disease, J. Pediatr. **88**:382, 1976.
144. Schlitt, L., and Keitil, H. G.: Pathogenesis of hyposthenuria in persons with sickle cell anemia or the sickle cell trait, Pediatrics **26**:249, 1960.
145. Schmid, R., Brecher, G., and Clemens, T.: Familial hemolytic anemia with erythrocyte inclusion bodies and a defect in pigment metabolism, Blood **14**:991, 1959.
146. Schwartz, A. D., and Pearson, H. A.: Impaired antibody response to intravenous immunization in sickle cell anemia, Pediatr. Res. **6**:145, 1972.
147. Schwartz, E., and McElfresh, A. E.: Treatment of painful crisis of sickle cell disease: a double blind study, J. Pediatr. **64**:132, 1964.
148. Seeler, R. A.: Intensive transfusion therapy for priapism in boys with sickle cell anemia, J. Urol. **110**:360, 1973.
149. Seeler, R. A., and Shwiaki, M. Z.: Acute splenic sequestration crisis (ASSC) in young children with sickle cell anemia, Clin. Pediatr. **11**:701, 1972.
150. Serjeant, G. R.: Leg ulceration in sickle cell anemia, Arch. Intern. Med. **133**:690, 1974.
151. Serjeant, G. R.: The clinical features of sickle cell disease, Amsterdam, 1974, North Holland Publishing Co.
152. Serjeant, G. R., Ashcroft, M. T., Serjeant, B. E., and Milner, P. F.: The clinical features of sickle cell β-thalassemia in Jamaica, Br. J. Haematol. **24**:19, 1973.
153. Serjeant, G. R., and Ashcroft, M. T.: Shortening of the digits in sickle cell anemia—a sequelae of the hand-foot syndrome, Trop. Geogr. Med. **23**:341, 1971.
154. Serjeant, G. R., Galloway, R. E., and Gueri, M.: Oral zinc sulfate in sickle cell ulcers, Lancet **2**:891, 1970.
155. Sexauer, C. L., Graham, H. L., Starling, K. A., and Fernbach, D. J.: A test for abnormal hemoglobins in umbilical cord blood, Am. J. Dis. Child. **130**:805, 1976.
156. Sharp, E. A., and Vonder Heide, E. C.: Eunuchoid habitus associated with sickle cell anemia and the sickling trait, J. Clin. Endocrinol. **4**:505, 1944.
157. Shibata, S., Miyaji, T., Kuchi, I., and Karita, K.: Hemoglobin M of the Japanese, Bull. Vamaguchi Med. Sch. **14**:141, 1967.
158. Shulman, S. T., Bartlett, J., Clyde, W. A., and Ayoub, E. M.: The unusual severity of mycoplasmal pneumonia in children with sickle cell disease, N. Engl. J. Med. **287**:164, 1973.
159. Silvestroni, E., and Bianco, I.: New data on microdrepanocytic disease, Blood **10**:623, 1955.
160. Singer, K., Motulsky, A. G., and Wile, S. A.: Aplastic

crisis in sickle cell anemia, J. Lab. Clin. Med. **33:**721, 1950.

161. Smith, E. W., and Conley, C. L.: Clinical manifestations of sickle cell disease, Publication No. 554, National Academy of Sciences–National Research Council, 1958.

162. Smith, E. W. and Conley, C. L.: Sicklemia and infarction of the spleen during aerial flight: electrophoreses of the hemoglobin in 15 cases, Bull. Johns Hopkins Hosp. **96:**35, 1955.

163. Smits, H. L., Oski, F. A., and Brody, J. I.: The hemolytic crisis of sickle cell disease: the role of glucose-6-phosphate dehydrogenase deficiency, J. Pediatr. **74:**544, 1969.

164. Snyder, G. B., and Wilson, C. A.: Surgical management of priapism and its sequelae in sickle cell disease, South. Med. J. **59:**1393, 1966.

165. Song, Y. S.: Hepatic lesions in sickle cell anemia, Am. J. Path. **33:**331, 1957.

166. Sproule, B. J., Halden, E. R., and Miller, W. F.: A study of cardiopulmonary alterations in patients with sickle cell disease and its variants, J. Clin. Invest. **37:**486, 1958.

167. Stamatoyannopoulos, G., and Fessas, P.: Thalassaemia, glucose-6-phosphate dehydrogenase deficiency, sickling, and malarial endemecity in Greece: a study of five areas, Br. Med. J. **1:**875, 1964.

168. Stamatoyannopoulos, G., Parer, J. R., and Finch, C. A.: Implications of a hemoglobin with decreased oxygen affinity, N. Engl. J. Med. **218:**915, 1969.

169. Stamatoyannopoulos, G., Wood, W. G., Papayannopoulou, T., and Nute, P. E.: A new form of hereditary persistence of fetal hemoglobin in blacks and its association with sickle cell trait, Blood **46:**683, 1975.

170. Statius, Van Eps, L. W., Pinedeo-Veels, C., DeVries, G. H., and De Koneng, K.: Nature of concentrating defect in sickle cell nephropathy microangiographic studies, Lancet **1:**450, 1970.

171. Stockman, J. A., Nigro, M. A., Mishkin, M. M., and Oski, F. A.: Occlusion of large cerebral vessels in sickle cell anemia, N. Engl. J. Med. **287:**846, 1972.

172. Strauss, R. G., Ashbrock, T., Foristal, J., and West, C. D.: Alternative pathway of complement in sickle cell disease, Ped. Res. **11:**285, 1977.

173. Suster, G., and Oski, F. A.: Enuresis in sickle cell anemia, Am. J. Dis. Child. **113:**311, 1967.

174. Sweeney, M. J., Dobbins, W. T., and Etteldorf, J. N.: Renal disease with elements of the nephrotic syndrome associated with sickle cell anemia, J. Pediatr. **60:**42, 1962.

175. Uzsoy, N. K.: Cardiovascular findings in patients with sickle cell anemia, Am. J. Cardiol. **13:**320, 1964.

176. Uzsby, N. K.: Coexistence of rheumatic heart disease and sickle cell anemia, Am. J. Med. Sci. **246:**462, 1963.

177. Van Enk, A., Lang, A., White, J. M., and Lehmann, H.: Benign obstetric history in women with sickle cell anemia associated with α-thalassaemia, Br. Med. J. **4:**524, 1972.

178. Watson, R. J., Burko, H., Megas, H., and Robinson, M.: The hand-foot syndrome in sickle cell disease in young children, Pediatrics **31:**975, 1963.

179. Weens, H. S.: Cholelithiasis in sickle cell anemia, Ann. Intern. Med. **22:**182, 1945.

180. Whitten, C. F.: Growth status of children with sickle cell anemia, Am. J. Dis. Child. **102:**355, 1961.

181. Winkelstein, J. A., and Drachman, R. H.: Deficiency of pneumococcal serum opsonizing activity in sickle cell disease, N. Engl. J. Med. **279:**459, 1968.

182. Zimmerman, S. L., and Barnett, R.: Sickle cell anemia simulating coronary occlusion, Am. Int. Med. **21:**1045, 1944.

15 □ Thalassemia syndromes

Howard A. Pearson

The thalassemias, a heterogeneous group of inherited disorders, are characterized by hypochromic anemia caused by deficient synthesis of one or more of the polypeptide chains of human hemoglobin. A variety of thalassemias involve different polypeptide chains, each of which has characteristic clinical and biochemical manifestations.

The most important forms of thalassemia result from autosomal mutant genes that reduce the rate of synthesis of the α- or β-polypeptide chains of Hb A, designated α- and β-thalassemia, respectively. Unlike the hemoglobinopathies, no abnormal hemoglobin variants are usually seen in the thalassemias although abnormal proportions of normal components, elongated or fusion hemoglobins, or tetrameric chain forms may be noted.

β-THALASSEMIA

In the homozygous state β-thalassemia genes result in a severe or total suppression of β-chain synthesis, clinically characterized as thalassemia major or Cooley's anemia. As a consequence of diminished Hb A synthesis the circulating red cells are small, thin, and misshapened, and they contain reduced amounts of hemoglobin. The anemia of thalassemia major is so severe that dependency on blood transfusions is established at an early age.

Historical perspective

In 1925 and 1927 Cooley et al.[19,20] culled a group of children with similar clinical and hematologic abnormalities from the heterogeneous classification of severe childhood disorders that at that time were designated Von Jaksch's anemia. The affected children were of Mediterranean ethnic background. They had striking skeletal and facial abnormalities and splenomegaly. They were profoundly anemic, and their blood contained large numbers of normoblasts, leading Cooley to designate this condition as erythroblastic anemia. In recognition of his observations, the eponym "Cooley's anemia" is used to describe the severe form of this disease. Whipple and Bradford,[142] in recognition of the fact that affected children were almost invariably of Italian or Greek ancestry, coined the term "thalassemia," or "anemia of the Mediterranean Sea."

Somewhat later, both in the United States and Italy, a mild microcytic anemia with morphologic abnormalities similar to those of Cooley's anemia was recognized in Mediterranean people.[143] This anemia was designated as familial microcytosis or target cell anemia. The relationship between the mild and severe anemias was clarified by the observation that both parents of children with severe Cooley's anemia had the mild microcytic anemia. Thus the concept was advanced that thalassemia is caused by a gene that in the heterozygous state produces thalassemia minor and in the homozygous state results in thalassemia major.[130]

Geographic distribution of the β-thalassemia gene

The β-thalassemia gene occurs commonly in countries bordering on the Mediterranean Sea. In Italy the highest frequency, approaching 5%, occurs in the Po valley, around Ferrara, and in southern Italy, Sicily, Sardenia, and Corsica.[116] In Greece prevalence varies considerably, ranging from less than 5% to nearly 15%.[79] An overall estimate of frequency in American Italian and Greek communities is 2.5% and 10%, respectively.[97] A so-called thalassemia belt extends along the shores of the Mediterranean and continues through Turkey, Iran, India, and into southeastern Asia and southern China.[76] (See Fig. 14-3.) β-thalassemia also occurs in African people, and the frequency of the gene in black Americans is 0.5% to 1.0%.[44]

Pathogenesis

The basic defect of β-thalassemia, impaired synthesis of β-polypeptide chains, can be most directly and convincingly demonstrated by in vitro hemoglobin synthesis techniques involving incubation of the patient's blood with a radioactive amino acid, usually ^{14}C-leucine. Reticulocytes, which actively synthesize hemoglobin, incorporate the radioactive amino acid into newly fabricated α- and β-polypeptide chains. These chains can then be chromatographically separated by a carboxymethyl cellulose column in the presence of 8M urea.[47,139] Chromatograms of globin from normal persons demonstrate that an equal amount of radioactivity is incorporated into α- and β-fractions, yielding a $\beta:\alpha$-ratio of approximately 1 (Fig. 15-1). When this procedure is performed using blood from β-thalassemia heterozygotes, reduced radioactivity is noted in β- compared to α-fractions, producing a reduced $\beta:\alpha$-ratio of 0.5 to 0.7. When this same type of incubation is performed with blood from a patient with β-thalassemia major, a marked reduction or even no β-chain synthesis is noted. α-Chain production is normal, re-

sulting in $\beta:\alpha$-ratio of 0.1 to 0.3. A small amount of γ-chain synthesis is also noted, presumably as a compensatory phenomenon (Fig. 15-1). Fig. 15-2 shows ranges for $\beta:\alpha$-synthesis in various thalassemia syndromes and for normal persons.

In about 10% of β-thalassemia homozygotes no β-chain synthesis occurs; this form has been called β^0-thalassemia. In other homozygotes small amounts of β-chain synthesis result in a $\beta:\alpha$

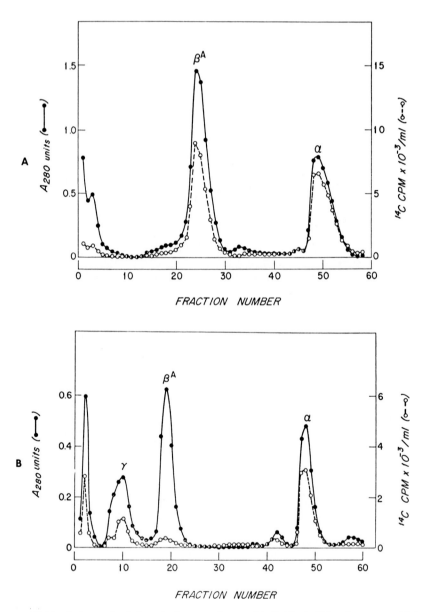

Fig. 15-1. Globin chain synthesis in reticulocytes of normal individuals **(A)** and persons with homozygous β^+-thalassemia **(B)**. Peripheral blood was incubated with ^{14}C-leucine. Globin was then prepared and fractionated by carboxymethylcellulose column chromatography. ●————● represents optical density of globin chains; ○— — —○ represents radioactivity incorporated into newly synthesized globin chains. (From Forget, B. G., and Kan, Y. W.: In Hematology of infancy and childhood, Philadelphia, 1974, W. B. Saunders Co.)

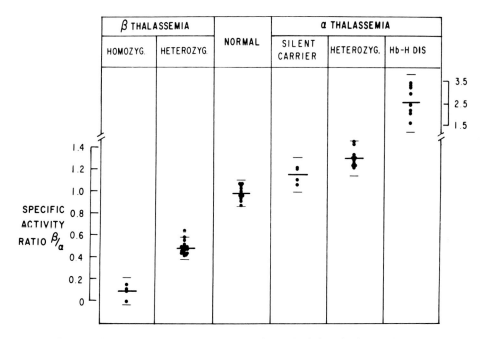

Fig. 15-2. Ranges of values for the ratio of β- to α-chain synthesis in reticulocytes in nonthalassemic and various thalassemic syndromes. (From Nathan, D. G.: N. Engl. J. Med. **286**:586, 1972. Reprinted by permission.)

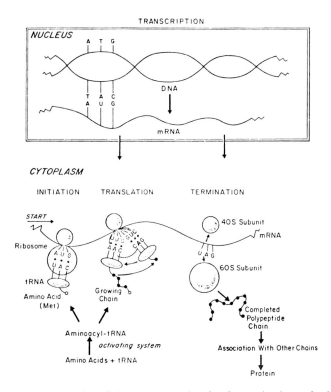

Fig. 15-3. Schematic representation of the sequence and molecular mechanisms of polypeptide chain synthesis. (From Forget, B. G., and Kan, Y. W.: In Hematology of infancy and childhood, Philadelphia, 1974, W. B. Saunders Co.)

synthetic ratio of 0.1 to 0.3, and this form has been designated β^+-thalassemia.[17,140] When in vitro globin chain synthesis is studied in nucleated red blood cells from bone marrow as opposed to peripheral blood reticulocytes, the discrepancy between β- and α-chain synthesis is less pronounced, but the significance of this observation is not clear.[9,110]

The fundamental cause of defective polypeptide chain synthesis in thalassemia has been elucidated by a series of sophisticated experiments examining the intracellular sequence of protein synthesis. The synthesis of proteins, including the polypeptide chains of hemoglobin, proceeds in a well-defined biologic sequence (Fig. 15-3).

The primary structure of a protein is determined by the genetic message encoded in DNA. The DNA sequence is transcribed into a complimentary sequence of a material designated messenger RNA (mRNA). The mRNA leaves the nucleus and becomes attached to ribosomes, where polypeptide chain synthesis actually occurs. A complicated series of reactions ensues resulting in the linking together of amino acid residues by peptide binding in a specific sequence that corresponds to the encoded sequence of triplets of base pairs in the original nuclear DNA message. Thus protein synthesis results from a series of steps: transcription of the nuclear message into mRNA and then sequential initiation, translation, and termination of peptide chain synthesis on the ribosomes.[135]

Because a defect of any of these steps could result in deficient protein synthesis, they have been carefully studied in thalassemia. The results of these studies have been summarized in recent reviews.[8,38] The mechanisms involved in all aspects of ribosomal activity have been found to be normal.[90] A number of investigators have demonstrated a quantitative deficiency of mRNA in thalassemic red cell precursors, but sophisticated studies have indicated that the mRNA present is structurally normal.[7,37,88,89] It has not been possible thus far to precisely determine the reason for the reduced amounts of mRNA in thalassemia. Alternatives include deficient synthesis per se and the production of an unstable mRNA that is rapidly denatured.[36]

The molecular genetic mechanism for β^0-thalassemia may be different than β^+-thalassemia. A gene deletion resulting in total absence of mRNA could explain the findings in this variant, but other mechanisms could be invoked.[38,129]

There are other β-thalassemias in addition to the β^+- and β^0-varieties. The so-called $\beta\delta$-variant is thought to be associated with a genetic deletion involving both β- and δ-loci.[124] Heterozygotes for $\beta\delta$-thalassemia have hematologic findings similar to the usual β-thalassemia trait. However, normal levels of Hb A_2 and elevated levels of Hb F are found. The Lepore hemoglobin gene is a fusion product of a crossover between β- and δ-genes replacing the normal loci of the chromosome.[3] Clinically and hematologically the Lepore trait resembles β-thalassemia but is characterized by the presence of the Lepore hemoglobin—a hemoglobin with Hb S–like mobility—in a concentration of 5% to 15%.[42]

Pathophysiology

Because of the profound deficiency of β-chains, total synthesis of Hb A ($\alpha_2\beta_2$) is markedly reduced or absent, and the patient with homozygous β-thalassemia is severely anemic. The red cells are hypochromic and microcytic. As a compensatory response to the severe hematologic processes, γ-chain synthesis remains activated and so the hemoglobin of the patient contains a relatively large proportion of Hb F.[118] However, since this γ-chain synthesis must operate postnatally against the so-called $\beta\gamma$-switch, it is ineffective and quantitatively insufficient. Furthermore, it tends to occur in an irregular clonal distribution in the red cell population.

Decreased hemoglobin synthesis alone does not explain some of the more striking biochemical and hematologic features of thalassemia major. These patients have evidence of a severe hemolytic process. The mechanism of severe hemolysis in thalassemia major is thought to result from unbalanced hemoglobin polypeptide chain synthesis.[84]

Synthesis of α-chains is not decreased in homozygous β-thalassemia; however, the total amount of non-α-chains (β, γ, and δ) is much less than total α-chain production. This *unbalanced* polypeptide chain synthesis results in an excess of free α-chains within nucleated red cells and reticulocytes. These free α-chains apparently aggregate into unstable units that precipitate within the red cell causing membrane damage and cell destruction within the bone marrow.[30,85] Thus the erythropoiesis in thalassemia is largely ineffective.[127] The red cells that gain entrance into the circulation are small and misshapen with a markedly decreased complement of hemoglobin—the classical hypochromic, microcytic, and poikilocytic blood smear of Cooley's anemia. Red cells containing a relatively large amount of Hb F have a somewhat longer survival.[40]

Clinical and laboratory findings

Blood. The anemia of thalassemia major is characterized by severe hypochromia and microcytosis. The child is not anemic at birth, but during the first months of life the hemoglobin level decreases progressively. When the child becomes symptomatic, the hemoglobin level may be as low as 3 to 4 gm/dl. The red cells' morphology is strikingly abnormal with many microcytes and bizarre poikilocytes and target cells. A characteristic finding is the presence of large, extraordinarily thin, often wrinkled and folded cells containing irregular clumps of hemoglobin (leptocytes).

Nucleated red cells are invariably found. A reticulocyte count of 2% to 8% is noted, which is lower than would be expected from the degree of marrow erythroid hyperplasia and hemolysis. A moderate polymorphonuclear leukocytosis and normal platelet count are usual unless hypersplenism has developed. The bone marrow shows marked hypercellularity resulting from a profound normoblastic hyperplasia. The red cell precursors also show defective hemoglobinization and reduced amounts of cytoplasm. Following splenectomy a prodigious outpouring of nucleated red blood cells sometimes reaches 50 to 100 × 10⁹/liter. Increased white count and thrombocytosis also are noted.

The osmotic fragility is strikingly abnormal. The red cells are markedly resistant to hemolysis in hypotonic sodium chloride solution so that they are not entirely hemolyzed even in distilled water. Decreased osmotic fragility occurs in thalassemia minor as well. The serum iron is increased and the iron-binding protein is fully saturated.[121]

The hemoglobin of the patient with thalassemia is predominantly Hb F. In patients with homozygous β^0-type no Hb A is found. In the newborn more than 90% is Hb F. With advancing age this tends to slowly decrease, but it is always considerably increased, in the range of 20% to 60%, unless transfusions confound exact Hb F quantitation.

Hb A_2 levels tend to parallel the levels of Hb A in thalassemia major, albeit at a much lower level. The ratio of $A_2:A_1$, which in the normal person is about 1:30, is increased to less than 1:20 in thalassemia major. Other biochemical abnormalities of the red cell in thalassemia major include a postnatal persistence of the i antigen and a decrease of red cell carbonic anhydrase.[43]

Fessas[30] described intraerythrocytic inclusions in the peripheral blood cells, especially after splenectomy. These inclusions, best seen with supravital staining with methylene blue or cresyl violet as well as with phase microscopy, are aggregates of precipitated, denatured α-chains.[31] They are also found in large numbers in erythroid precursors in the bone marrow.

The serum is icteric with elevated serum levels of unconjugated bilirubin ranging between 2.0 to 4.0 mg/dl. When the upper limit is exceeded, hepatitis, cholelithiasis, or a hemolytic crisis should be considered. Red cell survival in thalassemia major is variable but usually markedly decreased with ^{51}Cr $T_{1/2}$ ranging from 6.5 to 19.5 days compared to a normal of 25 to 35 days.[127] Increased plasma iron turnover and poor radio-iron utilization indicate ineffective erythropoiesis.

Frequent epistaxis in patients with thalassemia major often prompts a study of the coagulation mechanism. Coagulation data are similar to those found in patients with liver disease of any etiology (i.e., lowered levels of factors IX, XI, V, and VII and prothrombin).[48] The one abnormality that exists in a large number of patients is the decrease of factor XI. Patients who often had the most difficulty with epistaxis had no significant coagulation defects. Mild impairment of the coagulation mechanism appears in children between 7 and 10 years old. Only rarely are the coagulation abnormalities sufficient to require fresh-frozen plasma or specific concentrate therapy prior to surgery. A general correlation exists between the coagulation status and the other parameters of hepatic function, both deteriorating in older patients.[49]

Pathology. The anatomic and histologic changes observed in thalassemia major reflect a chronic, severe hemolytic anemia, the processes marshaled by the body in response to this, the long-term effects of hypoxia, and the consequences of therapy. Modern hypertransfusional therapy has somewhat delayed or ameliorated some of these abnormalities.

Skeletal changes. Skeletal abnormalities result primarily from hypertrophy and expansion of the erythroid marrow. This results in widening of the marrow space and thinning of the cortex with consequent osteoporosis.[11] Studies have suggested that the osteoporotic lesions in thalassemia are probably not actively related to the marrow hyperplasia but may result from faulty metabolism, which affects ossification.[14] Both hyperprolinemia and hyperprolinuria are found in thalassemic children.[75] Hydroxyproline constitutes approximately 14% of the amino acid residual of collagen, and 95% of collagen is found in bone. It is not yet clear whether an abnormality of proline metabolism is related to the osteoporosis in these patients.

Striking changes appear in the skull and facial bones. The frontal bone is thickened with prominent frontal bossing. The thickened, membranous bones of the skull do not expand adjacent to the sutures, resulting in a "hot-cross bun" appearance of the skull. Roentgenograms reveal the diploë to be widened. The skull at first has a granular appearance, but later perpendicular bony trabeculae appear, giving the classic "hair-on-end," or crew cut appearance (Fig. 15-4).

The maxilla is regularly involved. Pneumatization of the sinusoids is markedly delayed, and a

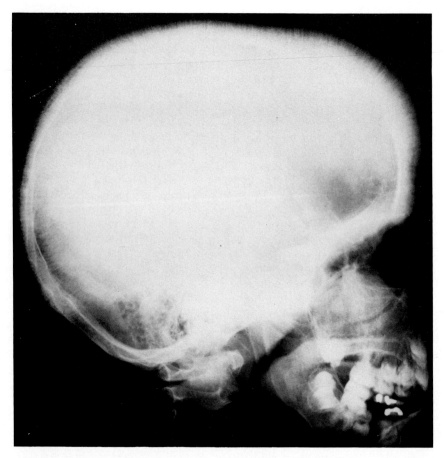

Fig. 15-4. Lateral skull roentgenogram of a patient with Cooley's anemia. The diploic spaces of the skull are thickened, with prominent ''hair-on-end'' appearance. There is marked overgrowth of the maxilla with overbite. The sinuses are not pneumatized.

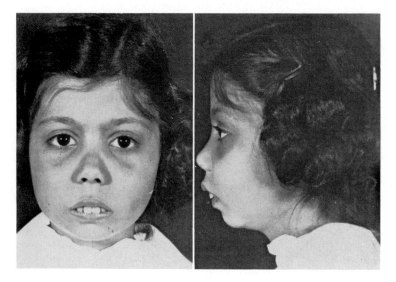

Fig. 15-5. Characteristic facies in severe Cooley's anemia (thalassemia major). Note prominent malar eminences, depression of the bridge of the nose, slight oblique appearance of eyes, and enlargement of superior maxilla with protrusion of lip upward exposing upper teeth.

marked overgrowth of the maxilla may result in severe malocclusion and jumbling of the upper incisors as well as prominence of the malar eminences.[2] These bony changes result in the classical Cooley's facies (Fig. 15-5). The earliest skeletal changes are observed in the metacarpals, metatarsals, and phalanges where expanded medullary cavities produce a rectangular and then a convex shape. Marked osteoporosis and cortical thinning may predispose to pathologic fractures of the extremities; compression fractures of the vertebrae may also occur. Premature fusion of the epiphyses of the long bones is common in patients who are more than 10 years old. Involvement of the epiphyses of the proximal humerus results in a characteristic shortening of the upper arms.[21]

The ribs may be very broad, especially at the point of attachment to the vertebral column, and may expand to the extent that they are visible as paravertebral masses (Fig. 15-6). An unusual and severe complication results from expansion of this paravertebral hematopoietic tissue into the spinal canal with resultant cord compression.[123] Decompressive laminectomy may be necessary to prevent permanent paralysis.

The character and degree of the bone changes are modified significantly with age. In older children the bone lesions regress in the more distal portions of the skeleton (hands, arms, and legs), whereas normally the red marrow is replaced with fatty marrow. The characteristic changes described in the hands and other peripheral areas are thus diminished and may disappear at puberty.[10,103] However, in the skull, spine, and pelvis (all sites of active, persistent erythropoiesis) the roentgenographic changes become more conspicuous.[10]

Liver and gallbladder. The livers of these patients are very enlarged. Initially this is in part a result of extramedullary hematopoiesis, and hepatomegaly can be reduced by hypertransfusion.[93] Later it is associated with extensive cirrhosis with nodular aggregates of regenerating hepatocytes, separated by broad bands of fibrous tissue. Iron deposition, initially present in the Kupfer cells, ultimately engorges the parenchymal cells, also resulting in findings that are indistinguishable from those in idiopathic hemochromatosis.[25,35] Many of these patients have also had homologous serum hepatitis, which may augment liver damage. The most important abnormalities of liver function include hyper-γ-globulinemia, hypoalbuminemia, and moderate decreases in the coagulation factors that are synthesized in the liver.[49]

Pigmentary gallstones are found increasingly in patients more than four years old, and two thirds of patients older than 15 years have multiple calculi.[23] Gallbladder surgery is not advocated unless biliary colic or obstructive jaundice has occurred. However, if gallstones are present at the time of splenectomy, cholecystectomy may be considered.

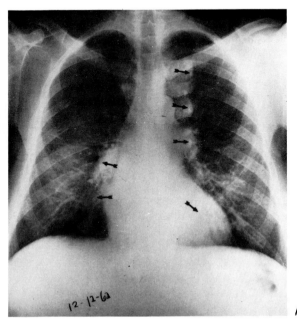
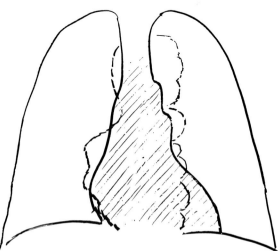

Fig. 15-6. Heterotropic bone marrow in thalassemia major. Intrathoracic masses of bone marrow occupy paravertebral spaces. The masses lie lateral to the vertebral bodies and project through the intercostal spaces. These masses consist of compensatory extramedullary hematopoietic tissue.

Heart. Cardiac abnormalities are frequent and important causes of morbidity and mortality in patients with thalassemia major. In the past cardiac dilatation secondary to severe anemia was frequently observed in young children. However, when hemoglobin levels are maintained above 9.0 gm/dl by hypertransfusion, cardiac size is normal during the first decade of life.

During the second decade of life myocardial hemosiderosis is inevitable, and serious cardiac disorders become frequent. The first electrocardiographic abnormalities noted include a prolonged P-R interval, first-degree heart block, and premature atrial contractions.[28]

Increasing attention is given to detection of abnormalities of cardiac function in these patients. Echocardiographic estimation of left ventricular function is a reliable, noninvasive indicator of myocardial dysfunction and may reveal abnormalities before there is other evidence of cardiac disease.

Episodes of sterile pericarditis manifested by pain, friction rub, and pericardial effusion are seen in about half of these patients, but cardiac tamponade has not been observed.[125] Although pericarditis is most often attributed to hemosiderosis, an association with β-hemolytic streptococcal infection has also been suggested.[133] Therapy is symptomatic, consisting of bed rest, treatment of associated infection, and management of superimposed congestive heart failure.

Cardiomegaly and left ventricular hypertrophy progress to chronic refractory congestive heart failure. Therapy at this point consists of careful maintenance of the hemoglobin level above 10 gm/dl, judicious use of digitalis and diuretics, dietary control and salt restriction, and bed rest. Management is difficult because the iron-overloaded myocardium is extremely sensitive to digitalis and has little capacity to improve its performance. Arrythmias may cause sudden death. Supraventricular tachycardia and atrial fibrillation may necessitate the use of agents such as quinidine and propranolol in conjunction with digitalis to reduce myocardial irritability. Electrical cardioversion may be necessary when arrythmias are life threatening. An expert cardiologist should manage these complications, which are the usual cause of death in patients with thalassemia major.

Kidneys. The kidneys are frequently enlarged in thalassemia major. Although this may in part reflect extramedullary hematopoiesis, marked dilatation of the renal tubules has also been described.[45] The urine is often dark brown because of the excretion of dipyrroles and mesofuchsins, reflecting a severe degree of ineffective erythropoiesis.[71] Large amounts of ureates and uric acid are noted in the urine.

Growth and endocrine status. In the past growth retardation was usual even in young children. This probably was a consequence of anemia, for hypertransfusion regimens are associated with relatively normal growth during the first decade of life. However, under any transfusion program the adolescent growth spurt is delayed or absent, and most patients do not attain normal stature.[57,77] Assays of growth hormone following insulin hypoglycemia reveal normal or exaggerated increases.[12] This finding suggests that end-organ nonresponsiveness or other peripheral factors are more important than primary pituitary failure.[74]

Menarche is frequently delayed. Breast development may be poor, and many girls are oligomenorrheic or amenorrheic. Small doses of estrogen and progesterone used to induce cyclic uterine bleeding may be of psychologic benefit. There are no reports of pregnancy in transfusion-dependent female patients.

Boys are frequently immature, with sparse facial and body hair. Although spermatogenesis may be normal, libido is often decreased. One patient was sexually active as a young man and fathered a child with thalassemia trait at 22 years of age. When lack of secondary sexual characteristics is emotionally disturbing, small doses of androgen may be used to produce phallic enlargement, deepening of the voice, and growth of facial and body hair. Any psychologic benefits derived from androgen therapy must be weighed against the potential risk of hepatic carcinoma (the incidence of which is higher in patients with hemosiderosis treated with androgens).

Evidence of abnormality of carbohydrate metabolism, ranging from chemical to overt diabetes mellitus, is common in older patients with thalassemia major. Glucagon secretion in response to alanine is blunted in contrast to the exaggerated response in hereditary diabetes mellitus.[73] Diabetes in these patients is thus associated with progressive obliteration of the islets affecting both α- and β-cells, and management may be somewhat difficult.

Multiple endocrine abnormalities (such as hypoparathyroidism, hypothyroidism, and pituitary and gonadal dysfunction) may be symptomatic or merely detectable by provocative tests.[74] Although generally ascribed to progressive iron deposition, chronic hypoxia may also be contributory. Definitive endocrine studies have not been described in groups of patients maintained from early life on hypertransfusion regimens.

Spleen and splenectomy. Most patients with thalassemia major ultimately require surgical removal of the spleen because the sheer size of the organ may cause mechanical discomfort. Thrombocytopenia and neutropenia may also result from hypersplenism, although infection and bleeding are unusual. With present management programs the most common indication for splenectomy is progressive shortening of the survival rate of transfused red blood cells evidenced by an increased transfusional requirement, making it difficult to maintain satisfactory hemoglobin levels. Occasionally serologic evidence of isoimmunization may be documented, permitting selection of compatible donor cells that have normal survival; however, sensitization cannot usually be detected in vitro. Red cell survival studies and determination of splenic sequestration by the ^{51}Cr method have been advocated to assist in a decision concerning the need for splenectomy,[122] but I believe that these data are of uncertain value in prediction of response. The observation of a significant, and especially progressive, increase in transfusion requirement is the most important indication for splenectomy. For reasons to be discussed subsequently, splenectomy should be deferred as long as possible—certainly until after 5 or 6 years of age.

Following splenectomy there is usually a significantly decreased requirement for blood transfusions.[16] Thrombocytosis, sometimes of a striking degree (platelet count > $1,000 \times 10^9$/liter), may occur, but this has not been associated with thromboembolic phenomena and anticoagulant therapy is not considered necessary. Increased numbers of nucleated red cells are noted in the blood, and "Fessas bodies" (precipitated masses of α-polypeptide chains) can be demonstrated in the circulating red cells. The urine may become considerably darker.

Patients with thalassemia major are at significant risk for developing acute, overwhelming, and often fatal infection after splenectomy. Fairly consistent bacteriologic and clinical features of the so-called postsplenectomy syndrome are age related, being most common in young children. The causative organisms are encapsulated pneumococci in two thirds of the cases and *Haemophilus influenzae* type B and meningococcus in the remaining patients. Clinically the disease is fulminant and may proceed from mild fever and headache to hyperpyrexia, prostration, shock, and death within 6 to 12 hours. As many as 10% to 30% of children with thalassemia major subjected to splenectomy may develop this complication.[117,119]

The basis of the increased susceptibility to infection is complex. The reticuloendothelial tissues of the spleen are unique in their capacity to clear bacteria from the blood in the absence of specific antibody.[112] In addition, there is evidence that the spleen actively participates in antibody formation in the early hours of an infection.[128] It may also be important in the properdin (alternate) pathway so important in opsonization when specific antibody is lacking.[13] In addition, levels of IgM are low in the splenectomized patients.[113] The high levels of serum iron and saturation of iron-binding protein seen in these patients may also predispose them to infection. When bacteria such as pneumococci gain entrance to the bloodstream of a young (and thus often nonimmune) splenectomized patient, they are not cleared and rapidly proliferate in the circulation, with a doubling time of 20 to 30 minutes. Enormous numbers of bacteria accumulate in a relatively short period of time, and hyperpyrexia, shock, disseminated intravascular coagulation, adrenal hemorrhage, and death may rapidly ensue.

Splenectomy should obviously be deferred as long as possible because the older patient is more likely to have developed humoral immunity to a broad range of bacteria. Oral penicillin therapy has been advocated as prophylaxis against postsplenectomy infection,[104,120] but there are no data to prove or disprove the effectiveness of this practice. When prophylactic antibiotics are used following splenectomy, parents should be instructed to seek medical attention immediately if the child develops significant fever (>101° F). If prophylactic antibiotics are not used, oral ampicillin should be started at the first sign of fever. Immunization with polyvalent pneumococcal and *Haemophilus influenzae* polysaccharide vaccines may prove to be of value in the future.[1]

Prognosis and therapy

General considerations. The prognosis of untreated homozygous thalassemia is in most cases grave. The infant with thalassemia major is not born with significant anemia, although deficient β-chain synthesis can be demonstrated at birth.[39] Symptoms are rarely noted in the first 6 months of life. Most affected children develop clear evidence of severe anemia by the end of the second year of life. Baty et al.[6] reported symptoms in thirteen of sixteen patients before the age of 2 years. In most untreated cases death occurs prior to 5 years of age.

In the past transfusions were given every 5 to 10 weeks. They were given only when symptoms of severe anemia, such as fatigue, weakness, and irritability, occurred. Because the hemoglobin level was permitted to fall to 5.0 to 6.0 gm/dl or even lower, the children were symptomatic much of the time. Further, because erythropoiesis was not suppressed, exuberant hypertrophy of erythroid tissue occurred in medullary and extramedullary sites as a response to the hemolysis and anemia. Marrow hypertrophy caused severe and progressive skeletal changes, producing osteoporosis and sometimes disfiguring facial changes. Severe splenomegaly, primarily caused by extramedul-

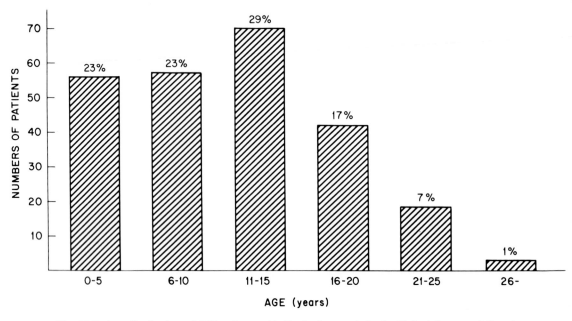

Fig. 15-7. Age distribution of 245 patients with Cooley's anemia in the United States and Canada determined in 1973. (From Pearson, H. A., and O'Brien, R. T.: Progr. Hematol. 1975. Used by permission.)

lary hematopoiesis, frequently necessitated splenectomy in early childhood.

Transfusions were used sparingly because of the recognition of the consequences of transfusional hemosiderosis. Each 500 ml of transfused blood results in tissue deposition of about 250 mg of iron that cannot be eliminated by physiologic processes. After hundreds of transfusions a massive iron burden causes dysfunction of many organ systems and tissues, resulting in endocrine abnormalities, growth retardation, diabetes mellitus, and cardiac failure. Life expectancy averages only 15 to 20 years (Fig. 15-7).

About 15 years ago Wolman convincingly proposed that transfusions in thalassemia major should be viewed as palliative therapy for an inevitably fatal disease.[131] If palliation is defined as the prevention of discomfort and the maintenance of as nearly normal life as possible, it was clear that the transfusion programs then in general use were unsatisfactory. The chronic and recurrent symptoms of anemia and the cosmetic consequences of overgrowth of erythropoietic tissue made life unpleasant and uncomfortable for these children. Because some of the problems of children with thalassemia major could be related to anemia per se, several centers initiated transfusion programs designed to ameliorate these symptoms. The minimal level varied somewhat, but in general hemoglobin levels were maintained above 9 to 10 gm/dl. These more vigorous regimens have been designated

hypertransfusion, although normotransfusion may be a more descriptive term.

The clinical benefits of hypertransfusion programs were dramatic. The growth of younger children, previously subnormal, returned to normal percentiles for height and weight.[67] Erythropoiesis was effectively suppressed, as evidenced by decreases in numbers of reticulocytes and normoblasts and marked reduction of the level of Hb F. Enlargement of the liver, and especially the spleen, receded. Changes in the facial appearance and osteoporosis of long bones either did not develop or regressed. Cardiac dilatation regressed, and normal age-appropriate activities were possible.[86,101]

Because hypertransfusion programs require an increase of 25% or more in the amount of blood to be administered, it was feared that this would result in accelerated iron overload, more rapid development of complications, and death at an earlier age. These concerns have not been realized, and the life expectancy of children on hypertransfusion programs does not appear to be significantly shortened. The amelioration of severe anemia is associated with significant reduction of gastrointestinal iron absorption, which somewhat offsets the increased transfusional load.

Hypertransfusion has proved so clearly clinically superior to older practices that most American centers have adopted this as standard management. Some complications of anemia and erythropoietic hypertrophy that were regularly encountered in the past have become uncommon. However, large numbers of patients managed from early life on hypertransfusion have not been followed long enough to permit solid conclusions concerning ultimate prognosis.[82,99] Most recently even more vigorous transfusional programs aimed at keeping hemoglobin levels above 12.0 gm/dl have been used to totally suppress erythropoiesis ("supertransfusion").

Before the first blood transfusion is given to an infant with thalassemia major, complete genotype of the red blood cells should be performed. This information may prove invaluable for identifying minor blood group incompatibility should isoimmunization develop later. Group- and type specific red cells that are compatible by the indirect antiglobulin reaction should be used, and the blood should be no more than 5 days old, preserved in CPD anticoagulant. Red cells are separated from the plasma and buffy coat and concentrated by centrifugation.

Febrile reactions are frequent in these patients who have had multiple transfusions. Because fever associated with transfusions is frequently caused by the development of leukoagglutinins, reactions can be minimized by the use of leukocyte-poor red cells. These can be prepared by repeated centrifugations and washing or by passing blood through nylon filters. If febrile reactions continue in spite of these precautions, pretransfusion therapy with aspirin and hydrocortisone (25 to 50 mg) may reduce the severity. Some centers use frozen red blood cell preparations that contain few leukocytes and produce few reactions. The use of some frozen red cell preparations may require somewhat larger amounts of blood than is necessary when using fresh blood.

A single transfusion consists of 15 ml/kg of packed red blood cells, which usually raises the patient's hemoglobin level by about 5 gm/dl (approximate predicted increase of Hb = ml/kg packed cells $\div$ 3). In more severely anemic patients several initial transfusions may be necessary to increase the hemoglobin level to 12 to 14 gm/dl, but no more than 15 ml/kg of packed red cells should be given in a 24-hour period. A regular and convenient outpatient schedule can usually be set up for transfusion. When it is well organized the entire process including cross matching and transfusion should take less than half a day.

Oxygen dissociation curves performed on patients with thalassemia major reveal a paradoxical shift to the left of the oxygen dissociation curve.[22] When substantial numbers of the patient's own red cells containing large amounts of Hb F are circulating, this may result from the decreased affinity between Hb F and 2,3-DPG. However, similar abnormalities are also noted in other patients receiving multiple transfusions. The apparent inability of the patient with severe thalassemia to respond to anemia by significantly increasing red blood cell 2,3-DPG and shifting the oxygen dissociation curve to the right may make the degree of functional anemia in the disease more severe than anticipated by the hemoglobin level.

Biochemical evidence of folic acid deficiency and occasional clinical benefit following treatment with this vitamin have been described.[56,78] Although significant changes in hemoglobin levels or transfusion requirements rarely occur, daily supplementation with 0.5 to 1.0 mg of folic acid is reasonable, especially if the diet is not optimal.

The large amounts of iron present in these patients' bodies and perhaps a degree of malabsorption secondary to pancreatic and hepatic fibrosis may lead to decreased levels of Vitamin E. Plasma levels of α-tocopherol are lower than normal and evidence of increased red cell membrane lipid peroxidation has been documented.[55,107] However, therapy with large doses of Vitamin E does not appear to improve survival of transfused red cells or decrease transfusion requirements.[55]

Hemosiderosis. The acquisition of the excessive iron burden in thalassemia major is cumulative and directly related to the number of blood transfusions received and the age of the patient.[18] Because the consequences of transfusional hemosiderosis are the basis of late morbidity and mortality in thalassemia major, a more favorable iron balance should lead to improved survival.

The daily acquisition of iron in the transfusion-dependent patient averages 8 to 16 mg of iron from the 250 to 500 ml of blood administered.[83] In addition, excessive gastrointestinal absorption of iron occurs although this is reduced when a hemoglobin level of more than 9 gm/dl is maintained.[29] There is no physiologic way to induce significant excretion of iron. Phlebotomy, the most efficient method of removing iron, is obviously useless in a disease in which regular transfusions are essential to sustain life. A pharmacologic approach requires development of specific chelating agents. A number of drugs with chelating properties have been synthesized or recovered from microorganisms, including penicillamine, EDTA, tricalcium diethylene triamine pentaacetate, DPTA, and desferrioxamine. Some of them lack specificity and efficiency; others carry significant toxicity.

Desferrioxamine B (Desferal), a siderophore isolated from cultures of *Streptomyces pilosus,* was introduced in 1960 as a nearly specific iron-chelating agent with low toxicity.[68] Increased iron excretion following administration of desferrioxamine is proportional to body iron stores.[33] In the patient with thalassemia major who is begun on regular transfusions during the first year of life, increased iron excretion following administration of desferrioxamine does not occur until after 4 or 5 years of age.[83,91] To offset the amount of iron received by way of transfusions (usually about 500 ml of packed red blood cells every 4 weeks in older children and adults) the chelating agent must effect the daily excretion of about 15 mg of iron. It has been found that this amount of iron excretion can only be attained in patients more than 5 to 10 years old who already have significant iron overload, perhaps because desferrioxamine interacts preferentially with iron within parenchymal tissues.[46]

Because of the apparently small impact of desferrioxamine on the total body iron burden and the discomfort and inconvenience of daily intramuscular injections, the use of this agent has not received wide or extensive use until recently. A 5-year controlled study from England demonstrated that intramuscular administration of 0.5 gm/day of desferrioxamine reduced the rate of hepatic iron accumulation and hepatic fibrosis in patients maintained on a hypertransfusion program.[4] Another uncontrolled study using an injection of 1.0 gm/day demonstrated decreases in cardiac and hepatic size and increased cardiac function in a small group of patients treated for 2 to 10 years.[114]

Studies prompted by the epidemiology of scurvy among the Bantu, which pointed out a relationship between iron overload and ascorbic acid depletion,[132] documented that ascorbic acid enhances desferrioxamine-induced urinary iron excretion in thalassemia major. The administration of 200 to 500 mg of oral ascorbic acid results in an approximate doubling of urinary iron excretion by the concurrent use of ascorbic acid and desferrioxamine. However, questions have been raised about possible increased cardiotoxicity resulting from the combination, and large doses (> 200 mg/day) should be used with caution.[87]

Even more exciting has been the observation that the iron excretion induced by desferrioxamine can be markedly enhanced by slow intravenous or subcutaneous injection of the drug.[106] Apparently a prolonged infusion period permits a longer exposure of the drug to a relatively small "chelatable" iron pool. In iron-overloaded, ascorbic acid–replete patients as much as 100 mg or more of daily urinary iron excretion is accomplished.[54] A multi-institutional program to assess the possible beneficial effects of chronic, constant subcutaneous infusions on cardiac and endocrine function is currently underway. It is possible to attain negative iron balance in most patients.[105]

Recent studies have described another chelating agent, 2,3-dihydrobenzoic acid (2,3-DHB). This drug also enhances iron excretion and has the advantage of being effective when given orally. It may work in a different way than desferrioxamine. With administration of oral 2,3-DHB iron excretion increased an average of 4.5 mg/day over control periods.[102]

THALASSEMIA INTERMEDIA

Approximately 10% of patients with homozygous β-thalassemia and some patients with the doubly heterozygous states for β-thalassemia and the Lepore or $\beta\delta$-thalassemia traits have a syndrome of intermediate hematologic severity. These exceptional patients, sometimes designated as having thalassemia intermedia, spontaneously maintain hemoglobin levels of 6 to 9 gm/dl. They do not require regular blood transfusions and so do not develop severe iron overload. Some have the potential for survival well into adult life, often with normal maturation and sexual development.[95]

However, patients with thalassemia intermedia may develop cardiomegaly, osteoporosis, fractures, and massive splenomegaly. Disfiguring facial changes may result in a grotesque appearance that causes considerable emotional and psychologic distress. These changes can be prevented by a transfusion program designed to suppress erythropoiesis; however, this program may not be warranted when the hemoglobin level is high enough to prevent symptoms. The risk of iron overload must be balanced against the other problems. Development of effective chelation may make this decision easier.

It has been noted that these patients may have a functional degree of anemia more severe than would be anticipated. Because of the high levels of Hb F and levels of 2,3-DPG, which are inappropriately low for the degree of anemia, the result is a left shift of the oxygen dissociation curve with P_{50} values of 20 to 26 mm/Hg.[22]

Reconstruction of the maxilla by a plastic surgeon may provide considerable cosmetic improvement of facial asymmetry and malocclusion.[58] Prevention of folic acid deficiency by regular supplementation may be more important in these patients with extreme marrow hyperplasia who do not require blood transfusions. Splenectomy is also usually required to eliminate significant degrees of secondary hypersplenism.

THALASSEMIA MINOR (THALASSEMIA TRAIT)

Heterozygous occurrence of a thalassemia gene usually results in a mild hypochromic microcytic anemia. The hemoglobin level on the average is 1 or 2 gm/dl lower than that seen in normal persons of the same age and sex. Osmotic fragility is decreased. The red cell count is in the normal or high normal range. The blood characteristically is hypochromic (MCH < 26 pg) and microcytosis (MCV < 75 fl); the smear shows in addition varying numbers of target cells, poikilocytes, ovalocytes, and basophilic stippling (see Plate 3).

A single thalassemia gene results in a partial deficiency of β-chain synthesis. As was previously mentioned, this defect is best demonstrated by in vitro globin synthetic studies in which a β:α ratio of 0.5 to 0.7 is noted. Ferrokinetic studies reveal impaired incorporation of iron into red cell hemoglobin.[98] The morphologic changes in thalassemia minor are more extreme than those seen in iron deficiency of a comparable degree of anemia. The reticulocyte count is normal or slightly elevated. Most patients are asymptomatic, and the blood abnormalities are incidentally discovered during a hematologic evaluation. In many instances a diagnosis of iron-deficiency anemia is entertained and iron therapy is given without significant improvement. Microcytic anemia refractory to iron therapy should always suggest the possibility of thalassemia trait. Mentzer has suggested a simple index based on electronic counter data to differentiate iron deficiency anemia and thalassemia. If the MCV:RBC ratio is greater than 12, iron-deficiency anemia is likely; in contrast if the MCV: RBC is less than 11, thalassemia trait is likely.[80]

A few persons with heterozygous β-thalassemia have more severe hematologic findings with chronic anemia and modest splenomegaly and osseous changes, the so-called malattia Rietti-Greppi-Mecheli of the Italian literature. Pigmentary gallstones and leg ulcers may be evident in later life.

There may be characteristic racial differences in the hematologic severity of β-thalassemia trait. In blacks the condition is invariably milder, red cell morphologic abnormalities less marked, and β:α-synthetic ratios higher than those observed in whites and Orientals with the trait.[137]

The diagnosis of β-thalassemia is established in most instances by demonstration of altered proportions of Hb A_2 and/or Hb F. The level of Hb A_2 in β-thalassemia trait averages 5.1% (range 3.5% to 7.0%), approximately twice the normal level (Fig. 15-8). The $A_1:A_2$ ratio is less than 1:20 instead of the normal 1:30. This increase is thought to reflect an actual increase in δ-chain synthesis. More than 95% of parents of children with thalassemia major (obligate heterozygotes) have elevated Hb A_2 levels. After the newborn period Hb A_2 levels do not change throughout life and tend to be constant in affected members of a pedigree.[41] However, if iron-deficiency anemia occurs, Hb A_2 levels are decreased sometimes into the normal range.[134]

Hb F levels are inconsistently elevated in β-thalassemia. In about half of the cases Hb F is in the normal range (<2.0%); in the remainder they are moderately elevated (2.1% to 5.0%). However, in almost every instance a minor population of red cells containing substantial amounts of Hb F can be demonstrated by the Kleihauer technique.[115]

OTHER FORMS OF β-THALASSEMIA

In addition to the common classic β-thalassemia trait associated with elevated levels of Hb A_2, other variants of thalassemia have been described with different biochemical characteristics.

βδ-Thalassemia (high–Hb F thalassemia)

The hematologic findings are those of a mild hypochromic microcytosis indistinguishable from those of β-thalassemia minor. Hb F is elevated from 5% to 20% but is heterogenously distributed in the red cells. As was previously mentioned, the doubly heterozygous state for high–Hb A_2 and βδ-thalassemia genes is usually associated with clinical thalassemia intermedia.[66] The homozygous

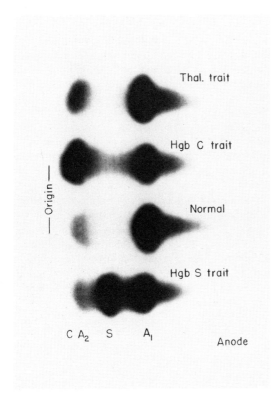

Fig. 15-8. Starch block electrophoresis of hemoglobin. The slow minor component, Hb A_2, is approximately two times increased in heterozygous thalassemia. Because Hb A_2 has a similar electrophoretic mobility to Hb C and E, it cannot be quantitated in the presence of these variants. (From Gerald, P. S., and Diamond, L. K.: Blood **13**:61, 1958. Used by permission.)

state for $\beta\delta$-thalassemia may also have intermediately severe clinical and hematologic findings.

Lepore hemoglobin ($\alpha_2\beta\delta_2{}^{Lepore}$)

Although as a rule no qualitatively abnormal hemoglobin species is found in thalassemia, the Lepore hemoglobin syndromes are exceptions to this generalization. The Lepore hemoglobin contains an unique kind of polypeptide chain that is a fusion of portions of both β- and δ-chains. The chains begin with a normal δ-chain and sequence at the N terminus and end with the β-chain sequence at the C terminus. The Lepore hemoglobin is hypothesized to be a consequence of unequal crossing over between the δ- and β-loci at meiosis. Three different Lepore hemoglobins have been described resulting from crossing over at different points. Because Hb Lepore is synthesized at a markedly reduced rate and accounts for only 5% to 15% of the total, the red cells have the typical microcytosis and hypochromia of thalassemia.

Heterozygosity for the Hb Lepore gene is associated with typical thalassemia minor and manifests as a mild hypochromic microcytosis.[42] The doubly heterozygous state for β-thalassemia and Lepore traits may be manifested as thalassemia intermedia.[96]

Silent carrier of β-thalassemia

Rarely persons who are obligate carriers of a β-thalassemia gene (identified because they parented a child with Cooley's anemia) have no hematologic evidence of thalassemia and normal levels of Hb A_2 and Hb F. Globin synthetic studies in such persons reveal reduced β-chain synthesis and a β:α-ratio of less than 1.[111]

DIAGNOSIS OF THALASSEMIA TRAIT

Thalassemia trait is one of the most common genetically determined defects in the world, affecting literally millions of people. Because the condition is frequently mistaken for iron-deficiency anemia and because it has important genetic implications, testing for thalassemia has clinical and epidemiologic implications.[108] Definitive methods for diagnosis of thalassemia trait include quantitative Hb A_2 determination and globin chain synthetic ratios. These are accurate but also expensive and therefore are not applicable to population screening. Since thalassemia is almost invariably associated with significant hypochromia (MCH < 26 pg) and microcytosis (MCV < 75 fl), determination of red cells indices by modern electronic equipment such as the Coulter Model S[100] has been used as a preliminary indicator of possible thalassemia trait. Iron deficiency must, of course, be excluded. A number of methods have been described for subsequent diagnostic tests. Stockman has suggested the value of free erythrocyte protoporphyrin (FEP) measurement in the evaluation of individuals with microcytosis. In thalassemia trait FEP is normal, whereas in iron deficiency and plumbism, FEP is elevated.[126]

Functions derived from Coulter counter indices have also been suggested as helpful in rapid differentiation between the microcytoses of thalassemia and iron deficiency. England and Fraser described a derived function (DF = MCV − RBC − [5 × Hb] − 3.4). Values of the DF in excess of 2 were indicative of iron deficiency, whereas values of less than 2 indicated thalassemia trait.[27] Mentzer showed that the ratio of MCV:RBC was also useful. Values of more than 12 indicated iron deficiency and those less than 11 were associated with thalassemia trait.[80]

PRENATAL DIAGNOSIS OF THALASSEMIA SYNDROMES

Development of techniques for the prenatal diagnosis of abnormalities of hemoglobin synthesis is being pursued vigorously in a number of centers.[24] Although it has been attempted less than 100 times as of this writing, a pattern of risk and reliability is becoming clear.

Because the β-chain-related hemoglobin genes are expressed and active only in cells actually producing hemoglobin, it is necessary to obtain an actual sample of fetal blood from the fetus in utero at 18 to 22 weeks of gestation. Although this is a formidable task, it has been accomplished by two methods. First, the location of placental attachment, anterior or posterior, on the uterus, is determined by ultrasound. If the placenta is predominantly posterior, a peripheral vein on the placenta can be punctured and aspirated under direct vision using a small fiberoptic amnioscope. Nearly pure fetal blood can be obtained for analysis with small risk to the fetus.[50] Alternatively, if the placenta is anterior, direct placental aspiration may be attempted. This generally results in a mixture of fetal and maternal blood. This mixed sample must be treated in various ways (anti-i antisera) to minimize the effects of maternal blood "contamination."[63]

The fetal blood sample is incubated with C^{14} leucine and then the relative rates of γ-, β-, and α-chain synthesis are determined by chromatography. In fetuses homozygous for β-thalassemia, β-chain synthesis is either absent or low. The β^+ γ:α-ratio is also low. There appears to be a discernable difference between normal and homozygous thalassemia genotypes.

Maternal risk and morbidity with either fetoscopy or placental aspiration is low. Placental aspiration has had a 10% risk of induced abortion. Although the laboratory results have generally been clear-cut and accurate, there have been occasional incorrect diagnoses.[24] The same methodology can be utilized to diagnose major β-chain abnormalities such as Hb SS disease.[61]

At the present time the only alternatives to couples at risk for having a child with thalassemia major are not to have children, to abort all pregnancies, or to take the 25% chance of having a child with a severe blood disease. Further experience with antenatal diagnosis may permit the option of selective abortion of affected fetuses. Should antenatal diagnosis become more reliable and widely available, widespread screening for thalassemia trait in populations at risk may become important.

Because the severe α-thalassemia (fetal hydrops syndrome) appears to result from gene deletions, fibroblasts contained in amniotic fluid have been used in tissue culture studies to diagnose fetal hydrops (Hb Bart's syndrome) (homozygous α-thalassemia).[60]

α-Thalassemia

The α-thalassemias are a group of familial microcytotic anemias resulting from decreased synthesis of α-polypeptide chains. They are difficult to diagnose and identify with certainty because there are no characteristic elevations in Hb S, Hb A_2, or Hb F. The α-thalassemias are more complex and difficult to explain because, at least in some ethnic groups, there are probably two sets of α-genes. This is somewhat controversial, and alternative hypotheses for the α-thalassemias based on one set or two sets of α-genes have been advanced.[65,70]

Silent carrier (α-thalassemia-2 trait)

α-Thalassemia-2 trait results from heterozygosity for α-thalassemia-2. There are no hematologic manifestations. The red cells are not microcytic; Hb A_2 and Hb F are normal. A mild decrease in α-chain synthesis with $\beta:\alpha$-ratios of about 1.2:1 is noted.[64] In the newborn period small amounts (1% to 3%) of Hb Bart's (γ_4) may be seen. After the newborn period this condition is most often diagnosed in the apparently hematologically normal parent of a patient with Hb H disease.

α-Thalassemia trait (α-thalassemia-1 trait)

α-Thalassemia trait is a mild, familial, microcytic anemia characterized by levels of Hb A_2 in the low to low normal range (1.5% to 2.5%) with $\beta:\alpha$-synthetic ratios averaging 1.4:1.[64] In the newborn period substantial amounts of Hb Bart's are noted (5% to 8%), and a relative microcytosis is present in cord blood erythrocytes.[69,109] When α-thalassemia-1 gene occurs in persons who are heterozygous for β-chain variant hemoglobins such as Hb S, Hb C, or Hb E, the proportion of the abnormal hemoglobin is lower (<30%) than seen in simple heterozygotes.[136] α-Thalassemia-1 is very common in Orientals and reaches a frequency of 20% in southeast Asiatic peoples, especially Thais. About 3% of blacks appear to have this trait.

Hb Constant Spring trait

There are usually no hemoglobin polypeptide chain variants in thalassemia. One exception to this generalization is Hb Lepore. A second exception is Hb Constant Spring, a minor hemoglobin

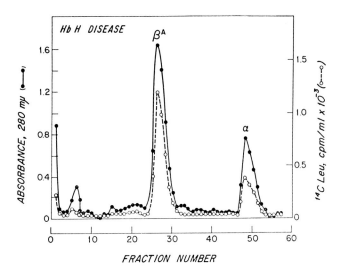

Fig. 15-9. Globin chain synthesis in reticulocytes of a patient with Hb H disease. A markedly reduced incorporation of radioactivity into newly synthesized α-chains is noted. (From Forget, B. G., and Kan, Y. W.: In Hematology of infancy and childhood, Philadelphia, 1974, W. B. Saunders Co.)

found in many Orientals and occasionally in whites with an α-thalassemia-like syndrome.[15,81] Hb Constant Spring has the structure $\alpha_2^{cs}\beta_2$ and is characterized by two elongated α-chains with either twenty-eight or thirty-one extra amino acids at the C terminal end. The heterozygous state has no hematologic abnormality other than 1% Hb Constant Spring and so resembles α-thalassemia-1 trait. A second type of elongated α-chain abnormal hemoglobin, Hb Icaria, has also been described in association with an α-thalassemia syndrome.[15]

Hb H disease

Hb H disease is a moderately severe but variable anemia resulting from combination of an α-thalassemia-2 gene and an α-thalassemia-1 or Hb Constant Spring gene. This results in a marked deficiency of α-chain synthesis with $\beta:\alpha$ synthesis ratios of 2.5 (Fig. 15-9). Therefore family studies reveal one parent who is hematologically normal and the other with microcytosis and hypochromia.[70] Hb H disease may resemble thalassemia intermedia with osseous changes and splenomegaly or be considerably milder. It occurs predominantly in Orientals, but also has been seen in whites; it is rare in blacks.

Because Hb H is unstable and precipitates within the red cell, a hemolytic component is evident. Hb H can be demonstrated by incubation of blood with supravital stains such as 1% brilliant cresyl blue. Multiple small inclusions form in the red cells (Fig. 15-10). Electrophoresis of freshly prepared hemolysate at alkali or neutral pH demonstrates a fast moving component that amounts to 10% to 30% of the total hemoglobin. Concomitant iron deficiency may reduce the amount of Hb

H in the patient's red cells.[92] In Hb H disease resulting from interaction of α-thalassemia-1 and Hb Constant Spring traits, slowly moving Hb Constant Spring bands are noted.[81]

Fetal hydrops syndrome

The homozygous state for an α-thalassemia-2 gene results in a lethal condition producing stillbirth or early neonatal death.[26] The clinical features of generalized edema (hydrops fetalis) and massive hepatosplenomegaly are noted. In contrast to severe erythroblastosis fetalis, the degree of anemia may be severe or only moderate (3 to 10 gm/dl), but marked normoblastemia and microcytosis are evident. Hemoglobin electrophoresis reveals a predominance of Hb Bart's (γ_4) with small amounts of Hb H and Hb Portland. Because α-chain synthesis is extremely low, little or no normal Hb F is evident.[141] Hb Bart's has a markedly increased affinity for oxygen. The oxygen dissociation curve is so shifted to the left that oxygen cannot be released at physiologic conditions; this results in severe hypoxia incompatible with life.[141]

$\gamma\beta$-Thalassemia

A family has been described in which a hemolytic microcytic anemia was documented in several newborn infants.[59] Globin chain synthetic studies revealed a marked deficiency of both γ- and β-chain synthesis. As one of the children matured, the hemolytic component subsided and by 1 year of age she had a mild hypochromic microcytic hematologic picture with normal levels of Hb A_2 and Hb F. β-Chain synthesis, however, remained decreased with $\beta:\alpha$-ratios of about 0.7. These findings suggested a heterozygous thalassemia

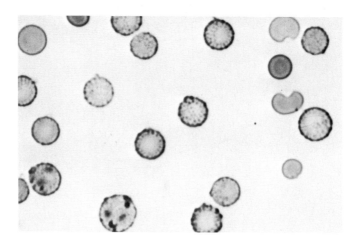

Fig. 15-10. Blood cells from patient with Hb H disease. Finely stippled and larger dense inclusion bodies consisting of precipitated Hb H (β_4) are identified after incubation with 1% brilliant cresyl blue.

syndrome involving both γ- and β-loci, which was more severe during the normal period of dependence on γ-chain synthesis.

$\alpha\beta$-Thalassemia

Because of the frequency of both α- and β-thalassemia genes in many populations, a number of various combinations have been observed. α-Thalassemia-1 trait plus β- or $\beta\delta$-thalassemia trait produced a mild microcytosis no more severe than either trait alone.[94] Inheritance of an α-thalassemia gene appeared to reduce the severity of homozygous β-thalassemia.[5]

Hereditary persistence of fetal hemoglobin (HPFH)

HPFH, although not strictly a thalassemia, is most conveniently discussed here. The genetic defect results in a hemoglobin synthetic state similar to that of the normal fetus. There is a failure to switch from γ- to β- (and δ-) chain synthesis. In the person heterozygous for a HPFH gene, there is a substantial amount of Hb F uniformly distributed in the red cell population. This uniform pattern is in contrast to the irregular distribution noted in thalassemia.[32]

There are ethnic differences in the HPFH. In blacks with heterozygous HPFH the Hb F ranges between 15% to 35% and contains γ^{gly} and γ^{ala} chains in a ratio of 2:3. In Greeks with HPFH Hb F levels are lower, between 10% and 20%, and contain only γ^{ala}.[52] Hb A_2 levels are lower than normal, but there are no other hematologic abnormalities in these persons.

A few black patients have been described with homozygous HPFH. All of the hemoglobin within their red cells was Hb F. Mild microcytosis and hypochromia of the red cells but no anemia were present. In fact, hemoglobin levels were mildly elevated, reflecting a left-shifted oxygen dissociation curve. Other interesting characteristics of the red cells of the homozygous person included persistence of fetal membrane characteristics (i antigen) and a deficiency of carbonic anhydrase.[138]

Persons doubly heterozygous for HPFH and a β-chain variant such as Hb S or Hb C lack normal Hb A in the red cells. Approximately 30% of the hemoglobin is Hb F, the remainder being Hb S or Hb C plus a small amount of Hb A_2. In the Hb S–HPFH person, despite the large amounts of Hb S, the uniform distribution within the red cell of Hb F inhibits sickling. Minimal gelling concentrations are high, and there are no hemolytic or vaso-occlusive manifestations. Mild targeting is the only morphologic finding. HPFH–β-thalassemia resembles $\beta\delta$-thalassemia except for a higher proportion and regular distribution of Hb F in the red cells.[52] A variant designated Hb Kenya results

from nonhomologous crossing over between γ- and β-genes, and in the heterozygous state resembles HPFH.[53]

REFERENCES

1. Amman, A. J., Addiego, J., Wara, D. W., et al.: Polyvalent pneumococal-polysaccharide immunization of patients with sickle cell anemia and patients with splenectomy, N. Engl. J. Med. **297**:897, 1977.
2. Asbell, M. B.: Orthodontic aspects of Cooley's anemia, Ann. N.Y. Acad. Sci. **119**:662, 1964.
3. Baglioni, C.: The fusion of two peptide chains in hemoglobin Lepore and its interpretation as a genetic deletion, Proc. Natl. Acad. Sci. **48**:1880, 1962.
4. Barry, M., Flynn, D. M., Letsky, E. A., and Rison, R. A.: Long-term chelation therapy in thalassemia major: effect on iron concentration, liver histology, and clinical progress, Br. Med. J. **2**:16, 1974.
5. Bate, C. M., and Humphries, G.: Alpha-beta thalassemia, Lancet **1**:1031, 1977.
6. Baty, J. M., Blackfan, K. D., and Diamond, L. K.: Blood studies in infants and in children. I. Erythroblastic anemia: a clinical and pathologic study, Am. J. Dis. Child. **43**:665, 1932.
7. Benz, E. J., Jr., and Forget, B. G.: Defect in messenger RNA for human hemoglobin syntheses in beta thalassemia, J. Clin. Invest. **50**:2755, 1971.
8. Benz, E. J., Jr., and Forget, B. Q.: The molecular genetics of the thalassemia syndrome, Progr. Hematol. **9**:107, 1975.
9. Braverman, A. S., and Bank, A.: Changing rates of globin chain synthesis during erythroid cell maturation in thalassemia, J. Mol. Biol. **42**:57, 1969.
10. Caffey, J.: Cooley's erythroblastic anemia: some skeletal findings on adolescents and young adults, Am. J. Roentgen. **65**:547, 1951.
11. Caffey, J.: Cooley's anemia: a review of the roentgenographic findings in the skeleton, Am. J. Roentgen. **78**:361, 1957.
12. Canale, V. C., Steinherz, P., New, M., and Erlandson, M.: Endocrine function in thalassemia major, Ann. N.Y. Acad. Sci. **232**:333, 1974.
13. Carlise, H. M., and Saslaw, S.: Properdin levels in splenectomized persons, Proc. Soc. Exp. Biol. Med. **102**:151, 1959.
14. Choremis, C., Liakakos, D., Tseghi, C., et al.: Pathogenesis of osseous lesions in thalassemia, J. Pediatr. **66**:962, 1965.
15. Clegg, J. B., Weatherall, D. J., Contopoulougriva, I.: Haemoglobin Icaria, a new chain termination mutant which causes alpha thalassemia, Nature **251**:245, 1974.
16. Clement, D. H., and Taffel, M.: Splenectomy in Mediterranean anemia, Pediatrics **16**:353, 1955.
17. Conconi, F., Bargellesi, A., Del Senno, L., Menegatti, E., Pontremoli, S., and Russo, G.: Globin chain synthesis in Sicilian thalassanemic subjects, Br. J. Haematol. **19**:469, 1970.
18. Constantoulakis, M., Economidou, J., Karagiorga, M., Katsantoni, A., and Gyftaki, E.: Combined long-term treatment of hemosiderosis with desferrioxamine and DTPA in homozygous β-thalassemia, Ann. N.Y. Acad. Sci. **232**:193, 1974.
19. Cooley, T. B., Lee, P.: A series of cases of splenomegaly in children with anemia and peculiar bone changes, Trans. Am. Pediatr. Soc. **37**:29, 1925.
20. Cooley, T. B., Witwer, E. R., and Lee, P.: Anemia in children with splenomegaly and peculiar changes in bones: report of cases, Am. J. Dis. Child. **34**:347, 1927.

21. Currarino, G., and Erlandson, M. E.: Premature fusion of epiphyses in Cooley's anemia, Radiology **83:**656, 1964.

22. de Furia, F. G., Miller, D. R., and Canale, V. C.: Red blood cell metabolism and function in transfused β-thalassemia, Ann. N.Y. Acad. Sci. **232:**323, 1974.

23. Dewey, K. W., Grossman, H., and Canale, V. C.: Cholelithiasis in thalassemia major, Radiology **96:**385, 1970.

24. Editorial: Antenatal diagnosis of the haemoglobinopathies, Lancet **1:**289, 1977.

25. Ellis, J. T., Schulman, I., and Smith, C. H.: Generalized siderosis with fibrosis of liver and pancreas in Cooley's (Mediterranean) anemia, Am. J. Pathol. **30:**287, 1954.

26. Eng, L.-I. L.: Alpha-chain thalassemia and hydrops fetalis in Malaya: report of five cases, Blood **20:**581, 1962.

27. England, J. M., and Fraser, P. M.: Differentiation of iron deficiency from thalassemia trait by routine blood count, Lancet **1:**449, 1973.

28. Engle, M. A.: Cardiac involvement in Cooley's anemia, Ann. N.Y. Acad. Sci. **119:**694, 1964.

29. Erlandson, M. E., Walden, B., Stern, G., Hilgartner, M. W., Wehman, J., and Smith, C. H.: Studies on congenital haemolytic syndromes. IV. Gastrointestinal absorption of iron, Blood **19:**359, 1962.

30. Fessas, P.: Inclusions of hemoglobin in erythroblasts and erythrocytes of thalassemia, Blood **21:**21, 1963.

31. Fessas, P., Loukopoulos, D., and Kaltsoya, A.: Peptide analysis of the inclusions of erythroid cells in β₆-thalassemia, Biochem. Biophys. Acta **124:**439, 1966.

32. Fessas, P., and Stamatoyannopoulos, G.: Hereditary persistence of fetal hemoglobin in Greece: a study and a comparison, Blood **24:**223, 1964.

33. Fielding, J.: Differential ferroxamine test for measuring chelatable body iron, J. Clin. Pathol. **20:**257, 1967.

34. Fielding, J.: Desferrioxamine chelatable body iron, J. Clin. Pathol. **20:**668, 1967.

35. Fink, H.: Transfusion hemochromatosis in Cooley's anemia, Ann. N.Y. Acad. Sci. **119:**680, 1964.

36. Forget, B. G., Baltimore, D., et al.: Globin messenger RNA in the thalassemia syndrome, Ann. N.Y. Acad. Sci. **232:**76, 1974.

37. Forget, B. G., Marotta, C. A., Weissman, S. M., et al.: Nucleotide sequences of human globin messenger RNA, Ann. N.Y. Acad. Sci. **241:**290, 1974.

38. Forget, B. G., and Nathan, D. G.: Molecular pathology of the thalassemias, Adv. Intern. Med. **21:**97, 1976.

39. Gaburro, D., Volpato, S., and Vigi, V.: Diagnosis of β-thalassaemia in the newborn by means of hemoglobin synthesis, Acta. Pediatr. Scand. **59:**523, 1970.

40. Gabuzda, T. G., Nathan, D. G., and Gardner, F. H.: The turnover of hemoglobins A, F, and A₂ in the peripheral blood of three patients with thalassemia, J. Clin. Invest. **42:**1678, 1963.

41. Gerald, P. S., and Diamond, L. K.: The diagnosis of thalassemia trait by starch block electrophoresis of the hemoglobin, Blood **13:**61, 1958.

42. Gerald, P. S., Efron, M. L., and Diamond, L. K.: A human mutation (the Lepore hemoglobinopathy) possibly involving two cistrons, Am. J. Dis. Child. **102:**514, 1961.

43. Giblett, E. R., and Crookston, M. C.: Agglutinability of red cells by anti-i in patients with thalassemia major and other hematological disorders, Nature **201:**1138, 1964.

44. Goldstein, M. A., Patpongpanij, N., and Minnick, V.: The incidence of elevated hemoglobin A₂ levels in the American Negro, Ann. Intern. Med. **60:**95, 1964.

45. Grossman, H., Dischi, M. R., Winchester, P. H., and Canali, V.: Renal enlargement in thalassemia major, Radiology **100:**645, 1971.

46. Hershiko, C., Cook, J. D., and Finch, C. A.: Storage iron kinetics. III. Study of desferrioxamine action by selective radio iron labels of R.E. and parenchymal cells, J. Lab. Clin. Med. **81:**876, 1973.

47. Heywood, J. D., Karon, M., and Weissman, S.: Amino acids: incorporation into alpha and beta chain of hemoglobin by normal and thalassemic reticulocytes, Science **146:**530, 1964.

48. Hilgartner, M. W., Erlandson, M. E., and Smith, C. H.: The coagulation mechanism in patients with thalassemia major, J. Pediatr. **63:**36, 1963.

49. Hilgartner, M. W., and Smith, C. H.: Coagulation studies as a measure of liver function in Cooley's anemia, Ann. N.Y. Acad. Sci. **119:**631, 1964.

50. Hobbins, J. C., and Mahoney, M. J.: In utero diagnosis of hemoglobinopathies: technic for obtaining fetal blood, N. Engl. J. Med. **290:**1065, 1974.

51. Horton, B. F., Thompson, R. B., Dozy, A. M., et al.: Inhomogeneity of hemoglobin, Blood **20:**302, 1962.

52. Huisman, T. H. J., Schroeder, W. A., et al.: Nature of fetal hemoglobin in the Greek type of hereditary persistence of fetal hemoglobin with and without concurrent β thalassemia, J. Clin. Invest. **49:**1035, 1970.

53. Huisman, T. H. J., and Wrightston, R. W., and Wilson, W. A.: Hemoglobin Kenya: the product of fusion of γ and β-polypeptide chains, Arch. Biochem. Biophys. **153:**850, 1972.

54. Hussain, M. A. M., Flynn, D. M., Green, N., and Hoffbrand, A. V.: Effect of dose, time, and ascorbate on iron excretion after subcutaneous desferrioxamine, Lancet **1:**977, 1977.

55. Hyman, C. B., Landing, B., Alfin-Slater, R., Kozak, L., Weitzman, J., and Ortega, J.: Dl- α-tocopherol, iron, and lipofuscin in thalassemia, Ann. N.Y. Acad. Sci. **232:**211, 1974.

56. Jandl, J. H., and Greenberg, M. S.: Bone marrow failure due to relative nutritional deficiency in Cooley's hemolytic anemia, N. Engl. J. Med. **266:**461, 1959.

57. Johnston, F. E., and Krogman, W. M.: Patterns of growth in children with thalassemia major, Ann. N.Y. Acad. Sci. **119:**667, 1964.

58. Jurkiewicz, M. J., Pearson, H. A., and Furlow, L. Y.: Reconstruction of the maxilla in thalassemia, Ann. N.Y. Acad. Sci. **165:**437, 1969.

59. Kan, Y. W., Forget, B. G., and Nathan, D. G.: Gamma-beta thalassemia: a cause of hemolytic disease of newborns, N. Engl. J. Med. **286:**129, 1972.

60. Kan, Y. W., Golbus, M. S., and Dozy, A. M.: Prenatal diagnosis of α-thalassemia, N. Engl. J. Med. **295:**1165, 1976.

61. Kan, Y. W., Golbus, M. S., Trecartin, R. F., et al.: Prenatal diagnosis of β-thalassemia and sickle cell anaemia, Lancet **1:**269, 1977.

62. Kan, Y. W., Holland, J. P., and Dozy, A. M.: Demonstration of nonfunctional β-globin MRNA in homozygous β-thalassemia, Proc. Natl. Acad. Sci. **72:**5140, 1975.

63. Kan, Y. W., Nathan, D. G., Cividalli, G., et al.: Concentration of fetal red blood cells from a mixture of maternal and fetal blood by anti-i serum and aid to prenatal diagnosis of hemoglobinopathies, Blood **43:**411, 1974.

64. Kan, Y. W., Schwartz, E., and Nathan, D. G.: Globin chain synthesis in the alpha thalassemia syndrome, J. Clin. Invest. **45:**2515, 1968.

65. Kattamis, C., and Lehman, H.: Duplication of alpha thalassaemia gene in thru Greek families with haemoglobin H disease, Lancet **2:**635, 1970.

66. Kattamis, C., Metaxotou-Mavromati, A., and Karamboula, K.: The clinical and haematological findings in children inheriting two types of thalassemia: high A₂ type β-thalassemia and high F type or βδ thalassemia, Br. J. Haematol. **25:**375, 1973.

67. Kattamis, C., Touliatos, N., Haidas, S., and Matsaniotis, N.: Growth of children with thalassemia and effect of different transfusion regimens, Arch. Dis. Child. **45:**502, 1970.

68. Keberle, H.: The biochemistry of desferrioxamine and its relation to iron metabolism, Ann. N.Y. Acad. Sci. **119:**758, 1964.

69. Koenig, H. M., and Vedvick, T. S.: Alpha thalassemia in American-born Filipino infants, J. Pediatr. **87:**756, 1975.

70. Koler, R. D., and Rigas, D. A.: Genetics of haemoglobin H, Ann. Hum. Genet. **25:**95, 1961.

70a. Konotey-Ahulu, F. I. D.: Hereditary qualitative and quantitative erythrocyte defects in Ghana: an historical and geographical survey, Ghana Med. J. **7:**118, 1968.

71. Krumer-Birnbaum, M., Pinkerton, P. H., and Bannerman, R. N.: Urinary dipyrroles: their occurrence and significance in thalassemia and other disorders, Blood **28:**933, 1966.

72. Kuo, B., Zaino, E., and Roginski, M. S.: Endocrine function in thalassemia major, J. Clin. Endocrin. Metab. **28:**805, 1968.

73. Lassman, M. N., Genel, M., Wis, J. K., Hendler, R., and Felig, P.: Carbohydrate homeostasis and pancreatic islet cell function in thalassemia, Am. J. Med. **80:**65, 1974.

74. Lassman, M. N., O'Brien, R. T., Pearson, H. A., Wise, J. K., Donabedian, R. K., Felig, P., and Genel, M.: Endocrine evaluation in thalassemia major, Ann. N.Y. Acad. Sci. **232:**226, 1974.

75. Liakakos, D., Karpouzas, J., and Agathopoulos, A.: Hyperprolinemia and hyperprolinuria in thalassemia, J. Pediatr. **73:**419, 1968.

76. Livingston, F. B.: Abnormal hemoglobins in human populations, Chicago, 1967, Aldine Publishing Co.

77. Logothetis, J., Loewenson, R. B., Augoustak, O., et al.: Body growth in Cooley's anemia (homozygous beta thalassemia) with a correlative study as to other aspects of the illness in 138 cases, Pediatrics **50:**92, 1972.

78. Luhby, A. L., and Cooperman, J. M.: Folic acid deficiency in thalassemia major, Lancet **2:**490, 1961.

79. Malamos, B., Fessas, P., and Stamatoyannopoulos, G.: Types of thalassemia trait carriers as revealed by a study of their incidence in Greece, Br. J. Haematol. **8:**5, 1962.

80. Mentzer, W. G., Jr.: Differentiation of iron deficiency from thalassemia trait, Lancet **1:**882, 1973.

81. Milner, P. F., Clegg, J. B., and Weatherall, D. J.: Haemoglobin H disease due to a unique haemoglobin variant with an elongated α chain, Lancet **1:**729, 1971.

82. Modell, B.: Management of thalassemia major, Br. Med. Bull. **32:**270, 1976.

83. Modell, C. B., and Beck, J.: Long-term desferrioxamine therapy in thalassemia, Ann. N.Y. Acad. Sci. **323:**201, 1974.

84. Nathan, D. G., and Gunn, R. B.: Thalassemia: the consequences of unbalanced hemoglobin synthesis, Am. J. Med. **41:**815, 1966.

85. Nathan, D. G., Stossel, T. B., Gunn, R. B., Zarkowsky, H. S., and Lafoiet, M. T.: Influence of hemoglobin precipitation on erythrocyte metabolism in alpha and beta thalassemia, J. Clin. Invest. **48:**33, 1969.

86. Necheles, T. F., Chung, S., Sabbah, R., and Whitten, D.: Intensive transfusion therapy in thalassemia major: an eight year follow up, Ann. N.Y. Acad. Sci. **232:**179, 1974.

87. Nienhuis, A. W.: Safety of intensive chelation therapy, N. Engl. J. Med. **296:**114, 1977.

88. Nienhuis, A. W., and Anderson, W. F.: Isolation and translation of hemoglobin messenger RNA from thalassemia, sickle cell anemia, and normal human reticulocytes, J. Clin. Invest. **50:**2458, 1971.

89. Nienhuis, A. W., Canfield, P. H., and Anderson, W. F.: Hemoglobin messenger RNA from human bone marrow: isolation and translation in homozygous and heterozygous β-thalassemia, J. Clin. Invest. **52:**1735, 1973.

90. Nienhuis, A. W., Laycock, D. G., and Anderson, A. F.: Translation of rabbit hemoglobin messenger RNA by thalassemia and non-thalassemic ribosomes, Nature (New Biol.) **231:**205, 1971.

91. O'Brien, R. T.: Ascorbic acid enhancement of desferroxamine-induced urinary iron escretion in thalassemia major, Ann. N.Y. Acad. Sci. **232:**221, 1974.

92. O'Brien, R. T.: The effect of iron deficiency on the expression of hemoglobin H, Blood **41:**853, 1973.

93. O'Brien, R. T., Pearson, H. A., and Spencer, R. P.: Transfusion induced decrease in spleen size in thalassemia major, J. Pediatr. **81:**105, 1972.

94. Pearson, H. A.: Alpha-beta thalassemia disease in a Negro family, N. Engl. J. Med. **275:**176, 1966.

95. Pearson, H. A.: Thalassemia intermedia: genetic and biochemical considerations, N.Y. Acad. Sci. **119:**390, 1964.

96. Pearson, H. A., Gerald, P. S., and Diamond, L. K.: Thalassemia intermedia due to interaction of Lepore trait with thalassemia trait, Am. J. Dis. Child. **97:**464, 1959.

97. Pearson, H. A., Guiliotis, D. K., O'Brien, R. T., McIntosh, S., and Aspores, G. T.: Thalassemia in Greek Americans, J. Pediatr. **86:**917, 1975.

98. Pearson, H. A., McFarland, W., and King, E. R.: Erythrokinetic studies in thalassemia trait, J. Lab. Clin. Med. **56:**866, 1960.

99. Pearson, H. A., and O'Brien, R. T.: The management of thalassemia major, Semin. Hematol. **12:**255, 1975.

100. Pearson, H. A., O'Brien, R. T., and McIntosh, S.: Screening for thalassemia trait by electronic measurements of mean corpuscular volume, N. Engl. J. Med. **288:**351, 1973.

101. Piomelli, A., Karpatkin, M. H., Arzanian, M., Zamani, M., Becker, M. H., Geneiser, N., Danoff, S. J., and Kuhns, W. J.: Hypertransfusion regimen in patients with Cooley's anemia, Ann. N.Y. Acad. Sci. **232:**186, 1974.

102. Peterson, C. M., Grazeani, J. H., Grady, R. W., Jones, R. L., Vdassara, H. V., Canale, V. C., Miller, D. R., and Cerami, A.: Chelation studies with 2,3-dehydrobenzoic acid in patients with β-thalassemia major, Br. J. Haematol. **33:**477, 1976.

103. Piomelli, S., Danoff, S. J., Becker, M. H., Pipera, M. J., and Travis, S. F.: Prevention of bone malformations and cardiomegaly in Cooley's anemia by early hypertransfusion regimen, Ann. N.Y. Acad. Sci. **165:**427, 1969.

104. Prevention of serious infections after splenectomy, Med. Lett. Drugs Ther. **19:**1, 1977.

105. Propper, R., Cooper, B., Rufo, R. R., et al.: Continuous subcutaneous administration of deferoxamine in patients with iron overload, N. Engl. J. Med. **297:**418, 1977.

106. Propper, R. D., Shurin, S. B., and Nathan, D. G.: Reassessment of the use of desferrioxamine B in iron overload, N. Engl. J. Med. **294:**1421, 1976.

107. Rachmilewitz, E. A., Lubin, B. H., and Shohet, S. B.: Lipid membrane peroxidation in β-thalassemia major, Blood **47:**495, 1976.

108. Rowley, P. T.: The diagnosis of beta thalassemia trait: a review, Am. J. Hematol. **1:**129, 1978.

109. Schmaier, A. A., Maurer, H. A., Johnston, C. L., and Scott, R. B.: Alpha thalassemia screening in neonates by mean corpuscular volume and mean corpuscular hemoglobin delineation, J. Pediatr. **83:**794, 1973.

110. Schwartz, E.: Heterozygous beta thalassemia: balance of globin synthesis in bone marrow cells, Science **167:**1513, 1970.

111. Schwartz, E.: The silent carrier of β-thalassemia, N. Engl. J. Med. **281:**1327, 1969.
112. Schulkind, M. L., Ellis, E. F., and Smith, R. J.: Effect of antibody on clearance of I^{125}-labeled pneumococci by the spleen and liver, Pediatr. Res. **1:**178, 1967.
113. Schumacker, M. J.: Serum immunoglobin and transferrin levels after childhood splenectomy, Arch. Dis. Child. **45:**114, 1970.
114. Seshadri, R., Colebatch, J. H., and Gordon, P.: Long-term administration of desferroxamine in thalassemia major, Arch. Dis. Child. **49:**8, 1974.
115. Shepard, M. K., Weatherall, D. J., and Conley, C. L.: Semiquantitative estimation of the distribution of fetal hemoglobin in red cell population, Bull. Johns Hopkins Hosp. **110:**293, 1962.
116. Silvestroni, E., and Bianco, I.: The distribution of the microcythaemias (or thalassemias) in Italy: some aspects of the haematological and haemoglobinic picture in these haemopathies. In Jonxis, J. H. P., and Delafreonaye, J. F., eds.: Abnormal haemoglobin, Oxford, 1959, Blackwell Scientific Publications.
117. Singer, D. B.: Postsplenectomy sepsis, Perspect. Pediatr. Pathol. **1:**285, 1973.
118. Singer, K., Chernoff, A. I., and Singer, L.: Studies on abnormal hemoglobins. I. Their demonstration in sickle-cell anemia and other hematological disorders by means of alkali denaturation, Blood **6:**413, 1951.
119. Smith, C. H., Erlandson, M. E., Schulman, I., and Stern, G.: Hazard of severe infections in splenectomized infants and children, Am. J. Med. **22:**390, 1957.
120. Smith, C. H., Erlandson, M. E., Stern, G., and Hilgartner, M. W.: Postsplenectomy infection in Cooley's anemia: an appraisal of the problem in this and other blood disorders with consideration of prophylaxis, N. Engl. J. Med. **266:**737, 1962.
121. Smith, C. H., Sisson, T. R. C., Floyd, W. H., Jr., et al.: Serum iron and iron-binding capacity of the serum in children with severe Mediterranean (Cooley's) anemia, Pediatrics **5:**799, 1950.
122. Smith, C. H., Schulman, I., Ando, R. E., and Stern, G.: Studies in Mediterranean (Cooley's) anemia: clinical and hematologic aspects of splenectomy with special reference to fetal hemoglobin synthesis, Blood **10:**582, 1955.
123. Sorsdahl, O. E., Taylor, P. E., and Noyes, W. D.: Extramedullary hematopoiesis mediastinal masses and spinal cord compression, J.A.M.A. **189:**343, 1964.
124. Stamatoyannopoulos, G., Pappyannopoulou, T., Fessas, P., et al.: The beta-delta thalassemia, Ann. N.Y. Acad. Sci. **165:**25, 1969.
125. Stanfield, J. B.: Acute benign pericarditis in thalassemia major, Proc. Roy. Soc. Med. **55:**236, 1962.
126. Stockman, J. A., III, Weiner, L. S., Simon, G. E., Stuart, M. J., and Oski, F. A.: The micromeasurement of free erythrocyte porphyrin (FEP) as a simple means of distinguishing iron deficiency from beta thalassemia trait in subjects with microcytosis, J. Lab. Clin. Med. **85:**113, 1975.
127. Sturgeon, P., and Finch, C. A.: Erythrokinetics in Cooley's anemia, Blood **12:**64, 1957.
128. Taliaferro, W. H., and Taliaferro, L. G.: The dynamics of hemolysin formation in intact and splenectomized rabbits, J. Inf. Dis. **87:**37, 1950.
129. Tolstoshev, P., Mitchell, J., Lanyon, G., et al.: Presence of gene for β-globin in homozygous β-thalassemia, Nature **259:**95, 1976.
130. Valentine, W. N., and Neel, J. V.: Hematologic and genetic study of transmission of thalassemia (Cooley's anemia: Mediterranean anemia), Arch. Int. Med. **74:**185, 1944.
131. Wolman, I. J.: Transfusion therapy in Cooley's anemia: growth and health as related to long range hemoglobin levels: a progress report, Ann. N.Y. Acad. Sci. **119:**736, 1964.
132. Wapnick, A. A., Lynch, S. R., Krawitz, P., et al.: Effects of iron overload on ascorbic acid metabolism, Br. Med. J. **3:**704, 1968.
133. Wasi, P.: Streptococcal infection leading to cardiac and renal involvement in thalassemia, Lancet **1:**949, 1971.
134. Wasi, P., Disthasongchan, P., and Nan-Nakorn, S.: The effect of iron deficiency on the levels of hemoglobins A_2 and E, J. Lab. Clin. Med. **71:**85, 1968.
135. Watson, J. D.: Molecular biology of the gene, ed. 2, New York, 1970, W. A. Benjamin Inc.
136. Weatherall, D. G.: The genetics of the thalassemias, Br. Med. Bull. **25:**24, 1969.
137. Weatherall, D. J.: Biochemical phenotypes of thalassemia in the American Negro population, Ann. N.Y. Acad. Sci. **119:**450, 1964.
138. Weatherall, D. J., and Clegg, J. B.: Hereditary persistence of fetal haemoglobin, Br. J. Haematol. **29:**191, 1975.
139. Weatherall, D. J., Clegg, J. B., and Naughton, M. A.: Globin synthesis in thalassaemia: an in vitro study, Nature **208:**1061, 1965.
140. Weatherall, D. J., Clegg, J. B., Na-Nakorn, S., and Wasi, P.: The pattern of disordered hemoglobin synthesis in homozygous and heterozygous β-thalassemia, Br. J. Haematol. **16:**251, 1969.
141. Weatherall, D. J., Clegg, J. B., and Wong, H. B.: The haemoglobin constitution of infants with the haemoglobin Bart's hydrops foetalis syndrome, Br. J. Haematol. **18:**357, 1970.
142. Whipple, G. H., and Bradford, W. L.: Mediterranean disease—thalassemia (erythroblastic anemia of Cooley): associated pigment abnormalities simulating hemochromatosis, J. Pediatr. **9:**279, 1936.
143. Wintrobe, M. M., Mathews, E., Pollack, R., and Dobyns, B. M.: A familial hemopoietic disorder in Italian adolescents and adults resembling Mediterranean disease (thalassemia), J.A.M.A. **114:**1530, 1940.

16 □ Hematologic manifestations of chronic systemic disease

Richard T. O'Brien

The hematopoietic system, by virtue of its function and distribution, often acts as a barometer of systemic homeostasis. Quantitative or qualitative abnormalities of the cellular elements of the peripheral blood almost invariably accompany systemic disorders whether they are of inflammatory, metabolic, or neoplastic origin. The severity of those hematologic changes in general parallels the course and stage of the underlying disease.

Hematologic equilibrium is the result of a balanced dynamic process of bone marrow production of the cellular elements of the blood and the removal of senescent cells by the reticuloendothelial system. In health this balance is accomplished with surprising precision so that hematologic values are fairly constant. The hematologic equilibrium can be profoundly altered by either acute or chronic systemic insults. The response to acute systemic disease is often volatile and unpredictable, particularly in the young infant. The child's hematologic responses to chronic systemic disorders do not differ significantly from those observed in adults, and certain clearly recognized patterns have been described. This chapter is restricted to a consideration of the hematologic manifestations of chronic systemic disease.

ANEMIA

Anemia is a common, if not inevitable, accompaniment to chronic systemic disease. In a patient with a chronic disorder the potential causes of anemia are numerous, and the possible mechanisms involved depend on the nature and extent of the underlying disease. The combined excretory and endocrine failure of the kidneys in the uremic state may have profound hematologic consequences. A variety of specific causes for anemia are found in malignant neoplastic diseases. Despite many potential contributory causes, there is a common mechanism for the anemia accompanying many chronic diseases. Although a variety of more descriptive phrases have been utilized to label that process, common usage and simplicity have favored the term "anemia of chronic disorders." Although it is a frequent cause of anemia, particularly in hospitalized patients, it is neither the only mechanism for anemia in chronic disease states nor is it invariably present.

In this section the nature and pathogenesis of the anemia of chronic disorders and other factors contributing to anemia in selected chronic diseases are considered.

Anemia of chronic disorders

The term "anemia of chronic disorders" describes a specific, albeit incompletely understood and probably complex mechanism for the anemia that occurs in many chronic conditions such as the following:

A. Chronic infections
  1. Tuberculosis
  2. Pyelonephritis
  3. Osteomyelitis
  4. Subacute bacterial endocarditis
  5. Chronic fungal disease
  6. Pelvic inflammatory disease
  7. Bronchiectasis
  8. Empyema
B. Chronic inflammatory disorders
  1. Rheumatoid arthritis
  2. Systemic lupus erythematosus
  3. Inflammatory bowel disease
  4. Sarcoidosis
  5. Burns
  6. Trauma
C. Malignant neoplastic disease
  1. Lymphoma
  2. Carcinoma

It is the single major mechanism responsible for the anemia associated with chronic infectious and inflammatory disorders and is also frequently observed in patients with malignant neoplastic diseases as well as many other chronic systemic conditions. This anemia is characterized by decreased levels of serum iron and iron-binding capacity, increased tissue iron stores, and relative bone marrow unresponsiveness to anemia. These typical features offer important clues to the pathogenesis of the disorder:

1. Mild to moderate anemia
2. Slightly decreased red blood cell survival

3. Decreased serum iron and iron-binding capacity
4. Increased tissue iron stores; increased serum ferritin
5. Decreased marrow sideroblasts
6. Increased free erythrocyte protoporphyrin
7. Relative bone marrow unresponsiveness

Description. The anemia of chronic disorders is generally mild or moderate. Hemoglobin concentrations are usually in the range of 7 to 10 gm/dl. Such levels of anemia by themselves are not sufficient to produce symptoms unless complicated by other factors that effect cardiovascular or pulmonary adaptation. In fact, the signs and symptoms of the underlying disease typically overshadow those of the anemia. The anemia develops fairly rapidly during the first 4 to 8 weeks of the illness but is not progressive thereafter.[14] The degree of anemia correlates roughly with the severity of the underlying disease as indicated by other hallmarks of inflammation such as fever, suppuration, or elevation of the erythrocyte sedimentation rate.[40]

The anemia is typically normocytic and either normochromic or hypochromic. Microcytosis may be present. Although in some instances this may be caused by concomitant iron deficiency, marked microcytosis in the absence of iron deficiency is frequently noted in severe inflammatory diseases such as juvenile rheumatoid arthritis (Still's disease). The reticulocyte count is either normal or slightly elevated, but when corrected for the degree of anemia the absolute number is normal or depressed.

The serum iron concentration is invariably decreased, as is the total iron-binding capacity. The percent saturation is usually normal or in the low-normal range. This is in contrast to iron-deficiency anemia, in which the transferrin saturation is markedly decreased ($<15\%$) because the low serum iron level is associated with an increased total iron-binding capacity. The bone marrow shows increased stainable iron, largely within reticuloendothelial cells.[4] Decreased numbers of sideroblasts, nucleated red blood cells with iron inclusions, are noted. Erythroid precursors in the bone marrow are usually present in normal numbers. Levels of serum ferritin are slightly to moderately increased.[53] The concentration of free erythrocyte protoporphyrin is also increased.[44]

Pathogenesis

Hemolysis. Mild to moderate shortening of red blood cell survival has been documented in the anemia of chronic disorders.[73] Cross-transfusion experiments in humans demonstrate that the shortened red cell survival is caused by extracorpuscular factors,[2,27] but as yet no specific factor has been identified. Because the rate of hemolysis is only mildly or moderately increased, it should be easily compensated for by a normal bone marrow (which can increase red cell production sixfold to eightfold). This makes it likely that inadequate erythropoietic compensation for a modest degree of hemolysis is the major determining factor in the anemia of chronic disorders.

Erythropoiesis. An inadequate erythropoietic response to anemia is most immediately apparent in the lack of reticulocytosis or increase in marrow erythroid compartment that would be expected from a normal bone marrow under similar stress. This is confirmed by ferrokinetic studies with ^{59}Fe that demonstrate normal or only slightly increased plasma iron clearance (PIDT ½) and iron uptake into newly synthesized red blood cells.[27,12] In absolute terms these normal values signal an impaired marrow erythropoietic response to anemia.

The causes of this inadequate marrow response to anemia are unclear. At one time it was thought that reduced erythropoietin production was the major mechanism involved. Low serum levels of erythropoietin have been reported in a number of patients.[84] Although marrow responsiveness to physiologic stimuli to erythropoietin production has been demonstrated in experimental animals[34] and humans,[75] erythropoietin production has usually been found subnormal for the degree of anemia.[56] One recent study, however, found that urinary erythropoietin excretion in some of these patients was appropriate for the degree of anemia.[3] Another recent study described a wide variation in both urinary and serum erythropoietin activity in a group of patients with the anemia of chronic disorders who were otherwise hematologically similar.[20] Newer in vitro culture techniques have shown that the marrow of patients with malignancy may not be as responsive to erythropoietin stimulation as that of normal persons or patients with inflammatory disease.[89] There is a general consensus that erythropoietin deficiency alone is an insufficient explanation for the failure of the erythroid marrow to respond to the anemic stimulus.

Another possible explanation could be a physiologic adaptation to reduced tissue oxygen requirements. Elevated levels of erythrocyte 2,3-DPG and whole blood P_{50}, however, were documented in all patients evaluated in one study,[20] indicating that the observed anemia was not merely a consequence of reduced oxygen demand.

A final factor, and perhaps the critical one in the pathogenesis of this hypoproliferative condition, is a lack of available iron for hemoglobin synthesis. Although the body iron burden (as indicated by elevated levels of serum ferritin[53] and increased reticuloendothelial iron)[4] is not depleted, there are obvious abnormalities in the distribution of iron. It appears that the iron in the tissues is not readily released, limiting its availability for hematopoiesis. This is reflected by the decreased sideroblasts in the marrow and the increased levels of free erythrocyte protoporphyrin.[44] Gastrointestinal iron absorption is also decreased.[14] Although the causes of this abnormal distribution of iron are not known, many investigators now consider a relative lack of available iron for hemoglobin synthesis as the major factor in the pathogenesis of the anemia of chronic disorders.

Management. Successful treatment of the underlying disease is the best and most direct form of therapy for the associated anemia. This, however, is not always possible. Since the degree of anemia is usually mild or moderate and generally well tolerated by the patient, no specific therapy is usually required. Blood transfusions are rarely indicated and at best would be merely of transient benefit. Superimposed causes of anemia (such as deficiency of hematinic substances, blood loss, or other complications) should be sought and treated appropriately when present. One should suspect such complicating factors when the degree of anemia is severe. Iron therapy is contraindicated.

Chronic renal disease and uremia

The hematologic changes of uremia are in many ways similar to those of other chronic systemic conditions. In addition, because the kidney is a major excretory organ, toxic hematologic effects may occur. Finally, by virtue of its secretion of erythropoietin, the kidney assumes a unique position in erythropoiesis.

Description. The anemia of chronic renal failure is clinically similar to that found in other chronic disorders. It is generally normochromic and normocytic, and the absolute reticulocyte count is normal or depressed. Bone marrow cellularity and myeloid:erythroid ratios are normal to increased.[13] Serum iron concentrations are variable but often reduced, as is the total iron-binding capacity.[54] The bone marrow usually reveals stainable iron and the serum ferritin is increased.

The degree of anemia correlates only roughly with the blood urea nitrogen[23] and the creatinine clearance[43] and somewhat better with inulin and para-aminohippuric acid clearances. Significant anemia occurs only when the glomerular filtration rate is reduced to lower than 25% to 30% of normal.[62]

Pathogenesis

Hemolysis. A mild to moderate shortening of the red blood cell life span occurs in approximately 70% of patients with uremia,[18] but does not correlate with the severity of the renal excretory impairment as measured by the blood urea nitrogen.[23] There are convincing in vivo and in vitro observations demonstrating extracorpuscular mecha-

nism(s) responsible for this hemolysis. Cross-transfusion studies have shown shortened survival rate of normal red cells in uremic patients and normal survival of uremic red cells in healthy recipients.[42,54] The in vitro autohemolysis of erythrocytes from uremic patients is increased, and this abnormality can be ameliorated by dialysis or washing of the red cells prior to incubation.[30,31] Red blood cells from healthy persons incubated in uremic serum also show increased autohemolysis. Although renal excretory failure yields an environment unfavorable to normal red blood cell survival, a specific toxin in uremic blood has thus far eluded detection.

Studies of the effect of uremia on erythrocyte glycolysis have yielded conflicting results.[64,67] Increased serum inorganic phosphates may stimulate glycolysis.[50,76] In addition, the extracellular inorganic phosphate concentration correlates directly with the level of erythrocyte 2,3-DPG and ATP in uremic patients (Fig. 16-1).[50] These glycolytic intermediates are particularly important in the anemic patient since they exert a major role in hemoglobin oxygen affinity.[81] However, red cell 2,3-DPG and shift to the right of the oxygen dissociation curve and P_{50} in patients with severe chronic renal disease are less than would be expected for the degree of anemia. This probably results from the concomitant large acid load[51] that tends to depress 2,3-DPG synthesis. The relationship between P_{50} of whole blood and 2,3-DPG in a variety of other clinical disorders is shown in Fig. 16-2.

Numerous studies have demonstrated many changes in the erythrocyte content of various gly-

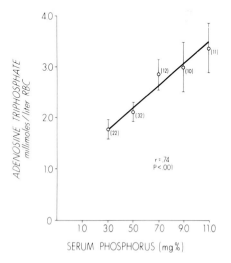

Fig. 16-1. Correlation of red cell ATP concentration and serum phosphorus concentration. The figures in parenthesis indicate the number of uremic patients studied. (From Lichtman, M. A., Miller, D. R., and Weed, R. I.: Trans. Assoc. Am. Physicians **82**:331, 1969.)

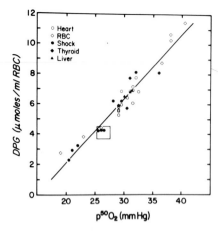

Fig. 16-2. Relationship between P_{50} of whole blood and red blood cell 2,3-DPG in a variety of clinical disorders. These include cyanotic heart disease (○), red blood enzyme defects (◇), septic shock (●), hyperthyroidism (◆), and chronic liver disease (▲). Square indicates normal range for P_{50} and red blood cell DPG. (From Oski, F. A., and Gottlieb, A. J.: Prog. Hematol. **7:**33, 1971. Used by permission.)

colytic enzyme activities. Pyruvate kinase and hexokinase activity is generally reduced, but G-6-PD activity is increased.[61] Most investigators attribute these changes to the slightly younger red cell population or to the effects of alterations in pH, ionic concentrate, or solute composition brought about by renal excretory impairment.

Alterations in red cell membrane ion transport resulting in increased K^+ loss[30] and Na^+ retention[86] have been noted among patients with uremia. Such abnormalities may be a consequence of a specific structural defect of the membrane or else a malfunction of the ATP-dependent cation pump of the membrane. A membrane abnormality could be secondary to acidosis with changes in phospholipids,[65] but a plasma factor has been found in some uremic patients that induces a reversible defect in the ouabain-sensitive ATPase of normal erythrocytes.[15]

Despite the array of functional metabolic alterations of the red blood cell described, a specific cause has not been identified for the increased hemolysis observed in the majority of patients with uremia. As in the anemia of chronic disorders, the rate of hemolysis should be easily compensated for by a normal bone marrow. It is likely that decreased red blood cell production rather than accelerated destruction is the major factor in the anemia of chronic renal insufficiency.

Erythropoiesis. Observations of the effects of hypoxemia in parabiotic rats[72] and in patients with differential cyanosis caused by a reverse-flow patent ductus arteriosus[80] suggested a humoral con-

trol of erythropoiesis. This was documented by studies demonstrating that plasma from anemic animals contains a substance that stimulates erythropoiesis when injected into nonanemic recipients.[21] This hormone, erythropoietin, is the primary regulator of erythropoiesis. A detailed review of the structure, production, metabolism, and action of this hormone is beyond the scope of this chapter, but is discussed in a recent article[29] and in Chapter 8.

The critical role of the kidney in the production of erythropoietin was documented in experiments demonstrating a lack of erythropoietic response to hypoxia in nephrectomized, uremic animals but not in their equally uremic, ureter-ligated littermates.[39] Removal of any other organ has no effect on obliterating the erythropoietic response to anemia or hypoxia. Whether the kidney secretes the erythropoietically active substance or a material that contributes to its production or activation is subject to debate, but a recent study indicates actual renal production of erythropoietin itself.[24] Regardless of the mechanism, the kidneys are essential for producing adequate levels of erythropoietin and maintaining normal erythropoiesis. In the anephric person erythropoietin production and erythropoiesis continue but at markedly reduced levels.[66-68] Extrarenal erythropoietin production accounts for only about 10% of the total erythropoietin produced. It is also responsive to hypoxic stimuli and is probably of hepatic origin.[28]

As in the anemia of chronic disorders, inadequate bone marrow response to anemia is clinically apparent in the lack of reticulocytosis or increase in marrow erythroid compartment. Ferrokinetic studies with ^{59}Fe show slow clearance of transferrin-bound iron from the plasma, decreased plasma iron turnover, and decreased incorporation of iron into red cells.[18,47,57]

It is likely that a relative deficiency of erythropoietin is primarily responsible for this inadequate bone marrow response, but assessment of erythropoietin levels may be difficult. Obviously urinary erythropoietin measurements are invalid in renal failure with oliguria. However, inappropriately low plasma erythropoietin levels are found in patients with uremia when compared to other conditions with comparable degrees of anemia.[9,58]

Even in uremia the kidney may exert some erythropoietic stimulating effect since the transfusion requirements of bilaterally nephrectomized patients on chronic dialysis are greater than those of comparable patients whose kidneys are left intact.[19,63] Ferrokinetic studies, however, have not shown any effect of bilateral nephrectomy on erythropoiesis.[67,68]

Although a specific toxic factor has not been identified, evidence suggests that the uremic milieu contributes to the suppression of red blood cell production. Amelioration of renal excretory failure by chronic dialysis often produces improvement in erythropoiesis without affecting renal endocrine function.[25,58] The response of nephrectomized animals to erythropoietin is subnormal and dependent on the severity of the uremia.[7,22] Recent in vitro studies have demonstrated that uremic serum inhibits heme synthesis.[26,83]

A potentially large number of secondary factors that influence the hematopoietic equilibrium may be superimposed on the already severely compromised situation induced by uremia. Chronic blood loss from the gastrointestinal tract or genitourinary system may lead to iron deficiency, as can the regular loss of blood during hemodialysis or from repeated venepunctures.[49] Urinary loss of transferrin in the nephrotic syndrome that could suppress erythropoiesis by making the availability of iron rate limiting has also been reported.[74] In addition, the chronic inflammatory state seen in collagen disease or chronic pyelonephritis may contribute to impaired iron utilization. Folic acid deficiency is common in chronic renal failure, particularly in patients receiving regular hemodialysis.[35,88]

In summary, the anemia of chronic renal insufficiency results from a combination of factors. The uremic environment is unfavorable for both red blood cell production and survival, but it is probably the inability of the severely compromised kidney to respond with an increase in erythropoietin production that is the major factor contributing to the anemia of chronic renal failure.

Management. A decision of whether to administer red cell transfusion should be guided by the patient's symptoms rather than arbitrary hemoglobin concentration. Patients usually tolerate even moderately severe degrees of anemia quite well, and increasing hemoglobin levels by transfusion has no effect on renal function.[8,60] Furthermore, transfusions have potentially harmful effects, for when the hemoglobin level is increased to more than 9 to 10 gm/dl suppression of the patient's own erythropoiesis ensues. Other complications and risks of transfusion that must also be considered include acute volume overload, hemolytic reactions, hepatitis, transfusional hemosiderosis, and sensitization to transplantation antigens.

The severity of the anemia generally parallels the course of the renal failure. Relief of the metabolic consequences of renal excretory impairment by dialysis is associated with increased erythropoiesis.[25,58] Hormonal replacement therapy could be expected to have a major beneficial effect on anemia of renal failure. Preparations of purified exogenous erythropoietin, however, are not available for clinical use. Stimulation of endogenous erythropoietin production can be accomplished with pharmacologic doses of androgens,[36] but the usefulness of these anabolic agents in chronic renal failure is limited because of the already compromised renal endocrine function and significant side effects of the compounds currently available.

Correction of both excretory and endocrine deficits may be accomplished by renal transplantation, and the effects of a successful graft on erythropoiesis are striking. A reticulocytosis followed by a rise in hemoglobin concentration is invariably seen when the transplant is successful, and this is generally associated with an elevation in the amount of erythropoietin detectable in the plasma and urine.[17,37]

Malignant neoplastic disease

Anemia is frequently associated with malignant neoplastic disease,[5,46] but the causes for anemia are more diverse than in other chronic diseases:
1. Anemia of chronic disorders
2. Blood loss
3. Bone marrow replacement or suppression
4. Leukoerythroblastic anemia
5. Pure red cell anemia
6. Immune hemolytic anemia
7. Hypersplenism
8. Microangiopathic hemolytic anemia
9. Dyserythropoietic anemia
10. Megaloblastic anemia
11. Refractory hypochromic anemia

Perhaps the most common cause, particularly in patients with widespread metastatic disease, is the same mechanism described earlier as the anemia of chronic disorders. Bone marrow replacement with malignant cells can produce anemia directly, as can the cytotoxic therapeutic modalities commonly employed in the management of those diseases. In addition, there are a number of other more specific causes for anemia found among patients with neoplastic disorders. This section deals with those causes for anemia other than the anemia of chronic disorders associated with neoplasia.

Blood loss. Acute or chronic blood loss is one of the more common causes of anemia, particularly in adults. Chronic blood loss produces the classical picture of iron-deficiency anemia. Bleeding may occur as the direct effect of local tumor invasion such as is commonly seen in carcinoma of the bowel or in genitourinary tract neoplasms. This is a less common phenomenon in pediatrics, but we have seen anemia secondary to blood loss in neuroblastoma and Wilms' tumor in which hemorrhage has occurred within the tumor itself.

A more common cause for blood loss in children with cancer is abnormalities in hemostasis. Thrombocytopenia secondary either to bone marrow replacement with malignant cells or to therapy-induced marrow suppression is quite common. In addition, chemotherapeutic agents such as L-asparaginase can produce a hemorrhagic diathesis through interference with the synthesis of coagulation factors in the liver.[33]

Direct bone marrow involvement. Extensive bone marrow replacement by malignant cells, as is typical in acute leukemias and sometimes seen in neuroblastoma, causes progressive pancytopenia. Another manifestation of direct bone marrow involvement with tumor cells is the so-called leukoerythroblastic anemia.[11,85] In that situation the anemia is associated with distinct morphologic abnormalities on peripheral blood smear, including the presence of immature myeloid cells, nucleated red blood cells, and teardrop-shaped red cells (Plate 3, *P*). Although this picture may be seen in other conditions, its appearance in a patient with malignant disease signals the presence of marrow involvement. Similar morphologic changes are observed in myelofibrosis and myeloid metaplasia, but those disorders are rare in children.

Pure red cell anemia. Pure red cell anemia is characterized by progressive anemia, reticulocytopenia, and a selective absence or marked diminution of red blood cell precursors in the bone marrow. It is distinguished from aplastic anemia by the normal cellularity and presence of normal numbers of other marrow cellular elements. Although it has been occasionally observed in association with other neoplasms, approximately half of adult patients with pure red cell aplasia have thymomas.[45] The association, however, is rare in childhood. In many of the patients the anemia resolves following removal of the thymoma. An immunoglobulin inhibitor to erythropoiesis has been demonstrated in the plasma of many of these patients. Other hypoplastic anemias are discussed in Chapter 8.

Immune hemolytic anemia. Coombs-positive hemolytic anemias are frequently associated with lymphoproliferative disorders, particularly chronic lymphatic leukemia and non-Hodgkin's lymphoma.[41,77] Such an association is common in adults but has also been reported in children.[10] The antibody may be either IgG or IgM, with variable specificity. The clinical course reflects that of the underlying disease. The peripheral blood smear typically reveals spherocytes in addition to polychromasia. Jaundice is frequently present. Other neoplastic processes have also been occasionally associated with this mechanism for anemia.[16]

Other causes of anemia. A variety of other types or causes of anemia can be found in association with malignancy. Hypersplenism, microangiopathic hemolytic anemia,[55] and dyserythropoietic anemia are occasionally seen. Megaloblastic morphologic changes in bone marrow and pe-

ripheral blood are common, particularly among patients receiving antineoplastic chemotherapy, but significant anemia secondary to folic acid or vitamin B_{12} deficiency is rare in children with neoplastic disease. A refractory hypochromic anemia has been described in association with lymphoid hyperplasia and malignant lymphoma.[59]

Endocrine diseases

Anemia is present in approximately one third of patients with hypothyroidism,[82] but many of those cases clearly have secondary causes such as iron deficiency[48] or pernicious anemia.[82] Iron deficiency is usually a coincidental problem, but there is an increased frequency of pernicious anemia among patients with hypothyroidism, probably secondary to a common autoimmune mechanism.

Even when deficiency states are excluded, anemia may occur in hypothyroid patients. Although it was at one time thought that thyroid hormone had a direct effect on erythropoiesis, it is now generally accepted that such an effect is largely indirect and induced by changes in oxygen consumption.[69,78] The lower hemoglobin concentration is a response to the decreased metabolic rate and oxygen consumption of hypothyroidism. The hemoglobin level observed in uncomplicated hypothyroidism is consistent with the oxygen supply and demand. The mild anemia is normochromic and normocytic. Red blood cell survival is normal and the reticulocyte count is normal or decreased. Erythropoietin activity is diminished and correlates directly with the hemoglobin concentration. Following thyroid replacement therapy there is a gradual return of hemoglobin levels to normal values. A similar mechanism has been invoked to explain the anemia sometimes observed in patients with hypopituitarism.

Lead poisoning

Lead poisoning remains a significant pediatric health problem, particularly among young children in poor urban areas.[52] A combination of socioeconomic, developmental, and physiologic factors contributes to the epidemiology of that health hazard. The old peeling paint of many poorly maintained dwellings in urban slums contains lead and represents the major source of exposure. The high incidence of pica among children also undoubtedly contributes to the frequency of lead poisoning, as does the greater absorption of ingested lead in young children than adults.[1] Iron deficiency, which commonly coexists in the same patient population, may predispose to lead intoxication. Experimental studies indicate that iron deficiency increases the retention of lead in the tissues.[79]

Anemia is common in lead poisoning. The degree of anemia varies and, although it is usually mild, correlates directly with the severity of the intoxication.[6] The red blood cell morphology is generally normocytic and hypochromic with prominent basophilic stippling and some polychromasia reflecting modest increases in the reticulocyte count (Plate 1, *E*). Concomitant iron deficiency yields a microcytic anemia.

Lead binds to the red blood cell membrane and also inhibits erythrocyte sodium and potassium ATPase resulting in potassium-loss.[87] Red blood cell survival is modestly shortened but of such a degree that the bone marrow should be able to fully compensate. The bone marrow shows normoblastic hyperplasia with ringed sideroblasts (Plate 3, *O*). Ferrokinetic studies indicate impaired hemoglobin production.

Lead inhibits amino levulinic acid synthetase and dehydrase, ferrochelatase, and coproporphyrinogen oxidase, which results in deficient heme synthesis and the accumulation and excretion of heme intermediates.[32] This forms the basis for the many screening tests for the detection of lead poisoning. The measurement of free erythrocyte porphyrins is currently the most popular and useful screening test.[71] Lead also inhibits globin synthesis, but the mechanism may be related to heme deficiency.[70]

Anemia, although common, is definitely of secondary importance compared to the potentially serious central nervous system effects of lead poisoning. Public health screening programs are aimed at the prevention of the significant central nervous system morbidity and mortality of lead poisoning through early detection and appropriate treatment.[38] Anemia is frequently detected during screening for lead poisoning; concomitant iron deficiency should also be suspected.

PLATELETS AND OTHER HEMOSTATIC FACTORS

Thrombocytopenia has been long recognized as a complication of chronic systemic disorders, but abnormalities of platelet function have been identified recently as a major factor contributing to a hemostatic defect accompanying many chronic diseases. Understanding of the structure, kinetics, and function of platelets has lagged considerably behind similar knowledge amassed concerning red blood cells. Much of this discrepancy can be attributed to technical problems related to the relatively brief survival of platelets in the circulation and their lability in vitro. New methods developed over the last decade have greatly facilitated the study of the platelet and resulted in a plethora of clinical and scientific papers relating to the structure and function of those cells in health and disease, including quantitative and qualitative ab-

normalities associated with chronic systemic diseases.[135,136]

Uremia

The prevalence of significant clinical bleeding in uremia varies widely in published reports but has definitely decreased since the advent of modern medical management of renal excretory failure. Although serious spontaneous hemorrhage is uncommon in patients with chronic renal insufficiency today, in vitro hemostatic defects are found in a majority of untreated patients and almost invariably among patients with clinical bleeding. Even in the absence of spontaneous bleeding, hemostatic defects may present potential management problems in the practice of modern nephrology in which an increasing number of invasive diagnostic and therapeutic maneuvers are utilized.

Mild or moderate thrombocytopenia caused by decreased platelet production is common in uremia, but platelet counts rarely fall below 50×10^9/liter, a level at which spontaneous hemorrhage is unlikely.[126] In addition, prolongation of the partial thromboplastin and prothrombin times, as well as depression of specific coagulation factor activity, has been reported in uremia, but those coagulation defects are uncommon and usually clinically insignificant.[95]

The most common and significant hemostatic defect in chronic uremia is abnormal platelet function demonstrable by a variety of tests. Prolongation of the bleeding time, poor clot retraction, decreased adhesiveness, impaired aggregation, and diminished activation of platelet factor 3 have all been reported.* Platelet functional defects are found in a majority of patients with chronic renal failure and almost invariably among those with clinical bleeding.

These platelet dysfunctions are induced by plasma factors, since they can be predictably reversed by peritoneal or hemodialysis,[127] and defects can be induced by incubating normal platelets with uremic plasma.[109] A number of substances that accumulate in renal excretory failure have been implicated, but considerable controversy persists over the relative importance of each. The effect of urea itself on platelet function has been the subject of a number of conflicting reports.†

Increased concentrations of guanidinosuccinic acid are found in uremic patients in sufficient amounts to inhibit adenosine diphosphate induced platelet factor 3 activation and to induce platelet morphologic changes in vitro.[110] Phenolic acids have been similarly implicated.[121] It seems likely that a number of dialyzable compounds are respon-

---

*References 94, 106, 114, 120.
†References 94, 95, 99, 100, 106, 120, 124.

sible for the reversible platelet dysfunction in uremia, but further investigations are necessary to define their relative importance and mechanism of action.

Bleeding difficulties in patients with uremia can be promptly and reliably reversed by successful dialysis. Clinical improvement may be noted as early as the first postdialysis day with correction of all laboratory evidence of a hemostatic defect within several days.[127,131]

Malignant neoplastic disease

Thrombocytopenia is a common complication of malignant neoplastic disease and is frequently severe, particularly in patients with hematologic malignancies. The mechanisms for thrombocytopenia are varied, but the most common is bone marrow replacement by malignant cells or bone marrow suppression induced by chemotherapy or radiation therapy. Shortened platelet survival in some patients may result from hypersplenism, disseminated intravascular coagulation, or immune mechanisms. Thrombocytosis has been noted in children with neoplastic disease,[91] and it has recently been reported to be a common presenting manifestation of histiocytosis X.[111]

Abnormalities in platelet function have been recently described in neoplastic diseases and related disorders. Defective platelet aggregation was reported in fourteen patients with acute leukemia before treatment was initiated.[98] Similar abnormalities have been noted in related disorders such as polycythemia vera,[90] myeloproliferative disease,[93] myelofibrosis,[103] and essential thrombocythemia.[125] A common denominator in many of those disorders, and in the patients described, has been thrombocytosis. Platelet dysfunction, however, is not found in secondary or transient thrombocytosis,[117] and many patients with myeloproliferative disease and abnormal platelet function have normal platelet counts.[129]

Inflammatory and infectious disease

Although thrombocytopenia is relatively common in acute infectious processes, thrombocytosis appears to be more frequent in chronic infectious and inflammatory conditions.[91,118] This is probably merely a reactive manifestation of a stimulated bone marrow and has little clinical significance because the elevation of platelet count is generally moderate and the platelets function normally.[117] Thrombocytopenia has been noted in sarcoidosis[102] and has been well recognized as a manifestation of systemic lupus erythematosus.[97] Antiplatelet antibody can be identified in a large majority of patients with systemic lupus whether they have thrombocytopenia or not.[112] These findings plus the presence of increased numbers of large plate-

lets suggest a compensated thrombocytolytic state.[107] Shortened platelet survival has been documented under those circumstances.

Of significance also has been the recent demonstration of qualitative platelet dysfunction induced by antiplatelet antibody in nonthrombocytopenic patients with idiopathic thrombocytopenic purpura[96] and systemic lupus erythematosus.[122] The mechanism by which antibody interferes with platelet function is incompletely understood, but treatment with steroids is associated with a return of platelet function to normal.

Cardiac disease

Hemostatic abnormalities are common among patients with congenital heart disease.[115] Prolongations of the prothrombin and partial thromboplastin times and depressions of specific coagulation factor activity have been reported in cyanotic congenital heart disease, but the mechanism responsible for these changes remains unclear. The possible role of disseminated intravascular coagulation has been contested in the literature.[105,113] These changes have been related to polycythemia and are corrected by relief of the polycythemia with regular phlebotomy therapy.[133] The frequency of the reported abnormalities of coagulation factors may be artificially high because of failure in some studies to consider the reduced amount of plasma in a given volume of whole blood from a polycythemic patient when it is added to a standard amount of anticoagulant for in vitro assays.

Thrombocytopenia with decreased platelet survival occurs in cyanotic congenital heart disease, correlates with the degree of polycythemia,[108,132] and is corrected by regular phlebotomy therapy.[133] Shortened platelet survival may also occur with prosthetic heart valves.[134]

The most common hemostatic abnormality in congenital heart disease, whether cyanotic or not, is qualitative platelet dysfunction manifested by prolonged bleeding times and abnormal platelet aggregation.[116] The cause of the abnormal platelet function is as yet unknown.

Other disorders

The availability of reliable in vitro techniques to evaluate platelet function has lead to descriptions of platelet functional abnormalities in an increasing number of clinical situations. The litany of disorders associated with platelet dysfunction is expanding and includes such diverse conditions as diabetes,[123] sickle cell anemia,[128] hypothyroidism,[104] liver disease,[130] postoperative states,[119] and emotional stress,[92] among others. A large number of drugs in addition to aspirin have also been implicated.[101] The clinical significance of each of these observations must await further study. It is conceivable that platelet dysfunction in some of these conditions may play a role in the pathophysiology of the disease, but it seems likely that in many it is merely a secondary effect with little or no clinical relevance.

NEUTROPHILS

The neutrophil is perhaps the most labile of the cellular elements of the peripheral blood, with a half-life in the circulation of only a few hours. Wide variations in neutrophil numbers accompany many acute systemic disorders, and neutrophilia is commonly observed in chronic inflammatory and infectious disease processes. Neutropenia has been well recognized in systemic lupus erythematosus[97] and, although specific studies are lacking, it is reasonable to assume that immune mechanisms are involved. Other causes for neutropenia, such as bone marrow replacement and hypersplenism, may occur in selected chronic disorders. A discussion of neutropenia appears in Chapter 18.

Recent advances in knowledge of neutrophil physiology have been followed by descriptions of various abnormalities in neutrophil function in a wide assortment of chronic disease states.*

1. Uremia[138,151]
2. Liver disease[140]
3. Diabetes[147,148,156]
4. Systemic lupus erythematosus[139]
5. Rheumatoid arthritis[149]
6. Crohn's disease[153]
7. Leukemias[142,143]
8. Hodgkin's disease[157]
9. Kwashiorkor[152]
10. Hypo-γ-globulinemia[155]
11. Sickle cell anemia[144]
12. Sarcoidosis[145]

Defects in chemotactic activity have been most frequently reported. The clinical significance of these functional changes and their role in the pathophysiology of each disease remains uncertain in most instances.

---

*References 137, 141, 146, 150, 154.

REFERENCES
Anemia

1. Alexander, F. W., Delves, H. T., and Clayton, B. E.: The uptake and excretion by children of lead and other contaminants. In proceedings of the International Symposium on Environmental Health Aspects of Lead, Amsterdam, October 2-6, 1972, Luxembourg Commission of the European Communities, May 1973.
2. Alexander, W. R. M., Richmond, J., Roy, L. M. H., et al.: Nature of anemia in rheumatoid arthritis. II. Survival of transfused erythrocytes in patients with rheumatoid arthritis, Ann. Rheum. Dis. **15:**12, 1956.
3. Alexanian, R.: Erythropoietin excretion in hemolytic anemia and in the hypoferremia of chronic disease, Blood **40:**946, 1972.
4. Bainton, D. F., and Finch, C. A.: The diagnosis of iron-deficiency anemia, Am. J. Med. **37:**62, 1964.
5. Banerjee, R. N., and Narang, R. M.: Haematologic changes in malignancy, Br. J. Haematol. **13:**829, 1967.
6. Betts, P. R., Astley, R., and Raine, D. N.: Lead intoxication in children in Birmingham, Br. Med. J. **1:**402, 1973.
7. Bozzini, E. E., Devoto, F. C. H., and Tomio, J. M.: Decreased responsiveness of hematopoietic tissue to erythropoietin in acutely uremic rats, J. Lab. Clin. Med. **68:**411, 1966.
8. Brod, J., and Hornych, A.: Effect of correction of anemia in the glomerular filtration rate in chronic renal failure, Isr. J. Med. Sci. **3:**53, 1967.
9. Brown, R.: Plasma erythropoietin in chronic uremia, Br. Med. J. **2:**1036, 1965.
10. Buchanan, G. R., Boxer, L. A., and Nathan, D. G.: The acute and transient nature of idiopathic immune hemolytic anemia in childhood, J. Pediatr. **88:**780, 1976.
11. Burkett, L. L., Cox, M. L., and Fields, M. L.: Leukoerythroblastosis in the adult, Am. J. Clin. Pathol. **44:**494, 1965.
12. Bush, J. A., Ashenbrucker, H., Cartwright, G. E., et al.: The anemia of infection. XX. The kinetics of iron metabolism in the anemia associated with chronic infection, J. Clin. Invest. **35:**89, 1956.
13. Callen, I. R., and Limarzi, L. R.: Blood and bone marrow studies in renal disease, Am. J. Clin. Pathol. **20:**3, 1950.
14. Cartwright, G. E.: The anemia of chronic disorders, Semin. Hematol. **3:**351, 1966.
15. Cole, C. H., Balfe, J. W., and Welt, L. G.: Induction of ouabain-sensitive ATPase defect by uremic plasma, Trans. Assoc. Am. Phys. **81:**213, 1968.
16. Dawson, M. A., Talbert, W., and Yarbro, J. W.: Hemolytic anemia associated with an ovarian tumor, Am. J. Med. **50:**552, 1971.
17. Denny, W. F., Flanigan, W. J., and Zukoski, C. F.: Serial erythropoietin studies in patients undergoing renal homotransplantation, J. Lab. Clin. Med. **67:**386, 1966.
18. Desforges, J. F., and Dawson, J. P.: The anemia of renal failure, Arch. Intern. Med. **101:**326, 1958.
19. DeStrihon, C. van Y., and Stragin, A.: Effects of bilateral nephrectomy on transfusion requirements of patients undergoing chronic renal dialysis, Lancet **2:**703, 1969.
20. Douglas, S. W., and Adamson, J. W.: The anemia of chronic disorders: studies of marrow regulation and iron metabolism, Blood **45:**55, 1975.
21. Erslev, A. J.: Humoral regulation of red cell production, Blood **8:**349, 1953.
22. Erslev, A. J.: Erythropoietic function in uremic rabbits, Arch. Intern. Med. **101:**407, 1958.
23. Erslev, A. J.: Anemia of chronic renal disease, Arch. Intern. Med. **126:**774, 1970.
24. Erslev, A. J.: In vitro production of erythropoietin by kidneys perfused with a serum-free solution, Blood **44:**77, 1974.
25. Eschbach, J. W., Funk, D., Adamson, J., et al.: Erythropoiesis in patients with renal failure undergoing chronic dialysis, N. Engl. J. Med. **276:**653, 1967.
26. Fisher, J. W., Lertora, J. L., Lindholm, D. D., et al.: Erythropoietin production and inhibitors in the anemia of uremia, Proc. Clin. Dial. Transplant. Forum **3:**22, 1973.
27. Freireich, E. J., Ross, J. F., Bayles, T. B., et al.: Radioactive iron metabolism and erythrocyte survival studies of the mechanism of the anemia associated with rheumatoid arthritis, J. Clin. Invest. **36:**1043, 1957.

28. Fried, W.: The liver as a source of extrarenal erythropoietin, Blood **40:**671, 1972.

29. Fried, W.: Erythropoietin, Arch. Intern. Med. **131:**929, 1973.

30. Giovannetti, S., Balestri, P. L., and Cioni, L.: Spontaneous in vitro autohaemolysis of blood from chronic uremic patients, Clin. Sci. **29:**407, 1965.

31. Giovannetti, S., Cioni, L., Balestri, P. L., et al.: Evidence that guanidines and some related compounds cause haemolysis in chronic uremia, Clin. Sci. **34:**141, 1968.

32. Goldberg, A.: Lead poisoning as a disorder of heme synthesis, Semin. Hematol. **5:**424, 1968.

33. Gralnick, H. R., and Henderson, E.: Hypofibrinogenemia and coagulation factor deficiencies with l-asparaginase treatment, Cancer **27:**1313, 1971.

34. Gutnisky, A., and Van Dyke, D.: Normal response to erythropoietin or hypoxia in rats made anemic with turpentine abscess, Proc. Soc. Exp. Biol. Med. **112:**75, 1963.

35. Hampers, C. L., Streiff, R., Nathan, D. G., et al.: Megaloblastic hematopoiesis in uremia and in patients on long-term dialysis, N. Engl. J. Med. **276:**551, 1967.

36. Hendler, E. D., Goffinet, J. A., Ross, S., et al.: Controlled study of androgen therapy in anemia of patients on maintenance hemodialysis, N. Engl. J. Med. **291:**1046, 1974.

37. Hoffman, G. S.: Human erythropoiesis following kidney transplantation, Ann. N.Y. Acad. Sci. **149:**504, 1968.

38. Increased lead absorption and lead poisoning in young children: a statement by the Center for Disease Control, J. Pediatr. **87:**824, 1975.

39. Jacobson, L. O., Goldwasser, E., Fried, W., et al.: Role of the kidney in erythropoiesis, Nature **179:**633, 1957.

40. Jeffrey, M. R.: Some observations on anemia in rheumatoid arthritis, Blood **8:**502, 1953.

41. Jones, S. E.: Autoimmune disorders and malignant lymphoma, Cancer **31:**1092, 1973.

42. Joske, R. A., McAlister, J. M., and Prankerd, T. A. J.: Isotope investigators of red cell production and destruction in chronic renal disease, Clin. Sci. **15:**511, 1956.

43. Kasanen, A., and Kalliomaki, J. L.: Correlation of some kidney function tests with hemoglobin in chronic nephropathies, Acta Med. Scand. **158:**213, 1957.

44. Krammer, B. A., Cartwright, G. E., and Wintrobe, M. M.: The anemia of infection. XIX. Studies of free erythrocyte coproporphyrin and protoporphyrin, Blood **9:**183, 1954.

45. Krantz, S. B.: Pure red cell aplasia, N. Engl. J. Med. **291:**345, 1974.

46. Kremer, W. B., and Laszlo, J.: Hematologic effects of cancer. In Holland, J. F., and Frei, E., III, (eds.): Cancer medicine, Philadelphia, 1973, Lea & Febiger.

47. Kurtides, E. S., Ramback, W. A., Alt, H. L., et al.: Effects of hemodialysis on erythrokinetics in anemia of uremia, J. Lab. Clin. Med. **63:**469, 1964.

48. Larsson, S. O.: Anemia and iron metabolism in hypothyroidism, Acta Med. Scand. **157:**349, 1959.

49. Lawson, D. H., Boddy, K., King, P. C., et al.: Iron metabolism in patients with chronic renal failure on regular dialysis treatment, Clin. Sci. **41:**345, 1971.

50. Lichtman, M. A., and Miller, D. R.: Erythrocyte glycolysis, 2,3-diphosphoglycerate and adenosine triphosphate concentration in uremic subjects: relationship to extracellular phosphate concentration, J. Lab. Clin. Med. **76:**267, 1970.

51. Lichtman, M. A., Murphy, M. S., Byer, B. J., et al.: Hemoglobin affinity for oxygen in chronic renal disease: the effect of hemodialysis, Blood **43:**417, 1974.

52. Lin-Fu, J. S.: Vulnerability of children to lead exposure and toxicity, N. Engl. J. Med. **289:**1289, 1973.

53. Lipschitz, D. A., Cook, J. D., and Finch, C. A.: A clinical evaluation of serum ferritin as an index of iron stores, N. Engl. J. Med. **290:**1213, 1974.

54. Loge, J. P., Lange, R. D., and Moore, C. V.: Characterization of the anemia associated with chronic renal insufficiency, Am. J. Med. **24:**4, 1958.

55. Lohrmann, H. P., Adam, W., Heymer, B., et al.: Microangiopathic hemolytic anemia in metastatic carcinoma: report of eight cases, Ann. Intern. Med. **79:**368, 1973.

56. Lukens, J. N.: Control of erythropoiesis in rats with adjuvant-induced chronic inflammation, Blood **41:**37, 1973.

57. Magid, E., and Hilden, M.: Ferrokinetics in patients suffering from chronic renal disease and anemia, Scand. J. Haematol. **4:**33, 1967.

58. Mann, D. L., Donati, R. M., and Gallagher, N. I.: Erythropoietin assay and ferrokinetic measurements in anemic uremic patients, J.A.M.A. **194:**1321, 1965.

59. Maron, B. J., and Shahidi, N. T.: Refractory hypochromic anemia in malignant lymphoma, J. Pediatr. **77:**93, 1970.

60. Melvin, K. E. W., Farrelly, R. O., and North, J. D. K.: Effect of blood transfusion on renal excretory function in chronic renal failure, Lancet **2:**537, 1963.

61. Merrill, J. P.: Uremia, N. Engl. J. Med. **282:**1014, 1970.

62. Mertz, D. P., and Koschnick, R.: Nephrogene anämie and Nierenhämodynamik, Schweiz. Med. Wochenschr. **95:**83, 1965.

63. Milman, N.: Blood transfusion requirements before and after bilateral nephrectomy in patients undergoing chronic hemodialysis, Acta Med. Scand. **195:**479, 1974.

64. Morgan, J. M., and Morgan, R. E.: Study of effect of uremia metabolites on erythrocyte glycolysis, Metabolism **13:**629, 1964.

65. Murphy, J. R.: Erythrocyte metabolism. V. Active cation transport glycolysis, J. Lab. Clin. Med. **61:**567, 1963.

66. Naets, J. P., and Wittek, M.: Erythropoiesis in anephric man, Lancet **1:**941, 1968.

67. Nathan, D. G., Beck, L. H., Hampers, C. L., et al.: Hematopoiesis in anephric man and the metabolism of the uremic erythrocyte, Ann. N.Y. Acad. Sci. **149:**539, 1968.

68. Nathan, D. G., Schupak, E., Stohlman, F., et al.: Erythropoiesis in anephric man, J. Clin. Invest. **43:**2158, 1964.

69. Peschle, C., Zanjani, E. D., Gidari, A. S., et al.: Mechanism of thyroxine action on erythropoiesis, Endocrinology **89:**609, 1971.

70. Piddington, S. K., and White, J. M.: The effect of lead on total globin and α- and β-chain synthesis: in vitro and in vivo, Br. J. Haematol. **27:**415, 1974.

71. Piomelli, S., Davidow, B., Guinee, V. F., et al.: The FEP (free erythrocyte porphyrins) test: a screening micromethod for lead poisoning, Pediatrics **51:**254, 1973.

72. Reissman, K. R.: Studies on the mechanism of erythropoietic stimulation in parabiotic rats during hypoxia, Blood **5:**372, 1950.

73. Richmond, J., Alexander, W. R. M., Potter, J. L., et al.: The nature of anemia in rheumatoid arthritis. V. Red cell survival measured by radioactive chromium, Ann. Rheum. Dis. **20:**133, 1961.

74. Rifkind, D., Kravetz, J., Knight, V., et al.: Urinary excretion of iron-binding protein in the nephrotic syndrome, N. Engl. J. Med. **265:**115, 1961.

75. Robinson, J. C., James, G. W., and Kark, R. M.: The effect of oral therapy with cobaltous chloride on the blood of patients suffering with chronic suppurative infection, N. Engl. J. Med. **240:**749, 1949.

76. Rose, I. A., Warms, J. V. B., and O'Connell, E. L.: Role of inorganic phosphate in stimulation glucose utilization of human red blood cells, Biochem. Biophys. Res. Commun. **15:**33, 1964.

77. Sacks, P. V.: Autoimmune hematologic complications in malignant lymphoproliferative disorders, Arch. Intern. Med. **134:**781, 1974.

78. Shalet, M., Coe, D., and Reissmann, K. R.: Mechanism of erythropoietic action of thyroid hormone, Proc. Soc. Exp. Biol. Med. **123:**443, 1966.

79. Six, K. M., and Goyer, R. A.: The influence of iron deficiency on tissue content and toxicity of ingested lead in the rat, J. Lab. Clin. Med. **79:**128, 1972.

80. Stohlman, F., Rath, C. E., and Rose, J. C.: Evidence for a humoral regulation of erythropoiesis: studies on a patient with polycythemia secondary to regional hypoxia, Blood **9:**721, 1954.

81. Thomas, H. M., Lefrak, S. S., Irwin, R. S., et al.: The oxyhemoglobin dissociation curve in health and disease: role of 2,3-diphosphoglycerate, Am. J. Med. **57:**331, 1974.

82. Tudhope, G. R., and Wilson, G. M.: Anaemia in hypothyroidism, Q. J. Med. **29:**513, 1960.

83. Wallner, S. F., Kurnick, J. E., Ward, H. P., et al.: The anemia of chronic renal failure and chronic diseases: in vitro studies of erythropoiesis, Blood **47:**561, 1976.

84. Ward, H. P., Kurnick, J. E., and Pisarczyk, M. I.: Serum level of erythropoietin in anemias associated with chronic infection, malignancy, and primary hematopoietic disease, J. Clin. Invest. **50:**332, 1971.

85. Weick, J. K., Hagedorn, A. B., and Linmann, J. W.: Leukoerythroblastosis: diagnostic and prognostic significance, Mayo Clin. Proc. **49:**110, 1974.

86. Welt, L. G., Sachs, J. R., and McManus, T. J.: An ion transport defect in erythrocytes from uremic patients, Trans. Assoc. Am. Physicians **77:**169, 1964.

87. White, J. M., and Selhi, H. S.: Lead and the red cell, Br. J. Haematol. **30:**133, 1975.

88. Whitehead, V. M., Comty, C. H., Posen, G. A., et al.: Homeostasis of folic acid in patients undergoing maintenance hemodialysis, N. Engl. J. Med. **279:**970, 1968.

89. Zucker, S., Friedman, S., and Lysik, R. M.: Bone marrow erythropoiesis in the anemia of infection, inflammation, and malignancy, J. Clin. Invest. **53:**1132, 1974.

Platelets and other hemostatic factors

90. Abraham, J. P., Johnson, S. A., and Ulutin, O. N.: Platelet function in polycythemia vera, J. Lab. Clin. Med. **54:**785, 1959.

91. Addiego, J. E., Mentzer, W. C., and Dallman, P. R.: Thrombocytosis in infants and children, J. Pediatr. **85:**805, 1974.

92. Arkel, Y. S.: Evaluation of platelet aggregation in disorders of hemostasis, Med. Clin. North Am. **60:**881, 1976.

93. Cardamone, J. M., Edson, J. R., McArthur, J. R., et al.: Abnormalities of platelet function in myeloproliferative disorders, J.A.M.A. **221:**270, 1972.

94. Castaldi, P. A., Rozenberg, M. C., and Stewart, J. H.: The bleeding disorder of uremia: a qualitative platelet defect, Lancet **2:**66, 1966.

95. Cheney, K., and Bonnin, J. A.: Haemorrhage, platelet dysfunction, and other coagulation defects in uremia, Br. J. Haematol. **8:**215, 1962.

96. Clancy, R., Jenkins, E., and Firkin, B.: Qualitative platelet abnormalities in idiopathic thrombocytopenic purpura, N. Engl. J. Med. **286:**622, 1972.

97. Cook, C. D., Wedgewood, R. J. P., Craig, J. M., et al.: Systemic lupus erythematosus: description of 37 cases in children and a discussion of endocrine therapy in 32 of the cases, Pediatrics **26:**570, 1960.

98. Cowan, D. H., and Haut, M. J.: Platelet function in acute leukemia, J. Lab. Clin. Med. **79:**893, 1972.

99. Cronberg, S.: Investigations in haemorrhagic disorders with prolonged bleeding time but normal number of platelets with special reference to platelet adhesiveness, Acta Med. Scand. **486**(suppl.):1, 1968.

100. Davis, J. W., McField, J. R., Phillips, P. E., et al.: Effects of exogenous urea, creatinine, and guanidinosuccinic acid on human platelet aggregation in vitro, Blood **39:**388, 1972.

101. De Gaetano, G., Donati, M. B., and Garattini, S.: Drugs affecting platelet function tests, Thromb. Diath. Haemorrh. **34:**285, 1975.

102. Dickerman, J. D., Holbrook, P. R., and Zinkham, W. H.: Etiology and therapy of thrombocytopenia associated with sarcoidosis, J. Pediatr. **81:**758, 1972.

103. Didisheim, P., and Bunting, D.: Abnormal platelet function in myelofibrosis, Am. J. Clin. Pathol. **45:**566, 1966.

104. Edson, J. R., Fecher, D. R., and Doe, R. P.: Low platelet adhesiveness and other hemostatic abnormalities in hyperthyroidism, Ann. Intern. Med. **82:**342, 1975.

105. Ekert, H., Gilchrist, G. S., and Stanton, R.: Hemostasis in cyanotic congenital heart disease, J. Pediatr. **76:**221, 1970.

106. Eknoyan, G., Wacksman, S. J., Glueck, H. I., et al.: Platelet function in renal failure, N. Engl. J. Med. **280:**677, 1969.

107. Garg, S. K., Amorosi, E. L., and Karpatkin, S.: Use of the megathrombocyte as an index of thrombopoiesis, N. Engl. J. Med. **284:**11, 1971.

108. Gross, S., Keefer, V., and Liebman, J.: The platelets in cyanotic congenital heart disease, Pediatrics **42:**651, 1968.

109. Horowitz, H. I., Cohen, B. D., Martinez, P., et al.: Defective ADP-induced platelet factor III activation in uremia, Blood **30:**331, 1967.

110. Horowitz, H. I., Stein, I. M., Cohen, B. D., et al.: Further studies on the platelet inhibitory effect of guanidinosuccinic acid and its role in uremic bleeding, Am. J. Med. **49:**336, 1970.

111. Kamalakar, P., Humbert, J. R., and Fitzpatrick, J. E.: Thrombocytosis in histiocytosis X, Pediatr. Res. **11:**473, 1977. (Abstract.)

112. Karpatkin, S., Strick, N., Karpatkin, M. B., et al.: Cumulative experience in the detection of antiplatelet antibody in 234 patients with idiopathic thrombocytopenic purpura, systemic lupus erythematosus, and other clinical disorders, Am. J. Med. **52:**776, 1972.

113. Komp, D. M., and Sparrow, A. W.: Polycythemia in cyanotic heart disease: a study of altered coagulation, J. Pediatr. **76:**231, 1970.

114. Larsson, S. O., Hedner, U., and Nilsson, I. M.: On coagulation and fibrinolysis in conservatively treated chronic uremia, Acta Med. Scand. **189:**433, 1971.

115. Maurer, H. M.: Hematologic effects of cardiac disease, Pediatr. Clin. North Am. **19:**1083, 1972.

116. Maurer, H. M., McCue, C. M., Caul, J., et al.: Impairment in platelet aggregation in congenital heart disease, Blood **40:**207, 1972.

117. McClure, P. D., Ingram, G. I. C., Stacey, R. S., et al.: Platelet function tests in thrombocythemia and thrombocytosis, Br. J. Haematol. **12:**478, 1966.

118. Morowitz, D. A., Allen, L. W., and Kirsner, J. B.: Thrombocytosis in chronic inflammatory bowel disease, Ann. Intern. Med. **68:**1013, 1968.

119. O'Brien, J. R., Etherington, M., and Jamieson, S.: Refractory state of platelet aggregation with major operations, Lancet **2:**741, 1971.

120. Rabiner, S. F., and Hrodek, O.: Platelet factor III in normal subjects and patients with renal failure, J. Clin. Invest. **47:**901, 1968.

121. Rabiner, S. F., and Molinas, F.: The role of phenol and phenolic acids on the thrombocytopathy and defective platelet aggregation of patients with renal failure, Am. J. Med. **49:**346, 1970.

122. Regan, M. G., Lackner, H., and Karpatkin, S.: Platelet function and coagulation profile in lupus erythematosus: studies in 50 patients, Ann. Intern. Med. **81:**462, 1974.
123. Sagel, J., Colwell, J. A., Crook, L., et al.: Increased platelet aggregation in early diabetes mellitus, Ann. Intern. Med. **82:**733, 1975.
124. Somer, J. B., Stewart, J. H., and Castaldi, P. A.: The effect of urea on the aggregation of normal human platelets, Thromb. Diath. Haemorrh. **19:**64, 1968.
125. Spaet, T. H., Lejnieks, I., Gaynor, E., et al.: Defective platelets in essential thrombocythemia, Arch. Intern. Med. **124:**135, 1969.
126. Stewart, J. H.: Platelet numbers and life span in acute and chronic renal failure, Thromb. Diath. Haemorrh. **17:**532, 1967.
127. Stewart, J. H., and Castaldi, P. A.: Uremic bleeding: a reversible platelet defect corrected by dialysis, Q. J. Med. **36:**409, 1967.
128. Stuart, M. J., Stockman, J. A., and Oski, F. A.: Abnormalities of platelet aggregation in vaso-occlusive crisis of sickle cell anemia, J. Pediatr. **85:**629, 1974.
129. Tangun, Y.: Platelet aggregation and platelet factor III activity in myeloproliferative disease, Thromb. Diath. Haemorrh. **25:**241, 1971.
130. Thomas, D. P., Ream, V. J., and Stuart, R. K.: Platelet aggregation in patients with Laennec's cirrhosis of the liver, N. Engl. J. Med. **276:**1344, 1967.
131. Von Kaulla, K. N., Von Kaulla, E., Wasantapruck, S., et al.: Blood coagulation in uremic patients before and after hemodialysis and transplantation of the kidney, Arch. Surg. **92:**184, 1966.
132. Waldman, J. D., Czapek, E. E., Paul, M. H., et al.: Shortened platelet survival in cyanotic heart disease, J. Pediatr. **87:**77, 1975.
133. Wedemeyer, A. L., and Lewis, J. H.: Improvement in hemostasis following phlebotomy in cyanotic patients with heart disease, J. Pediatr. **83:**46, 1973.
134. Weily, H. S., Steele, P. P., Davies, H., et al.: Platelet survival in patients with substitute heart valves, N. Engl. J. Med. **290:**534, 1974.
135. Weiss, H. J.: Platelet physiology and abnormalities of platelet function. Part 1, N. Engl. J. Med. **293:**531, 1975.
136. Weiss, H. J.: Platelet physiology and abnormalities of platelet function. Part 2, N. Engl. J. Med. **293:**580, 1975.

Neutrophils

137. Baehner, R. L.: Microbe ingestion and killing by neutrophils: normal mechanisms and abnormalities, Clin. Haematol. **4:**609, 1975.
138. Clark, R. A., Hamory, B. H., Ford, G. H., et al.: Chemotaxis in acute renal failure, J. Infect. Dis. **126:**460, 1972.
139. Clark, R. A., Kimball, H. R., and Decker, J. L.: Neutrophil chemotaxis in systemic lupus erythematosus, Ann. Rheum. Dis. **33:**167, 1974.

140. De Meo, A. N., Anderson, B. R.: Defective chemotaxis associated with a serum inhibitor in cirrhotic patients, N. Engl. J. Med. **286:**735, 1972.
141. Gallin, J. I., and Wolff, S. M.: Leukocyte chemotaxis: physiological considerations and abnormalities, Clin. Haematol. **4:**567, 1975.
142. Holland, J. F., Senn, H., and Banerjee, T.: Quantitative studies of localized leukocyte mobilization in acute leukemia, Blood **37:**499, 1971.
143. Humbert, J. R., Hutter, J. J., Thoren, C. H., et al.: Decreased neutrophil bactericidal activity in acute leukemia of childhood, Cancer **37:**2194, 1976.
144. Johnston, R. B., Newman, S. L., and Struth, A. G.: An abnormality of the alternate pathway of complement activation in sickle cell disease, N. Engl. J. Med. **288:**803, 1973.
145. Maderazo, E. G., Ward, P. A., Woronick, C. L., et al.: Leukotactic dysfunction in sarcoidosis, Ann. Intern. Med. **84:**414, 1976.
146. Miller, M. E.: Pathology of chemotaxis and random mobility, Semin. Hematol. **12:**59, 1975.
147. Miller, M. E., and Baker, L.: Leukocyte functions in juvenile diabetes mellitus: humoral and cellular aspects, J. Pediatr. **81:**979, 1972.
148. Mowat, A. G., and Baum, J.: Chemotaxis of polymorphonuclear leukocytes from patients with diabetes mellitus, N. Engl. J. Med. **284:**621, 1971.
149. Mowat, A. G., and Baum, J.: Chemotaxis of polymorphonuclear leukocytes from patients with rheumatoid arthritis, J. Clin. Invest. **50:**2541, 1971.
150. Quie, P. G.: Pathology of bactericidal power of neutrophils, Semin. Hematol. **12:**143, 1975.
151. Salant, D. J., Glover, A. M., Anderson, R., et al.: Depressed neutrophil chemotaxis in patients with chronic renal failure and after renal transplantation, J. Lab. Clin. Med. **88:**536, 1976.
152. Schopfer, K., and Douglas, S. D.: Neutrophil function in children with kwashiorkor, J. Lab. Clin. Med. **88:**450, 1976.
153. Segal, A. W., and Loewi, G.: Neutrophil dysfunction in Crohn's disease, Lancet **2:**219, 1976.
154. Senn, H. J., and Jungi, W. F.: Neutrophil migration in health and disease, Semin. Hematol. **12:**27, 1975.
155. Steerman, R. L., Snyderman, R., Leikin, S. L., et al.: Intrinsic defect of the polymorphonuclear leukocyte resulting in impaired chemotaxis and phagocytosis, Clin. Exper. Immunol. **9:**839, 1971.
156. Tan, J. S., Anderson, J. L., Watanakunakorn, C., et al.: Neutrophil dysfunction in diabetes mellitus, J. Lab. Clin. Med. **85:**26, 1975.
157. Ward, P. A., Berenberg, J. L.: Defective regulation of inflammatory mediators in Hodgkin's disease, Supernormal levels of chemotactic factor inactivator, N. Engl. J. Med. **290:**76, 1974.

PART THREE **WHITE BLOOD CELLS**

edited by

ROBERT L. BAEHNER

17 □ Aplastic anemia and bone marrow transplantation

Richard J. O'Reilly
Michael Sorell

Aplastic anemia is a disorder of hematopoiesis characterized by a severe and generalized reduction or depletion of erythroid, myeloid, and megakaryocytic elements in the marrow with resultant peripheral pancytopenia. The disorder exists in both constitutional and acquired forms in children. The disease is attributed to either a depletion of hematopoietic stem cells or an abnormality that severely limits their proliferative potential resulting from toxic or immunologic injury or infection.

In recent years the term "aregenerative anemia" has become a common synonym for aplastic anemia. In view of the fact that all three marrow precursor lines are involved, more descriptive terms would be aplastic or hypoplastic pancytopenia. However, such names are infrequently applied to the disorder. The term "hypoplastic anemia" is now usually applied to pure red cell aplasia rather than a mild form of aplastic anemia.

HISTORICAL PERSPECTIVE

Ehrlich[78] first described this disorder in 1888 and recognized many of its essential features. He noted fever, ulceration and bleeding of the mucous membranes, and a fat-filled acellular bone marrow. The term "aplastic anemia" was first used by Chauffard[47] in 1904. In the early decades of this century many patients were described with pancytopenia in whom cellular marrows were found at autopsy. Undoubtedly many of these patients were suffering from leukemia and peripheral pancytopenia. By the early 1940s the frequently encountered difficulties in distinguishing these two diseases were well appreciated.[30]

Exposure to benzene was associated with the development of aplasia as early as 1897.[34] Since then numerous drugs and chemicals have been implicated as etiologic agents. The association of chloramphenicol use and aplastic anemia[265,303] stimulated a great deal of interest in the disorder and its prevention, pathogenesis, and treatment. Aplasia following infectious hepatitis was first reported by Lorenz and Quaisar[188] in 1955. This early literature was the subject of an excellent review by Scott et al.[290] in 1959.

CLASSIFICATION

Aplastic anemia is initially classified according to whether it is congenital (constitutional) or acquired in origin.

The acquired form of aplastic anemia may develop as the result of exposure to radiation and to a variety of drugs or chemicals. It may also occur as a complication of infections such as infectious hepatitis or infectious mononucleosis. Aplastic anemia is also associated with other conditions such as paroxysmal nocturnal hemoglobinuria,[56,57,178] pancreatic disease,[297] and pregnancy.* A clear instance of an immunologic assault on the marrow is the aplastic anemia that develops in patients with severe combined immunodeficiency who develop lethal graft versus host disease following transfusions of nonirradiated blood products containing immunocompetent lymphocytes.† For most cases of aplastic anemia no etiology is determined. These cases are thus designated idiopathic.

The constitutional form of aplastic anemia may occur without or with multiple congenital anomalies (Fanconi's anemia). The following is a classification of alpastic anemia:

A. Acquired aplastic anemia
 1. Idiopathic acquired aplastic anemia
  a. Secondary to ionizing radiation or antineoplastic drugs
  b. Secondary to exposure to drugs or chemicals, e.g., chloramphenicol, benzene
  c. Following infectious hepatitis
  d. Secondary to paroxysmal nocturnal hemoglobinuria (PNH)
  e. Associated with other infections, e.g., tuberculosis, mononucleosis
  f. Associated with pregnancy
  g. Marrow hypoplasia associated with systemic disease, e.g., pancreatic disease
  h. Secondary to graft versus host disease
B. Constitutional aplastic anemia
 1. With multiple congenital anomalies (Fanconi's anemia)
 2. Without congenital anomalies

*References 87, 121, 164, 171, 275.
†References 136, 137, 203, 205, 226.

ACQUIRED APLASTIC ANEMIA
Incidence

The overall incidence of acquired aplastic anemia in the United States and Canada has been estimated as 3.5 to 5.4 cases/million persons/year, or about 1,000 new cases/year in the United States.[33,349] Two large autopsy series established the prevalence as 0.28% in the United States and 0.21% in Vienna.[52,163] This would be 5,600 fatalities yearly in the United States. However, both studies were performed at large referral centers and therefore probably overestimated the true incidence.

The idiopathic and drug-induced forms of aplastic anemia may occur at any age, but they predominantly affect children and young adults of both sexes.[290] Aplastic anemia developing as a complication of infectious hepatitis is rare after the age of 25; it occurs predominantly in males.[127] Acquired forms of aplastic anemia may occur in individuals of all racial groups. Furthermore, patients with acquired aplastic anemia can not be distinguished from the general population on the basis of prevalence of any one red cell or leukocyte (HLA) genetic phenotype.[8]

Etiology

For 30% to 50% of patients with aplastic anemia no etiology can be established despite extensive and detailed examination of the patient's history.[290,355] Of the known causes of aplastic anemia the most frequently cited is an exposure to drugs, chemicals, or toxins. A definite history of exposure to agents that may induce aplastic anemia has been reported in as many as 50% of pediatric and adult aplastic patients in large series.* However, the duration, intensity, and biologic significance of such exposures are generally difficult to establish. Aplastic anemia secondary to an identifiable agent or condition other than drug or chemical exposure occurs infrequently. In all, such cases constitute only 10% of 15% of the total population affected with this disorder.

In the following section we will discuss the more common causes of acquired aplastic anemia and review current evidence bearing on pathogenic mechanisms.

Chemical or drug-induced aplastic anemia. Certain drugs, such as the alkylating agents (e.g., cyclophosphamide) regularly produce bone marrow depression of a dose-related severity as an expected consequence of their pharmacologic action. The aplastic anemia induced by these agents as a complication of antineoplastic therapy may be profound but is usually transitory. With adequate supportive care the patient may be maintained until hematologic function recovers.

Many of the agents that have been associated with aplasia also produce other blood dyscrasias. Sometimes these reactions are the more common adverse effects of the drug. Since the pathogeneses of these disorders are poorly understood, there is no basis for the assumption that a drug-induced aplastic anemia develops via the same mechanism as the other dyscrasias commonly associated with the agent's use. Indeed, for some agents (e.g., chloramphenicol) there is indirect evidence suggesting that the pathologic basis for aplastic anemia is quite different from that contributing to the other dyscrasias.

Most pharmacologic agents that have been implicated in the etiology of aplastic anemia do not suppress marrow function at therapeutic doses. Aplastic anemia is a rare complication of normal use and generally not related to rate of administration or cumulative dosage. Because development of aplastic anemia cannot be attributed to the normal pharmacologic action of the suspected agent in such cases and may actually develop after exposure to the agent has ceased, this complication is usually attributed to what is termed an idiosyncratic drug reaction.

The following are agents that have been implicated in the pathogenesis of aplastic anemia (also given are other blood dyscrasias described as complications of their use*):

Acetaminophen (Ag, Th)	Hair dyes
Acetazolamide (Ag, Th)	Hydantoins (Ag, MA)
Allopurinol	Indomethacin (Th)
Amodiaquin (Ag)	Lithium
Amphotericin B	Meprobamate (Ag, Th)
Organic arsenicals (Ag, Th)	Mercury
Benzene and derivatives (see text)	Methicillin (Ag)
	Methyldopa (Ag, Th)
Bismuth	Methylmercaptoimidazole (Tapazol)
Carbamazepine (Tegretol)	
Carbethoxymethylglyoxaline (carbimazole) and methimazole [Thiamizole]) (Ag)	Oxytetracycline
	Parathion
	Penicillamine (Ag)
	Pentachlorophenol
Carbon tetrachloride	Phenacimide
Chloramphenicol (see text)	Phenylbutazone and oxyphenbutazone (Ag, Th)
Chlordiazepoxide (Librium) (Ag)	Potassium perchlorate
	Propylthiouracil (Ag)
Chlorophenothane (DDT)	Pyribenzamine (and certain other antihistamines) (Ag)
Chlorpromazine (and other phenothiazines) (Ag)	
Chlorpropamide (Ag, Th)	Pyrimethamine (Th, MA)
Chlortetracycline	Quinacrine (Th)
Colchicine (MA)	Quinidine (Ag, Th)
Colloidal silver	Streptomycin (Ag, Th)
Dinitrophenol (Ag)	Sulfonamides (Ag, Th)
Ethosuximide (Zarontin) (Ag)	Thiocyanate
	Tolbutamide (Ag, Th)
Gold salts (Th)	Trimethoprim-sulfamethoxazole (Ag, Th, MA)

---

*References 144, 162, 232, 290.

*Ag, agranulocytosis; Th, thrombocytopenia; MA, megaloblastic anemia.

The list above is based on the findings of the WHO Research Centre for International Monitoring of Adverse Reactions, which from 1968 to 1973 reported 257 cases of aplastic anemia, 1,294 of granulocytopenia or agranulocytosis, 948 of thrombocytopenia, 302 of hemolytic anemia, and 112 of macrocytic anemia associated with drug or chemical exposure.[260] The frequency with which the administration of certain agents (e.g., chloramphenicol and phenylbutazone) has been associated with the onset of aplastic anemia has clearly established their etiologic significance. However, for many of the agents listed, evidence for a causal relationship remains only suggestive and anecdotal.

The most common agents in most series are chloramphenicol, phenylbutazone and oxyphenbutazone, indomethacin, and gold salts. In areas where malaria is endemic quinacrine and its analogs are common causes.

Chloramphenicol. Chloramphenicol was the suspected etiologic agent in 163 of 408 cases of aplastic anemia reported to the Registry of Adverse Drug Reactions of the American Medical Association. The risk of aplastic anemia following chloramphenicol use has been estimated to be approximately 1/30,000.[173,297] Almost all published cases have developed after oral rather than parenteral administration of the drug. The reasons for this are not clear; bacterial degradation products of the drug have been suggested as etiologic agents.[147] Oral administration should not be employed except when specifically indicated.

Yunis and Bloomberg[366] concluded that there were two types of blood dyscrasia associated with chloramphenicol. The first is a true aplastic anemia and the second is a dose-related reversible suppression that principally affects erythropoiesis and less commonly involves thrombopoiesis and granulopoiesis. The reversible type of toxicity develops when the patient is receiving chloramphenicol therapy. Scott et al.[291] observed the relationship of dosage to toxicity. In this series the incidence rose from 10% in patients given doses of 2 gm daily to 90% in patients given 6 gm daily. Reversible toxicity usually occurred when serum levels of chloramphenicol were greater than 25 μg/ml.[291] A characteristic pathologic feature of this type of depression is vacuolization of the pronormoblasts and maturation arrest of red cell precursors without marrow hypoplasia.[273] The earliest sign of reversible toxicity is a fall in the reticulocyte count[168] and a rise in the serum iron level.[277,278] Rapid recovery from marrow suppression on withdrawal of the drug is the rule.

The onset of chloramphenicol-induced aplastic anemia usually does not occur until 6 to 10 weeks after exposure. The idiosyncratic nature of aplasia following chloramphenicol was inferred in an analysis of the cases reported in the AMA Registry of Adverse Drug Reactions.[23,260] The development of aplastic anemia was found to be independent of the dose of chloramphenicol administered or the duration of exposure. Indeed, 10% of the patients received chloramphenicol for 4 days or less. It is not known if withdrawal of the drug at the first sign of hematologic toxicity would diminish the chances of developing aplasia, but in view of these data it appears unlikely.

In vitro effects of chloramphenicol that might bear on the development of marrow aplasia have been analyzed extensively and were reviewed by Pisciotta[248] in 1971. Bacterial protein synthesis is inhibited by lower concentrations of the drug than the normal therapeutic levels.[357] Chloramphenicol binds to 50S ribosomal subunits, inhibits aminoacyl tRNA binding to the ribosome, and suppresses peptidyltransferase activity, which catalyzes formation of highly polymerized homopeptides from the small tRNA-associated peptides assembled on the 50S ribosomal subunit.* It appears that chloramphenicol has little effect on the cytoplasmic ribosomes of mature mammalian cells actively engaged in protein synthesis, since messenger RNA is already attached to ribosomes. In immature or undifferentiated cells, however, protein synthesis may be markedly affected. Similarly in a cell-free system chloramphenicol blocked the increase in protein synthesis usually seen when RNA, ribosomes, and amino acids are mixed in an energy-generating system.[353,354]

In mammalian cells chloramphenicol is a potent inhibitor of protein synthesis,[193,263] by mitochondrial ribosomes with the most obvious sign being a decrease in cytochrome aa_3 and a resultant decrease in the activity of cytochrome oxidase.[229] This may result in insufficient energy-generating capacity in certain cells.

Reduced ferrochelatase activity and a block in heme synthesis have also been described in dogs receiving chloramphenicol.[156,191,192] Drug-induced suppression of respiration by leukocytes involved in phagocytosis has been described.[159] Cellular division may also be directly inhibited at high doses.[272]

Although all of these effects of chloramphenicol may be relevant to the dose-related reversible bone marrow suppression, they do not explain why occasional patients develop severe, often irreversible aplastic anemia. Addressing this question, Yunis and Harrington[367] found that in patients who had recovered from chloramphenicol-induced aplasia, as little as 50 μg/ml of the drug was enough to inhibit DNA synthesis in marrow cells; in controls greater than 250 μg/ml was required. The latter doses are higher than those attained in the normal course of therapy. However, it must

---

*References 50a, 98, 173a, 245a.

still be determined whether this observation reflects an inherent difference between patients with chloramphenicol-induced aplasia and normal persons or rather reflects damage previously sustained by the marrow that led to the aplasia originally.[248]

Thiamphenicol, an analog of chloramphenicol with the same ring structure but with substitutions of a methylsulfonyl moiety for the *p*-nitro group, has been used extensively in Europe. This drug has not been associated with any cases of aplastic anemia (Keiser, cited by Yunis et al.[365]) although it produces reversible marrow toxicity as readily as chloramphenicol.[160] Furthermore, mitochondrial protein synthesis is inhibited to the same degree by chloramphenicol as by thiamphenicol. In contrast to chloramphenicol, thiamphenicol, even in high concentrations, does not inhibit DNA synthesis in dog marrow cells.[365] These experiments further support the hypothesis that reversible marrow depression and aplastic anemia are mediated by different pathogenic mechanisms and suggest that aplasia may be the result of a selective effect of chloramphenicol on DNA synthesis in certain susceptible individuals.

The susceptibility to drug-induced abnormalities in DNA synthetic mechanisms may be genetically influenced. Thus Yunis[364] demonstrated that unusual sensitivity to chloramphenicol-induced inhibition of formate uptake into DNA characterized not only patients with chloramphenicol-induced aplastic anemia but certain of their parents as well. Indeed, Nagao and Mauer[221] have reported aplastic anemia in identical twins following chloramphenicol use. However, similar reports of a familial incidence of this disorder are rare.

In the last decade awareness of hematologic complications has led to a sharp reduction in the use of chloramphenicol and a parallel decrease in the incidence of secondary aplastic anemia. Recently, however, the emergence of strains of *Haemophilus influenzae* B resistant to ampicillin has led to increased use of chloramphenicol for the treatment of sepsis and meningitis in children. In such cases the risk of aplasia must be considered secondary and should not deter the clinician from the parenteral use of chloramphenicol when it is indicated and after appropriate cultures have been performed.

Benzene and benzene derivatives. Benzene and benzene derivatives, which are widely used as organic solvents, were the earliest substances recognized to induce aplastic anemia,[34] and they remain a significant cause today. Benzene is volatile; toxic effects may result from inhalation. Anemia, thrombocytopenia, and leukopenia, either alone or in combination, are more common than aplastic anemia after benzene exposure. The anemia is often macrocytic.[122] Hematologic derange-

ments may occur shortly after exposure or be delayed for many years.[34] Intense proliferation may be seen in the bone marrow before the onset of aplasia. More than 100 cases of acute leukemia, mainly of nonlymphocytic types, have been reported after chronic exposure to benzene.[5,6,28,99,246] In many of these patients aplasia was documented before the onset of leukemia. Leukemia may develop as late as 10 years after cessation of exposure and recovery from aplasia. Chromosome damage has been documented in exposed workers even without obvious marrow damage.[346]

Recent studies in murine models suggest that susceptibility to aryl hydrocarbon–induced pancytopenia may be strongly influenced by the activity of certain enzymatic systems under genetic control.[269]

Phenylbutazone and oxyphenbutazone. Phenylbutazone and oxyphenbutazone are probably the most common causes of aplastic anemia at present, but they are rare causes in childhood because they are used infrequently in younger patients. The risk of aplasia is estimated to be about 1/24,000.[349] Aplasia most often follows prolonged use of the drug, frequently for periods of more than a year.[128] Agranulocytosis secondary to these drugs usually occurs within 3 months and is often associated with a rash, suggesting different mechanisms for the two dyscrasias.[100]

Patients with phenylbutazone-induced aplastic anemia, but not those with the idiopathic variety, show decreased ability to oxidize the drug.[180] To our knowledge similar studies have not been performed on their family members.

Quinacrine (Atabrine). Although rare as a cause of aplastic anemia in the United States today, quinacrine (Atabrine) is a significant etiologic agent in areas where malaria is endemic. During World War II the relative risk of aplasia secondary to this drug was assessed in United States servicemen. The incidence was about 1/20,000 for those who received the drug and 1/500,000 for those who did not. Prolonged usage seemed to increase the risk. In about half the cases the onset of aplasia was preceded by a rash.[55]

Anticonvulsants. The hydantoins, phenytoin (Dilantin) and mephenytoin (Mesantoin), are a significant cause of aplastic anemia, particularly in children. Examples can be found in most large series.[290,355] These drugs may also cause megaloblastic anemia and pure red cell aplasia. Onset may be as early as 2 weeks after treatment is begun or may not be seen for as long as 30 months. There appears to be no relation to age, sex, or dosage.[268] Trimethadione (Tridione), ethosuximide (Zarontin), and carbamazepine (Tegretol), nonhydantoin anticonvulsants, have also been associated with aplastic anemia.[88,105,114]

Agents presumed not to be associated with aplastic anemia. Although several agents have been the subject of reports associating their use with the development of aplasia, their widespread use and the paucity of such reports make their etiologic role unlikely. Among these agents are acetylsalicylic acid, barbiturates, chloral hydrate, narcotics, digitalis and its analogs, ephedrine, iron, and penicillin.

Total body irradiation exposure. The radiosensitivity of hematopoietic tissues has long been recognized.[141] Dose-response relationships for radiation effects are well documented in many mammalian species and, although data for humans (most of whom were victims of accidental radiation exposure) are incomplete in terms of dose, dose rate, and uniformity of exposure, the sensitivity of the human hematologic system appears to be comparable to that of other higher mammalian species.*

After total body exposure to more than 1,200 R death ensues in 4 to 5 days from damage to the gastrointestinal mucosa. Exposure to a smaller dose mainly affects hematopoietic and lymphoid tissue. The LD_{50} at 30 days for death from aplasia has been determined in various mammalian species, including the rat (800 rads), rabbit (750 R), mouse (600 R), and monkey (550 R). In humans an LD_{50} has been established to be 450 R.[31,224] Optimal supportive care may raise these values somewhat by allowing time for residual stem cells to repopulate the marrow.

Hematopoietic precursor cells are highly radiosensitive. In contrast, mature granulocytes, red cells, and platelets are functionally intact after doses in excess of 1,000 R. Mature lymphocytes, however, are sensitive to doses as small as 25 R.[129]

At doses up to 1,200 R aplasia is clearly secondary to damage to hematopoietic cells. Indeed, replacement by transplantation of normal marrow hematopoietic elements regularly produces reconstitution of hematopoietic function following 1,000 R total body irradiation.[327] At doses of 3,000 R and above, however, the stroma or microenvironment of the marrow may be damaged so that, even with a source of stem cells supplied, marrow function is permanently impaired in the irradiated area.[165,280]

In mice protection from an otherwise lethal dose of radiation could be obtained by shielding of the spleen or an entire femur.[150] Thus only a small proportion of stem cells need survive the radiation insult to repopulate all other bone marrow sites.

Infectious hepatitis. Aplastic anemia following viral hepatitis was first described in 1955.[188] Posthepatitic aplasia carries a poor prognosis. An overall mortality rate of 85.1% was noted in a literature review of 174 cases.[127] The mean age of onset is 19.9 years; approximately 60% of the patients are male.[43,127] Hepatitis B antigen has not been found in cases reported to date. The hepatitis is not usually severe, and at the time of diagnosis of pancytopenia, liver function studies or biopsies reveal subacute or resolving disease. The mean interval to the time of diagnosis of pancytopenia is about 9 weeks from the onset of hepatitis. In a series of 80 patients reported by Camitta et al.[43] median survival was only 11 weeks. Of the nine patients who survived without marrow transplantation, six showed evidence of improvement in less than 2 months.

The pathogenesis of aplasia following infectious hepatitis is unknown. Several hypotheses have been proposed. The hepatitis virus might be pantropic and infect and destroy hematopoietic stem cells. The result of this insult to the marrow would not be expressed until convalescence, when reductions in the viable pool of hematopoietic precursors would lead to an overall severe depression of hematologic function. It has also been proposed that during acute hepatitis the liver fails to clear compounds that are potentially harmful to the bone marrow.[61] This hypothesis seems unlikely since aplasia is uncommon following hepatocellular dysfunction of other etiologies. Virally induced autoimmune phenomena have been considered as a possible pathogenic mechanism for the development of aplasia.[76,77] Indeed, Burke et al.[42] found serum inhibitors of myeloid differentiation in some patients with posthepatitic aplasia but not in the sera of patients with idiopathic or drug-induced aplasia. Another possible mechanism is suggested from the studies of Festenstein et al.,[94,111] who have found that mouse cells infected with other viruses express new histocompatibility antigens that could provide a target for cell-mediated autoimmune reactions. An autoimmune mechanism is consistent with recent reports of recovery of autologous marrow function after treatment with immunosuppressive agents such as antithymocyte globulin[307] or cyclophosphamide.[239,292]

Other virus infections. At this date five cases of aplastic anemia have developed following infectious mononucleosis.[152,344,361] In addition, a group of dengue-like viruses that produce marrow depression during acute infection have been described in Thailand. Involvement is most pronounced in the granulocytic and megakaryocytic series, although erythroid precursors are also affected.[24,227]

Pregnancy. Thirty-two well-documented cases of aplastic anemia during pregnancy were reviewed by Knispel et al.[164] Eight patients had complete recovery after delivery. Three again

*References 3, 31, 214, 253, 348.

developed aplasia during subsequent pregnancies.

Paroxysmal nocturnal hemoglobinuria. Aplastic anemia is a well-documented complication of paroxysmal nocturnal hemoglobinuria.[56,57,178] It is fully discussed in Chapter 11.

Other causes. True aplastic anemia has not been reported as a complication of systemic lupus erythematosis. The myelosuppression that does occur in this disorder may represent an instance of immune assault, either on the precursor cells or on the microcirculatory system supporting their growth.[40,70]

Glue sniffing[256] and the use of synthetic hair dyes[18,130] have been associated with aplastic anemia. Overwhelming mycobacterial infection has been associated with aplasia.[83] Although marrow depression is common in such infections, aplasia is rare. The relative significance of the infection or its therapy in the pathogenesis of aplasia is unclear.

Pathophysiology and pathogenesis

Two hypotheses have been cited to explain the pathogenesis of drug- or chemical-induced aplastic anemia. The first proposes that the offending agent or a metabolite thereof exerts a direct toxic effect on hematopoietic precursors or their supporting milieu. The second suggests that the agent or its metabolite binds to the precursor cell and acts as a hapten, thereby engendering a humoral or cell-mediated immune reaction directed against hematopoietic progenitor cells.

For many agents (e.g., radiation, alkylating agents, and metabolic inhibitors) a direct toxic effect on marrow elements is the established mode of action. Other agents that produce aplastic anemia only rarely are presumed to produce marrow suppression only under selected host environmental conditions or in individuals of a restricted genetic type.[193,269,345]

The cellular targets of such toxic or immunologic reactions are, with few exceptions (e.g., the cell types affected by irradiation or alkylating agents), merely the subject of speculation. Radiation-, infection-, or chemical-induced functional defects hypothesized[29] to explain the development of aplastic anemia include the following:

A. Pluripotent stem cells
1. Reduced number of stem cells
2. Defective stem cells
B. Environment of pluripotent stem cells
1. Structural defect in the supporting microenvironment
2. Abnormality of chemical regulators of cell growth
3. Cellular or humoral inhibitors of marrow growth

Pluripotent stem cells. A reduction of the number of stem cells capable of generating normal numbers of circulating red cells, granulocytes, and platelets is the principal mechanism suggested in the pathogenesis of aplastic anemia. Although the marrow appears to have considerable reserve, as evidenced by recovery from repeated courses of antineoplastic therapy, in vitro and in vivo evidence now exists to suggest that all normal diploid cells have a capacity for only a finite number of divisions.[138,139] Indeed, treatment with large doses of alkylating agents such as busulfan or phenylalanine mustard permanently reduces the proliferative ability of mouse stem cells.[32,142] Restrictions in the regenerating potential of hematopoietic precursors are also indicated by the limited number of passages possible for marrow from a single donor transplanted serially into syngeneic lethally irradiated hosts.[202,362] Thus a severe insult to the marrow could severely limit the growth and differentiation of hematopoietic stem cells, leading to the development of aplasia in some patients. However, for those patients who recover spontaneously or after treatment with immunosuppressive drugs, another mechanism must be involved.

Defective stem cells. It has been proposed that stem cells divide asynchronously, with each cell giving rise to one daughter cell committed to differentiation and one daughter cell replenishing the stem cell pool. If replication and differentiation become unbalanced, a normal pool of stem cells might be maintained but production of mature hematologic elements might be grossly deficient.[29] How such an imbalance might occur is unknown.

Microenvironmental defects. For some years a defective microenvironment has been postulated as a possible cause of aplastic anemia.[166] Indeed, in rats it has been demonstrated that radiation doses of 4,000 rads to the femur may induce defects in the femoral marrow stroma that markedly reduce its capacity to support hematopoiesis.[165] Similar studies in patients receiving radiation to the sternum during treatment for Hodgkin's disease have also documented sustained local suppression of marrow function, apparently as a result of stromal injury.[280] Studies in murine systems suggest that high doses of alkylating agents such as cyclophosphamide and bulsulfan may suppress marrow stromal function.[102] The effects of other drugs known to cause aplastic anemia on the hematopoietic stroma are not known. Genetically defined abnormalities of the hematopoietic environment causing marrow hypofunction have also been described in murine model systems (e.g., congenital anemia of Sl/Sl^d mice).[198] However, no such condition has been described in humans.

The high frequency of reconstitution of marrow cellularity and function following marrow transplantation, particularly in patients receiving twin (isogeneic) grafts and in untransfused recipients of allogeneic marrow,[317,333] would suggest preservation of stromal function in most patients with aplastic anemia.

Deficiencies of humoral regulators. The humoral factors promoting hematopoiesis are multiple and poorly characterized. The circulating levels of erythropoietin, which stimulates proliferation and differentiation of erythroid precursors, are usually high in aplastic anemia. Concentrations of colony stimulating factor, which stimulates proliferation of myeloid precursors, are also normal or high.[242] Monocyte production of this factor is usually normal or increased.[65] To date no information is available regarding factors promoting differentiation of myeloid lines or proliferation and differentiation of megakaryocyte precursors.

Cellular inhibitors of hematopoiesis. A T lymphocyte suppressor of granulocyte colony formation (CFU-C) has been described in the marrow of certain patients with aplastic anemia;[157] when removed by treatment with antithymocyte globulin (ATG), myeloid precursors proliferate normally in vitro.[13,126,157] Lymphocyte suppressors of in vitro erythroid colony formation (CFU-E) have also been described in these patients.[146] The biologic significance of these observations has been questioned in a recent report[298] correlating the presence of such suppressors with transfusion history rather than underlying disease. However, methods used in this report differ markedly from those used in initial reports. Further studies will hopefully clarify the basis of these in vitro phenomena.

Several clinical reports add support to the hypothesis that cellular inhibitors of hematopoiesis may induce aplastic anemia. Transplants of isogeneic (identical twin) marrow have in certain cases failed to induce hematologic reconstitution.[93,108,276] Subsequent transplants following cyclophosphamide, however, have proved successful. A number of patients treated with antilymphocyte globulin or high-dose cyclophosphamide followed by a marrow transplant subsequently recovered their own marrow function.* Similarly we have recently reported autologous marrow recovery in a patient following high dose cyclophosphamide and transplants of fetal liver.[239]

Recovery following immunosuppressive therapy alone has also been described. Baran et al.[19] reported autologous marrow recovery in a patient treated with four daily doses of cyclophosphamide (30 mg/kg). Autologous recovery has also been described in a patient treated with ATG and

procarbazine.[154] Recently Speck et al.[307] have reported significant and sustained improvement in hematopoietic function in 60% of aplastic anemia patients prospectively analyzed following treatment with antithymocyte globulin and androgens with or without a subsequent transplant of hemiallogeneic marrow. Additional clinical trials are in progress to confirm these observations.

Humoral inhibitors of hematopoiesis. A number of endogenously produced mediators may inhibit marrow proliferation and differentiation. Prostaglandins produced by macrophages suppress generation of myeloid precursors and act as antagonists or regulators of the action of colony stimulating factor.[169] Both fibroblast- and immune lymphocyte–derived interferons may inhibit proliferation of hematopoietic precursors.[124,230,231] Endogenous chalones may also inhibit myeloid precursor proliferation.[186,245,281] An inhibitor of CFU-C proliferation derived from normal granulocytes has recently been described.[36] These and other peptides all participate in the regulation of hematopoiesis. Aberrations of such mechanisms might lead to aplasia. Autoimmune antibodies might also contribute. Ragab et al.[257] failed to detect serum inhibitors of in vitro granulopoiesis in eight children with aplastic anemia. However, in a larger series Burke et al.[40] found that the serum of patients with posthepatitic aplasia was either nonstimulatory or inhibitory to in vitro myeloid colony formation. In contrast, sera from patients with idiopathic aplastic anemia stimulated development of CFU-C. The significance of such findings is difficult to assess at this time. Since the in vitro targets employed for assessing inhibitor activity have been allogeneic marrow cells, alloantibodies stimulated by prior transfusion rather than autoreactive antibodies may be responsible for the inhibitory activity.

Clinical features

The clinical features of aplastic anemia are a direct result of the depressed hematopoietic function. Petechiae, ecchymoses, purpura, and epistaxes are the most common presenting manifestations. Anemia marked by pallor, fatigue, and dyspnea is the next most common sign of the disease. Patients may present with systemic or local infection accompanied by fever or mouth sores. A few patients are diagnosed as a result of routine blood counts. Most patients are diagnosed soon after the onset of symptoms.[181,355] Hepatomegaly or splenomegaly is absent in the great majority of the patients. Mild splenomegaly may develop after multiple transfusions. Adenopathy, if it occurs, is not related to the disease. The presence of these signs and marked hypocellularity of the marrow suggests the presence of a myeloprolifera-

---

*References 153, 292, 306, 326, 334.

tive disorder such as leukemia or non-Hodgkin's lymphoma.

Laboratory findings

Anemia is usually profound at the time of diagnosis, with the hemoglobin level ranging from 3 to 7 gm/dl. Red cells are most frequently normocytic. Macrocytosis may be seen in up to 40% of the cases, sometimes to an extreme degree.[355] At times only a portion of the cells are macrocytic. The reticulocyte count is usually less than 2% and even lower if corrected for the hemoglobin level. In many severe cases reticulocytes are completely absent. Leukopenia ($<4.3 \times 10^9$/liter) is observed in over 75% of cases, but is not necessarily present. Neutropenia ($<1.8 \times 10^9$/liter) is a constant finding in the course of this disorder and is detected at the time of clinical presentation in 90% of cases.[355] Thrombocytopenia is also a constant feature. More than 90% of patients have platelet counts less than 100×10^9/liter at presentation. Severe thrombocytopenia ($<20 \times 10^9$/liter) has been described in more than half of the patients at the time of initial diagnosis.[355] Some patients may present abnormalities of only one or two elements, but all usually become abnormal within a period of several months. There is often a direct relationship between blood neutrophil count and marrow myeloid cell content.[103]

Serum iron is increased and iron-binding capacity is usually saturated. Ferrokinetic studies usually show a delayed clearance of radiolabeled iron (^{59}Fe) from plasma and invariably show a decreased incorporation of iron into red cells.[116,117,223] Oral iron absorption is decreased; the amount of iron absorbed is not correlated with the degree of anemia.[287]

Iron isotopes, particularly ^{52}Fe, and indium (^{111}In), which are in the same family of elements, are biologically transported and utilized interchangeably with iron. They have been used to localize and monitor the sites of active iron incorporation in the marrow by scanning scintigraphy.[199] This method allows localization of active marrow and is a presumed indicator of marrow erythropoietic activity. In aplastic anemia indium chloride (^{111}InCl) scans usually reveal markedly decreased uptake in marrow sites. The degree of reduction in uptake varies directly with the severity of disease as monitored by morphologic indicators of decreased erythroid activity (e.g., reticulocyte count and marrow morphology) and long-term survival.[199]

Red cell survival usually is found to be normal early in the course of the disease[133,176,264] but may be significantly decreased in patients who have received multiple transfusions.[174]

Fetal hemoglobin is increased in some patients; the level is occasionally as high as 15%.[26,295] Red cell 2,3-DPG levels are decreased, suggesting a

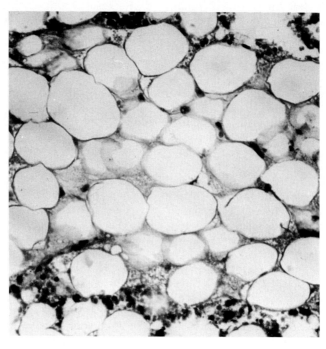

Fig. 17-1. Bone marrow biopsy from a 3½-year-old girl with idiopathic aplastic anemia, showing markedly hypocellular marrow with increased fat.

predominance of mature red cells and a proportional decrease in the fraction of newly generated red cells.[234] The red cells also exhibit enhanced susceptibility to lysis by antibody and complement, although not of the order characteristic for paroxysmal nocturnal hemoglobinuria.[179] This is a property of red cells late in their life span.

Expression of the I antigen on the surface of red cells is increased in aplastic anemia, leading to an increased susceptibility to cold-antibody lysis in the presence of anti-I and complement.[179] However, this cell surface characteristic is also seen in megaloblastic anemia, myelosclerosis, and leukemia. In paroxysmal nocturnal hemoglobinuria I antigen expression is normal but sensitivity to lysis by complement is markedly increased.

Neutrophils, although reduced in numbers, generally exhibit normal phagocytic and bactericidal activity. Responses to chemotactic stimuli may be reduced.[242a] Leukocyte alkaline phosphatase is usually high.[177]

Monocytopenia is usually present and is proportional to the degree of neutropenia.[338] Bactericidal and phagocytic functions of monocytes are normal. However, monocyte responses to lymphocyte-derived chemotactic factors are markedly reduced.[242a]

Lymphocyte counts and proportions of T and B lymphocytes in the circulation are generally normal. However, lymphopenia ($<1.0 \times 10^9$/liter) may also contribute to the profound leukopenia observed. Lymphocyte functions are normal as

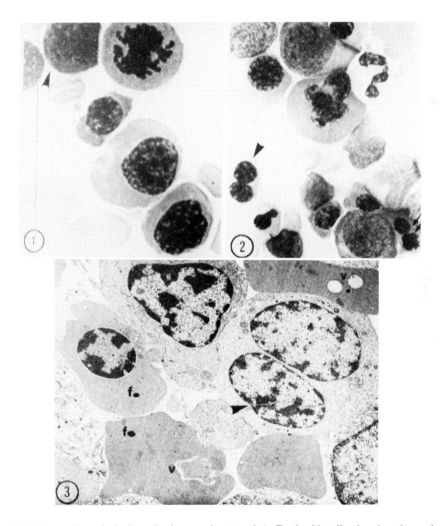

Fig. 17-2. Dyserythropoiesis in aplastic anemia. **1** and **2**, Erythroid cells showing dyserythropoietic features including megaloblasts, binucleate cells (arrows), chromatin bridge (double arrows), and irregular and mulberry-shaped nuclei. **3**, Low-power electron microscope field with binucleate erythroblast with nuclear cleft (arrow): accumulation of ferritin (*f*) and vesicles (*v*) in reticulocytes. ($<$6,000.) (From Frisch, B., Lewis, S. M., and Sherman, D.: Br. J. Haematol. **29:** 545, 1975.)

assayed by lymphocyte transformation and lymphokine generation in response to mitogens, antigens and allogeneic cells, skin tests for delayed-type hypersensitivity, and quantitative assays of immunoglobulins and antibodies.[80] Interestingly, although lymphocytes from aplastic anemia patients respond normally to allogeneic cells, they in turn frequently exhibit a reduced ability to stimulate allogeneic responder cells in mixed lymphocyte culture.[204] Twomey et al.[338] suggested that the monocytopenia observed might explain this phenomenon. However, monocytopenia has not been found to correlate with reduced stimulatory properties in large patient series.[206]

The marrow is hypoplastic, usually with marked reductions in all hematopoietic precursors (Fig. 17-1). In severe cases lymphocytes and plasma cells are the predominant nucleated cells.[103,181,190] Biopsy usually reveals markedly reduced cellularity with fatty infiltration of the marrow cavity. Aspirates and biopsies from multiple sites should be performed to establish the diagnosis and to rule out leukemia. Focal areas of normocellular, often megaloblastic marrow ("hot spots") may be observed, particularly early in the course of the disease.[158] These areas may suggest other etiologies for observed pancytopenia. Multiple biopsies, however, usually allow the correct diagnosis. Electron microscopic studies of marrow from patients with aplastic anemia have revealed many abnormalities in the erythroid series, including intercellular bridges, internuclear chromatin bridges, nuclear clefts, and nuclear inclusions[104] (Fig. 17-2).

In vitro assays of hematopoietic activity may further substantiate the diagnosis. Thus, although erythropoietin levels in plasma and urine are elevated,[9,168] the marrow contains markedly reduced numbers of hematopoietic progenitor cells capable of forming erythroid colonies in soft agar (CFU-E)[146] or of incorporating ^{59}Fe in suspension culture.[44] Production of colony stimulating factor by monocytes is normal or elevated.[65] However, the marrow concentration of precursors capable of forming myeloid colonies and clusters in soft agar (CFU-C) is profoundly reduced.* Normal or increased cluster formation with markedly depressed myeloid colony formation should suggest the diagnosis of myeloid leukemia rather than aplastic anemia.[211,212] In some patients cytogenetic studies have revealed an increased number of chromosome breaks,[134] but not as dramatically or as consistently as in patients with Fanconi's anemia.

Serum folate and B_{12} levels are usually normal

---

*References 65, 125, 126, 170, 257.

even in patients with focal megaloblastic changes. Coombs tests are negative. The acid hemolysis test is negative in acquired and constitutional forms of aplastic anemia but is positive in patients with aplasia secondary to paroxysmal nocturnal hemoglobinuria.

Differential diagnosis

Initial diagnosis may be difficult especially if only one or two blood elements are affected. Moreover, foci of residual hematopoietic activity may exist,[158] so that a single marrow aspiration is misleading. In all patients marrow biopsy should be performed in addition to aspiration to better gauge overall cellularity. Some reports emphasize the discrepancy between the findings on marrow aspirate and biopsy.[175] If initial biopsies and aspirates are cellular, several more at different sites should be performed.[175] If these are still cellular and remain so over a period of time, strong consideration should be given to another diagnosis, particularly leukemia or lymphoma. This is especially true if granulocyte counts are normal and sideroblastic changes are present.[262]

The diseases that must be considered in any child with pancytopenia are summarized below:

A. Leukemia with aleukemic blood picture
B. Aplastic anemia
C. Infiltration of the marrow
　　1. Malignant tumors
　　　　a. Non-Hodgkin's lymphoma
　　　　b. Neuroblastoma
　　　　c. Embryonal rhabdomyosarcoma
　　　　d. Metastatic carcinoma (rare in children)
　　2. Osteopetrosis (marble bone disease)
　　3. Myelofibrosis
D. Hypersplenic syndromes
　　1. Banti's disease
　　2. Lymphomas
　　3. Gaucher's disease
　　4. Niemann-Pick disease
　　5. Letterer-Siwe disease
　　6. Splenic panhematopenia
　　7. Disseminated lupus erythematosus
E. Paroxysmal nocturnal hemoglobinuria
F. Miscellaneous
　　1. Megaloblastic anemias
　　2. Overwhelming infections (e.g., tuberculosis)

Thrombocytopenia or chronic anemia may constitute the dominant feature of aplastic anemia early in the course. The diagnosis of idiopathic thrombocytopenic purpura, which may be considered early in the course of the disease, is associated with more than moderate anemia only as a result of blood loss. In the absence of overt hemorrhage anemia must therefore be explained on another basis.

Acute lymphoblastic leukemia in the leukopenic stage may simulate aplastic anemia, but microscopic study of aspirated marrow usually reveals the precise nature of the illness. With an acellular marrow, the use of concentrated and volumetric bone marrow aspiration facilitates the differentiation between the two diseases. Culture of marrow in soft agar may reveal increased clusters of less than forty cells in early myeloid forms of leukemia, whereas markedly diminished colony and cluster formation is characteristic of aplastic anemia.[211,212] Although occasional patients with well-documented, longstanding aplastic anemia develop acute leukemia,[182,210] this appears to be a rare event, even in long-term survivors.[175]

Splenomegaly and lymphadenopathy are frequent findings in patients with acute leukemia but are rarely detected in patients with aplastic anemia. Splenomegaly may develop in the hypertransfused patient. In patients with splenic panhematopenia and secondary hypersplenism the spleen is predominantly implicated in the pathogenesis of pancytopenia, and the bone marrow contains its full quota of each of the cellular elements. Myelofibrosis and neoplastic infiltration are also to be considered in the differential diagnosis. The acid hemolysis test should be performed serially, as it may be normal in the early stages of paroxysmal nocturnal hemoglobinuria.[178] The leukocyte alkaline phosphatase activity which is low in paroxysmal nocturnal hemoglobinuria, may also help distinguish this disorder.[175]

Treatment

Removal of causative agent. In any patient presenting with acquired aplastic anemia or progressive anemia, leukopenia, or thrombocytopenia, a careful history must be taken to determine exposure to potentially causative drugs, infections, or toxins. Such potentially noxious exposures should be immediately terminated. Elimination of exposure to agents directly toxic to the marrow may lead to hematopoietic recovery, in which case reexposure should be stringently avoided. Idiosyncratic reactions producing aplastic anemia are usually not dose related, and the resultant marrow injury may be appreciated long after exposure. Although elimination of exposure to such agents is appropriate, it is rarely beneficial.

Therapeutic approaches. Over the last 15 years four major approaches to the treatment of aplastic anemia have evolved. These include (1) supportive care, to include transfusions of red cells, platelets, and granulocytes, as needed for effective hematologic function and intensive antibiosis of intercurrent infections, (2) androgen and glucocorticosteroid therapy, (3) immunosuppressive therapy, and (4) marrow transplantation. Obviously the first approach, intensive supportive care, is also applied in each of the other treatment modes.

The choice of therapeutic approach should be made as early in the clinical course as possible, since the effectiveness of certain treatment modes, particularly marrow transplantation, may be dramatically reduced if certain guidelines are not observed in initial management. The selection process is currently determined by a careful assessment of the following: (1) disease etiology, (2) severity of disease and likely prognosis with or without therapy, and (3) availability of a histocompatible donor for marrow transplantation.

The prognosis for any one patient with aplastic anemia is difficult to assess because of the variability of the clinical course. Multiple factors have been examined for their prognostic significance. Those that have not proved useful include: idiopathic versus chemically induced aplasia,[173] age or sex of the patient (at least for individuals under 40 years of age),[144,173,181] and the presence or absence of "hot spots," i.e., foci of normal marrow cellularity.[173,187]

Elevated levels of fetal hemoglobin (>400 mg/dl) were initially thought to portend a good prognosis,[26] but this has not been confirmed in large series.[181] Factors that have been associated with a bad prognosis include profound neutropenia,[68,175] a high percentage of lymphocytes in the initial marrow aspirate,[103,144,181] and an absolute reticulocyte count of less than 10×10^9/liter.[185,190] Lynch et al.[190] examined clinical and laboratory data from ninety-nine cases of aplastic anemia. In this group the survival curve was clearly biphasic (Fig. 17-3). Forty-four percent of patients died within 4 months of diagnosis. Of the long-term survivors more than half died in the following 5 years. The remaining patients either recovered or maintained residual marrow stores sufficient for effective hematologic function with minimal transfusion support. The group of patients who died early in the course were generally characterized by short intervals between symptom onset and diagnosis, a high frequency of hemorrhage as a presenting symptom, profound neutropenia ($<0.6 \times 10^9$/liter) and thrombocytopenia ($<20 \times 10^9$/liter), a corrected reticulocyte count of less than 1%, and a profoundly hypoplastic marrow, with lymphocytes constituting more than 65% of the cellular elements.

Of patients presenting with the characteristics of severe disease, 71% died within 4 months of diagnosis, whereas 92% of patients presenting a less severe hematologic picture survived more than 4 months. Survival at 5 years was only 20% for the entire series and 30% in the group presenting with a less severe hematologic picture.

Aplastic anemia after hepatitis has a particularly grave prognosis, irrespective of initial presentation. Long-term survival is seen in only 15% of

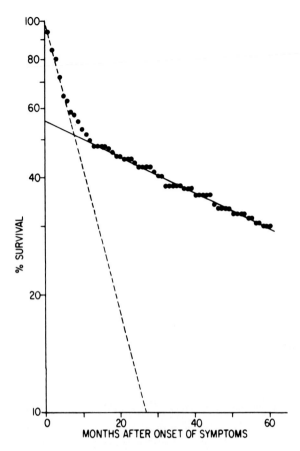

Fig. 17-3. Survival curve for aplastic anemia. (From Lynch, R. E., et al.: Blood **45:**517, 1975. Used by permission.)

cases. For patients with essentially acellular marrow biopsies 12-month survival is negligible.[43,127]

The prognostic features presented above may serve as a useful guide to the choice of a therapeutic approach. Thus for patients with a more favorable initial presentation a more conservative approach is warranted. For patients with severe disease therapeutic courses with a greater initial risk such as marrow transplantation or the use of immunosuppressive agents are indicated.

Because marrow transplantation is currently the treatment of choice for patients with severe aplastic anemia,[45,46,318] histocompatibility testing of the patient and his or her siblings and parents should be performed as soon as the diagnosis is established. Establishment of genetic evidence of engraftment is important in evaluating any transplant. Therefore samples for a complete red cell genetic phenotype should be drawn prior to initiation of transfusions, which render such analysis impossible.

Supportive care. Judicious use of transfusions is fundamental to the support of patients with aplastic anemia. Infusions of red cells, platelets, and granulocytes must be utilized when clinically indicated but must be planned carefully so that immediate benefits may be achieved with minimal detriment to future therapy.

Immunization to the surface alloantigens of blood cells is the major limitation to effective transfusion therapy, particularly for platelet and granulocyte replacement. Alloimmunization is especially important to the prognosis of a marrow transplant in those individuals who have a histocompatible sibling donor. Thus engraftment of marrow has been consistently achieved in aplastic patients who have not received transfusions prior to transplantation.[317] In contrast, 30% of aplastic patients with a history of prior transfusions prepared for transplantation with cyclophosphamide have rejected their marrow graft.[314,318] Transfusion of patients with blood products from parents or siblings generally precludes engraftment.[310]

Certain guidelines may serve to enhance the effectiveness of transfusion therapy in patients with aplastic anemia:

1. If a histocompatible family donor is available for marrow transplantation, transfusion from family members must be scrupulously avoided.
2. Transfusions of frozen or buffy-coat poor red cells for anemia *may* reduce the incidence of sensitization to leukocyte and platelet antigens.
3. Sensitization to platelet and leukocyte alloantigens may be restricted through the repeated use of a single donor or restricted group of donors for a given patient. The increasing use of cell separator systems for leukapheresis or platelet separations has provided this needed potential for obtaining large doses of platelets or granulocytes from individual donors.
4. Patients refractory to unrelated single- or random-donor platelets or granulocytes may be benefited by transfusions from HLA-matched unrelated donors.[7,209] Transfusions from HLA-matched unrelated donors are thought not to interfere with engraftment of marrow from HLA-identical siblings, since graft rejection in such cases is presumed to be caused by sensitization to alloantigens coded by genes not linked to the major histocompatibility region. Many large centers are developing computerized HLA-typed normal donor pools for this purpose. If donor nonavailability precludes consideration of marrow transplantation, family donors may be used for refractory individuals.

Red cell transfusions should be given as needed to maintain a hemoglobin concentration of 7 to

9 gm/dl, thereby circumventing symptoms of tissue hypoxia and congestive heart failure and ensuring relatively normal activity.

Infusions of platelet-rich plasma and platelet concentrates are indicated for active hemorrhage. If a patient is bleeding heavily, some replacement of coagulation factors may be needed in addition to red cell and platelet infusions. Administration of one unit of fresh frozen plasma for every three to four units of red cells will usually correct abnormal coagulation values.

It has been demonstrated that the risk of spontaneous hemorrage is high when platelet counts fall below 20×10^9/liter.[101] The use of prophylactic platelet transfusions to maintain platelet counts in excess of this number is controversial. The real risk of gastrointestinal or intracranial hemorrhage is usually outweighed by the immunologic restrictions on continued effectiveness of platelet transfusion therapy incurred by repeated platelet transfusions. In certain circumstances (e.g., infection or surgical procedure) in which acute reductions in the platelet counts may be anticipated, prophylactic administration of platelet concentrates is warranted.

In the thrombocytopenic patient certain measures should be incorporated into normal activities to reduce the risk of hemorrhage. Contact sports and other activities predisposing to trauma should be restricted. High-fiber diets, fecal softeners, and laxatives may be used to avoid constipation. Menstrual bleeding is usually not problematic except in the severely thrombocytopenic patient; in such cases hormonal suppression of the menses is indicated. The use of water picks or cotton swabs for oral hygiene may reduce the risk of gingival bleeding.

Patients with aplastic anemia have normal lymphoid function[80] and usually tolerate common viral infections well. Quantitative and functional abnormalities of the neutrophils and monocytes render the patient highly susceptible to disseminated bacterial and fungal infections.[359] The use of high-dose parenteral broad-spectrum antibiotics is thus indicated in any case of suspected sepsis and may be initiated as soon as appropriate diagnostic cultures have been obtained. However, for many of these agents, particularly the enteric pathogens and fungi, the neutrophil and the monocyte are the essential arbiters of host resistance,[50,363] providing the phagocytic and bactericidal activity needed to localize the infection and clear the invading pathogens. Without these cells such infections are often impossible to control, even with the use of intensive parenteral therapy with broad spectrum antibiotics (e.g., gentamicin and cephalothin [Keflin]) and/or antifungals (e.g., amphotericin and miconazole) to which

the agent or agents are sensitive. In randomized trials conducted in leukopenic leukemic patients, infusions of granulocytes have been shown to be an effective adjunct to antibiosis in the treatment of such infections.[7,123,143] In one study infusions of 0.2 to 0.8×10^{10} granulocytes/m^2 obtained by continuous flow centrifugation resulted in small increments of 0 to 100 granulocytes/μl of peripheral blood but a significant decrease in infection-associated mortality, particularly in individuals who failed to recover marrow function during the septicemic episode.[143] In this study transfusions of granulocytes obtained by continuous flow centrifugation were found to produce greater increments in peripheral counts than those obtained by filtration. Nevertheless, in a second study granulocytes obtained by filtration exclusively were found to be effective in reducing infection-associated mortality. Transfusions produced small rises in peripheral counts but significantly increased the cellularity of tissue inflammatory responses (as detected by Rebuck window).[7] Thus granulocyte transfusions are indicated in the treatment of sepsis in the profoundly leukopenic aplastic patient. Prophylactic granulocyte infusions might reduce the incidence of such infections but would be expected to shorten the time interval before the patient is refractory to transfusion support. At this time a functional advantage for the use of unrelated HLA-matched granulocytes has not been established, although data derived from studies of platelet function suggest this to be the case.

Androgens. Observations that androgenic hormones increased erythropoiesis to normal or polycythemic levels in patients with advanced breast cancer[2,161] and that these hormones are a specific stimulus to erythroid activity led to their use in aplastic anemia. Shahidi and Diamond[293,294] were the first to report improvement in hematopoiesis in patients with aplastic anemia following treatment with testosterone and related androgens. Subsequent early reports of improvement in small series of patients supported the utility of androgens in the therapy of aplastic anemia. The following are the agents that have been suggested to be useful and the dosages used:

1. Fluoxymesterone (Halotestin, Ultandren) oral (five times as potent as methyltestosterone)
2. Methyltestosterone, sublingual (i.e., Metandren), or testosterone propionate, sublingual (i.e., Oreton); dosage for either is 1 to 2 mg/kg, usually 30 to 50 mg daily in divided doses
3. Testosterone enanthate in oil, intramuscularly, 4 mg/kg once weekly[292a]
4. Testosterone cyclopentylpropionate (Depotestosterone), intramuscularly; dosage is under trial
5. Methandrostenolone (Dianabol), oral, 0.25 to 0.5 mg/kg

6. Oxymetholone (Dihydrotestosterone), oral, 2.0 to 6.5 mg/kg
7. Nandrolone decanoate, 1 to 1.5 mg/kg/week intramuscularly for no less than 4 months[58]

Corticosteroids such as prednisone in low doses have been combined with androgens to counteract the bone-maturing effects of the androgens. Corticosteroids have also been used as adjunctive therapy in older children and adults, ostensibly to increase capillary resistance, although no good evidence supports this contention.

The accumulation of reports of hematologic remissions associated with prolonged androgen administration led to widespread acceptance of this therapeutic modality. Unfortunately these studies* failed to discriminate between patients with severe and mild presentations of aplastic anemia, did not include control groups in therapeutic trials of any androgen preparation, and also failed to consider the contribution of recent improvements in supportive care to long-term survival. In 1969 Heyn et al.[144] reported a 51% long-term survival in aplastic patients treated with supportive care alone. However, the severity of disease presentation was not considered in the evaluation of results for comparisons with other studies. Nevertheless, subsequent analyses of large patient series by Li et al.[181] Davis and Rubin,[59] and others[35,46,213] failed to demonstrate a significant improvement in long-term survival associated with androgen therapy. Recognition that patients with aplastic anemia fell into at least two subgroups (severe and moderate forms of aplastic anemia) on the basis of survival[190] and that such patients could generally be differentiated at the time of diagnosis on the basis of disease presentation and morphologic and functional characteristics of marrow and peripheral blood (see above) provided a means for constructing meaningful prospective controlled randomized therapeutic trials. Recently Camitta et al.[46] reported such a trial comparing androgen therapy and supportive care with supportive care alone in patients with severe aplastic anemia; their results indicated that androgens were ineffective. Thus 28% of patients treated with oral oxymetholone (3 to 5mg/kg/day), 21% of those treated with parenteral nandrolone (3 to 5 mg/kg/week), and 26% of those treated with supportive care alone were alive at 30 months. Furthermore, no differences in the incidence of hematologic improvements or remission were recorded. It is possible that androgens will prove beneficial in patients with the moderate form of aplastic anemia and may be particularly useful in the constitutional forms of aplastic anemia, e.g., Fanconi's anemia. Unfortunately to date no controlled prospective trials have been reported to resolve this important issue.

In patients receiving androgens who do show hematologic improvement it is usually noted within 6 to 8 weeks of diagnosis and initiation of therapy, although periods of therapy of at least 3 months have been suggested to be necessary to detect many responses. The first evidence of recovery is a rise in the reticulocyte count. There is often an unexpected delay between reticulocytosis and a rise in hemoglobin. A shortened red cell survival has been demonstrated during this period. Anisocytosis is often present. An increase in neutrophil counts occurs later and is often not as dramatic as the rise in hemoglobin. The platelet response is highly variable. Once the hemoglobin rises to normal, androgen therapy can be discontinued. The hemoglobin level may drop during this period to 8 to 9 gm/dl but in most patients will spontaneously rise again. An occasional patient develops an absolute androgen dependence and must be maintained on these agents indefinitely. Some degree of virilization such as flushing of the skin, acne, deepening of the voice, and growth of pubic hair is expected. With the exception of the growth of pubic hair, these changes are reversible when the drug is discontinued.

Abnormal liver function, usually of a cholestatic nature, may be seen as a complication of androgen therapy.[69] Most often this is mild and consists of a slight hyperbilirubinemia. The most serious side effect, which has been reported in at least nine children, is the development of hepatocellular carcinoma.[200] The hepatotoxic action is more severe in the group of androgens containing a 17-α-methyl substitution, e.g., methyltestosterone, methandrostenolone, oxymetholone, and oxandrolone. If signs of hepatotoxicity occur, the patients may be switched to a non-17-α-substituted androgen, e.g., nandrolone. A rise in liver enzymes, e.g., SGPT or 5'-nucleotidase is probably a result of serum hepatitis, not androgen toxicity, in these patients. Some authorities recommend the use of sublingual preparations to avoid high concentrations of drugs in the liver.

Marrow transplantation. Marrow infusions for the treatment of aplastic anemia were first considered in the 1940s, but these attempts proved unsuccessful.[215,241] Subsequent studies demonstrated that mice could be protected from lethal hematologic effects of irradiation by infusion and subsequent engraftment of syngeneic marrow cells.* In 1957, Thomas et al.[329] administered al-

---

*References 10, 58, 62, 68, 162, 243, 283, 284, 293, 294, 300.

*References 97, 150, 151, 187.

logeneic marrow infusions to patients receiving radiation and chemotherapy and obtained transient engraftment of donor marrow cells. Subsequently Mathe et al.[194,196] administered allogeneic marrow grafts to six patients accidentally exposed to total body irradiation. Only transient engraftment was achieved, but some of these patients survived with autologous marrow recovery.

By 1967 at least five patients had been reported who had recovered from aplastic anemia following transplants of identical twin (syngeneic) marrow.[93,247] Successful hematologic reconstitution of patients receiving syngeneic marrow grafts has been regularly achieved, suggesting that defective or deficient hematopoietic stem cells, which are replaced through marrow transplantation, are the pathologic basis of most forms of aplastic anemia. Initial reports indicated that allogeneic transplants failed to engraft except in patients with severe combined immunodeficiency, in whom engraftment heralded the onset of what was later recognized as lethal graft versus host disease.[136,199,205]

Certain experimental observations proved essential to the development of marrow transplantation as a therapeutic modality. In murine systems certain genetically defined alloantigens expressed on the surface of lymphocytes and other cells were shown to be determinants of donor-host histocompatibility. One group of closely linked genes, termed the H-2 region, defined alloantigenic specificities necessarily shared by donor and host for successful organ or marrow transplantation.[81,299] Mismatching for these determinants invariably led to graft rejection by an immunocompetent host. Conversely engraftment of H-2-incompatible allogeneic marrow in an immunoincompetent host led to the development of severe, ultimately lethal graft versus host disease.[25,299] Analogous histocompatibility systems have been defined in humans (HLA), dogs (DLA), and other species.

Another major observation was that engraftment of allogeneic bone marrow in an immunocompetent host could only be achieved following intensive immunosuppressive treatment of the host. This led to the development of effective immunosuppressive regimens to prepare transplant recipients.[343] Total body irradiation,[343] cyclophosphamide,[285] procarbazine, and antithymocyte globulin[311] have been the agents most widely used.

In 1967 Epstein et al.[84] succeeded in correcting radiation-induced aplasia in dogs by transplantation of marrow from DLA-matched littermates. In 1968 Gatti, et al.[113] reported reconstitution of immunologic and hematopoietic function in a patient with severe combined immunodeficiency and graft versus host–induced aplasia following transplantation of marrow from an HLA-matched allogeneic sibling. In the ensuing decade marrow transplan-

tation has rapidly developed to become the current treatment of choice for severe combined immunodeficiency and aplastic anemia.*

Currently marrow transplantation is reserved for patients with severe aplastic anemia. Marrow transplantation is possible only if an HLA-matched sibling or relative is available to act as a marrow donor. Alloantigens of the HLA system are coded by a group of closely linked genes, termed the HLA complex, located on the sixth chromosome in man.† Expression of these alloantigenic specificities is dominantly inherited. Parental haplotypes are usually inherited en bloc (Fig. 17-4). Thus the probability that any one sibling of a patient will inherit the same two haplotypes is ¼. However, patients usually have more than one sibling. Empirically approximately 40% of individuals with aplastic anemia have been shown to be matched for HLA specificities with at least one sibling.[332,333]

The major histocompatibility complex, or the HLA complex, in humans is composed of a series of genes, each exhibiting a high degree of allelic polymorphism. A diagram of the HLA system and the specificities currently defined at each locus is presented in Fig. 17-4.[206] Lymphocyte alloantigens coded by the HLA-A, B, and C allelic groups may be identified serologically, utilizing complement-dependent microcytoxicity tests and antibodies to these specificities derived from multiparous women sensitized to paternal alloantigens through immunizations with fetal leukocytes.[204,336]

Histocompatibility between siblings at the HLA-D locus is defined by mutual nonresponsiveness in the mixed leukocyte culture reaction.[15-17,71,72] In this reaction lymphocytes from one individual (responders) are cultured with irradiated mononuclear cells from another individual (stimulators). Responder lymphocytes will transform and proliferate in the presence of incompatible HLA-D alloantigens on the stimulator cells. This response can be quantitated by measuring incorporation of radiolabeled thymidine into cellular DNA and compared with responses to autologous irradiated targets to determine identity or disparity for these specificites. An HLA-D phenotype may be assigned by examining the lymphocytes' reactions to a battery of irradiated lymphocytes, each homozygous for a given HLA-D specificity. Relative unresponsiveness to an HLA-D-homozygous cell indicates the responder possesses the stimulator lymphocytes' HLA-D specificity. At present, at least seven HLA-D alleles have been characterized.[71,72,132,206] The major histocompatibility complex and its significance to

---

*References 15-17, 71, 72, 336.
†References 4, 38, 45, 46, 73, 320.

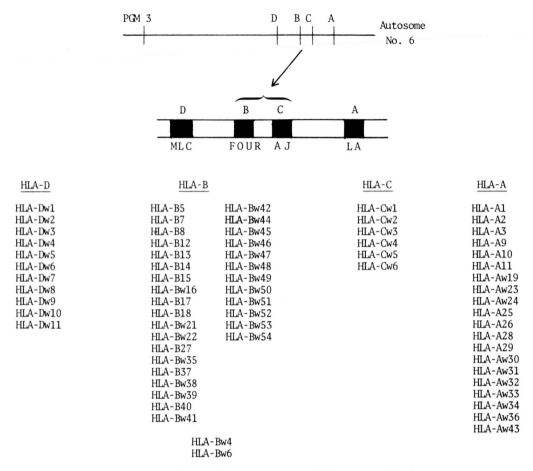

Fig. 17-4. The major human histocompatibility system (HLA).

transplantation and transfusion therapy have been the subjects of a number of recent reviews.*

In humans engraftment of HLA-haploidentical or fully mismatched marrow or blood containing immunocompetent thymus-dependent (T) lymphocytes in an immunoincompetent host has invariably led to fatal graft versus host disease.[38] However, as in mice, lethal graft versus host disease is only generated in response to alloantigenic disparities coded by genes within a restricted region of the major histocompatibility complex.[71,74] In mice the genes controlling alloantigens stimulating lethal graft versus host disease have been localized within the H-2 complex by analysis of transplants between congenic strains in which one strain is histoincompatible for certain determinants by virtue of crossover events within the major histocompatibility complex.[15-17,81] Similar recombinant events have been documented within the human HLA complex, providing instances in which marrow donor and host were identical for all

except a restricted group of HLA determinants within one parental haplotype.[51,113]

Successful lymphoid and hematopoietic reconstructions of patients with severe combined immunodeficiency or aplastic anemia have been achieved through transplantation of marrow mismatched for HLA-A or HLA-A and B determinants but compatible with the host by mixed leukocyte culture analysis.*

In contrast lethal graft versus host disease has almost invariably developed following engraftment of marrow transplanted from donors reactive against the host in mixed leukocyte culture.[38] Mutual unresponsiveness in mixed leukocyte culture has thus been considered to be the most important in vitro index of donor-host histocompatibility. Genes coding for the alloantigens stimulating graft versus host reactions are probably closely linked to, although distinct from, those coded by HLA-D, lying between the HLA-B and D loci. This hypothesis has been suggested

*References 15-17, 71, 132, 206, 336.

*References 51, 113, 236, 240.

by recent reports of two successful transplants without severe graft versus host disease from donors responsive to the host in mixed leukocyte culture but HLA-A and B identical by virtue of an apparent genetic recombination within the HLA complex.[235,322a]

Although histocompatibility for at least certain alloantigens coded by the major histocompatibility complex is required if lethal graft versus host disease is to be avoided, other alloantigenic systems also strongly influence donor-host interactions. This is evidenced both by the fact that individuals sensitized (through transfusion) to other alloantigens may reject a marrow graft from an HLA-identical sibling[314,318] and by the high incidence of morbidity and graft versus host disease in recipients of HLA-A, B, C, and D matched marrow allografts.[119,315] The alloantigenic systems contributing to the initiation of graft rejection or graft versus host disease are poorly defined.

Incompatibility for the ABO and Rh cell systems does not limit successful engraftment, nor does it lead to a greater incidence or severity of graft versus host disease.[109] To circumvent the potentially deleterious effects of host-derived isoagglutinins on the graft, extensive plasmapheresis of the host may be used following immunosuppression to remove circulating isoagglutinins. A four- to six-plasma volume exchange is usually sufficient.[109] Continued production of isoagglutinins by the host is aborted through lymphoablative immunosuppression; the lymphoid sytem following successful engraftment is of donor origin.

Sensitization to alloantigens expressed on leukocytes and platelets and coded by autosomal genes outside the major histocompatibility complex have been postulated to predispose to graft rejection. Parkman et al.[244] have described one such alloantigenic system detected by a cell-mediated lympholysis assay. Serum lymphotoxins directed against donor cells have been suggested as a measure of host sensitization, but this assay has not proved to be consistently useful as a prognostic indicator.[107,184,314] Alloantigens coded by the X and Y chromosomes have recently been implicated in the pathogenesis of graft versus host disease by the high incidence of this complication in sex-mismatched donor-host combinations.[315]

The technique of allogeneic marrow transplantation has been fully described.[331] Essential features of the procedure include ablation or profound suppression of the lymphoid system of the host to permit engraftment, intravenous infusion of donor marrow, intensive supportive care until hematologic function is reconstructed, and prophylaxis and treatment of graft versus host disease and infections. In transplants between identical twins engraftment may be achieved without immunosuppression, and graft versus host disease is not observed.

Cyclophosphamide in high dosage (50 mg/kg/day in four daily doses) has been the basic immunosuppressive regimen most widely used to prepare recipients for marrow transplantation. Procarbazine coupled with antithymocyte globulin have been used in combination with cyclophosphamide in patients presumed sensitized to their donors to reduce the potential for graft rejection.[311] Although the use of these adjunctive agents has resulted in some improvement in the rate of sustained engraftment, long-term survival has not been improved because of an increased incidence and severity of graft versus host disease and infectious complications.[259,320]

The marrow to be transplanted is obtained by multiple aspirations from the iliac crests, usually with the donor under general anesthesia. The marrow is then strained to remove bone chips and administered intravenously to the recipient. A large dose of marrow cells is a critical variable for successful engraftment. Thus in the Seattle experience marrow doses in excess of 3.0×10^8 nucleated cells/kg body weight have produced durable engraftment in 88% of cases; lower cell doses achieved this result in only 47% of patients.[314] Following marrow transplantation methotrexate in low dosage is given at defined intervals as a prophylaxis against graft versus host disease.[309,318] This measure is based on successful use of this agent for prevention and abrogation of graft versus host disease in canine marrow allograft recipients.[309] Antithymocyte and antilymphocyte globulins and/or high-dose corticosteroids have been used for the treatment of graft versus host disease.[106,312] The effectiveness of these agents in controlling visceral manifestations of graft versus host disease, particularly hepatitis, is not well established.[352] Chronic graft versus host disease of the skin, liver, and gastrointestinal tract has generally been refractory to combinations of conventional immunosuppressive drugs.

If an HLA-A, B, C, and D matched sibling donor is available, marrow transplantation is currently the treatment of choice for severe aplastic anemia. In an early series of patients with severe aplasia receiving transplants at varying stages of their disease, within 1 to 96 months after diagnosis thirty-one (43%) were alive and in complete hematologic remission 8 to 60 months after the transplant.[315] Appreciation of the role of sensitization by transfused platelets and leukocytes in enhancing the likelihood of graft rejection and graft versus host disease* has led to increasing use of transplantation early in the disease course

---

*References 310, 311, 316, 317.

with consequent improvement in results. In a recent prospective trial in which patients with severe aplastic anemia either received transplants within 6 weeks of diagnosis or were treated with either androgens and supportive therapy or supportive therapy alone, 55% of the transplanted group were alive in full hematologic remission 30 months after transplant. In contrast, 24% of the androgen-treated group and 26% of those treated with supportive care alone survived to 30 months, and less than half of the survivors have shown hematologic improvement.[45,46]

The persistent high morbidity and mortality associated with marrow transplantation is caused largely by three complications stemming from the allogeneic relationship between donor and host, namely graft rejection, graft versus host disease, and the infectious complications of immunologic suppression.

In the Seattle experience 30% of individuals with aplastic anemia who receive marrow transplants following immunosuppression with cyclophosphamide (50 mg/kg/day in four doses) ultimately reject the graft. Four mechanisms have been suggested to explain this phenomenon. These include (1) immune rejection by persistent host lymphocytes sensitized to donor marrow cells through prior transfusions with platelets or leukocytes,* (2) functional deficiencies in the marrow stroma inhibiting marrow growth, (3) a nonimmune cell-mediated resistance to allografts analogous to the phenomenon of allogeneic resistance described by Cudkowicz and Bennett[53,54] in mice, and (4) an autoimmune lymphocyte-mediated inhibition of both autologous and allogeneic marrow growth.†

An immunologic response by the sensitized host against the donor marrow graft probably accounts for most cases of graft rejection. In the Seattle experience[317] patients with aplastic anemia who have not received antecedent transfusions have uniformly achieved sustained engraftment. In contrast, patients with an extensive transfusion history have a high risk (>30%) of graft rejection.[314,318] In particular, transfusion of the potential marrow recipient with leukocytes or platelets from the matched sibling donor or other immediate family member may preclude sustained engraftment.[310] Recently pretransplant demonstrations of low-grade responses of donor lymphocytes against host leukocyte targets in mixed lymphocyte culture and in cell-mediated lympholysis assays has been found to correlate with a high incidence of graft rejection.[314] If such reactions are

indicators of immune presensitization of the host rather than the existing genetic disparities between donor and host, such results would further suggest that the host immune response is the predominant mediator of graft rejection.

Recent reports of failure to arrest the course of aplastic anemia through syngeneic (twin) marrow grafts suggest the possibility that stromal defects or autoimmune mechanisms may be operative in certain patients.* Since allogeneic resistance in mice is abrogated by pretreatment of the host with cyclophosphamide, the use of this agent to prepare aplastic patients for transplantation has been thought to preclude rejection through this mechanism. The validity of this assumption is untested. Development of in vitro correlates of allogeneic resistance[296] may provide means for assessing its importance in human marrow transplantation.

Graft versus host disease is a pathologic process initiated by the reaction of engrafted immunocompetent thymus-dependent donor lymphocytes against host cells and tissues expressing certain alloantigenic characteristics different from those of the donor.[25,81,299] Graft versus host disease of varying severity occurs in 70% of patients engrafted with HLA-matched allogeneic marrow. Acute graft versus host disease may be lethal in as many as 15% of marrow transplant recipients.[119] The onset of graft versus host disease occurs between 10 and 50 days after the transplant. It is characterized by one or more of the following signs and symptoms: skin rash; hepatitis; gastrointestinal lesions leading to diarrhea, and malabsorption; and suppression of lymphoid and hematopoietic function. Chronic graft versus host disease involving the skin, liver, and gastrointestinal tract may also produce long-term disability in a significant proportion of marrow transplant recipients. The pathology of acute and chronic graft versus host disease and methods for estimating its severity have recently been reviewed.[119,360] A number of immunosuppressive agents including antithymocyte globulin, corticosteroids, cyclophosphamide, methotrexate, and azathioprine have been utilized to treat acute and chronic graft versus host disease.† As noted earlier, results of such trials have been disappointing.

The state of immunodeficiency induced by pretransplant lymphoablative chemotherapy is profound and terminates late in the posttransplant period following functional engraftment of donor lymphocytes.‡ Graft versus host disease and its treatment intensify and further prolong this im-

---

*References 310, 311, 316, 317.
†References 13, 126, 146, 157.

*References 93, 108, 276, 351.
†References 108, 309, 312, 352.
‡References 80, 110, 225, 313.

munocompromised state.[313] During this interval the marrow transplant recipient is at high risk for severe infection. The causative agents are predominantly endogenous, opportunistic pathogens. Disseminated bacterial infections occur most frequently in the early posttransplant period when neutropenia is most profound. Enteric pathogens, particularly *E. coli* and *Pseudomonas,* are the agents most frequently isolated. The use of intensive parenteral antibiosis has reduced the mortality associated with such infections to 5% to 10% in large transplant series. However, disseminated fungal infections particularly, with *Candida albicans,* still constitute a major cause of death in transplant recipients.[356] Recently the introduction of techniques for preparatory skin and mucosol decontamination and sterile isolation has produced a significant reduction in the incidence of septic complications and associated morbidity and mortality. However, to date the use of such techniques has not been shown to significantly enhance long-term survival.[39]

Interstitial pneumonia is the most frequent lethal complication in the first 100 days following transplantation. In prospective studies the pathogens that have been most frequently isolated from the lung parenchyma are cytomegalovirus (46%), *Pneumocystis carinii* (21%), and herpes simplex virus (7%). However, in 40% of the cases no etiologic agent has been documented.[226] The pathogenesis of this disorder is complex. The incidence and severity are strongly influenced by the method of immunosuppression. For example, patients with leukemia or aplastic anemia receiving total body irradiation are particularly prone to severe interstitial pneumonia. Although total body irradiation and cyclophosphamide may produce direct injury to the lung parenchyma, the low incidence of interstitial pneumonia in leukemic patients transplanted with marrow from identical twins argues against such injury as a major precipitating factor. The importance of the allogeneic interaction between donor and host is indicated by the temporal association of graft versus host disease and interstitial pneumonia and the high incidence and severity of interstitial pneumonia in patients with this disorder. Neiman et al.[226] have reported an incidence of interstitial pneumonia of 78% with a mortality of 60% in transplant recipients with graft vs host disease. In contrast, in recipients without graft versus host disease interstitial pneumonia developed in 40% and was lethal in only 21%. The basis for the association between interstitial pneumonia, particularly that associated with cytomegalovirus infection, and graft versus host disease is still unclear. In vitro and in vivo studies in murine models suggest that graft versus host disease may activate latent cyto-

megalovirus infections of the lymphoid system or enhance lytic virus production in chronically infected hosts through infection of virus-susceptible, proliferating, alloreactive lymphocytes.[67,233] The possibility that virus-induced cell surface antigens may serve to intensify donor responses to host alloantigens and thereby contribute to graft versus host disease has also been suggested.[94,111]

At present the treatment of interstitial pneumonia is largely limited to respiratory support. Attempts at therapeutic intervention with antiviral agents, particularly adenine arabinoside (Ara-A) and interferon, have generally been disappointing.[48] Prophylaxis against viral interstitial pneumonia with adenine arabinoside or interferon has not been shown to be beneficial and may actually prove hazardous because of the myelosuppressive activity of these agents.[95,167,231] Methods for both active and passive immunization against cytomegalovirus are being developed and will be considered for clinical trials in a number of transplant centers.[79,249,254]

In summary, experience in marrow transplantation indicates this approach to be the current treatment of choice for patients with severe aplastic anemia for whom an HLA-A, B, C, and D histocompatible sibling donor is available. The morbidity associated with this therapeutic course is frequently severe, with lethal complications occurring in nearly half of the patients transplanted. Improved methods for preparing the patient for engraftment, particularly for reducing or eliminating the graft versus host disease-inducing potential of the donor marrow, should lead to significant improvement in results.

Recently a number of experimental approaches have been developed that may ultimately provide methods for extending the applicability of transplantation to the 60% of patients for whom a matched sibling donor is not available. Marrow transplants from nonsibling related donors who are HLA phenotypically identical to the host, at least for HLA-D specificities, have been successful in patients with severe combined immunodeficiency and in isolated patients with aplastic anemia.* Recently transplants from an HLA-A–nonidentical, HLA-B and D–identical unrelated donor have been used successfully to correct severe combined immunodeficiency and graft versus host–induced aplastic anemia,[236] indicating that the use of unrelated HLA-matched donors may be applicable in transplantation for lethal hematologic disorders. In canine models, however, transplants of unrelated HLA-compatible marrow are associated with a lower long-term survival because of an increased incidence and/

---

*References 113, 235, 238, 240.

or severity of complications such as graft rejection and graft versus host disease.[321] Newer techniques for selective elimination of alloreactive thymus-dependent lymphocytes from the marrow graft (involving pretreatment of the graft with specific antilymphocyte globulins,* selective suicide of alloreactive lymphocytes,† or immunochemical fractionation of marrow)[261] — and techniques for host preparation that potentiate graft-host tolerance (e.g., total nodal irradiation)[301] may reduce the incidence and severity of graft versus host disease and make possible the transplantation of histoincompatible marrow. Recent successes with transplants of HLA-mismatched fetal liver in the treatment of severe combined immunodeficiency indicate the potential of T lymphocyte–depleted grafts of hematopoietic precursor populations.[37,238] Techniques for long-term in vitro culture of hematopoietic stem cells from mouse, dog, and humans have recently been developed.[63] Preliminary studies in murine systems indicate that such cultured stem cells will reconstitute hematopoietic function when transplanted into lethally irradiated recipients. Thus the possibility of circumventing the problem of lethal graft versus host disease in recipients of HLA-mismatched grafts may soon be realized.

Immunosuppression. Recently interest in the use of immunosuppressive agents in the treatment of aplastic anemia has been spawned by multiple reports of autologous marrow recovery following treatment with high-dose cyclophosphamide or antithymocyte globulin used to prepare aplastic patients for marrow transplantation,‡ coupled with experimental observations suggesting the presence in the marrow of certain aplastic patients of cell populations of apparent lymphoid origin capable of suppressing proliferation of myeloid and erythroid precursors.§ Recently, Speck et al.[307] have reported significant hematologic improvement in 60% of patients with severe aplastic anemia treated with antithymocyte globulin and androgens with or without a subsequent transplant of hemiallogeneic marrow. The latter procedure, which may result in transient engraftment of donor marrow, is thought to improve results by providing additional inductive stimuli for autologous hematopoietic development. The role of androgens in this regimen is unclear, but their use is reported to improve long-term survival. In these studies and in preliminary experiments in animal models, clinical responses have been recorded most frequently in subjects whose marrow, when treated in vitro with antithymocyte globulin, demonstrates

improved generation of CFU-C.[304,305] Although neither the in vitro observations nor the clinical trials have incorporated suitable patient controls, the results are of such potential significance as to demand immediate initiation of suitably controlled prospective clinical trials. Such studies are currently in progress.

CONSTITUTIONAL APLASTIC ANEMIA

Included among the cases of bone marrow failure of unknown etiology are several distinctive familial syndromes. These are Fanconi's anemia (with congenital anomalies), dyskeratosis congenita with pancytopenia, and familial aplasia without congenital anomalies as described by Estren and Damashek[86] in 1947.

Fanconi's anemia is a familial disorder marked by the association of pancytopenia and marrow hypoplasia with a variable constellation of congenital anomalies of the skin, skeletal system, central nervous system, and genitourinary tract. Various chromosomal abnormalities may characterize the disorder even in the absence of congenital anomalies.[21] More than 200 cases of Fanconi's anemia have been reported.

Historical perspective

Fanconi[88] first described this disorder in three brothers who had microcephaly, intensive brown pigmentation, genital hypoplasia, internal strabismus, and strongly increased reflexes in addition to aplastic anemia. Uehlinger[341] proposed the term "familial hypoplastic pancytopenia" and Naegli[220] termed the disorder "Fanconi's anemia" in 1931. In recent years interest has centered on the spontaneous and induced chromosomal aberrations seen in the disorder and their relationship to the high incidence of malignancy seen in these patients and their relatives.

Classification

The following are the major types of constitutional aplastic anemia:
1. Constitutional aplastic anemia (delayed onset) with congenital anomalies or chromosome abnormalities (Fanconi's anemia)
2. Constitutional aplastic anemia without congenital anomalies (delayed onset) (Estren-Dameshek anemia)
3. Delayed onset aplasia with dyskeratosis congenita
4. Constitutional aplastic anemia (type II) — congenital thrombocytopenia with delayed-onset pancytopenia without congenital anomalies

Clinical features

For most patients with Fanconi's anemia the associated congenital anomalies are recognized at

---

*References 217, 218, 340, 342, 347.
†References 75, 266, 271, 282, 369.
‡References 153, 154, 239, 292, 306, 326, 334.
§References 13, 126, 146, 157.

birth or in early infancy. Hematologic abnormalities rarely become evident before 17 months of age and may not develop until the second decade. The asymptomatic period in a child with a skeletal defect before anemia becomes manifest has been unexplained. In an occasional patient studied during this period the bone marrow surprisingly has revealed erythroid hyperplasia with megaloblastoid changes.

A wide range of congenital anomalies may be present either singly or in combination. The anomalies that particularly contribute to the diagnosis of Fanconi's anemia are hyperpigmentation, skeletal malformations, small stature, and hypogonadism.

Skin pigmentation. A patchy hyperpigmentation is observed in 74% of patients with the disorder. It is most often central, involving the neck, axillae, areolae, abdomen, umbilicus, genitalia, and groin. The distal extremities and face are most often spared. Histologically increased melanin is seen in the basal layer.[228]

Short stature. Short stature is seen in 75% of cases. Characteristically the trunk is short and the legs are relatively long.[120] Several patients have been described with growth hormone deficiency.[49,251,368]

Skeletal anomalies. Skeletal anomalies are present in about 70% of the patients and most commonly involve the hands and forearms. They include absence of the thumb (Fig. 17-5), hypoplasia of the thumbnail, hypoplasia or absence of the first metacarpal, triphalangeal thumbs, and decreased number of ossification centers in the wrist.[250] Other anomalies include atrophy of the thenar eminence, immobility of one or both thumb joints, and a thumb attached to the hand only by soft tissue. Subtle anomalies including thinning of phalanges may be noted roentgenographically. The

radius may be absent bilaterally or unilaterally. In each of these cases the corresponding thumb is absent.[208] Other reported skeletal anomalies include congenital hip dislocation, webbing of the second and third toes, Klippel-Feil deformity, and Sprengel's deformity.

Renal anomalies. Renal anomalies are present in more than a quarter of the patients with Fanconi's anemia. The most common is absence of one kidney. Horseshoe kidneys and hydronephrosis have also been reported.[208]

Central nervous system anomalies. Microcephaly, low birth weight, microophthalmia, mental retardation, ptosis of the lid, lacrimal duct stenosis, deafness, external auditory canal atresia, strabismus, and nystagmus have all been reported. Hyperreflexia, however, is the most common central nervous system abnormality.

Other anomalies. Hypogenitalism has been reported in many instances but is difficult to evaluate in the younger patients. Atrophy of the spleen is frequently observed.[112]

Pancytopenia. The age of onset of pancytopenia in patients with Fanconi's anemia averages 6.6 years for boys and 8.8 years for girls and ranges from 17 months to 22 years.[120] Within families there is a tendency for the hematologic disorder to occur at about the same age in affected siblings.[90] The full expression of pancytopenia is variable in its temporal course, developing over a period of months or years. The factors contributing to its onset or progression are unknown.

The first abnormality to develop is usually thrombocytopenia,[208] with subsequent onset of granulocytopenia and anemia. In the early stages of the disease the marrow reveals erythroid hyperplasia and megaloblastosis. As the disease progresses, the marrow becomes progressively more

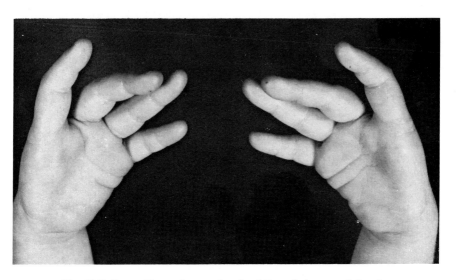

Fig. 17-5. Fanconi's syndrome, showing bilateral absence of thumbs.

hypoplastic with an increase in the number and proportion of lymphocytes, plasma cells, and reticulum cells.[270] When fully developed the pancytopenia is entirely similar to that seen in acquired forms of aplastic anemia and results in the same spectrum and severity of clinical expression. As in the acquired form, fetal hemoglobin levels are increased[295] and red cell G-6-PD levels decreased. Deficiencies of leukocyte hexokinase have been variably reported.[183] Red cell osmotic fragility has been reported to be abnormal.[252] Other parameters of hematologic function are consistent with those found in acquired aplastic anemia.

Occasional patients who with therapeutic intervention survive into the second or third decade often die of monocytic or myelomonocytic leukemia.[89]

Genetics. The genetic basis of inheritance of Fanconi's anemia is unclear. Certain characteristics suggest transmission by an autosomal recessive gene with variable penetrance. Affected individuals are frequently offspring of consanguineous marriages. In a compiled series[89] parental consanguineous marriages were observed in 20% of cases, far in excess of the frequency of 0.5% in the general population. Interestingly, even unrelated parents of patients with Fanconi's anemia are found to share certain genetic determinants. Thus mother and father frequently share determinants of the major histocompatibility system (HLA-D, chromosome 6) in one haplotype. This paternal haplotype is usually inherited by the proband so that mother and patient are HLA-D histocompati-

ble.[131] This finding suggests that at least restricted identity between multiple codons of the maternal and paternal genome may be necessary for the expression of disease. In many families multiple siblings are affected. However, vertical transmission of the hematologic features of the disease from parents to child has not been reported. Siblings of a proband may possess congenital anomalies without blood changes.[112] Furthermore, at least one patient has been reported whose father had one of the skeletal anomalies—radial aplasia.[11]

Several observations speak against a simple autosomal recessive mode of inheritance. The multiplicity of congenital anomalies and the variability of their expression are difficult to explain on the basis of a single gene. The ratio of affected to unaffected siblings is high (1:1.17). Maternal age at the time of delivery is higher than normal. Furthermore, approximately 66% of patients are male.[90] Thus other genetic and/or environmental factors may modulate the expression of disease.

Although lymphoreticular malignancies are a frequent late complication of Fanconi's anemia, the demonstration of a high incidence of leukemia in nonaffected family members is of particular interest. In one series[112] among forty-nine families in which Fanconi's anemia was found leukemia was reported four times, a rate of 1 in 12.2 cases, which is higher than the rate of familial leukemia (1 in 450) or the rate in the overall pediatric population (1 in 2,800). Swift[323] studied eight families with Fanconi's anemia and analyzed 102 deaths in nonaffected family members over a 40-year span.

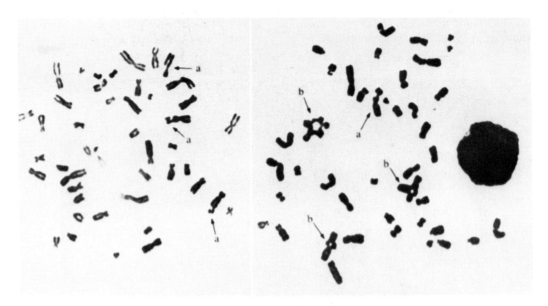

Fig. 17-6. Chromosomal abnormalities in Fanconi's anemia: *a,* breaks and gaps; *b,* chromatid exchanges. (From Beard, M. E. J., et al.: Fanconi's anaemia, Q. J. Med. **42:**403, 1973.)

Of these twenty-seven were secondary to malignancy. Prominent types were leukemia and carcinoma of the stomach or colon. With the frequency of heterozygotes for Fanconi's anemia estimated to be 1 in 300 in the normal population, Swift[323] hypothesizes that as much as 5% of all leukemia may occur in heterozygotes for this disorder.

Chromosomal abnormalities. Various spontaneous and induced chromosomal defects are seen and are probably an integral feature of the disorder. The usual abnormalities, seen in fibroblasts and in mitogen-transformed lymphocytes, include chromatid and chromosome breakages, gaps, constrictions, and occasionally translocations[288,289,324] (Fig. 17-6). Recent studies[74] suggest the breakages are not random, occurring most commonly in the interbands between R and Q bands of the longer chromosomal segments. Sister chromatid exchanges occur at normal, not increased, frequency.[74]

The cells of patients with Fanconi's anemia exhibit an abnormally high susceptibility to malignant transformation by SV40 virus.[337] Lymphocytes exhibit a fourfold (and fibroblasts a twofold) increase over normal in the incidence of chromosome damage following exposure to ionizing radiation.[145] Cells of these patients have a greater susceptibility to damage by DNA cross-linking agents[286] as well as by carcinogens.[14] They display defective DNA repair on exposure to ultraviolet light.[255, 258] Further evidence of defective cell replication is that the doubling time for cultured fibroblasts averages 30.3 hours as compared to 22.9 hours for normal cultures.[79] These findings may help explain the high incidence of malignancy seen in the patients with this disorder who survive aplastic anemia. Similarly the fact that chromosomal abnormalities as well as increased susceptibility to malignant transformation by SV40 virus have been observed in fibroblasts derived from the parents of some patients with Fanconi's anemia[66] may bear on the high incidence of malignancy in unaffected family members. No correlation has been established between any of the congenital anomalies or the severity of the anemia and the chromosomal disturbances.

Differential diagnosis

No difficulties should arise in patients with the typical stigmata of the disorder of if any siblings have previously been affected. Chromosome analysis and careful physical examination, skeletal survey, and intravenous pyelogram should help distinguish between Fanconi's anemia and acquired aplastic anemia. The following disorders may be considered in the differential diagnosis:

A. Without pancytopenia
  1. Triphalangeal thumb with hypoplastic anemia
  2. Thrombocytopenia and absent radii
B. With pancytopenia
  1. Fanconi's anemia
  2. Acquired aplastic anemia
  3. Dyskeratosis congenita
  4. Constitutional aplastic anemia without congenital anomalies (Estren-Damashek anemia)
  5. Constitutional aplastic anemia type II

Triphalangeal thumbs with hypoplastic anemia[1,155] and thrombocytopenia–absent radii syndromes both present their hematologic problems at birth and do not develop into full aplastic anemia. They should therefore not present any problem in differential diagnosis.

Constitutional aplastic anemia type II[27] consists of a megakaryocytic thrombocytopenia that is present at birth and the subsequent development of pancytopenia. Chromosomes are normal and congenital anomalies are absent.

Dyskeratosis congenita is a disorder that shares many features with Fanconi's anemia, including development of pancytopenia, increased skin pigmentation, mental retardation, and decreased growth. However, cutaneous telangiectatic erythema and atrophy, exocrine ungual and dental dysplasia, and esophageal diverticula may be present in dyskeratosis congenita and absent in Fanconi's anemia, whereas skeletal and renal abnormalities are present in Fanconi's anemia and absent in dyskeratosis congenita.[308] Chromosome abnormalities are usually absent in dyskeratosis congenita.[149] Other than leukemia and hepatoma, carcinoma of the anus, vulva, and gingiva are also seen in dyskeratosis congenita[308] and there may be difficulty in distinguishing the two disorders in certain patients.

Management

Management is similar to that of the acquired form: supportive care, androgens, and steroids. In these patients androgens usually must be given continuously, as relapses are the rule after discontinuance. Bone marrow transplants have produced full reconstitution in patients with Fanconi's anemia.[20] This approach may prove to be the treatment of choice for patients with Fanconi's anemia who prove refractory to androgen and steroid therapy. It is also possible that successful engraftment of normal hematopoietic precursors and elimination of host lymphoid elements may circumvent the problem of leukemia occurring late in the course of this disease. However, for host cells surviving this procedure, immunosuppression with cyclophosphamide may be expected to cause severe chromosome damage and may increase the likelihood of malignant change.

Prognosis

The use of steroids and androgens has resulted in long-term remission in the majority of the cases; prior to their use the disease was usually fatal within 2 years of diagnosis. Li and Alter[181] found that long-term survival was 45% in this disease. The possibility of increased proportion of malignancy in the survivor is a matter of great concern. At least seven cases of acute leukemia have occurred in patients with Fanconi's anemia and at least ten cases of solid tumors. Many more probably occurred and were unreported.[21]

REFERENCES

1. Aase, J. M., and Smith, D. W.: Congenital anemia and triphalangeal thumbs: a new syndrome. J. Pediatr. **74:** 471, 1969.
2. Adair, F. E., Mellors, R. C., et al.: The use of estrogens and androgens in advanced mammary cancer: clinical and laboratory study of 105 female patients, J.A.M.A. **140:** 1193, 1949.
3. Adelstein, S. J., and Dealy, J. B.: Hematologic responses to human whole body irradiation, Am. J. Roentgenol. **93:** 927, 1965.
4. Advisory Committee Bone Marrow Transplantation Registry: Bone marrow transplantation from donors with aplastic anemia, J.A.M.A. **236:** 1131, 1976.
5. Aksoy, M., Erdem, S., DinCol, G.: Leukemia in shoeworkers exposed chronically to benzene, Blood **44:** 837, 1974.
6. Aksoy, M., Erdem, S., Erdogan, G., et al.: Acute leukemia in 2 generations following chronic exposure to benzene, Hum. Hered. **24:** 70, 1974.
7. Alavi, J. B., Root, R. K., Djerassi, I., et al.: A randomized clinical trial of granulocytic transfusions for infection in acute leukemia, N. Engl. J. Med. **296:** 13, 1977.
8. Albert, E., Thomas, E. D., et al.: HLA-antigens and haplotype in 200 patients with aplastic anemia, Transplantation **22:** 528, 1976.
9. Alexanian, R.: Erythropoietin excretion in bone marrow failure and hemolytic anemia, J. Lab. Clin. Med. **82:** 438, 1973.
10. Allen, D. M., Fine, M. H., et al.: Oxymethalone therapy in aplastic anemia, Blood **32:** 83, 1968.
11. Altay, G., Sevgi, Y., and Pirnar, T.: Fanconi's anemia in offspring of patients with congenital radial and carpal hypoplasia, N. Engl. J. Med. **293:** 151, 1975.
12. Anderson, D. H.: Benzol poisoning with hyperplasia of the bone marrow, Am. J. Pathol. **10:** 101, 1934.
13. Ascensao, J., Pahwa, R., Kagan, W., et al.: Aplastic anemia: evidence for an immunologic mechanism, Lancet **1:** 669, 1976.
14. Auerbach, A. D., and Wolman, S. R.: Susceptibility of Fanconi's anemia fibroblasts to chromosome damage by carcinogens, Nature **261:** 494, 1976.
15. Bach, F. H., and van Rood, J. J.: The major histocompatibility complex. Part 1, N. Engl. J. Med. **295:** 806, 1976.
16. Bach, F. H., and van Rood, J. J.: The major histocompatibility complex. Part 2, N. Engl. J. Med. **295:** 872, 1976.
17. Bach, F. H., and van Rood, J. J.: The major histocompatibility complex. Part 3, N. Engl. J. Med. **295:** 927, 1976.
18. Baldrige, C. W.: Macrocytic anemia with aplastic features following the application of synthetic organic hair dye, Am. J. Med. Sci. **189:** 759, 1935.
19. Baran, D. T., Grimes, P. F., and Klemperer, M. R.: Recovery from aplastic anemia after treatment with cyclophosphamide, N. Engl. J. Med. **27:** 1522, 1976.
20. Barrett, A. J., Bridgen, W. D., et al.: Successful bone marrow transplant for Fanconi's anemia, Br. Med. J. **1:** 420, 1977.
21. Beard, M. E.: Fanconi's anemia. In Congenital disorders of erythropoiesis, Amsterdam, 1976, Elsevier.
22. Ben-Bassat, I., Brok-Simoni, F., and Ramot, B.: Complement-sensitive red cells in aplastic anemia, Blood **46:** 357, 1975.
23. Best, W. R.: Chloramphenicol-associated blood dyscrasias, J.A.M.A. **201:** 99, 1967.
24. Bierman, H. R., and Nelson, E. R.: Hematodepressive virus diseases of Thailand, Ann. Intern. Med. **62:** 867, 1965.
25. Billingham, E. R.: Reactions of grafts against their hosts, Science **130:** 947, 1959.
26. Bloom, G. E., and Diamond, L. K.: Prognostic value of fetal Hgb levels in acquired aplastic anemia, N. Engl. J. Med. **278:** 304, 1968.
27. Bloom, G. E., Warner, S., Gerald, P. S., and Diamond, L. K.: Chromosomal abnormalities in constitutional aplastic anemia, N. Engl. J. Med. **274:** 8, 1976.
28. Bloomfield, C. D., and Brunning, R. D.: Acute leukemia as a terminal event in nonleukemic hematopoietic disorders, Semin. Oncol. **3:** 297, 1976.
29. Boggs, D. R., and Boggs, S. S.: The pathogenesis of aplastic anemia: a defective pluripotent hematopoietic stem cell with inappropriate balance of differentiation and self replication, Blood **48:** 71, 1976.
30. Bomford, R. A., and Rhoads, O. P.: Refractory anemia, Q. J. Med. **10:** 175, 1941.
31. Bond, V. P., Fliedner, T. M., Archambeau, J. O.: Mammalian radiation lethality, New York, 1965, Academic Press, Inc.
32. Botnick, L. E., Hannon, E. C., and Hellman, S.: Limited proliferation of stem cells surviving alkylating agents, Nature **262:** 68, 1976.
33. Bottiger, L. E., and Westerholm, B.: Aplastic anemia. III. Aplastic anemia and infectious hepatitis, Acta Med. Scand. **192:** 323, 1972.
34. Bowditch, M., et al.: Chronic exposure to benzene, J. Ind. Hyg. Toxicol. **21:** 331, 1939.
35. Brands, R. F., Amsden, T. W., and Jacob, H. S.: Randomized study of nandrolone therapy for anemias due to bone marrow failure, Arch Intern. Med. **137:** 65, 1977.
36. Broxmeyer, H. E., Moore, M. A. S., and Ralph, P.: Cell-free granulocyte colony inhibiting activity derived from human polymorphonuclear neutrophils, Exp. Hematol. **5**(2):87, 1977.
37. Buckley, R. H., Winsnant, J. K., et al.: Correction of severe combined immunodeficiency by fetal liver cells, N. Engl. J. Med. **294:** 1076, 1976.
38. Buckley, R. J.: Reconstitution: grafting of bone marrow and thymus. In Amos B., ed.: Progress in immunology, New York, 1971, Academic Press, Inc.
39. Buckner, C. D., Clift, R. A., Sanders, J. E., and Thomas, E. D.: The role of protective environment and prophylactic granulocyte transfusions in marrow transformation, Transplant. Proc. **10:** 255, 1978.
40. Budman, D. R., and Steinberg, A. D.: Hematologic aspects of systemic lupus erythematosus: current concepts, Ann. Intern. Med. **86:** 220, 1977.
41. Reference deleted in proofs.
42. Burke, P. J., Karp, J. E., and Schacter, L. P.: Evidence for an etiologic role of serum inhibitor factors in patients with hepatitis related aplastic anemia, Exp. Hematol. **5**(suppl. 2):103, 1977.
43. Camitta, B. M., Nathan, D., et al.: Posthepatitic severe aplastic anemia: an indication for early bone marrow transplantation, Blood **43:** 473, 1974.

44. Camitta, B. M., Rappaport, J. M., et al.: Selection of patients for bone marrow transplantation in severe aplastic anemia, Blood **45:**355, 1975.

45. Camitta, B. M., and Thomas, E. D.: Severe aplastic anemia: a prospective study of the effect of early marrow transplantation on acute mortality, Blood **48:**63, 1976.

46. Camitta, B. M., Thomas, E. D., Nathan, G., et al.: Severe aplastic anemia: effect of androgens on survival, Blood **50:**313, 1977.

47. Chauffard, M.: Un cas di'anemie perniceuse aplastique, Bull. Sco. Med. d'Hop. **21:**313, 1904.

48. Chien, L. T., Cannon, N. J., et al.: Effect of adanine arabinoside on cytomegalovirus infections, J. Inf. Dis. **130:**32, 1974.

49. Clarke, W. L., and Weldon, U. U.: Growth hormone deficiency and Fanconi's anemia, J. Pediatr. **86:**814, 1975.

50. Cline, M. J.: Defective mononuclear phagocyte function in patients with myelomonocytic leukemia and in some patients with lymphoma, J. Clin. Invest. **52:**2185, 1973.

50a. Condliffe, E., and McQuillen, K.: Bacterial protein synthesis: the effects of antibiotics, J. Med. Biol. **30:**137, 1967.

51. Copenhagen Study Group of Immunodeficiencies: Bone-marrow transplantation from and HL-A non-identical but mixed-lymphocyte-culture identical donor, Lancet **1:**1146, 1973.

52. Corrigan, G. E.: An autopsy survey of aplastic anemia, Am. J. Clin. Pathol. **62:**488, 1974.

53. Cudkowicz, G., and Bennett, M.: Peculiar immunobiology of bone marrow allografts, J. Exp. Med. **134:**1513, 1971.

54. Cudkowicz, G., and Bennett, M.: Peculiar immunobiology of bone marrow allografts. I. graft rejection by irradiated responder mice, J. Exp. Med. **134:**83, 1971.

55. Custer, R. P.: Aplastic anemia in soldiers treated with atabrine, Am. J. Med. Sci. **212:**211, 1946.

56. Dacie, J. V.: Paroxysmal nocturnal haemoglobinuria, Proc. R. Soc. Med. **56:**587, 1963.

57. Dacie, J. V., and Lewis, S. M.: Paroxysmal nocturnal haemoglobinuria: variation in clinical severity and association with bone marrow hypoplasia, Br. J. Haematol. **7:**442, 1961.

58. Daiber, A., et al.: Treatment of aplastic anemia with nandrolone decanoate, Blood **36:**748, 1970.

59. Davis, S., and Rubin, A. D.: Treatment and prognosis in aplastic anemia, Lancet **1:**871, 1972.

60. de Gruchy, G. C.: In Drug induced blood disorders, Oxford, 1975, Blackwell Scientific Publications, Ltd.

61. Dellez, J. J., Cirkeena, W. J., and Marcarelli, J.: Fatal pancytopenia associated with viral hepatitis, N. Engl. J. Med. **266:**297, 1971.

62. Deposito, F., Akatsuka, Y., et al.: Bone marrow failure in pediatric patients. I. Cortisone and testosterone treatment, J. Pediatr. **64:**683, 1964.

63. Dexter, T. M., Moore, M. A. S., and Sheridan, A. P. C.: Maintenance of hemopoietic stem cells and production of differentiated progeny in allogeneic and semiallogeneic bone marrow chimeras in vitro, J. Exp. Med. **145:**1612, 1977.

64. Diamond, L. K., and Shahidi, N. T.: Treatment of aplastic anemia in children, Semin. Hematol. **4:**278, 1967.

65. Dicke, K. A., van Putten, L. M., et al.: Standardization of human bone marrow cultures (Robinson assay) and its application in aplastic anaemia. In Proceedings of the International Symposium on Leukaemia and Aplastic Anemia, Naples, 1974.

66. Dosik, N., Hsu, L. Y., Todaro, G. J., et al.: Leukemia in Fanconi's anemia: cytogenetic and tumor virus susceptibility studies, Blood **36:**341, 1970.

67. Dowling, J. N., Wu, B. C., et al.: Enhancement of murine cytomegalovirus infection during graft vs. host reaction, J. Inf. Dis. **135:**990, 1977.

68. Duarte, L., Lopez Sandoval, R., et al.: Androstane therapy of aplastic anemia, Acta Haematol. **47:**140, 1972.

69. Duarte, L., Sanchez-Medal, L., Cordova, M. S., et al.: Alteraciones hepaticas por anabolios, Rev. Invest. Clin. **21:**415, 1969.

70. Dubois, E. L., and Tuffanelli, D. L.: Clinical manifestations of systemic lupus erythematosus, J.A.M.A. **190:**104, 1964.

71. Dupont, B., Hansen, J. A., Good, R. A., and O'Reilly, R. J.: In Ferrara, G. B., ed.: HLA system-new aspects, Amsterdam, 1977, Elsevier/North-Holland Biomedical Press.

72. Dupont, B., Hansen, J. A., and Yunis, E. J.: Human mixed-lymphocyte culture reaction: genetics, specificity, and biological implications, Adv. Immunol. **23:**107, 1976.

73. Dupont, B., O'Reilly, R. J., Jersild, C., et al.: Transplantation of immunocompetent cells, Progr. Immunol. **5:**203, 1974.

74. Dutrillaux, B., Couturier, J., and Viegas Pequignot, E.: Localization chromatid breaks in Fanconis Anemia, using three consecutive stains, Hum. Genet. **37**(1):65, 1977.

75. Dutton, R. W., and Mishell, R. I.: Cell populations and cell proliferation in the in vitro response of normal mouse spleen to heterologous erythrocytes, J. Exp. Med. **126:**443, 1967.

76. Editorial: Aplastic anemia after hepatitis, N. Engl. J. Med. **273:**1165, 1965.

77. Editorial: Infection hepatitis following aplastic anemia, Lancet **1:**844, 1971.

78. Ehrlich, P.: Ueber einen fall von anamie mit bemerkungen uber regenerative veranderungen des knochanmarks, Charite Ann. **13:**300, 1888.

79. Elek, S. D., and Stern, H.: Development of a vaccine against mental retardation caused by cytomegalovirus infection in utero, Lancet **1:**1, 1974.

80. Elfenbein, G. H., Anderson, P. N., et al.: Immune system reconstitution following allogeneic bone marrow transplantation in man: multiparameter analysis, Transplant. Proc. **8:**641, 1976.

81. Elkins, W. L.: Cellular immunology and the pathogenesis of graft versus host reactions, Prog. Allergy **15:**78, 1971.

82. Elmore, E., and Swift, M.: Growth of cultured cells from patients with Fanconi's anemia, J. Cell Physiol. **87:**229, 1975.

83. Engstrom, P., et al.: Disseminated *Mycobacterium kansasii* infection, Am. J. Med. **52:**533, 1972.

84. Epstein, R. B., Storb, R., Ragde, H., et al.: Cytotoxic typing antisera for marrow grafting in littermate dogs, Transplantation **6:**45, 1968.

85. Erslev, A. J., Iverson, C. K., and Laurason, F. D.: Cortisone and ACTH in hypoplastic anemia, Yale J. Biol. Med. **25:**44, 1952.

86. Estren, S., and Dameshek, W.: Familial hypoplastic anemia of childhood: report of eight cases in 2 families with beneficial effects of splenectomy in 1 case, Am. J. Dis. Child. **73:**671, 1943.

87. Evans, J. L.: Aplastic anemia in pregnancy remitting after abortion, Br. Med. J. **3:**166, 1968.

88. Fanconi, G.: Familiare infantile periziosaartige anamie (Pernizioses blutbild und knostitution) J. Kinderheilik **117:**257, 1927.

89. Fanconi, G.: Die hypothese einer chromosomentranslokation zur Erklärung Genetik ker Familiaren Konstitutionellen Panmyelopathic Typus Fanconi, Helv. Paediatr. Acta. **19:**29, 1964.

90. Fanconi, G.: Familial constitutional panmyelocytopathy, Fanconi's anemia (F.A.). I. clinical aspects, Semin. Hematol. **4:**233, 1967.
91. Fefer, A., et al.: Cure of hematologic neoplasia with transplantation of marrow from identical twins, N. Engl. J. Med. **296:**61, 1977.
92. Fellows, W. R.: A case of aplastic anemia and pancytopenia with tegretol therapy, Headache **9:**92, 1969.
93. Fernbach, D. J., and Trentin, J. J.: Isologous bone marrow transplantation in identical twin with aplastic anemia, In: Proceedings of 8th International Congress of Hematology, Tokyo, 1960, Pan Pacific Press.
94. Festenstein, H., Garrido, F., et al.: The major histocompatibility system, tumors, and viruses. In Ferrara, G. B., ed.: HLA system: new aspects, Amsterdam, 1977, North Holland Publishing Co.
95. Fleming, W. A., McNeill, T. A., and Killen, M.: The effects of an inhibiting factor (interferon) on the in vitro growth of granulocyte macrophase, Immunology **23:**429, 1972.
96. Floersheim, G. L.: Treatment of hyperactue graft versus host disease in mice with cytosine arabinoside, Transplantation **14:**325, 1972.
97. Ford, C. E., Hamerton, J. L., et al.: Cytological identification of radiation chimaeras, Nature **177:**452, 1956.
98. Forget, B. G., and Jordan, B.: 5S RNA synthesized by *Escherichia coli* in presence of chloramphenicol: different 5′-terminal sequences, Science **167:**382, 1970.
99. Forni, A., and Vigliani, E. C.: Chemical leukemogenesis in man, Semin. Haematol. **7:**211, 1974.
100. Fowler, P. D.: Marrow toxicity of pyrazoles, Ann. Rheum. Dis. **26:**344, 1967.
101. Freireich, E. J.: Effectiveness of platelet transfusion in leukemia and aplastic anemia, Transfusion **6:**50, 1966.
102. Fried, W., Kedo, A., and Barone, J.: Effect of cyclophosphamide and of busulfan on spleen colony-forming units and on hematopoietic stroma, Cancer Res. **37:**1205, 1977.
103. Frisch, B., and Lewis, S. M.: The bone marrow in aplastic anemia: diagnostic and prognostic features, J. Clin. Pathol. **27:**231, 1974.
104. Frisch, B., et al.: The ultrastructure of dyserythropoiesis in aplastic anemia, Br. J. Haematol. **29:**545, 1975.
105. Gabriel, B., Gabriel, S. J., and Olner, J.: Aplaises medullaires au cour des traitments anti-epileptiques, Marseille Med. **103:**935, 1966.
106. Gale, R. P.: Bone marrow transplantation in severe aplastic anemia, UCLA Bone Marrow Transplantation Team, Lancet **2:**921, 1976.
107. Gale, R. P., Cahan, M., Cline, M. J., et al.: Pretransplant lymphocytotoxins and bone marrow graft rejection, Lancet **1:**170, 1978.
108. Gale, R. P., Falk. P., et al.: Failure of recovery following syngeneic marrow graft in aplastic anemia, UCLA Bone Marrow Transplantation Team, Exp. Hematol. **5:**103, 1977.
109. Gale, R. P., Feig, S. A., et al.: ABO blood group system and bone marrow transplantation, Blood **50:**185, 1977.
110. Gale, R. P., Opelz, G., Mickey, M. R., et al.: Immunodeficiency following allogeneic bone marrow transplantation, UCLA Bone Marrow Transplantation Team, Transplant. Proc. **10:**223, 1978.
111. Garrido, F., Schirrmacher, V., and Festenstein, H.: H-2 like specificities of foreign haplotypes appearing on a mouse sarcoma after vaccinia virus infection, Nature **259:**228, 1976.
112. Garriga, S., and Crosby, W. H.: The incidence of leukemia in families of patients with hypoplasia of the marrow, Blood **14:**1008, 1959.
113. Gatti, R. A., Meuwissen, H. J., Allen, H. D., et al.: Immunological reconstitution of sex-linked lymphopenic immunological deficiency, Lancet **2:**1366, 1968.
114. Gayford, J. J., and Redpath, J. H.: The side effects of carbamezepine, Proc. R. Soc. Med. **61:**615, 1969.
115. Geraedts, J. P., et al.: Trisomy 6 associated with aplastic anemia, Hum. Genet. **35:**113, 1976.
116. Gevirtz, N. R., and Berlin, N. I.: Erythrokinetic studies in severe bone marrow failure of diverse etiology, Blood **18:**637, 1961.
117. Giblett, E. R., Colemna, D. H., et al.: Erythrokinetics: quantitative measurements of red cell production and destruction in normal subjects and patients with anemia, Blood **11:**291, 1956.
118. Giblett, E. R., and Crookston, M. C.: Agglutinability of red cells by anti-i in patients with thalassemia major and other hematological disorders, Nature **201:**1138, 1964.
119. Glucksberg, H., Storb, R., Fefer, A., et al.: Clinical manifestations of GVHD in human recipients of marrow from HL-A matched sibling donors, Transplantation **18:**295, 1974.
120. Gmyrek, D., and Sylm-Rappaport, L.: Analysis of 129 reported cases of Fanconi's anemia, Kinderheilik **91:**297, 1964.
121. Goldstein, J. M., and Coller, B. S.: Aplastic anemia in pregnancy: recovery after normal spontaneous delivery, Ann. Intern. Med. **82:**537, 1975.
122. Goldwater, L. J.: Disturbances in the blood following exposure to benzol, J. Lab. Clin. Med. **26:**957, 1941.
123. Graw, R. G., Herzig, G., Perry, S., et al.: Normal granulocyte transfusion therapy: treatment of septicemia due to gram-negative bacteria, N. Engl. J. Med. **287:**367, 1972.
124. Greenberg, P. L., and Mosny, S. A.: Cytotoxic effects of interferon in vitro on granulocytic progenitor cells, Cancer Res. **37:**1794, 1977.
125. Greenberg, P. L., and Schrier, S. L.: Granulopoiesis in neutropenic disorders, Blood **41:**753, 1973.
126. Haak, H. L., Goselink, H. M., et al.: Acquired aplastic anemia in adults. IV. Histological and CFu studies in transplanted and non-transplanted patients, Scand. J. Haematol. **19:**159, 1977.
127. Hagler, L., Pastore, R. A., and Borgin, J. V.: Aplastic anemia following viral hepatitis: report of two fatal cases and literature, Rev. Med. **54:**139, 1975.
128. Hale, G. S., and de Gruchy, G. C.: Aplastic anemia following the administration of phenylbutazone, Med. J. Aust. **2:**449, 1960.
129. Haley, T. J.: In Szirmai, E., ed.: Nuclear hematology, New York, 1965, Academic Press, Inc.
130. Hamilton, S., and Sheridan, J.: Aplastic anemia and hair dye, Br. Med. J. **1:**834, 1976. (Letter.)
131. Hansen, J. A., Good, R. A., Dupont, B., et al.: HLA-D compatibility between parent and child, Transplantation **23:**366, 1977.
132. Hansen, J. A., O'Reilly, R. J., Good, R. A., and Dupont, B.: Relevance of major human histocompatibility determinants in clinical bone marrow transplantation, Transplant. Proc. **8:**581, 1976.
133. Harris, J. W., and Kellermeyer, R. A.: The red cells, Cambridge, Mass., 1970, Harvard University Press.
134. Hashimoto, Y., Takaku, F., Kosaha, K.: Damaged DNA in lymphocytes of aplastic anemia, Blood **46:**735, 1975.
135. Hast, R., Skorberg, K. O., et al.: Oxymetholone treatment in aregenerative anemia. II. Remission and survival, a prospective study, Scand. J. Haematol. **16:**90, 1976.
136. Hathaway, W. E., Fulginiti, V. A., et al.: Graft vs. host reaction (human runt disease) following a single blood transfusion, J.A.M.A. **201:**1015, 1967.
137. Hathaway, W. E., Githens, J. H., et al.: Aplastic anemia, histiocytosis and erythrodermia in immunologically deficient children, N. Engl. J. Med. **273:**953, 1965.
138. Hayflick, L.: The cell biology of human aging, N. Eng. J. Med. **295:**1302, 1976.
139. Hayflick, L., and Moorhead, P. S.: The serial cultivation of human diploid cell strains, Exp. Cell Res. **25:**585, 1961.

140. Heaton, L. D., Crosby, W. H., and Cohen, A.: Splenectomy in the treatment of hypoplasia of the bone marrow, with a report of twelve cases, Ann. Surg. **146:**637, 1957.

141. Heinecke, H.: Experimentelle untersuchung en uber die einwirkung des roentgenstrahlen aud das knochenmark, nebst einigen bemerkungen uber die roentgentherapie der leukaemie und pseudoleukaemia und das sarkoma, Deut. Z. Chr. **78:**196, 1905.

142. Hellman, S., and Botnick, L. E.: Stem cell depletion: an explanation of the late effects of cytotoxins, Int. J. Radiat. Oncol. Biol. Phys. **2:**181, 1977.

143. Herzig, R. H., Herzig, G. P., et al.: Successful granulocyte transfusion therapy for gram-negative septicemia, N. Engl. J. Med. **296:**701, 1977.

144. Heyn, R. M., Ertel, I. J., and Tuberger, D. G.: Course of acquired aplastic anemia in children treated with supportive care, J.A.M.A. **208:**1372, 1969.

145. Higuroshi, M., and Conen, P. E.: In vitro chromosmal radiosensitivity in Fanconi's anemia, Blood **38:**336, 1971.

146. Hoffman, R., Zanjani, E. D., et al.: Suppression of erythroid-colony formation by lymphocytes from patients with aplastic anemia, N. Engl. J. Med. **296:**10, 1977.

147. Holt, R.: The bacterial degradation of chloramphenicol, Lancet **1:**1259, 1967.

148. Hotta, T., and Yamada, H.: In vitro response of bone marrow cells to erythropoietin in aplastic anemia, Acta Haematol. **52:**265, 1974.

149. Inoue, S., Mekanik, G., Mahallati, M., et al.: Dyskeratosis congenita with pancytopenia, Am. J. Dis. Child **126:**389, 1973.

150. Jacobsen, L. O., Marks, E. K., Robson, M. J., Gaston, E. O., and Zirkle, R. E.: Spleen protection on mortality following X-irradiation, J. Lab. Clin. Med. **34:**1538, 1949.

151. Jacobsen, L. O., Simmons, E. L., et al.: Recovery from radiation injury, Science **113:**510, 1951.

152. Jain, S., and Sherlock, S.: Infectious mononucleosis with jaundice, anaemia and encephalopathy, Br. Med. J. **3:**138, 1975.

153. Jeannet, M., Speck, B., et al.: Autologous marrow reconstitutions in severe aplastic anemia after ALG pretreatment and HL-A semi-incompatible bone marrow cell transfusion, Acta Haematol. **55:**129, 1976.

154. Jeannet, M., Rubinstein, A., et al.: Prolonged remission of severe aplastic anemia after ALG pretreatment and HL-A semi-incompatible bone marrow cell transfusion, Transplant. Proc. **4:**359, 1974.

155. Jones, B., and Thompson, H.: Triphalangeal thumbs associated with hypoplastic anemia, Pediatrics **52:**609, 1973.

156. Jones, M. S., and Jones, O. T. G.: The structural organization of haem synthesis in rat liver mitochondria, Biochem. J. **113:**507, 1969.

157. Kagan, W. A., Ascensao, J., et al.: Aplastic anemia: presence in human bone marrow of cells that suppress myelopoiesis, Proc. Natl. Acad. Sci. **73:**2890, 1976.

158. Kamsu, E., and Erslev, A. J.: Aplastic anemia with "hotpockets," Scand. J. Haematol. **17:**326, 1976.

159. Kaplan, S., Perillie, P. E., and Finch, S. C.: The effect of chloramphenicol on human leukocyte phagocytosis and respiration, Proc. Soc. Exp. Biol. Med. **130:**839, 1969.

160. Katlwasser, J. P., Simmon, G., Werner, E., et al.: Unter suchungen zur hamatotoxizitent von thiamphenicol, Arzneim. Forsch. **24:**343, 1973.

161. Kennedy, B. J., and Nathanson, I. T.: Effects of intensive sex steroid hormone therapy in advanced breast cancer, J.A.M.A. **152:**1135, 1953.

162. Killander, A., Lundmark, K. M., and Sjolin, S.: Idiopathic aplastic anemia in children: results of androgen treatment, Acta Paediatr. Scand. **58:**10, 1969.

163. Kletter, G.: Aplastiche anemien im obduktionsvgut, Wien. Klin. Wochenschr. **84:**145, 1972.

164. Knispel, J. W., et al.: Aplastic anemia in pregnancy: a case report, review of the literature and a re-evaluation of management, Obstet. Gynecol. Surv. **31:**523, 1976.

165. Knospe, W. H., Blom, J., et al.: Regeneration of locally irradiated bone marrow. I. Dose dependent, long-term changes in the rat, with particular emphasis upon vascular and stromal reaction, Blood **28:**398, 1966.

166. Knospe, W. H., and Crosby, W. H.: Aplastic anemia: a disorder of the bone marrow sinusoidal microcirculation rather than stem cell failure, Lancet **2:**20, 1971.

167. Kraemer, K. G., Neiman, P. E., Reeves, W. C., and Thomas, E. D.: Prophylactic adenine arabinoside following marrow transplantation, Transplant, Proc. **10:**237, 1978.

168. Krakoff, I. H., Karnofsky, D. A., and Burchenal, J. H.: Effect of large doses of chloramphenicol on human subjects, N. Engl. J. Med. **253:**7, 1955.

169. Kurland, J., and Moore, M. A.: Modulation of hemopoiesis by prostaglandins, Exp. Hematol. **5:**357, 1977.

170. Kurnick, J. E., Robinson, W. A., and Dickey, C. A.: In vitro granulocytic colony-forming potential of bone marrow from patients with granulocytopenia and aplastic anemia, Proc. Soc. Exp. Biol. Med. **137:**917, 1977.

171. Lachman, A., Lund, E., and Uinther-Poulsen, N.: Severe refractory anemia in pregnancy, Acta Obstet. Gynecol. Scand. **33:**395, 1954.

172. Lange, R. D., McCarthy, J. M., and Gallagher, N. J.: Plasma and urinary erythropoietin in bone marrow failure, Arch. Intern. Med. **108:**850, 1961.

173. Leiken, S. L., Welch, H., and Guin, G. H.: Aplastic anemia due to chloramphenicol, Clin. Proc. Child. Hosp. D.C. **17:**171, 1961.

173a. Lessard, J. L., and Pestka, S.: Studies on the formation of transfer ribonucleic acid–ribosome complexes. XXIII. Chloramphenicol, aminocyte-oligonucleotides, and *Escherichia coli* ribosomes, J. Biol. Chem. **247:**6909, 1972.

174. Lewis, S. M.: Red cell abnormalities and hemolysis in aplastic anemia, Br. J. Haematol. **8:**322, 1962.

175. Lewis, S. M.: Course and prognosis in aplastic anaemia, Br. Med. J. **1:**1027, 1965.

176. Lewis, S. M.: Studies of the erythrocyte in aplastic anemia and other dyserythropoietic disorders, Nouv. Rev. Fr. Hematol. **9:**49, 1969.

177. Lewis, S. M., and Dacie, J. V.: Neutrophil (leucocyte) alkaline phosphatase in paroxysmal nocturnal hemoglobinuria, Br. J. Haemat. **11:**549, 1962.

178. Lewis, S. M., and Dacie, J. V.: The aplastic anemia—paroxysmal nocturnal hemoglobinuria syndrome, Br. J. Haematol. **13:**236, 1967.

179. Lewis, S. M., Grammaticos, P., and Dacie, J. V.: Lysis by anti-I in dyserythropoietic anemias: role of increased uptake of antibody, Br. J. Haematol. **18:**465, 1970.

180. Leyland, M. J., Cunningham, J. L., et al.: A pharmacokinetic study of phenyl butazone-associated hypoplastic anemia, Br. J. Haematol. **28:**142, 1974.

181. Li, F. P., Alter, B. P., and Nathan, D. G.: The mortality of acquired aplastic anemia in children, Blood **40:**153, 1972.

182. Li, F. P., and Nathan, D. G.: Therapy-linked leukaemia, Br. Med. J. **3:**765, 1971.

183. Lohr, G. W., Waller, H. D., et al.: Hexokinasemangel in blutzellen bei einer Sippe mit familiarer Panmyelopathie (Typ Fanconi), Klin. Wochenschr. **43:**870, 1975.

184. Lohrmann, H. P., Kern, P., Nathammer, D., and Hempel, H.: Allogeneic bone marrow transplantation, Lancet **2:**647, 1976.

185. Lohrmann, H. P., Kern, P., et al.: Identification of high risk patients with aplastic anemia in selection for allo-

geneic bone marrow transplantation, Lancet 647, 1976.

186. Lord, B. I., Cercek, L., et al.: Inhibitors of haemo-poietic cell proliferation: specificity of action within the haemopoietic system, Br. J. Cancer **29:**168, 1974.

187. Lorenz, E., and Congdon, C. C.: Modification of lethal irradiation injury in mice by injection of homologous and heterologous bone, J. Natl. Cancer Inst. **14:**955, 1954.

188. Lorenz, E., and Quaisar, K.: Panmyelopathie nach Hepatitis epidemica, Wien Med. Wochenschr. **105:**11, 1955.

189. Lowenthal, R. M., Grossman, L., and Goldman, J. M.: Granulocyte transfusions in treatment of infections in patients with acute leukemia and aplastic anemia, Lancet **1:**353, 1975.

190. Lynch, R. E., Williams, D. M., et al.: The prognosis in aplastic anemia, Blood **45:**517, 1975.

191. Manyan, D. R., Arinura, G. K., and Yunis, A. A.: Chloramphenicol induced erythroid suppression and bone marrow fenochelatase activity in dogs, J. Lab Clin. Med. **79:**137, 1972.

192. Manyan, D. R., and Yunis, A.: The effect of chloramphenicol treatment on ferrochelatase activity in dogs, Biochem. Biophys. Res. Commun. **41:**926, 1970.

193. Martelo, O. J., Manyan, D. R., Smith, V. S., and Yunis, A. A.: Chloramphenicol and bone marrow mitochondria, J. Lab. Clin. Med. **74:**927, 1969.

194. Mathé, G.: Total body irradiation injury: a review of the disorders of the blood and hematopoietic tissues and their therapy. In Szirmai, E., ed.: Nuclear hematology, New York, 1965, Academic Press, Inc.

195. Mathé, G., and Amiel, J. L.: A haematologists approach to modern grafting problems, Br. Med. J. **2:**527, 1964.

196. Mathé, G., Jammet, H., et al.: Transfusions et greffes de moelle osseuse homologue chez des humains irradies a' haute dose accidentellement, Rev. Fr. Etud. Clin. Biol. **4:**226, 1959.

197. Mathé, G., Schwarzenburg, L., Amiel, J. L., et al.: Immunogenetic and immunological proglems of allogeneic haemopoietic radio-chimeras in man, Scand. J. Hematol. **4:**193, 1967.

198. McCulloch, E. A., Siminovitch, L., Till, J. E., et al.: The cellular basis of the genetically determined hemopoietic defect in anemic mice of the genotype Sl-Sld, Blood **26:**399, 1965.

199. McNeil, B. S., et al.: Indium chloride scintigraphy, an index of severity in patients with aplastic anemia, Br. J. Haematol. **34:**599, 1976.

200. Meadows, A. T., Haiman, J. L., and Valdes-Dapena, M.: Hepatoma associated with androgen therapy for aplastic anemia, J. Pediatr. **84:**109, 1974.

201. Mella, B., and Lang, D. J.: Leukocyte mitosis: Suppression in vitro associated with acute infectious hepatitis, Science **155:**80, 1967.

202. Metcalf, D., and Moore, M. A. S.: Senescence of haemopoietic tissues. In frontiers of biology: haemopoietic cells, Amsterdam, 1971, North Holland, Publishing Co.

203. Meuwissen, H. K., Gatti, R. A., Terasaki, P. J., Hong, R., and Good, R. A.: Treatment of lymphopenic hypogammaglobulinemia and bone marrow aplasia by transplantation of allogenic marrow: crucial role of histocompatibility matching, N. Engl. J. Med. **281:**691, 1969.

204. Mickelson, E. M., Fefer, A., and Thomas, E. D.: Aplastic anemia: failure of patient leukocytes to stimulate cells in mixed leukocyte culture, Blood **47:**793, 1976.

205. Miller, M. E.: Thymic dysplasia ("Swiss agammaglobinemia"). I. Graft vs. host reaction following bone marrow transfusion, J. Pediatr. **70:**730, 1967.

206. Miller, W. V., and Grumet, F. C., eds.: HLA typing. Washington, D.C., 1976, American Association of Blood Banks.

207. Mills, S. D., Kyle, R. A., et al.: Bone marrow transplant in an identical twin, J.A.M.A. **188:**1037, 1964.

208. Minagi, H. J., and Steinbach, H.: Roentgen appearance of anomalies associated with hypoplastic anemia of childhood: Fanconi's anemai and congenital hypoplastic anemia (erythrogenesis imperfecta), Am. J. Roentgenol. **97:**100, 1966.

209. Mittal, K. K., Ruder, E. A., and Green, D.: Matching of histocompatibility (HL-A) antigens for platelet transfusion, Blood **47:**31, 1976.

210. Mohler, D. N., and Learell, B. S.: Aplastic anemia: an analysis of 50 cases, Ann. Intern. Med. **49:**326, 1958.

211. Moore, M. A. S., and Spitzer, G.: In vitro studies in the myeloproliferative disorders. In Lymphocyte recognition and effector mechanisms. In Proceedings of the 8th leukocyte culture congress, New York, 1974, Academic Press, Inc.

212. Moore, M. A. S., Spitzer, G., Williams, N., et al.: Agar culture studies in 127 cases of untreated acute leukemia: the prognostic value of reclassification of leukemia according to in vitro growth characteristics, Blood **44:**1, 1974.

213. Morely, A., Remes, J., and Trainor, K.: A controlled trial of androgen therapy in experimental chronic hypoplastic marrow failure, Br. J. Haematol. **32:**533, 1976.

214. Morgan, K. Z., and Turner, J. E.: Principles of radiation protection, New York, 1967, John Wiley & Sons, Inc.

215. Morrison, M., and Samwick, A. A.: Intramedullary (sternal) transfusion of human bone marrow, J.A.M.A. **115:**1708, 1940.

216. Muller-Berat, C. N., van Putten, L. M., and van Bekkum, D. W.: Cytostatic drugs in the treatment of secondary disease following homologous bone marrow transplantation: extrapolation from the mouse to the primate, Ann. N.Y. Acad. Sci. **129:**340, 1966.

217. Muller-Ruchholtz, W., Wottge, H. U., and Muller-Hermelink, H. K.: Modulation of immune reactions by antilymphocyte serum, Transplant. Proc. **10:**23, 1978.

218. Muller-Ruchholtz, H., Wottge, H.-U., and Muller-Hermelink, H. K.: Bone marrow transplantation in rats across strong histocompatibility barriers by selective elimination of lymphoid cells in donor marrow, Transpl. Proc. **8:**537, 1976.

219. Murphy, S., and Lubin, B.: Triphalangeal thumbs and congenital erythroid hypoplasia: report of a case with unusual features, J. Pediatr. **81:**987, 1972.

220. Naegli, O.: Blutkrankheiten und blutdiagnostik, 5 Augl., Julius Springer, 1931.

221. Nagao, T., Mauer, A. M.: Concordance for drug induced aplastic anemia in identical twins, N. Engl. J. Med. **261:**119, 1959.

222. Naiman, J. L., Punnett, H. H., Lischner, H. W., et al.: Possible graft-versus-host reaction after intrauterine transfusion for HR erythroblastosis foetalis, N. Engl. J. Med. **281:**697, 1969.

223. Najean, Y., Meens-Bith, L., et al.: Isotopic study of erythrokinetics in 31 cases of chronic idiopathic pancytopenia with histologically normal or rich marrow, Sang **30:**101, 1959.

224. National Council on Radiation Protection and Measurements: N.C.R.P. Report, p. 33, 1969.

225. Neely, J. E., Neely, A. N., and Kersey, J. H.: Immunodeficiency following human marrow transplantation: in vitro studies, Transpl. Proc. **10:**229, 1978.

226. Neiman, P. E., Reeves, W., Ray, G., Flournoy, N., Lerner, K. G., et al.: A prospective analysis of interstitial pneumonia and opportunistic viral infection among recipients of allogeneic bone marrow grafts, J. Infect. Dis. **136:**754, 1977.

227. Nelson, E. R., and Bierman, H. R.: Dengue feur: a thrombocytopenic disease, J.A.M.A. **190**:99, 1964.
228. Nelson, M., Levy, J., and Robertson, J.: Fanconi's aplastic anemia, Ir. J. Med. **6**:119, 1964.
229. Nijhof, W., and Krron, A. M.: The interference of chloramphenicol and thiamphenicol with the biogenesis of mitochondria on animal tissues: a possible clue to the toxic action, Postgrad. Med. J. **50**(suppl. 5):53, 1974.
230. Nissen, C., Emodi, G., et al.: In vitro cytotoxicity of human interferon, Exp. Hematol. **4**:21A, 1976.
231. Nissen, C., Speck, B., Emodi, G., et al.: Toxicity of human leucocyte interferon preparation in human bone marrow cultures, Lancet **1**:203, 1977. (Letter.)
232. O'Gorman-Hughes, D. W.: Aplastic anemia in childhood: a reappraisal, classification and assessment, Med. J. Aust. **1**:1059, 1969.
233. Olding, L. B., Jensen, F. C., and Oldstone, M. B. A.: Pathogenesis of cytomegalovirus infection. I. Activation of virus from bone marrow-derived lymphocytes by in vitro allogenic reaction, J. Exp. Med. **141**:561, 1975.
234. Opalinski, A., and Beutler, E.: Creatinine, 2,3-diphosphoglycerate and anemia, N. Engl. J. Med. **285**:483, 1971.
235. Opelz, G., Gale, R. P., et al.: Significance of HLA and non-HLA antigens in bone marrow transplantation, Transplant. Proc. **10**:43, 1978.
236. O'Reilly, R. J., Dupont, B., et al.: Reconstitution in severe combined immunodeficiency by transplantation of marrow from an unrelated donor, N. Engl. J. Med. **297**:1311, 1977.
237. O'Reilly, R. J., Everson, L. K., et al.: Effects of exogenous interferon on cytomegalovirus infections complicating bone marrow transplantation, Clin. Immunol. Immunopathol. **6**:51, 1976.
238. O'Reilly, R. J., Pahwa, R., Dupont, B., and Good, R. A.: Severe combined immunodeficiency: transplantation approaches for patients lacking an HLA genotypically identical sibling, Transplant. Proc. **10**:187, 1978.
239. O'Reilly, R. J., Pawha, R., Kagan, W., et al.: Reconstitution of hematopoietic function in posthepatic aplasia following high-dose cyclophosphamide and allogeneic fetal liver, Exp. Hematol. **5**(suppl. 2):46, 1977.
240. O'Reilly, R. J., Pahwa, R., Kirkpatrick, D., et al.: Sustained engraftment and hematologic reconstitution following transplantation of marrow from an HLA-A, B mismatched, HLA-D heterozygous sibling donor into an HLA-D homozygous patient with aplastic anemia, Proc. 7th Int. Congr. Transplant. Soc., Rome, 1978.
241. Osgood, E. E., Riddle, M. C., Mathews, T. J.: Aplastic anemia treated with daily transfusions and intravenous marrow, Ann. Intern. Med. **13**:357, 1939.
242. Pagliardi, G. L., Agiletta, M., Foa, R., et al.: Colony stimulating activity (CSA) in aplastic anemia, Exp. Hematol. **5**(suppl. 2):98, 1977.
242a. Pahwa, S. G., et al.: Phagocytic function in aplastic anemia: studies before and after bone marrow transplantation (BMT), Exp. Hematol. **5**(suppl. 2):83, 1977.
243. Palva, I. P., and Wasastjerna, C.: Treatment of aplastic anemia with methenolone, Acta Haematol. **47**:13, 1972.
244. Parkman, R., Rosen, F. S., Rappaport, J., et al.: Detection of genetically determined histocompatibility antigen differences between HL-A identical and MLC nonreactive siblings, Transplantation **21**:110, 1976.
245. Paukovits, W. R.: Granulopoiesis-inhibiting factor: demonstration and preliminary chemical and biological characterization of a specific polypeptide (chalone), Nat. Cancer Inst. Monogr. **38**:147, 1973.
245a. Pestka, S.: Studies on the formation of transfer ribonucleic acid–ribosome complexes. VIII. Survey of the effect of antibiotics on N-acetyl-phenylalanyl-puromycin formation: possible mechanism of chloramphenicol action, Arch. Biochem. Biophys. **136**:80, 1970.
246. Pierre, R. V.: Pre-leukemic state, Semin. Hematol. **11**:73, 1974.
247. Pillow, R. P., Epstein, R. B., et al.: Treatment of bone marrow failure by isogeneic marrow infusion, N. Engl. J. Med. **275**:94, 1966.
248. Pisciotta, A. V.: Drug-induced leukopenia and aplastic anemia, Clin. Pharmacol. Ther. **12**:13, 1971.
249. Plotkin, S. A., Farquhar, J., and Hornberger, E.: Clinical trials of immunization with the Towne 125 strain of human cytomegalovirus, J. Infect. Dis. **134**:470, 1976.
250. Pochedly, C.: Fanconi's anemia: clues to early recognition, Clin. Pediatr. **11**:20, 1972.
251. Pochedly, C., Collipp, P. J., Wolman, S. R., et al.: Fanconi's anemia with growth hormone deficiency, J. Pediatr. **79**:93, 1971.
252. Pochedly, C., Vernick, S., Collipp, P. J., et al.: Red cell defects in Fanconi's anemia, Mt. Sinai J. Med. **39**:592, 1972.
253. Pollard, E. C.: The biological action of ionizing radiation, Ann. Sci. **57**:206, 1967.
254. Pollard, R. B., and Merigan, T. C.: Perspectives for the control of cytomegalovirus infections in bone marrow transplant recipients, Transplant. Proc. **10**:241, 1978.
255. Poon, P. K., O'Brien, R. L., and Parker, J. W.: Defective DNA repair in Fanconi's anemia, Nature **250**:223, 1974.
256. Powars, D.: Aplastic anemia secondary to glue sniffing, N. Engl. J. Med. **273**:700, 1965.
257. Ragab, A. H., Gilberson, F., et al.: Granulopoiesis in childhood aplastic anemia, J. Pediatr. **88**:790, 1976.
258. Rainbow, A. J., and Howes, M.: Defective repair of ultraviolet and gamma-ray damaged DNA in Fanconi's anemia, Int. J. Radiat. Biol. **31**:191, 1977.
259. Rappeport, J., Parkman, R., et al.: Successful bone marrow transplantation of presensitized recipients with severe aplastic anemia after multi-agent immunosuppression, Blood **50**:315, 1977.
260. Registry of Adverse Reactions, Panel on Hematology, Council on Drugs, April-May 1965, June 1967, American Medical Association.
261. Reisner, Y., Itzkovitch, L., Meshorer, A., and Sharon, N.: Fractionation of murine spleen and bone marrow cells by lectins: a new approach for blood transplantation. (In press.)
262. Reizenstein, P., and Lagarlof, B.: Aregenerative anemia with hypercellular sideroblastic marrow: a preleukemic condition, Acta Haematol. **47**:1, 1972.
263. Rendi, R.: The effect of chloramphenicol on the incorporation of labelled amino acids into proteins by isolated subcellular fractions from rat liver, Exp. Cell Res. **18**:187, 1959.
264. Reynafarje, C., and Faura, J.: Erythrokinetics in the treatment of aplastic anemia with methandrostenolone, Arch. Intern. Med. **120**:654, 1967.
265. Rich, M. L., Ritterhof, R. J., and Hoffman, R. J.: A fatal case of aplastic anemia following chloramphenicol (chloromycetin) therapy, Ann. Intern. Med. **33**:1459, 1950.
266. Rich, R. R., Kilpatrick, C. H., and Smith, T. K.: Simultaneous suppression of responses to allogeneic tissue in vitro and in vivo, Cell Immunol. **5**:190, 1972.
267. Richie, E. R., Gallagher, M. T., and Trentin, J. J.: Inhibition of the graft-versus-host reactions, Transplantation **15**:486, 1973.
268. Robbins, M. M.: Aplastic anemia secondary to anticonvulsant, Am. J. Dis. Child **104**:614, 1962.
269. Robinson, J. R., Felton, J. S., Levitt, R. C., et al.: Relationship between ''aromatic hydrocarbon responsiveness'' and the survival times in mice treated with various drugs and environmental compounds, Molecular Pharm. **11**:850, 1975.

270. Rohr, K.: Familial panmyelophthisis, Blood **4:**130, 1949.
271. Romano, T. J., Nowakowski, M., Bloom, B. R., et al.: Selective viral immunosuppression of the graft-versus-host reaction, J. Exp. Med. **145:**666, 1977.
272. Rondanelli, E. G., Gorni, P., and Magliurlo, E.: Chloramphenicol and erythropoiesis, Acta Haematol. **34:**321, 1965.
273. Rosenbach, L., Caviles, A., and Mteus, W. J.: Chloramphenicol toxicity: reversible vacuolation of erythroid cells, N. Engl. J. Med. **263:**724, 1960.
274. Rosse, W., and Dacie, J. V.: Immune lysis of normal human and paroxysmal nocturnal hemoglobinuria (PNH) red blood cells. I. The sensitivity of PNH red cells to lysis by complement and specific antibody, J. Clin. Invest. **45:**736, 1966.
275. Rovinsky, J. J.: Primary refractory anemia complicating pregnancy and delivery, Obstet. Gynecol. Surv. **14:**149, 1959.
276. Royal Marsden Hospital Bone Marrow Transplantation Team: Lancet **2:**742, 1977.
277. Rubin, D., Weissberger, A. S., and Clark, D. R.: Early detection of drug induced erythropoietic depression, J. Lab. Clin. Med. **56:**453, 1960.
278. Rubin, D., Weissberger, A. A., et al.: Changes in iron metabolism in early chloramphenicol toxicity, J. Clin. Invest. **37:**1286, 1958.
279. Rubin, E., Gottlieb, C., and Vogel, P.: Syndrome of hepatitis and aplastic anemia, Am. J. Med. **45:**88, 1968.
280. Rubin, P., Landman, S., Mayer, E., et al.: Bone marrow regeneration and extension after extended field irradiation in hodgkin's disease, Cancer **32:**699, 1973.
281. Rytömaa, T.: Role of chalone in granulopoiesis, Br. J. Hematol. **24:**141, 1973. (Annotation.)
282. Salmon, S. E., Krakauer, R. S., and Whitmore, W. F.: Lymphocyte stimulation: selective destruction of cells during blastogenic response to transplantation antigens, Science **172:**490, 1971.
283. Sanchez-Medal, L., and Gomez-Leal, A.: Anabolic androgenic steroids in the treatment of acquired aplastic anemia, Blood **34:**283, 1969.
284. Sanchez-Medal, L., Pizzuto, J., et al.: Effect of oxymethalone in refractory anemia, Arch. Intern. Med. **113:**721, 1964.
285. Santos, G. W.: Immunosuppression for clinical marrow transplantation, Semin. Hematol. **11:**341, 1974.
286. Sasli, M. S., and Tonomura, A.: A high susceptibility of fanconi's anemia to chromosome breaks by DNA cross linking agents, Cancer Res. **33:**1829, 1973.
287. Schiffer, L. M., Brann, I., et al.: Iron absorption and excretion in aregenerative anemia, Acta Haematol. **35:**80, 1966.
288. Schmid, W.: Familial constitutional panmyelocytopathy, Fanconi's anemia (F.A.). II. A discussion of the cytogenetic findings in Fanconi's anemia, Semin Hematol. **4:**241, 1967.
289. Schroeder, T. M., Anshinitz, F., and Knopp, A.: Spontane chromosomen aberrationen bei familiares panmyelopathie, Humangenetik **1:**194, 1964.
290. Scott, J. L., Cartwright, G. E., and Wintrobe, M. M.: Acquired aplastic anemia: an analysis of 39 cases and review of the pertinent literature, Medicine **38:**119, 1959.
291. Scott, J. L., Feingold, S. M., Belkin, G. A., et al.: A controlled double blind study of the hematologic toxicity of chloramphenicol, N. Engl. J. Med. **272:**1137, 1965.
292. Sensenbrenner, L. L., Steele, D. A., and Santos, G. W.: Recovery of hematologic competence without engraftment following attempted bone marrow transplantation for aplastic anemia: report of a case with diffusion chamber studies, Exp. Hematol. **5:**51, 1977.
292a. Shahidi, N. T.: Aplastic and congenital hypoplastic anemias. In Gellis, S. S., and Kagan, B. M., eds.: Current pediatric therapy, Philadelphia, 1964, W. B. Saunders Co.
293. Shahidi, N. T., and Diamond, L. K.: Testosterone-induced remission in aplastic anemia of both acquired and congenital types, N. Engl. J. Med. **264:**953, 1961.
294. Shahidi, N. T., and Diamond, L. K.: Testosterone induced remission in aplastic anemia, Am. J. Dis. Child. **98:**293, 1959.
295. Shahidi, N. T., Gerald, P. S., and Diamond, L. K.: Alkali resistant hemoglobin in aplastic anemia of both acquired and congenital type, N. Engl. J. Med. **266:**117, 1962.
296. Shearer, G. M., Cudkowicz, G., Schmitt-Verhulst, A. M., et al.: F₁ hybrid anti-parental cell-mediated lympholysis to alloantigens. In Forty-first Cold Spring Harbor Symposium on Lymphocyte Diversity, June, 1976.
297. Shwachman, H., Diamond, L. K., Oski, F. A., and Khaw, K. T.: The syndrome of pancreatic insufficiency and bone marrow dysfunction, J. Pediatr. **65:**645, 1964.
298. Singer, J. W., Brown, J. E., James, M. C., et al.: The effect of lymphocytes from patients with aplastic anemia on marrow granulocytic colony growth from HLA matched and mismatched marrows: the effect of transfusion sensitization. (In press.)
299. Simonson, J.: Graft versus host reactions. Their natural history, and applicability as tools of research, Prog. Allergy **6:**349, 1962.
300. Skorberg, K. O., Engstedt, L., et al.: Oxymethalone treatment in hypoproliferate anemia, Acta Haematol. **49:**321, 1973.
301. Slavin, S., Fuks, Z., Kaplan, H. S., and Strober, S.: Transplantation of allogeneic bone marrow without graft versus host disease using total lymphoid irradiation, J. Exp. Med. **147:**963, 1978.
302. Smick, K., Conpit, P. K., et al.: Fatal aplastic anemia: an epidemiological study of its relationship to the drug chloramphenicol, J. Chron. Dis. **17:**899, 1964.
303. Smiley, R. K., Cartwright, G. E., and Wintrobe, M. M.: Fatal aplastic anemia following chloramphenicol (chloromyetin) administration, J.A.M.A. **149:**914, 1952.
304. Speck, B., Cornu, P., Nissen, C., et al.: On the immune pathogenesis of aplastic anemia, Exp. Hematol. **5**(suppl. 2):2, 1977.
305. Speck, B., Cornu, J., et al.: Immunologic aspects of aplasia, Transplant. Proc. **10:**131, 1978.
306. Speck, B., Cornu, P., et al.: Autologous marrow recovery following allogeneic marrow transplantation in a patient with severe aplastic anemia, Exp. Haematol. **4:**131, 1976.
307. Speck, B., Gluckman, E., et al.: Treatment of aplastic anemia by antilymphocyte globulin with and without allogeneic bone marrow infusions, Lancet **2:**1145, 1977.
308. Stier, W., Van Voolen, G. A., and Selmanowitz, U. J.: Dyskeratosis congenita: relationship to Fanconi's anemia, Blood **39:**510, 1972.
309. Storb, R., Epstein, R. B., et al.: Methotrexate regimens for control of graft-versus-host disease in dogs with allogeneic marrow grafts, Transplantation **9:**240, 1970.
310. Storb, R., Epstein, R. B., Rudolph, R. H., et al.: The effect of prior transfusions on marrow grafts between histocompatible canine siblings, J. Immunol. **105:**627, 1970.
311. Storb, R., Floersheim, G. L., Weiden, P. L., et al.: Effect of prior blood transfusions on marrow grafts: abrogation of sensitization by procarbazine and anti-thymocyte serum, J. Immunol. **112:**1508, 1974.
312. Storb, R., Gluckman, E., et al.: Treatment of established graft-versus-host disease by antithymocyte globulin, Blood **44:**57, 1974.
313. Storb, R., Ochs, H. D., Weiden, P. L., and Thomas,

E. D.: Immunologic reactivity in marrow graft recipients. Transplant. Proc. **8:**637, 1976.

314. Storb, R., Prentice, R. L., and Thomas, E. D.: Marrow transplantation for aplastic anemia: factors associated with rejection, N. Engl. J. Med. **296:**61, 1977.

315. Storb, R., Prentice, R. L., and Thomas, E. D.: Treatment of aplastic anemia by marrow transplantation from HLA identical siblings: prognostic factors associated with GVHD and survival, J. Clin. Invest. **59:**625, 1977.

316. Storb, R., Rudolph, R. H., Graham, T. C., et al.: The influence of transfusions from unrelated donors upon marrow grafts between histocompatible canine siblings, J. Immunol. **107:**409, 1971.

317. Storb, R., Thomas, E. D., et al.: Marrow transplantation in untransfused patients with severe aplastic anemia. Blood **50:**316, 1977.

318. Storb, R., Thomas, E. D., et al.: Aplastic anemia treated by allogeneic bone marrow transplantation: a report on 49 new cases from Seattle, Blood **48:**817, 1976.

319. Storb, R., Thomas, E. D., Buckner, C. D., et al.: Allogeneic marrow grafting for treatment of aplastic anemia: a follow-up on long-term survivors, Blood **48:**485, 1976.

320. Storb, R., Thomas, E. D., Weiden, P. L., et al.: One hundred-ten patients with aplastic anemia treated by marrow transplantation in Seattle, Transplant. Proc. **10:** 135, 1978.

321. Storb, R., Weiden, P. L., Graham, T. C., et al.: Marrow grafts between unrelated dogs homozygous and identical for DLA antigens, Transplant. Proc. **9:**281, 1977.

322. Storb, R., Weiden, P. L., Graham, T. C., et al.: Hemopoietic grafts between DLA-identical canine littermates following dimethyl myleran: evidence for resistance to grafts not associated with DLA and abrogated by antithymocyte serum, Transplantation **24:**349, 1977.

322a. Storb, R., et al.: Personal communication.

323. Swift, M.: Fanconi's anemia in the genetics of neoplasia, Nature **230:**371, 1971.

324. Swift, M. R., and Hirschhorn, K.: Fanconi's anemia inherited susceptibility to chromosome breakage in various tissues, Ann. Intern. Med. **65:**495, 1966.

325. Swift, M., Sholman, L., and Gilmour, D.: Diabetes mellatus and the gene for Fanconi's anemia, Science **178:**308, 1971.

326. Territo, M. C.: Autologous bone marrow repopulation following high dose cyclophosphamide and allogeneic marrow transplantation in aplastic anemia (for the UCLA Bone Marrow Transplant Team), Br. J. Haematol. **36:** 305, 1977.

327. Thomas, E. D., Buckner, C. D., et al.: One hundred patients with acute leukemia treated by chemotherapy, total body irradiation, and allogeneic marrow transplantation, Blood **49:**511, 1977.

328. Thomas, E. D., Collins, J. A., Herman, E. C., and Ferrebee, J. W.: Marrow transplants in lethally irradiated dogs given methotrexate, Blood **19:**217, 1962.

329. Thomas, E. D., Lochte, H. L., and Ferrebee, J. W.: Irradiation of the entire body and marrow transplantation: some observations and comments, Blood **14:**1, 1959.

330. Thomas, E. D., Lochte, H. L., et al.: Treatment of acute leukemia by supralethal whole-body irradiation and isolgous marrow transplantation, J. Clin. Invest. **38:**1048, 1959.

331. Thomas, E. D., and Storb, R.: Technique for human marrow grafting, Blood **36:**507, 1970.

332. Thomas, E. D., Storb, R., Clift, R. A., et al.: Bone marrow transplantation. Part 2, N. Engl. J. Med. **292:**895, 1975.

333. Thomas, E. D., Storb, R., Clift, R. A., et al.: Bone marrow transplantation. N. Engl. J. Med. **292:**832, 1975.

334. Thomas, E. D., Storb, R., et al.: Recovery from A.A. following attempted marrow transplantation, Exp. Hematol. **4:**97, 1976.

335. Thompson, W. P., Richter, M. N., and Edsall, K. S.: An analysis of so called aplastic anemia, Am. J. Med. Sci. **187:**77, 1934.

336. Thorsby, E.: The human major histocompatibility system, Transplant. Rev. **18:**51, 1974.

337. Todaro, G., Green, H., and Swift, M. D.: Susceptibility of human diploid fibroblast strains to transformation by SV 40 virus, Science **153:**1252, 1966.

338. Twomey, J. J., Douglas, C. C., and Starkey, O.: The monocytopenia of aplastic anemia, Blood **41:**187, 1973.

339. Tyan, M. L.: Modification of bone marrow induced GVH disease with heterologous antisera to γ globulin or whole serum, Immunology **106:**586, 1971.

340. Tyan, M. L.: Modification of severe graft-versus-host disease with antisera to the θ antigen or to whole serum, Transplantation **15:**601, 1973.

341. Uehlinger, E.: Konstitutionelle infantile (pernicasaartige) anamie, Klin. Wochenschr. **82:**1501, 1929.

342. van Bekkum, D. A., Balner, H., et al.: The effect of pretreatment of allogeneic bone marrow graft recipients with antilymphocytic serum on the acute graft-versus-host reactions in monkeys, Transplantation **13:**400, 1972.

343. van Bekkum, D. W., and DeVries, M. J.: In Radiation chimaeras, London, 1967, Logos Press.

344. van Doornik, M. C., van de Veer-Kortuf, E. T., et al.: Fatal aplastic anemia complicating infectious mononucleosis, Scand. J. Haematol **20:**52, 1978.

345. Verhest, A., et al.: Specificity of the 5_q-chromosome in a distinct type of refractory anemia, J. Natl. Cancer Inst. **56:**1053, 1976.

346. Vigliani, E. C., and Forni, A.: Benzene chromosome changes and leukemia, J. Occup. Med. **11:**148, 1969.

347. von Boehmer, H., Sprent, J., and Nabholz, M.: Tolerance to histocompatibility determinants in tetraparental bone marrow chimeras, J. Exp. Med. **141:**322, 1975.

348. Wald, W., Thoma, F. E., and Brown, G.: Hematologic manifestations of radiation exposure in man, Prog. Hematol. **3:**1, 1962.

349. Wallerstein, R. O., Condit, P. K., et al.: Statewide study of chloramphenicol therapy and aplastic anemia, J.A.M.A. **208:**2045, 1969.

350. Warren, R. P., Storb, R., Weiden, P. L., et al.: Direct and antibody-dependent cell-mediated cytotoxicity against HLA identical sibling lymphocytes: correlation with marrow graft rejection. (In press.)

351. Weber, W., Speck, B., Cornu, P., et al.: Failure of isogenic marrow engraftment in a patient with acute leukemia, Acta. Hematol. **56:**338, 1976.

352. Weiden, P. L., Doney, K., Storb, R., and Thomas, E. D.: Anti-human thymocyte globulin (ATG) for prophylaxis and treatment of graft-versus-host disease in recipients of allogeneic marrow grafts, Transplant. Proc. **10:**213, 1978.

353. Weisberger, A. S., and Wolfe, S.: Effect of chloramphenicol on protein synthesis, Fed. Proc. **23:**976, 1964.

354. Weisberger, A. S., Wolfe, S., and Armentrout, S.: Inhibition of protein synthesis in mammalian cell free systems by chloramphenicol, J. Exp. Med. **120:**A161, 1964.

355. Williams, D. M., Lynch, R. E., et al.: Drug-induced aplastic anemia, Semin. Hematol. **10:**195, 1973.

356. Winston, D. J., Meyer, D. V., Gale, R. P., et al.: Further experience with infections in bone marrow transplant recipients, Transplant. Proc. **10:**247, 1978.

357. Wissman, C. L., Jr., Smadel, J. E., et al.: Mode of action of chloramphenicol. I. Activity of chloramphenicol on assimilation of ammonia and/or synthesis of proteins and nucleic acids in *Escherichia coli,* J. Bacteriol. **67:**662, 1954.

358. Witherspoon, R., Noel, D., Storb, R., et al.: The effect of graft-versus-host disease on reconstitution of the immune system following marrow transplantation for aplastic anemia or leukemia, Transplant. Proc. **10**:233, 1978.

359. Wolf, J. A.: Anemias caused by infections and toxins, idiopathic aplastic anemia caused by renal disease, Pediatr. Clin. North Am. **4**:469, 1957.

360. Woodruff, J. M., Hansen, J. A., Good, R. A., et al.: The pathology of the graft-versus-host reaction (GVHR) in adults receiving bone marrow transplants, Transplant. Proc. **8**:675, 1976.

361. Worlledge, S. M., and Dacie, J. V.: Haemolytic and other anaemias in infectious mononucleosis. In Carter, R. L., and Penman, H. G., eds.: Infectious mononucleosis, Oxford, 1969, Blackwell Scientific Publications, Ltd.

362. Worton, R. G., McCullogh, E. A., and Till, J. E.: Physical separation of hemopoietic stem cells differing in their capacity for self renewal, J. Exp. Med. **130**:91, 1969.

363. Young, L. S., and Armstrong, D.: Human immunity to *Pseudomonas aeruginosa*. I. In-vitro interaction of bacteria, polymorphonuclear leukocytes, and serum factors, J. Infect. Dis. **126**:257, 1972.

364. Yunis, A. A.: Chloramphenicol toxicity. In Blood disorders due to drugs and other agents. In Goodwood, R. H., ed.: Amsterdam, 1973, Excerpta Medica.

365. Yunis, A. A., Arimura, G. K., et al.: Comparative metabolic effects of chloramphenicol and thiamphenicol in mammalian cells, Postgrad. Med. J. **50**(suppl. 5):60, 1974.

366. Yunis, A. A., and Bloomberg, G. R.: Chloramphenicol toxicity: clinical feature and pathogenesis, Prog. Haematol. **4**:138, 1964.

367. Yunis, A. A., and Harrington, W. J.: Patterns of inhibition of chloramphenicol of nucleic acid synthesis in human bone marrow and leukemic cells, J. Lab. Clin. Med. **56**:831, 1960.

368. Zachman, M., Illig, R., and Prader, A.: Fanconi's anemia with isolated growth hormone deficiency, J. Pediatr. **80**:159, 1972.

369. Zoschke, D. C., and Bach, F. H.: Specificity of antigen recognition by human lymphocytes in vitro, Science **170**:1404, 1970.

18 □ Disorders of granulopoiesis

Robert L. Baehner

GRANULOCYTE MORPHOLOGY
Stem cell

The proliferation of the committed stem cell in the bone marrow in a variety of environmental and intrinsic conditions leads to the generation of three recognizable granulocytic cell lines—the neutrophil, the eosinophil, and the basophil—as well as to monocyte.[58] Although neither the pleuripotent stem cell nor the committed stem cell are clearly recognizable, these cells have been found in association with the population of small mononuclear leukocytes resembling lymphocytes in the bone marrow.[197] The basis for pleuripotency and committed potency of certain stem cells was first confirmed by Till and McCulloch[290] who injected syngeneic bone marrow into lethally irradiated mice and then observed colonies arising from single progenitor cells to be either mixtures or pure colonies of granulocytes, erythrocytes, and megakaryocytes. More evidence for pluripotency stems from the observation that the Philadelphia chromosome of chronic myelogenous leukemia has been noted in dividing granulocytic, erythroid, and megakaryocytic precursors.[312] The stem cell continually renews its own compartment while proliferating daughter cells of additional maturity.

Neutrophil

The myeloblast, the earliest recognizable myeloid precursor, is identified by a large, round to slightly oval nucleus relative to the volume of the cytoplasm with one or more prominent nucleoli. The nuclear membrane is smooth without condensation of chromatin; the cytoplasm is dark blue and lacks cytoplasmic organelles. Less than 5% of the myeloid cells are myeloblasts. The myeloblast proliferates during the next 24 hours, giving rise to promyelocytes that contain cytoplasmic azurophilic or pink granules, often overlaying and obscuring the nucleus. The nucleoli remain but the chromatin network of the nucleus is coarse. Cytoplasmic basophilia is still prominent because of a rich complement of ribosomes. Azurophilic granules contain myeloperoxidase, arginine-rich basic cationic protein, sulfated mucopolysaccharides, acid phosphatase, and other hydrolases.[15] Subsequent cell divisions reduce the concentration of primary azurophilic granules as they are parceled out to the daughter myelocytes, which in turn undergo three divisions. The maturing myelocytic nucleus becomes smaller and oval and assumes an eccentric position; nucleoli are no longer visible and the nuclear chromatin is even more condensed. The cytoplasm loses its basophilia, and specific or secondary granules containing lactoferrin and lysozyme (muramidase) become evident. Alkaline phosphatase, a specific granule enzyme in the rabbit heterophil, is found in the microsomal fraction of human polymorphonuclear neutrophils.[16] The granulocytic maturational pool consists of the metamyelocyte with its indented nucleus, which elongates to a horseshoe bilobed shape in the band form and finally to the trilobed and quadralobed neutrophils. A bone marrow aspirate fixed and stained with Wright's stain reveals a predominance of granulocytic precursors relative to nucleated erythroid cells; the myeloid:erythroid ratio ranges between 2:1 and 4:1.

Eosinophil

The eosinophil shares morphologic features with the neutrophil, but their surface antigenicity, enzymes, and longevity in the circulation differ.[8,58] The eosinophil was first described by Jones more than 125 years ago.[142] In 1879 Ehrlich noted the affinity of the coarse granules for acid dyes and coined the term "eosinophil." Eosinophils and neutrophils are derived from a common hematopoietic precursor cell type and have similar bone marrow maturation characteristics.[71] The eosinophilic promyelocyte is the earliest identifiable cell of this series. As maturation proceeds, the eosinophilic granules become more prominent and numerous; by the myelocyte stage of development azurophilic granules are no longer seen and only the characteristic eosinophilic granules remain. The eosinophilic metamyelocyte and band forms are slightly smaller than their antecedent myelocytes and generally contain fewer granules. The mature eosinophil has a bilobed nucleus[325] with prominent eosinophilic granules containing peroxidase, PAS-reactive material, acid phosphatase, β-glucuronidase, cathepsin, aryl sulfatase, ribonuclease and deoxyribonuclease, and kininase but not alkaline phosphatase, lysozyme, or histamine.[7,58]

By transmission electron microscopy the crystalloid granules are shown to have peroxidase activity rimming the core that is antigenically and spectrographically different from neutrophil and monocyte peroxidase. More recently genetic dissociation of peroxidase was shown in two siblings whose eosinophils lacked peroxidase although their neutrophils and monocytes stained positive for it. Conversely patients with myeloperoxidase deficiency of the polymorphonuclear neutrophil have normal eosinophil peroxidase activity.[46,110,246] Eosinophil granules also contain zinc and basic protein high in arginine content, accounting for 55% of the total granule protein, but the isolated granules lack antihistamine activity and antibacterial activity and do not increase vascular permeability or contract guinea pig ileum. Between 1% and 3% of myeloid cells are eosinophils in the blood, and there are three times more eosinophils in the bone marrow compared to the relative numbers in the blood.[227]

Basophil

The basophil shares many characteristics with tissue mast cells. In Wright's stained preparations basophils are distinguished by the purple or bluish granules that fill the cytoplasm and partially cover the nucleus. The precursor of the blood basophil generally has been presumed to reside in the bone marrow. Although less clear than that of eosinophils, basophilic differentiation from a pleuripotent granulocyte precursor probably occurs at the promyelocyte stage of development when large, round granules first appear.

Basophil granules contain abundant acid mucopolysaccharides, including heparin and histamine; however, the acid hydrolases, alkaline phosphatase and peroxidase, have not been found in basophil granules.[83] Basophils are the least numerous granulocytes, accounting for 0.5% to 1.0% of blood leukocytes and bone marrow nucleated cells.[146]

GRANULOCYTE DIFFERENTIATION AND KINETICS
Stem cell

Recent studies using the in vitro agar culture technique provide evidence that the committed stem cell is under hormonal control. The double layer technique for culture of human bone marrow is provided in Fig. 18-1.[74,136] The more solid underlayer contains cells or fluid known to elaborate or contain colony stimulating activity, or factor (CSA, or CSF).[137,196] Single cell suspensions from bone marrow are dispersed in the softer overlayer. Proliferation begins and discreet colonies are evident after a 10- to 14-day period of in-

cubation. Colonies may be of granulocytic lines or monocyte-macrophage lines with some colonies being mixed in nature. The committed stem cell that gives rise to these colonies is known as the colony forming unit cell (CFU-C), while the pleuripotent stem cell populating the spleen and bone marrow of lethally irradiated rats is known as the colony forming unit spleen cells (CFU-S). Approximately one colony arises from every 500 to 1,000 bone marrow cells planted.

Colony stimulating activity (CSA) is elaborated from blood monocytes and from fixed tissue macrophages, stimulating the formation of neutrophil colonies while sensitized lymphocytes stimulate production of eosinophilic colonies in vitro.[257] CSA has been partially purified as a glycoprotein with relative stability, resisting heat at 60° C for 30 minutes, and it has an estimated molecular weight between 50,000 and 100,000 daltons. The role of CSA either as a specific growth-promoting substance or as an essential metabolite for bone marrow growth in vivo has not been well defined. Studies with cells cultured in sealed chambers to allow soluble diffusion in vivo suggest that the circulating neutrophil exerts a negative feedback on the proliferating compartments of bone marrow cells.[253] Other in vivo regulators include a neutrophil releasing factor demonstrated in the plasma of dogs rendered leukopenic, inciting a release of cells from the bone marrow reserve pool similar to that caused by an injection of endotoxin.[35]

Neutrophil

It is convenient to consider granulocyte movement between a number of intraconnected compartments as outlined in Table 18-1: the bone marrow, blood, and the tissue. The marrow compartment is comprised almost equally of the mitotic and the storage reserve. Assessment of DNA replication with tritiated thymidine shows that only myeloblasts, promyelocytes, and myelocytes are labeled in the mitotic pool. Myelocytes predominate since their replication is three times that of the single replications of earlier progenitors.[308] The mean time for replication is approximately 24 hours, and the labeled population reaches the circulation in 4 to 8 days.[10,33,34] Clinically the bone marrow reserve contains one hundredfold more granulocytes than the blood and is assessed by the ability of administered endotoxin or hydrocortisone to mobilize granulocytes into the peripheral blood.[11,189]

The blood phase is comparised of the circulating and marginating granulocyte pools. Proof for this comes from the observation that when labeled polymorphonuclear neutrophils are injected into normal subjects, a mean of 44% can be accounted

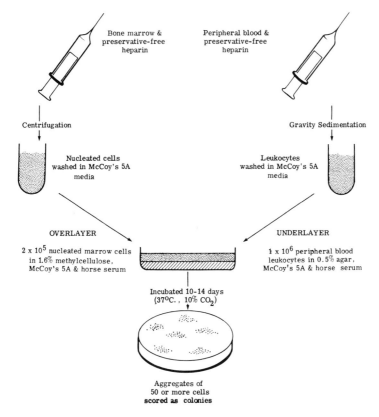

Fig. 18-1. Procedure for in vitro assay of colony forming unit cells, CFU-C, from human bone marrow and for assay of colony stimulating activity (CSA) or colony stimulating factor (CSF) from human blood.

Table 18-1. Kinetics of neutrophils, eosinophils, and monocytes

	Bone marrow	Blood	Tissue
Pools	Mitotic, storage	Circulating, marginating	Extravascular
Time			
Neutrophils	4-8 days	6-8 hours	Hours
Eosinophils	3-6 days	5-24 hours	Days
Monocytes	1-2 days	8 hours	Months to years
Relative distribution			
Neutrophils	+ + + +	+	± (increased in infection)
Eosinophils	+ +	±	+ (increased in allergic states)
Monocytes	±	±	+ + + (RES macrophages)

for in the circulation.[11] Stress and adrenaline release the adherent polymorphonuclear neutrophils from the vascular endothelium to allow almost 100% of the injected polymorphonuclear neutrophils to be recovered in the circulation.[10] Granulocytes labeled with diisopropyl phosphate (DFP[32]) disappear randomly from the blood at a mean half-life of 6 to 7 hours on a one-way passage to tissue sites.[10] The loss is even more rapid when inflammation, infection, or fever occurs.

Eosinophil

Current concepts of the control mechanism for eosinophil differentiation are based on animal studies. The eosinophilia produced in rats and mice by *Trichinella* larvae is dependent on functional lymphocytes.[21,304] Animals whose pools of recirculating lymphocytes are depleted or inactivated by irradiation, neonatal thymectomy, administration of antilymphocyte serum, or thoracic duct drainage are not able to mount an eosinophilic response to intravenously administered larvae but do generate a neutrophilia in response to pyogenic infection. The eosinophilic response of normal animals to larval infestation can be transmitted to uninfected animals by large lymphocytes from peripheral blood or thoracic duct but not by plasma or lymphocyte-free cells. The potency of the active lymphocytes is not impaired by enclosing them in cell-tight diffusion chambers. Furthermore, the in vitro cell culture of granulocytes show that lymphocytes release a CSA that differentiates stem cells to eosinophilic lines of production.[257]

Kinetic properties of eosinophils in humans are qualitatively similar to those of neutrophils.[106] After 3 to 6 days of maturation from precursor cells the eosinophil is released from the bone marrow in response to eosinophilic factors and hypoxia,[134] and the half-disappearance time from the blood varies between 5 and 24 hours.[50,122] Pharmacologic doses of corticosteroids or epinephrine block the mobilization of eosinophils from the bone marrow and induce a temporary eosinopenia[289]; the latter effect can be blocked by propranolol, suggesting that its action is mediated by β-adrenergic receptors.[157] ^{51}Cr-labeled cells from patients with hypereosinophilic syndromes transiently leave the circulating pool for the first 3 hours after infusion, then reenter the circulating pool, and finally disappear from the circulation with a mean half-life of 44 ± 2 hours in contrast to neutrophils of normal persons, which leave the circulation progressively with an estimated blood half-life of 12.4 ± 2 hours. However, under normal conditions, once the eosinophil leaves the circulation and enters tissue, it probably does not return to the bloodstream. The peripheral blood contains only a small fraction of the total eosinophil pool. For each circulating eosinophil there is a bone marrow reserve of 300 mature and immature cells and between 100 and 300 eosinophils in tissues.[133] Eosinophils can survive for 8 to 12 days in tissue culture in comparison to 2- to 4-day survival of neutrophils; this in vitro observation correlates with their prolonged residence at tissue sites.[228]

Basophil

Limited information is available on the kinetics of the blood basophil, although a single dose of ACTH is reported to reduce the number of circulating basophils in humans and in rabbits.

MONOCYTE MORPHOLOGY, DIFFERENTIATION, AND KINETICS

The blood monocyte is an intermediate in the cell line, the youngest identifiable forms in the bone marrow are monoblasts and promonocytes and the most mature are found in the tissue as the resident macrophage population of the reticuloendothelial system. Coincident with this matura-

tion is not only a shift in morphologic features, but also metabolic and cytoarchitectural changes.[62] Monoblasts are not easily identifiable in normal bone marrow because there is no storage pool. The immediate progenitor of the monocyte remains in the bone marrow for only about 18 hours after the last DNA synthesis. Evidence for monocyte progenitors exists in the in vitro culture system, suggesting that the granulocytic series and the mononuclear series share a common stem cell.[196]

Studies of monoblastic leukemia reveal cells 15 to 25 μ in diameter with a round or oval nucleus with fine chromatin structure and prominent nucleoli. They show little motility, are not adhesive to glass surfaces, and are rarely phagocytic. A more adherent promonocyte has a larger cytoplasmic ratio with basophilic cytoplasm, faint granule peroxidase activity, some glass adherence, and a capability to incorporate tritiated thymidine. Monocytes in Wright's stained blood smears appear as large cells, 10 to 18 μ in diameter, with gray-blue cytoplasm frequently containing small numbers of faint azurophilic granules. The centrally located nucleus is indented or is horseshoe shaped and has a fine, lacy chromatin structure.

The total blood monocyte pool is comprised of a circulating and a marginating pool with the latter about three times the size of the former. Monocytes leave the vascular space exponentially with a T½ of 8.4 hours, but this is prolonged in patients with moncytosis and shortened in those with acute infection or splenomegaly.[198] Once the monocyte leaves the circulation it does not return. The monocyte is more slowly motile and arrives at inflammatory sites hours after the polymorphonuclear neutrophil, as illustrated in Rebuck skin window preparations, in which polymorphonuclear neutrophils occur in abundance within 3 hours to become mixed with monocytes by 6 to 8 hours. Monocytes adhere to glass, are capable of phagocytosis, stain positive with naphthol ASD esterase, which can be inhibited with fluoride,[59,294] and contain Fc receptors to bind immunoglobulin-coated blood cells.

In the tissues the monocyte undergoes transformation to a macrophage; it may live there for many months, perhaps even years.[273] These tissue macrophages take on a variety of forms, depending on the organ in which they reside. The lung contains alveolar macrophages, the liver has Kupffer cell macrophages, and the bone marrow, spleen, and serosal surfaces of the pleura, peritoneal, and joint cavities contain their own resident macrophages.

ABNORMAL NEUTROPHIL MORPHOLOGY
Inherited abnormalities

Hereditary hypersegmentation and hereditary macropolycytes. Hereditary hypersegmen-

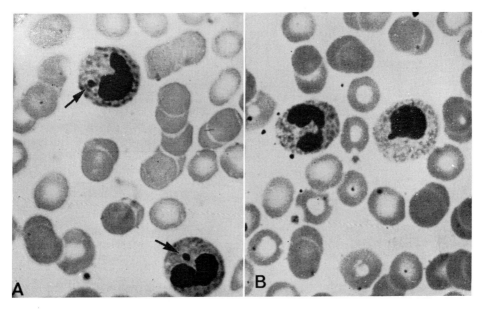

Fig. 18-2. Pelger-Huët anomaly in blood smear of 5-year-old girl. Note the characteristic bilobed nucleus of granulocytes in both illustrations. The nuclei have a rodlike, dumbbell, or "pince-nez" appearance and possess a coarse and lumpy chromatin structure. Arrows in **A** point to sex chromatin appendage, demonstrating its occurrence in this anomaly. (Courtesy Dr. Philip Lanzkowsky, New York, N.Y.)

tation and hereditary macropolycytes constitute an autosomal dominant disorder not associated with clinical disease. A similar condition of eosinophils exists. In each case the cells are abnormally large with more than five lobes to the nucleus in the absence of any recognizable defect or deficiency of DNA synthesis.[293]

Pelger-Huët anomaly. Pelger-Huët anomaly, an autosomal dominant disorder, occurs with an incidence of 1/6,000 persons. It is characterized by a neutrophil anomaly in which the nuclear lobes fail to develop completely. The heterozygous condition is identified from mature neutrophils with bilobed nuclei, whereas homozygotes have mature neutrophils with round nuclei containing clumped chromatin[23] (Fig. 18-2). The morphologically abnormal neutrophils have no apparent functional impairment. Neutrophils resembling those of the Pelger-Huët anomaly may be seen in several acquired diseases such as myeloproliferative disorders, severe myxedema, and influenza and in association with sulfa therapy.[266]

May-Hegglin anomaly. The autosomal dominant May-Hegglin anomaly is characterized by large bizarre platelets, leukopenia, and neutrophils containing one or two large intracytoplasmic inclusions known as Döhle bodies that consist of aggregates of ribosomal material.[145] One third of the patients have thrombocytopenia and many of them are asymptomatic. Other patients have hemorrhagic diathesis possibly ascribed to abnor-

malities of platelet function, in addition to the thrombocytopenia.[170]

Alder-Reilly anomaly. Metachromatic granules occur in the lymphocytes of 10% to 60% of patients with the mucopolysaccharide syndromes, including type I (Hunter's syndrome), type II (Hurler's syndrome), and type III (Sanfilippo syndrome). Less common are the abnormal azurophilic granules in their polymorphonuclear neutrophils as first pointed out by Alder. Patients with type V (Scheie syndrome) do not have abnormalities of lymphocytes or polymorphonuclear granules.

Chediak-Higashi syndrome. Chediak-Higashi syndrome is transmitted as an autosomal recessive trait and is characterized by giant lysosomes in polymorphonuclear neutrophils and other leukocytes as well as other cells throughout the body (Fig. 18-3). Patients present with oculocutaneous albinism, fine light hair, an increased susceptibility to infection, neurologic dysfunction, and at times a bleeding diathesis. The disease culminates in an accelerated phase characterized by pancytopenia and hepatosplenomegaly, usually ending in death. This disorder is discussed in detail in Chapter 19.

Acquired abnormalities

Toxic granulation and vacuolization. Morphologic alteration of the neutrophil occurs with severe bacterial infection. Toxic neutrophils are characterized by the presence of Döhle bodies,

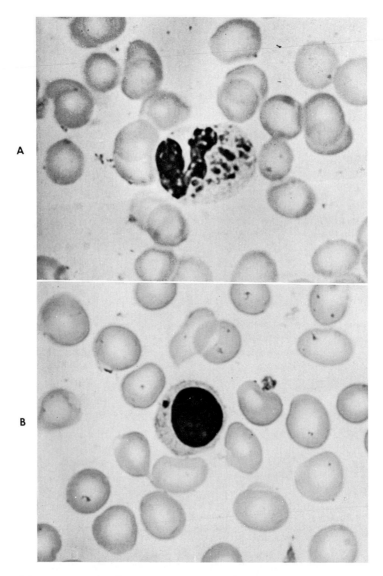

Fig. 18-3. Blood smear in Chediak-Higashi syndrome. **A,** Note pyknotic nucleus of polymorphonu-
clear leukocyte and abnormally large oval, fusiform, and irregularly shaped cytoplasmic granules.
B, One such granule is also present in lymphocyte. (Courtesy Dr. Frederick H. von Hofe, East
Orange, N.J.)

heavy granulation, and cytoplasmic vacuoles.[1]
Döhle bodies are not specific for this condition
and have also been noted in the polymorphonuclear neutrophils from pregnant females,[1] in familial
thrombocytopenia with giant platelets (May-
Hegglin anomaly), and in patients given cyclophosphamide chemotherapy.[138] Toxic granules are
identified by Wright's stain as heavy azurophilic
granules (Fig. 18-4); electron microscopy reveals
large, electron-dense, peroxidase-positive granules. Polymorphonuclear neutrophils that contain
toxic granules have increased alkaline phosphatase
activity but normal hydrolytic enzyme activity.
Toxic granules have been seen in a variety of disorders characterized by acute and chronic inflam-

mation such as infection, severe burns, and acute
inflammatory diseases.[104]

**Hypersegmentation and macrocytic neutro-
phils.** Hypersegmentation of mature neutrophils
and larger than normal neutrophils occur at all
levels of maturation in patients with folic acid or
vitamin B_{12} deficiency. Similar changes can occur
in the use of chemotherapeutic agents such as
6-mercaptopurine, cytosine arabinoside, methotrexate, and vincristine.

NEUTROPENIA

Neutropenia is a reduction in circulating neutrophils. The term "granulocytopenia" is often used,
but in a true sense this includes neutrophils, eosin-

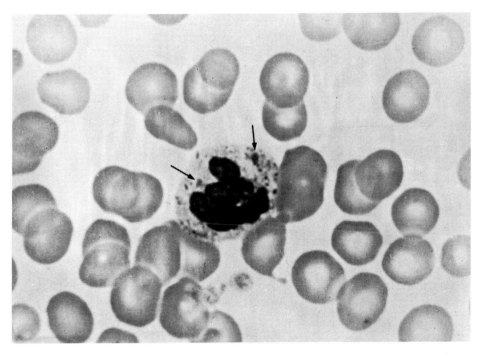

Fig. 18-4. Blood smear from an infant with meningitis. Arrows point to two Döhle inclusion bodies in neutrophil. These are small localized areas of bluish cytoplasm and probably represent defective maturation. (×2,000.) (Courtesy Dr. Julius Rutzky, Pontiac, Mich.)

ophils, and basophils. Agranulocytosis indicates a severe degree of neutropenia. The absolute neutrophil count is calculated as a product of the total leukocyte count and the percentage of neutrophils in the differential count. Normal absolute neutrophil counts usually exceed 1.5×10^9/liter but the risk of infection is only a problem when levels fall below 0.5×10^9/liter. Neutropenia can be considered from a kinetic viewpoint: (1) failure or ineffective leukocyte production in the bone marrow, (2) excessive neutrophil destruction in the peripheral blood and tissues, or (3) combinations of these abnormalities.

The range for total white blood cell counts as well as for the distribution of the granulocytes varies during the first 4 years of life. There is a leukocytosis to 40×10^9/liter at birth, which decreases to 20×10^9/liter during the first week of life, generally returning to the normal range of 5 to 10×10^9/liter by a few weeks of life. A predominance of polymorphonuclear neutrophils at birth is replaced by an equal distribution of lymphocytes and polymorphonuclear leukocytes by the end of the first week. Thereafter lymphocytes predominate until about age 4 years, but by 8 years of age there is a predominance of polymorphonuclear leukocytes in the blood.

Patients with neutropenia experience variable extents of infection with pyogenic and enteric bacteria, but viral and fungal infections are unusual except in the host otherwise suppressed by cyto-

toxic drugs. Since the era of antibiotics, *Diplococcus* pneumonia and streptococcal infections are rarely encountered. As expected, *Staphylococcus aureus, Pseudomonas* species, *E. coli,* and other enteric species were most frequently isolated from the blood and from skin and soft tissue abcesses.[131]

Cyclic neutropenia

Cyclic neutropenia is one of the periodic diseases with regularly recurring manifestations reflecting an underlying intrinsic body rhythm. Oscillations are based on cyclic changes in bone marrow production and release of neutrophils. The periodicity is generally between 19 and 21 days but may be as short as 14 days or as long as 30 days.

Historical perspective. Cyclic neutropenia was first described by Leale[169] in 1910. Morley et al.[211] described 20 more patients in 1967. Usually the disorder is familial, and it may be occasionally associated with an underlying hematologic malignancy.

Etiology. Experimental models of cyclic neutropenia have been developed by using immunosuppressive drugs such as cyclophosphamide, which dampen the feedback pool of bone marrow myeloid cells and thus accentuate the normal fluctuation of granulocyte proliferation.[212] Cycles of leukocytosis and leukopenia occur in some cases of chronic myelogenous leukemia. An animal model exists for this disease in the gray collie dog; an autosomal recessive disorder with hair-coat abnormalities, recurrent infection, and cyclic neutropenia occurs in the affected animals.[73] Recent studies of affected humans and animals show that the entire stem cell pool is involved with this periodic disease since alterations in reticulocyte and platelet numbers parallel the fluctuations in neutrophils.[212] Serum muramidase and blood CSA activity as well as urinary excretion of CSF parallel blood monocytosis, which often precedes the rise in blood neutrophils.[113,187] The level of erythropoietin is also increased in the period of neutropenia preceding the periodic reticulocytosis.

Agar culture of marrow cells shows higher CFU-C levels during periods of profound neutropenia; counts return to normal during periods of normal levels of blood neutrophils.[108] Serum myeloperoxidase levels vary inversely with the blood neutrophil count.[40] A model of granulopoiesis has been proposed on the basis of these observations in which a positive stimulus for granulopoiesis is provided by CSA and elaborated by monocytes and a negative or neutral influence is exerted by mature granulocytes.[210]

Clinical features. Clinical manifestations nearly always appear before patients reach 10 years of age. The disease generally runs a benign course although death from infection has occurred in a few cases. Fever, oral ulcerations, and skin infections are the predominant features. Periodontal disease occurs in most families but symptoms are rarely seen when the neutrophil count is more than 0.5×10^9/liter. During periods of adequate blood neutrophil levels patients are asymptomatic, but this is interrupted by intervals of fever, malaise, headache, lymphadenitis, arthritis, and mouth sores. I have encountered an infant in the newborn nursery with minor skin infections who was proved to have cyclic neutropenia for the first 3 months of his life; another infant who also had the disease had a labial ulceration at age 7 months that recurred on a monthly basis for several months.

Laboratory features. The total white blood count and differential count may be normal during periods when patients are asymptomatic. During symptomatic periods the absolute granulocyte count may fall to zero with monocytosis and eosinophilia occurring in some patients. The metabolic and phagocytic function of these cells is normal. Fluctuations in the percentage of reticulocytes and platelet numbers also parallel the fall in neutrophil numbers. Cyclic neutropenia has been associated with immunologic dysfunction including agammaglobulinemia, dysgammaglobulinemia, and cartilage-hair hypoplasia. Leukoagglutinins are not found.[206] Serial evaluations of the bone marrow during the cycle demonstrated that granulocyte precursors disappear prior to the onset of neutropenia. Their reappearance prior to the return of neutrophils to the blood is consistent with the idea that the cycles are caused by quantitatively decreased entry of granulocyte progenitor cells into granulopoiesis.

Treatment. Cyclic neutropenia generally runs a benign course. Case reports of colon necrosis, peritonitis, and clostridial sepsis emphasize the potential severity of this usually benign condition.[95] Splenectomy and adrenocorticosteroids have produced systematic improvement in some cases, but long-term treatment has not been helpful in most cases. Frequent washes with saline or glycerin–hydrogen peroxide solution offer modest relief from the discomfort of mouth sores.

Chronic neutropenia

Hereditary neutropenia
Infantile genetic agranulocytosis of Kostmann. During the past two decades twenty-one of twenty-two infants and toddlers in the isolated northern parish of Overkalix, Norrbotten, Sweden have died from repeated infections resulting from severe granulocytopenia, which was proved to be present on the first day of life in two instances.[160] Another thirty-two cases have been reported from Scandinavia, England, and the North American continent. As Kostmann points out, the lack of finding more than one affected child in most families outside Sweden is not surprising since it is extremely difficult to trace rare autosomal recessive genes except in isolated geographic areas where inbreeding is excessive and affected homozygotes accumulate.

CLINICAL FEATURES. The clinical signs in all cases are quite similar. During the first few months of life, irritability, fever, and skin boils as well as omphalitis occur; they are associated with and immediately followed by otitis media, pneumonia, lymphadenitis, gingivitis, and perianal and urinary infections. Septicemia, lung and liver abscesses, peritonitis, or severe enteritis with chronic diarrhea and vomiting are more frequently associated with the terminal stages of the illness. *Staphylococcus aureus, E. coli,* and *Pseudomonas* in the late stages are common pathogens although all varieties of gram-positive and gram-negative bacteria may be isolated from infected sites.

LABORATORY FEATURES. Granulocytopenia is severe and persists in most cases throughout the entire illness. Eosinophil and monocyte maturation is usually not affected. Blood neutrophil counts range betweeen 0 and 0.8×10^9/liter. Eosinophil counts range from 0 to 1.4×10^9/liter, and monocytosis reaches levels approaching 10×10^9/liter in some cases. Anemia of chronic inflammation is frequently present in severely infected patients, but thrombocytopenia does not occur. Normal to elevated levels of serum immunoglobulins reflect the degree of chronic infection present. The neutropenia is severe, although total leukocyte counts are often normal because of monocytosis. Absolute neutropenia with less than 0.3×10^9 neutrophils/liter is the rule.

The bone marrow is usually depleted of a reserve of mature granulocytes and shows a predominance of vacuolated promyelocytes and myelocytes with large azurophilic granules, as well as an increased in monocytes, eosinophilic granulocytes, histiocytes, and reactive plasma cells. Cellularity of the bone marrow varies.[22,159,320] Chromosome analysis has been normal in most cases.

In vitro cell culture shows that the precursor stem cell in the bone marrow is capable of proliferating, with colonies of normal size and number, but the prior observations that the colonies contain normal neutrophils has recently been challenged.[174,326] The electron microscopic study of these colonies shows markedly aberrant cells rarely containing mature neutrophils and exhibiting bizarre nuclei, excessive cytoplasm, and a dearth of granules. Monocyte and eosinophil colonies are differentiated normally and the patient's cells and sera support growth of normal colonies. Epinephrine stimulation tests and endotoxin or hydrocortisone infusions confirm the lack of a marginating pool or a bone marrow reserve pool, respectively, in these children.[326]

Normal neutrophils transfused into affected patients leave the blood at approximately normal rates, suggesting a defect in stem cell production rather than increased destruction and, indeed, infusion of normal plasma does not alleviate the neutropenia or alter the appearance of the bone marrow. Treatment with steroids, testosterone, or splenectomy has not been helpful. If the congenital neutropenia appears to result from an intrinsically defective committed stem cell, attempts at bone marrow transplantation are warranted.

Familial benign chronic neutropenia. Familial benign chronic neutropenia, an autosomal dominant disorder, is associated with mild to moderate chronic degrees of neutropenia and is usually not associated with significant leukopenia. The occurrence of neutropenia in successive generations of families has been observed in people of African origin,[267] in certain Jewish families of Yemenite origin,[79] and in German, French, American, and South African families.[36,72,94] In an isolated case this relatively benign condition may be confused with more severe forms of neutropenic disorders. The true incidence of this condition is unknown because of the mild nature of the defect.

CLINICAL FEATURES. Most patients have no symptoms, especially the Yemenite Jews and South Africans. A few develop mild skin furuncles and mouth sores with gingivitis; however, there is no periodicity to these symptoms or signs. The physical examination is otherwise normal.

LABORATORY FEATURES. Laboratory studies reveal total white blood cell counts between 1.5 and 6×10^9/liter with neutrophils ranging between 10% and 30%, monocytes ranging between 5% and 20%, and eosinophils usually less than 10%. There is no anemia or thrombocytopenia. The neutropenia is not cyclic. The bone marrow is normal in the Yemenites, but the cloning efficiency in cell culture in vitro is increased. Bone marrow cells from eight patients gave an average of about twice the number of granulocyte colonies compared to nonneutropenic patients with iron-deficiency anemia.[204] The American patients had myeloid hyperplasia with reduction of mature granulocytes. On the basis of these studies it has been suggested that the neutropenia is caused by a defect in the release of mature granulocytes from the bone marrow to the peripheral blood.

TREATMENT. Recognition of this disease in a family is important because its benign nature does not require therapy such as splenectomy or corticosteroids and is compatible with a normal life.[140]

Pseudoneutropenia. Following the description of genetic neutropenia in Africans from Kampala a report from the United States confirmed that the mean absolute neutrophil counts in black American men and women were significantly lower than those of age-matched white men and women: black men, $3.356 \pm 1.554 \times 10^9$/liter, white men, $5.60 \pm 1.381 \times 10^9$/liter ($p < .01$); black women, $3.129 \pm 1.469 \times 10^9$/liter, white women, $4.633 \pm 1.413 \times 10^9$/liter ($p < .01$). More than 30% of black men and 40% of black women had total white blood counts of less than 5×10^9/liter compared to 7% of white men and women. This fact must be kept in mind when evaluating possible neutropenia in blacks.[148]

Familial severe neutropenia. It is uncertain whether familial severe neutropenia represents a distinct genetic disorder or whether it is the more severe form of the autosomal dominant benign disorder described above. These patients experience more severe infections, particularly mouth infections, and the degree of neutropenia is more pronounced with monocytosis. Bone marrows show depletion of the mature granulocyte pool, giving the impression of a maturation arrest.[126]

Neutropenia associated with immunoglobulin abnormality. Although it is not frequently emphasized, one third of boys with X-linked agammaglobulinemia have associated neutropenia. Twenty-five cases of transient, persistent, or cyclic neutropenia have been described in seventy-five cases reported from three major immunology centers.[45,100,103] The neutropenia often gives way to leukocytosis in the later course of infection.

In 1961 Rosen described dysgammaglobulinemia type I, which is characterized by the absence of IgA, marked deficiency of IgG, and normal to elevated IgM levels in serum. All affected children are boys and almost all have recurrent, cyclic, or persistent neutropenia.[256] Hemolytic anemia, thrombocytopenia, and other manifestations of autoimmune disease are frequently encountered in these patients. Isolated deficiency of IgA in serum and saliva with normal levels of IgG and IgM (dysgammaglobulinemia type III) has been associated with severe neutropenia, recurrent respiratory and skin infections, and lymph node abscesses. Total leukocyte counts ranged from 2.1 to 5.6×10^9/liter, with neutrophils ranging between 1% and 15% and monocytes between 18% and 56%. The bone marrow in one case was cellular with fewer mature neutrophils than normal but with a normal myeloid:erythroid ratio. There was an associated Coombs-positive hemolytic anemia. IgA was absent in the serum and saliva of the mother but her neutrophil count and Coombs test were negative, suggesting the true nature of the neutropenia to be due to autoantibodies.[261]

Another similar case has recently been described in a 14-year-old boy with a history of thrombocytopenia, lymphadenopathy, and splenomegaly. After splenectomy he developed recurrent attacks of bronchopneumonia and otitis media and was found to have low IgA with normal IgG and elevated IgM levels.[220]

Three brothers were described with IgG levels of 252 to 372 mg/dl but two of them had normal IgM and depressed IgA; all had severe neutropenia with mild responses of increased blood granulocyte to as high as 6.5×10^9/liter with infection. Their two sisters and parents were healthy. Onset of symptoms occurred between 9 months and 39 months with repeated episodes of ulcerative stomatitis, pneumonia, and otitis media. Physical examination showed prominent lymphadenopathy, splenomegaly, and moderate anemia. The bone marrow was cellular with few mature granulocytes. The lymph nodes showed a lack of germinal centers, but plasma cells were present. All three boys died of progressive infection.[179] These patients are similar to those described by Canale and Smith[52] with chronic lymphadenopathy simulating lymphoma.

TREATMENT. The neutropenia in most patients with dysgammaglobulinemia has not responded to γ-globulin replacement. However, three boys with type I dysgammaglobulinemia have had a restoration of their neutrophil counts from a range of 0.068 to 0.48×10^9/liter to levels as high as 6×10^9/liter after infusions of plasma and injections of high doses of γ-globulin (up to 1.6 ml/kg initially and 0.8 ml/kg every 2 weeks) to maintain IgG levels above 200 mg/dl. As the neutrophil count returned to normal, mouth ulcers also cleared.[251] Corticosteroids may be useful if the neutropenia is associated with an antineutrophil antibody.

Neutropenia associated with defective cell-mediated immunity. Four siblings (three girls and a boy) suffered recurrent bacterial infections (eczema, polyarthralgias, pneumonias, and otitis media) with neutropenia and eosinophilia. Physical examination revealed eczema (sometimes generalized) and often secondary infection of the skin. Serum IgA levels were markedly elevated and antibody responses to tetanus and polio vaccinations were blunted. Leukocytes were elevated during periods of infection but both in vivo inflammatory skin windows, as described by Rebuck, and in vitro chemotaxis were impaired. A defect of cell-mediated immunity was demonstrated by an absence of reactivity to various skin test antigens and disseminated varicella infection in two of the children.[29]

Reticular dysgenesis. Reticular dysgenesis appears to be a defect in the development of the hematopoietic stem cells. Affected infants not only have failure of thymus development and moderate to severe lymphopenia and agammaglobulinemia but also hypoplasia of bone marrow and blood granulocytes with marked neutropenia, while erythroid and megakaryocytic development is normal. A postmortem examination of twin boys who died from this condition showed complete absence of lymph nodes, tonsils, and Peyer's patches; there were no lymphocytes, plasma cells, or follicles in the spleen.[76]

Neutropenias associated with phenotypic abnormalities

METAPHYSEAL CHONDRODYSPLASIA, DWARFISM, PANCREATIC EXOCRINE INSUFFICIENCY, AND NEUTROPENIA. A syndrome of metaphyseal chrondrodysplasia, dwarfism, variable neutropenia, and exocrine pancreatic insufficiency with normal sweat electrolytes has been described.

HISTORICAL PERSPECTIVE. In 1963 Shwachman et al.[270] reported pancreatic exocrine insufficiency occurring in six children with neutropenia or pancytopenia with normal lungs and normal sweat electrolytes. One year later Bodian et al.[32] reported two similar cases with failure to thrive and the onset of bulky, foul-smelling stools occurring at 9 weeks and 12 weeks of age. Their absolute neutrophil counts were 0.871 and 0.369×10^9/liter. The pancreatic biopsies revealed severe lipomatosis and pancreatic hypoplasia. An additional eighteen cases were added from the literature.[32] Three years later radiographic bone lesions, one of epiphyseal dysostosis of the knees and two with rib changes, were described in three of eleven newly discovered cases.[47] An additional three cases with severe bilateral metaphyseal dysostosis of the hips and dwarfism were described in 1968.[98] This syndrome is the most common form of exocrine pancreatic insufficiency in infants and children excluding cystic fibrosis of the pancreas. Thirty-six cases were described in the span of 5 years after its initial discovery.

GENETICS. Both sexes are equally affected. Assuming an autosomal recessive mode of transmission, it can be concluded that the gene frequency in the population is probably quite high. The disease is likely hereditary because more than one affected sibling has been found in six of thirty families.[81,269]

IMMUNOLOGY. Two brothers, ages 22 and 25 years, and another 16-year-old boy and his 19-year-old sister, all with pancreatic insufficiency and neutropenia, were noted to have dysgammaglobulinemia with normal to slightly decreased serum IgG levels and low levels of both IgM and IgA. Usually immunoglobulin levels are normal.

CLINICAL FEATURES. The onset of symptoms occurs as early as 3 weeks of age with diarrhea, weight loss, and failure to thrive. A few infants experience eczema and otitis media. Although pneumonia does occur, it is uncommon. Diabetes mellitus has occurred, but usually there is a positive family history of it. Growth failure and dwarfism are usually noted between the first and second years of life. Infections of the skin and respiratory tract and sinuses recur, and vertebral and hip abnormalities accentuate the growth failure.

LABORATORY FEATURES. In thirty-five of thirty-six published cases neutropenia was present, with absolute neutrophil counts below 1×10^9/liter in about two thirds of the patients. Usually the neutropenia is chronic, but cyclic neutropenia has occurred. Anemia with a low reticulocyte count occurs in slightly more than half of the cases (nineteen of thirty-six), and mild to moderate degrees of thrombocytopenia were found in twenty-nine. Raised levels of Hb F have been noted in some cases. Bone marrow is usually hypocellular but does not significantly contribute to the diagnosis. Although sweat chloride tests are consistently normal following a test meal or secretin stimulation, the duodenal juice and stool lack pancreatic trypsin, lipase, and amylase activity. Fecal fat exceeds 4.0 gm/day, but xylose excretion and peroral intestinal biopsies are normal. Pancreatic tissue obtained by surgical biopsy or autopsy is replaced by adipose tissue with preservation of islets embedded in the fat. No fibrosis of pancreatic acinar, duct, or adipose tissue occurs. The chest x-ray film is usually normal, and the chronic lung changes so characteristic of cystic fibrosis do not occur.

Severe structural changes of the neck of the femurs (metaphyseal chondroplasia) lead to coxa vara from downward slipping of the femoral head.

These changes differ from the metaphyseal dysostosis of the knees and other joints seen with cartilage-hair hypoplasia in the Amish population. Metaphyseal chondroplasia of the ribs, wrists, knees, vertebrae, and upper humerus may also occur.[277] Unusual generalized osteoporosis, impaired tubulation of long bones, shortening of the fibulas and ulnas, and subluxation of the radial heads have been noted in one case.[87] Electron microscopic examination of cartilage shows failure of chondrocytes to undergo hypertrophy and also signs of degeneration. Cytoplasmic inclusions may be seen in some of the chrondrocytes.[276]

Bone age is not decreased as much as is height age.

TREATMENT. The malabsorption can be improved with high doses of pancreatic extract and medium chain triglyceride oil supplementation. Neither the neutropenia nor the dwarfism is significantly improved by this therapy. Respiratory and sinus infections should be treated with appropriate antibiotics if cultures are positive for pathogenic bacteria. Hip dysostosis requires prompt orthopedic consultation.

PROGNOSIS. Twenty-five percent of the patients die during infancy or childhood. Mental retardation has been noted in a few cases. The malabsorption problem seems to improve with age in some cases. Infections continue to recur throughout life and disability results primarily from marked joint deformity, especially in the hip.

Cartilage-hair hypoplasia. Cartilage-hair hypoplasia is an autosomal recessive disorder occurring in the Amish population characterized by short-limb dwarfism, fine silky hair, and undue susceptibility to infections.[195] There are variable immunologic alterations with attrition of T cell function and neutropenia well documented in two patients.[184] (See Chapter 20.)

Neutropenia and syndrome of onychotricho dysplasia. An infant with fine, dry, short, curly, sparse hair of the scalp, eyelashes, and eyebrows; nail hypoplasia; koilonychia and onychorrhexis of all fingers and toes; and mild generalized hypotonia and psychomotor retardation has recently been described.[50] This child had chronic neutropenia with neutrophil counts in the range between 0 and 1×10^9/liter. Minor infections accompanied by fever were frequently observed. Although this is an isolated case, the parents were half–first cousins with a common grandmother, which suggests that the syndrome could have been inherited as an autosomal recessive trait.

Congenital neutropenia
Chronic idiopathic granulocytopenia with bone marrow myelokathexis. A case of chronic granulocytopenia in a 10-year-old girl who suffered repeated infections and persistent neutropenia since infancy was the subject of two separate

reports,[163,326] and a new case has recently been reported.[226] Numerous bone marrow examinations revealed the presence of a large reservoir of segmented neutrophils with peculiar morphology. The neutrophils in the bone marrow contained pyknotic nuclei and cytoplasmic nuclei with long, thin intrasegmental chromatin strands separating nuclear lobes. A leukokinetic study with [^{32}P]DFP showed the T½ of the patient's neutrophils to be shortened in her own circulation and in the circulation of a normal recipient; normal cells survived normally in the patient's circulation. Granulocytes were released from the bone marrow into the blood after stimulation with endotoxin as well as in response to infection, but the patient's neutrophils in the circulation exhibited decreased motility, decreased phagocytic capacity, and increased permeability to dyes. These findings seem to support the hypothesis that the mature granulocytes were functionally and morphologically inferior and that they were retained for long periods in the bone marrow where they underwent senescence and intramedullary death.

Chronic granulocytopenia of childhood.
Chronic granulocytopenia of childhood, a nonfamilial, relatively benign disorder, is characterized by repeated pyogenic infections beginning soon after birth. In some patients complete recovery eventually takes place. Although total white blood cell counts are usually normal, absolute granulocyte counts have ranged between 0 and 0.2×10^9/liter, and monocytosis is common. The bone marrow shows normal to increased cellularity, and neutrophilic bands and metamyelocytes have been plentiful, but mature neutrophils have been absent. In contrast to patients with hereditary infantile genetic agranulocytosis, the blood neutrophils of children with chronic granulocytopenia of childhood increase in the circulation in response to infection or to endotoxin.[328] Whether this represents a different disorder from similar cases observed primarily in adults is purely speculative at this point.[165] Sporadic cases of chronic neutropenia associated with a remarkable hypoplasia of the entire granulocytic series in the bone marrow have been reported in adults and called chronic hypoplastic neutropenia.[271] However, it has been pointed out in a recent review of chronic neutropenia of childhood that the prognosis could not be predicted from the bone marrow morphology nor from the presence or absence of reactive blood monocytosis or the pattern of genetic transmission. Even the results of special neutrophil function studies were not helpful. The authors suggest that the complex nomenclature associated with chronic neutropenic states may best be put aside until a better basis for classification becomes available.[239] The possible role of lymphocyte-mediated sup-

pression of granulopoiesis remains to be determined, but this will be a fruitful area of clinical investigation.

Acquired neutropenic disorders. A variety of exogenous factors can be associated with neutropenia. These include agents that produce bone marrow injury such as cytotoxic drugs, drugs interfering with the metabolism of precursor cells, and immunologic injury and irradiation. Replacement of the bone marrow with tumor cells and fibrosis of the bone marrow may be other causes. Vitamin B_{12} and folic acid deficiencies causing defects of DNA synthesis have been associated with neutropenia. The most common of all causes of neutropenia is that associated with intercurrent infections, usually viral in origin.

Drugs. Cytotoxic drugs and irradiation administered in high enough concentrations regularly produce depression of bone marrow and circulating leukocyte counts. Noncytotoxic drugs only irregularly produce neutropenia and are not ordinarily considered cytotoxic. Cytotoxic drugs are frequently used in cancer chemotherapy and in treating disorders related to other immune disorders that require immunosuppression. They interrupt normal replication of the bone marrow cells with resultant neutropenia, thrombocytopenia, or anemia. The commonly used agents that produce these effects are alkylating agents such as cyclophosphamide and nitrogen mustard; antimetabolites such as 6-mercaptopurine, 6-thioguanine, and methotrexate; cytosine arabinoside and its analogs; the nitrosureas, BCNU, CCNU, and methyl CCNU; vinca alkaloids; and antibiotics, including actinomycin D, procarbazine, daunomycin, and adriamycin.

Irradiation of the bone marrow has a similar effect to that of cytotoxic drugs; usually the effects on the replicating hematopoietic cells are transient, although ablating doses to the bone marrow occur if the dose is sufficiently high, such as that used in preparing patients for bone marrow transplantation. The noncytotoxic drugs most frequently associated with neutropenia and other evidence of myelosuppression include phenothiazine, chloramphenicol, thiouracil derivatives, methimazole, sulfonamides, phenylbutazone, and anticonvulsants. The mechanism of myelosuppression of these drugs is not known.[241] The drugs listed below lead to neutropenia in certain persons:

Drugs	*References*
Antimicrobial agents	
Chloramphenicol	116, 263, 324, 325
Sulfonamides	193, 281
Ampicillin	105, 111
Streptomycin	225
Ristocetin	219
Gentamicin	43, 54

Drugs	References
Lincomycin	223
Griseofulvin	84
Cephalothin	77
Dapsone	143, 175, 288, 298
Nitrofurantoin	177, 230
Amphotericin	181
Silver sulfadiazine	53
Clindamycin	90
Trimethoprim-sulfamethoxazole	229, 265, 318
Nafcillin	188, 260
Penicillin	254
Cephapirin	176
Benzylpenicillin	64
Phenothiazines (mepazine, promazine, etc.)	89, 130, 155, 186, 240, 243, 284, 309
Dibenzazepine compounds (imipramine, etc.)	69, 156
Antihistamines (tripelennamine [Pyribenzamine], etc.)	49, 119
Anticonvulsants	
Trimethadione (Tridione)	199, 272
Phenytoin (Dilantin)	233, 292
Antithyroid drugs (Methimazole, thiouracil derivatives)	6, 194, 315
Anti-inflammatory agents	
Indomethacin	55, 203
Phenylbutazone	91, 190, 192, 252
Gold salts	132, 153, 154, 171, 311
Ibuprofen	112
Diuretics	
Thiazide	120
Ethacrynic acid	303
Mercurial diuretics	161
Acetazolamide (Diamox)	237
Hypoglycemic agents	
Tolbutamide	5
Chlorpropamide	278
Miscellaneous	
Penicillamine	66
Phenindione	287
Cinchophen	115, 280
Hydroxychloroquine	50, 244, 247
Quinidine	20
Procaine amide	114, 123, 158, 164, 286, 305
Allopurinol	3, 107
Propranolol	217

Possible causes might relate to a genetically acquired lack of drug detoxification systems, lack of alternate metabolic pathways around the drug block, unusual drug binding, or kinetics of distribution and excretion. Perhaps other still undefined mechanisms are also involved.[214] It is clear that pyrazolone derivatives and antithyroid drugs have been shown to have a direct suppressive effect on bone marrow function.[257] An immunologic mechanism for agranulocytosis should be suspected when a patient develops precipitous agranulocytosis. In this case a search for leukoagglutinins or antineutrophil antibodies would be indicated. Since drugs are chemically and pharmacologically different, the mechanism for the bone marrow suppression (either toxic direct effects on marrow stem cells or increased peripheral destruction by antibodies) should be sought in every case.[242]

Chemical toxins. Certain chemical compounds have been associated with agranulocytosis. These include benzol, benzene,[279] arsenic,[166,313] nitrous oxide,[232] thioglycolic acid,[68] dinitrophenol[102] thiocyanate,[93] bismuth,[264] carbon tetrachloride and other solvents,[258,283] and thorotrast.[221]

Bacterial infections. Typhoid and paratyphoid fever and sometimes tularemia cause leukopenia. Early in the course of typhoid fever mild leukocytosis and neutrophilia may predominate,[78] but during bacteremia neutropenia is the rule.[13] During paratyphoid fever from *Salmonella* infection, a similar clinical and laboratory picture occurs. In tularemia during the fever or pulmonary phase an absence of leukocytosis is also the rule, although generally leukopenia is not present.[248] Neutropenia sometimes results from overwhelming infection such as tuberculosis[17] and septicemia.[26]

Viral infections. A wide variety of viral diseases commonly produce leukopenia and neutropenia and are the most common cause for this acquired condition in children. Some of the common viral infections known to be associated with neutropenia are the following: infectious hepatitis,[216] infectious mononucleosis, influenza, poliomyelitis, rubeola,[24] rubella,[124] roseola, smallpox,[128] psittacosis, Colorado tick fever,[141] dengue, yellow fever,[25] sandfly fever, and varicella.[82]

Rickettsial infections. Leukopenia and neutropenia may occur with variable frequency in most rickettsial infections, usually during the first week of the disease. Leukopenia is common in rickettsialpox but less common in epidemic typhus, scrub typhus, Rocky Mountain spotted fever, and rickettsial typhus.*

Protozoa infestations. Slight leukocytosis may occur with malaria for a short time during the parasitism, but as parasitemia progresses, leukopenia and shift neutropenia develop.[75] In relapsing fever the leukopenia is found between periods of fever; during febrile periods the leukocyte count may be quite elevated.

Bone marrow infiltration. Neutropenia resulting from diminished production can be seen in a number of malignant diseases in which the bone marrow is infiltrated with tumor. This phenomenon is known as myelophthisis. The bone marrow replacement resulting in neutropenia is more often seen in hematologic malignancies such as acute leukemia, lymphomatous conversion of the bone

---

*References 81, 118, 255, 319.

marrow to leukemia, metastatic neuroblastoma, and rhabdomyosarcoma as well as myelofibrosis with myeloid metaplasia in which normal hematopoietic elements of the bone marrow are replaced by fibrous tissue.

Nutritional deficiencies. Generalized nutritional deficiencies that occur with starvation and with anorexia nervosa, a peculiar psychogenic disorder of teenage girls, may produce pancytopenia or selective neutropenia.[236,268] Bone marrow is usually hypocellular. Deficiencies of vitamin B_{12} and folate interfering with nucleic acid synthesis of myeloid precursors in the bone marrow lead to an inadequate granulopoiesis that often is ineffective, resulting in intermedullary destruction of young granulocytes.[88] Neutrophils with more than five lobed nucleii are common in abnormal DNA synthesis resulting from nutritional deficiency of vitamin B_{12} or folic acid or from administration of antimetabolite drugs such as cytosine arabinoside, methotrexate, or 6-mercaptopurine.

Immune neutropenia

Felty's syndrome and systemic lupus erythematosis (SLE). In one series of 258 patients with SLE 66% developed leukopenia. In Felty's syndrome, a condition characterized by arthritis, splenomegaly, and leukopenia, not only is there variable reduction in neutrophils and total leukocyte counts but also increased susceptibility to infection is not uncommon.[180] Two possible mechanisms to explain the neturopenia in these conditions are a circulating leukoagglutinin and splenomegaly with hypersplenism.[35,85] In both Felty's

syndrome and SLE granulocyte survival in the circulation may be reduced. In Felty's syndrome there may be a low ratio of the circulating granulocyte pool compared to the total body granulocyte pool, indicating sequestration of granulocytes in the spleen.[300] In some patients with either condition, diminished granulopoiesis contributes to the development of neutropenia.[28]

Neonatal isoimmune neutropenia. Neonatal isoimmune neutropenia is similar in its pathogenesis to Rh hemolytic disease of newborns from Rh-negative mothers in whom Rh-positive antigens are present on their unborn infant's red cells. Antigens specifically derived from fetal neutrophils gain access to maternal circulation where they incite the production of IgG antibodies. The maternal antibodies then cross the placenta and cause transient neonatal neutropenia. Frequently the neutropenia is associated with perinatal infection. As indicated in the following list, the antibody is directed against polymorphonuclear neutrophil–specific antigens, such as NA1, NA2, NB1, or NC1:

A. Antineutrophil-specific IgG, rarely IgM
   1. NA1, NA2, NB1, NC1
   2. Antigen found on myelocytes, metamyelocytes, bands, and polymorphonuclear neutrophils
B. Antihistocompatibility antigen (HLA): not specific for polymorphonuclear neutrophils
C. Drug-dependent leukoagglutinins: antigen + hapten ↔ antibody
D. Drug-associated leukoagglutanins: antigen ↔ antibody

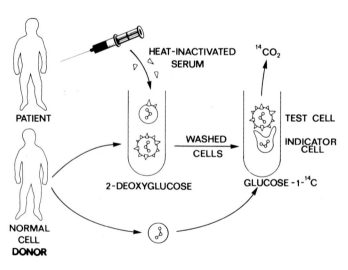

Fig. 18-5. Procedure for assay of antineutrophil antibody from human heat-inactivated serum. In this procedure normal donor neutrophils are incubated with test serum, and 2-deoxyglucose antibody, if present, will bind to donor cells made nonphagocytic by 2-deoxyglucose. After cells are washed normal neutrophils and glucose-1-^{14}C are added. $^{14}CO_2$ is evolved if phagocytosis of the test cell occurs, indicating the presence of antineutrophil antibody on the cell surface.

The neutropenia is frequently severe with absolute granulocyte counts of 0 to 0.5×10^9/liter that last from 2 weeks to as long as 17 weeks from the time of birth. Eosinophil percentages range between 3% and 8% and monocytes range between 10% and 57% with total white blood cell counts ranging between 1.5 and 12.3×10^9/liter.

The clinical manifestations include recurrent fevers and serious infections such as pneumonia, skin and scalp abscesses, staphylococcal pustules, pyoderma caused by β-hemolytic streptococci, omphalitis, otitis media, and septicemia. The majority of infants have clinical manifestations, and death resulting from overwhelming infection occurs in 10% of cases.[168]

Laboratory detection and confirmation of this disease rests on the ability to determine neutrophil antibodies specific for the infant's antigenic cell type in the serum of the mother. The leukocyte agglutinin test is insensitive and requires large volumes of antisera and cell suspensions. Other modifications include a microagglutination test and a capillary agglutination test.[168] Recently Boxer and Stossel[38] have developed a more sensitive functional assay for determining the presence of antineutrophil antibodies as outlined in Fig. 18-5. Human neutrophils are incubated with heat-inactivated sera containing antineutrophil antibody and then incubated for one hour with 1 mM 2-deoxyglucose to render the sensitized polymorphonuclear neutrophil nonphagocytic. The indicator cells are normal polymorphonuclear neutrophils that readily phagocytize the sensitized polymorphonuclear neutrophil, which is reflected by the increased evolution of $^{14}CO_2$ from glucose-1-^{14}C.

The original test used rabbit macrophages as the phagocytic cell and nitroblue tetrazolium as the indicator. Neutrophils treated with rabbit anti-human leukocyte antiserum or IgG with the sera from mothers of infants with neonatal isoimmune neutropenia and with sera from frequently transfused patients promote a rapid ingestion of sensitized neutrophils by alveolar macrophages with subsequent reduction of nitroblue tetrazolium. This method is currently the most sensitive assay for detecting antineutrophil antibodies.[302]

Neonatal neutropenia caused by passive transfer of maternal antibody. Profound neutropenia caused by the passive transfer of IgG antineutrophil antibody from the mother to the infant is a self-limiting problem of the newborn. In contrast to neonatal isoimmune neutropenia, there is no specific sensitization but rather a shared antigenicity between the inciting antigen for the disease and the mother and that present on the neutrophil of the infant. The disorder in the newborn is usually 2 to 4 weeks in duration.

Autoimmune neutropenia. With the recent development of the functional opsonic antibody assay,[38] cases of chronic neutropenia of unexplained etiology have been found to be caused by autoantibody. The clinical symptoms of these patients are variable and relatively mild. They include malaise, pharyngitis, cellulitis, and mucosal ulcerations. This disease is caused by an endogenous development of either a 7S IgG

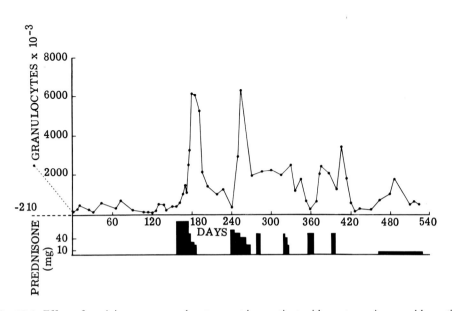

Fig. 18-6. Effect of prednisone on granulocyte count in a patient with neutropenia caused by antineutrophil antibodies.

or a 19S IgM antibody. A recent report describes an acquired neutropenia caused by autoimmune antineutrophil antibody in an 8-month-old infant with chronic benign neutropenia. This type of immunoneutropenia appears to be analagous to the immunohematologic abnormalities such as idiopathic thrombocytopenia purpura and autoimmune hemolytic anemia. Affected children have generally been able to respond to bacterial infection with some increase in peripheral granulocytes. The bone marrow is normally cellular. The cases seem similar to five cases described earlier by Zuelzer and Bajoghli,[328] described in the discussion of nonhereditary-type chronic benign neutropenia. The clear dependence and prompt response to prednisone therapy in raising the absolute granulocyte counts to normal levels are demonstrated in Fig. 18-6. A recent analysis of chronic autoimmune neutropenia has shown the defect to be caused by a neutrophil-specific anti-NA2 antibody.[167]

Transfusion reactions. Development of febrile transfusion reactions from the presence of leukocyte agglutinins is now a familiar complication. The reaction is considered to be related to the release of pyrogen from neutrophils following antigen-antibody reaction. Antibodies may be directed against HLA as well as to specific antineutrophil and antilymphocyte antigens. In addition to febrile responses, recently recognized complications include the development of pulmonary manifestations with severe dyspnea and large pulmonary infiltrates.[306] Approximately one third of sera from frequently transfused patients contains antineutrophil antibody. Transfusion reactions are discussed in greater detail in Chapter 4.

Drugs. The classic example for drug-dependent immunologic injury of neutrophils is aminopyrine, a drug no longer in common use.[208] The drug acts as a hapten linking to the leukocyte surface, and the antibody made is directed against the hapten. The antibody to the drug may be present in the circulation without deleterious effects until the drug is administered; then the interaction of the antibody with the leukocyte-bound drug results in cell agglutination and sequestration in the pulmonary capillary bed and probably other vascular filtrations beds such as the spleen. Drug-induced immunologic neutropenia occurs by at least three mechanisms: (1) the antibody interacts directly with the drug, which is bound to the cell surface; (2) the antibody interacts with antigen in the fluid phase of the blood, and the immune complex absorbs to the surface of the cell; and (3) the antibody coats the cell surface and then reacts with administered antigen. Certain drugs have been linked to immunologic injury and the development of antibody. These include mercurial diuretics,

phenylbutazone, chlorpromazine, and α-methyldopa.

Evaluation of a child with neutropenia

The clinical evaluation of a child with suspected neutropenia should first document the degree of neutropenia and establish whether its pattern is chronic or cyclic. Generally an absolute granulocyte count of less than 1.5×10^9/liter is considered the criterion for diagnosis of neutropenia, but attributing symptoms of recurrent infections to it requires the absolute neutrophil count to be less than 0.5×10^9/liter. As indicated in the following list, serial complete blood counts done three times per week for a minimum of 6 weeks are required to rule out the diagnosis of cyclic neutropenia.

1. Complete blood count, platelet count, absolute granulocyte count, and reticulocyte count three times weekly for at least 6 weeks
2. Bone marrow aspiration and biopsy
3. Epinephrine stimulation test[11]
4. Endotoxin[189] and/or hydrocortisone stimulation tests
5. Rebuck skin window test[249]
6. Diisopropyl fluorophosphate ([^{32}P]DFP) or ^{51}Cr survival study
7. Antineutrophil antibody assay[38]
8. Colony forming unit (CFU-C) assay, colony stimulating factor (CSF) assay[238]
9. Immunologic evaluation (quantitative immunoglobulins, skin test reactivity, T and B cell evaluation)
10. Pancreatic exocrine, folate, vitamin B_{12}, and copper levels and metabolic deficiency screening evaluation
11. Collagen vascular disease evaluation with studies of antinuclear antibodies, C3 and C4, LE cell preparation, and rheumatoid factor
12. Evaluation of other family members for evidence of neutropenia and chest and long bone x-ray films to rule out phenotypic skeletal expressions of neutropenic diseases

Although bone marrow aspiration and biopsy are usually not particularly helpful in predicting the severity of the neutropenia, it is useful to perform them for an estimation of the bone marrow reserve pool, bone marrow morphology of the granulocytes, maturational status of the cells, and in vitro colony formation. The marginating pool of granulocytes can be assessed by an epinephrine stimulation test. After a single subcutaneous injection of 0.1 to 0.3 ml aqueous epinephrine (1:1,000) white blood counts and differential counts are obtained at zero time and at 5, 10, 15, and 30 minutes. Normally there is a twofold increase in polymorphonuclear neutrophils compared to the preinjection value. The bone marrow reserve pool can be evaluated by either an endotoxin stimulation test or a hydrocortisone stimulation test. The administration of endotoxin from *Salmonella enteritidis* (0.8 ng/kg intravenously) or typhoid vaccine (0.5 ml subcutaneously) with white blood cell and differential counts obtained over the next 6 to 24 hours will assess the bone marrow reserve. The mean increase of polymorphonuclear neutrophils is $6 \pm 0.8 \times 10^9$/liter. A single intravenous injection of 200 mg of hydrocortisone sodium succinate can also be used, and white blood cell counts and differential counts are obtained during the next 6 to 24 hours; the maximal increase in polymorphonuclear neutrophils occurs during the 6-hour period, with absolute mean increases to $4 \pm 0.3 \times 10^9$/liter.

The Rebuck skin window assesses the in vivo inflammatory response and will be discussed in Chapter 19.

[^{32}P]DFP is rarely used today to study granulocyte survival. ^{51}Cr offers an alternative, but both of these tests are extremely difficult to perform unless research facilities are available. The neutrophil antibody assay is necessary to rule out an immune basis. The in vitro cell culture system is useful to assess CFU-C activity as well as CSA in selected cases.

An immunologic evaluation including quantitative immunoglobulins should be done in every case of neutropenia because of the close association of neutropenia and immunoglobin deficiencies. A careful search for viral, bacterial, rickettsial, and fungal infections is usually indicated. Evaluations of pancreatic exocrine function should be included. Total nutritional assessment, vitamin B$_{12}$, folate, and copper levels and urinary amino acid screening tests are necessary. Collagen vascular disease should be ruled out with antinuclear antibody tests, serum C3 and C4 quantitation, and a determination of rheumatoid factor. Serum muramidase testing may be useful in patients with marked elevation and destruction of mononuclear cells as occurs in monocytic and myelomonocytic leukemia.

An evaluation of the family members and a careful family history are necessary to rule in or out hereditary neutropenic syndromes. X-ray studies of the long bones and chest are indicated if the patient is thought to have an associated phenotypic abnormality of the skeletal system.

NEUTROPHILIA
Acute infections

Neutrophilia may be the result of acute infections, especially those caused by pyogenic microorganisms (staphylucuccus, streptococcus, pneumococcus, gonococcus, meningococcus, *E. coli,* and *Pseudomonas aeruginosa*), *Corynebacterium diphtheriae, Pasteurella pestis,* fungi (*Actinomyces*), *Leptospira icterohaemorrhagiae,* viruses (rabies, poliomyelitis, herpes zoster, smallpox, and varicella), and rickettsiae (typhus and paratyphus). Neutrophilia is found in association with localized infections (such as furuncles, carbuncles, abscesses, tonsillitis, otitis media, and osteomyelitis) and with widespread infections (such as pneumonia, meningitis, peritonitis, pleuritis, pericarditis, arthritis, and acute appendicitis). In acute infection total leukocyte counts of 15 to 25 $\times 10^9$/liter are common; counts may reach as high as 50×10^9/liter.

Leukemoid reactions

Total leukocyte counts in excess of 50×10^9/liter are usually associated with a "shift to the left" of more immature myeloid cells including occasional myeloblasts and promyelocytes as well as myelocytes and metamyelocytes in the peripheral blood. Although any of the pyogenic bacteria that cause neutrophilia may produce a leukemoid reaction, it is more commonly associated with staphylococcal abscesses and pneumonia.[129] Tuberculosis, brucellosis, and toxoplasmosis have also been reported to cause myeloid leukemoid reactions. Tumor invasion of the bone marrow space results in the appearance of immature myeloid and nucleated red cells in the blood smear. This latter finding can be a useful sign in the course and management of patients with malignancies that metastasize to bone marrow such as lymphoma, neuroblastoma, and rhabdomyosarcoma. Leukemoid reactions have been described in acute glomerulonephritis, acute liver failure, and as a response to intramuscular injections of iron-dextran complexes.[173,259] Patients with acute episodes of rheumatoid arthritis or patients with polyserositis from any cause may also have leukemoid reactions.[129]

Differential diagnosis of leukemoid reactions includes chronic myelocytic leukemia of the adult type. Patients with chronic myelogenous leukemia have a myeloid proliferation including eosinophils and basophils in the peripheral blood in addition to immature neutrophils. The activity of leukocyte alkaline phosphatase (LAP) is increased in the polymorphonuclear neutrophils of leukemoid reactions and decreased in those of chronic myelocytic leukemia.[173] Generally, massive splenomegaly is a more characteristic feature in chronic myelogenous leukemia. If the blood findings persist for more than a few days or no specific cause for the extreme leukocytosis can be found, bone marrow studies should be obtained for Philadelphia chromosome. Infants with Down's syndrome may develop a myeloproliferative response associated with a leukemoid reaction in the blood. The condition resembles acute leukemia because of the large number of circulating blast cells. Generally the reaction subsides spontaneously during the first year of life.[139]

Noninfectious neutrophilia

Noninfectious causes of neutrophilia include burns, postoperative states, ischemic tissue necrosis, metabolic uremia, diabetic acidosis, acute hemorrhage, acute hemolysis, disseminated malignant neoplasms, stress caused by exercise, and injections of adrenocorticosteroids.

EOSINOPHILIA

Normal eosinophil counts. At birth and during the immediate postnatal period peripheral blood eosinophils are decreased in number. Thereafter they increase progressively and reach peak values in boys and in girls at 6 to 8 years of age. On the average boys have higher eosinophil counts than girls.[70] Average values for children are 0.24×10^9 /liter (range 0 to 0.74×10^9/liter); average values for adults are 0.15 to 0.20×10^9/liter (range 0 to 0.7×10^9/liter). A definite diurnal variation occurs, with a midmorning nadir approximately 20% less than the 8:00 A.M. level and a maximum nocturnal peak approximately 30% greater than the 8:00 A.M. level. This diurnal variation is not observed in patients with adrenal insufficiency. Estimates of eosinophil numbers based on differential counts and stained blood smears are subject to error because the natural stickiness or adherence of eosinophils prevents their even distribution. Three percent to 6% of bone marrow nucleated cells are eosinophils. Of these approximately half are mature, bilobed cells similar to those seen in the peripheral blood.[67,183]

Tissue eosinophilia. Several eosinophilic chemotactic factors are responsible for tissue and often blood eosinophilia. Complement fragments C3a and C5a cleaved during the complement cascade attract eosinophils as well as polymorphonuclear neutrophils.[151,307] An eosinophilic chemotactic precursor substance elaborated by antigen-stimulated lymphocytes might explain eosinophilia accompanying some autoimmune and collagen vascular diseases.[61] Allergic disorders characterized by eosinophilia appear to result from the reaction of antigen and antibody of IgE class fixed to the surface of the tissue mast cell or blood basophil resulting in the liberation of vasoactive histamine, which renders blood vessel walls permeable, allowing circulating eosinophils to escape nonspecifically and migrate with other leukocytes. Another mast cell–releasing component is the eosinophilic chemotactic factor of anaphylaxis, which selectively attracts eosinophils.[152] There are many likely nonimmunologic causes for eosinophilia, considering the molecular arrangement of proteins, polysaccharides, and macromolecules that can simulate antigen-antibody complexes.[101]

Function of eosinophils. There is no marked difference between neutrophils and eosinophils in terms of the type of particles they ingest, their rates of engulfment, their modes of degranulation, or the types of microorganisms they kill. If anything, the eosinophil is more sluggish than the neutrophil in its rate of ingestion and bacterial killing; yet parodoxically it has a higher metabolic activity in terms of hydrogen peroxide production, oxidative response, and iodination.[14,60,200]

Purified eosinophil populations, in contrast to neutrophil or mononuclear preparations, release ^{51}Cr from labeled immature schistosomes, which suggests that eosinophils can selectively destroy parasites. The eosinophils from normal subjects but not from patients with eosinophilia were most effective in this system, suggesting the possibility that eosinophilic surface receptors were altered by circulating antigen-antibody complexes.[48] Recent scanning and transmission electron microscopic studies of eosinophils show that the surface architecture is spherical and resembles that of lymphocytes.[245] In an in vivo system using mice with *Schistosoma mansoni* infection partial immunity was provided from specific antibody made in a rabbit against the schistosomes. The protective effect of this antibody was abrogated by prior treatment of the mice with antieosinophil serum but not with antisera directed against lymphocytes, monocytes, or neutrophils. Thus eosinophils seemed to have parasiticidal properties.

The eosinophil may also function in the immediate type of allergic or anaphylactic hypersensitivity reactions. Here all stages of the allergic response, i.e., mediator release, mediator inactivation, and mediator replenishment, are regulated. Since tissue mast cells sensitized by IgE release chemical mediators of anaphylaxis including histamine, slow-reacting substance of anaphylaxis (SRS-A), and eosinophilic chemotactic factor of anaphylaxis, the eosinophil moves to the tissue site and then releases an eosinophil-derived inhibitor of histamine as well as an eosinophil histaminase, an aryl sulfatase that selectively inhibits histamine and SRS-A.[150]

Clinical disorders associated with eosinophilia

As can be seen in the following list, a wide variety of disorders are associated with mild to moderate eosinophilia; however, only a few conditions provide extreme degrees of eosinophilia and will be discussed in more detail. The following conditions are associated with eosinophilia:

A. Allergic disorders
   1. Bronchial asthma
   2. Urticaria
   3. Angioneurotic edema
   4. Hay fever
B. Parasitic infestations
   1. *Toxocara* infestation
   2. Trichinosis
   3. *Echinococcus* infestation
   4. *Strongyloides* infestation
   5. *Ascaris* infestation
   6. Hookworm infestation
   7. Filariasis
   8. Tropical eosinophilia
C. Idiopathic hypereosinophilic syndrome
D. Drugs
E. Infections
   1. Scarlet fever
   2. Chorea
   3. Erythema multiforme
   4. Histoplasmosis, coccidioidomycosis, tuberculosis
F. Hematopoietic disorders
   1. Acute lymphocytic leukemia
   2. Chronic myelocytic leukemia
   3. Acute granulocytic leukemia
   4. Hodgkin's disease
   5. Malignant histiocytosis
   6. Postsplenectomy
   7. Hyperimmunoglobulin E
   8. X-linked agammaglobulinemia with *Pneumocystis carinii* pneumonia
   9. Severe combined immunodeficiency syndrome with reticuloendotheliosis and eosinophilia
   10. Postirradiation
G. Skin diseases
   1. Atopic dermatitis
   2. Pemphigus
   3. Dermatitis herpetiformis
H. Miscellaneous disorders characterized by chronic inflammation
   1. Periarteritis nodosa
   2. Rheumatoid arthritis
   3. Chronic hepatitis
   4. Regional enteritis
   5. Eosinophilic gastroenteritis
   6. Eosinophilic cystitis
   7. Infected ventricular-peritoneal or ventricular-pleural shunt
   8. Chronic peritoneal dialysis

Allergy. Allergy is probably the most common cause of eosinophilia in children in the United States.[282] Approximately 85% of children with bronchial asthma have eosinophil counts in excess of 0.6×10^9/liter. The eosinophilia associated with asthma is persistent and does not correlate with symptoms or with measurement of pulmonary function. Urticaria, infantile eczema, serum sickness, and angioneurotic edema are usually associated with moderate to mild eosinophilia.

Evaluating nasal secretions for eosinophils appears useful in patients with certain forms of allergic rhinitis. Children with allergic rhinitis seen during the grass pollinating season universally have abnormal smears (defined as 10 eosinophils/high-power field in any two high-power fields). Children with allergic rhinitis from house dust, dogs, or cats also usually have eosinophils in nasal secretions, but eosinophils are seldom found in the nasal secretions of children with allergic rhinitis caused by food alone.[215] Nasal smears are also useful in differentiating an allergic rhinitis from viral upper respiratory infections.[317]

Patients with air pollution bronchitis characterized by wheezing display eosinophil counts of more than 0.4×10^9/liter.[292] Inhaled *Aspergillus* spores may induce eosinophilia and an eosinophilic pneumonia with wheezing, cough, and transient pulmonary infiltrates.[144]

Parasitic infestations. Parasitic infestations are present in one third of the world's population and are the most common cause of eosinophilia outside the United States. In general an increase in blood eosinophils is observed in helminthic but not protozoan infestations. Helminths that invade tissue induce a greater eosinophilia than those that remain in the intestinal lumen. Infestations of the small intestine are more often associated with significant eosinophilia than those restricted to the duodenum or colon. This may explain the lack of eosinophilia in *Giardia lamblia* enteropathy and in anorectal pruritis caused by pinworms (*Enterobius vermicularis*). Eosinophilia is most marked during the stages of acute invasion, larval development, and migration. As a result eggs and larvae may not be easily identified in feces at the time of maximal eosinophilia. Some parasites such as *Trichinella spiralis* and *Toxocara canis* and *cati* are never identified by stool analysis. Thus parasitic infestations as the cause of eosinophilia cannot be excluded by failure to demonstrate eggs or larvae in feces, nor can parasitic infestations be dismissed because of the absence of eosinophilia.

During the tissue migration of *Trichinella spiralis* 20% or more of the blood leukocytes are eosinophils. Maximal eosinophilia with *Ascaris* and hookworm disease parallels the pulmonary infiltrates produced by their migrating larvae. In a recent study in which four male students were exposed to massive doses of *Ascaris suum*, a parasite endemic to pigs, the students manifested a clinical picture of pulmonary infiltrates with eosinophilia and asthma. The two patients with the most widespread pulmonary infiltrates also had the most marked eosinophilia and elevated levels of IgE, plus IgM precipitating antibodies to *Ascaris suum* antigen. The immune response may also have had a protective function since the students with the most marked immune response to the *Ascaris* antigen also more effectively eradicated the parasites.

Eosinophilia is demonstrated in only 20% to 25% of patients with hydatid disease. Mild to moderate eosinophilia is observed with several variants of tapeworm infestation. *Giardia lamblia,* a parasitic infestation of the duodenum and upper gastrointestinal tract, does not produce eosinophilia. Malaria is the only exception to the generalization that protozoan infections fail to produce an increase in eosinophilia. A moderate eosinophilia is frequently observed during the convalescent phase of malarial attacks.[182]

Visceral larva migrans. By far the most common of the hypereosinophilic syndromes in children is visceral larva migrans.[125,135,208] Visceral larva migrans is characterized by hepatomegaly, pulmonary infiltrates, eosinophilic leukocytosis, anemia, and hyperglobulinemia. The etiologic agents are *Toxocara canis* and *Toxocara cati,* the common roundworms of dogs and cats. They are ubiquitous in their geographic distribution and, because of their thick shells, they remain viable in soil for years. When ingested by humans, the eggs hatch in the upper gastrointestinal tract and the released larvae gain access to the portal circulation, lodging themselves in the liver parenchyma. Some larvae migrate from the liver to the lung and from there to the heart, from which they are disseminated in the systemic circulation. The larvae rarely mature and the eggs are not identified in fecal specimens.

CLINICAL FEATURES. In some cases the condition is totally asymptomatic, save for the eosinophilia. However, more frequently medical attention is sought because of a febrile illness associated with cough, occasional wheezing, and demonstrable pulmonary infiltrates in approximately 50% of children. Liver enlargement often associated with splenic enlargement is observed in 60% to 90% of affected children. Seizures and encephalitis are rare complications. The retinal lesion caused by *Toxocara* larvae may be indistinguishable from that produced by retinoblastoma. Consequently, when a diagnosis of retinoblastoma is entertained, *Toxocara* infestation should be carefully considered. Skin lesions have been described, including tender nodules on the palms and soles, erythema nodosum, urticaria, and purpura. Rarely myocarditis is associated with refractory congestive heart failure.

LABORATORY FEATURES. Leukocyte counts in excess of 100×10^9/liter with 80% to 90% mature eosinophils are not uncommon. In most children eosinophils comprise more than 50% of the circulating leukocytes. Eosinophilia may persist for months to years after other manifestations of infection have resolved. Mild anemia secondary to

chronic inflammation is often noted. Severe anemia results from coexistent iron deficiency. Hyperglobulinemia is a frequent finding, resulting in part from increased isohemagglutinins, which suggests a cross-reactivity between the antibody directed against the infecting parasite and group A and group B substances on the red blood cell. Recent surveys have documented increased titers of anti-A and anti-B in schistosomiasis, malaria, and other parasitic infestations.[183] A hemagglutinin test is available but lacks the sensitivity and specificity to confirm the diagnosis in some instances.[147] An immunoprecipitation immunodiffusion test is also available. In addition to elevations of IgM, IgG, and IgA, IgE has been reported to be increased in visceral larva migrans.[127]

CLINICAL COURSE. The prognosis for children with visceral larva migrans is almost always favorable. The clinical expressions of the larval infestations subside within weeks. The ocular pseudotumor formation occurs some months later after inflammation has subsided. A few fatalities have been reported from extensive central nervous system and myocardial involvement. Generally no treatment is needed. Thiabendazole, a broad-spectrum antihelmenthic agent, is reported to have relieved symptoms and shortened the convalescence of a small group of children with visceral larva migrans.[12] However, because the course of the infection is one of spontaneous improvement, control studies will be needed to evaluate the usefulness of any agent with therapeutic potential.

Tropical eosinophilia. Tropical eosinophilia, a syndrome seen with greatest frequency in India and Southeast Asia, is characterized by chronic or recurrent pulmonary infiltrations with asthmalike symptoms, lymphadenopathy, and eosinophilia.[304] Serum levels of IgA and IgD are normal with slightly increased levels of IgG and IgM; however, the serum IgE levels are increased 30 to 270 times the mean normal level.[85,301] Treatment with other antihelmenthic agents also has been effective and, because of these dramatic responses, a filarial parasite has been proposed as the major causative agent.

Idiopathic hypereosinophilic syndromes. Idiopathic hypereosinophilic syndrome has been described under a number of designations including, disseminated eosinophilic collagen disease, Löffler's disease, endocarditis with endomyocardial fibrosis, pulmonary infiltration with eosinophilia (PIE syndrome), and eosinophilic pneumonopathy. There are those who suggest that this is a syndrome that comprises a continuum from Löffler's pneumonia at one extreme to eosinophilic leukemia at the other.[117] A variety of drugs has also been incriminated as the cause of the PIE syndrome. The pulmonary disease associated with the use of nitrofurantoin is the most common and best characterized.[2]

Clinical manifestations. Although the idiopathic hypereosinophilic syndrome has been documented in children as young as 5 months of age,[250] most reports of the descriptions of the disorder are in men from 20 to 40 years of age.[42] Clinical symptoms usually result from congestive heart failure. In addition to cardiomegaly, murmurs of mitral insufficiency and less frequently murmurs of mitral stenosis and tricuspid insufficiency develop. Both pulmonary infiltrates and pleural effusion may be observed. Although the liver and spleen are enlarged, hepatic function is preserved. As a rule, organ enlargement is progressive, and congestive heart failure is intractable. The constrictive cardiomyopathy may result from the prolonged release of products from degranulated eosinophils.[275]

The differential diagnosis includes eosinophilic leukemia. The peripheral blood and visceral eosinophils are mature, and there is no disturbance in eosinophilic maturation in the aspirates of the bone marrow from patients with idiopathic hypereosinophilic syndrome. Anemia and thrombocytopenia are not seen and the clinical picture is dominated by cardiopulmonary decompensation. The differential diagnosis of eosinophilic lung disease also includes Löffler's pulmonary eosinophilia caused by parasites or drugs, producing migratory peripheral infiltrates that clear without treatment within a month; allergic aspergillosis causing infiltrates in the course of chronic asthma, producing a picture of recurrent pneumonia and atelectasis with eosinophilia; polyarteritis nodosa and the other variants of hypersensitivity angiitis, producing severe symptoms with pulmonary involvement and usually occurring before multisystem disease; Wegener's granulomatosis, producing large pulmonary nodules; and cavitation with modest eosinophilia.[57]

Drugs. Drug-induced eosinophilia may be associated with other expressions of hypersensitivity reactions but more commonly occurs as an isolated phenomenon. Penicillin, ampicillin, cephalosporins, nitrofurantoin, para-aminosalicylic acid, phenytoin, hydralazine, and chlorpromazine may produce a moderate increase in blood eosinophils.

Hematopoietic disorders. Eosinophilia has been described in association with both acute lymphocytic leukemia and acute granulocytic leukemia. The degree of eosinophilia when the patient is originally seen may suggest the diagnosis of eosinophilic leukemia.[250] However, recent studies suggest that the eosinophilia is reactive to the leukemic process rather than a part of it.[274] The association of eosinophilia and Löffler's endomyocardiofibrosis has occurred in acute lymphoblastic leukemia.[30] There does appear to be a clear-cut

condition of acute eosinophilic leukemia; however, it must be differentiated from the reactive eosinophilia of acute lymphoblastic leukemia and the eosinophilic predominance noted in some patients with chronic myelogenous leukemia with the Philadelphia chromosome.[310,321] Chronic myelocytic leukemia occurs in less than 2% of children with leukemia and characteristically is associated with a mild eosinophilia and basophilia. Levels of transcobalamin I, derived from granulocytes, are elevated in patients with eosinophilic leukemia,[63] in contrast to transcobalamin II, which is derived from liver.

Lymphopenia and slight eosinophilia occur in untreated Hodgkin's disease. Patients with a progressive form of malignant histiocytosis are known to have eosinophilia as part of their clinical picture. They have fever and histiocytic infiltration of skin, lymph nodes, liver, and spleen. This disease is rapidly progressive and usually patients die within a period of months. Pathologically there is a systemic proliferation of nonphagocytic immature histiocytes in all affected organs. The disease process shares certain clinical and pathologic features with histiocytic medullary reticulosis and partly with histiocytosis X. The progressive nature of the disease and the cutaneous skin involvement as well as the immaturity of the histiocytes involved in the infiltrative process set this disease apart from them.[18,178]

Immune disorders. A variety of immune disorders are associated with eosinophilia. Rapidly fatal familial histiocytosis has occurred in patients with severe combined immunodeficiency syndrome. These infants develop an erythematous, maculopapular skin eruption associated with failure to thrive, hepatomegaly, lymphadenopathy, and eosinophilia with a rapidly fatal course resulting from infection and diarrhea.[19,222,224] These patients should be differentiated from infants with classical Letterer-Siwe syndrome, the syndrome of familial malignant histiocytosis, and the runting syndrome of chronic graft versus host reaction.[202]

Eosinophilia has been noted in three male siblings with infantile X-linked agammaglobulinemia who developed fatal *Pneumocystis carinii* pneumonia. On the other hand, *Pneumocystis carinii* pneumonia in patients who have normal immunoglobulins is not associated with eosinophilia.

Massive polyclonal hyperimmunoglobulinemia E associated with an increase in peripheral blood lymphocytes that stain for surface IgE and eosinophil counts in excess of 18×10^9/liter has been reported. The affected patient had no evidence of hematologic, parasitic, immunodeficiency, hypersensitivity, or allergic disease.[235]

Postirradiation eosinophilia. The occurrence of eosinophilia following radiotherapy or exposure to ionizing radiation is common. The first demonstration of this occurred in cyclotron workers exposed to excessive radiation who then developed an increase in total circulating eosinophils.[213] Large field ^{58}Co radiation is associated with eosinophilia in 30% of all cases and seems to be unrelated to the type of disease treated. Typically the eosinophilia peaks in the fourth week. Improved prognosis in adults with ovarian and endometrial cancer has been noted in the group who developed significant radiation-related eosinophilia, but the prognostic implication of eosinophilia remains untested in children.[97]

Chronic inflammation. Miscellaneous disorders characterized by chronic inflammation also have been associated with mild to moderate eosinophilia. These include periarteritis nodosa, rheumatoid arthritis, chronic hepatitis, regional enteritis, eosinophilic cystitis, gastroenteritis, infected ventricular-peritoneal or ventricular-pleural shunts,* and chronic peritoneal dialysis.[172,297]

EOSINOPENIA

In contrast to the large number of clinical conditions associated with eosinophilia, the frequency and significance of eosinopenia is less well differentiated. A decrease of eosinophils has been observed immediately postnatally. Pharmacologic doses of corticosteroids produce a temporary eosinopenia by blocking the mobilization of eosinophils from the bone marrow. A decrease in bone marrow and blood eosinophils has been described in a few patients with Down's syndrome.[8]

BASOPHILIA

Basophils are the least numerous of human granulocytes, accounting for 0.5% to 1% of circulating leukocytes and less than 1% of nucleated cells in the bone marrow. Modest variation in basophil frequency has been noted with age and sex. Young adult females are likely to have slightly higher basophil counts than men. Because of their relative paucity, estimates of basophil number based on ordinary differential Wright's stain blood smears are subject to substantial error. Basophil enumeration is best approached by using a direct counting method in which basophils are selectively stained and enumerated with Fuchs-Rosenthal chambers.[205,322]

Blood basophil levels are depressed by corticosteroids, thyrotropic hormone, and thyroxin. Basophil levels are elevated in myxedema and lowered in thyrotoxicosis. Basophilia is common in myeloproliferative disorders, particularly chronic granulocytic leukemia in which basophils may number more than 90×10^9/liter and on occasion

*References 92, 231, 282, 285.

can account for 90% or more of circulating leukocytes.[322] Basophilia is the earliest sign of developing chronic myelogenous leukemia.[210] Elevated basophil levels have also been reported in polycythemia vera, chronic hemolytic anemia, Hodgkin's disease, smallpox, chickenpox, some cases of cirrhosis, ulcerative colitis, and various allergic states such as asthma and after radiation or splenectomy. Blood histamine levels rise in proportion to the number of circulating basophils. Recent studies have shown a close association between histamine release and circulating IgE. The tissue counterpart to the basophil is the mast cell, which releases histamine by contact with specific antigen or by anti-IgE antibody. Basophil and mast cell release of histamine contributes to cell-mediated hypersensitivity reactions observed by skin testing and to increased vascular permeability.[83]

MONOCYTOSIS

A variety of factors influence the number of circulating monocytes. In the normal child and adult the relative monocyte percentage is between 1% and 6% of the total leukocyte count and rarely exceeds 10%. The absolute monocyte count in the adult ranges between 0.285 and 0.5×10^9 cells/liter of blood. In children the absolute number ranges up to 0.75 to 0.8 cells/liter. Of those disease states that characteristically produce monocytosis are those associated with chronic long-standing bacterial infection, certain malignancies, and a variety of other disorders.[185] Relative monocytosis is normal in the neonate and may persist for several weeks.

The infections with intracellular microorganisms and parasites that have been associated with monocytosis are the following: subacute bacterial endocarditis, tuberculosis, typhoid fever, rickettsial disease, syphilis, brucellosis, malaria, trypanosomiasis, leishmaniasis, and *Listeria monocytogenes* infection. Monocytosis and abnormal monocytes may be associated with a variety of malignant diseases but especially with lymphoproliferative and histiocytic proliferative disorders. For example, chronic monocytosis may antedate the development of acute leukemia. It has also been described in myelomonocytic leukemia, Hodgkin's disease, non-Hodgkin's lymphoma, and multiple myeloma. Relative monocytosis occurs in some forms of granulocytopenia, after splenectomy, and in some hemolytic anemias. Patients with collagen vascular diseases such as rheumatic endocarditis, SLE, and rheumatoid arthritis may have monocytosis. Chronic inflammatory gastrointestinal diseases such as ulcerative colitis, Crohn's disease, and serositis have also been associated with monocytosis.

MONOCYTOPENIA

Administration of endotoxin results in monocytopenia followed by a recovery phase that is slow and incomplete relative to the granulocyte response. Glucocorticoid administration may induce monocytopenia. In contrast to the profound granulocytopenia and leukopenia associated with irradiation, monocytes and their progeny appear to be relatively insensitive to radiation.

REFERENCES

1. Abernathy, M. R.: Döhle bodies associated with uncomplicated pregnancy, Blood **27**:380, 1966.
2. Adickman, M. A., and Tuthill, T. M.: Pulmonary infiltrates and eosinophilia associated with drug reactions and parasitic infections, Post-Grad. Med. **60**(9):143, 1976.
3. Allopurinol and cytotoxic drugs: interaction in relation to bone marrow depression, Boston Collaborative Drug Surveillance Program, J.A.M.A. **227**:1036, 1974.
4. A.M.A. Council on Drugs: Evaluation of a new oral diuretic agent: ethacrynic acid and ethacrynate sodium (edecrin and edecrin sodium), J.A.M.A. **208**:2327, 1969.
5. A.M.A. Council on Drugs: Registry on adverse reactions, tabulation of reports, panel on hematology, Chicago, 1964, American Medical Association.
6. Amrhein, J. A., Kenny, F. M., and Ross, D.: Granulocytopenia, lupus-like syndrome, and other complications of propylthiouracil therapy, J. Pediatr. **76**:54, 1970.
7. Archer, G. T., and Hirsch, J. G.: Isolation of granules from eosinophil leucocytes and study of their enzyme content, J. Exp. Med. **118**:277, 1963.
8. Archer, R. K., English, H. J. C., Gaha, T., and Ruxton, J.: The eosinophil leucocytes in the blood and bone marrow of patients with Down's anomaly, Br. J. Haematol. **21**:271, 1971.
9. Arrowsmith, W. R., Binkley, B., and Moore, C. V.: Fatal agranulocytosis following the intra-peritoneal implantation of sulfanilamide crystals, Ann. Intern. Med. **21**:323, 1944.
10. Athens, J. W.: Neutrophilic granulocyte kinetics and granulocytopoiesis. In Gordon, A. S., ed.: Regulation of hematopoiesis, New York, 1970, Appleton-Century-Crofts.
11. Athens, J. W., Haab, O. P., Raab, S. O., et al.: Leukokinetic studies. IV. The total blood, circulating and marginal granulocyte pools, and the granulocyte turnover rate in normal subjects, J. Clin. Invest. **40**:989, 1961.
12. Aur, J. A., Pratt, C. B., and Johnson, W. W.: Thiabendazole and visceral larva migrans, Am. J. Dis. Child. **121**:226, 1971.
13. Austin, J. H., and Leopoid, S. S.: An extraordinary polymorphonuclear leukopenia in typhoid fever, J.A.M.A. **66**:1084, 1916.
14. Baehner, R. L., and Johnston, R. B., Jr.: Metabolic and bactericidal activity of human eosinophils, Br. J. Haematol. **20**:277, 1971.
15. Baggiolini, M.: The enzymes of the granules of polymorphonuclear leukocytes and their functions, Enzyme **13**:132, 1972.
16. Bainton, D. F., and Farquhar, M. G.: Differences in enzyme content of azurophil and specific granules of polymorphonuclear leukocytes. II. Cytochemistry and electron microscopy of bone marrow cells, J. Cell. Biol. **39**:299, 1968.
17. Ball, K., Joules, H., and Pagel, W.: Acute tuberculous septicaemia with leucopenia, Br. Med. J. **2**:869, 1951.
18. Ballard, J. O., Binder, R. A., Rath, C. E., and Powell, D.: Malignant histiocytosis in a patient presenting with leukocytosis, eosinophilia, and lymph node granuloma, Cancer **35**:1444, 1975.
19. Barth, R. F., Khurana, S. K., Vergara, G. G., et al.: Rapidly fatal familial histiocytosis associated with eosinophilia and primary immunological deficiency, Lancet **2**:503, 1972.
20. Barzel, U. S.: Quinidine-sulfate-induced hypoplastic anemia and agranulocytosis, J.A.M.A. **201**:325, 1967.
21. Basten, A., and Beeson, P. B.: Mechanism of eosinophilia. II. Role of the lymphocyte, J. Exp. Med. **131**:1288, 1970.
22. Beard, M. E. J., Newmark, P., Smith, M. E., and Franklin, A. W.: Infantile genetic agranulocytosis associated with changes in serum vitamin B_{12} binding proteins, Acta Paediatr. Scand. **61**:526, 1972.
23. Begemann, N. H., and Campagne, A. Van L.: Homozygous form of Pelger-Huët's nuclear anomaly in man, Acta Haematol. **7**:295, 1952.
24. Benjamin, B., and Ward, S. M.: Leukocytic response to measles, Am. J. Dis. Child. **44**:921, 1932.
25. Berry, G. P., and Kitcheness, F.: Yellow fever accidentally contracted in the laboratory, Am. J. Trop. Med. **11**:365, 1931.
26. Bethell, F. H.: The response to infection in bone marrow dyscrasias, J. Lab. Clin. Med. **20**:362, 1935.
27. Bilezikian, S. B., Laleli, Y., Tsan, M. F., et al.: Immunological reactions involving leukocytes. III. Agranulocytosis induced by antithyroid drugs, Johns Hopkins Med. J. **138**:124, 1976.
28. Bishop, C. R., Rothstein, G., Ashenbrucker, H. E., and Athens, J. W.: Leukokinetics studies. XIV. Blood neutrophil kinetics in chronic, stead-state neutropenia, J. Clin. Invest. **50**:1678, 1971.
29. Björkstén, B., and Lundmark, K. M.: Recurrent bacterial infections in four siblings with neutropenia, eosinophilia, hyperimmunoglobulinemia A, and defective neutrophil chemotaxis, J. Infect. Dis. **133**:63, 1976.
30. Blatt, P. M., Rothstein, G., Miller, H. L., and Cathey, W. J.: Loeffler's endomyocardio fibrosis with eosinophilia in association with acute lymphoblastic leukemia, Blood **44**:489, 1974.
31. Blendis, L. M., Ansell, I. D., Jones, K. L., et al.: Liver in Felty's syndrome, Br. Med. J. **1**:131, 1970.
32. Bodian, M., Sheldon, W., and Lightwood, R. L.: Congenital hypoplasia of the exocrine pancreas, Acta Paediatr. **53**:282, 1964.
33. Boggs, D. R.: The kinetics of neutrophilic leukocytes in health and in disease, Semin. Hematol. **4**:359, 1967.
34. Boggs, D. R., and Chervenick, P. A.: Hematopoietic stem cells. In Greenwalt, T. J., and Jamieson, G. A. eds.: Formation and destruction of blood cells, Philadelphia, 1970, J. B. Lippincott Co.
35. Boggs, D. R., Marsh, J. C., Chervenick, P. A., et al.: Neutrophil releasing activity in plasma of normal human subjects when injected with endotoxin, Proc. Soc. Exp. Biol. Med. **127**:689, 1968.
36. Bousser, J., and Neyde, R.: La neutropénie familiale, Sang **18**:521, 1947.
37. Boxer, L. A., Greenberg, M. S., Boxer, G. J., and Stossel, T. P.: Autoimmune neutropenia, N. Engl. J. Med. **293**:748, 1975.
38. Boxer, L. A., and Stossel, T. P.: Effects of anti-human neutrophil antibodies in vitro: quantitative studies, J. Clin. Invest. **53**:1534, 1974.
39. Bradley, T. R., and Metcalf, D.: The growth of mouse bone marrow cells in vitro, Austr. J. Exp. Biol. Med. Sci. **44**:287, 1966.
40. Brandt, L., Forssman, O., Mitelman, F., et al.: Cell production and cell function in human cyclic neutropenia, Scand. J. Haematol. **15**:228, 1975.

41. Breese, T. J., and Solomon, I. L.: Granulocytopenia and hemolytic anemia as complications of propylthiouracil therapy, J. Pediatr. **86:**117, 1975.
42. Brink, A. J., and Weber, H. W.: Fibroplastic parietal endocarditis with eosinophilia, Am. J. Med. **34:**52, 1963.
43. Brun, J., Perrin-Fayolle, M., and Sedallian, A.: La gentamycine en pneumologie: etude clinique et bacteriologique, Lyon Med. **218:**1263, 1967.
44. Buchanan, J. G., Pearce, L., and Wetherley-Mein, G.: The May-Hegglin Anomaly: a family report and chromosome study, Br. J. Haematol. **10:**508, 1964.
45. Buckley, R. H., and Rowlands, D. T., Jr.: Agammaglobulinemia, neutropenia, fever, and abdominal pain, J. Allergy Clin. Immunol. **51:**308, 1973.
46. Bujak, J. S., and Root, R. K.: The role of peroxidase in the bactericidal activity of human blood eosinophils, Blood **43:**727, 1974.
47. Burke, V., Colebatch, J. H., Anderson, C. M., and Simons, M. J.: Association of pancreatic insufficiency and chronic neutropenia in childhood, Arch. Dis. Child. **42:**147, 1967.
48. Butterworth, A. E., Sturrock, R. F., Houba, V., et al.: Eosinophils as mediators of antibody-dependent damage to schistosomula, Nature **256:**727, 1975.
49. Cahan, A. M., Meilman, E., and Jacobson, B. M.: Agranulocytosis following pyrabenzamine, N. Engl. J. Med. **241:**865, 1949.
50. Carper, H. A., and Hoffman, P. L.: The intravascular survival of transfused canine Pelger-Huet neutrophils and eosinophils, Blood **27:**739, 1966.
51. Catalano, P. M.: Dapsone agranulocytosis, Arch. Dermatol. **104:**675, 1971.
52. Cavale, V. C., and Smith, C.: Chronic lymphadenopathy simulating malignant lymphoma, J. Pediatr. **70:**891, 1967.
53. Chan, C. K., Jarrett, F., and Moylan, J. A.: Acute leukopenia as an allergic reaction to silver sulfadiazine in burn patients, J. Trauma **16:**395, 1976.
54. Chang, J. C., and Reyes, B.: Agranulocytosis associated with gentamycin, J.A.M.A. **232:**1154, 1975.
55. Chapman, R. A.: Suspected adverse reactions to indomethacin, Can. Med. Assoc. J. **95:**1156, 1966.
56. Chernof, D., and Taylor, K. S.: Hydroxychloroquine-induced agranulocytosis, Arch. Dermatol. **97:**163, 1968.
57. Citro, L. A., Gordon, M. E., and Miller, W. T.: Eosinophilic lung disease (or how to slice PIE), Am. J. Roentgenol. Radium Ther. Nucl. Med. **117:**787, 1973.
58. Cline, M. J.: The white cell, Cambridge, Mass., 1975, Harvard University Press.
59. Cline, M. J., and Golde, D. W.: A review and re-evaluation of the histiocytic disorders, Am. J. Med. **55:**49, 1973.
60. Cline, M. J., Hanifin, J., and Lehrer, R. I.: Phagocytosis by human eosinophils, Blood **32:**922, 1968.
61. Cohen, S., and Ward, P. A.: In vitro and in vivo activity of a lymphocyte and immune complex-dependent chemotactic factor for eosinophils, J. Exp. Med. **133:**133, 1971.
62. Cohn, Z. A., and Benson, B.: The differentiation of mononuclear phagocytes, morphology, cytochemistry, and biochemistry, J. Exp. Med. **121:**153, 1965.
63. Coltman, C. A., Jr., Panettiere, F., and Carmel, R.: Serum Vitamin B_{12}-binding proteins in a case of eosinophilic leukemia, Med. Ped. Oncol. **1:**185, 1975.
64. Colvin, B., Rogers, M., and Layton, C.: Benzylpenicillin-induced leucopenia: complication of treatment of bacterial endocarditis, Br. Heart J. **36:**216, 1974.
65. Cooper, J. R., and Cruickshank, C. N. D.: Improved method for direct counting of basophil leucocytes, J. Clin. Pathol. **19:**402, 1966.
66. Corcos, J. M., Soler-Bechara, J., Mayer, K., et al.: Neutrophilic agranulocytosis during administration of penicillamine, J.A.M.A. **189:**265, 1964.
67. Costello, R. T.: An unopette for eosinophil counts, Am. J. Clin. Pathol. **54:**249, 1970.
68. Cotter, L. H.: Thioglycolic acid poisoning in connection with the "cold ware" process, J.A.M.A. **131:**592, 1946.
69. Crammer, J. L., and Elkes, A.: Agranulocytosis after desipramine, Lancet **1:**105, 1967.
70. Cunningham, A. S.: Eosinophil counts: age and sex differences, J. Pediatr. **87:**426, 1975.
71. Curry, J. L., and Trentin, J. J.: Hemopoietic spleen colony studies. I. Growth and differentiation, Dev. Biol. **15:**395, 1967.
72. Cutting, H. O., and Lang, J. E.: Familial benign chronic neutropenia, Ann. Intern. Med. **61:**876, 1964.
73. Dale, D. C., Alling, D. W., and Wolff, S. M.: Cyclic hematopoiesis: the mechanism of cyclic neutropenia in grey collie dogs, J. Clin. Invest. **51:**2197, 1972.
74. Dale, D. C., Hubert, R. T., and Fauci, A.: Eosinophil kinetics in the hypereosinophilic syndrome, J. Lab. Clin. Med. **87:**487, 1976.
75. Dale, D. C., and Wolff, S. M.: Studies of the neutropenia of acute malaria, Blood **41:**197, 1973.
76. DeVaal, O. M., and Seynhaeve, V.: Reticular dysgenesis, Lancet **2:**1123, 1959.
77. Dicato, M. A., and Ellman, L.: Cephalothin-induced granulocytopenia, Ann. Intern. Med. **83:**671, 1975.
78. Dietrich, H. F.: Typhoid fever in children: a study of 60 cases, J. Pediatr. **10:**191, 1937.
79. Djaldetti, M., Joshua, H., and Kalderon, M.: Familial leukopenia-neutropenia in Yemenite Jews, Bull. Res. Council Isr. E **9:**24, 1961.
80. Doe, W. F.: Two brothers with congenital pancreatic exocrine insufficiency, neutropenia, and dysgammaglobulinaemia, Proc. R. Soc. Med. **66:**1125, 1973.
81. Doherty, R. L.: A clinical study of scrub typhus in North Queensland, Med. J. Aust. **2:**212, 1956.
82. Douglas, R. G., Jr., Alford, R. H., Cate, T. R., and Couch, R. B.: The leukocyte response during viral respiratory illness in man, Ann. Intern. Med. **64:**521, 1966.
83. Dvorak, H. F., and Dvorak, A. M.: Basophilic leucocytes: structure, function, and role in disease, Clin. Haematol. **4:**651, 1975.
84. Elgart, M. L.: Griseofulvin: a review of the literature and summary of present usage, Med. Ann. D.C. **36:**331, 1967.
85. Ezeoke, A., Perera, B. V., and Hobbs, J. R.: Serum IgE elevation with tropical eosinophilia, Clin. Allergy **3:**33, 1973.
86. Faber, V., and Pribin, E.: Leukocyte-specific antinuclear factors in patients with Felty's syndrome, rheumatoid arthritis, systemic lupus erythematosus, and other diseases, Acta Medica Scand. **179:**257, 1966.
87. Fellman, K., Kozlowski, K., and Senger, A.: Unusual bone changes in exocrine pancreas insufficiency with cyclic neutropenia, Acta Radiol. **12:**428, 1972.
88. Finch, S. C.: Granulocytopenia. In Williams, W. J., Boiler, E., Erslev, A. J., and Reynolds, R. W., eds.: Hematology, New York, 1972, McGraw-Hill Book Co.
89. Fiore, J. M., and Noonan, F. M.: Agranulocytosis due to mepazine (phenothiazine), N. Engl. J. Med. **260:**375, 1959.
90. Fleming, G. F., and Crowe, G. R.: Granulocytopenia due to a clindamycin, Med. J. Aust. **1:**70, 1976. (Letter.)
91. Fraumeni, J. F., Jr.: Bone marrow depression induced by chloramphenicol or phenylbutazone: leukemia and other sequelae, J.A.M.A. **201:**828, 1967.
92. Frensilli, F. J., Sacher, E. C., and Keegan, G. T.:

Eosinophilic cystitis: observations on etiology, J. Urol. **107**:595, 1972.

93. Frohman, L. A., and Klocke, F. J.: Recurrent thiocyanate intoxication, with pancytopenia, hypothyroidism and psychosis. N. Engl. J. Med. **268**:701, 1963.

94. Gänsslen, M.: Konstitutionelle familiäre leukopenie (neutropenie), Klin. Wochenschr. **20**:922, 1941.

95. Geelhoed, G. W., Kane, M. A., Dale, D. C., and Wells, S. A.: Colon ulceration and perforation in cyclic neutropenia, J. Pediatr. Surg. **8**:379, 1973.

96. Gershwin, M. E., Fajardo, L. P., Gurwith, M., and Kosek, J. C.: Eosinophilia terminating in myeloblastoma, Am. J. Med. **53**:348, 1972.

97. Ghossein, N. A., and Stacey, P.: The prognostic significance of radiation-related eosinophilia, Radiology **107**:631, 1973.

98. Giedion, A., Prader, A., Hadorn, B., et al.: Metaphysäre dysostose und angeborene pankreasinsuffizienz, Fortschr. Rontgenstr. **108**:51, 1968.

99. Gilman, P. A., Jackson, D. P., and Guild, H. G.: Congenital granulocytopenia, prolonged survival, and terminal acute leukemia, Blood **36**:576, 1970.

100. Gitlin, D., Janeway, C. A., Apt, L., and Craig, J. M.: Agammaglobulinemia. In Lawrence, H. S., ed.: Cellular and humoral aspects of the hypersensitive states, New York, 1959, Paul B. Hoeber, Inc.

101. Gleich, G. J., Loegering, D. A., and Maldonado, J. E.: Identification of a major basic protein in guinea pig eosinophil granules, J. Exp. Med. **137**:1459, 1973.

102. Goldman, A., and Haber, M.: Acute complete granulopenia with death due to dinitrophenol poisoning, J.A.M.A. **107**:2115, 1936.

103. Good, R. A., Kelly, W. D., Röstein, J., and Varco, R. L.: Immunological deficiency diseases. In Kallós, P., and Waksman, B. H., eds.: Progress in allergy, vol. 6, New York, 1962.

104. Gordin, R.: Toxic granulation in leukocytes, Acta Med. Scand. **143**(suppl.):270, 1952.

105. Graf, M., and Tarlov, A.: Agranulocytosis with monhistiocytosis associated with ampicillin therapy, Ann. Intern. Med. **69**:91, 1968.

106. Greenberg, M. L., and Chikkappa, G.: Eosinophil production and survival in a patient with eosinophilia (leukemia?), Blood **38**:826, 1971.

107. Greenberg, M. S., and Zambrano, S. S.: Aplastic agranulocytosis after allopurinol therapy, Arthritis Rheu. **15**:413, 1972.

108. Greenberg, P. L., Bax, I., Levin, J., and Andrews, T. M.: Alteration of colony stimulating factor output, endotoxemia, and granulopoiesis in cyclic neutropenia, Am. J. Hematol. **1**:375, 1976.

109. Gresser, I., and Lang, D. J.: Relationships between viruses and leukocytes, Prog. Med. Virol. **8**:62, 1966.

110. Grignaschi, V. J., Sperperato, A. M., Etcheverry, M. J., and Macario, A. J.: A new cytochemical picture: spontaneous negativity of the peroxidase, oxidase, and lipid reactions in a neutrophil progeny and in the monocytes of two siblings, Rev. Asoc. Med. Argent. **77**:218, 1963.

111. Grossman, E. R.: Ampicillin reaction, Am. J. Dis. Child. **112**:609, 1966.

112. Gryfe, C. I., Rubenzahl, S.: Agranulocytosis and aplastic anemia possibly due to ibuprofen, Can. Med. Assoc. J. **114**:877, 1976.

113. Guerry, D., Adamson, J. W., Dale, D. C., and Wolff, S. M.: Human cyclic neutropenia: urinary colony stimulating factor in the erythropoietin levels, Blood **44**:257, 1974.

114. Gunay, U., and Honig, G. R.: Agranulocytosis in a 12-year-old girl treated with procainamide, Clin. Pediatr. **13**:728, 1974.

115. Gupta, M. C., Kumar, S., Tyagi, S. P., and Srivastava, S. S.: Stomatitis agranulocytosis and hepatitis due to phenindione sensitivity, J. Indiana Med. Assoc. **63**:324, 1974.

116. Gussoff, B. D., and Lee, S. L.: Chloramphenicol-induced hematopoietic depression: a controlled comparison with tetracycline, Am. J. Med. Sci. **251**:8, 1966.

117. Hardy, W. R., and Anderson, R. E.: The hypereosinophilic syndromes, Ann. Intern. Med. **68**:1220, 1968.

118. Harrell, G. T.: Rocky mountain spotted fever, Medicine **28**:333, 1949.

119. Harter, J. G.: Antihistaminics: tailoring dosage to suit patients, Clin. Pharmacol. Ther. **6**:553, 1965.

120. Havard, C. W. H.: A reappraisal of the thiazide diuretics, Curr. Med. Drugs **7**:14, 1966.

121. Heiner, D. C., and Kevy, S. V.: Visceral larva migrans: report of the syndrome in three siblings, N. Engl. J. Med. **254**:629, 1956.

122. Herion, J. C., Glaser, R. M., Walker, R. I., and Palmer, J. G.: Eosinophil kinetics in two patients with eosinophilia, Blood **36**:361, 1970.

123. Hickson, B., Davidson, R. J., and Walker, W.: Agranulocytosis caused by procainamide, Scot. Med. J. **17**:165, 1972.

124. Hillenbrand, F. K. M.: The blood picture in rubella, Lancet **2**:66, 1956.

125. Hilts, S. V., and Shaw, C. C.: Leukemoid blood reactions, N. Engl. J. Med. **249**:434, 1953.

126. Hitzig, W. H.: Familiäre neutropenie mit dominantem Erbgang und hypergammaglobulinämie, Helv. Med. Acta **26**:779, 1959.

127. Hogarth-Scott, R. S., Johansson, S. G. O., and Bennich, H.: Antibodies to toxocara in the sera of visceral larva migrans patients: the significance of raised levels of IgE, Clin. Exp. Immunol. **5**:619, 1969.

128. Holbrook, A. A.: The blood picture in chicken pox, Arch. Intern. Med. **68**:294, 1941.

129. Holland, P., and Mauer, A. M.: Myeloid leukemoid reactions in children, Am. J. Dis. Child. **105**:568, 1963.

130. Hollister, L. E., Caffey, E. M., Jr., and Klett, C. J.: Abnormal symptoms, signs, and laboratory tests during treatment with phenothiazine derivatives, Clin. Pharmacol. Ther. **1**:284, 1960.

131. Howard, M. W., Strauss, R. G., and Johnston, R. B., Jr.: Infections in patients with neutropenia, Am. J. Dis. Child. **131**:788, 1977.

132. Howell, A., Gumpel, J. M., and Watts, R. W. E.: Depression of bone marrow colony formation in gold-induced neutropenia, Br. Med. J. **1**:432, 1975.

133. Hudson, G.: Quantitative study of the eosinophil granulocytes, Semin. Hematol. **5**:166, 1968.

134. Hudson, G., Chin, K. M., and Moffatt, D. J.: Changes in eosinophil granulocyte kinetics in severe hypoxia, Acta Haematol. **48**:58, 1972.

135. Huntley, C. C., Costas, M. C., and Lyerly, A.: Visceral larva migrans syndrome: clinical characteristics and immunologic studies in 51 patients, Pediatrics **36**:523, 1965.

136. Ichikawa, Y., Pluznik, D. H., and Sachs, L.: In vitro control of the development of macrophage and granulocytic colonies, Proc. Natl. Acad. Sci. **56**:488, 1966.

137. Iscove, N. N., Senn, J. E., Till, J. E., and McCulloch, E. A.: Colony formation by normal and leukemic human marrow cells in culture: effect of conditioned medium from human leukocytes, Blood **37**:1, 1971.

138. Itoga, T., and Laszlo, J.: Döhle bodies and other granulocytic alterations during chemotherapy with cyclophosphamide, Blood **20**:668, 1962.

139. Jackson, E. W., Turner, J. H., Klauber, M. R., Norris, F. D.: Down's syndrome: variation of leukemia occurrence in institutionalized populations, J. Chronic Dis. **21**:247, 1968.

140. Jacobs, P.: Familial benign chronic neutropenia, S. Afr. Med. J. **49:**692, 1975.
141. Johnson, E. S., Napoli, V. M., and White, W. C.: Colorado tick fever as a hematologic problem, Am. J. Clin. Pathol. **34:**118, 1960.
142. Jones, T. W.: The blood corpuscle considered in its different phases of development in the animal series, Memoir I, Vertebrate Phil. Trans. R. Soc. Lond. **136:**63, 1846.
143. Jopling, W. H.: Why agranulocytosis from dapsone? Ann. Intern. Med. **77:**153, 1972.
144. Jordan, M. C., Bierman, C. W., and Van Arsdel, P. P., Jr.: Allergic bronchopulmonary aspergillosis, Arch. Intern. Med. **128:**576, 1971.
145. Jordan, S. W., and Larsen, W. E.: Ultrastructural studies of the May-Hegglin anomaly, Blood **25:**921, 1965.
146. Juhlin, L.: Basophil leukocyte differential in blood and bone marrow, Acta Haematol. **29:**89, 1963.
147. Kagan, I. G.: Serologic diagnosis of visceral larva migrans, Clin. Pediatr. **7:**508, 1968.
148. Karayalcin, G., Rosner, F., and Sawitsky, A.: Pseudoneutropenia in American Negroes, Lancet **1:**387, 1972.
149. Kato, K.: Leucocytes in infancy and childhood: a statistical analysis of 1,081 total and differential counts from birth to 15 years, J. Pediatr. **7:**7, 1935.
150. Kay, A. B.: Functions of the eosinophil leukocyte, Br. J. Haematol. **33:**313, 1976.
151. Kay, A. B.: Studies on eosinophil leucocyte migration. II. Factors specifically chemotactic for eosinophils and neutrophils generated from guinea pig serum by antigen-antibody complexes, Clin. Exp. Immunol. **7:**723, 1970.
152. Kay, A. B., Stechschulte, D. J., and Austen, K. F.: An eosinophil leukocyte chemotactic factor of anaphylaxis, J. Exp. Med. **133:**602, 1971.
153. Kay, A. L.: Myelotoxicity of gold, Br. Med. J. **1:**1266, 1976.
154. Kiczak, J., and Wichert, K.: A cured case of agranulocytosis caused by gold therapy, Pol. Arch. Med. Wewn. **33:**85, 1963.
155. Kinross-Wright, J.: The current status of phenothiazines, J.A.M.A. **200:**461, 1967.
156. Klerman, G. L., and Cole, J. O.: Clinical pharmacology of imipramine and related antidepressant compounds, Pharmacol. Rev. **17:**101, 1965.
157. Koch-Weser, J.: Beta adrenergic blockade and circulating eosinophils, Arch. Intern. Med. **121:**255, 1968.
158. Konttinin, Y. P., and Tuominen, L.: Reversible procainamide-induced agranulocytosis twice in one patient, Lancet **2:**925, 1971.
159. Kostmann, R.: Infantile genetic agranulocytosis (agranulocytosis infantalis hereditaria): a new recessive lethal disease in man, Acta Paediatr. **105:**45, 1956.
160. Kostmann, R.: Infantile genetic agranulocytosis: a review with presentation of ten new cases, Acta Paediatr. Scand. **64:**362, 1975.
161. Koszewski, B. J., and Hubbard, T. F.: Immunologic agranulocytosis due to mercurial diuretics, Am. J. Med. **20:**958, 1956.
162. Krill, C. E., Jr., and Mauer, A. M.: Congenital agranulocytosis, J. Pediatr. **68:**361, 1966.
163. Krill, C. E., Jr., Smith, H. D., and Mauer, A. M.: Chronic idiopathic granulocytopenia, N. Engl. J. Med. **270:**973, 1964.
164. Kwan, V. W.: Procaine amide-induced leukopenia, J. Am. Geriatr. Soc. **17:**404, 1969.
165. Kyle, R. A., and Linman, J. W.: Chronic idiopathic neutropenia, N. Engl. J. Med. **279:**1015, 1968.
166. Kyle, R. A., and Pease, G. L.: Hematologic aspects of arsenic intoxication, N. Engl. J. Med. **273:**18, 1965.
167. Lalezari, P., Jiang, A. F., Yegen, L., and Santorineou, M.: Chronic autoimmune neutropenia due to anti-NA2 antibody, N. Engl. J. Med. **293:**744, 1975.
168. Lalezari, P., and Radel, E.: Neutrophil specific antigens: immunology and clinical significance, Semin. Hematol. **11:**281, 1974.
169. Leale, M.: Recurrent furunculosis in an infant showing an unusual blood picture, J.A.M.A. **54:**1854, 1910.
170. Lechner, K., Breddin, K., Moser, K., et al.: May-Hegglinsche anomalie, Acta. Haematol. **42:**303, 1969.
171. Lee, J. C., Dushkin, M., Eyring, E. J., et al.: Renal lesions associated with gold therapy light and electron microscopic studies, Arthritis Rheum. **8:**1, 1965.
172. Lee, S., and Schoen, I.: Eosinophilia of peritoneal fluid and peripheral blood associated with chronic peritoneal dialysis, Am. J. Clin. Pathol. **47:**638, 1967.
173. Leonard, B. J., Israëls, M. C. G., and Wilkinson, J. F.: Alkaline phosphatase in the white cells in leukaemia and leukaemoid reactions, Lancet **1:**289, 1958.
174. L'Esperance, P. E., Brunning, R., and Good, R. A.: Congenital neutropenia: in vitro growth of colonies mimicking the disease, Proc. Natl. Acad. Sci. U.S.A. **70:**669, 1973.
175. Levine, P. H., and Weintraub, L. W.: Pseudoleukemia during recovery from dapsone-induced agranulocytosis, Ann. Intern. Med. **68:**1060, 1968.
176. Levison, M. E., Bran, J. L., Jepson, J. H., and Kaye, D.: Neutropenia associated with cephapirin therapy, Antimicrob. Agents Chemother. **1:**174, 1972.
177. Levy, S. B., Meyers, B., and Mellin, H.: Reversible granulocytopenia in a patient with polycythemia vera taking nitrofurantoin: report of a case, J. Mt. Sinai Hosp. **36:**26, 1969.
178. Liao, K. T., Rosai, J., and Daneshbod, K.: Malignant histiocytosis with cutaneous involvement and eosinophilia, Am. J. Clin. Pathol. **57:**438, 1972.
179. Lonsdale, D., Deodhar, S. D., and Mercer, R. D.: Familial granulocytopenia and associated immunoglobulin abnormality, J. Pediatr. **71:**790, 1967.
180. Louie, J. S., and Pearson, C. M.: Felty's syndrome, Semin. Hematol. **8:**216, 1971.
181. Louria, D. B.: The treatment of endocarditis, Am. Heart J. **66:**429, 1963.
182. Lowe, T. E.: Eosinophilia in tropical disease: experiences at an Australian general hospital, Med. J. Aust. **1:**453, 1944.
183. Lukens, J. N.: Eosinophilia in children, Pediatr. Clin. North Am. **19:**969, 1972.
184. Lux, S. E., Johnston, R. B., Jr., August, C. S., et al.: Chronic neutropenia and abnormal cellular immunity in cartilage-hair hypoplasia, N. Engl. J. Med. **282:**231, 1970.
185. Maldonado, J. E., and Hanlon, D. G.: Monocytosis: a current appraisal, Mayo Clin. Proc. **40:**248, 1965.
186. Mandel, A., and Gross, M.: Agranulocytosis and phenothiazines, Dis. Nerv. Syst. **29:**32, 1968.
187. Mangalik, A., and Robinson, W. A.: Cyclic neutropenia: the right relationship between urine and granulocyte colony stimulating activity and neutrophil count, Blood **41:**79, 1973.
188. Markowitz, S. M., Rothkopf, M., Holden, F. D., et al.: Nafcillin-induced agranulocytosis, J.A.M.A. **232:**1150, 1975.
189. Marsh, J. C., and Perry, S.: The granulocyte response to endotoxin in patients with hematologic disorders, Blood **23:**581, 1964.
190. Mauer, E. F.: The toxic effects of phenylbutazone (Butazolidin): review of the literature and report of the twenty-third death following its use, N. Engl. J. Med. **253:**404, 1955.
191. McCall, C. E., Katayama, I., Cotran, R. S., and Finland,

M.: Lysosomal and ultrastructural changes in human "toxic" neutrophils during bacterial infection, J. Exp. Med. **129**:267, 1969.

192. McCarthy, D. D., and Chalmers, T. M.: Hematological complications of phenylbutazone therapy: review of the literature and report of 2 cases, Can. Med. Assoc. J. **90**:1061, 1964.

193. McCluskey, H. B.: Corticotropin (ACTH) in treatment of agranulocytosis following sulfisoxazole therapy; J.A.M.A. **152**:232, 1953.

194. McGavack, T. H., and Chevalley, J.: Untoward hematologic responses to the antithyroid compounds, Am. J. Med. **17**:36, 1954.

195. McKusick, V. A., Eldridge, R., Hostetler, J. A., Ruangwit, U., and Egeland, J. A.: Dwarfism in the Amish. II. Cartilage-hair hypoplasia, Bull. Johns Hopkins Hosp. **116**:285, 1965.

196. Metcalf, D.: Regulation by colony-stimulating factor of granulocyte and macrophage colony formation in vitro by normal and leukemic cells. In Clarkson, B., and Baserga, R., eds.: Control of proliferation in animal cells, Cold Springs Harbor Conference on Cell Proliferation **1**:887, 1974.

197. Metcalf, D., Moore, M. A. S., and Shortman, K.: Adherence column and buoyant density separation of bone marrow stem cells and more differentiated cells, J. Cell. Physiol. **78**:441, 1971.

198. Meuret, G., and Hoffmann, G.: Monocyte kinetic studies in normal and disease states, Br. J. Hematol. **24**:275, 1973.

199. Michelstein, I., and Weiser, N. J.: Fatal agranulocytosis due to trimethadione (Tridione), Arch. Neurol. Psychiatr. **62**:358, 1949.

200. Mickenberg, I. D., Root, R. K., and Wolff, S. M.: Bactericidal and metabolic properties of human eosinophils, Blood **39**:67, 1972.

201. Miller, D. R., Freed, B. A., and La Pey, J. D.: Congenital neutropenia: report of a fatal case in a Negro infant with leukocyte function studies, Am. J. Dis. Child. **115**:337, 1968.

202. Miller, M. E.: Thymic dysplasia: swiss agammaglobulinemia. I. Graft vs. host reaction following bone marrow transfusion, J. Pediatr. **70**:730, 1967.

203. Millington, D.: Leucopenia and indomethacin, Br. Med. J. **5478**:49, 1966.

204. Mintz, U., and Sachs, L.: Normal granulocyte colony-forming cells in the bone marrow of Yemenite Jews with genetic neutropenia, Blood **41**:745, 1973.

205. Mitchell, R. G.: Basophilic leukocytes in children in health and disease, Arch. Dis. Child. **33**:193, 1958.

206. Miyazaki, S.: Immunologic studies on cyclic neutropenia, Acta Hematol. Jpn. **37**:276, 1974.

207. Mok, C. H.: Visceral larva migrans: a discussion based on review of the literature, Clin. Pediatr. **7**:565, 1968.

208. Moloney, W. C., and Lange, R. D.: Cytologic and biochemical studies on the granulocytes in early leukemia among atomic bomb survivors, Tex. Rep. Biol. Med. **12**:887, 1954.

209. Moore, M. A. S., Spitzer, G., Metcalf, D., and Pennington, D. G.: Monocyte production of colony stimulating factor in familial cyclic neutropenia, Br. J. Haematol. **27**:47, 1974.

210. Mooschlin, S., and Wagner, K.: Agranulocytosis due to the occurrence of leukocyte-agglutinins, Acta Haematol. **8**:29, 1952.

211. Morley, A. A., Carew, J. P., and Baikie, A. G.: Familial cyclic neutropenia, Br. J. Hematol. **13**:719, 1967.

212. Morley, A., and Stohlman, F., Jr.: Cyclophosphamide-induced cyclical neutropenia: an animal model of a human periodic disease, N. Engl. J. Med. **282**:643, 1970.

213. Moses, C., and Platt, M.: Changes in the total circulating eosinophile count in Cyclotron workers, Science **113**:676, 1951.

214. Motulsky, A. G.: Drug reactions, enzymes, and biochemical genetics, J.A.M.A. **165**:835, 1957.

215. Murray, A. B.: Nasal secretion eosinophilia in children with allergic rhinitis, Ann. Allergy **28**:142, 1970.

216. Nagaraju, M., Weitzman, S., and Baumann, G.: Viral hepatitis and agranulocytosis, Am. J. Dig. Dis. **18**:247, 1973.

217. Nawabi, I. U., and Ritz, N. B.: Agranulocytosis due to propranolol, J.A.M.A. **223**:1376, 1973.

218. Nesarajah, M. S.: Pulmonary function in tropical eosinophilia before and after treatment with diethylcarbamazine, Thorax **30**:574, 1975.

219. Newton, R. M., and Ward, V. G.: Leukopenia associated with ristocetin (Spontin) administration, J.A.M.A. **166**:1956, 1958.

220. Ng, R. P., and Prankerd, T. A.: IgA deficiency and neutropenia, Br. Med. J. **1**:563, 1976.

221. Oberling, J. M., Lang, J. M., Fabre, M., Liautaud, M., Mayer, G., and Waitz, R.: Thorotrastose post-angiographique et agranulocytose chronique, Nouv. Rev. Fr. Hematol. **13**:291, 1973.

222. Ochs, H. D., Davis, S. D., Mickelson, E., et al.: Combined immunodeficiency and reticuloendotheliosis with eosinophilia, J. Pediatr. **85**:463, 1974.

223. O'Connell, C. J., and Plaut, M. E.: Intravenous lincomycin in high doses, Curr. Ther. Res. **11**:478, 1969.

224. Omenn, G. S.: Familial reticuloendotheliosis with eosinophilia, N. Engl. J. Med. **273**:427, 1965.

225. Oppenheim, M., and de Myyer, G.: Granulo-und thrombocytopenie infolge streptomycin-behandlung, Schweiz. Med. Wochenschr. **79**:1187, 1949.

226. O'Regan, S., Newman, A. J., and Graham, R. C.: "Myelokathexis" neutropenia with marrow hypoplasia, Am. J. Dis. Child. **131**:655, 1977.

227. Organakis, N. G., Ostlund, R. E., Bishop, C. R., and Athens, J. W.: Normal blood leukocyte concentration values, Am. J. Clin. Pathol. **53**:647, 1970.

228. Osgood, E. E.: Culture of human marrow: length of life of the neutrophil, eosinophils, and basophils of normal blood as determined by comparative cultures of blood and sternal marrow from healthy persons, J.A.M.A. **109**:933, 1937.

229. Palva, I. P., and Koivisto, O.: Agranulocytosis associated with trimethoprim sulfamethoxazole, Br. Med. J. **4**:301, 1971.

230. Palva, I. P., and Lehmola, U.: Agranulocytosis caused by nitrofurantoin, Acta Med. Scand. **194**:575, 1973.

231. Panush, R. S., Wilkinson, L. S., and Fagin, R. R.: Chronic active hepatitis associated with eosinophilia and Coombs'-positive hemolytic anemia, Gastroenterology **64**:1015, 1973.

232. Parbrook, G. D.: Leucopenic effects of prolonged nitrous oxide treatment, Br. J. Anaesth. **39**:119, 1967.

233. Parker, W. A., Pharm, D., and Gumnit, R. J.: Diphenylhydantoin toxicity: dose-dependent blood dyscrasia, Neurology **24**:1178, 1974.

234. Parmley, R. T., Ogawa, M., Darby, C. P., Jr., and Spicer, S. S.: Congenital neutropenia: neutrophil proliferation with abnormal maturation, Blood **46**:723, 1975.

235. Patterson, R., Soo, H. O., Roberts, M., and Hsu, C. C. S.: Massive polyclonal hyperimmunoglobulinemia E, eosinophilia, and increased IgE-bearing lymphocytes, Am. J. Med. **58**:553, 1975.

236. Pearson, H. A.: Marrow hypoplasia in anorexia nervosa, J. Pediatr. **71**:211, 1967.

237. Pearson, J. R.: Binder, C. I., and Neber, J.: Agranulo-

cytosis following Diamox therapy, J.A.M.A. **157**:339, 1955.

238. Pike, B. L., and Robinson, W. A.: Human bone marrow colony growth in agar-gel, J. Cell. Physiol. **76**:77, 1970.

239. Pincus, S. H., Boxer, L. A., and Stossel, T. P.: Chronic neutropenia in childhood: analysis of 16 cases and a review of the literature, Am. J. Med. **61**:849, 1976.

240. Pisciotta, A. V.: Agranulocytosis induced by certain phenothiazine derivatives, J.A.M.A. **208**:1862, 1969.

241. Pisciotta, A. V.: Drug induced leukopenia in aplastic anemia, Clin. Pharmacol. Ther. **12**:13, 1971.

242. Pisciotta, A. V.: Immune and toxic mechanisms in drug-induced agranulocytosis, Semin. Hematol. **10**:279, 1973.

243. Pisciotta, A. V.: Studies on agranulocytosis. IX. A biochemical defect in chlorpromazine-sensitive marrow cells, J. Lab. Clin. Med. **78**:435, 1971.

244. Polano, M. K., Cats, A., and Olden, G. A.: Agranulocytosis following treatment with hydroxychloroquine sulphate, Lancet **1**:1275, 1965.

245. Polliack, A., and Douglas, S. D.: Surface features of human eosinophils: a scanning and transmission electron microscopic study of a case of eosinophilia, Br. J. Haematol. **30**:303, 1975.

246. Presentey, B. Z.: A new anomaly of eosinophilic granulocytes, Tech. Bull. Regist. Med. Tech. **38**:131, 1968.

247. Propp, R. P., and Stillman, J. S.: Agranulocytosis and hydroxychloroquine, N. Engl. J. Med. **277**:492, 1967.

248. Pullen, R. L., and Stuart, B. M.: Tularemia, J.A.M.A. **129**:495, 1945.

249. Rebuck, J. W., and Crowley, J. H.: A method of studying leukocyte functions in vivo, Ann. N.Y. Acad. Sci. **59**:757, 1955.

250. Rickles, F. R., and Miller, D. R.: Eosinophilic leukemoid reaction: report of a case, its relationship to eosinophilic leukemia, and review of the pediatric literature, J. Pediatr. **80**:418, 1972.

251. Rieger, C. H. L., Moohr, J. W., and Rothberg, R. M.: Correction of neutropenia associated with dysgammaglobulinemia, Pediatrics **54**:508, 1974.

252. Ries, C. A., and Sahud, M. A.: Agranulocytosis caused by Chinese herbal medicines: dangers of medications containing aminopyrine and phenylbutazone, J.A.M.A. **231**:352, 1975.

253. Robinson, W. A., and Mangalik, A.: Regulation of granulopoiesis: positive feed-back, Lancet **2**:742, 1972.

254. Romig, D. A., and Voth, D. W.: Neutropenia: therapy with penicillin and its congeners, J. Kans. Med. Soc. **76**:8, 1975.

255. Rose, H. M.: The clinical manifestations and laboratory diagnosis of rickettsialpox, Ann. Intern. Med. **31**:871, 1949.

256. Rosen, F. S., Craig, J., Vawter, G., and Janeway, C. A.: The dysgammaglobulinemias and sex-linked thymic hypoplasia, Birth Defects **4**:67, 1968.

257. Ruscetti, F. W., Cypess, R. H., and Chervenick, P. A.: Specific release of neutrophilic- and eosinophilic-stimulating factors from sensitized lymphocytes, Blood **47**:757, 1976.

258. Ruvidie, R., and Jelic, S.: Haematological aspects of drug-induced agranulocytosis, Scand. J. Haematol. **9**:18, 1972.

259. Samuels, L. D.: Leukemoid reaction to parenteral iron-dextran complex: a case report, J.A.M.A. **182**:1334, 1962.

260. Sandberg, M., Tuazon, C. U., and Sheagren, J. N.: Neutropenia probably resulting from nafcillin, J.A.M.A. **232**:1152, 1975.

261. Schreiber, Z. A., Rosner, F., Alter, A. A., et al.: Severe persistent neutropenia, direct positive antiglobulin reaction, and familial IgA deficiency, Isr. J. Med. Sci. **8**:613, 1972.

262. Scott, J. L., Cartwright, G. E., and Wintrobe, M. M.: Acquired aplastic anemia: an analysis of thirty-nine cases and review of the pertinent literature, Medicine **38**:119, 1959.

263. Scott, J. L., Finegold, S. M., Belkin, G. A., and Lawrence, J. S.: A controlled double-blind study of the hematologic toxicity of chloramphenicol, N. Engl. J. Med. **272**:1137, 1965.

264. Sezary, A., and Boucher, G.: Agranulocytose bismuthique, Bull. Mem. Soc. Med. Hosp. Paris **47**:1795, 1931.

265. Shah, C. P., Sanghavi, N. G., and Amin, V. C.: Efficacy and toxicity of trimethoprime sulfamethoxazole in typhoid fever, J. Assoc. Physicians India **23**:317, 1975.

266. Shanbrom, E., Collins, Z., and Miller, S.: "Acquired" Pelger-Huet cells in blood dyscrasias, Am. J. Med. Sci. **240**:732, 1960.

267. Shaper, A. G., and Lewis, P.: Genetic neutropenia in people of African origin, Lancet **2**:1021, 1971.

268. Shapiro, Y. L.: Changes in differential leukocyte counts prolonged total alimentary starvation, Fed. Proc. **23**(suppl.):447, 1964.

269. Shmerling, D. H., Prader, A., Hitzig, W. H., Giedion, A., Hadorn, B., and Kuhri, M.: The syndrome of exocrine pancreatic insufficiency, neutropenia, metaphyseal dysostosis, and dwarfism, Helv. Paediatr. Acta **24**:547, 1969.

270. Shwachman, H., Diamond, L. K., Oski, F. A., and Khaw, K. T.: The syndrome of pancreatic insufficiency and bone marrow dysfunction, J. Pediatr. **65**:645, 1964.

271. Spaet, T. H., and Dameshek, W.: Chronic hypoplastic neutropenia, Am. J. Med. **13**:35, 1952.

272. Sparberg, M.: Diagnostically confusing complications of diphenylhydantoin therapy: a review, Ann. Intern. Med. **59**:914, 1963.

273. Spector, W. G., and Ryan, G. B.: New evidence for the existence of long-lived macrophages, Nature **221**:860, 1969.

274. Spitzer, G., and Garson, O. M.: Lymphoblastic leukemia with marked eosinophilia: a report of two cases, Blood **42**:377, 1973.

275. Spry, C. J., and Tai, P. C.: Studies on blood eosinophils. II. Patients with Loffler's cardiomyopathy, Clin. Exp. Immunol. **24**:423, 1976.

276. Spycher, M. A., Giedion, A., Shmerling, D. H., and Ruttner, J. R.: Electron microscopic examination of cartilage in the syndrome of exocrine pancreatic insufficiency, neutropenia, metaphyseal dysostotis, and dwarfism, Helv. Paediatr. Acta **29**:471, 1974.

277. Stanley, P., and Sutcliffe, J.: Metaphyseal chondrodysplasia with dwarfism, pancreatic insufficiency, and neutropenia, Pediatr. Radiol. **1**:119, 1973.

278. Stein, J. H., Hamilton, H. E., and Sheets, R. F.: Agranulocytosis caused by chlorpropamide: a case report with confirmation by leukoagglutination studies, Arch. Intern. Med. **113**:186, 1964.

279. Steinberg, B.: Bone marrow regeneration in experimental benzene intoxication, Blood **4**:550, 1949.

280. Sternlieb, P., and Eisman, S. H.: Toxic hepatitis and agranulocytosis due to cinchophen, Ann. Intern. Med. **47**:826, 1957.

281. Stevens, A. R., Jr.: Agranulocytosis induced by sulfaguanidine: the danger of an antibacterial drug in a symptomatic remedy, Arch. Intern. Med. **123**:428, 1969.

282. Stickney, J. M., and Heck, F. J.: The clinical occurrence of eosinophilia, Med. Clin. North Am. **28:**915, 1944.

283. Strauss, B.: Aplastic anemia following exposure to carbon tetrachloride, J.A.M.A. **155:**737, 1954.

284. Swett, C., Jr.: Outpatient phenothiazine use and bone marrow depression: a report from the drug epidemiology unit and the Boston Collaborative Drug Surveillance Program, Arch. Gen. Psychiatry **32:**1416, 1975.

285. Sylvester, R. A., and Pinals, R. S.: Eosinophilia in rheumatoid arthritis, Ann. Allergy **28:**565, 1970.

286. Talmers, F. N., and Telmos, A. J.: A case report: procaine amide hydrochloride (Pronestyl) induced agranulocytosis, Mich. Med. **64:**655, 1965.

287. Tashjian, A. H., Jr., and Leddy, J. P.: Agranulocytosis associated with phenindione: A case report with review of the literature. Arch. Intern. Med. **105:**121, 1960.

288. Ten Broeke, J. E., and Cunningham, L. D.: Agranulocytosis during dapsone administration, Dermatologica **146:**21, 1973.

289. Thevathasan, O. I., and Gordon, A. S.: Adrenocortical-medullary interactions on the blood eosinophils, Acta Haematol. **19:**162, 1958.

290. Till, J. E., and McCulloch, E. A.: A direct measurement of the radiation sensitivity of normal mouse bone marrow cells, Radiat. Res. **14:**213, 1961.

291. Tremonti, L. P.: Eosinophilia in Tokyo Yokohama asthma, Ann. Allergy **30:**524, 1972.

292. Tsan, M. F., Mehlman, D. J., Green, R. S., and Bell, W. R.: Dilantin, agranulocytosis, and phagocytic marrow histocytes, Ann. Intern. Med. **84:**710, 1976.

293. Undirtz, E.: Les malformations hereditaires dez elements figures, LeSang **25:**296, 1954.

294. van Furth, R.: Origin and kinetics of monocytes and macrophages, Semin. Hematol. **7:**125, 1970.

295. van Furth, R., and Cohn, Z. A.: The origin and kinetics of mononuclear phagocytes, J. Exp. Med. **128:**415, 1968.

296. van Furth, R., Cohn, Z. A., Hirsch, J. G., Humphrey, J. H., et al.: A mononuclear phagocyte system: a new classification of macrophages, monocytes, and their precursor cells, Bull. W.H.O. **46:**845, 1972.

297. Venes, J. L.: Pleural fluid effusion and eosinophilia following ventriculopleural shunting, Dev. Med. Child. Neurol. **16:**72, 1974.

298. Viani, H., and Holland, P. D. J.: The control of Dapsone Heinz-body anaemia with adrenal corticosteroids, Br. J. Dermatol. **76:**63, 1964.

299. Vigliani, E. C., and Saita, G.: Benzene and leukemia, N. Engl. J. Med. **271:**872, 1964.

300. Vincent, P. C., Levi, J. A., and MacQueen, A.: The mechanism of neutropenia in Felty's syndrome, Br. J. Haematol. **27:**463, 1974.

301. Viswanathan, R.: Immunoglobulins in pulmonary eosinophilosis (tropical eosinophilia), Acta Med. Scand. **193:**219, 1973.

302. Volkman, A., and Collins, F. M.: Recovery of delayed-type hypersensitivity in mice following suppressive doses of x-radiation, J. Immunol. **101:**846, 1968.

303. Walker, J. G.: Fatal agranulocytosis complicating treatment with ethacrynic acid: report of a case, Ann. Intern. Med. **64:**1303, 1966.

304. Walls, R. S., Basten, A., Leuchars, E., and Davies, A. J. S.: Mechanisms for eosinophilic and neutrophilic leucocytoses, Br. Med. J. **3:**157, 1971.

305. Wang, R. I., and Schuller, G.: Agranulocytosis following procainamide administration, Am. Heart J. **78:**282, 1969.

306. Ward, H. N.: Pulmonary infiltrates associated with leukoagglutinin transfusion reactions, Ann. Intern. Med. **73:**689, 1970.

307. Ward, P. A.: Chemotaxis of human eosinophils, Am. J. Pathol. **54:**121, 1969.

308. Warner, H. R., and Athens, J. W.: An analysis of granulocyte kinetics in blood and bone marrow, Ann. N.Y. Acad. Sci. **113:**523, 1964.

309. Weiden, P. L., and Buckner, C. D.: Thioridazine toxicity: agranulocytosis and hepatitis with encephalopathy, J.A.M.A. **224:**518, 1973.

310. Weinger, R. S., Andre-Schwartz, J., Desforges, J. F., and Baker, M.: Acute leukemia with eosinophilia or acute eosinophilic leukemia: a dilemma, Br. J. Haematol. **30:**65, 1975.

311. Westwick, W. J., Allsop, J., Gumpel, J. M., and Watts, R. W. E.: Studies on pyrimidine biosynthesis in the granulocytes of patients receiving gold therapy for rheumatoid arthritis, Q. J. Med. **43:**231, 1974.

312. Whang, J., Frei, E., III, Tijo, J. H., et al.: The distribution of the Philadelphia chromosome in patients with chronic myelogenous leukemia, Blood **22:**664, 1963.

313. Wheelihan, R. Y.: Granulocytic aplasia of the bone marrow following the use of arsenic, Am. J. Dis. Child. **35:**1032, 1928.

314. Wiberg, J. J., and Nuttall, F. Q.: Methimazole toxicity from high doses, Ann. Intern. Med. **77:**414, 1972.

315. Willcox, P. H.: Antithyroid treatment: a personal series, Postgrad. Med. J. **43:**146, 1967.

316. Willett, E. M., and Oppenheim, E.: Pulmonary infiltrations with associated eosinophilia, Am. J. Med. Sci. **212:**608, 1946.

317. Williams, R. B. III, and Gwaltney, J. M., Jr.: Allergic rhinitis or virus cold? Nasal smear eosinophilia in differential diagnosis, Ann. Allergy **30:**189, 1972.

318. Williamson, G. D., and Crowe, G. R.: Trimethoprim-sulphamethoxazole mixtures and agranulocytosis, Med. J. Aust. **2:**1506, 1972.

319. Woodward, T. E., and Bland, E. F.: Clinical observations in typhus fever, J.A.M.A. **126:**287, 1944.

320. Wriedt, K., Kauder, E., and Mauer, A. M.: Defective myelopoiesis in congenital neutropenia, N. Engl. J. Med. **283:**1072, 1970.

321. Yam, L. T., Li, C. Y., Necheles, T. F., and Kayayama, I.: Pseudoeosinophilia, eosinophilic endocarditis in eosinophilic leukemia, Am. J. Med. **53:**193, 1972.

322. Youman, J. D., Taddeini, L., and Cooper, T.: Histamine excess symptoms in basophilic chronic granulocytic leukemia, Arch. Intern. Med. **131:**560, 1973.

323. Yunis, A. A., and Bloomberg, G. R.: Chloramphenicol toxicity: clinical features and pathogenesis. In Moore, C. V., and Brown, E. B., eds.: Progress in hematology, vol. 4, New York, 1964, Grune & Stratton, Inc.

324. Yunis, A. A., and Harrington, W. J.: Patterns of inhibition by chloramphenicol of nucleic acid synthesis in human bone marrow and leukemic cells, J. Lab. Clin. Med. **56:**831, 1960.

325. Zucker-Franklin, D.: Electron microscopic studies of human granulocytes: structural variations related to function, Semin. Hematol. **5:**109, 1968.

326. Zucker-Franklin, D. Z., L'Esperance, P. E., and Good, R. A.: Congenital neutropenia: an intrinsic cell defect demonstrated by electron microscopy of soft agar colonies, Blood **49:**425, 1977.

327. Zuelzer, W. W.: "Myelokathexis": a new form of chronic granulocytopenia, N. Engl. J. Med. **270:**699, 1964.

328. Zuelzer, W. W., and Bajoghli, M.: Chronic granulocytopenia in childhood, Blood **23:**359, 1964.

19 □ Disorders of granulocyte function

Robert L. Baehner

HISTORICAL PERSPECTIVE

Patients with granulocyte disorders have frequent infections and their clinical manifestations are quite similar, whether the disorder results from insufficient numbers of cells or cell dysfunction. In either case, infections tend to be prolonged, there is a poor response to appropriate antibiotics, and recurrent infections are the rule. Infection results from the invasion of tissue by bacteria, fungi, protozoa, viruses, or parasites. Infected tissues usually become inflamed, displaying the four major signs of inflammation as first described by the Roman writer of the first century Cornelius Celsus: *rubor et tumor, cum calore et delore* (redness and swelling with heat and pain).[150] Cohnheim noted a series of changes in blood vessels in the inflamed area initiated by dilatation of the arterioles, leading to an accelerated blood flow in the entire vascular network, followed by a slowing of that flow and then the appearance of white blood cells lining the walls of the venules. Finally the white cells move across the wall of the venules and into the extravascular tissues by a process called diapedesis.

The Russian biologist Elie Metchnikoff,[162] in describing the process of phagocytosis, reasoned that this unique cellular event is the ultimate purpose of the inflammatory response. He observed that leukocytes leave the circulation and move toward the area of tissue infection where they engulf invading bacteria or any other foreign matter. In 1882 Metchnikoff introduced a thorn into a starfish larva, and by the next morning he noted that the thorn was surrounded by clusters of phagocytic cells. That experiment formed the basis of the phagocyte theory, a counterview to the common belief of the times that leukocytes spread rather than contained infection.

The phagocyte theory met opposition from the proponents of the humoral hypothesis, which attributed bacterial killing solely to the effects of substances present in the plasma. Eventually it was realized that collaboration is required between humoral factors and phagocytes. The mobilization of neutrophils to the inflamed area is signaled by a variety of humoral factors through a process termed chemotaxis.[89]

Sir Almroth Wright found that phagocytosis of bacteria by leukocytes usually requires the presence of serum.[209] He proposed that the bacteria need to be coated with certain serum factors called opsonins before phagocytosis can occur. For bacteria this special coating, or opsonization, is now known to consist of two main groups of serum factors: specific antibody and the complement system. The opsonized bacteria can attach to the advancing neutrophil's surface, which in turn bifurcates into two embracing pseudopodia, engulfing and entrapping the bacteria within the cell in a phagocytic vacuole. Next the granules converge around the phagocytic vacuole and discharge their contents into it through a process termed degranulation. Finally the bacteria are killed and digested. During the past two decades extensive studies of phagocytic morphology, function, and oxidative metabolism* have provided clearer insight into normal and abnormal cellular and humoral mechanisms as they relate to defense of the host against pyogenic infection.

HUMORAL MEDIATORS OF INFLAMMATION

As noted in Table 19-1, humoral substances inciting inflammation are derived from bacteria, plasma, and tissue. Chemical messengers (mediators) of inflammation include bacterial products that directly cause vascular leakage as well as attraction of leukocytes to the site of infection. Both bacterial filtrates and formyl-methionyl tripeptides derived from bacteria are chemotactic for neutrophils and monocytes.

Plasma contains three interconnected mediator-producing systems: (1) the kinin system product bradykinin, (2) complement-derived C3 and C5 fragments and C567 complex, and (3) fibrinopeptides and fibrin degradation products. Bradykinin in low doses causes a slow contraction of certain kinds of smooth muscles in vitro, dilatation of blood vessels in vivo, and pain when applied to the base of a blister or when injected into the skin, and it increases vascular permeability at sites of injection. It does not attract leukocytes when tested

---

*References 16, 17, 57, 120.

Table 19-1. Humoral mediators of inflammation

Source	Mediator	Action
Bacteria	Formyl-methionyl peptides and filtrates	Chemotactic
Plasma	Bradykinin, C3 and C5 fragments and C567 complex, fibrinopeptides and fibrin split products	Dilates vessel; increase vascular permeability; chemotactic
Tissue	Histamine, 5-hydroxytryptamine	Increase vascular permeability; chemotactic for polymorphonuclear neutrophils and eosinophils
	Slow-reacting substance of anaphylaxis	Contracts vessels
	Prostaglandins and thromboxanes	Increase vascular permeability, induce histamine release from mast cells; chemotactic
	Lysosomal enzymes	Digest proteins and injured tissues
	Lymphocyte-derived lymphokines	Chemotactic; inhibit macrophages; cytotoxic; skin reactivity

by in vitro chemotactic systems. The generation of bradykinin involves a cascade of reactions similar to those involved in clotting, in which there is progressive amplification in the number of molecules involved. The cascade reaction is initiated when Hageman factor is activated by contact with any of a number of substances including glass, kaolin, collagen, basement membrane, cartilage, sodium urate crystals, trypsin, kallikrein (a later component of the kinin system), plasmin (the enzyme that dissolves fibrin), coagulation factor XI, and bacterial lipopolysaccharides (endotoxin). Hageman factor, when activated, normally triggers the coagulation and fibrinolytic system to generate fibrin and plasmin, respectively, but it also triggers the prekallikrein activator that converts prekallikrein to kallikrein, which in turn activates kininogen to form kinin or bradykinin. Bradykinin is inactivated by kininase.[163]

The complement cascade is activated by antigen-antibody complexes. The by-product of this reaction, low molecular weight fragments of C3 and C5, a high molecular weight complex of C5, C6, and C7, and possibly another cleavage product of C2 (C-kinin) all play a role in inflammation. Both C3a and C5a fragments induce the release of histamine from tissue cells and are known as anaphylatoxins. Their most important effect is to serve as chemotactic attractants to neutrophils and monocytes.

Two potential inflammatory mediators derived from the coagulation system are (1) fibrinopeptides released from fibrinogen molecules by the action of thrombin during clotting, which induce vascular leakage and are chemotactic for neutrophils, and (2) fibrin degradation products released from fibrin by the proteolytic action of plasmin, which may well be chemotactic for neutrophils.

Tissue-derived inflammatory mediators include (1) vasoactive amines (histamine and 5-hydroxytryptamine), (2) slow-reacting substance of anaphylaxis (SRS-A), (3) lysosomal enzymes, and

(4) lymphocyte-derived lymphokines. Histamine is present in the granules of mast cells, basophils, and platelets, whereas 5-hydroxytryptamine (serotonin) is present in mast cells and platelets. Amines are released from mast cells residing in loose connective tissues. Mast cells contain chemical mediators preformed in granules, including (1) histamine, which increases vascular permeability and eosinophilic migration, (2) eosinophil chemotactic factor, (3) neutrophil chemotactic factor, and (4) heparin, without significant anticoagulant antithrombin III activity. Mast cells also release SRS-A, an acidic sulfur-containing lipid, which contracts smooth muscle, causes vascular leakage, and induces platelets to aggregate.[13,104,151]

Various groups of prostaglandins (E, F, A, and B) and their counterpart thromboxanes are released from phagocytic cells and have been identified in inflammatory exudates. The prostaglandins PGE_1 and PGE_2 induce vascular leakage when injected into human skin, perhaps inducing histamine release from mast cells, and PGE_1 possesses chemotactic activity for neutrophils in vitro.[241,249] Anti-inflammatory compounds such as indomethacin, phenylbutazone, salicylates, and corticosteroids inhibit the release of prostaglandins from cells.[236] Another important role for prostaglandin may reside in its capacity to inhibit certain inflammatory processes: PGE_1 causes accumulation of intracellular cyclic AMP by activating adenylcyclase, leading to inhibition of leukocyte locomotion, inhibition of release of SRS-A from mast cells, and inhibition of lysosomal enzyme release from neutrophils during phagocytosis.[38]

Lysosomal components from neutrophils, platelets, and tissue cells are likely mediators of inflammation. Cationic proteins and proteins active at neutral and acid pH are released from cells during phagocytosis or on their death. Sensitized thymus-dependent lymphocytes release an array of mediators called lymphokines, including the following:

1. Migration inhibitory factor (MIF), which

inhibits the migration of macrophages and thereby presumably acts to retain immuno-reactive monocytes in the area

2. Lymphocyte-derived chemotactic factors specific for macrophages, neutrophils, basophils, eosinophils, and even lymphocytes
3. Lymphotoxin nonspecifically toxic to other cells
4. Skin reactive factors, which can be found in the supernatants from stimulated lymphocytes and which provoke delayed hypersensitivity reactions when injected into the skin of normal guinea pigs
5. Mitogenic factors inducing proliferation of unsensitized lymphocytes[65]

Other lymphokines that may have a role in inflammation include a factor that triggers leukocytes to release endogenous pyrogen and another with colony stimulating activity that may play a role in granulopoiesis.

CELLULAR ADHERENCE AND DIRECTED LOCOMOTION (CHEMOTAXIS)

Blood neutrophils react to inflammatory mediators by adhering to the walls of blood vessels,[143] then emigrating between endothelial cells and out to tissues, where the provocative stimulus may have originated. This process of directional locomotion is called chemotaxis. Neutrophils become less adherent when exposed to substances that inhibit cell metabolism, disassemble microtubules, or alter certain surface properties of the cell.[79] Colchicine, drugs that oxidize sulfhydryl proteins including microtubules, EDTA (which chelates calcium), and agents that raise cyclic AMP levels in the leukocyte decrease neutrophil adhesiveness, whereas ascorbic acid and reduced glutathione polymerize tubulin protein and restore to normal the adhesiveness of cells previously altered by colchicine. Recently a test to quantify granulocyte adherence using nylon filters contained in micropipettes has been described.[148]

Neutrophils predominate in tissues during the early phases of the inflammatory response. After a day or so the intensity of the response subsides when the mononuclear phagocytes predominate. If tissues are infected with pyogenic bacteria, the influx of neutrophils is greatly enhanced and sustained to the extent of frank abscess formation. A simple superficial scraping of skin surfaces followed by application of glass coverslips on the abraded area serves as a convenient clinical method for following the inflammatory response.[201] The peak neutrophil immigration occurs between 3 and 6 hours.

The in vitro assay for chemotaxis consists of a chamber with two compartments separated by a filter membrane with a 5 μ pore size. Leukocytes placed in the upper compartment crawl through the pores of the filter when the chemotactic solution is placed in the lower compartment. The chemotactic activity of the fluid in the lower compartment is evaluated by counting the number of cells on the lower side of the filter or the extent of penetration of cells into the filter after a certain time.[39] Leukocytes move randomly until they are exposed to chemotactic gradients; then they uniformly align to move toward the chemotactic source, indicating the capacity to sense differences in concentrations of chemotactic molecules.[259,260]

Phagocyte movement requires the expenditure of energy as the actin-myosin apparatus of the cell contracts in an orderly sequence to move it.[228] Recent studies have shown that G-actin polymerizes to F-actin in the presence of salt solutions and F-actin can be transformed from a sol to a gel after activation by a high molecular weight protein (actin-binding protein).[42] Contraction of this gel requires the activation of magnesium ATPase present in the myosin head. Although calcium is not required for activation, a cofactor is essential. It is likely that microtubule assembly may also be required for cell movement since treatment of neutrophils with colchicine or other agents that disassemble microtubules leads to decreased cell movement.[178]

OPSONIZATION AND RECOGNITION

The attachment of particles to the oncoming phagocytic cell involves alteration of the surface of the particle or bacteria as well as the presence of receptor sites on the surface of the phagocytic cell. For bacteria, it is apparent that special coating, or opsonization, of the particles is required for attachment to the phagocyte. There are two main groups of opsonic serum factors: (1) heat-stable IgG1 and IgG3, specific antibodies directed against antigenic components of the microorganism, and (2) heat-labile opsonic fragments from the third component of serum complement.[254] After opsonic molecules of IgG are bound to the particle's surface, the phagocyte recognizes and binds them to surface receptors that attach to the Fc portion of the antibody molecule. However, in most clinical situations opsonization of bacteria requires the additional activation of the complement system by IgG or IgM antibodies and the surface antigens of the bacteria. The direct complement activation of C1 generates C42 (C3 convertase), which cleaves C3 to form two small fragments: C3a, a chemotactic and anaphylatoxic peptide, and C3b fragment, which attaches to bacterial surfaces. Small amounts of C3 convertase can generate hundreds of molecules of C3b.[112] Receptor sites for bacteria opsonized by complement are also present on the surface of neutrophils and monocytes.[103,137]

In contrast to particles opsonized with specific antibody, the binding of bacteria opsonized by complement to neutrophils is less stable in hypothermic conditions or in the presence of oxidant drugs.[42] C3b may also be generated and used as an opsonin through activation of the alternative pathway of the complement system and bypassing the direct activation of C3 through C142. This system appears to be operative in nonimmune and germ-free animals and in responses to specific polysaccharide antigens such as activation of *Pneumococcus* antigen.[219] The alternative pathway involves the properdin system, consisting of factors A and B, properdin, magnesium, and other less well-characterized proteins.[190]

In contrast to the direct complement pathway, activation of the alternate pathway does not depend on specific antibodies and likely plays an important role in the early preantibody stages of infection. Ingestion of bacteria by neutrophils and monocytes requires an expenditure of energy from ATP made available predominantly from anaerobic glycolysis, whereas the resident macrophage population of the lung depends largely on oxidative phosphorylation for ATP generation.[183] As the phagocytic cell approaches the particle to be ingested, hyaline pseudopodia, formed from the bifurcating front end of the phagocyte, embrace and ultimately entrap the opsonized bacteria by fusing the tips of the pseudopodia.[250] This process of cytoplasmic movement and pseudopod formation almost certainly involves actin-myosin microfilaments.[227] Pseudopodia are devoid of organelles but appear rich in actin filaments when studied by the transmission electron microscope. Furthermore, treatment of neutrophils with the antibiotic

cytochalasin B inhibits the gelation of polymerized microfilaments and blocks ingestion of paraffin oil particles opsonized with either C3 or aggregated IgG, indicating the requirement of microfilaments for ingestion of opsonized particles. A sensitive in vitro assay to measure the rate of uptake of opsonized particles by phagocytic cells employs paraffin oil droplets stained with oil red O and coated with *E. coli* lipopolysaccharide.[230]

DEGRANULATION

After the phagocytic vacuole containing the entrapped bacteria has been created within the neutrophil or monocyte, the primary and secondary lysosomal granules in the cell move to the vacuole and their membranes fuse as a variety of hydrolytic, peroxidative, and cationic proteins are deposited onto the bacteria. This process of degranulation appears to be controlled by microtubules since treatment of cells with the microtubule-disassembly agent colchicine partially inhibits it. The lateral displacement of homogenously distributed surface membrane receptors by concanavalin A (capping) also is associated with inhibition of microtubule assembly. Agents that elevate intracellular levels of cyclic GMP tend to enhance degranulation, whereas those that elevate levels of cyclic AMP retard this process. Cellular adhesiveness and directed cell movement are potentiated by cholinergic agonists or cyclic GMP but are retarded by β-adrenergic stimulants as well as by cyclic AMP and colchicine. Capped neutrophils are less adherent. Thus the cytoplasmic microtubular system appears to regulate processes in addition to degranulation, including movement, adherence, and the distribution of concanavalin A

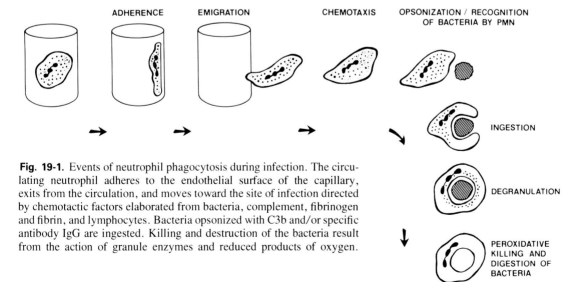

Fig. 19-1. Events of neutrophil phagocytosis during infection. The circulating neutrophil adheres to the endothelial surface of the capillary, exits from the circulation, and moves toward the site of infection directed by chemotactic factors elaborated from bacteria, complement, fibrinogen and fibrin, and lymphocytes. Bacteria opsonized with C3b and/or specific antibody IgG are ingested. Killing and destruction of the bacteria result from the action of granule enzymes and reduced products of oxygen.

receptors on the surface membranes of neutrophils. These cellular events are illustrated in Fig. 19-1.

OXIDATIVE METABOLISM OF PHAGOCYTIZING LEUKOCYTES

Coincident with binding of particles to the surface of the neutrophil or monocyte, there occurs an activation of membrane oxidases leading to cyanide-insensitive increased oxygen consumption,[120] and release of a variety of reduced products of oxygen from the cell. Reduction of oxygen by phagocytizing leukocytes occurs by one electron transfer to oxygen from reduced pyridine nucleotides (NADPH and NADH) formed from the hexose monophosphate shunt and from the anaerobic glycolytic pathway, respectively.[213] The univalent reduction product of oxygen is superoxide anion (O_2^-),[15,76] which rapidly dismutates to the bivalent product hydrogen peroxide.[106] Hydrogen peroxide may acquire another electron from O_2^- or from other sources to form hydroxyl radical OH, a potent oxidant that is finally reduced by another electron to water. Singlet oxygen ($^1O_2$) is formed when an absorption of energy shifts a valence electron to an orbital of higher energy with an inversion of spin[121] (Fig. 19-2). Oxidative activity occurs not only by particle contact, but also when the membrane is perturbed by C3b, C5a, antigen-antibody complexes, and endotoxin.[83] Superoxide anion generated by phagocytizing neutrophils can be quantified spectrophotometrically by determining the amount of nitroblue tetrazolium or ferricytochrome c reduced before and after the addition of superoxide dismutase (SOD), an enzyme that effectively irradicates O_2^- by rapidly dismutating two molecules to hydrogen peroxide.[15] Methionol is converted to ethylene by hydroxyl radical, which can be scavenged with sodium benzoate or mannitol.[31] On the other hand, singlet oxygen can be scavenged by 2,5-diphenylfuran, converting it to *cis*-dibenzoyl ethylene.[124]

Phagocytizing leukocytes emit light, reaching

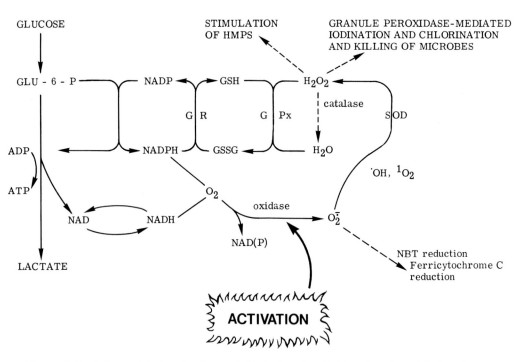

Fig. 19-2. Oxidative metabolism in phagocytizing leukocytes. Oxidase is activated during phagocytosis and this results in the reduction of oxygen by NADH generated during reduction of glucose to lactate and NADPH made in the hexose monophosphate shunt (HMPS) to form superoxide anion (O_2^-). Superoxide dismutase (SOD) aids in the dismutation of O_2^- to hydrogen peroxide (H_2O_2). NBT reduction and ferricytochrome c reduction are convenient tests to quantitate O_2^-. H_2O_2 is required for stimulation of HMPS and for granule peroxidase-mediated iodination and chlorination and killing microbes. Excessive hydrogen peroxide is destroyed by catalase and is used by glutathione peroxidase (GPx) to oxidize reduced glutathione (GSH) to its oxidized form (GSSG). Glutathione reductase (GR) is required to maintain GSH levels in the reduced state by the oxidation of NADPH and NADP.

maximal intensity 10 minutes after they are incubated with opsonized particles.[3] The quantity of light emitted, called chemiluminescence, is detectable by a liquid scintillation spectrometer. Although earlier studies favored singlet oxygen as the main cause for light emission, more recent studies suggest that superoxide anion and granule myeloperoxidase more likely contribute to this interesting reaction.[206]

The oxidation of NADPH either directly by oxidase or indirectly by hydrogen peroxide through the glutathione peroxidase–glutathione system leads to the coupled reduction of oxidized glutathione (GSSG) by NADPH, alters the NADPH-NADP ratio, and activates the hexose monophosphate shunt (Fig. 19-2). The activity of the shunt is determined by the rate of $^{14}CO_2$ evolved from glucose-1-^{14}C during the decarboxylation of the six-carbon phosphorylated sugar to ribose-5-phosphate.[205] The oxidation of formic acid by neutrophils requires intracellular hydrogen peroxide and is catalyzed by cytoplasmic catalase. This serves as an indirect quantitation of intracellular hydrogen peroxide produced during phagocytosis.[20,106]

PHAGOCYTIC PEROXIDATIVE BACTERIAL KILLING AND OTHER RELATED MICROBICIDAL REACTIONS IN LEUKOCYTES

The bacterial killing within the phagocytic vesicle of the neutrophil depends largely on the generation of hydrogen peroxide, which can destroy the bacteria either directly or indirectly through a mechanism involving the peroxidative iodination or chlorination of bacteria by myeloperoxidase, hydrogen peroxide, and iodide or chloride.[127,128] This system requires the efficient transfer of granule myeloperoxidase into the phagocytic vesicle that serves as a substrate for hydrogen peroxide to complete this important bactericidal reaction. Microorganisms can serve as their own source of hydrogen peroxide for the myeloperoxidase-mediated antimicrobial system. These organisms lack catalase and thus accumulate hydrogen peroxide.[160] Among the peroxide-producing bacteria are included pneumococci, streptococci, and lactobacilli.[14]

Evidence for involvement of granule myeloperoxidase in the killing reaction stems from observations on myeloperoxidase-deficient leukocytes as well as on inhibition of myeloperoxidase activity by exposure of normal intact neutrophils to azide or cyanide, which totally inhibits their myeloperoxidase activity.[128,129] Hydroxyl radicals, O_2^-, and $^1O_2$ generated during phagocytosis also may be involved in the microbicidal event.[111]

An array of other intraleukocyte factors independent of oxygen and its reduced products may also contribute to the ultimate killing and digestion of bacteria. These include (1) the acid pH within the phagocytic vesicle, (2) granular cationic proteins, (3) lysozyme and lactoferrin content of specific granules, and (4) hydrolytic enzymes from azurophilic granules.[127] A fall in the pH in the vicinity of the phagocytic vacuole may be microbicidal for certain ingested organisms. Pneumococci are highly acid sensitive[14] and may be killed in phagocytic vacuoles by acid alone. A fall in the pH creates conditions favorable for the activity of other leukocytic antimicrobial systems within the phagocytic vesicle and also facilitates the digestion of killed intracellular organisms by the lysosomal acid hydrolases.[248] The maintenance of a transmembrane hydrogen ion concentration gradient by carbonic anhydrase in the neutrophil has been proposed, based on the presence of this enzyme in the cell and on the inhibition in both the fall in pH and in the digestion of phagocytized particles by carbonic anhydrase inhibitors.[56,153] The cationic proteins in human granulocytes are heat stabile and acid resistant and can be separated into at least seven bands, five of which have been extensively purified.[182] These proteins can be separated by electrophoretic techniques into a number of fractions, each with a different antimicrobial specificity.[258] They are released into the phagocytic vacuole where they can be visualized histochemically at the surface of the ingested organisms. Despite their potent antimicrobial activity in isolated fractions, their precise role in bacterial killing in human leukocytes is yet to be defined. To date there have been no specific defects in cationic proteins noted in humans.

Lysozyme (muramidase), a basic protein of relatively low molecular weight, is known to lyse the bacterial cell walls consisting of linear polysaccharide chains. Pathogenic organisms are not killed by lysozyme under conditions of testing.[9] However, on exposure of the organisms to heat, lipid solvents, chelating agents, polybasic antibiotics, or ascorbic acid plus hydrogen peroxide or antibody plus complement, lysozyme may then serve as a digestive enzyme to already killed bacteria within the phagocytic vesicle. Lysozyme is discharged into the vesicle from secondary granules.[9]

Lactoferrin is an iron-binding protein similar to transferrin and is present in neutrophil granules and presumably released into the phagocytic vesicles.[139] It has the capacity to inhibit growth of proliferating bacteria by binding the iron required as an essential nutrient. Recently it was demonstrated that *Streptococcus mutans,* an etiologic agent of dental carries in humans and animals, and *Vibrio cholerae,* the causitive agent of Asiatic cholera—but not *Escherichia coli*—were killed by incubation of the microorganisms with purified human lactoferrin, stripped of its iron. This bactericidal effect was contingent on the chelating properties of the lactoferrin molecule.[12] The antimicrobial systems of the neutrophil are listed below*:

A. Oxygen-dependent
 1. Myeloperoxidase-H_2O_2-iodide
 2. Myeloperoxidase-H_2O_2-chloride
 3. Hydrogen peroxide-H_2O_2
 4. Hydroxyl radical ($\cdot$OH)
 5. Superoxide anion (O_2^-)
 6. Singlet oxygen ($^1O_2$)
B. Oxygen-independent
 1. Acid
 2. Cationic proteins
 3. Lysozyme
 4. Lactoferrin

CLINICAL CONDITIONS ASSOCIATED WITH DEFECTIVE POLYMORPHONUCLEAR LEUKOCYTE CHEMOTAXIS

An impressive number of clinical conditions in patients with abnormal neutrophil chemotactic responsiveness have been documented in the past decade.[168,220] The defect may arise in the neutrophil itself or may be the result of a defective chemotactic capacity in the serum. Often these defects are a part of a larger spectrum of related functional abnormalities of either the cell or serum systems, i.e., microtubule dysfunction leads to altered cell movement, adherence, degranulation, and bacterial killing, whereas complement depletion renders the serum devoid of chemotactic and opsonic function. The serum may also contain inhibitors to the neutrophil response to normal chemotactic gradients. Most clinical situations result from intrinsic neutrophil dysfunction. In these instances neutrophils isolated from patients function abnormally even when suspended in normal fresh serum, and patient serum or plasma does not compromise the chemotaxis of normal neutrophils.

Clinical features

Patients with chemotactic disorders may be infected by any of a wide spectrum of microorganisms. *Staphylococcus aureus* is the most common bacterial species identified in infectious lesions, but gram-negative enteric bacteria, certain fungal species, and *Staphylococcus epidermidis* are frequently responsible for recurrent and prolonged disease. Infections most typically involve the skin and regional lymph nodes. The dermatosis is usually eczematoid with episodes of pyoderma and furuncles involving the scalp, face, and skin fold areas. The lymph nodes are usually large, especially in regions draining areas of skin inflammation, and may progress to suppuration requiring incision and drainage. Pneumonia occurs frequently but bacteremia and septicemia are uncommon. In contrast to patients with opsonic defects caused by abnormal immunoglobulin responses, patients with chemotactic disorders frequently have infections with *Streptococcus pneumoniae, Haemophilus influenzae,* and group A streptococci; septicemia or meningitis with these organisms is common in comparison to the rarity with which it is observed in patients with other types of neutrophil dysfunction.

Even though patients with defective leukocyte chemotaxis have cells that move slowly in vitro in the Boyden chamber test, as well as in vivo with the inflammatory skin window technique, these patients are capable of forming purulent lesions. Copius fluid abscesses involving lungs or subcutaneous tissue do occur. However, the usual physical signs of inflammation so evident by physical examination or by radiograph and radionuclide scanning in established infections may not occur in the early phases of infection in these patients because of the delay in accumulation of leukocytes in tissues. Subsequent systemic spread may be prevented by the eventual migration of neutrophils and monocytic cells to the inflamed and infected areas. The following are conditions associated with defects of granulocyte chemotaxis in which the defect appears to be related to the increased susceptibility to infection:

A. Cellular defect of chemotaxis
 1. Newborns
 2. Dermatitis with elevated serum IgE (including Job's syndrome)
 3. Dermatitis and respiratory infections with elevated serum IgA
 4. Lazy leukocyte syndrome
 5. Congenital ichthyosis and recurrent infection
 6. Allergic rhinitis and furunculosis
 7. Chronic renal failure
 8. Diabetes mellitus
 9. Rheumatoid arthritis
 10. Bone marrow transplantation
 11. Malnutrition
 12. Infection
B. Cellular defect of chemotaxis in addition to other immune defects
 1. Chediak-Higashi syndrome
 2. Hypogammaglobulinemia
 3. Chronic mucocutaneous candidiasis
 4. Wiscott-Aldrich syndrome
 5. Actin dysfunction
 6. Chronic granulomatous disease
C. Serum defect of chemotactic activity
 1. C3 deficiency
 2. C5 deficiency
 3. Inhibitors
 4. Deficiency of antagonist to inhibitors
 5. Newborns

*Modified from Klebanoff, S. J.: Semin. Hematol. **12:**117, 1975.

Newborn infants. Not only do polymorphonuclear neutrophils from newborns fail to migrate normally toward chemotactic attractants, but their serum fails to generate normal chemotactic activity.[164] In addition, neonatal monocytes also are impaired in their response to chemotactic signal.[131] These cellular chemotactic defects may be related either to decreased membrane deformability as noted in newborns or to other intracellular factors that regulate cell movement.[165] Although abnormal leukocyte locomotion may contribute to the newborn's decreased ability to localize infections, most newborns acquire a resident microbial flora uneventfully despite a generally immature inflammatory response. The inability of newborns to mount a delayed hypersensitivity response may be related to their in vitro monocyte chemotactic defect.

Syndrome of elevated serum IgE with depressed neutrophil chemotaxis including Job's syndrome

Clinical findings. The syndrome of elevated serum IgE with depressed neutrophil chemotaxis is not uncommon. It is characterized by the early onset of pustular, chronic, atopic dematitis during the first few months of life. The skin may become the site of infection with *Staphylococcus aureus* or group A *Streptococcus*. In contrast to the chronic nature of the dermatitis, which can involve the scalp, face, and flexor surfaces, abscesses of lymph nodes, lungs, deep soft tissue structures, and retroperitoneal spaces occur on a sporadic basis and generally respond to appropriate antistaphylococcal antibiotic therapy. Some patients suffer oral moniliasis. The majority of these patients also experience monilial mouth lesions and occasionally monilial skin infections. Rarely dermatophytes and *Herpesvirus hominis* may be cultured from the skin and appear to be the cause of the infection.[239]

Genetics. Some but not all cases appear to be genetically transmitted. In one family the mother and her daughter were both affected with chronic eczema; the daughter experienced staphylococcal lung abscesses at the age of 18 months and later a retropharyngeal abscess, while the mother was troubled with recurrent breast abscesses.[239] Females with fair skin and red hair are plagued with recurrent "cold" *Staphylococcus* skin abscesses. The classical features of inflammation are lacking and the abscesses are not associated with local pain, tenderness, heat, or redness. This disorder has been likened to the biblical experiences recorded by Job and is known as Job's syndrome.[95]

Laboratory abnormalities. Patients with Job's syndrome may have marked elevation in serum IgE levels, a marked depression of neutrophil chemotaxis in vitro, or both. The degree of the chemotactic defect seems to parallel the severity

of the skin infections in patients with or without Job's syndrome.[64] In other patients without Job's syndrome but with elevated serum IgE levels and defects of neutrophil chemotaxis, humoral immunity is normal and neutrophil phagocytic and bactericidal tests are also normal.[96] In one patient so studied who had monilial mouth lesions, monilial skin test reactivity and lymphocyte uptake of tritiated thymidine in response to monilial antigen were markedly diminished.[55] Although the molecular basis for the chemotactic defect has not been clearly elucidated, histamine released from tissue mast cells and involved in severe atopic dermatitis has also been demonstrated to inhibit release of lysosomal enzymes from leukocytes involved in the inflammatory response. In addition, histamines can raise intracellular levels of cyclic AMP, a biochemical condition that is known to retard the movement of neutrophils and inhibit the secretion of lysosomal enzymes from the cell.[123]

Treatment. The antihelminthic drug levamisole hydrochloride improved chemotactic responses of neutrophils and monocytes and increased cyclic GMP levels in monocytes in vitro at concentrations comparable with blood levels observed after oral administration. More important, when patients were given 150 mg of the drug for two successive days a similar improvement in chemotactic function was noted.[257] Even though early reports suggest that clinical improvement has occurred,[68] the usefulness of levamisole for elevated IgE syndrome and other chemotactic disorders will require controlled clinical trials. Other agents known to improve chemotactic function are ascorbic acid, carbamylcholine (the cholinergic agonist) (see discussion of Chediak-Higashi syndrome), and serotonin.[210]

Elevated serum IgA levels and recurrent skin and upper respiratory infections. Four siblings have had increased levels of circulating IgA, recurrent pneumonia, recurrent skin infections, otitis media, and staphylococcal abscesses. All of these patients had depressed neutrophil chemotactic responsiveness, neutropenia, and marked eosinophilia.[35] Recent studies show that polymers of human IgA isolated from the sera of patients with multiple myeloma are cytophilic to human neutrophils and suppress their movement in response to chemotactic signals.[238]

"Lazy leukocyte" syndrome and related disorders. Patients with "lazy leukocyte" syndrome and related disorders experience mild infection similar to patients with benign forms of neutropenia. The clinical manifestations of gingivitis, dermatitis, otitis media, and low grade fever are associated with severe neutropenia. Because the polymorphonuclear neutrophils from these patients have limited migration into Rebuck skin windows, it is difficult to determine whether the in vitro defect is chemotactic or results from the neutropenia per se. Humoral and cellular immunity are normal. Although neutrophils phagocytize and kill bacteria normally, their in vitro random motility in vertically positioned microhematocrit tubes and their response to chemotactic factors generated from normal serum when studied in a Boyden chamber are diminished.[169]

Congenital ichthyosis and recurrent infection. Two kindreds of children afflicted with congenital ichthyosis and recurrent infections particularly with *Trichophyton rubrum* have been described. In contrast to the patients with "lazy leukocyte" syndrome, these patients were not neutropenic and had a normal Rebuck skin window response.[168] Their neutrophils did demonstrate a cellular chemotactic defect in vitro. At times patients with laboratory features of hyperimmunoglobulinemia and skin abscesses may experience severe forms of ichthyosis, and striking defects in neutrophil chemotaxis can be documented.[192]

Allergic rhinitis and furunculosis. A transient depression of leukocyte chemotactic responsiveness occurs in patients with allergic rhinitis who subsequently develop recurrent staphylococcal furunculosis.[98] Their serum contains normal concentrations of IgE and chemotaxis returns to normal when the patients become clinically well. In these patients the onset of allergic symptoms is associated almost predictably with decreased neutrophil chemotaxis and staphylococcal skin abscesses.

Chronic renal failure. Depressed chemotactic responsiveness occurs in patients with chronic renal failure, especially after prolonged hemodialysis.[85] This is not a constant phenomenon of all patients on chronic dialysis, but there is a direct correlation between the number of dialysis treatments and the degree of depression of neutrophil chemotactic responsiveness. Patients receiving long-term hemodialysis are unusually susceptible to severe infections. Although several predisposing factors provide ready access for bacteria and fungi, defective neutrophil function may contribute to their susceptibility to infection.

Diabetes mellitus. Patients with diabetes mellitus have mildly depressed neutrophil chemotaxis.[172] Although chemotaxis in most diabetic patients is nearly normal, many patients demonstrate neutrophil chemotactic responsiveness that is two standard deviations lower than normal. A similar depression of chemotactic responsiveness occurs in children with diabetes mellitus.[97] The presence or absence of this chemotactic defect does not correlate with age, degree of control, or serum concentration of glucose, cholesterol, triglycerides, or creatinine. However, incubation of diabetic leukocytes in 100 units of insulin in a glu-

cose-containing medium does improve the responsiveness of cells to chemotactic stimulants. The fact that similar defects have been found in first-degree relatives of patients with diabetes suggests that a cellular membrane defect associated with diabetes may also be associated with abnormal neutrophil chemotactic responsiveness.[172]

Rheumatoid arthritis. Patients with rheumatoid arthritis have blood neutrophils that are less responsive to chemotactic stimulation in Millipore chambers. Five-day treatment of such patients with appropriate doses of corticosteroids corrects the neutrophils' chemotactic defect, whereas in vitro incubation of neutrophils with the drug does not improve this function. Prior incubation of normal neutrophils with purified rheumatoid factor complexes, serum, or macromolecules of iron-dextran complex also impairs chemotaxis. This observation suggests that the phagocytosis of complexes in vivo may explain in part the observed cellular defect in chemotaxis.[173]

Bone marrow transplantation. Certain patients who have undergone bone marrow transplantation for leukemia or aplastic anemia have severely depressed chemotactic responsiveness of their engrafted neutrophils. Generally these patients are undergoing marked graft versus host reactions or receiving antithymocyte globulin. Patients with graft versus host disease suffer significantly more severe bacterial infections than those patients with normal neutrophil chemotaxis and minimal to absent graft versus host disease. Whether this in vitro defect contributes to their increased risk of severe respiratory and generalized infections remains to be proved.[53]

Malnutrition and diminished chemotaxis. Delayed chemotactic responsiveness is noted in children with kwashiorkor. These children have marked reduction in body weight, apathy, irritability, edema, hepatomegaly, and necrotizing skin lesions. They are susceptible to bacterial, fungal, and viral infections and frequently the inflammatory response present within their infected lesions is minimal. Although these patients' neutrophils have diminished chemotactic activity at early times when studied in Boyden chambers, normal numbers of neutrophils migrate completely through the filters by 180 minutes of incubation.[214]

Infection. A transient depression of granulocyte chemotaxis and random migration has been found in children with measles.[11] Chemotactic function returns to normal approximately 10 days after the onset of the measles rash. The improvement of leukocyte function coincides with the patient's clinical improvement. During acute bacterial infection neutrophils have both increased chemotactic activity and increased spontaneous reduction of nitroblue tetrazolium. Both of these activities return to normal following appropriate therapy.[93]

CELLULAR DEFECTS OF CHEMOTAXIS IN ADDITION TO OTHER DEFECTS IN LEUKOCYTE FUNCTION

Clear-cut defects of chemotaxis in vitro as well as in vivo are part of more generalized defects of phagocytic function in the following conditions, which are described in more detail in other sections: Chediak-Higashi syndrome,[54] hypogammaglobulinemia,[222] chronic mucocutaneous candidiasis,[78] Wiskott-Aldrich syndrome,[8] actin dysfunction,[41] and chronic granulomatous disease.[244]

DEFECTS OF SERUM CHEMOTACTIC FACTORS

Abnormal chemotaxis may also result from abnormality of serum factors that generate chemotactic factors. Defects of complement components, especially C3 and C5, as well as inhibitors in the serum directed against these chemotactic factors or against the oncoming phagocytic cell may all be responsible for recurrent infection.

Complement deficiencies

Although defects in the early components of the complement system such as C1r-deficient serum may generate chemotactic activity more slowly, there has been no increase in susceptibility to infection in these instances.[78] However, serious infections with encapsulated gram-positive and gram-negative bacteria have occurred in patients with low levels of serum C3.[4,29] Deficiency of C5 has occurred in some patients with lupus erythematosis who have been plagued with oral and vaginal moniliasis, infected cutaneous and subcutaneous ulcers, chronically draining sinus tracts, sepsis, and meningitis. Family members who are heterozygous for C5 deficiency remain asymptomatic and are able to generate normal chemotactic activity.[207] A dysfunction of C5 has also been described in patients with recurrent infections whose sera were incapable of generating normal chemotactic activity.[167]

Inhibitors to chemotaxis

Serum inhibitors may be directed against chemotactic factors. The long list of clinical conditions associated with these inhibitors continues to expand. Patients with cirrhosis, sarcoidosis,[149] leprosy,[243] Hodgkin's disease,[242] and uremia have had inhibitors in their serum. These inhibitors may be naturally occurring plasma proteins or products of an inflammatory response. Chemotaxis is decreased only when high concentrations of these substances are present in the serum. Generally these patients are incapable of developing delayed hypersensitivity responses, which may be related to circulating inhibitors preventing the migration of leukocytes to inflammatory sites. They are highly susceptible to bacterial, fungal, and viral infections. Circulating serum inhibitors directed against phagocytic cells can be documented by isolating patient neutrophils and demonstrating depressed chemotaxis in vitro when the neutrophils are incubated with autologous serum but normal chemotaxis after the cells have been washed and suspended in normal serum.

Deficiency of antagonist to serum inhibitors to chemotaxis

One patient had a lifelong respiratory and skin infection with elevated levels of circulating IgA and IgG and a high titer of rheumatoid factor. An 8-month-old child had cytomogelovirus infection, recurrent pneumonia, and staphylococcal skin infections. When plasma was given to the latter patient there was a striking clinical improvement, suggesting that both patients lacked a normal antagonist to their respective serum inhibitors of chemotaxis.[218,221] Sixteen patients have been described with serum chemotactic inhibitors directed against phagocytic cells during acute illnesses associated with leukocytosis and negative skin test response to recall antigens.[237] In these situations the chemotactic defect was transient and cleared following irradication of the acute infection, and the inhibitor was associated with the serum IgA component.

Wiskott-Aldrich syndrome

Children with Wiskott-Aldrich syndrome have plasma that inhibits chemotaxis of normal monocytes. The lymphocytes from these patients produce much more lymphocyte-derived chemotactic factor than normal phagocytes, and it is possible that the monocytes in these patients are constantly exposed to high levels of lymphocyte-derived chemotactic factor, which deactivates them, causing them to become less chemotactic.[8]

CLINICAL DISORDERS OF OPSONIZATION
Newborn infants

The serum of low birth weight infants appears compromised in its capacity to completely opsonize *Escherichia coli, Pseudomonas aeruginosa, Serratia marcescens,* and *Staphylococcus aureus.*[75,158] In these infants the opsonic activity correlates with their serum C3 levels, which in turn correlate with gestational age. The concentration of C3 and C5 in newborn serum is approximately 50% of adult levels.[1] Even a full-term infant's serum is deficient in its opsonic activity for *Escherichia coli* and *Serratia marcescens.*[72] Opsonization of gram-negative organisms requires IgM specific antibody for activation of the complement system, and the lack of transplacentally transferred IgM may be the cause for the decreased opsonization. On the other hand, IgG crosses the placenta and offers the full-term newborn infant opsonic defense against streptococci, *Haemophilus influenzae,* and *Staphylococcus aureus,* presuming that maternal levels are adequate.

The basis for the high incidence of group B β-hemolytic *Streptococcus* infection may be related to this idea. It has recently been demonstrated that women with low levels of IgG antibody to capsular polysaccharide antigen isolated from type III group B *Streptococcus* deliver infants who have a statistically significant risk for development of clinical infection with the same type of group B *Streptococcus.*[28]

In certain respects the newborn is similar to the nonimmune animal and may depend on the alternate complement pathway for C3b generation. Factor B, glycine-rich-β-glycoprotein (GBG), a component of the alternate pathway, does not cross the placenta and is deficient in more than half of the blood samples.[6]

Congenital disorders of opsonin system

Profound deficiency of C3 produces lifelong bacterial infection. A teenage girl was found to have only 0.001 of the normal amount of C3 in her serum; her parents and some of her other family members had C3 levels approximately half of normal, indicating an autosomal recessive inheritance pattern.[7] The defect was attributed to a decreased synthetic rate. On the other hand, a man with increased susceptibility to infection and low C3 levels was found to have an increased catabolic rate of C3. Normal serum but not purified C3 restored to normal his serum complement-mediated functions of chemotaxis, opsonization of pneumococci, and serum microbicidal activity against gram-negative organisms.[4,5]

Two unrelated infants have been described with dysfunction of C5[107,167] and clinical features of Leiner's disease consisting of generalized seborrheic dermatitis, intractable severe diarrhea, recurrent infections with *Candida albicans,* and marked wasting of body tissues. Although levels of C5 as determined by immunochemical methods were normal, there was faulty generation of chemotactic factor and opsonic activity in the serum as determined by phagocytosis of yeast particles, which requires C5. In these cases phagocytosis of yeast was diminished but ingestion of sensitized red cells, pneumococci, and polystyrene particles was normal. Therapy with fresh plasma or blood stored less than 5 days improved the patients' clinical course.

Serum from three patients with complete selective deficiency of C2 did not promote optimal killing of *Staphylococcus aureus* by neutrophils in vitro. The defect was corrected by addition of C2 to the patients' serum, which supports the idea that the classical pathway of complement activation was required for opsonization of *Staphylococcus aureus.* Patients with C2 deficiency generally experience recurrent bacterial upper respiratory infections and have chronic vasculitis.[202]

Deficiency of specific antibodies as opsonins are found in patients with defects of humoral immunity. Thus the many patients with deficient immunoglobulin develop recurrent and chronic pyogenic infections on this basis.[108]

Sickle cell disease

Bacterial infection is the leading cause of death in children with sickle cell disease.[30] The sera of some children who are at risk of developing life-threatening pneumococcal septicemia and meningitis have been found to be markedly deficient in heat-labile opsonin for pneumococcus.[255] The clinical observations that the frequency of infection with certain type-specific pneumococci has drastically diminished in the normal population with acquired type-specific antibodies[116] suggests that the alternative pathway may be critical for opsonization in those circumstances in which type-specific antipneumococcal antibody is lacking. Sera from patients with sickle cell disease promoted phagocytosis of pneumococci normally, but only when the bacteria had previously been sensitized with an excess of antibody. However, phagocytosis of the same type-specific pneumococci did not occur when specific antibody was omitted, shifting the requirement for opsonic function to the alternative pathway to fix the essential opsonin, C3b, to the bacteria; this may explain in part the increased susceptibility to pneumococcal infection in these patients.[114,132] This observation does not exclude the importance of the phagocytic function of the spleen in children with sickle cell disease since it is likely that a coordinated opsonin-reticuloendothelial function is necessary for adequate host defense against such microorganisms.

DISORDERS OF NEUTROPHIL INGESTION
Actin dysfunction

Intrinsic abnormalities of neutrophil ingestion must be extremely rare or incompatible with life beyond the neonatal period. One infant who had onset of recurrent pyogenic infections at birth was observed to have nonmotile neutrophils deficient in chemotaxis and ingestion of opsonized paraffin oil particles. Despite a white cell count of 50×10^9/liter, the infant died of overwhelming infection. Isolation of the infant's neutrophil actin revealed that the actin did not polymerize under conditions that fully polymerized the actin of normal neutrophils. These findings constitute evidence that the state of actin polymerization is relevent for ingestion.[41]

Phagocytic immaturity

Clinical conditions associated with the lack of mature circulating neutrophils include acute lymphocytic and nonlymphocytic leukemia, aplastic anemia, and neutropenic syndromes. Each condition is associated with severe bacterial life-threatening infection. Although metamyelocytes and myelocytes as well as eosinophils and monocytes are capable of ingesting microorganisms and other particulate debris, they are not as efficient phagocytic cells as are neutrophils. That the microfilament system is responsible for ingestion is inferred by the ability of the microfilament disassembly agent cytochalasin B to inhibit the ingestion process.[261]

Modification of ingestion rates

Phagocytic rates can be modified by the antioxidant α-tocopherol (vitamin E), which protects the cell membrane against the peroxidative effects of hydrogen peroxide generated during phagocytosis.[18] Depression of glycolysis from low intracellular phosphate concentrations noted in the sera of malnourished patients receiving intravenous hyperalimentation produces an ingestion defect in these affected cells.[60] In patients with congenital enzymatic defects of glycolysis, compensatory shifts in neutrophil cell metabolism may occur. For example, the neutrophils from a patient with phosphoglycerate kinase deficiency[19] depended on microchondrial phosphorylation for ATP generation to compensate for the lack of ATP generation from anaerobic glycolysis.

DISORDERS OF DEFECTIVE DEGRANULATION
Chediak-Higashi syndrome

The Chediak-Higashi syndrome occurs in humans, mink, mice, cows, cats, and white killer whales.* This syndrome consists of partial oculocutaneous albinism with photophobia and rotatory nystagmus, frequent pyogenic infections, intermittent febrile episodes, and abnormally large granules in blood leukocytes and many other body cells. A mild bleeding diathesis has been described in some patients. An accelerated phase of the disorder develops with widespread lymphoid and histiocytic infiltrates of lymphoreticular organs, producing pancytopenia, lymphadenopathy, and hepatosplenomegaly. Death usually occurs at an early age during the accelerated phase of the illness from

---

*References 133, 134, 185, 234.

infection or less commonly from hemorrhage.

Historical perspective. Beguez-Cesar[32] first noted the giant granules in blood neutrophils from patients in 1943, and Steinbrinck[223] described another case in 1948. Higashi[91] reported on the maldistribution of myeloperoxidase in the granules of patients' neutrophils. Chediak extended the observations on the family originally described by Beguez-Cesar.[52] In 1955 Sato[211] recognized the similarity between Chediak's and Higashi's data and coined the eponym "Chediak-Higashi" in honor of the astute observations of the Cuban pathologist and the Japanese pediatrician.

Incidence. An extensive review of fifty-nine cases of the Chediak-Higashi syndrome has recently been reported.[37] The Chediak-Higashi syndrome is widely distributed throughout the world. Cases have been described in North America, Latin America, Europe, and Asia. Among fifty-seven cases of neutrophil dysfunction in Japan, eleven cases of Chediak-Higashi syndrome and forty cases of chronic granulomatous disease were identified.[90] It is of interest that there have been no reported cases in blacks.

Genetics. The involvement of four of thirteen siblings from the first family ever described suggested that this syndrome is inherited as an autosomal recessive disorder.[59] All further cases reported both in humans and animals would support this original observation. The observed twenty-seven cases from ninety-eight children (27%), excluding propositi from the analysis to reduce the sampling bias, is close to the expected 25% for an autosomal recessive condition. A high percentage of marriages producing affected children are known to be consanguineous. Experimental breeding in cattle, mice, and mink, including an introduction in each species of a gene into different strains than that in which it originated, has shown that genetic transmission of Chediak-Higashi syndrome also behaves as a single autosomal recessive trait in these studies.[186]

Etiology. More than a decade ago it was postulated that Chediak-Higashi syndrome is caused by an abnormal fusion of lysosomes and possibly represents a lysosomal disease.[246] Most of the clinical manifestations of the disease can be explained by the abnormal dispersion of lysosomal enzymes into giant lysosomes within body cells.

The photophobia and albinism result from the abnormal dispersion and distribution of melanosomes within retinal and skin cells.[253] Similarly microscopic analysis of hair obtained from affected patients reveals the presence of giant melanin granules abnormally dispersed in the pulp, and this pigmentary dilution explains the clinical observation that the hair color is several shades lighter than the original phenotypic strain.

The increased incidence of pyogenic infection in these patients can be explained by a failure of the giant lysosomes to transfer their peroxidative and lysosomal enzymes into phagocytic vesicles of blood neutrophils containing the ingested bacteria. This results in a delayed killing of ingested bacteria.[205]

The bleeding diathesis, which is mild in most cases, can be ascribed to a failure of normal platelet function in these cells. The platelets from Chediak-Higashi patients do not aggregate on exposure to collagen and thrombin but respond normally to ADP.[40] Striking lysosomal abnormalities with giant granule formation have been found in neural connective tissue cells and may in part account for the progressive neurologic abnormalities seen in this disease.[232] Abnormal granules have also been described in the adrenal cortex, anterior pituitary gland, capillary endothelium, and thyroid gland. Unfortunately the nature of the lymphoreticular infiltrate associated with the accelerated phase and the reason for its occurrence have not yet been adequately explained.

An extensive search for underlying unusual infections such as toxoplasmosis, cytomegalic inclusion disease, and herpesvirus and Epstein-Barr virus infections has been unrewarding. On the other hand, Aleutian disease of mink (slow virus type), to which mink with Chediak-Higashi syndrome are more susceptible, is associated with extensive lymphoid and plasma cell infiltration and immune deposition throughout the vascular tree.[193]

Immunology. Recent studies have shown conclusively that the granulocytes from these patients have an intrinsic chemotactic defect.[54] Skin window preparations demonstrate less migration of leukocytes into abraded tissues, and in vitro movement of human Chediak-Higashi syndrome granulocytes through micropore membranes is slower than normal. Delayed hypersensitivity skin reactivity is probably normal although occasionally a patient has failed both to develop sensitivity to recall skin test antigens and to be sensitized to new antigenic stimuli. As in other patients with chronic and recurrent infections, immunoglobulin levels generally are elevated, especially IgG and IgA. Macrophage phagocytosis assessed by the ability to clear intravenously administered microaggregated particles is not impaired and may even be accelerated in some cases.[37]

Studies of patients and animals with Chediak-Higashi syndrome have documented an impairment in bactericidal activity of blood-derived neutrophils. Opsonized bacteria are ingested normally, but the rate of killing is delayed until 60 minutes have passed in the in vitro incubation system. This impaired bactericidal activity appears related to delayed delivery of lysosomal contents into the phagosome.[230]

Clinical features. The partial oculocutaneous albinism is manifested in at least one of three organ systems: hair, skin, and eyes. The hair color varies from blond to dark brown but exhibits in each case a silvery tint that is particularly noticeable in strong light and after a thorough washing of the hair. Comparison with the unaffected siblings or parents within the same family often reveals this subtle but definite feature of the disease caused by dilution of melanin pigment of the hair.

An increase in red reflex, photophobia, and rotatory nystagmus in bright light are expressions of the ocular pigmentary dilution.[187] Pigmentation is less in the affected patients than in their parents and siblings. They are also susceptible to severe sunburns and often pyoderma develops thereafter. Nevi and lentigines have been noted as irregular areas of increased pigmentation.[253] Thus the pigmentary disturbance is not caused by an absence of melanin; as mentioned earlier in microscopic analysis of these tissues, it is caused by abnormal aggregation of melanin-containing lysosomes.

Episodes of fever are common in these patients and most often can be ascribed to pyogenic infections, which occur repeatedly and regularly. Particularly likely infections include infections of the upper and lower respiratory tract with otitis media, sinusitis, pharyngitis, bronchitis, bronchial pneumonia, and lobar pneumonia. Skin surface infections including pyoderma, impetigo, subcutaneous abscesses, and orbital cellulitis are common. Gastrointestinal infections, gingivitis, urinary tract infections, and sepsis occur less frequently. Table 19-3 (p. 546) records the sites of infection and organisms cultured from these infected sites in the sixty-three cases reported from the literature.

In contrast to chronic granulomatous disease, peroxide-producing bacteria such as *Diplococcus pneumoniae*, *Streptococcus*, and *Haemophilus influenzae* all cause infection in Chediak-Higashi syndrome. Fever has been noted in the accelerated phase of the disease in the absence of infection in approximately one third of the cases. The accelerated phase is characterized by enlargement of the liver, spleen, and lymph nodes associated with depression of granulocyte and platelet counts. Hemolytic anemia may or may not be evident. Except for extremity petechiae, bleeding is not a problem until the accelerated phase when severe gastrointestinal hemorrhage occurs frequently.[185] Hypogammaglobulinemia has been associated with a few cases. Pronounced neurologic abnormalities occur in these patients with longstanding disease. Loss of deep tendon reflexes, paresis or weakness, sensory loss, cerebellar clumsiness, seizures, behavior disturbances, and peripheral neuropathy have all been noted. In addition, nine of the sixty-three patients have been observed to be mentally retarded.[37]

Laboratory features. The diagnosis is often established by an astute laboratory worker who notices the giant granules within the bone marrow or peripheral blood leukocytes. (See Fig. 18-3, p. 503.) The giant granules stain positive for myeloperoxidase and are easily demonstrable on a Wright's stained blood smear. Cultured fibroblast cells also contain the giant lysosomes. Although the patients may have mild anemia related to their infection, severe anemia is not evident until the accelerated phase of the disease. Hemolysis caused by splenic sequestration is the principle cause for the profound anemia. The direct Coombs test is usually negative, and iron and folic acid deficiencies are rarely evident. Neutropenia almost always accompanies the accelerated phase of the disease, whereas thrombocytopenia is evident in more than one half of the cases. Inspection of the bone marrow aspirate confirms the presence of giant lysosomes in the precursor granulocytes, eosinophils, and mononuclear cells. Granulocyte precursors are increased and many contain degenerative vacuoles coinciding with the markedly elevated serum muramidase activity indicative of the increased intramedullary destruction of granulocytes known to occur in this disease.[37]

Platelet counts, plasma coagulation factors, and fibrinolytic systems are normal, although thrombocytopenia is noted during the accelerated phase. Throughout the illness the cutaneous bleeding time is prolonged. Platelet aggregation and response to collagen and thrombin are markedly abnormal, response to ADP is normal, suggesting a decreased storage of ADP. The platelets from one infant with Chediak-Higashi syndrome demonstrated decreased release of nonmetabolic adenine nucleotides and 5-hydroxytryptamine in response to aggregating agents; this is similar to the findings previously described for storage pool disease patients.[245] In contrast to storage pool disease without albinism and the Hermansky-Pudlak syndrome,[247] in which the platelet dense bodies are consistently reduced in numbers, electron microscopic studies of Chediak-Higashi platelets demonstrate a normal number of platelet dense bodies. In storage pool disease associated with albinism, platelet dense bodies are normal.[145]

Light microscopic and electron microscopic studies of lymph nodes and other affected tissues during the accelerated phase show the nodes to be infiltrated with mature lymphocytes and histiocytes. Plasma cells are prominent. The architecture of the organs involved is usually spared, although at times marked histiocytic hyperplasia with erythrophagocytosis is evident. In some cases circulating atypical cells of a nonmalignant nature are noted.

Differential diagnosis. Patients with Chediak-Higashi syndrome must be differentiated from those with true albinism in which a depletion rather than an abnormal dispersion of melanosomes occurs. The content of neutrophil lysosomal enzymes in Chediak-Higashi syndrome, although decreased, does not represent a true deficiency of the enzymes.

No other condition is known to present with such dramatic coalescence of lysosomes in most body cells, including reticuloendothelial cells, fibroblasts, kidney cells, bone marrow, and blood leukocytes. The accelerated phase may resemble either lymphoma or infectious mononucleosis. Serologic tests for toxoplasmosis, cytomegalic inclusion disease, and infectious mononucleosis show no evidence for these etiologic agents as the basis for the lymphoid hypertrophy. On the other hand, typical lymphoid malignancies usually show distortion of the lymph node architecture and invasion of the lymph node capsule with immature blast cells, which is not the case in these patients' tissues.

Pathophysiology. The abnormal lysosomal function in these cells likely represents a fundamental defect in microtubule control within these cells. A relationship of microtubule function and cyclic nucleotide concentration, although unclear, is supported by the observation that peripheral blood monocytes isolated from two patients, as well as fibroblasts obtained in mice with Chediak-Higashi syndrome when grown in the presence of the cholinergic agonist carbamyl methylcholine, contain significantly fewer abnormal lysosomes.[177] Similarly the functional defects of polymorphonuclear neutrophils may arise because of impaired microtubular assembly from cytoplasmic tubulin.[176] Microtubules are linear structures involved in secretory and degranulation function of cells. In a cell-free system, assembly is promoted by guanosine triphosphate (GTP), magnesium, glycerol, heat, and several high molecular weight microtubule-associated proteins, whereas the process is inhibited by calcium.[181] Reduced glutathione and ascorbic acid further enhance tubulin polymerization in an independent and additive fashion.[235]

Microtubule assembly in neutrophils is promoted by perturbation of the cell membrane with ingestible particles or lectins such as concanavalin A (Con A).[176] Fluoresceinated Con A is bound homogenously over the neutrophil membrane by receptors that are connected to cytoplasmic microtubules. Inhibiting microtubule assembly by colchicine or drugs that oxidize sulfhydryl groups on tubulin results in displacement of Con A to polar regions (caps) in the membrane. Lysosomal enzyme secretion and degranulation are triggered by opsonized particles and potentiated by agents that raise cyclic GMP levels,[152] but elevations in cyclic AMP retard this process.

Table 19-2. Leukocyte function tests

Function	Principle of test	Purpose of test	Normal values	Reference
Microtubule				
Adherence	Granulocytes are passed over a microcolumn of nylon fiber packed in a Pasteur pipette and the percentage of cells adhering is calculated.	Measures surface adherence of neutrophil or monocyte.	60% to 80%	146
Chemotaxis	Neutrophils are sedimented on Millipore filter, placed in Boyden chamber, and incubated 3 hr at 37° C, with a source of chemotactic factor placed on the opposite side of the filter. Chemotactic index is calculated by assessing the number of neutrophils migrating completely through the filter.	Assay studies directed neutrophil movement in response to a variety of chemotactic factors. Test can be adapted to study cells, serum, or the effects of pharmacologic agents on chemotaxis.	Chemotactic index: 13 ± 5 (without chemotactic factor), 67 ± 16 (with chemotactic factor)	96
Fluorescein-con-canavalin A capping	PMN incubated with fluorescein-Con A; the movement of fluorescence into polar aggregates represents microtubule depoly-merization.	Tests for factors that control microtubule polymerization in neu-trophils. Drugs (e.g., colchicine) and diseases (e.g., Chediak-Higashi syndrome) that interfere with microtubule assem-bly increase number of capped neutrophils.	Fluorescence distribution: random >90%; capped <10%	178
Degranulation of lysosomal en-zymes into phagolyso-somes	Emulsified liquid petro-latum, containing oil red O is phagocytized by neutrophils. Phagocytic vesicles are isolated from homogenized cells on a density gradient. Vesicles float to the top of the gradient, and the other cell components sediment.	Assesses lysosomal move-ment in neutrophils, de-pendent in part on nor-mal microtubular as-sembly.	$14.5 \pm 2.2\%$ of total β-glucuronidase released into phagocytic vesicles in 45 min	227
Degranulation of lysosomal en-zymes into media	Cytochalasin B inhibits ingestion and converts PMN to "secretory" cells releasing lysosomal enzymes during incuba-tion with opsonized zymosan particles.	Assesses lysosomal move-ment in neutrophils, de-pendent in part on nor-mal microtubule assembly.	20% of total β-glucoroni-dase released in 30 min	260
Microfilament				
Phagocytic up-take of oil red O particles	Liquid petroleum, stained by oil red O dye and emulsified by sonica-tion, is coated with *Escherichia coli* lipo-polysaccharide, requir-ing opsonification by alternative pathway for efficient uptake by PMN.	Measures the rate of uptake of particles by neutro-phils; also measures functional alternative pathway opsonic ca-pacity.	0.138 (0.121-0.157) mg liquid petrolatum taken up/min/10^7 cells	223

Table 19-2. Leukocyte function tests—cont'd

Function	Principle of test	Purpose of test	Normal values	Reference
Oxidase				
Oxygen consumption	Cyanide-insensitive O_2 consumption is associated with, but is not required for, phagocytosis by neutrophils and monocytes.	Phagocytic blood cells reduce oxygen to hydrogen peroxide (H_2O_2), superoxide anion (O_2^-), singlet oxygen ($^1O_2$), and hydroxyl radical ($\cdot OH$). Some or all of these reduction products are required for intraleukocyte bacterial killing.	Resting: 7.4 ± 3.8 μl O_2 consumed/hr/10^7 cells Phagocytosis: 37.6 ± 22.5 μl O_2 consumed/hr/10^7 cells	101
Superoxide release	Univalent reduction product of oxygen is O_2^-; it and other substances reduce ferricytochrome c and that amount of ferricytochrome c inhibited by purified superoxide dismutase (SOD) is due only to O_2^-.	Measures release of O_2^- from neutrophils and monocytes at rest and during phagocytosis.	Resting: 0.50 nmole O_2^-/min/10^7 cells Phagocytosis: 1.0 nmoles/15 min/10^7 cells	15
Nitroblue tetrazolium (NBT) reduction	Solubilized redox dyes of tetrazolium salts when incubated with neutrophils are reduced to insoluble formazan. Reduction occurs to a larger extent during phagocytosis. Addition of superoxide dismutase (SOD) decreases amount of formazan formed, indicating that NBT reduction, in large part, reflects O_2^- generated by neutrophils.	Detects carriers of the X-linked form of chronic granulomatous disease (CGD); detects all affected patients with CGD.	Resting: 0.088 ± 0.040 OD/15 min/10^7 cells Phagocytosis: 0.319 ± 0.112 OD/15 min/10^7 cells	24
Glucose-1-^{14}C $\rightarrow$ $^{14}CO_2$	Oxidation of glucose through the hexose monophosphate shunt is stimulated in neutrophils and monocytes during phagocytosis.	NADPH oxidation by O_2 and/or H_2O_2 occurs in neutrophils with an intact NADPH/NADH oxidase system activated during phagocytosis.	Resting: 62.6 ± 10 nmoles glucose oxidized/30 min/5×10^6 cells Phagocytosis 169 ± 28 nmoles glucose oxidized/30 min/5×10^6 cells	204
Formate ^{14}C $\rightarrow$ $^{14}CO_2$	Oxidation of formic acid by neutrophils requires H_2O_2 and is catalyzed by catalase.	This is an indirect quantitation of H_2O_2 produced during phagocytosis by neutrophils.	Resting: 0.6 (0.2-1.1) nmoles formate oxidized/hr/mg protein Phagocytosis: 2.8 (1.1-5.9) nmoles formate oxidized/hr/mg protein	26
Hydrogen peroxide release	Scopoletin fluorescence is extinguished when oxidized by H_2O_2 in presence of horseradish peroxidase.	Provides sensitive, direct quantitation of release of H_2O_2 from neutrophils during phagocytosis.	Resting: 0.012 ± 0.003 nmole H_2O_2 released/min/2.5×10^6 cells Phagocytosis: 0.445 ± 0.064 nmole H_2O_2 released/min/2.5×10^6 cells	203

Continued.

Table 19-2. Leukocyte function tests — cont'd

Function	Principle of test	Purpose of test	Normal values	Reference
Oxidase — cont'd				
Iodination	Bacteria and other particulate proteins are iodinated following their ingestion by neutrophils and monocytes. Biochemical requirements are halide ion, peroxidase, and hydrogen peroxide.	Measures capacity of specific granule peroxidase in blood phagocytes (neutrophils and monocytes) to be discharged into phagolysosomes and assesses available pool of H_2O_2 in region of phagolysosomes to iodinate ingested particles.	Resting 0.04 ± 0.03 nmole iodide consumed/ hour/10^7 cells Phagocytosis: 3.95 ± 0.82 nmoles iodide consumed/hr/10^7 cells	189
Chemiluminescence	Measures light produced by neutrophils and monocytes during phagocytosis of zymosan.	Measures capacity of neutrophils and monocytes to reduce O_2 to H_2O_2, O_2^-, and $'O_2$; all three are required for optimal chemoluminescence.	142.5 ± 64 × 10^3 counts/ min/13 min/10^7 cells	3
Bactericidal				
Bacterial killing	Opsonized live bacteria are ingested and killed by phagocytic blood cells.	Measures capacity of blood phagocytes to kill opsonized bacteria; may also be used to measure opsonic activity of sera.	Less than 10% of most bacterial species viable after 60 min at 37° C incubation with an equal number of neutrophils	198

Treatment of Chediak-Higashi syndrome leukocytes in vitro with agents that increase cyclic GMP levels improves microtubular function. The quantitation of cyclic GMP and cyclic AMP levels in Chediak-Higashi syndrome neutrophils has documented a marked elevation of cyclic AMP levels in neutrophils of three patients. Thus the abnormal elevation of cyclic AMP may be directly impairing the motility of the granules by inhibiting microtubule assembly. There is evidence that two cyclic nucleotides, cyclic AMP and cyclic GMP, may produce functionally opposite effects in cells. The correction in leukocyte function in vitro obtained by dibutyl cyclic GMP in Chediak-Higashi syndrome cells may relate to the antagonizing effect of the excessive cyclic AMP concentrations.[82] This observation correlates with the improvement of monocyte granule morphology in mice with the Chediak-Higashi syndrome treated by mouth with cholinergic agents.[179] Chemotaxis is also thought to be dependent on microtubule as well as microfilament function.[226] The addition of cyclic AMP to normal leukocytes impairs their movement, whereas the effect of cyclic GMP is to potentiate movement.[210]

Diminished chemotaxis in Chediak-Higashi syndrome may also be caused by impaired microtubule function mediated by the abnormal cyclic nucleotide levels. Ascorbic acid enhances chemotaxis of normal neutrophils[210] and can directly enhance the polymerization of purified bovine brain tubulin, suggesting that correction of the functional defects in Chediak-Higashi syndrome could be ascribed to this effect rather than to an effect from cyclic nucleotide alteration.[235] In addition, the abnormal Con A cap formation on the surface membranes of polymorphonuclear leukocytes of animals and patients with Chediak-Higashi syndrome can also be corrected by incubation of these cells in vitro with cyclic GMP and cholinergic agents.[180]

Still another microtubule-related function of the surface membrane of polymorphonuclear neutrophils has recently been correlated with capping. Cellular adherence to nylon wool fibers in vitro is decreased in capped neutrophils. The Chediak-Higashi syndrome neutrophils demonstrate a high degree of spontaneous cap formation and are less adherent. This may explain their failure to be mobilized into tissue sites in vivo. Ascorbic acid both in vitro and in vivo will correct the abnormal cap formation, improve the cellular adherence of these cells, and restore the other microtubule-related functions of degranulation and bactericidal killing to normal in the Chediak-Higashi syndrome neutrophils from mice, mink, and humans.[44,195]

Treatment and management. Recently it was demonstrated that 200 mg of ascorbic acid given daily corrected the in vitro microtubule-related defects of leukocyte adherence, chemotaxis, degranulation, and bacterial killing. Whether such treatment will prevent the morphologic alterations in the cells and prevent the accelerated phase and neurologic complications of the disease remains to be seen.

Careful attention should be given to the extreme photophobia and skin sensitivity to direct sunlight by shielding the eyes and skin from direct sunlight. Wearing tinted glasses and covering the skin are useful ways to prevent the annoying side effects of this disease.

Fever generally means that the patient has active infection; a careful search for the source must be made by obtaining bacteriologic cultures and sensitivity studies to select proper antibiotic therapy. The response to infection is slower than normal in these patients. Patients with gastrointestinal bleeding may require platelet transfusions. Cytotoxic drugs utilized for treating lymphoma have not been effective in reducing the size of the lymphoid and organ hyperplasia. It does appear that the hepatosplenomegaly, lymphadenopathy, and pancytopenia are somewhat responsive to high doses of prednisone therapy, albeit for a temporary period of time in these cases. Patients with severe hemolysis require multiple blood transfusions in the accelerated phase of the disease. Progressive granulocytopenia with proved septicemia may also require granulocyte transfusions to combat the infection.

Prognosis. There is some evidence that the worsening of the neuropathy is coincident with an increase in the accelerated phase of the disease.[232] In more than 85% of patients the disease progresses to the accelerated phase with death following shortly thereafter. In the past few patients survived beyond the teenage period.

Future research will be directed to ways to alter the morphologic aberrations within the body cells so that the abnormal lysosomal fusion no longer occurs. It remains to be seen whether long-term ascorbic acid treatment will provide total correction of the disease.

DISORDERS OF DEFECTIVE PEROXIDATIVE KILLING OF BACTERIA AND FUNGI BY PHAGOCYTES
Chronic granulomatous disease (CGD)

The term "chronic granulomatous disease" has been applied to a syndrome occurring in infants and children who experience chronic and lifelong recurrent, purulent infections of the skin, lymph nodes, upper and lower respiratory tracts, bones, and gastrointestinal tract, ranging from ulcerative stomatitis to granulomatous colitis with perianal abscesses and fistulas. The infected organs become the site of granulomatous reactions containing pigmented lipid histiocytes.

A variety of gram-positive and gram-negative bacteria lacking the capacity to produce hydrogen peroxide can be cultured from the infected tissues. The patient's peripheral blood leukocytes ingest but fail to kill those bacteria that cause infection in them. The killing defect is associated with a metabolic defect of the cell, resulting in a failure of the leukocyte to reduce oxygen to form superoxide anion, hydroxyl radical, singlet oxygen, and the important bactericidal product, hydrogen peroxide.

Historical perspective. The historical aspects of this disease were the subject of a recent review.[17] In the mid-1950s pediatric immunologists became aware of a group of boys with recurrent pyogenic infections similar to those caused by agammaglobulinemia except that their serum contained normal to elevated levels of immunoglobulins.[109] In 1957 Berendes et al.[34] defined this condition as a distinct clinical entity and coined the term "fatal granulomatous disease of childhood" to describe the clinical severity of the disease as well as the histopathology of the involved organs. These investigators noted the frequent association of infections by *Staphylococcus aureus* and *Serratia marcescens* and that the infected tissue contained peculiar granulomata that were often infiltrated by pigmented lipid histiocytes. In that same year Landing and Shirkey[136] provided the first definitive series of pathologic studies of the disease. One year later Carson et al.[48] documented the genetic transmission to be X linked.

Fundamental understanding of the pathogenesis of the disease began with studies published in 1967. Holmes et al.[102,199] reported that leukocytes from affected patients could ingest but could not kill bacteria that infected them. The association of the disease to a defect in leukocyte oxidase activity was first suggested in 1967.[23,100] The significance of the metabolic defect, and especially the absence of hydrogen peroxide generation, was clarified by the important studies of Klebanoff. Klebanoff[130] showed that peroxidative iodination of catalase-positive bacteria, e.g., *Staphylococcus aureus* and other microorganisms that infect patients with chronic granulomatous disease, did not occur in patients' neutrophils, whereas catalase-negative bacteria, e.g., *Lactobacillus* sp., were iodinated and killed. The species specificity of the in vitro intracellular microbicidal defect was first described by Quie who noted that chronic granulomatous disease leukocytes could kill ingested streptococci and *Escherichia coli* but failed to kill *Staphylococcus aureus,* a bacterium known to contain a potent catalase system leading to a failure to generate endogenous peroxide.[117] The nitroblue tetrazolium (NBT) test was introduced as a simple laboratory test to establish the diagnosis and to define the carrier state.[24]

Incidence. From 1967 until 1971 ninety-two cases were described[110] and by 1977 an additional seventy-six cases were reported in the literature, bringing the total to 168 cases.[113] The disease occurs in all parts of the world, including North America, South America, Europe, Asia, Japan, and England, and has been described in blacks, whites, and Orientals.

Etiology. The cause of this disease appears to be a failure of the blood phagocytic cells, including neutrophils, eosinophils, and monocytes, to reduce oxygen to the bactericidal product hydrogen peroxide. In addition, the free radicals formed during the univalent reduction of oxygen include superoxide anion (O_2^-), hydroxyl radical ($\cdot OH$), and singlet oxygen ($^1O_2$). Although the phagocytic cells take up bacteria normally, catalase-positive bacteria that do not elaborate their own hydrogen peroxide survive in these cells. Compared to normal neutrophil killing in which less than 10% of the bacteria remain viable at the end of a 60-minute incubation, after incubation with an equal number of cells more than 80% of bacteria survive within the neutrophils of patients with chronic granulomatous disease.[199] Similarly chronic granulomatous disease neutrophils also lack normal fungicidal capacity.[140] Thus the viable microorganisms within the phagocytic cells of the blood circulate to tissues throughout the body where they incite abscess formation or chronic granulomatous reactions.

The bactericidal and metabolic defects evident in these phagocytic cells can be explained by a failure to activate one or more oxidases required for enhanced cyanide-insensitive oxygen consumption and reduction.[23,100] The rate of reduction of oxygen to superoxide anion can be quantified by reduction of NBT to insoluble purple formazan[174] or by the differential reduction of ferricytochrome *c* before and after addition of superoxide dismutase, an enzyme that effectively removes or dismutates O_2^- to hydrogen peroxide.[63] The neutrophils and monocytes from children with chronic granulomatous disease fail to reduce nitroblue tetrazolium and ferricytochrome *c*. In addition, hydrogen peroxide is not generated, leading to a failure to stimulate the hexose monophosphate shunt as measured by increased rates of glucose-1-^{14}C oxidation.[204] Hydrogen peroxide also is required for the iodination and chlorination reactions that normally result in the effective killing of catalase-positive bacteria.[126] These reactions do not occur in CGD neutrophils.

The exact enzymatic basis for the oxidative deficiency in chronic granulomatous disease is still unclear. NADH and NADPH oxidase have been reported to be either normal or reduced in neutrophils of patients with chronic granulomatous disease.[22,62,215] Recent electron micrographic studies indicate that NADH oxidase generates hydrogen peroxide on the surface membrane of normal human neutrophils as well as on membranes of the phagocytic vesicle.[45] Spectrophotometric studies indicate that NADPH oxidase on granule membranes isolated from phagocytic neutrophils requires manganese for stimulation of activity.[99] Further proof for the importance of oxidase deficiency in leukocytes in chronic granulomatous disease comes from the observation that replacement of glucose oxidase bound to latex particles in these defective cells restores their peroxide-generating, iodination, and bactericidal capacities toward normal.[46] The activity of the cytoplasmic enzyme glutathione peroxidase was found to be about one third of the normal value when tested in cells from two girls and two boys with chronic granulomatous disease, including one brother-sister pair,[101,157] but normal activity of this enzyme has been described in seven other patients.[67,251] Although this enzyme appears to be an important means for removing excess cellular hydrogen peroxide, it is difficult to assign it a primary role for initiating the phagocytic respiratory burst.

Genetics. There is evidence for at least two distinct genetic forms of chronic granulomatous disease. Of a total of 168 patients with chronic granulomatous disease 144 are boys and 24 are girls, a ratio of 6:1. This in itself favors the X-linked transmission as the predominant mode of inheritance. In a recent study leukocytes from nineteen of twenty-three mothers of males with chronic granulomatous disease had intermediate defective neutrophil function that identified the heterozygote carrier state.

Sisters and female maternal relatives of affected males also have been identified as carriers, and at least two mothers have delivered defective offspring from different fathers. A carrier state cannot be detected in families of most female patients with the disease.[24] Besides the occurrence in girls, the disease has been reported in sisters, siblings of both sexes, and some boys without demonstrable leukocyte defects in either parent. Consanguinity has been documented in at least three sets of parents. In addition, the lack of a suspected or defined relative with chronic granulomatous disease in these families points to an autosomal genetic transmission, but other mechanisms are possible, including spontaneous gene mutations.

In one study an autosomal recessive pattern of inheritance with sex modification leading to more severe disease in boys was postulated. Abnormality of neutrophil bactericidal function was found in both mothers and fathers.[50] However, clinical experience indicates there is no difference in the severity of the disease in boys with the sex-linked form and in girls or boys without detectable family member carriers.[197] The NBT test has been used to detect the carrier state. Mothers, grandmothers, and sisters of affected boys with chronic granulomatous disease have abnormal NBT test results.[24]

Other quantitative metabolic tests, such as the release of superoxide anion from phagocytizing cells using ferricytochrome *c* are also useful to discriminate the carrier state.[111] Both the quantitative NBT test and a slide test adaptation of it indicate that approximately half the phagocytizing cells from female carriers reduce NBT, compared to a consistent absence of dye reduction in cells from boys with the disease.[24] Histochemical identification of two metabolically different cell populations provides evidence that random inactivation of the X chromosome in female cells has occurred.[248] Although a mild neutrophil bactericidal defect may be demonstrated in vitro in female carriers, they remain free from recurrent infection. One carrier had persistent *Salmonella* infection.[170] Several mothers of boys with chronic granulomatous disease demonstrated lesions of the skin diagnosed as discoid lupus erythematosis.[147]

Red blood cells from some boys with chronic granulomatous disease carry a rare null Kell blood group phenotype, K_0, in which all antigenic products of the Kell antigen are absent.[80] More recently it has been reported that neutrophils from fifty normal persons possess a Kell group antigen designated K_x whereas all five boys with chronic granulomatous disease who were tested lacked this antigen.[156] This highly significant association raises the possibility that the absence of membrane antigen on neutrophils in chronic granulomatous disease may be linked to the abnormal membrane function and points to a single gene mutation on the membrane.

Clinical signs and symptoms. Most patients develop signs and symptoms of infection during the first 2 years of life. Of 140 patients whose age at the onset of disease was known, 109 developed their first symptoms by 1 year of age, and 125 by 2 years of age.[113] Rarely clinical problems are delayed until school age. Adult patients have been described with signs and symptoms of chronic granulomatous disease.[29] The age of onset has not been appreciably different in boys and girls, and at least fourteen children had their first definite symptom of chronic granulomatous disease in the first week of life.[86]

Most of the clinical features reflect involvement of the reticuloendothelial and integumentary systems. Lymphadenopathy occurs in almost all cases and generally is one of the first manifestations of the disease. A common presentation is enlargement of lymph nodes about the head and neck, which often require repeated incision and drainage. Generalized lymphadenopathy may also be present. Hepatomegaly and splenomegaly occur later and often signify hepatic and perihepatic abscesses. At times abscess formation within the liver may be quite silent and require nuclide scans to confirm their presence.

The second major group of symptoms reflects the inability of circulating phagocytic cells to kill invading bacteria at sites of penetration below the skin and mucous membranes. Thus pneumonia, lung, and subcutaneous abscesses and recurrent skin furunculosis all occur sooner or later in most patients with chronic granulomatous disease. The rash may mimic eczematoid dermatitis. Impetiginous lesions occur around the mouth and nose and often progress to granulomatous skin reactions. Ulcerative stomatitis may recur in these patients.

Less frequently observed but more resistant to treatment is osteomyelitis. Osteomyelitis usually involves small bones of the hands and feet. The infected bones become enlarged and often considerable destruction of the bone occurs. There is gradual resolution after many weeks[256] and new bone lesions may develop while patients are receiving high-dose antibiotic therapy intravenously.

Lesions of the gastrointestinal tract are relatively common in patients with chronic granulomatous disease. A history of persistent diarrhea may indicate granulomatous colitis. Perianal abscesses and rectal fistula tracts are found in nearly one third of the patients. Biopsy of the bowel has shown microabscesses and abnormal histiocytes in several patients.[10] As indicated in Table 19-3, every organ system may be involved in patients with this disease, and healing progresses slowly so that lesions persist for many weeks. At times unusual symptoms may develop. A diagnosis of chronic granulomatous disease was established in a patient with hyperthyroidism and *Aspergillus fumigatus* infection of the thyroid gland.[88] In one study three of fourteen patients with chronic granulomatous disease had secondary cardiac failure as a result of pulmonary hypertension, mitral stenosis, or stenosis of the descending aorta.[229] Obstructive uropathy secondary to tissue granulomas was present in four patients and other patients had granulomatous lesions of the bladder wall. Choroid and retinal lesions have also been noted in chronic granulomatous disease.

Laboratory features. Total leukocyte and differential counts reflect responses to acute and

Table 19-3. Infections in patients with Chediak-Higashi syndrome and chronic granulomatous disease

	No. of patients	
	Chediak-Higashi syndrome	Chronic granulomatous disease
Site of infection		
Bronchopulmonary	37	134
Nodes	*	137
Nasopharynx	20	27
Ears	10	3
Skin	28	120
Eye	1	27
Gingival stomatitis	7	26
Gastrointestinal	9	34
Sepsis/meningitis	5	29
Urinary tract	1	11
Liver (parahepatic abscesses)	—	63
Perianal abscesses	—	28
Bone	—	54
Total number of patients	63	168
Organisms cultured		
Staphylococcus aureus	24	87
Staphylococcus albus	—	13
Streptococcus pyogenes	4	9
Diplococcus pneumoniae	3	—
Haemophilus influenzae	2	—
Escherichia coli	—	26
Shigella-Salmonella	1	10
Klebsiella-Aerobacter	2	29
Pseudomonas aeruginosa	1	15
Proteus sp.	1	9
Neisseria sp.	1	—
Serratia marcescens	—	16
Aspergillus	2	13
Candida albicans	1	12
Nocardia	—	4
Mycobacterium	—	4
Paracolobactrum	—	4
Actinomyces	—	2
Other enteric bacteria	—	9
Total number of patients	63	125

*Greater than 80% lymphohistiocytic infiltration.

chronic infection. There may be neutrophilic, monocytic, or eosinophilic leukocytosis. The morphology of the leukocyte is normal. Neutrophils often show ''toxic'' changes with heavy granulation, vacuoles, and Döhle bodies. Often the white blood cell count is normal. A normocytic normochromic or microcytic hypochromic anemia reflects the chronic infection; serum iron and total iron-binding transferrin levels are low. The serum ferritin level is elevated. Serum concentrations of IgM, IgG, and IgA are usually elevated and at times extreme elevations are observed. Delayed hypersensitivity skin tests and lymphocyte T cell function are normal.

Renal function and liver function are usually preserved. Most patients have abnormalities on chest x-ray films that represent the high incidence of acute and chronic pneumonia leading to granulomatous reactions and/or pulmonary fibrosis.[81] Diffuse and miliary lesions may occur with few respiratory symptoms. Calcifications in soft tissues and organs are often evident. Other radiologic manifestations of chronic granulomatous disease include gastric antral narrowing on barium swallow,[87] evidence of granulomatous colitis on barium enema, and abnormal liver-spleen scans showing liver abscesses.[194] Bone pain or tenderness usually signifies osteomyelitis, which can be documented by radiographs of bone or bone scans.

Information about infecting organisms in 125 of 168 patients is given in Table 19-3. All organisms are pathogens since they were cultured from blood, spinal fluid, or exudates from an abscess or osteomyelitis. The predominance of staphylococci and enteric bacteria is striking but the fungi, *Aspergillus,* and *Candida* have also been common pathogens. The high incidence of *Serratia marcescens* infections is also evident. *Salmonella* caused septicemia or meningitis in ten patients. Five patients were infected with mycobacteria and two patients experienced disseminated disease as a result of BCG vaccine given in the neonatal period.[240] The absence of *Haemophilus influenzae* and pneumococci and the relative infrequency of streptococci from cultures of patients correlates with the in vitro ability of the patients' phagocytes to kill these catalase-negative, peroxide-producing organisms.[110,154]

Differential diagnosis. During the early phases of the illness the skin rash may be confused with infantile eczema, impetigo, moniliasis, or erythema multiforme. Persistent lymphadenopathy suggests lymphoma, histiocytosis X, or tuberculous lymphadenitis. Some patients have pronounced fever and arthralgias that may be mistaken for juvenile rheumatoid arthritis or other collagen vascular diseases. The diagnosis must be established by performing functional phagocytic tests on the blood leukocytes.

Pathology. Biopsy and autopsy material from infected sites and organs showed the characteristic granulomas containing histiocytes, some filled with pigmented lipid material, usually yellow or tan.[136] The origin of this material remains unknown but most likely it represents remnants of bacterial components.

Treatment and management. Although specific therapy for chronic granulomatous disease is still not available, clinical experience over the past decade has indicated that long-term antibiotic therapy prolongs infection-free intervals and decreases the severity of infection in most patients. The choice of antibiotic treatment is based on results of in vitro bacterial cultures and sensitivity studies. The theoretical advantage of a lipid-soluble antibiotic such as rifampin is unfortunately dismissed by the rapid resistance to it developed by *Staphylococcus aureus.*[155] Continuous long-term therapy with nafcillin may eliminate the problem of recurrent liver abscesses in patients with chronic granulomatous disease. Nafcillin has the advantage of being primarily excreted by the liver and it is effective against nearly all strains of *Staphylococcus aureus.*[189] Another rationale for therapy is the use of sulfonamides and sulfone compounds that generate free radical products of reduced oxygen. The idea is to attempt to restore normal intracellular bactericidal activity in these cells.[105,115]

Although restoration of deficient oxidase activity into neutrophils in chronic granulomatous disease has been accomplished in vitro, total biochemical correction of the defect still remains a therapeutic challenge of the future.[26] Most acute systemic infections must be treated with intravenous antibiotics. The selection of specific antibiotics depends on the results of the cultures for bacteria and fungi as well as their in vitro sensitivity to antibiotics. The patient response to antibiotics is generally slow and requires about two to three times the treatment interval required by a normal child with the same infection. Transfusion of granulocytes from healthy donors constitutes emergency short-term therapy for patients with severe infection and neutropenia and may be of some use in treating patients with chronic granulomatous disease during acute episodes of overwhelming or unrelenting infection. Transfusions of leukocytes from 58 units of blood appeared to significantly improve the condition of a child with *Aspergillus* pneumonia. Neutrophils with normal metabolic activity could be demonstrated in a patient's circulation after leukocyte transfusions in this case.[200] One boy with chronic granulomatous disease has been treated with a bone marrow transplant from his histocompatible sister. Engraftment occurred and skin lesions cleared for a period of 3 months. Afterwards the transplanted cells were apparently rejected and infection returned.[69]

Prognosis. Forty-nine of the fifty-nine reported deaths have occurred before the patient reached the age of 7 years. Survival has improved during the past few years. In addition, milder forms of the disease have been identified. One report documented chronic granulomatous disease in four brothers who are alive at ages 28, 30, 32, and 40 years.[71] Two female patients are alive in their fourth decade of life. Pulmonary disease is the primary cause of death in more than half of the patients and one third of the deaths are associated with septicemia or meningitis.

G-6-PD deficiency

Blacks with erythrocyte G-6-PD deficiency have normal levels of neutrophil enzyme and the vast majority of whites with red cell deficiency have 20% to 50% of normal G-6-PD activity in their neutrophils. Bactericidal capacity is normal in vitro and the patients do not experience recurrent infections. However, patients with less than 1% G-6-PD activity in their leukocytes have a disease that resembles chronic granulomatous disease.[59,84] Three brothers and a 52-year-old woman have experienced recurrent infection similar to that observed in children with chronic granulomatous disease. There was evidence of a carrier state in the mother of the three boys, suggesting sex-linked genetic transmission of the disease. These patients' cells do not reduce NBT nor do they generate hydrogen peroxide. This has been attributed to a lack of substrate NADH and NADPH for the enzymatic reduction of oxygen to superoxide anion and peroxide. Neutrophils from patients with a total deficiency of G-6-PD do not kill *Staphylococcus aureus* or *Escherichia coli* but do kill *Streptococcus faecalis* normally. Patients with levels of G-6-PD that are deficient but greater than 5% have normal neutrophil bactericidal activity both in vitro and in vivo, whereas one boy with approximately 5% of normal activity was asymptomatic but had leukocytes with abnormal in vitro activity. Patients with red cell G-6-PD deficiency may be more vulnerable to in vivo hemolysis during infection when hydrogen peroxide is released from phagocytizing neutrophils. Studies suggest that red cell reduced glutathione levels decrease and red cell survival in vivo shortens after G-6-PD-deficient red cells are exposed to phagocytizing neutrophils in vitro.[25] Increased lability of G-6-PD and altered levels of G-6-PD stabilizing factors have been described in chronic granulomatous disease but do not represent the primary underlying defect in these cells.[33,73]

Myeloperoxidase deficiency

The first report of the absence of normal peroxidase staining of neutrophils was by Sato and Yoshimatsu[212] in 1925. Myeloperoxidase is a heme-containing enzyme found in the primary or azurophilic granules of neutrophils. Blood monocytes contain about one-third the amount of myeloperoxidase found in neutrophils.[21] Eosinophil peroxidase is contained in granules of that cell type but it is biochemically and genetically distinct since the activity is not inhibited by chemical blockers of neutrophil peroxidase, nor is it deficient in patients with neutrophil peroxidase deficiency. Although myeloperoxidase contributes to the myeloperoxidase–hydrogen peroxide–halide bactericidal and fungicidal systems of neutrophils, most patients with this deficiency do not experience increased susceptibility to infection. Chicken neutrophils are devoid of myeloperoxidase, lending additional support to the idea that this enzyme is not critical for host defense against bacterial and fungal infection.[188]

Since 1969 more than ten patients have been described with congenital or acquired deficiencies of granule myeloperoxidase. One patient with myeloperoxidase deficiency was reported to suffer from chronic *Candida albicans* infections, and his neutrophils were completely incapable of killing intracellular *Candida albicans* in vitro.[141] The leukocytes from the members of this family also lacked myeloperoxidase and the capacity to kill *Candida albicans;* however, they did not develop *Candida*

infections, suggesting that their anatomic barriers against fungal infections were intact. Another case of myeloperoxidase deficiency occurred in a patient with generalized pustular psoriasis, although eight other patients with psoriasis had normal myeloperoxidase activity in their neutrophils.[224] Patients with acute myelocytic and myelomonocytic leukemia, refractory megaloblastic anemia, and preleukemic states may have neutrophils that lack myeloperoxidase activity.* One such patient was studied who had *Candida* infections and pneumonia. His neutrophils demonstrated a decreased capacity to kill intracellular *Staphylococcus aureus* and *Escherichia coli* during the first 60 minutes of incubation, but after 4 hours more than 90% of the bacteria were killed.[66]

The in vitro abnormality of bactericidal function in patients with myeloperoxidase deficiency is similar to that observed in patients with Chediak-Higashi syndrome. In both conditions there is a delay in the intracellular killing of catalase-positive and catalase-negative bacteria during the first 30 to 40 minutes of the incubation. However, after 60 minutes of incubation the rate of bacterial killing is equal in myeloperoxidase-deficient and control neutrophils. Oxidative activities, including oxygen uptake and hexose monophosphate shunt activity, are exaggerated in myeloperoxidase-deficient leukocytes during phagocytosis. The diagnosis can be established from a blood smear by demonstrating the absence of enzyme activity in the neutrophils with a histochemical stain for myeloperoxidase.[119]

ACQUIRED DISORDERS OF PHAGOCYTIC DYSFUNCTION
Iron deficiency and iron metabolism

The role of iron in leukocyte function has only recently received attention. Although infections do occur in patients with iron-deficiency anemia, it has been difficult to establish a clear cause-and-effect relationship in these patients.[146] The bactericidal function of neutrophils in iron-deficient children without protein-calorie malnutrition has been studied in thirty-eight children from three separate centers throughout the world. The mean number of viable *Staphylococcus aureus* organisms present after 140 minutes of incubation was compared to the number of viable organisms present at 20 minutes in an in vitro study.[52] Controls demonstrated approximately a 1 log reduction in viable bacteria from 20 to 140 minutes, whereas patient neutrophils reduced the number of viable bacteria by only ½ log during the same period. After treatment with parenteral iron, all patients showed a rapid return of bactericidal killing to normal. A

---

*References 45, 48, 96, 142.

similar finding was observed in another study using *Staphylococcus albus*.[81] On the other hand, neutrophils from iron-deficient patients effectively killed opsonized *Escherichia coli*. Recently, depressed phagocytic function was exhibited by polymorphonuclear leukocytes from chronically iron-deficient animals.[144]

There is some evidence that excessive iron may have an adverse effect on phagocytic function. Patients with active hemolysis seem more susceptible to bacterial infection than normal persons. The addition of ferric sulfate to intact neutrophils causes decreased release of hydrogen peroxide and diminished stimulation of the hexose monophosphate shunt.[118] A correlation between serum transferrin levels and death from bacterial infection following treatment of patients with kwashiorkor with iron was found. It has been postulated that the decreased transferrin levels allowed ferrous iron to circulate freely; free iron may contribute to the increased susceptibility of these patients to bacterial infections.[159] Ferric or ferrous iron in concentrations of more than 0.1 μ inhibits the intracellular killing of staphylococci by rabbit neutrophils either by its inhibitory action on leukocyte cationic protein or by inhibition of leukocyte oxidative metabolism.[77]

Protein-calorie malnutrition

The greatly increased susceptibility to infection in children with protein-calorie malnutrition may in part be related to phagocytic defects. However, depressed synthesis of essential humoral factors for antibody formation is probably of primary importance. A deficiency of C3 proactivator in patients with protein-calorie malnutrition and recurrent infections has recently been documented.[217] In experimental animals and in patients long-term total parenteral nutrition has been shown to result in reduced chemotactic responses of neutrophils and in hypophosphatemia. This metabolic abnormality results in diminished ATP content of neutrophils, which is necessary for their motility.[61] Defective leukocyte mobilization has been observed in children with kwashiorkor.[135] Glycolytic activities supplying the necessary energy for particle uptake were found to be decreased in phagocytizing leukocytes isolated from children suffering from protein-calorie malnutrition, indicating either decreased phagocytosis or a metabolic defect. Stimulation of glycolytic activity seen in normal leukocytes in the presence of particles was also absent in patients with protein-calorie malnutrition. Stimulation of the hexose monophosphate shunt occurred but to a lesser extent than in leukocytes obtained from controls. Following treatment these metabolic parameters change toward a normal pattern. Bactericidal activity of

leukocytes against *Escherichia coli* isolated from patients with protein-calorie malnutrition was also significantly lower than normal and showed considerable improvement after treatment.[216]

Malignancy and decreased phagocytic activity

Neutrophil dysfunction has been reported as a consequence of leukemia.[27,231] However, neutrophils from patients with acute lymphocytic leukemia in early remission have normal bactericidal capacity, but during the period when cranial–spinal axis irradiation is given to prevent leukemic involvement of the central nervous system, blood leukocytes from these patients have diminished capacity to kill *Staphylococcus aureus*, *Pseudomonas*, and *Diplococcus pneumoniae*. This transient defect clears within 2 to 4 weeks after cessation of irradiation therapy and was not observed in patients receiving cranial irradiation with intrathecal methotrexate. The combination of neutropenia and lymphopenia observed after irradiation renders the patients more susceptible to both bacterial and nonbacterial infections.[27]

Burns

Patients with severe thermal injuries acquire an intracellular bactericidal defect.[2] These patients are susceptible to septic complications. The burn injury is associated with a decrease in leukocyte content of three granular enzymes, β-glucuronidase, acid phosphatase, and lysozyme, suggesting lysosomal depletion in these cells.

Evaluation of patients with suspected phagocytic dysfunction

Patients with a history of chronic or recurrent pyogenic or fungal infections should be considered to have a phagocytic dysfunction if there is no evidence for immunoglobulin deficiency or neutropenia. Defects are liable to occur at each step of the phagocytic process and may be responsible for the signs and symptoms observed in the patient. Obviously not all of the tests provided in Table 19-2 are necessary, but rather one of each group should be selected to evaluate a particular neutrophil function. The patient should be instructed to discontinue taking all medication for a period of 1 week prior to the studies. Blood is collected from a peripheral vein into a syringe containing heparin as the anticoagulant and mixed. The syringe is inverted and allowed to stand upright for 30 to 60 minutes. If the patient has an active infection and an elevated sedimentation rate of red cells, leukocytes will remain in the supernatant red cell free layer as the red cells aggregate and settle to the bottom of the syringe. At times 6% dextran, fibrinogen, or Plasma-gel is added to enhance sedimentation of the red cells.

Since chemotactic defects are quite common, the patient's neutrophils and serum should be studied separately using the Boyden chamber. If the test indicates a serum chemotactic defect, the fresh serum should be assayed for total hemolytic complement activity and quantified for IgG, IgA, IgM, and IgE. The recently developed leukocyte adherence test is easy to perform and gives additional information about surface properties of the cells. The capacity of leukocytes to phagocytize particles is best studied employing the oil red O particle uptake assay. The NBT test measures oxidase-mediated superoxide anion generation and is an excellent screening test for disorders of oxidative metabolism, principally chronic granulomatous disease. The in vitro bactericidal assay using patient's cells and both control and patient serum as separate sources of opsonin is probably the most important assay in evaluating a patient for recurrent infection. Careful inspection of the peripheral blood smear for presence of giant granules as noted in Chediak-Higashi syndrome and histiochemical stains for myeloperoxidase are simple and direct assays to evaluate the patient with recurrent infection. Usually this group of tests is sufficient to rule out a disorder of phagocytic dysfunction. If further pursuit is necessary, the additional tests listed in Table 19-2 can be performed.

REFERENCES

1. Adinolfi, M.: Levels of two components of complement (C4 and C3) in human fetal and newborn sera, Dev. Med. Child. Neurol. **12:**306, 1970.
2. Alexander, J. W., and Wilson, D.: Neutrophil dysfunction in sepsis in burn injury, Surg. Gynecol. Obstet. **130:**431, 1970.
3. Allen, R. C., Stjernholm, R. L., and Steele, R. H.: Evidence of the generation of an electronic excitation state(s) in human PMN's and its participation in bactericidal activity, Biochem. Biophys. Res. Comm. **47:**679, 1972.
4. Alper, C. A., Abramson, N., Johnston, R. B., Jr., et al.: Increased susceptibility to infection associated with abnormalities of complement-mediated functions and of the third component of complement, (C3), N. Engl. J. Med. **282:**350, 1970.
5. Alper, C. A., Abramson, N., Johnston, R. B., Jr., et al.: Studies in vivo and in vitro on an abnormality in the metabolism of C3 in a patient with increased susceptibility to infection, J. Clin. Invest. **49:**1975, 1970.
6. Alper, C. A., Boenisch, T., and Watson, L.: Genetic polymorphism in human glycine-rich beta-glycoprotein, J. Exp. Med. **135:**68, 1972.
7. Alper, C. A., Colten, H. R., Rosen, F. S., et al.: Homozygous deficiency of C3 in a patient with repeated infections, Lancet **2:**1179, 1972.
8. Altman, L. C., Snyderman, R., and Blaese, R. N.: The rise of chemotactic lymphokine synthesis in mononuclear leukocyte chemotaxis in Wiskott-Aldrich syndrome, J. Clin. Invest. **54:**486, 1974.
9. Amano, T., Inai, S., and Seki, Y.: Studies on the immune bacteriolysis. I. Accelerating effect on the immune bacteriolysis by lysozyme-like substances of leukocytes and egg white lysozyme, Med. J. Osaka Univ. **4:**41, 1954.
10. Ament, M. E., and Ochs, H. D.: Gastrointestinal manifestations of chronic granulomatous disease, N. Engl. J. Med. **288:**382, 1973.
11. Anderson, R., Sher, R., Rabson, A. R., et al.: Defective chemotaxis in measles patients, South Afr. Med. J. **48:**1819, 1974.
12. Arnold, R. R., Cole, M. F., and McGhee, J. R.: A bactericidal effect for human lactoferrin, Science **197:**263, 1977.
13. Austin, K. S.: The role of mast cells as mediators of inflammation. In Austin, K. S., Becker, E. L., eds.: Biochemistry of the acute allergic reactions, second international symposium, Oxford, 1971, Blackwell Scientific Publications, Ltd.
14. Avery, O. T., and Morgan, H. J.: The occurrence of peroxide in cultures of pneumococcus, J. Exp. Med. **39:**275, 1924.
15. Babior, B. M., Kipnes, R. S., and Curnutte, J. T.: Biological defense mechanisms: the production by leukocytes of superoxide, a potential bactericidal agent, J. Clin. Invest. **52:**741, 1973.
16. Baehner, R. L.: Molecular basis for functional disorders of phagocytes, J. Pediatr. **84:**317, 1974.
17. Baehner, R. L.: The growth and development of our understanding of chronic granulomatous disease. In Bellanti, J. A., and Dayton, D. H., eds.: The phagocytic cell and host resistance, New York, 1975, Raven Press.
18. Baehner, R. L., Boxer, L. A., and Allen, J. M.: Autooxidation as a basis for altered function of polymorphonuclear leukocytes, Blood **50:**327, 1977.
19. Baehner, R. L., Feig, S. A., Seigel, G. V., et al.: Metabolic phagocytic and bactericidal properties of phosphoglycerate kinase-deficient PGK polymorphonuclear leukocytes (PMN), Blood **39:**833, 1970.
20. Baehner, R. L., Gilman, N., and Karnovsky, M. L.: Respiration and glucose oxidation in human and guinea pig leukocytes: Comparative studies, J. Clin. Invest. **49:**692, 1970.
21. Baehner, R. L., and Johnston, R. B., Jr.: Monocyte function in children with neutropenia and chronic infections, Blood **40:**1, 1972.
22. Baehner, R. L., and Karnovsky, M. L.: Deficiency of reduced nicotinimide adenine dinucleotide oxidase in chronic granulomatous disease, Science **162:**1277, 1968.
23. Baehner, R. L., and Nathan, D. G.: Leukocyte oxidase: defective activity in chronic granulomatous disease, Science **155:**835, 1967.
24. Baehner, R. L., and Nathan, D. G.: Quantitative nitroblue tetrazolium test in chronic granulomatous disease, N. Engl. J. Med. **278:**971, 1968.
25. Baehner, R. L., Nathan, D. G., and Castle, W. B.: Oxidation injury of caucasian G-6-PD deficient red blood cells by phagocytizing leukocytes during infection, J. Clin. Invest. **50:**2466, 1971.
26. Baehner, R. L., Nathan, D. G., and Karnovsky, M. L.: Correction of metabolic deficiencies in the leukocytes of patients with chronic granulomatous disesae, J. Clin. Invest. **49:**692, 1970.
27. Baehner, R. L., Neiburger, R. G., Johnson, D. E., and Murrmann, S. M.: Transient bactericidal defect of peripheral blood phagocytes from children with acute lymphocytic leukemia receiving craniospinal irradiation, N. Engl. J. Med. **289:**1209, 1973.
28. Baker, C. J., Kasper, D. L., Tager, I. B., et al.: Quantitative determination of antibody to capsular polysaccharide in infection with type III strains of Group B streptococcus, J. Clin. Invest. **59:**810, 1977.

29. Ballow, M., Shira, J. E., Harden, L., et al.: Complete absence of the third component of complement in man, J. Clin. Invest. **56:**703, 1975.

30. Barrett-Conner, E.: Bacterial infection and sickle cell anemia: an analysis of 250 infections in 166 patients and a review of the literature, Medicine **50:**97, 1971.

31. Beauchamp, C., and Friedovich, I.: A mechanism for the production of ethylene from methionol, J. Biol. Chem. **245:**4641, 1970.

32. Beguez-Cesar, A. B.: Neutropenia cronica maligna familiar con granulaciones atipicas de los leucocitos, Bol. Soc. Cubana Pediatr. **15:**900, 1943.

33. Bellanti, J. A., Cantz, B. E., and Schlegel, R. J.: Accelerated decay of G-6-PD dehydrogenase activity in chronic granulomatous disease, Pediatr. Res. **4:**405, 1970.

34. Berendes, H., Bridges, R. A., and Good, R. A.: A fatal granulomatous of childhood. The clinical study of a new syndrome, Minn. Med. **40:**309, 1957.

35. Björksten, B., and Lundmark, K. M.: Recurrent bacterial infection in 4 siblings with neutropenia, eosinophilia, hyperimmunoglobulinemia A, and defective neutrophil chemotaxis, J. Infect. Dis. **133:**63, 1976.

36. Blume, R. S., Bennett, J. M., Yankee, R. A., and Wolff, S. M.: Defective granulocyte regulation in the Chediak-Higashi syndrome, N. Engl. J. Med. **279:**1009, 1968.

37. Blume, R. S., and Wolff, S. M.: The Chediak-Higashi syndrome: studies in four patients and a review of the literature, Medicine **51:**247, 1972.

38. Bourne, H. R., Lichtenstein, L. M., Melmon, K. L., et al.: Modulation of the inflammation in immunity by cyclic AMP, Science **184:**19, 1974.

39. Boyden, S.: Chemotactic effect of mixtures of antibody and antigen on polymorphonuclear leukocytes, J. Exp. Med. **115:**453, 1962.

40. Boxer, G. J., Holmsen, H., Robkin, L., et al.: Abnormal platelet function in Chediak-Higashi syndrome, Br. J. Haematol. **35:**521, 1977.

41. Boxer, L. A., Hedley-Whyte, E. T., and Stossel, T. P.: Neutrophil actin dysfunction and abnormal neutrophil behavior, N. Engl. J. Med. **291:**1093, 1974.

42. Boxer, L. A., Richardson, S. B., and Baehner, R. L.: Effects of surface active agents on neutrophil receptors, Fed. Proc. 1976.

43. Boxer, L. A., and Stossel, T. P.: Interactions of actin, myosin, and an actin-binding protein of chronic myelogenous leukemia leukocytes, J. Clin. Invest. **57:**964, 1976.

44. Boxer, L. A., Watanabe, A. M., Rister, M., et al.: Correction of leukocyte function in Chediak-Higashi syndrome by ascorbate, N. Engl. J. Med. **295:**1041, 1976.

45. Breton-Gorius, J., Houssay, D., and Dreyfus, B.: Partial myeloperoxidase deficiency in a case of preleukemia. I. Studies of fine structure and peroxidase synthesis of promyelocytes, Br. J. Haematol. **30:**273, 1976.

46. Briggs, R. T., Karnovsky, M. L., and Karnovsky, M. J.: Hydrogen peroxide production in chronic granulomatous disease: a cytochemical study of reduced pyridine nucleotide oxidases, J. Clin. Invest. **59:**1088, 1977.

47. Caldicott, W. J. H., and Baehner, R. L.: Chronic granulomatous disease of childhood: radiologic manifestations. Am. J. Roentgenol. **103:**133, 1968.

48. Carson, M. J., Chadwick, D. L., Brubaker, C. A., et al.: Thirteen boys with progressive septic granulomatosis, Pediatrics **35:**405, 1968.

49. Catovsky, D., Galton, D. A. G., and Robinson, J.: Myeloperoxidase-deficient neutrophils in acute myeloid leukaemia, Scand. J. Hematol. **9:**142, 1972.

50. Chandra, R. K., Cope, W. A., and Soothill, J. F.: Chronic granulomatous disease: evidence for an autosomal mode of inheritance, Lancet **2:**71, 1969.

51. Chandra, R. K., and Saraya, A. K.: Impaired immuno-

52. competence associated with iron deficiency, J. Pediatr. **86:**899, 1975.

52. Chediak, M.: Nouvelle anomalie leucocytaire de caractere constitutional et familial, Rev. Hematol. **7:**362, 1952.

53. Clark, R. A., Johnson, F. L., Klebanoff, S. J., and Thomas, E. D.: Defective neutrophil chemotaxis in bone marrow transplantation patients, J. Clin. Invest. **58:**22, 1976.

54. Clark, R. A., and Kimball, H. R.: Defective granulocyte chemotaxis in the Chediak-Higashi syndrome, J. Clin. Invest. **50:**2645, 1971.

55. Clark, R. A., Root, R. K., Kimball, H. R., and Kirkpatrick, C. H.: Defective neutrophil chemotaxis and cellular immunity in a child with recurrent infections, Ann. Intern. Med. **78:**515, 1973.

56. Cline, M. J.: Mechanism of acidification of the human leukocyte phagocytic vacuole, Clin. Res. **21:**595, 1973.

57. Cohn, Z. A., and Hirsch, J. G.: The influence of phagocytosis on the intracellular distribution of granule-associated components of polymorphonuclear leukocytes, J. Exp. Med. **112:**1015, 1960.

58. Cohn, Z. A., and Hirsch, J. G.: The isolation of properties of the specific cytoplasmic granules of rabbit polymorphonuclear leukocytes, J. Exp. Med. **112:**983, 1960.

59. Cooper, M. R., De Chatelet, L. R., McCall, C. E., et al.: Complete deficiency of leukocyte glucose-6-phosphate hydrogenase with defective bactericidal activity, J. Clin. Invest. **51:**769, 1972.

60. Craddock, P. R., Yawata, Y., Silvus, S., and Jacob, H.: Phagocytic dysfunction induced by intravenous hyperalimentation, Clin. Res. **21:**597, 1973.

61. Craddock, P. R., Yawata, Y., Vansanten, L., et al.: Acquired phagocyte dysfunction: a complication of hypophosphotemia due to parenteral hyperalimentation, N. Engl. J. Med. **290:**1402, 1974.

62. Curnutte, J. T., Kipnes, R. S., and Babior, B. M.: Defect in pyridine nucleotide-dependent superoxide production by a particulate fraction from the granulocytes of patients with chronic granulomatous disease, N. Engl. J. Med. **293:**628, 1975.

63. Curnutte, J. T., Whitten, D. M., and Babior, B. M.: Effective superoxide production by granulocytes from patients with chronic granulomatous disease, N. Engl. J. Med. **290:**593, 1974.

64. Dahl, M. V., Greene, W. H., Jr., and Quie, P. G.: Infection, dermatitis, increased IgE, and impaired neutrophil chemotaxis, Arch. Derm. **112:**1387, 1976.

65. David, J. R.: Lymphocyte mediators in cellular hypersensitivity, N. Engl. J. Med. **288:**143, 1973.

66. Davis, A. T., Brunning, R. D., and Quie, P. G.: Polymorphonuclear myeloperoxidase deficiency in a patient with myelomonocyte leukemia, N. Engl. J. Med. **35:**789, 1971.

67. De Chatelet, L. R., Shirley, P. S., McPhail, L. C.: Normal leukocyte glutathione peroxidase activity in patients with chronic granulomatous disease, J. Pediatr. **89:**598, 1976.

68. DeCree, J. H., Verhaegen, W., DeCock, R., et al.: Impaired neutrophil phagocytosis, Lancet **2:**294, 1974.

69. Delmas, Y., Goudemand, J., and Farriaux, J. P.: La granulomatose familiale chronique traitement par greffe de moelle (une observation), Nouv. Presse Med. **4:**2334, 1975.

70. De Meo, A. N., and Anderson, B. R.: Defective chemotaxis associated with a serum inhibitor in cirrhotic patients, N. Engl. J. Med. **286:**735, 1972.

71. Dilworth, J. A., and Mandell, G. L.: Adults with chronic granulomatous disease of childhood, Am. J. Med. **63:**233, 1977.

72. Dossett, J. H., Williams, R. C., and Quie, P. G.: Studies

on interaction of bacteria, serum factors, and polymorphonuclear luekocytes in mothers and newborns, Pediatrics **44:**49, 1969.

73. Erickson, R. P., Stites, D. P., Fudenberg, H. H., and Epstein, C. J.: Altered levels of G6PD dehydrogenase stabilizing factors in X-linked chronic granulomatous disease, J. Lab. Clin. Med. **80:**644, 1972.

74. Estensen, R. D., Hill, H. R., Quie, P. G., et al.: Cyclic GMP and cell movement, Nature **245:**458, 1973.

75. Forman, M. L., and Steihm, E. R.: Impaired opsonic activity but normal phagocytosis in low birth weight infants, N. Engl. J. Med. **281:**926, 1969.

76. Fridovich, I.: Superoxide dismutases, Ann. Rev. Biochem. **44:**147, 1975.

77. Galdstone, J. P., and Walton, E.: The effect of iron and haematin on the killing of staphylococci by rabbit polymorphs, Br. J. Exp. Pathol. **52:**452, 1971.

78. Gallin, J. I.: Abnormal chemotaxis: cellular and humoral components. In Bellanti, J. H., and Dayton, D. H., eds.: The phagocytic cell in host resistance, New York, 1975, Raven Press.

79. Gallin, J. I., Durocher, J. R., and Kaplan, A. P.: Interaction of leukocyte chemotactic factors with the cells surface. I. Chemotactic factor-induced changes in human granulocyte surface charges, J. Clin. Invest. **55:**967, 1975.

80. Giblett, E. R., Klebanoff, S. J., Pincus, S. H., et al.: Kell phenotypes in chronic granulomatous disease: a potential transfusion hazard, Lancet **1:**1235, 1971.

81. Gold, R. H., Douglas, S. O., Preger, L., et al.: Roentgenographic features of the neutrophil dysfunction syndromes, Radiology **92:**1045, 1969.

82. Goldberg, N. D., Haddox, M. K., Dunham, E., et al.: The yin-yang hypothesis of biological control: opposing influences of cyclic GMP and cyclic AMP in the regulation of cell proliferation and other biological processes. In Clarkson, B., and Baserga, R., eds.: Control of proliferation and animal cells, Cold Spring Harbor Conference on Cell Proliferation, vol. 1, 1974.

83. Goldstein, I. M., Roos, D., Kaplan, H. B., and Weissmann, G.: Complement and immunoglobulins stimulate superoxide production by human leukocytes independently of phagocytosis, J. Clin. Invest. **56:**1155, 1975.

84. Gray, G. R., Stamatoyannopoulos, G., Naiman, S. C., et al.: Neutrophil dysfunction: chronic granulomatous disease in nonspherocytic hemolytic anemia caused by complete deficiency of glucose-6-phosphate dehydrogenase, Lancet **2:**530, 1973.

85. Greene, W. H., Ray, C., Mauer, S. M., and Quie, P. G.: The effect of hemodialysis on neutrophil chemotactic responsiveness, J. Lab. Clin. Med. **88:**971, 1976.

86. Griscelli, C., and Tchernia, G.: Granulamtose septique chronique: Etude granulacytaire et immunologique de six garcons, Arch. Fr. Pediatr. **29:**345, 1972.

87. Griscom, N. T., Kirkpatrick, J. A., Girdany, B. R., et al.: Gastric antral narrowing in chronic granulomatous disease of childhood, Pediatrics **54:**456, 1974.

88. Halazun, J. F., Anast, C. S., and Lukens, J. N.: Thyrotoxicosis associated with aspergillus thyroiditis in chronic granulomatous disease, J. Pediatr. **80:**106, 1972.

89. Harris, H.: Chemotaxis of granulocytes, J. Pathol. Bacteriol. **66:**135, 1953.

90. Hayakawa, H., Iizuka, N., and Kobayashi, N.: Chronic granulomatous disease and some other neutrophil dysfunction syndromes in Japan, International Symposium on Phagocytosis, Tokyo, 1977.

91. Higashi, O.: Congenital gigantism of peroxidase granules. The first case ever reported of qualitative abnormality of peroxidase, Tohoku J. Exp. Med. **59:**315, 1954.

92. Higashi, O., Katsuyama, N., and Satodate, R.: A case

with hematological abnormality characterized by the absence of peroxidase activity in blood polymorphonuclear leukocytes, Tohoku J. Exp. Med. **87:**77, 1965.

93. Hill, H. R., Gerrard, J. M., Hogan, N. A., and Quie, P. G.: Hyperactivity of neutrophil leukotactic responses during active bacterial infection, J. Clin. Invest. **53:**996, 1974.

94. Hill, H. R., Hogan, N. A., Thomas, G. M., and Quie, P. G.: Evaluation of a cytocentrifuge method for measuring neutrophil granulocyte chemotaxis, J. Lab. Clin. Med. **86:**703, 1975.

95. Hill, H. R., Ochs, H. D., Quie, P. G., et al.: Defect in neutrophil granulocyte chemotaxis in Job's syndrome of recurrent "cold" staphylococcal abscesses, Lancet **2:** 617, 1974.

96. Hill, H. R., and Quie, P. G.: Raised serum IgE levels and defective neutrophil chemotaxis in three children with eczema and recurrent bacterial infections, Lancet **1:**183, 1974.

97. Hill, H. R., Sauls, H. S., Dettloff, J. L., and Quie, P. G.: Impaired leukotactic responsiveness in patients with juvenile diabetes mellitus, Clin. Immunol. Immunopathol. **2:**395, 1974.

98. Hill, H. R., Williams, P. B., Krueger, G. G., and Janis, B.: Recurrent staphylococcal abscesses associated with defective neutrophil chemotaxis and allergic rhinitis, Ann. Intern. Med. **85:**39, 1976.

99. Hohn, D. C., and Lehrer, R. I.: NADPH oxidase deficiency in X-linked chronic granulomatous disease, J. Clin. Invest. **55:**707, 1975.

100. Holmes, B., Page, A. R., and Good, R. A.: Studies of the metabolic activity of leukocytes from patients with a genetic abnormality of phagocytic function, J. Clin. Invest. **46:**1422, 1967.

101. Holmes, B., Park, B. H., Malawista, S. E., et al.: Chronic granulomatous disease in females: a deficiency of leukocyte glutathione peroxidase, N. Engl. J. Med. **283:** 217, 1970.

102. Holmes, B., Quie, P. G., Windhorst, D. B., and Good, R. A.: Fatal granulomatous disease of childhood: an inborn abnormality of phagocytic function, Lancet **1:**1225, 1966.

103. Huber, H., Polley, M. J., Linscott, W. D., et al.: Human monocytes: distinct receptor sites for the third component of complement and for immunoglobulin G, Science **162:** 1281, 1968.

104. Hurley, J. V., Edwards, B., and Ham, K. N.: The response of newly formed blood vessels in healing wounds to histamines and other permeability factors, Pathology **2:**133, 1970.

105. Ismail, G., Boxer, L. A., Allen, J. M., and Baehner, R. L.: Improvement of PMN oxidative and bactericidal functions in chronic granulomatous disease with 4-amino-4′-hydroxylaminodiphenyl sulfone, J. Reticuloendothel. Soc. 1977.

106. Iyer, G. Y., Islam, M. F., and Quastel, J. H.: Biochemical aspects of phagocytosis, Nature **192:**535, 1961.

107. Jacobs, J. D., and Miller, M. E.: Fatal familial Leiner's disease: a deficiency of the opsonic activity of serum complement, Pediatrics **49:**225, 1972.

108. Janeway, C. A.: Progress in immunology. Syndromes of diminished resistance to infection, J. Pediatr. **72:**885, 1968.

109. Janeway, C. A., Craig, J., Davidson, M., et al.: Hypergammaglobulinemia associated with severe recurrent and chronic nonspecific infection, Am. J. Dis. Child. **88:** 388, 1954.

110. Johnston, R. B., Jr., and Baehner, R. L.: Chronic granulomatous disease: correlation between pathogenesis and clinical findings, Pediatrics **48:**730, 1971.

111. Johnston, R. B., Jr., Keele, B. B., Misra, H. P., et al.:

The role of superoxide anion generation in phagocytic bactericidal activity: studies with normal and chronic granulomatous disease leukocytes, J. Clin. Invest. **55:** 1357, 1975.

112. Johnston, R. B., Jr., Klemperer, M. R., Alper, C. A., and Rosen, F. S.: The enhancement of bacterial phagocytosis by serum: the role of complement components and two cofactors, J. Exp. Med. **129:**1275, 1969.

113. Johnston, R. B., Jr., and Newman, S. L.: Chronic granulomatous disease, Pediatr. Clin. North Am. **24:**365, 1977.

114. Johnston, R. B., Jr., Newman, S. L., and Struth, A. G.: An abnormality of the alternate pathway of complement activation in sickle cell disease, N. Engl. J. Med. **288:** 803, 1973.

115. Johnston, R. B., Jr., Wilfert, C. M., Buckley, R. H., et al.: Enhanced bactericidal activity of phagocytes from patients with chronic granulomatous disease in the presence of sulphisoxazole, Lancet **1:**824, 1975.

116. Kamme, C., Ageberg, M., and Lundgren, K.: Distribution of *Diplococcus pneumoniae* types in acute otitis media in children and influence of the types on the clinical course in penicillin V therapy, Scand. J. Infect. Dis. **2:**183, 1970.

117. Kaplan, E. L., Laxdal, T., Quie, P. G.: Studies of polymorphonuclear leukocytes in patients with chronic granulomatous disease of childhood: bactericidal capacities for streptococci, Pediatrics **41:**591, 1968.

118. Kaplan, S. S., Quie, P. G., and Basford, R. E.: Effect of iron on leukocyte function: inactivation of H_2O_2 by iron, Infect. Immun. **12:**303, 1975.

119. Kaplow, L. S.: Simplified myeloperoxidase stain using benzidine dihydrothyloxide, Blood **26:**215, 1965.

120. Karnovsky, J. L.: Metabolic basis of phagocytic activity, Physiol. Rev. **42:**143, 1962.

121. Kearns, D. R.: Physical and chemical properties of singlet molecular oxygen, Chem. Rev. **71:**395, 1971.

122. Kellogg, E. N. III, and Fridovich, I.: Superoxide hydrogen peroxide and singlet oxygen in lipid peroxidation by a xanthine oxidase system, J. Biol. Chem. **250:**8812, 1975.

123. Kelly, M. T., and White, A.: Histamine release induced by human leukocyte lysates. Reabsorption of previously released histamine after exposure to cyclic AMP-active agents, J. Clin. Invest. **52:**1834, 1973.

124. King, M. M., Lai, E. K., and McKay, P. B.: Singlet oxygen production associated with enzyme-catalyzed lipid peroxidation in liver microsomes, J. Biol. Chem. **250:**6496, 1975.

125. Klebanoff, S. J.: Antimicrobial mechanisms in neutrophilic PMN's, Semin. Hematol. **12:**117, 1975.

126. Klebanoff, S. J.: Intraleukocytic microbicidal defects, Ann. Rev. Med. **22:**39, 1971.

127. Klebanoff, S. J.: Iodination of bacteria: a bactericidal mechanism, J. Exp. Med. **126:**1063, 1967.

128. Klebanoff, S. J.: Myeloperoxidase: contribution to the microbicidal activity of intact leukocytes, Science **169:** 1095, 1970.

129. Klebanoff, S. J., and Pincus, S. H.: Hydrogen peroxide utilization in myeloperoxidase-deficient leukocytes: a possible microbicidal control mechanism, J. Clin. Invest. **50:**2226, 1971.

130. Klebanoff, S. J., and White, L. R.: Iodination defect in the leukocytes of a patient with chronic granulomatous disease of childhood, N. Engl. J. Med. **280:**460, 1969.

131. Klein, R. B., Fisher, T. J., Gard, S. E., et al.: Decreased mononuclear and polymorphonuclear chemotaxis in human newborns, infants, and young children, Pediatrics **60:**467, 1977.

132. Koethe, S. M., Casper, J. T., and Rodey, G. E.: Alternative complement pathway activity in sera from patients with sickle cell disease, Clin. Exp. Immunol. **23:**56, 1976.

133. Kramer, J. W., Davis, W. C., and Prieur, D. J.: An inherited condition of enlarged leukocytic and melanin granules in cats: probable homology with the Chediak-Higashi syndrome, Fed. Proc. **34:**861, 1975.

134. Kritzler, R. A., Turner, J. Y., Lindenbaum, J., et al.: Chediak-Higashi syndrome: cytologic and serum lipid observations in a case and family, Am. J. Med. **36:**583, 1964.

135. Kulapongs, P., Edelman, R., Suskind, R., and Oslon, R. E.: Defective local leukocyte mobilization in children with kwashiorkor, Am. J. Clin. Nutr. **30:**367, 1977.

136. Landing, B. H., and Shireky, H. S.: A syndrome of recurrent infection and infiltration of viscera by pigmented lipid histiocytes, Pediatrics **20:**431, 1957.

137. Lay, W. H., and Nussenzweig, V.: Receptors for complement on leukocytes, J. Exp. Med. **128:**991, 1968.

138. Leader, R. W., Padgett, G. A., and Gorham, J. R.: Studies of abnormal leukocyte bodies in the mink, Blood **22:**477, 1963.

139. Leffell, M. S., and Spitznagel, J. K.: Association of lactoferrin with lysozyme in granules of human polymorphonuclear leukocytes. Infect. Immunol. **6:**671, 1972.

140. Lehrer, R. I.: Measurement of candidal activity of specific leukocyte types in mixed cell populations. II. Normal and chronic granulomatous disease eosinophils, Infect. Immunol. **3:**800, 1971.

141. Lehrer, R. I., and Cline, M. J.: Leukocyte myeloperoxidase deficiency in disseminated candidiasis: the role of myeloperoxidase in resistance to candida infections, J. Clin. Invest. **48:**1478, 1969.

142. Lehrer, R. I., Goldberg, L. S., Apple, M. A., and Rosenthal, T.: Refractory megaloblastic anemia with myeloperoxidase deficient neutrophils, Ann. Intern. Med. **76:** 447, 1972.

143. Lichtman, M. A., and Weed, R. I.: Electrophoretic mobility and N-acetyl neuraminic acid content of human normal and leukemic lymphocytes and granulocytes, Blood **32:**12, 1970.

144. Likhite, V., Rodvien, R., and Crosby, W. H., Jr.: Depressed phagocytic function exhibited by polymorphonuclear leukocytes from chronically iron-deficient rabbits, Br. J. Haematol. **34:**251, 1976.

145. Logan, L. J., Rapaport, S. I., and Maher, B. S.: Albinism and abnormal platelet function, N. Engl. J. Med. **284:**1340, 1971.

146. Lukens, J. N.: Iron deficiency and infection: fact or fable? Am. J. Dis. Child. **129:**160, 1975.

147. MacFarlane, P. S., Speirs, S., and Sommerville, R. G.: Fatal CGD of childhood and benign lymphocytic infiltration of the skin (congenital dysphagocytosis), Lancet **1:**408, 1967.

148. MacGregor, R. R., Spagnuolo, R. J., and Lentnek, A. L.: Inhibition of granulocyte adherence by ethanol, prednisone, and aspirin measured with an assay system, N. Engl. J. Med. **291:**642, 1974.

149. Maderazo, E. G., Ward, P. A., Woronick, C. L., et al.: Leukotactic dysfunction in sarcoidosis, Ann. Intern. Med. **84:**414, 1976.

150. Majno, G.: The healing hand: man and wound in the ancient world, Cambridge, Mass., 1975, Harvard University Press.

151. Majno, G., and Palade, G. E.: Studies of inflammation. I. The effect of histamine and serotonin on vascular permeability: an electron microscopic study, J. Biophys. Biochem. Cytol. **11:**571, 1961.

152. Malawista, S. E.: Microtubules and the mobilization of lysosomes and phagocytizing human leukocytes, Ann. Am. Acad. Sci. **253:**738, 1975.

153. Mandell, G. L.: Intraphagocomal pH of human polymorphonuclear neutrophils, Proc. Soc. Exp. Biol. Med. **134:**447, 1970.

154. Mandell, G. L., and Hook, E. W.: Leukocyte bactericidal activity in chronic granulomatous disease: correlation of bacterial hydrogen peroxide production and susceptibility to intracellular killing, J. Bacteriol. **100:**531, 1969.

155. Mandell, G. L., and Vest, T. K.: Killing of intraleukocytic *Staphylococcus aureus* by rifampin, J. Infect. Dis. **125:**486, 1972.

156. Marsh, W. L., Oyen, R., Nichols, M. E., and Allen, F. H., Jr.: Chronic granulomatous disease in the Kell blood groups, Br. J. Haematol. **29:**247, 1975.

157. Matsuda, I., Oka, Y., Taniguchi, N., et al.: Leukocyte glutathione peroxidase deficiency in a male patient with chronic granulomatous disease, J. Pediatr. **88:**581, 1976.

158. McCraken, G. H., Jr., and Eichenwald, H. F.: Leukocyte function and the development of opsonic and complement activity in the neonate, Am. J. Dis. Child. **121:**120, 1971.

159. McFarlane, H., Reddy, S., Adcock, K. J., et al.: Immunity, transferrin, and survival in kwashiorkor, Br. Med. J. **4:**268, 1970.

160. McLeod, J. W., and Gordon, J.: Production of hydrogen peroxide by bacteria, Biochem. J. **16:**499, 1922.

161. Messner, R. P., and Jelinek, J.: Receptors for human gamma globulin on human neutrophils, J. Clin. Invest. **49:**2165, 1970.

162. Metchnikoff, E.: Lectures on the comparative pathology of inflammation, New York, 1968, Dover Publications, Inc.

163. Miles, A.: The kinin system: a history and review of the kinin system, Proc. R. Soc. Lond. **173:**341, 1969.

164. Miller, M. E.: Chemotactic function in the human neonate: humoral and cellular aspects, Pediatr. Res. **5:**487, 1971.

165. Miller, M. E.: Development maturation of human neutrophil motility and its relationship to membrane deformability In Bellanti, J. A., and Dayton, D. H., eds.: The phagocytic cell in host resistance, New York, 1975, Raven Press.

166. Miller, M. E.: Pathology of chemotaxis and random mobility. Semin. Hematol. **12:**59, 1975.

167. Miller, M. E., and Nilsson, V. R.: A familial deficiency of the phagocytosis enhancing activity of serum related to a dysfunction of the fifth component of complement (C5), N. Engl. J. Med. **282:**354, 1970.

168. Miller, M. E., Norman, M. E., Koblenzer, P. J., and Schonauer, T.: A new familial defect of neutrophil movement, J. Lab. Clin. Med. **82:**1, 1973.

169. Miller, M. E., Oski, F. A., and Harris, M. B.: "Lazy leukocyte" syndrome: a new disorder of neutrophil function, Lancet **1:**665, 1971.

170. Moellering, R. C., Jr., and Weinberg, A. N.: Persistent *Salmonella* infection in a female carrier for CGD, Ann. Intern. Med. **73:**595, 1970.

171. Molenaar, D. M., Palumbo, P. J., Wilson, W. R., and Ritts, R. E., Jr.: Leukocyte chemotaxis in diabetic patients and their nondiabetic first degree relatives, Diabetes **25**(suppl. 2):880, 1976.

172. Mowat, A. G., and Baum, J.: Chemotaxis of polymorphonuclear leukocytes from patients with diabetes mellitus, N. Engl. J. Med. **284:**621, 1971.

173. Mowat, A. G., and Baum, J.: Chemotaxis of polymorphonuclear leukocytes from patients with rheumatoid arthritis, J. Clin. Invest. **50:**2541, 1971.

174. Nathan, D. G., Baehner, R. L., and Weaver, D. K.: Failure of nitroblue tetrazolium reduction in the phagocytic vacuoles of leukocytes in chronic granulomatous disease, J. Clin. Invest. **48:**1895, 1969.

175. Oh, M. H. K., Rodey, G. E., Good, R. A., et al.: Defective candidal capacity of polymorphonuclear leukocytes in chronic granulomatous disease of childhood, J. Pediatr. **75:**300, 1969.

176. Oliver, J. M.: Impaired microtubular function correctable by cyclic GMP and cholinergic agonists in the Chediak-Higashi syndrome, Am. J. Pathol. **85:**395, 1976.

177. Oliver, J. M., Krawiec, J. A., Berlin, R. D.: Carbamyl choline prevents giant granule formation in cultured fibroblasts from beige (Chediak-Higashi) mice, J. Cell. Biol. **69:**205, 1976.

178. Oliver, J. M., Ukena, T. E., and Berlin, R. D.: Effects of phagocytosis and colchicine on the distribution of lectin-binding sites on cell surfaces, Proc. Natl. Acad. Sci. **71:**394, 1974.

179. Oliver, J. M., and Zurier, R. B.: Correction of characteristic abnormalities in microtubular function in granulomorphology in Chediak-Higashi syndrome with cholinergic agonists. Studies in vitro in man and in vivo in the beige mice, J. Clin. Invest. **57:**1239, 1976.

180. Oliver, J. M., Zurier, R. B., and Berlin, R. D.: Concanavalin A cap formation on polymorphonuclear leukocytes of normal and beige (Chediak-Higashi) mice, Nature **253:**471, 1975.

181. Olmstead, J. B.: The role of divalent cations and nucleotides in microtubule assembly in vitro, Cold Spring Harbor Conf. Cell Prolif. **3:**1081, 1976.

182. Olsson, I., and Venge, P.: Cationic proteins of human granulocytes. I. Isolation of the cationic proteins from the granules of leukaemic myeloid cells, Scand. J. Haematol. **9:**204, 1972.

183. Oren, R., Farnhan, A. E., Saito, K., et al.: Metabolic patterns in three types of phagocytizing cells, J. Cell Biol. **17:**487, 1963.

184. Orlowski, J. P., Sieger, L., and Anthony, B. F.: Bactericidal capacity of monocytes of newborn infants, J. Pediatr. **89:**797, 1976.

185. Padgett, G. A.: The Chediak-Higashi syndrome, Adv. Vet. Sci. **12:**239, 1968.

186. Padgett, G. A., Leader, R. W., Gorham, J. R., and O'Mary, C. C.: The familial occurence of the Chediak-Higashi syndrome in mink and cattle, Genetics **49:**505, 1964.

187. Page, A. R., Berrendes, H., Warner, J., and Good, R. A.: The Chediak-Higashi syndrome, Blood **20:**330, 1962.

188. Penniall, R., and Spitznagel, J. K.: Chicken neutrophils: oxidative metabolism in phagocytic cells devoid of myeloperoxidase, Proc. Natl. Acad. Sci. **72:**5012, 1975.

189. Philippart, A. I., Colodny, A. H., and Baehner, R. L.: Continuous antibiotic therapy in chronic granulomatous disease preliminary communication, Pediatrics **50:**923, 1972.

190. Pillemer, L., Blum, L., Lepow, I. H., et al.: The properdin system and immunity. I. Demonstration and isolation of a new serum protein, properdin, and its role in immune phenomena, Science **120:**279, 1954.

191. Pincus, S. H., and Klebanoff, S. J.: Quantitative leukocyte iodination, N. Engl. J. Med. **284:**744, 1971.

192. Pincus, S. H., Thomas, I. T., Clark, R. A., and Ochs, H. D.: Defective neutrophil chemotaxis with variant ichthyosis, hyperimmunoglobulinemia E, and recurrent infections, J. Pediatr. **87:**908, 1976.

193. Porter, D. D., and Larsen, A. E.: Aleutian disease of mink: infectious virus-antibody complexes in the serum, Proc. Soc. Exp. Biol. Med. **126:**680, 1967.

194. Preimesberger, K. F., and Goldberg, M. E.: Acute liver abscess in chronic granulomatous disease of childhood, Radiology **110:**147, 1974.

195. Provisor, D., Boxer, L. A., Strawbridge, R., et al.: Granulocyte adherence in the Chediak-Higashi syndrome, Clin. Res. **25:**382A, 1977.

196. Quie, P. G.: Pathology of bactericidal powerer of neutrophils, Semin. Hematol. **12:**143, 1975.

197. Quie, P. G., and Hill, H. R.: Granulocytopathies. In Disease in lungs, Year Book Chicago, 1973, Medical Publishers, Inc.

198. Quie, P. G., Messner, R. P., and Williams, R. C., Jr.: Phagocytosis in subacute bacterial endocarditis: localization of the primary opsonic site to Fc fragment, J. Exp. Med. **128:**553, 1968.

199. Quie, P. G., White, J. G., Holmes, B., and Good, R. A.: In vitro bactericidal capacity of human polymorphonuclear leukocytes: diminished activity in chronic granulomatous disease of childhood, J. Clin. Invest. **46:**668, 1967.

200. Raubitschek, A. A., Levin, A. S., Stites, D. P., et al.: Normal granulocyte infusion therapy for aspergillosis in chronic granulomatous disease, Pediatrics **51:**230, 1973.

201. Rebuck, J. W., and Crowley, J. H.: A method of studying leukocytic functions in vivo, Ann. N.Y. Acad. Sci. **59:**757, 1955.

202. Repine, J. E., Clawson, C. C., and Friend, P. S.: Influence of a deficiency of the second component of complement on the bactericidal activity of neutrophils in vitro, J. Clin. Invest. **59:**802, 1977.

203. Rogge, J. L., and Hanifin, J. M.: Immunodeficiencies in severe atopic dermatitis: Depressed chemotaxis and lymphocyte transformation, Arch. Dermatol. **112:**1391, 1976.

204. Root, R. K., Medcalf, J., Oshino, N., and Chance, B.: H_2O_2 release from human granulocytes during phagocytosis: documentation, quantitation, and some regulatory factors, J. Clin. Invest. **55:**945, 1975.

205. Root, R. R., Rosenthal, A. S., and Balestine, D. J.: Abnormal bactericidal, metabolic, and lysosomal function of Chediak-Higashi syndrome leukocytes, J. Clin. Invest. **51:**649, 1972.

206. Rosen, H., and Klebanoff, S. J.: Chemiluminescence and superoxide production by myeloperoxidase-deficient leukocytes, J. Clin. Invest. **58:**50, 1976.

207. Rosenfeld, S. I., Kelly, M. E., and Leddy, J. P.: Hereditary deficiency of the fifth component of complement in man. I. Clinical, immunochemical, and family studies, J. Clin. Invest. **57:**1626, 1976.

208. Rosner, F., Valmont, I., Kozinn, P. J., and Caroline, L.: Leukocyte function in patients with leukemia, Cancer **25:**835, 1970.

209. Ryan, G. B., and Majno, G.: Inflammation. In Thomas, B. A., ed.: Kalamazoo, Mich., 1977, Upjohn,

210. Sandler, J. A., Gallin, J. I., and Vaughn, M.: Effects of serotonin, carbamylcholine, and ascorbic acid on leukocyte cyclic AMP and chemotaxis, J. Cell Biol. **67:**480, 1975.

211. Sato, A.: Chediak and Higashi's disease: probable identity of "a new leucocytal anomaly (Chediak)" and "congenital gigantism of peroxidase granules (Higashi)," Tohoku J. Exp. Med. **61:**201, 1955.

212. Sato, A., and Yoshimatsu, S.: The peroxidase reaction in epidemic encephalitis, Am. J. Dis. Child. **29:**301, 1925.

213. Sbarra, A. J., and Karnovsky, M. L.: The biochemical basis of phagocytosis. I. Metabolic changes during the ingestion of particles by polymorphonuclear leukocytes, J. Biol. Chem. **234:**1355, 1959.

214. Schopfer, K., and Douglas, S. D.: Neutrophil function in children with kwashiorkor, J. Lab. Clin. Med. **88:**450, 1976.

215. Segal, A. W., and Peters, T. J.: Characterization of the enzyme defects in chronic granulomatous disease, Lancet **1:**1363, 1976.

216. Selvaraj, R. J., and Bhat, K. S.: Metabolic and bactericidal activities of leukocytes in protein-calorie malnutrition, Am. J. Clin. Nutr. **25:**166, 1972.

217. Sirisinha, S., Suskind, R., Edelman, R., et al.: Complement and C3-proactivator levels in children with protein calorie malnutrition and effect of dietary treatment, Lancet **1:**1016, 1973.

218. Smith, C. W., Hollers, J. C., Dupree, E., et al.: A serum inhibitor of leukotaxis in a child with recurrent infections, J. Lab. Clin. Med. **79:**878, 1972.

219. Smith, M. R., and Wood, W. B., Jr.: Heat Labile opsonins to pneumococcus. I. Participation of complement, J. Exp. Med. **130:**1209, 1969.

220. Snyderman, R., and Pike, M. C.: Disorders of leukocyte chemotaxis, Pediatr. Clin. North Am. **24:**377, 1977.

221. Soriano, R. B., South, M. A., Goldman, A. S., and Smith, C. W.: Defect of neutrophil motility in a child with recurrent bacterial infections and disseminated cytomegalovirus infection, J. Pediatr. **83:**951, 1973.

222. Steerman, R. L., Snyderman, R., Leikin, S. L., and Colten, H. R.: Intrinsic defect of the polymorphonuclear leucocyte resulting in impaired chemotaxis and phagocytosis, Clin. Exp. Immunol. **9:**939, 1971.

223. Steinbrinck, W.: Uber Eine neue granulations anomalie der leukocyten, Dtsch. Arch. Klin. Med. **193:**577, 1948.

224. Stendahl, O., and Lindgren, S.: Function of granulocytes with deficient myeloperoxidase-mediated iodination in a patient with generalized pustular psoriasis, Scand. J. Haematol. **16:**144, 1976.

225. Stossel, T. P.: Evaluation of opsonic and leukocyte function with a spectrophotometric test in patients with infection and phagocytic disorders, Blood **42:**121, 1973.

226. Stossel, T. P.: Phagocytosis, N. Engl. J. Med. **290:**717, 1974.

227. Stossel, T. P., and Hartwig, J. H.: Interaction of actin, myocin, and a new actin-binding protein of rabbit pulmonary macrophages. II. Role of cytoplasmic movement in phagocytosis, J. Cell. Biol. **68:**602, 1976.

228. Stossel, T. P., and Pollard, T. D.: Myosin in polymorphonuclear leukocytes, J. Biol. Chem. **248:**8288, 1973.

229. Stossel, T. P., Pollard, R. D., and Mason, J. D.: Isolation and properties of phagocytic vesicles from polymorphonuclear leukocytes, J. Clin. Invest. **51:**604, 1972.

230. Stossel, T. P., Root, R. K., and Vaughan, M.: Phagocytosis in chronic granulomatous disease and the Chediak-Higashi syndrome, N. Engl. J. Med. **286:**120, 1972.

231. Strauss, R. R., Paul, B. B., Jacobs, A. A., et al.: The metabolic and phagocytic activities of leukocytes from children with acute leukemia, Cancer Res. **30:**480, 1970.

232. Sung, J. H., Meyers, J. P., Stadlan, E. M., et al.: Neuropathological changes in Chediak-Higashi disease, J. Neuropathol. Exp. Neurol. **28:**86, 1969.

233. Sutcliffe, J., and Chrispin, A. R.: Chronic granulomatous disease, Br. J. Radiol. **43:**110, 1970.

234. Taylor, R. F., and Farrell, R. K.: Light and electron microscopy of peripheral blood neutrophils in a killer whale affected with Chediak-Higashi syndrome, Fed. Proc. **32:**822, 1973.

235. Vanderbuilt, B. L., Boxer, L. A., Yang, H. H., and Baehner, R. L.: Effects of ascorbic acid on polymorphonuclear leukocyte microtubule function and on polymerization of isolated bovine brain tubulin, Clin. Res. **25:**481, 1977.

236. Vane, J. R.: Inhibition of prostaglandin synthesis as a mechanism of action for aspirin-like drugs, Nature (New Biol.) **231:**232, 1971.

237. Van Epps, D. E., Palmer, D. L., and Williams, R. C., Jr.: Characterization of serum inhibitors of neutrophil chemotaxis associated with energy, J. Immunol. **113:**189, 1974.

238. Van Epps, D. E., and Williams, R. C., Jr.: Suppression of leukocyte chemotaxis by human IgA myeloma components, J. Exp. Med. **144:**1227, 1976.

239. Van Scoy, R. E., Hill, H. R., Ritts, R. E., Jr., and Quie, P. G.: Familial neutrophil chemotaxis defect, recurrent bacterial infections, mucocutaneous candidiasis, and

hyperimmunoglobulinemia E, Ann. Intern. Med. **82:** 766, 1975.

240. Verronen, P.: Presumed disseminated BCG in a boy with chronic granulomatous disease of childhood, Acta Pediatr. Scand. **63:**627, 1974.

241. Ward, P. A.: Leukotactic factors in health and disease, Am. J. Pathol. **64:**521, 1971.

242. Ward, P. A., and Berenberg, J. L.: Defective regulation of inflammatory mediators in Hodgkin's disease, N. Engl. J. Med. **290:**76, 1974.

243. Ward, P. A., Goralnick, S., and Bullock, W. E.: Defective leukotaxis in patients with lepromatous leprosy, J. Lab. Clin. Med. **87:**1025, 1976.

244. Ward, P. A., and Schlegel, R. J.: Impaired leucotactic responsiveness in a child with recurrent infections, Lancet **2:**344, 1969.

245. Weiss, H. J., Tschopp, D. B., Rogers, J., and Brand, H.: Studies of platelet 5-hydroxytryptamine (serotonin) in storage pool disease in albinism, J. Clin. Invest. **54:** 421, 1974.

246. White, J. G.: The Chediak-Higashi syndrome: a possible lysosomal disease, Blood **28:**143, 1966.

247. White, J. G., Edson, J. R., Desnick, S. J., and Witkop, C. J.: Studies of platelets in a variant of the Hermansky-Pudlak syndrome, Am. J. Pathol. **63:**319, 1971.

248. Whittenbury, R.: Hydrogen peroxide formation and catalase activity in the lactic acid bacteria, J. Gen. Microbiol. **35:**13, 1964.

249. Wilkinson, P. C.: Chemotaxis and inflammation, Edinburgh, 1974, Churchill Livingstone.

250. Wilkinson, P. C.: Recognition and response in mononuclear and granular phagocytes, Clin. Exp. Immunol. **25:**355, 1976.

251. Windhorst, D. B., and Katz. E. D.: Normal enzyme activities in chronic granulomatous leukocytes, J. Reticuloendothel. Soc. **11:**400, 1972.

252. Windhorst, D. B., Page, A. R., Holmes, B., et al.: The pattern of genetic transmission of the leukocyte defect in fatal granulomatous disease of childhood, J. Clin. Invest. **47:**1026, 1968.

253. Windhorst, D. B., Zelickson, A. S., and Good, R. A.: A human pigmentary dilution based on a heritable subcellular structural defect—the Chediak-Higashi syndrome, J. Invest. Dermatol. **50:**9, 1968.

254. Winkelstein, J. A.: Opsonins: the function, identity, and clinical significance, J. Pediatr. **2:**747, 1973.

255. Winkelstein, J. A., and Drachman, R. H.: Deficiency of pneumococcal serum opsonizing activity in sickle cell disease, N. Engl. J. Med. **279:**459, 1968.

256. Wolfson, J. J., Kane, W. J., Laxdal, S. D., et al.: Bone findings in chronic granulomatous disease of childhood, J. Bone Joint Surg. **51A:**1573, 1969.

257. Wright, D. G., Kirkpatrick, C. H., and Gallin, J. I.: Effects of levamisole on normal and abnormal leukocyte locomotion, J. Clin. Invest. **59:**941, 1977.

258. Zeya, H. I., and Spitznagel, J. K.: Arginine-rich proteins of polymorphonuclear leukocyte lysosomes, antimicrobial specificity, and biochemical heterogeneity, J. Exp. Med. **127:**927, 1968.

259. Zigmond, S. H.: Mechanisms of sensing chemical gradients by polymorphonuclear leukocytes, Nature **249:**450, 1974.

260. Zigmond, S. H., and Hirsch, J. G.: Leukocyte locomotion in chemotaxis: new methods for evaluation and demonstration of a cell-derived chemotactic factor, J. Exp. Med. **137:**387, 1973.

261. Zurier, R. B., Hoffstein, S., and Weissmann, G.: Cytochalasin B: effect on lysosomal enzyme release from human leukocytes, Proc. Natl. Acad. Sci. **70:**844, 1973.

262. Zurier, R. B., Weissmann, G., Hoffstein, S., et al.: Mechanisms of lysosomal enzyme release from human leukocytes, J. Clin. Invest. **53:**297, 1974.

20 □ Lymphocytes

Robert L. Baehner

Immune disorders

STRUCTURE-FUNCTION RELATIONS IN THE LYMPHOID SYSTEM
Development of the two component lymphoid systems

Fig. 20-1 depicts our current concept of the lymphoid cellular system. During embryologic development some cells of the yolk sac and fetal liver containing the precursors of all the hematopoietic elements function as prethymic cells capable of differentiating under the influence of the thymus into a population of postthymic T cells that maintain cellular immunity and elaborate lymphokines. In humans blood-borne stem cells enter the thymus and begin differentiation during the eighth week of gestation. Other cells develop into different populations to function in antibody and immunoglobulin synthesis and secretion. In birds the organ that subserves this differentiative function is a lymphoepithelial organ located at the posterior end of the gastrointestinal tract called the bursa of Fabricius.[29] The possibility that bone marrow subserves this function in humans and other mammals has been considered. In mice both mature marrow and spleen provide the milieu for differentiation of either yolk sac or fetal liver cells to immunoglobulin-producing B cells.[4]

Function and distribution of T cells

Experimental studies utilizing neonatal extirpation of thymus in mice with or without lethal irradiation and reconstitution employing fetal liver cells from neonatal, adult, and genetically athymic mice have provided models of thymic system deficiency.[42] T cells are responsible for delayed allergic reactions, allograft rejection reactions, and detection and destruction of malignant cells, and they provide a defense against many viruses, fungi, and facultative intracellular pyogenic bacterial pathogens. T cells may be both short- and long-lived; in humans their life span may approach 10 years[20,34] and may explain why removal of the thymus produces no immediate immunologic deficit. T cells tend to be distributed selectively in certain regions of peripheral lymphoid sites, occupying the deep cortical regions of lymph nodes and perifollicular and perivascular areas in the malpighian white matter of the spleen (Fig. 20-2). They circulate in the blood and lymph nodes as small and medium-sized lymphocytes.

Cells of the T and B cells system can be identi-

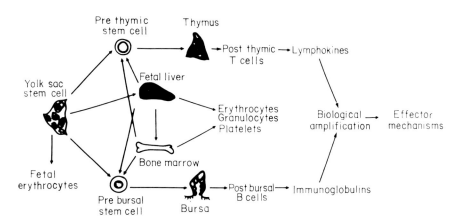

Fig. 20-1. Current concepts of development of the two immunity systems. (From Good, R. A., and Bach, F. H.: In Bach, F. H., and Good, R. A., eds.: Clinical immunobiology, New York, 1974, Academic Press, Inc.)

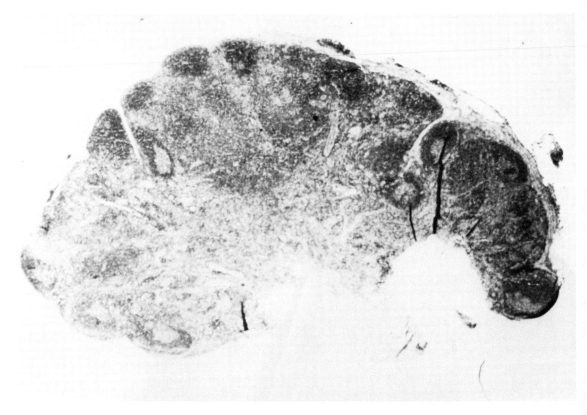

Fig. 20-2. Normal lymph node of a child showing germinal centers, deep cortical areas, and medullary cords. T cells are located in the deep cortical areas, whereas B cells are located in germinal centers and medullary cords. (Courtesy Dr. Richard O'Reilly, New York, N.Y.)

fied and precisely enumerated. T cells are identified by their capacity to form rosettes spontaneously when incubated with sheep red blood cells.[71] Cells of the B cell line can be detected and their number quantitated by using an elegant immunofluorescent technique.[83,85] The immunoglobulins demonstrable at the surfaces of B cells represent secretory products from the cell binding at selective sites on the plasma membrane. Other markers for B cells include the identification of C3 surface receptors and receptors for Epstein-Barr virus. The distribution of B and T cells in blood, bone marrow, lymph nodes, appendix, thymus, and spleen of children and adults are listed in Table 20-1.[71,113]

Fully differentiated T cells are the only cells that respond by blast transformation, nucleic acid synthesis, and proliferation in vitro culture to kidney bean extract phytohemagglutinin (PHA), concanavalin A, or mismatched lymphoid cells previously irradiated or mitomycin-treated (the mixed lymphocyte culture, or MLC); pokeweed mitogen stimulates both T and B cells.[53] In vitro stimulation of lymphocytes by PHA is presumed to correlate with T cell function and does not require previous sensitization of the patient's lymphocytes,

which is necessary when specific antigens are used.[70] Stimulated lymphocytes in vitro release a variety of soluble factors (lymphokines) that are also presumed to correlate with T cell function.[86] These include macrophage inhibitory factor (MIF), interferon, macrophage activating factor (MAF), chemotactic factors for polymorphonuclear leukocytes and monocytes, cytotoxic factors, lymphocyte blastogenesis factor, and T cell helper function.[68] They contribute to the enhanced cooperative function between T cells with phagocytic macrophages, monocytes, polymorphonuclear leukocytes, and B cells. Another subset of T cells can suppress B cell function. Diagnostic studies for patients with suspected immunodeficiency syndromes are listed below:

A. Humoral (B cell) immunity
    1. Serum immunoglobulin quantitation (IgG, IgA, IgM, IgD, IgE)
    2. Specific antibody responses
        a. Schick test
        b. Antibody titers after typhoid, diphtheria, tetanus, pertussis, and poliomyelitis immunization
        c. Serum isohemagglutinin titers
        d. Secretory antibodies

Table 20-1. Distribution of T and B lymphocytes

	T cells (%)	B cells (%)			
		IgG	IgA	IgM	Total
Peripheral blood					
Adult	46.3 ± 1.8	16.1 ± 0.9	5.2 ± 0.4	7.5 ± 0.5	26.5 ± 2.3
Children	44.0 ± 4.2	14.9 ± 3.1	3.3 ± 2.3	7.5 ± 1.4	30.4 ± 3.1
Bone marrow	11.6 ± 1.4	12.4 ± 2.3	1.9 ± 0.3	6.3 ± 1.5	20.6 ± 2.4
Lymph nodes	32.4 ± 2.7	5.0 ± 0.6	2.4 ± 0.4	10.4 ± 1.0	17.8 ± 1.6
Appendix	19.4 ± 3.5*	6.0 ± 2.7	2.1 ± 0.9	14.7 ± 3.8	22.3 ± 6.5
Thymus	42.4†	0.5	0.0	0.3	0.8
Spleen	16.0	15.0	6.0	34.0	55.0

*Mean ± standard error of the mean.
†Mean.

B. Cell-mediated (T cell) immunity
1. Total blood lymphocyte count
2. Antigen skin tests
   a. Recall: streptokinase-streptodornase, *Candida, Trichophyton,* mumps
   b. Sensitization and response: dinitrochlorobenzene
3. In vitro lymphocyte response to phytohemagglutinin, allogeneic cells, or antigens
4. Posteroanterior and lateral chest x-ray films for thymus shadow
5. T cell percentage and number in blood
6. Skin homograft
7. Lymphokine assays
8. Lymph node biopsy

Function, development, and distribution of B cells

Bursa-derived cells in birds and marrow-derived cells of mammals comprise a population of lymphocytes and plasma cells that produce and secrete immunoglobulins and antibody into interstitial tissues, lymph, blood, and alimentary and respiratory passages. They are more sessile than T cells and may leave lymph nodes and enter lymph and blood following antigenic challenge. A single B cell and its clone produce only one class of immunoglobulins (IgM, IgG, IgA, IgD, or IgE) and further populations of B cells are encountered with selective IgG subclass specificity (IgG1, IgG2, IgG3, and IgG4).[67,111]

In the human fetus B cells bearing IgM, IgG, and IgA surface immunoglobulin determinants have been demonstrated in peripheral blood, bone marrow, liver, and spleen at 11½ weeks of gestation.[60] By 14 weeks the percentage of cells in the circulation having each class of receptors is equivalent to that in adults but the capacity of these fetal cells to synthesize and secrete immunoglobulin cannot be detected until about 20 weeks.[109] There appears to be an orderly progression for the clonal development of B cells as each uncommitted stem cell proliferates, differentiates, and secretes IgM and then may or may not give rise to B cells with a genetic commitment to synthesize IgG; some of the latter cells remain true to their new commitment while others go on to become B cells with the genetic commitment to synthesize IgA.[28] Thus the development of the B cell pool is independent of exogenous antigenic stimulation but the terminal response of B cells to plasma cell differentiation and antibody synthesis requires that these cells be able to recognize and respond to specific antigenic challenge.

Electron microscopic study of a fully differentiated plasma cell reveals extraordinary cytoplasmic development including striking granular endoplasmic reticulum and a well-developed Golgi apparatus essential to the secretory process (Fig. 20-3). In lymph nodes B cells are concentrated in the far cortical areas of the node and make up the majority of cells in the medullary cord of the node (Fig. 20-2). One to 2 weeks following antigenic stimulation B cells differentiate into plasma cells and become prominent in the hyperplastic germinal follicles of the reactive lymph node. The various immunoglobulin subclasses of B cells have a somewhat different distribution. IgA- and IgE-producing B cells are concentrated in the subepithelial regions, the lamina propria and glands of the gastrointestinal tract, Peyer's patches, and the pharyngeal tonsils. Although fully differentiated plasma cells are found in bone marrow, they rarely appear in the blood.

Structure and function of immunoglobulins

There are five known major immunoglobulin classes in humans; each class is designated by the letter G, A, M, D, or E. The basic linear immunoglobulin structure consists of two heavy and two light polypeptide chains. As noted in Table 20-2, each immunoglobulin molecule is made up of two identical pairs of heavy chains, which determine

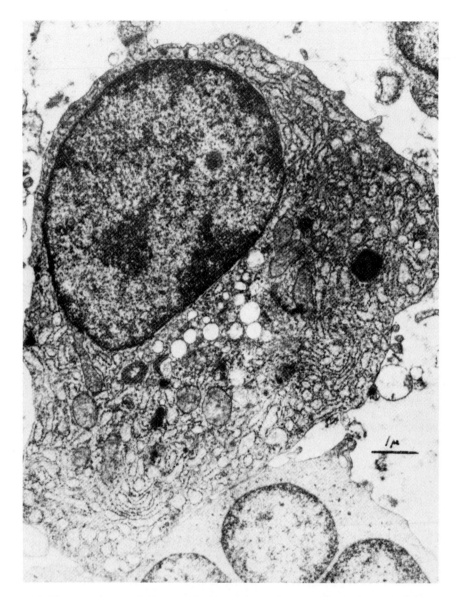

Fig. 20-3. Electron micrograph of mature human plasma cell. (From Good, R. A.: In Bach, F. H., and Good, R. A., eds.: Clinical immunobiology, vol. 1, New York, 1972, Academic Press, Inc.)

the type of monomer immunoglobulin formed (IgG, IgA, IgD, or IgE) and two identical pairs of light chains of either κ or λ type. These are held together by disulfide bonds and weak noncovalent forces.

The variable region of each heavy and light chain determines the immunoglobulin type. The dimeric form of IgA contains a subunit secretory component, whereas the polymeric form of IgM contains five subunits held together by disulfide bonds. The enzyme papain cleaves the IgG molecule into thirds, two identical portions (Fab) containing antigen-combining sites and a remaining Fc portion, which controls metabolic decay,

body distribution, antigenic uniqueness, cytotrophic tendency, and whether or not the molecule crosses the placenta, fixes complement, polymerizes, and fixes to skin. Thus for each immunoglobulin monomer there are four antigen-combining sites consisting of a portion of the heavy and light chains at each end of the molecule close to the variable region of the chain (Fig. 20-4). Antigenic markers of light chains are κ and λ and a given immunoglobulin molecule can be antigenically described as being of the κ or λ class. Of all the immunoglobulins, approximately two-thirds bear κ determinants and the remainder are of the λ class.

The major heavy-chain antigens are designated

Table 20-2. Nomenclature of immunoglobulins

Polypeptide chains			Formula for whole molecule	Name
Heavy chain	Light chain	Other		
Monomers				
γ	κ		$\gamma_2\kappa_2$	IgG, γG-globulin
	λ		$\gamma_2\lambda_2$	
α	κ		$\alpha_2\kappa_2$	IgA, γA-globulin
	λ		$\alpha_2\lambda_2$	
δ	κ		$\delta_2\kappa_2$	IgD, γD-globulin
	λ		$\delta_2\lambda_2$	
ϵ	κ		$\epsilon_2\kappa_2$	IgE, γE-globulin
	λ		$\epsilon_2\lambda_2$	
Polymers				
α	κ	SC, J	$(\alpha_2\kappa_2)_2 SC \cdot J$	Secretory IgA
	λ	SC, J	$(\alpha_2\kappa_2)_2 SC \cdot J$	
μ	κ	J	$(\mu_2\kappa_2)_5 \cdot J$	IgM, γM-globulin
	λ	J	$(\mu_2\lambda_2)_5 \cdot J$	

*From Hong R: In Bach, F. H., and Good, R. A., eds.: Clinical immunobiology, vol. 1, New York, 1972, Academic Press, Inc.

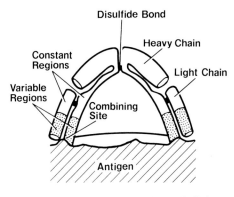

Fig. 20-4. Diagrammatic model of the IgG immunoglobulin molecules in combination with antigen. The two heavy chains and light chains are held together with disulfide bonds. The variable portions of the heavy and light chains (darker shading) are about equal in length and contain the antigen combining site. (From Stiehm, E. R.: In Stiehm, E. R., and Fulginiti, V. A.: Immunologic disorders in infants and children, Philadelphia, 1973, W. B. Saunders Co.; modified from Nisonoff, A.: Hosp. Pract. **2**:19, 1967.)

by the Greek letters γ, α, μ, δ, and ϵ, and within each of the major classes, subgroups known as types have been described. There are four for IgG (G1, G2, G3, and G4) and two each for IgA and IgM. Most antigens of the heavy-chain class are localized to the Fc half of the chain (G2 and G4 do not fix complement). Further subdivision of the immunoglobulins can be made on the basis of genetic factors called allotypes. These are termed the Gm, Inv, and Am factors. Unlike subtypes and subclasses, these factors are present only in certain individuals as determined by mendelian genetics. IgG and IgM are assembled within lymph nodes and lymphoid aggregations of the spleen.

Eighty-five percent of cells in the lamina propria of the gastrointestinal tract synthesize IgA, the major immunoglobulin constituent of saliva, tears, and gastrointestinal secretions. IgE is the reaginic antibody largely responsible for symptoms of hay fever and asthma. Competent immunoglobulin production is indicated by an abundance of lymphoid tissue arranged in follicle formation associated with plasma cells. IgM-producing plasma cells are morphologically distinct from other immunoglobulin-producing cells since they have scanty cytoplasm and a poorly developed endoplasmic reticulum resembling a large lymphocyte. They are often termed lymphocytoid plasma cells and are found in abundance in patients with Waldenström's macroglobulinemia. There are no morphologic differences between plasma cells producing the other classes of immunoglobulins because multiple myelomas of the IgA, IgG, IgD, and IgE varieties are not distinguishable morphologically. Heavy and light chains are synthesized separately on polyribosomes of plasma cells and accumulate between membranes of the endoplasmic reticulum, producing inclusions called Russell bodies (Plate 4, *M*). They are combined prior to release, and the entire process takes only 30 minutes.

It is estimated that each immunoglobulin-producing cell synthesizes 2,000 molecules of γ-globulin/second and 1.7×10^8 molecules daily. Based

Table 20-3. Metabolic properties of the immunoglobulin classes*

	IgG	IgM	IgA	IgD	IgE
Mean adult serum concentration (mg/100 ml)	1,200	150	300	3	0.03
Percent of total immunoglobulin	70-80	5-10	10-15	<1	<0.01
Biologic half-life (days)	25	5	7	2.8	2.3
Distribution (% intravascular)	45	80	45	75	50
Total body pool (mg/kg)	1,150	49	230	1.5	0.04
Synthetic rate (mg/kg/day)	35	7	25	0.4	0.02
Placental transfer	+	−	−	−	−
Fractional catabolic rate (% body content catabolized/day)	3	14	12	35	89

*From Stiehm, E. R.: In Stiehm, E. R., and Fulginiti, V. A., eds.: Immunologic disorders in infants and children, Philadelphia, 1973, W. B. Saunders Co.

on an IgG synthetic rate of 35 mg/kg/day, the total volume of plasma cells required for this production is 10 ml.[109] The half-life of circulating immunoglobulins has been measured using purified trace-labeled molecules. In addition, by careful quantitation of its dilution into the plasma, the rate of excretion in urine and stool, the intravascular and extravascular distribution, the total body pool, the synthetic rate, and the amount of the total body pool synthesized per day (fractional catabolic rate)[110] have also been determined. These data are summarized in Table 20-3.

DISORDERS CAUSED BY LOSS OR ALTERATION OF LYMPHOCYTE FUNCTION
B cell dysfunction

Transient hypogammaglobulinemia of infancy. Normally the full-term newborn is the recipient of sufficient maternal IgG to the extent that umbilical cord and maternal serum contain similar concentrations of IgG. The maternal IgG is slowly catabolized so that the infant's serum IgG level reaches its low point of approximately 300 mg/dl by the end of the second month of life when the infant begins to synthesize IgG. Serum levels of IgG rapidly rise toward normal adult values by the age of 1 year. The normal newborn starts synthesizing IgM antibodies at birth so that by 1 year IgM values are 75% of adult values. IgA is synthesized by the third week and reaches 75% of adult values by the end of the second year of life. Table 20-4 provides normal values for infants and children.

Perhaps the most widely diagnosed immunodeficiency disease is transient hypogammaglobulinemia of infancy, which occurs equally in males and females. Premature infants are especially prone to this disorder during the first few months of life. During this period immunoglobulin levels are often less than 200 mg/dl. Their own immunoglobulin synthesis is delayed until 9 to 15

months of age, and normal levels are not reached until between 2 and 4 years of age.[92,93]

The etiology is unknown and familial occurrences have been recorded.[112] One proposal was maternal isoimmunization to an IgG allotype of the infant, resulting in transplacental passage of maternal antibodies against the infant's γ-globulin to effect either destruction or suppression of γ-globulin synthesis.[37] However, infants of pregnancies with proven fetal-maternal incompatibility of γ-globulin and maternal sensitization have not had immunodeficiency states.[69]

Presenting signs and symptoms include an undue susceptibility to infections with gram-positive bacteria of the skin and respiratory tract. Recurrent otitis media, bronchiolitis, and bronchitis are the most common infections. Bacterial meningitis is also more common in this group of infants. Suggestive features in the history include failure to thrive with poor weight and height gain. If total immunoglobulin levels (IgG, IgM, and IgA) exceed 400 mg/dl, the diagnosis can usually be excluded. At times the condition must be differentiated from X-linked infantile agammaglobulinemia.

Rectal biopsy of infants with transient hypogammaglobulinemia shows plasma cells in the lamina propria of the rectal mucosa, and lymph node biopsy reveals normal lymph node architecture. Antibody response to protein antigens such as diphtheria, tetanus, and pertussis antigens is normal and cellular immunity is intact. Even when levels fall below these values, unless the infant is experiencing repeated infections that are interferring with normal growth, γ-globulin injections are not required since excessive therapy may lead to prolongation of the syndrome.

X-linked agammaglobulinemia. X-linked agammaglobulinemia was the first reported immunodeficiency described by Bruton[17] in 1952. Study of large numbers of kindreds with mutliple

Table 20-4. Levels of immune globulins in serum of normal subjects at different ages*

Age	No. of subjects	Level of γG† mg/100 ml (range)	% of adult level	Level of γM† mg/100 ml (range)	% of adult level	Level of γA† mg/100 ml (range)	% of adult level	Level of total γ-globulin† mg/100 ml (range)	% of adult level
Newborn	22	1,031 ± 200 (645-1,244)	89 ± 17	11 ± 5 (5-30)	11 ± 5	2 ± 3 (0-11)	1 ± 2	1,044 ± 201 (660-1,439)	67 ± 13
1-3 mo	29	430 ± 119 (272-762)	37 ± 10	30 ± 11 (16-67)	30 ± 11	21 ± 13 (6-56)	11 ± 7	481 ± 127 (324-699)	31 ± 9
4-6 mo	33	427 ± 186 (206-1,125)	37 ± 16	43 ± 17 (10-83)	43 ± 17	28 ± 18 (8-93)	14 ± 9	498 ± 204 (228-1,232)	32 ± 13
7-12 mo	56	661 ± 219 (279-1,533)	58 ± 19	54 ± 23 (22-147)	55 ± 23	37 ± 18 (16-98)	19 ± 9	752 ± 242 (327-1,687)	48 ± 15
13-24 mo	59	762 ± 209 (258-1,393)	66 ± 18	58 ± 23 (14-114)	59 ± 23	50 ± 24 (19-119)	25 ± 12	870 ± 258 (398-1,586)	56 ± 16
25-36 mo	33	892 ± 183 (419-1,274)	77 ± 16	61 ± 19 (28-113)	62 ± 19	71 ± 37 (19-235)	36 ± 19	1,024 ± 205 (499-1,418)	65 ± 14
3-5 yr	28	929 ± 228 (569-1,597)	80 ± 20	56 ± 18 (22-100)	57 ± 18	93 ± 27 (55-152)	47 ± 14	1,078 ± 245 (730-1,771)	69 ± 17
6-8 yr	18	923 ± 256 (559-1,492)	80 ± 22	65 ± 25 (27-118)	66 ± 25	124 ± 45 (54-221)	62 ± 23	1,112 ± 293 (640-1,725)	71 ± 20
9-11 yr	9	1,124 ± 235 (779-1,456)	97 ± 20	79 ± 33 (35-132)	80 ± 33	131 ± 60 (12-208)	66 ± 30	1,334 ± 254 (966-1,639)	85 ± 17
12-16 yr	9	946 ± 124 (726-1,085)	82 ± 11	59 ± 20 (35-72)	60 ± 20	148 ± 63 (70-229)	74 ± 32	1,153 ± 169 (833-1,284)	74 ± 12
Adults	30	1,158 ± 305 (569-1,919)	100 ± 26	99 ± 27 (47-147)	100 ± 27	200 ± 61 (61-330)	100 ± 31	1,457 ± 353 (730-2,365)	100 ± 24

*From Stiehm, E. R., and Fudenberg, H. H.: Pediatrics **37:**715, 1966. Copyright American Academy of Pediatrics, 1966.
†Mean is ±1 S.D.

occurrences of congenital agammaglobulinemia has documented an X-linked pattern of inheritance. A positive family history is obtained in less than half of the cases. The disease is manifested by recurrent infections with pyogenic bacteria, e.g., staphylococci, streptococci, pneumococci, and *Haemophilus influenzae*. Purulent sinusitis, pneumonia, sepsis, meningitis, and furunculosis are the most common types of infections. Many of these boys later develop bronchiectasis and ultimately die of pulmonary complications. They can sustain measles, mumps, varicella, and rubella in ordinary fashion. The prognosis has improved with the development of better antibiotic drugs and the administration of γ-globulin. Nevertheless, patients do succumb to overwhelming infections by pathogens that are difficult to treat such as *Pneumocystis carinii,* fungi, *Pseudomonas,* and *Proteus.* Physical examination findings are not always helpful in establishing the diagnosis. Most patients lack palpable lymph nodes, but occasionally nodes may be enlarged. Liver and spleen enlargement does not occur. The absence of adenoid tissue can be shown by a lateral x-ray film of the nasopharynx.

The diagnosis is established by observing a serum IgG of less than 100 mg/ml and IgA and IgM concentrations of less than 1% of normal adult values. The absence of isohemagglutinins in an infant not of the AB blood type serves as a good diagnostic screen. The Schick test remains positive after diphtheria-pertussis-tetanus immunization. No antibody response is detected after immunization with typhoid, influenza, poliomyelitis, or other vaccines.

Peripheral white blood cell counts are usually normal. Lymphopenia is unusual, but circulating B lymphocytes are reduced in numbers and percentage.[40] The diagnosis can be confirmed pathologically by the demonstration of an absence of plasma cells, lymphoid follicles, and germinal centers from a lymph node (Fig. 20-5). Since plasma cells are sparse in bone marrow of infants and preschool children,[100] bone marrow examination is not a useful test to aid in establishing the diagno-

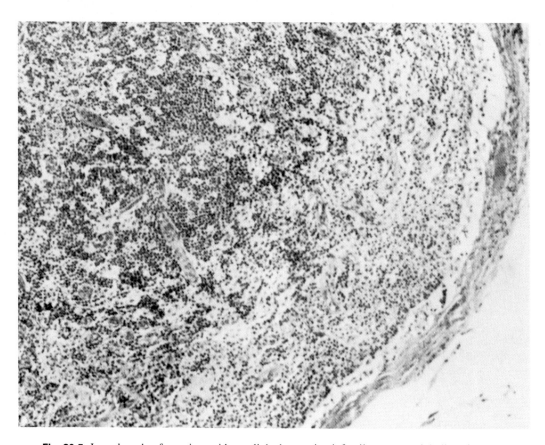

Fig. 20-5. Lymph node of a patient with sex-linked recessive infantile agammaglobulinemia. Note the well-populated deep cortical regions (T cells), the absence of germinal centers, and the deficiency of cells in the far cortical regions. (From Good, R. A.: In Kagan, B. M., and Stiehm, E. R., eds.: Immunologic incompetence, Copyright © 1971, by Year Book Medical Publishers, Inc., Chicago. Used by permission.)

sis. Rectal biopsy is rewarding and shows absence of plasma cells in the lamina propria.[32] A convenient way to make the diagnosis is with a regional node biopsy 1 week after three weekly injections of 0.25 ml typhoid vaccine plus a determination of serum anti-H titers showing a titer of less than 1:5, in comparison to the normal titer response of 1:160 or more.

The injection of γ-globulin has been effective in preventing severe infections if the serum level is raised by approximately 200 mg/dl. γ-Globulin as a 16.5% solution is available at cost from the American Red Cross. A newly diagnosed patient is given 1.8 ml (300 mg)/kg in three divided doses and this usually raises the serum γ-globulin level to 300 mg/dl. Because the half-life of injected γ-globulin is 30 days, a monthly maintenance dose of 0.6 mg (100 mg)/kg is usually required to maintain the desired level of approximately 200 mg/dl. No commercial preparation of IgA or IgM is currently available for clinical use. If the disorder is diagnosed before chronic infection is established in the respiratory tract, there is no need to administer prophylactic antibiotics. Patients with bronchiectasis require antibiotics and vigorous pulmonary therapy including postural drainage. Chronic otitis media often results in hearing loss.

The majority of affected boys develop arthritis of the large joints that abates once γ-globulin replacement therapy has begun.[44] A rare but progressively fatal complication is a syndrome resembling dermatomyositis with edema, muscle induration and weakness, a rash over the extensor surfaces of the joints, and occasionally a fatal neurologic disorder[90] with amyloidosis.[114] Although typical virus infections are no problem, adenovirus type 12 and echovirus types 9 and 30 have been cultured from older boys dying of this syndrome.

Drug eruptions, atopic eczema, poison ivy, allergic rhinitis, and asthma occur with high frequency but the dermatographic wheal-and-flare reaction after stroking the skin that is typical of allergic patients cannot be elicited. Autoimmune hemolytic anemia has been described.[87] Although chronic diarrhea is rare, a malabsorption syndrome caused by *Giardia lamblia* occurs in a variety of immunodeficient states.[74]

Immunodeficiency with increased IgM. One of the more common partial immunoglobulin defects, first reported in 1961, is characterized by a deficiency of IgG and humoral and secretory IgA with normal to elevated levels of IgM.[91] The secretory component of IgA is present in the secretions. Generally the onset of pyogenic infections is delayed until after the first year of life when recurrent tonsillitis, otitis media, pneumonia, and cervical adenitis occur. The disorder is inherited with an X-linked pattern and has frequently been asso-

ciated with congenital rubella. An acquired form occurs in older boys and girls. Many patients develop a combination of thrombocytopenia, neutropenia, aplastic or hemolytic anemia, and renal disease, presumably on an autoimmune basis.

Physical examination often reveals enlargement of the liver and spleen. Serum IgM levels range between 150 and 1,000 mg/dl with IgG levels less than 100 mg/dl and IgA levels less than 10 mg/dl. Isohemagglutinin titers are usually elevated, patients may have antibody responses to some immunizations, and the Schick test may become negative after repeated immunizations. However, impaired antibody response to a wide variety of antigens is the rule. Lymph node architecture is abnormal with few or no lymphoid follicles, no germinal centers, and few or no typical plasma cells. Peripheral lymphocyte numbers are normal. A 2-year-old boy studied by our laboratory had 27%, 10%, and 18% IgM, IgA, and IgG cells, respectively, and his cellular immunity was intact. In the so-called acquired form, lymphoid follicles and germinal centers are present in lymph nodes.

Administration of γ-globulin monthly has reduced serum IgM levels and improved neutropenia in some cases. Deaths due to *Pseudomonas* sepsis, *Pneumocystis carinii* pneumonia, and a progressive infiltrative process of IgM-producing lymphocytes of the gastrointestinal tract, liver, spleen, and lymph nodes have been recorded.[30,90,101]

Immunodeficiency with normal levels or hyperimmunoglobulinemia

IgA deficiency. The most common partial immunoglobulin defect is IgA deficiency, which occurs in 1 of 500 to 1 of 900 persons.[8] Usually selective serum IgA deficiency is associated with secretory IgA deficiency. Serum IgA levels are less than 5 mg/dl while all other serum immunoglobulins are normal. Both antibody-mediated immunity and cell-mediated immunity are intact, and the subclass of IgA-bearing B cells in the blood is normal.[38] Patients with selective IgA deficiency have a high incidence of autoimmune diseases including systemic lupus erythematosis, rheumatoid arthritis, dermatomyositis, pernicious anemia, thyroiditis, cerebral vasculitis, idiopathic Addison's disease, Sjögren's syndrome, lupoid hepatitis, transfusion reactions, idiopathic thrombocytopenic purpura, Coombs-positive hemolytic anemia, pulmonary hemosiderosis, regional enteritis, and ulcerative colitis.[3] The incidence of IgA deficiency among allergic patients is 1/200 and they seem to experience more gastrointestinal and upper respiratory tract problems.[19] Chronic and recurrent pulmonary disease is also more frequent and presents as chronic bronchitis, obstructive lung disease, or recurrent pneumonia. Despite the lack of a consistent correlation between selective IgA deficiency and chromosome 18 defects, a familial inheritance pattern that is either autosomal dominant or recessive has been noted, and many of the relatives of patients have increases or decreases of other immunoglobulins.[72]

IgM deficiency. Selective IgM deficiency has been reported in a few patients with septicemia, malabsorption, hemolytic anemia, and eczema. IgA and IgG levels have ranged from low normal to elevated in different patients. Results of investigations of production of antibody to a variety of antigens (e.g., typhoid, poliomyelitis) in patients with recurrent infection and growth failure despite normal immunoglobulin levels emphasize the point that patients suspected of having immunodeficiency diseases cannot be adequately evaluated simply by determining concentrations of immunoglobulins but must have antibody-stimulation tests.

T cell dysfunction

Congenital thymic hypoplasia (DiGeorge's syndrome). Congenital thymic hypoplasia (DiGeorge's syndrome) is a congenital immunodeficiency caused by a failure of embryogenesis of the entodermal derivatives of the third and fourth pharyngeal pouches resulting in aplasia of the parathyroid and thymus glands.[31,88] It usually is not familial, and both sexes are equally affected.

As a result of thymic aplasia the cellular immune system remains undifferentiated, leading to a lack of delayed hypersensitivity to skin test antigens, diminished or absent responses of lymphocytes in vitro to mitogenic and antigenic substances, delayed rejection of a heterologous skin graft, and a depletion of lymphocytes from the subcortical thymic-dependent portion of lymph nodes and from the periarteriolar sheaths of the spleen but with retention of cortical germinal centers of lymph nodes and spleen (Fig. 20-6).

As a result of aplasia of the parathyroid gland infants have a characteristic clinical picture of hypocalcemic tetany in the first few hours of life. The serum calcium level is lowered to 5 to 7 mg/dl and serum phosphorous is attenuated. These infants resemble each other because they have hypertelorism and mongoloid slant of the eyes; shortened philtrum of the lip; low-set, notched ear pinnas, and micrognathia. They may manifest sensorineural, conductive, or mixed hearing losses of widely varying degrees.[13] More than 80% (nineteen of twenty-three patients) were found to have aortic arch and/or intracardiac anomalies such as tetrology of Fallot, truncus arteriosus, pulmonary and aortic valve defects, and patent ductus and ventricular septal defects.[36] They fail to thrive and are susceptible to chronic rhinitis, otitis media,

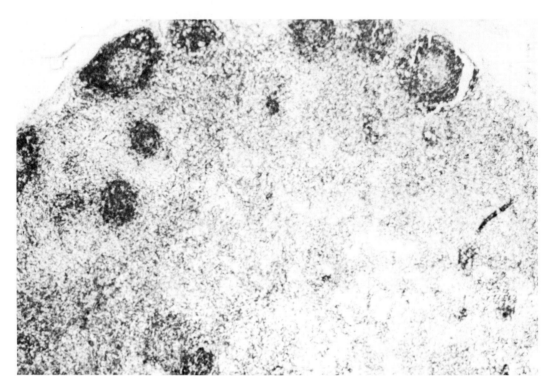

Fig. 20-6. Lymph node in patient with DiGeorge's syndrome lacking paracortical cells (T cells) but with normal germinal centers. (Courtesy Dr. Richard O'Reilly, New York, N.Y.)

pneumonia, oral and anal candidiasis, diarrhea, and sudden death. Other noted defects have been bifid uvula, esophageal atresia, nephrocalcinosis, and urinary tract infections.

Laboratory evaluation reveals absence of a thymic shadow on posterior-anterior and lateral chest x-ray films, normal to slightly decreased numbers of circulating lymphocytes, normal immunoglobulin levels and antibody function but a decrease of circulating T lymphocytes,[27] and absence of all T cell–mediated responses. After in vitro incubation with normal thymus extracts, bone marrow cells differentiate into T lymphocytes.[108]

Treatment in the nursery is to control hypocalcemic tetany. Intravenous calcium gluconate (2 to 86 mg/day) is required followed by a low-phosphorous diet and large doses of vitamin D (50,000 to 250,000 units/day). Thymus transplantation is the recommended treatment of choice.[6,24] The source has been a fetus between 12 and 20 weeks of gestation. The thymus is implanted under the rectus abdominus sheath or injected intraperitoneally. In contrast to bone marrow transplantation, ABO, Rh, and HLA typing are not crucial. Successful thymic transplants result in restoration of cellular immunity for as long as 6 years,[23] but sometimes a second transplant is required because of gradual loss of thymic-dependent immune function. Some infants have only a partial thymic deficiency, denoted by diminution in thymic mass demonstrable by direct exploration or indirect clinical means, and they die of cardiac anomalies rather than from infection.[62]

Chronic mucocutaneous candidiasis. Chronic mucocutaneous candidiasis is characterized by chronic diarrhea, polyendocrinopathies, and persistent *Candida albicans* infection of the mucous membranes and skin that often extends to the nails. The age of onset is variable; infants often have severe *Candida* dermatitis of the diaper area and scalp, whereas older children may be afflicted with one or more endocrine disorders before *Candida* infections become evident. Diabetes mellitus, hypoparathyroidism, hypothyroidism, and hypoadrenalism may occur. Multiple cases may occur within families.

The in vitro response of lymphocytes to phytohemagglutinin is normal, but in most patients there is diminished response of cultured lymphocytes to *Candida* antigen. Cutaneous anergy to many antigens as well as to *Candida* antigen has been observed, and attempts to sensitize patients with 2,4-dinitrofluorobenzene have been unsuccessful.[57] An almost consistent abnormality in all case reports is the persistence of *Candida* antibody in high titers in the serum of these patients during remissions as well as exacerbations.[7,106]

Treatment with topical antifungal agents has not usually been effective, but both topical and oral administration of clotrimazole has resulted in dramatic clearing of skin and mouth lesions in a few cases.[61,81] Intravenous therapy with amphotericin B as well as 5-fluorocytosine has resulted in transient improvement and occasionally in complete amelioration of the disease. The use of transfer factor in some but not all subjects has resulted in clearing of *Candida* infections and reversal of cutaneous anergy.[57,89] Administration of transfer factor, which had previously failed, was successful after a fetal thymus transplant in a 9-year-old boy, suggesting that thymus-derived cells were required for acquisition of transfer factor–induced cellular immunity.[56] Correction of iron deficiency in patients with familial disease has improved nail and tongue disease.[48]

The ultimate prognosis is guarded. Disfiguring aspects of facial disease cause significant psychologic disturbance. Sudden death from unsuspected adrenal insufficiency may occur. Affected patients usually do not survive beyond the third decade, with death occurring from infection or hepatic or endocrine failure.

Combined immunodeficiencies

Severe combined immunodeficiency syndrome (SCIDS). Severe combined immunodeficiency syndrome (SCIDS) is a congenital and usually hereditary deficiency involving both humoral and cell-mediated immunity; it is characterized clinically by the early onset of severe infections with a rapid progressive course and early death. Pathologically it is characterized by lymphoid and plasma cell aplasia and thymic dysplasia. Next to selective IgA deficiency, it is the most common immunodeficiency. Inheritance patterns are either X linked or autosomal recessive, and isolated cases do occur. Deficiency of adenosine deaminase has been associated with the autosomal recessive form.[41,66a,78] The ratio of males to females affected is 3:1.

Illness begins in the first month of life when oral thrush becomes evident and often disseminates to the gastrointestinal tract and skin. A morbilliform exanthematous rash is another usual feature of the disease and frequently follows transfusion of nonfrozen or irradiated blood. Extensive exfoliative dermatitis is a result of graft versus host disease in these cases. The skin may closely resemble the infiltrative eczema of Letterer-Siwe disease.[22] Nearly all the patients have diarrhea with loose, watery stools. Cystic fibrosis, celiac disease, food allergy, or feeding problems are often suspected. Another common manifestation is the presence of cough and clinical evidence of bronchopneumonia. *Pneumocystis carinii* infection is a frequent pulmonary problem. Intermittent febrile episodes caused by sepsis, sometimes involving specific areas such as the meninges, occur. Infections associated with varicella, measles, and cytomegalovirus and adenovirus infections are usually life threatening.

Laboratory findings show evidence of profound absence of humoral and cell-mediated immunity. Immunoglobulin levels are consistently low. IgG, if present, may limit heterogeneity with an excess of one subclass and a deficiency of another. Isohemagglutinins are absent, as are antibodies to previously administered vaccine antigens. The Schick test is positive despite previous diphtheria immunizations. Lymphopenia with total lymphocyte counts below 2×10^9/liter is common but not invariably present. Large mononuclear lymphocytes may be present in normal or increased numbers but small lymphocytes are depleted. The myeloid series and platelet numbers are usually normal. Eosinophilia is common. The bone marrow shows a deficiency in plasma cells, lymphocytes, and lymphoblasts. The bone marrow in normal infants contains up to 20% cells in the lymphocytic series. This deficiency may well be the primary defect in the disease, resulting from the failure to form an immunopotential cell that originates in the bone marrow. Lymph node biopsy exhibits a complete lack of plasma cells and lymphocytes in the germinal element (Fig. 20-7). Only

the stroma of the node is seen to contain occasional mast cells and eosinophils or rarely small collections of lymphoid cells without any apparent organization. Skin test reactivity to recall antigens is negative. Infants cannot be sensitized to dinitrochlorobenzene. Peripheral blood lymphocytes are completely unresponsive to phytohemagglutinin or antigenic stimulation. Skin grafts are accepted with no microscopic or macroscopic signs of rejection. The thymus gland is absent on chest x-ray films. The autopsy specimens show absence of lymphoid tissue in spleen, tonsils, appendix, and intestines. The thymus gland, when found with difficulty, has usually failed to descend in the normal manner into the anterior mediastinum, weighs less than 1 gm, and is composed of primordial spindle-shaped cells occurring occasionally in swirls or rosettes. No Hassall's corpuscles and few if any lymphocytes are present.

In adenosine deaminase deficiency Hassall's corpuscles and differentiated germinal epithelium are present in an involuted thymus. The enzyme is lacking in lymphocytes, erythrocytes, fibroblasts, and amniotic-fluid cells.[66a] A 5-year-old girl with clinical and laboratory findings of severe T cell deficiency and normal B cell immunity had erythrocytes lacking nucleoside-phosphorylase activity, required for converting inosine to hypoxanthine, which is only one metabolic step beyond the con-

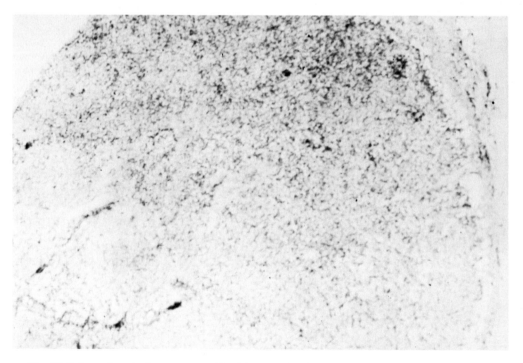

Fig. 20-7. Lymph node in severe combined immunodeficiency disease (SCID) with absence of germinal centers and virtually acellular paracortical areas. (Courtesy Dr. Richard O'Reilly, New York, N.Y.)

version of adenosine to inosine catalyzed by adenosine deaminase.[41a]

Unless the patient received irradiated or frozen red cells, he or she is in constant danger of engraftment of the transfused cells with a resultant fatal graft versus host reaction. The characteristic maculopapular rash starting on the face about 7 days after the administration of the immunocompetent cells hails the onset of graft versus host disease. The rash spreads ultimately to all skin surfaces including palms and soles. Thrombocytopenia, leukopenia, jaundice, and anasarca follow in quick succession, and the bone marrow aplasia leads to death from massive hemorrhage by the twelfth or fourteenth day.

The treatment of choice is bone marrow transplantation using HLA- and mixed lymphocyte culture–(MCL-) compatible donor marrow, usually from a sibling. Even in these conditions a mild to serious graft versus host reaction develops in the majority of these patients. Some patients have had complete restoration of T and B cell function, whereas others have had only partial correction of their immunologic defects. A review of sixty-nine patients with SCIDS showed that ten of sixteen (63%) infants receiving HLA- and MLC-compatible bone marrow and nine of twenty-one (43%) receiving fetal liver and/or thymus are alive with a functioning graft 6 months after time of transplantation. Survival was related to development of graft versus host disease, which was mild in nine of fourteen HLA- and MLC-compatible transplants but was severe in seven of ten who received HLA-compatible but MLC-incompatible marrow.[43]

Fetal liver cells have also been employed to correct the immune defects of infants with SCIDS.[19a,86a] Transfusion of irradiated frozen red blood cells containing the enzyme restored humoral and cell-mediated immunity in one patient with adenosine deaminase deficiency and SCIDS.[82] Another autosomal recessive variant of SCIDS with lymphopenia and normal immunoglobulin of one or all classes was first described by Nezelof et al.[73] Although the onset of symptoms may be delayed until the end of the second or third year, the clinical features are similar to those of SCIDS. Plasma cells are abundant, but antigenic stimulation does not result in a detectable antibody rise and Coombs-positive hemolytic anemia is common. A half dozen infants with reticular dysgenesis have had severe neutropenia with complete or incomplete absence of myeloid precursors and no erythroid cells or megakaryocytes in the bone marrow, in addition to all of the other clinical and pathologic findings in SCIDS.[1,76] They failed to survive beyond 3 months of age.

Wiskott-Aldrich syndrome. Wiskott-Aldrich syndrome is a sex-linked recessive immunologic deficiency disorder characterized by thrombocytopenia, eczema, and recurrent infection. The child usually experiences bleeding episodes caused by thrombocytopenia as one initial manifestation of the disease. A characteristic eczematous rash appears by several months of age and becomes progressively more severe and difficult to control. This is combined with an excessive number of infections of the skin, middle ear, and respiratory tract, frequently accompanied by recurrent *Herpesvirus hominis* infection. Life-threatening infections with cytomegalovirus and *Pneumocystis carinii* have also been recorded. Both gram-positive and gram-negative bacteria, as well as viruses and fungi, cause these severe infections. Except for the eczema, the affected boys do not have other manifestations of allergy such as asthma or sensitivity to pollens.

Clinical and laboratory features. Physical examination reveals only eczema and petechiae during the first few months of life; however, as the child ages, eczema may involve the arms, legs, and scalp as well as the more typical antecubital and popliteal fossa areas. Splenomegaly and hepatomegaly are frequently present. The tympanic membranes are dull, and a chronic purulent discharge is frequently seen in the ears. The lungs become chronically infected and rales and rhonchi are often observed. Conjunctivitis and chronic keratitis caused by herpesvirus infection of the eye are another feature frequently observed in the physical examination.

The serum IgM concentration is usually low, but the IgG level is normal and IgA and IgE levels are usually elevated. Isohemagglutinins are regularly absent from the serum,[58] reflecting the most consistent defect in synthesis of specific antibody to polysaccharide antigens.[34] Antibody responses to Vi antigen of *Escherichia coli* and pneumococcal polysaccharide types I and II are almost totally absent. In addition to absence of polysaccharide antigenic responses, responses to protein antigens including keyhole limpet hemocyanin (KLH); poliovirus types I, II, and III; and diphtheria and tetanus toxoids are suppressed, whereas responses to complex antigens having adjuvant properties such as *Brucella abortus,* tularemia antigen, and typhoid vaccine are normal.[15] There is hypercatabolism of immunoglobulin proteins resulting in an increased synthetic rate.[14] Transient uncontrolled clonal proliferation of IgG-producing cells results in production of paraproteins.[84]

Lymphocyte counts as well as total circulating B lymphocyte counts are normal.[46] Circulating T lymphocytes have been variably described as normal to decreased.[97] The children are anergic with failure to demonstrate delayed-type hypersensitivity to common microbial antigens such as *Candida albicans, Trichophyton,* streptokinase-streptodornase, mumps, purified protein derivative, diphtheria or tetanus toxoids, or foreign antigens such as dinitrocholorobenzene or KLH.[26] However, even during the first few months of life their blood lymphocytes will proliferate in response to mitogenic agents such as phytohemagglutinin.[75] These stimulated lymphocytes elaborate lymphokines including MIF, lymphotoxin, and monocyte chemotactic factor. Cytotoxic effector and killer T and B lymphocyte function in vitro are normal.[97] Complement levels are normal or elevated. Response to hepatitis B virus infection is normal, as evidenced by the ability to make antibody to hepatitis B surface antigen and a lack of chronic hepatitis B antigen carrier state. Blood neutrophils reduce NBT and kill bacteria normally, although adherence to nylon fibers and chemotaxis is decreased. Lymphocyte-derived chemotactic factor production was increased; this was thought to explain the diminished chemotactic responsiveness of mononuclear leukocytes in patients with the Wiskott-Aldrich syndrome.[2] Interferon production is also normal.

Thrombocytopenia is always present, although it varies in degree. Autologous platelets labeled with ^{51}Cr have a shortened life span.[9] Platelets from normal donors, on the other hand, survive normally in affected children.[59,79] Platelet adhesiveness to collagen is defective and platelet aggregation with ADP, collagen, or epinephrine is severely depressed. Platelets are somewhat smaller than normal and their glycogen content is one-third to one-half normal. The number of megakaryocytes in the bone marrow is usually normal to only slightly decreased. Anemia is variable and depends on the degree of gastrointestinal bleeding. There is a 5% to 10% incidence of immunoglobulin-positive hemolytic anemia that may occur concomitant with viral infections or during transfer factor therapy.[10] Variable degrees of eosinophilia occur.

Pathology. Thymus and lymphoid tissue is variably involved. Younger children's lymph nodes show only slight depletion of thymic-dependent areas, and follicular formation is normal. In contrast, older patients have marked depletion of both thymic-dependent and thymic-independent areas and follicle formation is poor or nonexistent. Children with longer survival and young adults are prone to develop malignant neoplasms of the reticuloendothelial system, including histiocytic and lymphocytic lymphoma, myelogenous leukemia, and multiple myeloma.[39] Recent cases include histiocytic lymphoma of the skin in an 18-year-old receiving transfer factor and of the brain in a 19-year-old.[47,96]

Treatment. Bleeding, especially of the gastrointestinal tract, usually responds to platelet transfusions. Splenectomy is contraindicated because of the increased risk of fulminant septicemia after splenectomy.[52] Prednisone and other steroids have failed to increase platelet levels. Antibiotics have been useful to control bacterial infections of the respiratory tract and blood as well as eczematoid skin infections. The long-term use of penicillin to eradicate β-hemolytic *Streptococcus,* often a pathogen in the skin, seems of use in this disease. Frozen or irradiated plasma from a single donor given every 3 weeks to supply passive antibody may be of some value.[102]

Bone marrow transplantation has been performed in four patients, with clinical improvement and partial restoration of immune function in two[5] and complete correction in the other two.[78a]

Transfer factor, a low molecular weight substance found in lymphocytes, has the capacity to transfer delayed hypersensitivity to an unsensitized recipient. Therapy with transfer factor has restored skin test reactivity and improved the clinical status of certain patients with Wiskott-Aldrich syndrome, especially the group lacking monocyte-macrophage receptors for IgG.[99] After one or more treatment courses those patients who respond to transfer factor showed reduction in frequency and severity of infections, clearing of eczema, regression of splenomegaly, and in some cases improved control of bleeding. Controlled studies to determine the efficacy of transfer factor are still needed.

PREPARATION OF TRANSFER FACTOR. Transfer factor is prepared from 450 ml of blood collected in 50 ml syringes and mixed with sodium EDTA and 10% dextran. The plasma buffy coat layer is collected, pooled, and centrifuged at 1,000 rpm for 10 minutes at 4° C to provide a total volume of approximately 1.5 ml packed cells and a total count of 1.5×10^9 cells. The cells are resuspended in 4 ml pyrogen-free saline and alternately frozen and thawed ten times. Magnesium and DNase* are added to the mixture, which is incubated at 37° for 30 minutes. The resultant cell lysate is dialyzed against 500 ml distilled water in the cold for 2 days and redialyzed by the same procedure. The dialysate containing transfer factor is lyophilized and stored at −20° C. Before use it is dissolved in 200 ml of sterile distilled water at room temperature and passed through a 0.45 μ Millipore filter. On use 1 ml of transfer factor preparation, representing the extract from 7.5×10^8 white cells, is injected subcutaneously into the deltoid area. Another 0.1 ml is injected intradermally in the forearm to test for local transfer.

Prognosis. Early death is primarily related to massive bleeding episodes or overwhelming infections. Survival to puberty is rare, and with in-

---

*Worthington Biochemical Corp., Freehold, N.J.

creasing age the development of lymphoreticular malignancy, a common cause of death, becomes more likely.[55]

Ataxia telangiectasia. Ataxia telangiectasia is a complex disorder characterized by the appearance in early childhood of cerebellar ataxia, ocular and cutaneous telangiectasia, and frequent severe respiratory infections associated with lymphoid tissue abnormalities and an immune deficiency state. IgA, the chief immunoglobulin in external secretions, is usually absent in the serum,[107] but low molecular weight IgM is usually present.[103] Defects of humoral and cellular immunity may coexist. The thymus gland may be abnormal or entirely absent.

Clinical and laboratory features. The presenting symptoms usually are recognized when the child begins to walk. At that time the gait becomes ataxic and speech becomes increasingly dysarthnic, and with time choreoathetosis, myoclonic jerks, and intention tremors develop. Many but not all patients have an increased incidence of bacterial infections of the upper and lower respiratory system, including the nasal sinuses and middle ears, with onset between the ages of 3 and 8 years. Skin infections are less common. The third major clinical manifestation, conjunctival telangiectasia, appears between the ages of 2 and 8 years or even later. Fifty percent of patients subsequently have telangiectasia of the skin exposed to friction and trauma, such as the nasal bridge, the ear, and the flexure folds of the neck and extremities, but typically the mucous membranes are spared.

A positive family history is obtained in more than 50% of cases and is thought to follow an autosomal recessive inheritance pattern. Malignancy is more commonly encountered with increasing age, especially reticulum cell sarcoma, malignant lymphomas, leukemia, Hodgkin's disease, and certain brain tumors.[80] Since the gene frequency of heterozytes in the population is about 1%, study showed relatives of homozygotes to have a five-fold greater risk than the general population for development of malignant neoplasms before 45 years of age, especially ovarian, gastric, and biliary system carcinomas, leukemias, and lymphomas.[104]

Approximately 50% of affected children are short statured, falling below the third percentile for height and weight. Telangiectasias confined to the conjunctiva or extending to other skin surfaces are present in the majority. Gray hair is present; seborrheic dermatitis, pigmented nevi, café au lait spots, and vitiligo are occasionally noted. Associated with chronic bronchiectasis is the development of pulmonary osteoarthropathy or clubbing. Lymphoid tissue is reduced in most patients and lymphadenopathy and hepatosplenomegaly

are not usually seen.[65] Findings in the neurologic examination vary, depending on the progress of the neurologic function. Earliest findings are cerebellar ataxia and nystagmus. Ocular motor dyspraxia, choreoathetosis, myoclonic jerks, and loss of deep tendon reflexes are occasionally seen. Older patients tend to have distal weakness accompanied by wasting and loss of vibration and poor perception. Half of the patients have low intellectual abilities.

One third of the patients have lymphocytopenia with absolute lymphocyte counts of less than 1.5×10^9/liter. Despite chronic pulmonary disease and cyanosis, polycythemia is rare. Hepatic dysfunction with elevations in serum alkaline phosphatase, SGOT, SGPT, and LDH occur in almost half of the patients. About half of the patients have abnormal carbohydrate metabolism with glucose intolerance, elevated fasting levels of plasma insulin, excessive insulin production, and failure of insulin to reduce blood sugar levels. Glucosuria and ketosis are not seen. On the other hand, growth hormone levels, as well as the response to hypoglycemia, appear to be normal.[95] Secretion of urinary gonadotropins in postpubertal patients and thyroid function are generally normal.

Seventy percent to 80% have undetectable or deficient quantities of IgA in their serum, respiratory tract, and intestinal secretions. However, levels of circulating IgA-bearing lymphocytes are normal or increased but reduced along the respiratory and intestinal tract. Serum IgE is undetectable in more than 90% of the patients. Serum IgM levels tend to be elevated, and IgG and IgD levels are normal. The serum antibody response to antigenic challenge is below average and local secretory antibody responses are uniformly impaired.

Pathology and pathogenesis. Lymph nodes are small with decreased numbers of follicles and germinal centers. Plasma cells may be normal or diminished in the medullary cords. Reticulum cell hyperplasia is pronounced even in the severely lymphocyte-depleted lymph nodes. Lymph nodes along the gastrointestinal tract are hypocellular and underdeveloped. The thymus is often absent or very small. Lymphocytes are sparse and there is no differentiation between cortex and medulla with few exceptions. Hassall's corpuscles are absent.[12,54] Chromosomal studies of patients' and family members' peripheral blood lymphocytes and cultured skin fibroblasts reveal an apparently abnormal chromosome possessing a large acrocentric marker chromosome, $14Q+$.[25,77] More recent studies on the DNA repair mechanisms of x-ray–damaged human fibroblasts in ataxia telangiectasia show that these cells lack functional endonuclease and thus fail to initiate repair of DNA[11]; this is similar to the observed effect of actinomycin D.[50]

Treatment. Plasma infusions provide missing IgA and have been of modest help in decreasing the frequency of infections. Thymic gland transplantation to reconstitute T cells has been less successful in the United States than in the Soviet Union.[63] The use of transfer factor has recently shown promise in clinical trials in Switzerland.[35] There have been few attempts at immunologic reconstitution. Transplantation of thymus and spleens from fetuses aged 27 to 36 weeks have failed to improve immune function in patients.[45] Recent attempts at bone marrow transplantation without immunosuppression of the patients produced only transient improvement of skin test reactivity thought to be related to transfer factor activity rather than to bone marrow transplantation per se.[18] One patient treated with dantrolene experienced a dramatic response to his neurologic deficits.[21]

Cartilage-hair hypoplasia with immunodeficiency. Cartilage-hair hypoplasia is a form of short-limb dwarfism characterized clinically by sparse and fine scalp hair, eyebrows, and eyelashes with shortened long bones, loose joints producing hyperextension at the elbows, shortened and pudgy hands, and hypoplastic nails.[66] This disease is thought to be autosomal recessive. Immunodeficiency is characterized by defective cell-mediated immunity. These patients may suffer malabsorption and are susceptible to fulminant and fatal varicella infections. X-ray films reveal irregular sclerosis, cystic changes, and a scalloped appearance of the metaphyseal portion of the long bones. The skull and spine are usually normal, in contrast to those of patients with achondroplasia.

Laboratory studies reveal significant lymphopenia, abnormal delayed hypersensitive skin test reactions, failure to be sensitized to 2,4-dinitrochlorobenzene, diminished peripheral blood response to phytohemagglutinin, and delayed rejection of skin homografts. Additional patients with cyclic neutropenia have been reported.[64] In patients with antibody-mediated immune defects γ-globulin replacement may be of benefit. Thymic transplant has resulted in partial immunologic reconstitution of one patient.[51] Although most patients lack severe responses to live viral vaccines and do not have deficient antibody-mediated immunity, patients with these features have also been described.[93]

Disorders related to infection
INFECTIOUS MONONUCLEOSIS

Infectious mononucleosis is a disease that has fascinated clinicians as well as laboratory investigators for more than half a century. Today the disease is well recognized by its clinical manifestations, the appearance of atypical lymphocytes in the peripheral blood, and the development of heterophile and Epstein-Barr virus antibody responses in affected patients.

Historical perspective

Sprunt and Evans[190] were the first to call attention to the three types of atypical lymphocytes occurring in the blood of patients with infectious mononucleosis. Laboratory confirmation of the disease was placed on firm ground by the great work of Paul and Bunnell[169] and Davidsohn[129] who recognized in the serum of patients with infectious mononucleosis an antibody that regularly agglutinated sheep red blood cells, which they termed heterophil antibodies. The gamut of clinical manifestations was compiled by Hoagland[148] from 200 cases occurring in the military.

Etiology

In 1964 Epstein et al.[135] cultured a herpeslike virus from lymphoblasts in patients with East African Burkitt's lymphoma, a malignant tumor involving lymphoid tissue that most often affects children in East Africa and tropical areas of the West Indies, New Guinea, and parts of South America. Two years later intracellular viral antigens were identified by use of a fluorescent antibody directed against Epstein-Barr virus (EBV).[142] A year later a laboratory technician who had previously been shown to have serum devoid of antibodies to EBV and in whom attempts to culture leukocytes had been unsuccessful, developed infectious mononucleosis. Following her illness, not only did she develop EBV antibodies, but it also became possible to culture her leukocytes. One percent to 3% of these cultured leukocytes contained EBV antigen.[141,142,143] This chance observation led to examination of sequentially collected sera obtained from freshmen at Yale University and stored in the expectation that some of these students would develop infectious mononucleosis. All students who contracted infectious mononucleosis developed significant rises in antibody titer to EBV. Although their heterophil antibodies declined to undetectable levels within 2 to 3 months, EBV antibodies persisted.[138]

Several distinct groups of EBV-related antigens can be differentiated by immunofluorescence or other serologic procedures. These groups include EBV capsid antigen (VCA), EBV cell membrane antigen (MA), EBV-induced early antigen (EA) (both diffuse [D] and restricted [R] components), and EBV nuclear antigen (NA), as well as soluble complement fixing (S-CF) antigens and neutralizing (N) antigens unrelated to the other groups. After EBV infection levels of IgM antibody to VCA and EA rise temporarily, whereas IgG antibodies to VCA, MA, NA, S-CF, and N persist for life. Detection of IgM VCA antibody probably will prove to be the best system for proving recent or current infection, although the IgG VCA antibody is more available at present.

There is now complete agreement that EBV causes infectious mononucleosis. The virus can be recovered from peripheral leukocytes and throat washings of patients with infectious mononucleosis,[144] and specific receptors for EBV have been found on B lymphocytes.[151] Exudative tonsillitis and heterophile antibodies have been reproduced experimentally in monkeys inoculated with EBV.[164,185]

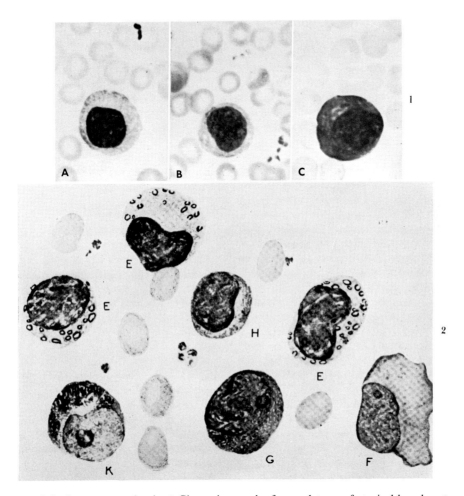

Fig. 20-8. Infectious mononucleosis. **1,** Photomicrograph of several types of atypical lymphocytes found in the blood smear of patients with infectious mononucleosis. **A** and **C** posses a finely vacuolated cytoplasm giving a foamy appearance, exaggerated in **C** by the deep basophilia. The color of the cytoplasm with Wright's stain varies from a slate color to the deep blue of a plasma cell. The nuclear pattern in **B** is not so coarse as that in the other cells and is more immature, with finer strands of lighter staining chromatin. Several nucleoli are present. This cell resembles somewhat the lymphoblast and is often referred to as the Downey type III cell (see **K** in **2**). (Courtesy Dr. Ralph L. Engle, Jr., New York, N.Y.)

2, Drawings of representative cells in the blood smear of patients with infectious mononucleosis. Although a number of different cell types usually appear in the blood smear at one time, especially at the height of the disease, all of these cells were not found together in any single case. **F** is a cell with irregular edges, eccentric nucleus, abundant cytoplasm, and concentration of basophilia in the periphery. A lightly staining perinuclear zone is observed in **K**. Deep basophilia of the cytoplasm is noticeable in **G, H,** and **K**. Vacuolation of the cytoplasm is present in **E** and **G**. The finer vacuoles and deep basophilia in **G** give the cytoplasm a foamy appearance, an important diagnostic feature. Cells of type K occurred most infrequently. The nucleus of the K-type cell stains lightly and approaches in immaturity the nucleus of the lymphoblasts. (From Smith, C. H.: Am. J. Dis. Child. **62:**231, 1941.)

Clinical features

Symptoms. The onset of the disease usually begins with subtle prodromata such as excessive fatigue, malaise, sweating, fever, headache, and anorexia; nausea, vomiting, and photophobia occasionally occur. The most common symptom and the usual presenting complaint is a sore throat, which develops several days after the onset of nonspecific symptoms and then increases in severity over the next week.

Physical signs. Fever is uniformly present and usually persists for several weeks. The pharynx, uvula, and soft palate are edematous and erythematous. A tonsillar and pharyngeal exudate is present in one third to one half of the cases and often cannot be distinguished from typical group A β-hemolytic streptococcal tonsillitis or diphtheria. Sharply circumscribed red spots up to 1 mm in diameter occur at the junction of the soft and hard palate during the second and third week of illness in one third to one half of the cases. Lymphadenopathy is invariably present and reaches a maximum by 10 days after the onset of symptoms. The posterior cervical nodes are the most commonly involved but axillary, inguinal, occipital, postauricular, and epitroclear nodes may also be prominent. Enlargement of anterior cervical nodes without posterior cervical node enlargement is unusual. The lymph nodes are slightly painful and tender, but they are not matted and are fairly movable. Splenomegaly has been reported in 50% to 75% of cases and in most instances the enlargement is not massive. Hepatomegaly is detected in 25% of the cases and may be associated with slight liver tenderness. Mild clinical jaundice is present in 5% to 10% of cases. A rash is observed in 5% to 10% of cases; it may be erythematous, macular, scarlatiniform, urticarial, or petechial in appearance. Ten percent of normal children administered ampicillin develop rashes, but when the drug is administered to patients with infectious mononucleosis the incidence of rashes has been reported to be between 69% and 100%.[154]

Laboratory findings

Leukopenia caused by a reduction in total numbers of circulating granulocytes may be present at the onset, but the total white blood cell count usually rises during the febrile stage of the illness. A range of 15 to 25 × 10⁹/liter is usual; total leukocyte counts above 40 × 10⁹/liters are unusual.[122] During the first 48 hours of the illness polymorphonuclear leukocytes predominate, but by the end of the first week a mononuclear leukocytosis with an array of atypical lymphocytes becomes evident. Patients with infectious mononucleosis have more than 25% atypical lymphocytes, whereas patients with other illnesses such as acquired cytomegalovirus disease, acquired

toxoplasmosis, viral hepatitis, viral pneumonia, herpes zoster, herpes simplex, roseola, rubella, adenovirus infection, and influenza type B have fewer than 25% atypical lymphocytes in their blood. Both T and B lymphocytes can be identified in the atypical lymphocyte population.[140,168] Atypical lymphocytes contain either dark, basophilic cytoplasm with vacuolization, a perinuclear clear zone, and an indented mature nucleus with dense nuclear chromatin (type I Downey cell) or lighter blue cytoplasm with less vacuolization and a round nucleus with coarse chromatin (type II Downey cell). Rarely a frank lymphoblast without abundant cytoplasm and a nucleus containing fine chromatin and an occasional nucleolus as noted in leukemia is also seen (type III Downey cell)[131] (Fig. 20-8). Electron microscopic studies of atypical lymphocytes in mononucleosis show an increase in cytoplasmic ribosomes as also noted in normal lymphocytes after stimulation by phytohemagglutinin.[184] The bone marrow of individuals with infectious mononucleosis usually demonstrates myeloid hyperplasia, and atypical lymphocytes are only rarely noted.[162]

The original serologic test for infectious mononucleosis was the Paul-Bunnell test, in which sera from patients with the disease agglutinated suspensions of sheep red blood cells.[169] The heterophil antibody is an IgM antibody produced against a variety of antigens and is absorbed by beef red blood cells but not guinea pig kidney cells.[129] Heterophil antibody rises after the first week of illness, reaches a maximum titer at 2 to 3 weeks, and falls at 6 to 8 weeks. Contrary to a popular idea,[193] children younger than 5 years are capable of developing a positive heterophil titer.[115] It is now clear that a spectrum of diseases can be associated with EBV infection in small children, ranging from a nonspecific febrile illness and illnesses associated with diarrhea and vomiting to classical infectious mononucleosis.

The presumptive agglutination test employs nonabsorbed serum and sheep erythrocytes and may be positive in patients with viral hepatitis, viral pneumonia, lymphoma, leukemia, tuberculosis, or serum sickness and after immunizations with A and B blood group antigens, as occurs in

Table 20-5. Scheme of differential heterophil agglutination

Serum	Heterophil agglutinins after absorption by	
	Guinea pig kidney	Beef red cells
Infectious mononucleosis	Present	Absent
Normal	Absent	Present
Serum sickness	Absent	Absent

mismatched blood transfusions. However, these antibodies, but not true heterophil antibodies, will be absorbed completely by Forssman antigens. Serum heterophil titers of 1:56 or greater for the presumptive or Paul-Bunnell test and 1:28 or greater after guinea pig absorption are generally accepted as positive indication of infectious mononucleosis[148] (Table 20-5). Commercial simplifications of the test are now available. The Monospot test* utilizes the patient's serum treated either with beef red cell stroma or guinea pig kidney and the more sensitive formalinized horse red cell agglutination as indicator. The slide test is positive when agglutination occurs in the presence of sera treated with guinea pig kidney and does not occur in the presence of sera treated with beef red cell stroma. Unlike the original test, which requires a 24-hour laboratory procedure, the spot test can be done in 2 minutes as an office procedure with the reagents conveniently provided in a kit; it is 96% to 99% accurate.

Clinical course

The illness generally is milder in younger children. In young adults the illness lasts 2 to 3 weeks but may be more prolonged when liver involvement is more severe. Postconvalescent lethargy may last for several months. Recurrences are rare, although nonspecific viral illness may cause an anamnestic heterophil response.[147]

Complications

Although a variety of complications can occur with infectious mononucleosis, they are rare. The incidence of neurologic involvement ranges from 0.37% to 7.3%[186] and includes Guillain-Barré syndrome, facial nerve palsy, meningoencephalitis, aseptic meningitis, transverse myelitis, seizures, peripheral neuritis, optic neuritis, acute psychoses, diplopia, and Reye's syndrome.[174] Although pericarditis with friction rub and chest pain is rare,[189] transient ECG abnormalities have been observed in up to 6% of cases.[146] Spontaneous rupture of the spleen occurs in less than 1% of cases, usually in the second to third week of illness[119,180,183] with sudden shock or with abdominal or left shoulder pain. Interstitial pneumonia and pleural effusions occur in less than 5% of cases.[136] Airway obstruction by pharyngeal edema and massive tonsillar enlargement has occurred. Intravenous hydrocortisone may be of value but nasotracheal or orotracheal intubation or tracheostomy is occasionally required to relieve the obstruction.[141]

Although abnormal urinary findings have been recorded,[191] renal function has been reported to be impaired and the entity of infectious mononucle-

osis nephritis has been challenged by many authors who ascribe its real cause to poststreptococcal complications. Throat cultures from patients with infectious mononucleosis are positive for β-hemolytic streptococci only as frequently as those from a control group of patients. Thus the inflamed pharynx and necrotic tonsils are seldom subject to bacterial superinfection and there is no indication for routine use of antibiotics when infectious mononucleosis is diagnosed.[124]

Hematologic complications include autoimmune hemolytic anemia in 3% of cases.[120] About 70% of the patients with hemolytic anemia have a positive direct Coombs test and a similar number have increased titers of cold agglutinins. The latter antibodies usually have anti-i specificity but anti-N and anti-I antibodies have also been demonstrated.[121,150] The hemolytic anemia is generally transient with a good prognosis. Modest degrees of thrombocytopenia are common, but bleeding is rare.[123] Most instances of mild thrombocytopenia are probably related to either platelet trapping or immune destruction in the spleen. Immunologic dysfunction of both the T and B cell systems include acquired agammaglobulinemia and acquired T cell dysfunction leading to a fatal outcome in some.[116,172] Fatal infectious mononucleosis has been described in twenty patients; nine deaths were the result of neurologic manifestations, three of splenic rupture, three of secondary infection, two of hepatic failure, one of myocarditis, and two of causes unrelated to the disease.[174]

Treatment

Treatment is symptomatic. Most patients prefer to establish their own degree of ambulation depending on the severity of the illness. Antipyretics will suffice to reduce the degree of fever, but salicylates should be avoided if thrombocytopenia is present. Severe respiratory distress as a result of hypertrophy of the nasopharyngeal airway occurs in some cases and seems to respond rather dramatically to corticosteroid therapy. Endotracheal intubation or tracheostomy may be required in some cases. Antibiotics are not indicated in most cases since superinfection with bacteria is extremely rare. Severe autoimmune hemolytic anemia or rapidly progressing hemorrhage caused by thrombocytopenic purpura is an indication for corticosteroid therapy. A reasonable dosage schedule of prednisone is 1 to 2 mg/kg/day for 1 to 2 weeks, depending on the response, with rapid tapering of the drug over the next week.

HETEROPHIL-NEGATIVE MONONUCLEOSIS SYNDROMES
Acquired cytomegalovirus infection

The classic clinical and hematologic picture of infectious mononucleosis with negative heterophil

---

*Wampole Diagnostics, Inc., Stamford, Conn.

White blood cells*

antibody is usually not associated with EBV infection. Cytomegalovirus appears to be the most common cause of heterophil-negative mononucleosis.[126,152] The clinical picture resembles that of EBV infection. The patient experiences the onset of fever, malaise, and fatigue, but sore throat is unusual. Physical examination generally reveals hepatosplenomegaly and lymphadenopathy, but the limited degree of lymphadenopathy and the absence of tonsillar pharyngitis distinguish it from EBV infection.[155] The percentage of atypical lymphocytes in the blood rarely exceeds 15%. The diagnosis can be established by demonstrating a significant rise in cytomegalovirus antibody in the blood. Although the virus can be isolated from the pharynx and urine, it may be shed chronically and its relationship with the acute disease is more difficult to establish.

Postperfusion syndrome

The advent of the cardiopulmonary bypass technique employed in open heart surgery has resulted in the recognition of an infectious mononucleosis–like syndrome characterized by fever, splenomegaly, and the appearance of atypical lymphocytes in the blood 3 to 6 weeks after operation.[118,156] The disorder has become known as the postperfusion syndrome, and its incidence varies from 1% to as high as 20% of patients undergoing open heart surgery. Cytomegalovirus has been recovered from these patients, and complement-fixing antibody to cytomegalovirus can also be detected.[159] Antibodies to EBV have been found in 8% of patients undergoing open heart surgery with or without extracorporeal circulation. Only a few of the EBV infections are clinically expressed and only rarely is heterophil antibody present.[145] Since both EBV and cytomegalovirus are carried chronically in circulating white blood cells, transfusion of virus is a logical explanation for the pathogenesis of the postperfusion syndrome. The course is benign, and symptoms subside within 3 to 7 weeks. Its recognition is helpful from a management and prognosis point of view since it may prevent unnecessary investigation and antibiotic therapy for possible subacute bacterial endocarditis following open heart surgery.

This condition is to be differentiated from the postcardiotomy syndrome, which is an uncommon complication of heart surgery occurring after a latent period. It is identified by fever and pleuro-pericarditis,[133,177] elevated erythrocyte sedimentation rate, and spontaneous resolution. Arthralgia and tendency to relapse are less common features. Atypical cells are only rarely noted. Corticosteroid administration rapidly suppresses the disorder and when used prophylactically prevents its appearance. A hypersensitivity reaction in an immuno-

logic sense, with positive tests for heart antibodies, has been demonstrated.[177]

Acquired toxoplasmosis infection

Another cause of the infectious mononucleosis syndrome is acquired infection with *Toxoplasma gondii*. Generalized lymphadenopathy is prominent and is often associated with generalized muscle pains. A modest increase in atypical circulating lymphocytes is noted and a rise in complement-fixing Sabin-Feldman dye test hemagglutination or immunofluorescent antibody can be demonstrated.[175]

Other virus infections

The infectious mononucleosis syndrome has been described in patients in whom adenovirus infection, rubella, and herpes simplex have been found.[137,160] Infectious and serum hepatitis may be associated with the presence of atypical lymphocytes; however, in all cases the percentage usually does not exceed 15%.

Noninfectious systemic diseases

Patients receiving drugs such as para-amino-salicylic acid (PAS), phenytoin (Dilantin), and diaminodiphenylsulfone (dapsone) have been reported to develop an infectious mononucleosis–like picture.[160] Hypersensitivity reactions and serum sickness–like reactions may also provoke atypical lymphocytosis.[182]

LYMPHOCYTOSIS

The relative number of each type of leukocyte is calculated from the leukocyte count and the percentage found in the peripheral smear. When for some reason the polymorphonuclear leukocyte percentage is decreased, the numbers of lymphocytes appear elevated. A relative lymphocytosis is thus associated with a neutropenia and should be differentiated from an absolute increase. An absolute lymphocytosis is found in patients with (1) acute infectious lymphocytosis, (2) chronic (nonspecific) infectious lymphocytosis, (3) pertussis and related infections, and (4) syphilis, tuberculosis, and hyperthyroidism. A relative increase in lymphocytes is common in patients with conditions with a decreased number of granulocytes, such as the leukopenia of measles, rubella, exanthem subitum, and brucellosis. It will be recalled that following the first week of life lymphocytes normally predominate until the fourth or fifth year of life, and a lymphocytosis occurring during this period must be elevated from this level (Fig. 20-9). Occasionally in infancy a marked lymphocytosis transiently accompanies an infectious or post-infectious state that cannot be attributed to a specific cause.

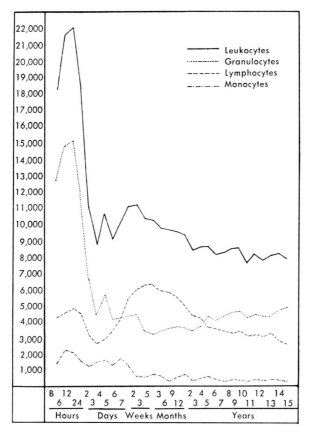

Fig. 20-9. Curves of average leukocyte counts from birth to 15 years of age. (From Kato, K.: J. Pediatr. **7**:7, 1935.)

Acute infectious lymphocytosis

Acute infectious lymphocytosis* is a specific entity of unknown etiology that is both infectious and contagious. It may occur sporadically or in epidemic form. The incubation period has been estimated to be between 12 and 21 days. It is characterized by hyperleukocytosis caused by an increase in small mature lymphocytes; the elevated blood levels persist for approximately 2 to 7 weeks. It is a benign infection, distinct from infectious mononucleosis, acute lymphoblastic and chronic lymphocytic leukemia, and miscellaneous infections associated with a lymphocytosis. The clinical signs and symptoms may be so mild as to escape attention, or the onset may be marked by varying degrees of constitutional reaction. A noteworthy feature is the absence of lymphadenopathy and enlargement of the spleen.

Incidence. The highest incidence is in children from 1 to 14 years of age, with most of the recorded cases occurring during the first 10 years of life.[134] In general the height of the leukocyte

count tends to vary inversely with the age of the patient.

Etiology. Attempts to identify a causative agent have thus far met with inconclusive results. Organisms obtained from routine nasopharyngeal cultures probably represent normal inhabitants or secondary invaders. They do not differ from the flora of patients exhibiting the usual hematologic response with similar respiratory infections. A bacterial or viral etiology has been postulated.[158] An adenovirus type 12 has been isolated from the upper respiratory tract of four children with a pertussis-like lymphocytosis.[166] In one of the patients the white cell count rose to 168×10^9/liter with a predominance of small mature lymphocytes. The additional finding of eosinophilia implicated acute infectious lymphocytosis rather than pertussis. The studies in this small series suggested that this agent is responsible for a pertussis-like illness with hematologic findings indistinguishable from and diagnostic of acute infectious lymphocytosis. This finding awaits confirmation in other cases.

In an epidemic[149] in a state school for retarded children, in whom white blood counts ranged be-

---

*References 127, 132, 166, 179, 187, 188.

tween 26 and 93 × 10^9/liter, a search was made for infectious and noninfectious agents. An enterovirus, untyped but resembling coxsackie virus A subgroup in physical, chemical, and host specificity, was isolated in 21% of the patients' stool specimens. Fourfold rises in neutralizing antibody against this enterovirus occurred in the sera of a significantly greater proportion of patients than in patient contacts. Recently this enterovirus (EVU-16) has been further characterized. It has a single-stranded RNA genome and contains a procapsid similar to other enteroviruses. However, attempts to induce lymphocytosis by the inoculation of EVU-16 into various animals, including immunologically aberrant "nude" mice, were unsuccessful. Since the disease often terminates with eosinophilia, stools were examined for intestinal parasites as an etiologic factor. *Giardia lamblia* was not an uncommon finding, but since it is a parasite that is ubiquitous in institutionalized children, its relationship to lymphocytosis remains in doubt.

Epidemiology. The disease occurs sporadically as multiple cases in families and in institutional epidemics.* It is therefore contagious but of a low degree of infectivity. It has been reported in North, Central, and South America, Europe, and Africa. In the epidemic reports the majority of patients had no positive physical findings. According to some reports, the patients had signs of respiratory infection or gastrointestinal distress, principally diarrhea.[171] In a large epidemic,[149] 4 months after investigation of the first case hyperleukocytosis with lymphocytosis had developed in twenty-seven children.

Incubation period. Because the abnormal white cell counts are unexpectedly encountered in the course of routine blood examinations, the exact onset and duration of the leukocytic changes are unknown. It is therefore difficult to designate a precise incubation period. From the available cases thus far reported, it has been possible to fix the approximate length of the incubation period between 12 and 21 days.

Pathology. Microscopic examination of lymph nodes in the few patients studied[188] revealed the striking proliferation of the lining reticuloendothelium with almost complete blockage of the sinuses by masses of these cells and degeneration of the lymph follicles. In a 14-year-old boy complaining of recurring abdominal pain, surgical exploration revealed a normal appendix. One of a group of shotty nodes in the ileocecal mesentery revealed hyperplasia of the follicles, some of which showed hyalinization and prominence of the cells lining the sinuses.[179]

Clinical features. The condition at times may be so mild as to escape attention, or the onset may be

marked in individual patients by varying degrees of constitutional reaction. Fever, upper respiratory infections, skin rashes, abdominal complaints, and meningoencephalitic manifestations may be present. Accidental discovery as the result of routine blood examinations is not uncommon, particularly in institutional epidemics. No consistent correlation is evident between the degree of leukocytosis and the severity of symptoms.

Nasopharynx. Mild infection of the upper respiratory tract is a common feature in symptomatic patients. The throat may be deeply injected at the time of the initial examination, and a history of recent infection of the upper respiratory tract frequently is elicited.

Nervous system. Increasing experience has shown that acute infectious lymphocytosis should be considered in the diagnosis of an acute febrile illness in which there are symptoms suggestive of central nervous system involvement. Headache, irritability, vertigo, and pain and slight stiffness of the back of the neck may occur without other signs of meningitis. The spinal fluid may show a slight pleocytosis with variations in the type of predominating cells,[192] although a slight increase in lymphocytes has been reported when the spinal fluid count was positive. This disease may simulate poliomyelitis and meningoencephalitis[127] since headache, stiffness of the neck, restlessness, fever, malaise, vomiting, sore throat, and identical spinal fluid changes may occur at the onset of both conditions. The blood counts readily separate both diseases. Differentiation between these conditions assumes particular importance when the symptoms occur during the summer and early fall.

Skin. A generalized morbilliform eruption and less commonly a herpetic eruption have been observed in patients during the first week of the disease.

Abdomen. Signs may be sufficiently pronounced to suggest an acute surgical condition with an elevated temperature, vomiting, and severe abdominal pain.[179] Diarrhea was the most prominent symptom in sixteen of twenty-eight patients in one epidemic.[171]

Spleen and lymph nodes. An important diagnostic criterion of infectious lymphocytosis is absence of significant enlargement of the spleen and lymph nodes. Preexisting cervical nodes, especially of the posterior chain, are usually sequelae of previous attacks of nasopharyngitis and are not directly related to the development of acute infectious lymphocytosis. Lymphadenopathy and enlargement of the spleen are absent, unless they existed prior to the onset of the disease.

Laboratory findings

Blood. The red cell count, hemoglobin content, platelet count, and sedimentation rate are normal if the disease is uncomplicated. When the constitu-

---

*References 117, 139, 161, 171, 176, 181.

tional reaction is severe, the hemoglobin content and the red blood cell count may drop to the lower limit of normal. The absence of anemia is an important feature in differentiating this ailment from acute lymphoblastic and chronic lymphatic leukemia and from the lymphocytosis occurring in prolonged postinfectious states. No deviations in hemostatic function have been observed.

The outstanding feature in patients with acute infectious lymphocytosis is the hyperleukocytosis with a relative and absolute increase in normal small mature lymphocytes (Figs. 20-10 and 20-11). White blood cell counts at the height of the disease are usually over 40 to 50 $\times$ 10^9/liter with a maximum recorded level over 100 $\times$ 10^9/liter. In the reported institutional epidemics the peak white blood cell counts in the individual patients ranged from 15 to 147 $\times$ 10^9/liter and lympho-

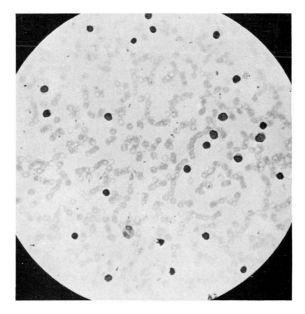

Fig. 20-10. Typical blood smear from a patient with acute infectious lymphocytosis. ($\times$400.)

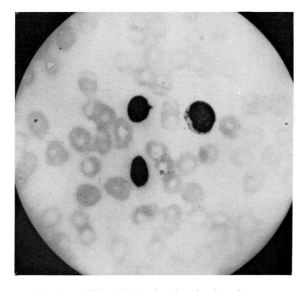

Fig. 20-11. Higher magnification of Fig. 20-10, showing that lymphocytes are mainly of the small variety and of uniform size and structure. Only occasionally are slightly larger or intermediate types encountered, but these are also mature. ($\times$1,000.) (From Smith, C. H.: J.A.M.A. **125:** 342, 1944.)

cytes from 60% to 97%.[181] The lymphocytes are mainly the small variety and are of uniform size and normal structure. Only occasionally are slightly larger or intermediate types encountered, but these are also mature cells. The nucleus in these cells is condensed and possesses the coarse chromatin masses of the normal mature lymphocytes. These lymphocytes have also been referred to as overripe and have been described as being smaller than normal with a dark purple chromatic material in the nucleus and with very little cytoplasm.[163]

A recent study of peripheral lymphocytes isolated from a 15-month-old boy with acute infectious lymphocytosis by the Ficoll-Hypaque density gradient technique revealed that 46% of the proliferating lymphocytes formed rosettes with sheep red blood cells, identifying them as T cells, whereas only 2% of the cells had surface immunoglobulins stained by the immunofluorescent technique, identifying them as B cells. Since the white blood count was 178 × 10^9/liter with 96% small lymphocytes, of which 2% were B cells, 46% T cells, and 52% null cells, the results show that the absolute number of T and null cells was remarkably increased, whereas the absolute number of B cells remained normal.[128]

The duration of the markedly abnormal leukocytic reaction is usually 3 to 5 weeks and occasionally 7 weeks. An elevation in the percentage of eosinophilic leukocytes occurs frequently during the course of the disease, usually at or following the peak of leukocytosis.

Bone marrow. The myeloid elements and nucleated red cells are normal in number. In many patients the bone marrow shows an increase in the total number of nucleated cells and in the percentage of small mature lymphocytes; otherwise it is not abnormal.

Heterophil agglutination (Paul-Bunnell) test. The heterophil agglutination test is uniformly negative.

Differential diagnosis (Table 20-6). Lymphocytic reactions in childhood are difficult to interpret because a predominance of lymphocytes and a greater lability of the blood-forming mechanism are common to this age period. In the differentiation of acute infectious lymphocytosis, these physiologic hematopoietic responses, as well as certain specific conditions in which the lymphocytes or their precursors are known to be increased, must be evaluated.

Infectious mononucleosis. Infectious mononucleosis is usually more severe and characterized by fever, sore throat, rash, rarely jaundice, enlargement and tenderness of the lymph nodes, and often splenomegaly. The febrile phase lasts for 1 to 3 weeks, but enlargement of the glands and spleen may persist. Acute infectious lymphocytosis, on the other hand, may run an asymptomatic course, or there may be transient sore throat, fever, and constitutional symptoms. Lymph nodes and spleen are not enlarged. The heterophil antibody reaction is usually positive in patients with infectious mononucleosis but is consistently negative in those with acute infectious lymphocytosis.

The blood picture constitutes the most important differential feature. In patients with infectious mononucleosis the total white blood cell count usually does not exceed 20 × 10^9/liter, whereas acute infectious lymphocytosis is characterized by a

Table 20-6. Differential diagnosis of acute infectious lymphocytosis*

	Acute infectious lymphocytosis	Infectious mononucleosis	Acute lymphoblastic leukemia	Chronic lymphocytic leukemia
Age (usual incidence)	First decade	First 3 decades	First and second decades	After 45 yr
Fever and systemic symptoms	Occasionally present	Usually present	Variably present	Infrequent
Enlarged lymph nodes	Absent	Present	Present	Present
Splenomegaly	Absent	Present in 50%	Present	Present
Leukocytosis	Extreme	Moderate	Leukopenia to marked	Usually pronounced
Lymphocytosis	Present	Present	Present	Present
Types of lymphocytes, diagnostic cells	Normal, small	Atypical, abnormal	Lymphoblasts	Mature, small
Anemia	Absent	Rare	Present	Late in course
Thrombocytopenia	Absent	Rare	Present	Present
Bone marrow lymphocytes	Increased in number; normal, small	Occasionally atypical	Lymphoblasts predominate	Lymphocytes predominate
Heterophil agglutination	Negative	Positive	Negative	Negative
Prognosis	Uniformly favorable	Favorable with few exceptions	Median survival, 5 years	Uniformly fatal

*From Smith, C. H.: Advances in pediatrics, vol. 2, Chicago, 1947, Year Book Medical Publishers, Inc.

hyperleukocytosis, with maximal levels frequently exceeding 50×10^9/liter. A more important feature of a hematologic differentiation rests in the morphologic appearance of the lymphocytes in the two conditions. In patients with acute infectious lymphocytosis the hyperleukocytosis is associated with a preponderance of small lymphocytes possessing a normal cytologic appearance. In those with infectious mononucleosis, however, the distinctive feature is the presence of characteristic atypical mononuclear cells. The variability of atypical lymphocytes and monocytes in persons with this disease contrasts sharply with the uniform size and normal structure of the cells in those with acute infectious lymphocytosis.

Acute lymphoblastic leukemia. The extreme leukocytosis and the predominance of lymphocytes in patients with acute infectious lymphocytosis have occasionally led to the erroneous diagnosis of acute lymphoblastic leukemia. Identification of the blast cell, which is invariably found in a careful search of the blood smear of patients with leukemia, is the distinguishing feature. The size of these cells varies from that of a small lymphocyte to twice that size. Lymphoblasts are usually readily distinguishable from small mature lymphocytes, which occasionally may resemble microlymphoblasts.

In patients with acute leukemia with a hyperleukocytosis of the magnitude found in those with acute infectious lymphocytosis, the blood exhibits not only large numbers of lymphoblasts but also a severe anemia and a decrease in platelets, and the spleen and lymph nodes are enlarged.

Examination of the bone marrow also serves to differentiate the two diseases. In acute lymphoblastic leukemia in children, bone marrow aspiration usually shows complete replacement of the bone marrow by blast cells. In children with acute infectious lymphocytosis, on the other hand, the myeloid and erythroblastic elements are present in normal proportions, and the chief abnormality in many patients consists of an increased percentage of normal lymphocytes.

Chronic lymphocytic leukemia. The blood picture of patients with acute infectious lymphocytosis resembles that of those with chronic lymphocytic leukemia in respect to the white blood cells. In patients with either of these diseases there is a hyperleukocytosis with a preponderance of small mature lymphocytes and the bone marrow shows increased percentages of normal small lymphocytes and is cellular. The age incidence of the two diseases, however, is very different since chronic lymphocytic leukemia is a disease of older persons. In patients with chronic lymphocytic leukemia the spleen and lymph nodes are enlarged, anemia and thrombocytopenia eventually develop,

and the outcome is uniformly fatal, in contrast to the negative physical and hematologic findings and favorable prognosis in patients with acute infectious lymphocytosis.

Leukemoid reactions. The hyperleukocytosis of infectious lymphocytosis cannot be regarded as a leukemoid reaction of the lymphoid type. The absence of immature and atypical cells in the blood and bone marrow precludes this designation. Moreover, the leukemoid reaction resulting from infection is transitory; the lymphocytic response in patients with acute infectious lymphocytosis is protracted. Pertussis as a cause of the extreme leukocytosis and lymphocytosis can be excluded by the absence of cough and characteristic clinical manifestations.

Miscellaneous infections. A number of specific infections are associated with lymphocytosis. Typhoid fever, brucellosis, and tuberculosis should be excluded by appropriate tests.

Pertussis. During the latter part of the catarrhal period or early paroxysmal stage, the total leukocyte count rises to a level from 15 to 50×10^9/liter. Lymphocytes account for 70% to 90% of the total increase in the number of leukocytes. The leukocytosis and lymphocytosis exceed those of any other febrile illness except infectious lymphocytosis. In one series[191] marked leukocytosis of more than 50×10^9/liter was found in only eight cases.

Available data render invalid the view that the lymphocytosis represents a peculiar individual response, the so-called constitutional lymphatic reaction. Patients with acute infectious lymphocytosis afflicted with antecedent, concurrent, or subsequent illnesses such as acute otitis media or pneumonia exhibit a neutrophilic response.

Treatment and prognosis. There is no specific therapy. Treatment is symptomatic and similar to that in patients with other acute infections of the upper respiratory tract. Because of the low infectivity of the condition, the large number of asymptomatic cases, and the brief span of constitutional reactions in the febrile cases, no isolation seems necessary. The prognosis in all cases has been uniformly excellent, and no sequelae have been observed.

It has been suggested that infectious lymphocytosis, which affects the hematopoietic system and in which the lymphatic system has at one time experienced such an extreme proliferative response, might be associated with long-term sequelae such as leukemia. A follow-up 19 years after a thirty-one–case epidemic of infectious lymphocytosis in Wisconsin showed that, in the twenty-five persons located and examined, no significant after-effects could be associated with this illness.[125,173]

Chronic nonspecific infectious lymphocytosis (low-grade fever syndrome)

Clinical features. The symptom complex of chronic nonspecific infectious lymphocytosis is characterized by a persistent slight to moderate leukocytosis and a preponderance of lymphocytes. It is frequently encountered in pediatric practice[178] and is distinct from acute infectious lymphocytosis. Difficulties in diagnosis arise when an acute infection of the upper respiratory tract is followed for prolonged periods by a low-grade fever, with the temperature ranging from 38° C up to and usually not exceeding 39° C. In addition to the protracted fever the symptom complex includes anorexia, pallor, irritability, fatigability, and abdominal pain localized to the region of the umbilicus. The fauces are injected, the tonsils, when present, are usually greatly hypertrophied, and postnasal discharge is frequent. At times, the superficial cervical lymph nodes are slightly enlarged. The heart and lungs are normal; there are no murmurs or other cardiac abnormalities. In infants and young children the spleen may be palpable, but this finding is inconstant, especially in older children. The age of incidence is usually from 6 months through 10 years, especially in the period from 3 to 6 years. Cases are less commonly observed between 3 and 6 months of age. In these infants moderate elevations of temperature (39° to 40° C) frequently interrupt the usual course of low-grade fever (temperature up to 39° C). Although these episodes are usually related to exacerbations of infection of the nasopharynx, other causes of lymphocytosis must be eliminated.

Laboratory findings. The accompanying slight to moderate leukocytosis and lymphocytosis usually persist for periods of months and sometimes a year or more. The total white blood cell counts usually range from 8 to 18×10^9/liter, rarely reaching 20×10^9/liter, with 60% to 80% lymphocytes. White blood cell counts reaching 25×10^9/liter are frequently observed in infants under 6 months of age. The hemoglobin ranges between 10 and 11 gm/dl, and the platelets are normal in number. Lymphocytosis in this group of patients with chronic disease resembles that in postinfectious states in infants and children. Most of the lymphocytes are of the small mature type, structurally similar to those in patients with acute infectious lymphocytosis. Occasionally cells of the larger variety are seen, which are of normal shape and possess a deeply basophilic cytoplasm and an eccentric nucleus that stains more intensely than that of the normal lymphocyte. The same depth of staining is observed in another type of lymphocyte, which is about 1½ times the size of a red cell and whose nucleus is round, oval, or slightly indented. In infants the zone of cellular cytoplasm is often wider and the basophilia deeper than in the corresponding cells of blood in older children. These larger cells are not specific, since they appear in increased numbers in the blood of young children during the active stage and convalescence of a large variety of infections and may occasionally be found in the blood of normal infants.

Differential diagnosis. Chronic nonspecific infectious lymphocytosis is not contagious and does not appear in epidemic form, in contrast to acute infectious lymphocytosis. Moreover, the acute disease is usually asymptomatic, the blood reaction is comparatively short and well defined, hyperleukocytosis is marked, and the disease is not characterized at any age period by either lymphadenopathy or splenomegaly.

Chronic nonspecific infectious lymphocytosis is often confused with infectious mononucleosis (especially in young children), acute lymphoblastic leukemia, and acute rheumatic fever. Not only is the heterophil agglutinin test negative in the patient with chronic infectious lymphocytosis, but the lymphocytes lack the irregularity of shape and the abundant, frequently vacuolated, and foamy cytoplasm that are distinctive features of the cells of patients with infectious mononucleosis.

Acute lymphoblastic leukemia is differentiated by the presence of lymphoblasts, hyperleukocytosis, often leukopenia, anemia (hemoglobin level below 10 gm/dl), and thrombocytopenia. Marked lymphadenopathy and splenomegaly are additional confirmatory features but may be absent in the patient with early disease. Examination of the bone marrow serves to differentiate the two diseases unequivocally, although this procedure is rarely necessary.

Many of the patients are referred with a diagnosis of acute rheumatic fever because of a more or less continuous low-grade fever, a failure to gain weight or a loss of weight, fatigability, and abdominal pain. From the hematologic standpoint, acute rheumatic fever is usually associated with moderate leukocytosis with polymorphonuclear leukocytes as the predominant cell in contrast to chronic nonspecific infectious lymphocytosis in which lymphocytosis characterizes the blood smear. The sedimentation rate is markedly increased in patients with rheumatic fever and does not approach normal until some time after the fever and clinical signs have abated, whereas in those with chronic lymphocytosis the sedimentation rate is normal or only slightly increased for short intervals. Nosebleeds; the development of carditis; pains in the arms, legs, and joints; subcutaneous nodules; and erythematous rashes are other features present in patients with rheumatic fever and absent in those with lymphocytic diseases.

A disease identical with or similar to chronic

infectious lymphocytosis has been reported as lymphocytic fever.[178] It occurs chiefly in children under 2 years of age with enlargement of the liver and spleen, slight lymphadenopathy, and a leukocytosis with a preponderance of small lymphocytes persisting for months and occasionally a year or more.

The lymphocytic blood picture in patients with chronic infectious lymphocytosis is a useful diagnostic aid in differentiating the abdominal pain, which may occur in both diseases, from surgical conditions and from nonspecific mesenteric lymphadenitis, which are associated with a neutrophilic response.

Treatment and prognosis. Chronic nonspecific infectious lymphocytosis may be a source of anxiety to both parents and physician. It is therefore desirable to emphasize that the prognosis is entirely favorable, that treatment is symptomatic, and that subsidence of the disease depends on relief of infection in the nasopharynx. Striking improvement often follows tonsillectomy, but tonsillectomy is not advocated as a routine measure.

Repeated temperature readings are unnecessary, and antibiotics are futile in altering the pattern of low-grade fever. Once the diagnosis is established, restriction of activities is unnecessary.

REFERENCES
Immune disorders

1. Alonso, K., Dew, J. M., and Starke, W. R.: Thymic alymphoplasia and congenital aleukocytosis (reticular dysgenesis), Arch. Pathol. **94:**179, 1972.
2. Altman, L. C., Snyderman, R., and Blaese, R. M.: Abnormalities of chemotactic lymphokine synthesis and mononuclear chemotaxis in Wiskott-Aldrich syndrome, J. Clin. Invest. **54:**486, 1974.
3. Ammann, A. J., and Hong, R.: Selective IgA deficiency. In Stiehm, E. R., and Fulginiti, V. A., eds.: Immunologic disorders in infants and children, Philadelphia, 1973, W. B. Saunders Co.
4. Anderson, J., Buxbaum, J., Citronbaum, R., et al.: IgM producing tumors in the BALB/c mouse: a model for B-cell maturation, J. Exp. Med. **140:**742, 1974.
5. August, C. S., Hathaway, W. E., Githens, J. H., et al.: Improved platelet function following bone marrow transplantation in an infant with the Wiskott-Aldrich syndrome, J. Pediatr. **82:**58, 1973.
6. August, C. S., Rosen, F. S., Filer, R. M., et al.: Implantation of a foetal thymus restoring immunological competence in a patient with thymic aplasia (DiGeorge's syndrome), Lancet **2:**1210, 1968.
7. Axelsen, N. H., Kirpatrick, C. H., and Buckley, R.H.: Precipitins to *Candida albicans* in chronic mucocutaneous candidiasis studied by crossed immunoelectrophoresis with intermediate gel, Clin. Exp. Immunol. **17:**385, 1974.
8. Bachmann, R.: Studies on the serum γ-A globulin level. III. The frequence of a-γ-A-globulinemia, Scand. J. Clin. Lab. Invest. **17:**316, 1965.
9. Baldini, M. G.: The nature of the platelet defect in the Wiskott-Aldrich syndrome, Ann. N.Y. Acad. Sci. **201:**437, 1972.
10. Ballow, M., and DuPont, B., and Good, R. A.: Autoimmune hemolytic anemia in Wiskott-Aldrich syndrome

during treatment with transfer factor, J. Pediatr. **83:**772, 1973.
11. Baterson, M. C., Smith, B. P., Lohman, B., et al.: Defective excision repair of gamma ray induced DNA in human (ataxia telangiectasia) fibroblasts, Nature **260:**444, 1976.
12. Biggar, W. D., and Good, R. A.: Immunodeficiency in ataxia telangiectasia, Birth Defects **11:**271, 1975.
13. Black, F. O., Spanier, S. S., and Kohut, R. I.: Aural abnormalities in partial DiGeorge syndrome, Arch. Otolaryngol. **101:**129, 1975.
14. Blaese, R. M., Strober, W., Levy, A. L., and Waldmann, T. A.: Hypercatabolism of IgG, IgA, IgM and albumin in the Wiskott-Aldrich syndrome, J. Clin. Invest. **50:**2331, 1971.
15. Blaese, R. M., Strober, W., and Waldmann, T. A.: Immunodeficiency in the Wiskott-Aldrich syndrome, Birth Defects **11:**254, 1975.
16. Boyse, E. A., Old, L. J., and Stockert, E.: An approach to the mapping of antigen on the cell surface, Proc. Natl. Acad. Sci. **60:**886, 1968.
17. Bruton, O. C.: Agammaglobulinemia, Pediatrics **9:**722, 1952.
18. Buckley, R. H.: Bone marrow and thymus transplantation in ataxia telangiectasia, Birth Defects **11:**421, 1975.
19. Buckley, R. H., and Dees, S. C.: Correlation of milk precipitins with IgA deficiency, N. Engl. J. Med. **281:**465, 1969.
19a. Buckley, R. H., Whisnant, K. J., Schiff, R. I., et al.: Correction of severe combined immunodeficiency by fetal liver cells, N. Engl. J. Med. **294:**1076, 1976.
20. Buckton, K. E., and Pike, M. C.: Chromosome investigations on lymphocytes from irradiated patients: effect of time in culture, Nature **202:**714, 1964.
21. Case records of Massachusetts General Hospital, weekly CPC exercises, N. Engl. J. Med. **292:**1231, 1975.
22. Cederbaum, S. D., Niwayama, G., Stiehm, E. R., et al.: Combined immunodeficiency manifested by the Letterer-Siwe syndrome, Lancet **1:**958, 1972.
23. Cleveland, W. W.: Immunologic reconstitution in the DiGeorge's syndrome by fetal thymic transplant, Birth Defects **11:**352, 1976.
24. Cleveland, W. W., Fogel, B. J., Brown, W. T., and Kay, H. E. M.: Foetal thymic transplant in a case of DiGeorge's syndrome, Lancet **2:**1211, 1968.
25. Cohen, M. M., Shaham, M., Dagan, G., et al.: Cytogenetic investigations in families with ataxia telangiectasia, Cytogenet. Cell Genet. **15:**338, 1975.
26. Cooper, M. D., Chase, H. T., Lohman, J. T., et al.: Wiskott-Aldrich syndrome: an immunologic deficiency disease involving the afferent limb of immunity, Am. J. Med. **44:**499, 1968.
27. Cooper, M. D., and Lawton, A. R.: Circulating B-cells in patients with immunodeficiency, Am. J. Pathol. **69:**513, 1972.
28. Cooper, M. D., Lawton, A. R., and Kincade, P. W.: A two stage model for development of antibody-producing cells, Clin. Exp. Immunol. **11:**143, 1972.
29. Cooper, M. D., Peterson, R. D. A., and Good, R. A.: Delineation of the thymic and bursal lymphoid systems in the chicken, Nature **205:**143, 1965.
30. Davis, S. D.: Antibody deficiency diseases. In Stiehm, E. R., and Fulginiti, V. A., eds.: Immunologic disorders of infants and children, Philadelphia, 1973, W. B. Saunders Co.
31. DiGeorge, A. M.: Congenital absence of the thymus and its immunologic consequences: concurrence with congenital hypothyroidism. In Bergsma, D., and Good, R. A., eds.: immunologic deficiency diseases in man, Baltimore, 1968, The Williams & Wilkins Co.
32. Eidelman, S., and Davis, S. D.: Immunoglobulin content

of intestional mucosal plasma cells in ataxia-telangiec-tasia, Lancet **1:**884, 1968.

33. Engle, R. L., Jr., and Wallis, L. A.: Immunoglobulin-opathies, Springfield, 1969, Charles C Thomas, Publisher.

34. Everett, N. B., Caffery, R. W., and Rieke, W. O.: Recirculation of lymphocytes, Ann. N.Y. Acad. Sci. **113:** 887, 1964.

35. Francki, C. H., and Grob, P. J.: Transfer factor therapy, Schweiz. Med. Wochenschr. **104:**146, 1974.

36. Freedom, R. M., Rosen, F. S., and Nadas, A. S.: Congenital cardiovascular disease and anomalies of third and fourth pharyngeal pouch, Circulation **46:**165, 1972.

37. Fudenberg, H. H., and Fudenberg, B. R.: Antibody to hereditary human gamma globulin (CM) factor resulting from maternal-fetal incompatibility, Science **145:**170, 1964.

38. Gatti, R. A.: On the classification of patients with primary immunodeficiency disorders, Clin. Immunol. Immunopathol. **3:**243, 1974.

39. Gatti, R. A., and Good, R. A.: Occurrence of malignancy in immunodeficiency diseases: a literature review, Cancer **28:**89, 1971.

40. Geha, R. S., Scheeberger, E., Merler, E., and Rosen, F. S.: Heterogeneity of "acquired or common variable agammaglobulinemia, N. Engl. J. Med. **291:**1, 1974.

41. Giblett, E. R., Anderson, J. E., and Cohen, F.: Adenosine-deaminase deficiency in two patients with severely impaired cellular immunity, Lancet **2:**1067, 1972.

41a. Giblett, E. R., Ammann, A. J., Wara, D. W., et al.: Nucleoside-phosphorylase deficiency in a child with severely defective T-cell immunity and normal B-cell immunity, Lancet **1:**1010, 1975.

42. Good, R. A.: Morphological basis of the immune response and hypersensitivity. In Felton, H., et al., eds.: Host parasite relationships in living cells, Springfield, 1957, Charles C Thomas, Publisher.

43. Good, R. A., Bach, F. H., VanBekkum, D. W., et al.: Severe combined immunodeficiency disease: characterization of the disease and results of transplantation, J.A.M.A. (In press.)

44. Good, R. A., and Rötstein, J.: Rheumatoid arthritis and agammaglobulinemia, Bull. Rheumatol. Dis. **10:**203, 1960.

45. Goya, N., Kodata, S., Kuroko, Y., and Sumiyoshi, A.: Influence of transplantation of thymus and spleen cells on patients with ataxia telangiectasia. In Kagan, B. M., and Stiehm, E. R., eds.: Immunologic incompetence, Chicago, 1971, Year Book Medial Publishers, Inc.

46. Grey, H. M., Rabellino, E., and Pirofsky, B.: Immunoglobulins on the surface of lymphocytes. IV. Distribution in hypogammaglobulinemia, cellular immune deficiency, and chronic lymphatic leukemia, J. Clin. Invest. **50:**2368, 1971.

47. Heidelberger, K. T., and LeGoldan, D. P.: Wiskott-Aldrich syndrome and cerebral neoplasia: report of a case with localized reticulum cell cell sarcoma, Cancer **33:** 280, 1974.

48. Higgs, J. M., and Wells, R. S.: Chronic mucocutaneous candidiasis: new approaches to treatment, Br. J. Dermatol. **89:**179, 1973.

49. Hitzig, W. H., and Willi, H.: Heterogeneity of phenotypic expression in a family with Swiss type agammaglobulinemia: observations on the acquisition of agammaglobulinemia, J. Pediatr. **78:**968, 1971.

50. Hoar, D. I., and Sargent, P.: Chemical mutagen hypersensitivity in ataxia telangiectasia, Nature **261:**590, 1976.

51. Hong, R., Huang, S. W., Levy, R. L., et al.: Cartilage-hair hypoplasia: effect of thymus transplants, Cell. Immunol. Immunopathol. **1:**15, 1972.

52. Huntly, C. C., and Dees, S. C.: Age associated with thrombocytopenic purpura and purulent hepatitis media: report of five fatal cases, Pediatrics **19:**351, 1957.

53. Janossy, G., Greaves, M. F., Doenhoff, M. J., and Snajdr, J.: Lymphocyte activation. V. Quantitation of the proliferative responses to mitogens using defined T and B cell populations, Clin. Exp. Immunol. **14:**581, 1973.

54. Karan, O., Yalaz, K., Taysi, K., and Say, B.: Immunological studies in ataxia telangiectasia, Clin. Genet. **5:** 40, 1974.

55. Kersey, J. H., Specter, D. D., and Good, R. A.: Primary immunodeficiency diseases in cancer. The immunodeficiency cancer registry, Int. J. Cancer **12:**333, 1973.

56. Kirpatrick, C. H., Ottenson, E. A., Smith, T. K., et al.: Reconstitution of defective cellular immunity with foetal thymus and dialysable transfer factor: long-term studies in a patient with chronic mucocutaneous candidiasis, Clin. Exp. Immunol. **23:**414, 1976.

57. Kirpatrick, C. H., Rich, R. R., and Bennett, J. E.: Chronic mucocutaneous candidiasis: model building of cellular immunity, Ann. Intern. Med. **74:**955, 1971.

58. Krivit, W., and Good, R. A.: Aldrich's syndrome (thrombocytopenia, eczema and infection in infants), Am. J. Dis. Child. **97:**137, 1959.

59. Krivit, W., Yunis, E., and White, J.: Platelet survival studies in Aldrich syndrome, Pediatrics **37:**339, 1966.

60. Lawton, A. R., Self, K. S., Royal, S. A., and Cooper, M. D.: Ontogeny of B-lymphocytes in the human fetus, Clin. Immunol. Immunopathol. **1:**84, 1972.

61. Leiken, S., Parrott, R., and Randolph, J.: Clotrimazole treatment of chronic mucocutaneous candidiasis, J. Pediatr. **88:**864, 1976.

62. Lischner, H. W.: DiGeorge syndrome(s), J. Pediatr. **81:**1042, 1972.

63. Lopukhin, Y., Moroso, V. Y., and Petrov, R.: Transplantation of a neonate thymus sternum: complex in ataxia telangiectasia, Transplant. Proc. **5:**823, 1973.

64. Lux, S. E., Johnston, R. B., August, C. S., et al.: Chronic neutropenia and abnormal cellular immunity: Cartilage-hair hypoplasia, N. Engl. J. Med. **282:**234, 1970.

65. McFarlin, D. E., Strober, W., and Waldmann, T. A.: Ataxia telangiectasia, Medicine **51:**281, 1972.

66. McKusick, V. A., Eldridge, R., Hostetler, J. A., et al.: Dwarfism in the Amish: cartilage-hair hypoplasia, Bull. Johns Hopkins Hosp. **116:**285, 1976.

66a. Meuwissen, H. J., Pollara, B., and Pickering, R.: Combined immunodeficiency disease associated with adenosine deaminase deficiency. J. Pediatr. **86:**169, 1975.

67. Miller, H. C., and Cudkowicz, G.: Density gradient separation of marrow cells restricted for antibody class, Science **171:**913, 1971.

68. Morley, J., Wolstencroft, R. A., and Dumonde, D. C.: The measurement of lymphokines. In Weir, D. M., ed.: Cellular immunology, Oxford, 1973, Blackwell Scientific Publications, Ltd.

69. Nathenson, G., Schorr, J. B., and Litwin, S. D.: Gm factor fetomaternal gamma globulin incompatibility, Pediatr. Res. **5:**2, 1971.

70. Napitz, C. K., and Richter, M.: The action of phytohemmagglutinin in vivo and in vitro: a review, Prog. Allergy **12:**1, 1968.

71. Neiburger, J. B., Neiburger, R. G., Richardson, S. T., et al.: Distribution of T and B lymphocytes in lymphoid tissues of infants and children, Infect. Immun. **14:**118, 1976.

72. Nell, P. A., Ammann, A. J., Hong, R., and Stiehm, E. R.: Familial selective IgA deficiency, Pediatrics **49:**71, 1972.

73. Nezelof, C., Jammet, M. L., Lortholary, P., et al.: L'hypoplasie héréditaire du thymus: sa place et sa respon-

sabilité dans une observation d'aplasie lympocytaire, normoplasmocytaire et normoglobulinémique du nourrisson, Arch. Fr. Pediatr. **21:**897, 1964.

74. Ochs, H. D., Ament, M. E., and Davis, S. D.: Giardiasis with malabsorption in X-linked agammaglobulinemia, N. Engl. J. Med. **287:**341, 1972.

75. Oppenheim, J. J., Blaese, R. M., and Waldmann, T. A.: Defective lymphocyte transformation and delayed hypersensitivity in the Wiskott-Aldrich syndrome, J. Immunol. **104:**835, 1970.

76. Ownby, D. R., Pizzo, S., Blackmon, L., et al.: Severe combined immunodeficiency with leukopenia (reticular dysgenesis) in siblings: immunologic and histopathologic findings, J. Pediatr. **89:**382, 1976.

77. Oxford, J. M., Harnden, D. G., Parrington, J. M., and Delhanty, J. D.: Specific chromosome aberrations in ataxia telangiectasia, J. Med. Genet. **12:**251, 1975.

78. Parkman, R., Gelfand, E. W., and Rosen, F. S.: Severe combined immunodeficiency and adenosine deaminase deficiency, N. Engl. J. Med. **292:**717, 1975.

78a. Parkman, R., Rappeport, J., Geha, R., et al.: Complete correction of the Wiskoff Aldrich Syndrome by allogenic bone marrow transplantation, N. Engl. J. Med. **298:** 921, 1978.

79. Pearson, H. A., Schuman, N. R., Oski, F. A., and Eitzman, D. B.: Platelet survival in Wiskott Aldrich syndrome, J. Pediatr. **68:**754, 1966.

80. Peterson, R. D. A., Cooper, M. D., and Good, R. A.: Lymphoid tissue abnormalities associated with ataxia telangiectasia, Am. J. Med. **41:**342, 1966.

81. Piamphongsant, T., and Yavapolkul, V.: Diffuse chronic granulomatous mucocutaneous candidiasis, Int. J. Dermatol. **15:**219, 1976.

82. Polmar, S. H., Stern, R. C., Schwartz, A. L., et al.: Enzyme replacement therapy for adenosine deaminase deficiency and severe combined immunodeficiency, N. Engl. J. Med. **295:**1337, 1976.

83. Rabellino, E., Colon, S., Grey, H. M., and Unanue, E. R.: Immunoglobulins on the surface of lymphocytes. I. Distribution and quantitation, J. Exp. Med. **133:**156, 1971.

84. Radl, J., Dorren, L. J., Morell, A., et al.: Immunoglobulins in transit paraproteins in sera of patients with Wiskott Aldrich syndrome: a follow-up study, Clin. Exp. Immunol. **25:**256, 1976.

85. Raff, M. C.: Two distinct populations of peripheral lymphocytes in mice distinguishable by immunofluorescence, Immunology **19:**637, 1970.

86. Remold, H. G., and David, J. R.: Migration inhibition factor and other mediators in cell-mediated immunity. In McCluskey, R. T., and Cohen, S., eds.: Mechanisms of cell-mediated immunity, New York, 1974, John Wiley & Sons, Inc.

86a. Rieger, C. H., Lustig, J. V., Hirschhorn, R., and Rothberg, R. M.: Reconstitution of T-cell function in severe combined immunodeficiency disease following transplantation of early embryonic liver cells, J. Pediatr. **90:**707, 1977.

87. Robbins, J. B., Skinner, R. G., and Pearson, H. A.: Autoimmune hemolytic anemia in a child with congenital x-linked hypogammaglobulinemia, N. Engl. J. Med. **280:** 75, 1969.

88. Robinson, H. B., Jr.: DiGeorge's or the III-IV pharyngeal pouch syndrome: Pathology and a theory of pathogenesis, Perspect. Pediatr. Pathol. **2:**173, 1975.

89. Rocklin, R. E.: Use of transfer factor in patients with depressed cellular immunity and chronic infection, Birth Defects **11:**431, 1975.

90. Rosen, F. S.: Immunological deficiency disease. In Bach, F. H., and Good, R. A., eds.: Clinical immunobiology, vol. 1, New York, 1972, Academic Press, Inc.

91. Rosen, F. S., Kevy, S. V., Merler, E., et al.: Recurrent bacterial infections and dysgammaglobulinemia: deficiency of 7S gamma-globulins in the presence of elevated 19S gamma-globulins, Pediatrics **28:**182, 1961.

92. Rosen, F. S., and Janeway, C. A.: The gamma globulins. III. The antibody deficiency syndrome, N. Engl. J. Med. **275:**709, 1966.

93. Rosen, F. S., and Janeway, C. A.: The gamma globulins. III. The antibody deficiency syndrome, N. Engl. J. Med. **275:**769, 1966.

94. Saulsbury, F. T., Winklestein, J. A., Davis, L. E., et al.: Combined immunodeficiency in vaccine-related poliomyelitis in a child with cartilage-hair hypoplasia, J. Pediatr. **86:**868, 1975.

95. Schalck, D. S., McFarlin, D. E., and Barlow, M. H.: An unusual form of diabetes mellitus in ataxia telangiectasia, N. Engl. J. Med. **282:**1396, 1970.

96. Sellars, W. A., and South, M. A.: Wiskott-Aldrich syndrome with 18 year survival, Am. J. Dis. Child. **129:** 622, 1975.

97. Sherwood, G., and Blaese, R. M.: Phytohaemagglutinin-induced cytotoxic effector lymphocyte function in patients with the Wiskott-Aldrich syndrome (WAS), Clin. Exp. Immunol. **13:**515, 1973.

98. Smith, R. W., Blaese, R. M., Hathcock, K. S., and Edelson, R. L.: T and B lymphocyte markers in lymphoid cell research and in human disease. In Proceedings of the eighth leukocyte culture conference, New York, 1976, Academic Press, Inc.

99. Spitler, L. E., Levin, A. S., Stites, D. P., et al.: The Wiskott-Aldrich syndrome results of transfer factor therapy, J. Clin. Invest. **51:**3216, 1972.

100. Steiner, M. L., and Pearson, H. A.: Bone marrow plasmacyte values in childhood: morphologic correlation in developmental immunology, J. Pediatr. **68:**562, 1966.

101. Stiehm, E. R., and Fudenberg, H. H.: Clinical and immunologic features of dysgammaglobulinemia type I, Am. J. Med. **40:**805, 1966.

102. Stiehm, E. R., and McAntosh, R. M.: Wiskott-Aldrich syndrome: a review and report of a large family, Clin. Exp. Immunol. **2:**179, 1967.

103. Stobo, J. D., and Thomasa, T. B., Jr.: A low molecular weight immunoglobulin antigenetically related to 19S IgM, J. Clin. Invest **46:**1329, 1967.

104. Swift, M., Sholman, L., Perry, M., and Chase, C.: Malignant neoplasm in the family of patients with ataxia telangiectasia, Cancer Res. **30:**209, 1976.

105. Takahashi, T., Old, L. J., McIntire, K. R., and Boyse, E. A.: Immunoglobulin and other surface antigens of cells of the immune system, J. Exp. Med. **134:**815, 1971.

106. Takeya, K., Nomoto, K., Matsumoto, T., Miyake, T., and Himeno, K.: Chronic mucocutaneous candidiasis accompanied by enhanced antibody production, Clin. Exp. Immunol. **25:**497, 1976.

107. Thieffry, S. T., Arthuis, M., Aicardi, J., and Lyon, G.: L'ataxie telangiéctasia, Rev. Neurol. **105:**390, 1961.

108. Touraine, J. L., Touraine, F., Dutruge, J., et al.: Immunodeficiency diseases. I. T-lymphocyte precursors and T-lymphocyte differentiation in partial DiGeorge syndrome, Clin. Exp. Immunol. **21:**39, 1975.

109. VanFurth, R., Schuit, H. R. E., and Hijamans, W.: The immunological development of the human fetus, J. Exp. Med. **122:**1173, 1965.

110. Waldmann, T. A., and Stoker, N.: Metabolism of immunoglobulins, Prog. Allergy **13:**1, 1969.

111. Walters, C. S., and Wigzell, H.: Demonstration of heavy and light chain antigenic determinants on the cell-bound receptor for antigen: similarities between membrane-attached and humoral antibodies produced by the same cell, J. Exp. Med. **132:**1233, 1970.

112. Willenbockel, U.: Transitorisch-protahiertes Antikor-

permengelsyndrom bei zweieiigen Zwillingen, Z. Kinderheilk. **84:**477, 1960.
113. Wolff, L. J., Richardson, S. T., Neiburger, J. B., et al.: Poor prognosis of children with acute lymphocytic leukemia and increased B cell markers, J. Pediatr. **89:**956, 1976.
114. Ziegler, J. B., and Penny, R.: Fatal ECHO 30 virus infection and anyloidosis in x-linked hypogammaglobulinemia, Clin. Immunol. Immunopathol. **3:**347, 1975.

Disorders related to infection

115. Baehner, R. L., and Shuler, S. E.: Infectious mononucleosis in childhood: clinical expressions, serologic findings, complications and prognosis, Clin. Pediatr. **6:**393, 1967.
116. Bar, R. S., DeLor, C. J., Clausen, K. P., et al.: Fatal infectious mononucleosis in a family, N. Engl. J. Med. **290:**363, 1974.
117. Barnes, G. R., Jr., Yannet, H., and Lieberman, R.: A clinical study of an institutional outbreak of infectious lymphocytosis, Am. J. Med. Sci. **218:**646, 1949.
118. Battle, J. E., Jr., and Hewlett, J. S.: Hematologic changes observed after extracorporeal circulation during open heart surgery, Cleve. Clin. Q. **25:**112, 1958.
119. Bender, C. E.: The value of corticosteroids in the treatment of infectious mononucleosis, J.A.M.A. **119:**529, 1967.
120. Boughton, C. R.: Glanular fever: the study of a hospital series in Sidney, Med. J. Aust. **2:**529, 1970.
121. Bowman, H. S., Marsh, W. L., Schumacher, H. R., et al.: Auto anti-N immunohemolytic anemia in infectious mononucleosis, Am. J. Clin. Pathol. **61:**465, 1974.
122. Cantow, E. F., and Kostinas, J. E.: Studies on infectious mononucleosis. IV. Changes in the granulocytic series, J. Clin. Pathol. **46:**43, 1966.
123. Carter, R. L.: Platelet levels in infectious mononucleosis, Blood **25:**817, 1965.
124. Chretien, J. H., and Esswein, J. G.: How frequent is bacterial superfection of the pharynx in infectious mononucleosis? Clin. Pediatr. **15:**424, 1976.
125. Clement, D. H.: Reassurance regarding infectious lymphocytosis, Pediatrics **41:**597, 1968.
126. Clizer, E. E.: Cytomegalovirus mononucleosis, J.A.M.A. **228:**606, 1974.
127. Crisalli, M., and Terragna, A.: La malattia diSmith (linfocitosi infettiva acuta), revisione della letterature e presentazione di tre casi, Minerva Pediatr. **10:**849, 1958.
128. Dadash-Zadeh, M., Hsu, C. C., and Schwartz, A. D.: T and null cell proliferation in a patient with acute infectious lymphocytosis, J. Pediatr. **88:**520, 1976.
129. Davidsohn, I.: Serologic diagnosis of infectious mononucleosis, J.A.M.A. **108:**289, 1937.
130. Dirckx, J. H.: Infectious mononucleosis, J.A.M.A. **226:**78, 1973.
131. Downey, H., and McKinlay, C. A.: Acute lymphadenosis compared with acute leukemia, Arch. Intern. Med. **32:**82, 1923.
132. Drescovich, C., and Santarsierg, M.: La malattia di Smith (linfocitosi infettiva acuta), contributo clinico ed osservazioni su vertisette casi, Clin. Pediatr. Bologne **45:**233, 1963.
133. Dresdale, D. T., Ripstein, C. B., Guzman, S. V., and Greene, M. A.: Postcardiotomy syndrome in patients with rheumatic heart disease: cortisone as a prophylactic and therapeutic agent, Am. J. Med. **21:**57, 1956.
134. Duncan, P. A.: Acute infectious lymphocytosis in young adults, N. Engl. J. Med. **233:**177, 1945.
135. Epstein, M. A., Achong, B. G., and Barr, Y. M.: Virus particles in cultured lymphoblasts from Burkitt's lymphoma, Lancet **7:**702, 1964.

136. Evans, A. S.: Infectious mononucleosis in University of Wisconsin students: report of a 5 year investigation, Am. J. Hygiene **71:**342, 1960.
137. Evans, A. S.: Infectious mononucleosis and other mono-like syndromes, N. Engl. J. Med. **286:**836, 1972.
138. Evans, A. S., Niederman, J. C., and McCollum, R. W.: Seroepidemiologic studies of infectious mononucleosis with EB virus, N. Engl. J. Med. **279:**1121, 1968.
139. Finucane, D. L., and Philips, R. S.: Infectious lymphocytosis, Am. J. Dis. Child. **68:**301, 1944.
140. Giuliano, V. J., Jasin, H. E., and Ziff, M.: The nature of the atypical lymphocyte in infectious mononucleosis, Clin. Immunol. Immunopathol. **3:**90, 1974.
141. Gutgesell, H. P., Jr.: Acute airway obstruction in infectious mononucleosis, Pediatrics **47:**141, 1967.
142. Henle, G., and Henle, W.: Immunofluorescence in cells derived from Burkitt's lymphoma, J. Bacteriol. **91:**1248, 1966.
143. Henle, G., Henle, W., and Diehl, V.: Relation of Burkitt's tumor-associated herpes-type virus to infectious mononucleosis, Proc. Natl. Acad. Sci. **59:**94, 1968.
144. Henle, G., Henle, W., and Horwitz, C. A.: Antibodies to Epstein-Barr virus-associated nuclear antigen in infectious mononucleosis, J. Infect. Dis. **130:**231, 1974.
145. Henle, W., and Henle, G.: Antibody responses to the Epstein-Barr virus and cytomegalovirus after open heart and other surgery, N. Engl. J. Med. **282:**1068, 1970.
146. Hoagland, R. J.: Mononucleosis and heart disease, Am. J. Med. Sci. **248:**1, 1964.
147. Hoagland, R. J.: Resurgent heterophile-antibody reaction after mononucleosis, N. Engl. J. Med. **269:**1307, 1963.
148. Hoagland, R. J.: The clinical manifestations of infectious mononucleosis: a report of 200 cases, Am. J. Med. Sci. **240:**21, 1960.
149. Horowitz, M. S., and Moore, G. T.: Acute infectious lymphocytosis; and epidemiologic study of an outbreak, N. Engl. J. Med. **279:**399, 1968.
150. Jenkins, W. J., Koster, G. H., Marsh, W. L., and Carter, R. L.: Infectious mononucleosis: an unsuspected source of anti-i, Br. J. Haematol. **11:**480, 1965.
151. Jondal, M., and Klein, G.: Surface markers on human B and T lymphocytes. II. Presence of Epstein-Barr virus receptors on B lymphocytes, J. Exp. Med. **138:**1365, 1973.
152. Jordan, M. C., Rousseaw, W. E., Stewart, J. A., et al.: Spontaneous cytomegalovirus mononucleosis: clinical and laboratory observations in 9 cases, Ann. Intern. Med. **79:**153, 1973.
153. Karzon, D. T.: Infectious mononucleosis, Adv. Pediatr. **22:**231, 1976.
154. Kerns, D. S., Shira, G. E., Go, S., et al.: Ampicillin rash in children: relationship to penicillin allergy and infectious mononucleosis, Am. J. Dis. Child. **125:**187, 1973.
155. Klemola, E., BonEssen, R., and Henle, G.: Infectious mononucleosis-like disease with negative heterophile agglutination test: clinical features and relation to Epstein-Barr virus and cytomegalovirus antibodies, J. Infect. Dis. **121:**608, 1970.
156. Kreel, I., Zaroff, L. I., Canter, J. W., et al.: A syndrome following total body perfusion, Surg. Gynecol. Obstet. **111:**317, 1960.
157. Lagergren, J.: The white blood cell count and the erythrocyte sedimentation rate in pertussis, Acta Paediatr. **52:**405, 1963.
158. Landolt, R. F.: Akute infektiose Lymphocytosen in Kindesalter, Helv. Paediatr. Acta **2:**377, 1947.
159. Lang, D. J., and Anshaw, J. B.: Cytomegalic virus infection in the post perfusion syndrome: recognition of primary infections in four patients, N. Engl. J. Med. **280:**1145, 1969.

160. Lascari, A. D., and Bapat, B. R.: Syndromes of infectious mononucleosis, Clin. Pediatr. **9**:300, 1970.

161. Lemon, B. K., and Kaump, D. H.: Infectious lymphocytosis: report of epidemic in children, J. Pediatr. **36**:61, 1950.

162. Linarzi, L. R., Paul, J. T., and Poncher, H. G.: Blood and bone marrow in infectious mononucleosis, J. Lab. Clin. Med. **31**:1079, 1946.

163. Meyer, L. M.: Acute infectious lymphocytosis, Am. J. Clin. Pathol. **16**:244, 1946.

164. Miller, G., Niederman, J. C., and Andrews, L. L.: Prolonged oropharyngeal excretion of Epstein-Barr virus after infectious mononucleosis, N. Engl. J. Med. **288**:229, 1973.

165. Myers, E. F., and Crupin, B.: Anesthetic management of emergence tonsillectomy and adenoidectomy in infectious mononucleosis, Anesthesiology **42**:490, 1975.

166. Olson, L. C., Miller, G., and Hanshaw, J. B.: Acute infectious lymphocytosis presenting as a pertussis-like illness: its association with adenovirus type 12, Lancet **1**:20, 1964.

167. Ottesen, J.: On the age of human white cells in the peripheral blood, Acta Physiol. Scand. **32**:75, 1959.

168. Papamichail, M., Sheldon, P. J., and Holborow, E. J.: T and B cell subpopulations in infectious mononucleosis, Clin. Exp. Immunol. **18**:1, 1974.

169. Paul, J. R., and Bunnell, W. W.: The presence of heterophile antibodies in infectious mononucleosis, Am. J. Med. Sci. **183**:90, 1932.

170. Penman, H. G.: Fatal infectious mononucleosis: a critical review, J. Clin. Pathol. **23**:765, 1970.

171. Peterman, M. G., Kaster, J. D., Gecht, E. A., and Lembert, G. L.: Epidemic of acute infectious lymphocytosis with diarrhea, Pediatrics **3**:214, 1949.

172. Provisor, A. J., Iacuone, J. J., Chilcote, R. R., et al.: Acquired agammaglobulinemia after a life-threatening illness with clinical and laboratory features of infectious mononucleosis in three related male children, N. Engl. J. Med. **293**:62, 1975.

173. Putnam, S. M., Moore, G. T., and Mitchell, D. W.: Infectious lymphocytosis: long-term follow-up of one epidemic, Pediatrics **41**:588, 1968.

174. Rahal, J. J., Jr., and Henle, G.: Infectious mononucleosis in Reye's syndrome: a fatal case with studies for Epstein-Barr virus, Pediatrics **46**:776, 1970.

175. Remington, J. S., Barnett, C. G., Meikel, M., and Lunde, M. N.: Toxoplasmosis and infectious mononucleosis, Arch. Intern. Med. **110**:744, 1962.

176. Reyersbach, G., and Lenert, T. F.: Infectious mononucleosis without clinical signs or symptoms, Am. J. Dis. Child. **61**:237, 1941.

177. Robinson, J., and Bridgen, W.: Immunological studies in the postcardiotomy syndrome, Br. Med. J. **2**:706, 1963.

178. Rosenbaum, S.: Febris lymphocytotica, Ann. Paediatr. **162**:117, 1938.

179. Ryder, R. J. W.: Acute infectious lymphocytosis, Am. J. Dis. Child. **110**:299, 1965.

180. Sakulsky, S. B., Wallace, R. B., Silverstein, M. N., and Dockerty, M. B.: Ruptured spleen in infectious mononucleosis, Arch. Surg. **94**:349, 1967.

181. Scalettar, H. E., Maisel, J. E., and Bramson, M.: Acute infectious lymphocytosis, Am. J. Dis. Child. **88**:15, 1954.

182. Schmidt, J. J., Robinson, H. J., and Pennypacker, C. S.: Peripheral plasmacytosis in serum sickness, Ann. Intern. Med. **59**:542, 1963.

183. Schumacher, H. R., Jacobson, W. A., and Bemiller, C. R.: Treatment of infectious mononucleosis, Ann. Intern. Med. **58**:217, 1963.

184. Schumacher, H. R., McFeely, A. E., and Maugel, T. K.: The mononucleosis cell. II Electron microscopy, Blood **33**:833, 1969.

185. Shope, T., and Miller, G.: Epstein-Barr virus: heterophile responses in squirrel monkeys inoculated with virus-transformed autologous leukocytes, J. Exp. Med. **137**:140, 1973.

186. Silverstein, A., Steinberg, G., and Nathanson, M.: Nervous system involvement in infectious mononucleosis: the heralding and/or major manifestations, Arch. Neurol. **26**:353, 1972.

187. Smith, C. H.: Infectious lymphocytosis, Am. J. Dis. Child. **62**:231, 1941.

188. Smith, C. H.: Acute infectious lymphocytosis: specific infection: report of four cases showing its communicability, J.A.M.A. **125**:342, 1944.

189. Smith, J. N.: Complications of infectious mononucleosis, Ann. Intern. Med. **44**:861, 1956.

190. Sprunt, T. P., and Evans, F. A.: Mononuclear leukocytosis in relation to acute infectious ("infectious mononucleosis"), Bull. Johns Hopkins Hosp. **31**:410, 1920.

191. Tennant, F. S.: The glomerulonephritis in infectious mononucleosis, Rep. Biol. Med. **26**:603, 1968.

192. Thelander, H. E., and Shaw, E. B.: Infectious mononucleosis, with specific reference to cerebral complications, Am. J. Dis. Child. **61**:1131, 1941.

193. Vahlquist, B., Ekelund, H., and Tveteras, E.: Infectious mononucleosis and pseudomononucleosis in childhood, Acta Paediatr. **47**:120, 1957.

21 □ Hematologic malignancies: leukemia and lymphoma

Robert L. Baehner

Leukemia

Acute leukemia is a primary malignancy of bone marrow leading to replacement of normal bone marrow and blood elements by immature or undifferentiated blast cells and their accumulation in other tissues (lymph nodes, liver, spleen, kidneys, brain and meninges, testes and ovaries, lungs, and subcutaneous tissue). The diagnosis is established by observing an increased percentage of blast cells in bone marrow obtained by needle aspiration or biopsy, then smeared on glass slides and stained with a Romanowsky stain containing methylene blue and eosin, e.g., May-Grünwald or Wright-Giemsa stain. Normal bone marrow is cellular and contains less than 5% blast cells, and myeloid, erythroid, and megakaryocyte proliferation and maturation should be evident. In the majority of new cases of acute leukemia there are more than 80% blast cells in the bone marrow associated with decreased numbers of myeloid, erythroid, and megakaryocyte precursors. Chronic myelocytic or granulocytic leukemia is a malignant proliferation of differentiated myeloid elements in the bone marrow and blood that terminates in death caused by a blastic crisis in more than 70% of cases. Chronic lymphatic leukemia is a malignant proliferation of differentiated lymphocytes in the bone marrow and blood associated with a long life expectancy. Chronic lymphatic leukemia does not occur in children.

The following are common terms used to describe the response to treatment: A *complete remission* means that bone marrow and blood morphology is normal and that the physical examination is also normal.[45] The persistence of increased numbers of blast cells in the bone marrow and/or lymphadenopathy, hepatosplenomegaly, pallor, bruising, and/or petechiae indicate an *incomplete remission*. The same findings occurring after complete remission indicate a *relapse*. Relapse may occur independently in the bone marrow or in extramedullary sites. *Central nervous system relapse* means that leukemic blast cells can be identified in the brain and in the spinal fluid. *Testicular relapse* is the second most common type of extramedullary relapse.

HISTORICAL PERSPECTIVE[60]

Classification. Leukemia was first described in 1845 by the physiologist Bennett in Scotland and by the pathologist Virchow in Germany in independent publications. The postmortem appearance of the blood, which Virchow termed weisses Blut (white blood), the "yellowish white almost greenish mass" within the blood vessels, and the massive size of the spleen were distinct features of these first case descriptions. Owing to the exceedingly crude hematologic methods then available, it was possible to make only the most superficial examination of the blood, and although it was realized that there was more than one variety of white blood cells, they could not be characterized morphologically. It remained for Neumann to point out in 1870 that the bone marrow was the likely origin of the leukemic cell and surmise that there might be three forms of leukemia: "myelogenous," splenic, and lymphatic. Following Ehrlich's discovery of staining methods in 1891 it became possible to describe accurately the cytologic features of the leukemias. In a remarkable farsighted paper in 1903 Turk grouped together the lymphatic leukemias, both chronic and acute, and the lymphosarcomas in one system of "lymphomatoses"; he stated that this included benign (chronic lymphocytic leukemia), acute, either benign or malignant (acute leukemia and chloroma), and chronic malignant (lymphosarcoma) forms, which differed from each other in only two ways: (1) by the degree of proliferation and invasion of tissue by lymphoid cells and (2) by the presence or absence of blood invasion.

The discovery of the myeloblast by Naegeli in 1905 ushered in an era of interest in the precise nature of the immature leukocytes of acute leukemia. Hirschfeld in 1914 first described acute granulocytic leukemia and noted that in some cases the red cell precursors were involved in the leukemic process, i.e., erythroleukemia. Reschad and Schilling in 1913 reported another new form of acute leukemia with involvement of the "splenocyte," the forerunner of the monocyte.

Thus by 1914 the distinct entities of chronic lymphocytic, chronic granulocytic, and acute lymphocytic, myeloblastic, monoblastic leukemia and erythroleukemia had all been described. Despite improved methods of classification, progress toward determining its cause and treatment remained dormant until the past several decades.

Treatment. Antibiotics and immunization procedures developed during the past several decades have controlled infectious disease to the level that, excluding accidents, malignancy is now the leading cause of death in children between the ages of 1 and 14 years.[91] The median duration of survival of children with acute leukemia prior to the era of chemotherapy was only 2 to 4 months. The introduction of the folic acid antagonist aminopterin by Farber et al. in 1948 initiated the era of chemotherapy, which has dramatically influenced survival in acute leukemia by improving the induction-remission rate as well as the duration of remission.[96] Remission-induction rates with 6-mercaptopurine, methotrexate, cytosine arabinoside (Ara-C), daunomycin, and cyclophosphamide used alone range between 22% and 40%, compared to 57% to 67% with vincristine, prednisone, and L-asparaginase used as single agents. Induction-remission rates of 90% were achieved by combining the most active drugs.[129] The mean duration of remissions with placebo, vincristine, prednisone, cyclophosphamide, methotrexate, and 6-mercaptopurine used alone ranged from 2 to 8 months, respectively; increased to 11 to 16 months when drugs were given in cycles; and was extended to between 24 and 33 months when they were administered in combination.[287] As the duration of bone marrow remission was extended beyond 1 year, central nervous system relapse occurred in 50% of these children.[77] Prophylactic treatment of the central nervous system has reduced the incidence of central nervous system leukemia to less than 5% and has extended the length of initial bone marrow remission to 5 years or longer in 50% of children with acute lymphocytic leukemia.

The results of treatment of nonlymphocytic leukemia in childhood are not as good. Similar to the experience in adults, successful induction of a remission in nonlymphocytic leukemia occurs in approximately 60% to 70% of cases, and the duration of remission is generally no more than 1 year.[98] The best results have been obtained with combinations of cytosine arabinoside, daunomycin, 6-mercaptopurine, and 5-azacytidine.[44]

The mortality in patients with hematologic malignancy is not directly related to the leukemic or lymphomatous process per se but rather is a result of the sequelae of bleeding and infection.[192] In 450 patients autopsied at the National Cancer Institute from 1965 to 1971 hemorrhage was the cause of death in 21% and infection in 79%. Improved management of these complications of chemotherapy was a challenge of the past and still poses a major problem for the future.

CLASSIFICATION

Acute leukemia accounts for approximately 50% of childhood cancer; of these cases 78% to 86% are lymphocytic and the remainder are nonlymphocytic[240,305] (Table 21-1). The nonlymphocytic types include myeloblastic, promyelocytic, monoblastic, myelomonoblastic, and erythroid leukemia. When cell morphology is studied carefully with special stains, 32% to 34% of all the cases of acute leukemia in children cannot be classified with certainty; these are considered undifferentiated or stem cell type but are treated as acute lymphocytic leukemia. Chronic myelocytic leukemia, accounting for less than 1% of childhood leukemia, may be either the juvenile or adult type. Chronic lymphocytic leukemia is not a disease of childhood.

The classification of acute leukemia is based on morphologic characteristics of blast cells in smears of bone marrow stained with May-Grünwald-Giemsa and histochemical stains (Table 21-2). Bone marrow slides should be freshly made without anticoagulants since EDTA or heparin may produce morphologic distortions within a few

Table 21-1. Incidence and classification of childhood leukemias

Classification	Children's Cancer Study Group (% of 1,770 cases)[240]	Southwest Cancer Chemotherapy Study Group (% of 745 cases)[305]
Acute lymphocytic	78	86
Lymphoblastic	44	54
Undifferentiated–stem cell	34	32
Acute nonlymphocytic	19	13
Myeloblastic-promyelocytic	8	9
Monoblastic-histiocytic	8	2
Myelomonoblastic	—	2
Erythroleukemia	1	—
Chronic		
Myelocytic (juvenile and adult types)	1	<1
Lymphocytic	—	—
Classification not stated	2	1

Table 21-2. Morphologic criteria for classification of cell types in acute leukemias

Stain	Lymphoblast	Myeloblast	Monoblast	Erythroblast
May-Grünwald-Giemsa				
Cell size	Variable	Regular	Regular	Regular
Nucleus	Round, clefted	Irregular, indented	Lobulated	Round, immature
Nucleolus	0-1	2-4	1-3	0-1
Cytoplasm	Scanty, basophilic	Moderate, basophilic	Large, sky blue	Basophilic
PAS	Coarse, granular (50%)	Faint, diffuse, or negative	Negative	Diffuse, strongly positive
Peroxidase	Negative	Positive	Positive	Negative
Sudan black	Negative	Positive	Positive	Negative
Esterase				
Naphthol AS-D acetate	Weakly positive	Positive	Positive	Negative
After fluoride	Positive	Positive	Negative	Negative

minutes. (See Chapter 2.) Lymphoblasts appear small (approximately 11 μ), the size of small lymphocytes, or large (larger than 11 μ), and they contain scanty basophilic cytoplasm, a round nucleus with coarse to clumped chromatin, and only rare nucleoli.

Rieder cells, although not diagnostic of acute lymphocytic leukemia, are identified by deep nuclear clefts suggesting lobulation of the nucleus.

Myeloblasts generally are more regular in size than lymphoblasts and have moderate basophilic cytoplasm and delicate azurophilic granules. Auer bodies appear as elongated red rods in myeloblasts, representing coalescence of azurophilic granules[94]; they are noted in myeloblastic and myelomonoblastic leukemia but are not found in normal myeloblasts. The myeloblastic nucleus is indented or shaped irregularly and contains fine chromatin and two to four distinct nucleoli. Malignant promyelocytes filled with azurophilic granules predominate in the bone marrow of patients with promyelocytic leukemia.

Monoblasts have relatively abundant, mildly basophilic cytoplasm; a folded or indented nucleus containing coarse chromatin; and several nucleoli. Historically monocytic leukemias were divided into the pure type of Schilling[264] and the mixed type of Naegeli,[228] on the basis of the misconception that monocytes originated either from the reticuloendothelial system (Schilling type) or the bone marrow (Naegeli type). Recent evidence indicates that blood monocytes originate solely from bone marrow monoblasts and in turn give rise to fixed tissue macrophages of the reticuloendothelial system.[316]

Erythroid leukemia (erythremic myelosis, or Di Guglielmo's disease) is characterized by excessive erythroid precursors with abnormal morphology both in the bone marrow and blood. Dis-

ordered myeloid proliferation is almost always evident, and the ratio of each cell type varies widely. Proerythroblasts, polychromatophilic erythroblasts, and orthochromic erythroblasts all show vacuolization of the cytoplasm and nucleus, with some degree of megaloblastic dysmaturity.

Histochemical stains most useful to aid in classification are periodic acid–Schiff (PAS),[126] Sudan black[283] and/or peroxidase,[154] and naphthol AS-D acetate esterase inhibition by fluoride.[86] PAS positivity was noted in forty-two of seventy-seven cases of acute lymphocytic leukemia under 18 years of age; the pattern was finely granular in six and coarsely granular in thirty-six.[88] This granular pattern is never seen in nonlymphoblasts. The PAS stain may be weakly positive with a diffuse pattern in one third of acute myeloblastic leukemias and is progressively more positive in differentiating myeloid cells. Since 18% of the dry weight of mature polymorphonuclear leukocytes is glycogen, PAS is strongly positive in them.[156] The bone marrow erythroblasts of erythroid leukemia and thalassemia major stain positive, whereas those of megaloblastic and sideroachrestic anemias and of normal persons are negative.[195] Although the peroxidase reaction is more sensitive than Romanowsky stains to identify azurophilic granules in diagnosing a myeloid origin of acute leukemia, its main value is to add certainty to the diagnosis; the peroxidase reaction is always negative in lymphoblasts and lymphocytes. Sudan black stain provides results that are similar in distribution and sensitivity to those of the peroxidase stain. Naphthol AS-D chloroacetate esterase stains granulocytes with less sensitivity than peroxidase and Sudan black and is always positive in acute monocytic leukemia. The naphthol AS-D acetate esterase distinguishes acute monocytic leukemia from other acute leukemias since only monocyte

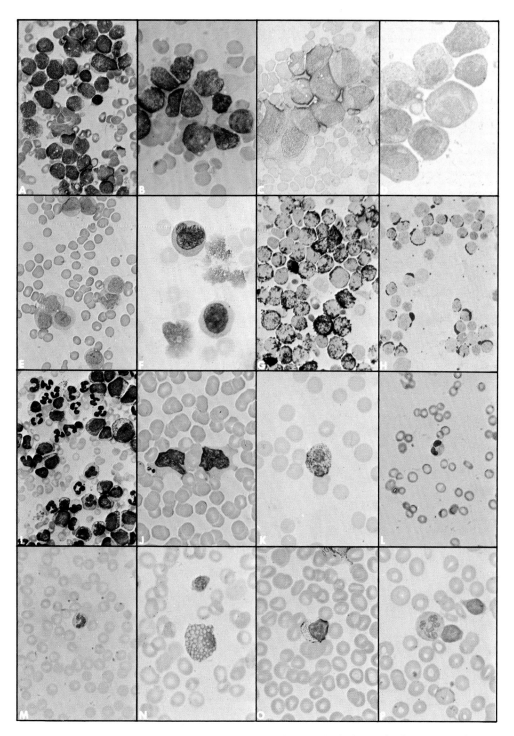

Plate 4. Leukemia and leukocyte disorders. **A,** Acute lymphoblastic leukemia (L1 type). **B,** Acute lymphoblastic leukemia (L2 or sarcoma type). **C,** Acute myeloblastic leukemia. **D,** Auer rods. **E,** Acute monomyeloblastic leukemia. **F,** Acute monoblastic leukemia. **G,** Peroxidase-positive myeloblasts. **H,** Periodic acid–Schiff–positive lymphoblasts. **I,** Chronic granulocytic leukemia. **J,** Atypical lymphocytes in infectious mononucleosis. **K,** Alder's anomaly. **L,** Pelger-Huet anomaly. **M,** D_1 trisomy syndrome. **N,** Plasma cell with Russel bodies. **O,** Lymphocytes in Hunter's syndrome. **P,** Hypersegmented neutrophils.

esterase activity is inhibited by 1.5 mg/ml sodium fluoride.[86] Ultrastructural studies are of no added benefit in classification of acute leukemia.[28]

New approaches to the subclassification of acute lymphocytic leukemia have recently been attempted. One approach is based on the size of the lymphoblast, determined by light and electron microscopy.[200,223] Four distinctive subgroups have been suggested; in order of decreasing cell size and presumed increased differentiation they are prolymphoblastic, macrolymphoblastic, prolymphocytic, and microlymphoblastic. A fifth subtype, immunoblastic,[198] or Burkitt's, leukemia has been recognized. In one study children with acute macrolymphoblastic leukemia had poorer responses to therapy than those with microlymphoblasts.[199] There are many uncontrolled variables in such a study, including smear and staining techniques, and it is not surprising that other similar studies have produced conflicting results.[150,234] A more useful and reproducible subclassification has been proposed by a collaborative group of French, American, and British investigators[24] who defined three types of lymphoblasts, on the basis of differentiation, the number of nucleoli, vacuolization, and the amount of cytoplasm. Lee et al.[189] found that a poor prognosis was associated with lymphoblasts containing abundant cytoplasm and two or more distinct nucleoli. Similarly Bloomfield and Brunning[32] and Flandrin and Bernard[87] have defined nonsarcomatous and sarcomatous lymphoblasts, the latter associated with a poorer prognosis. The PAS reactivity of lymphoblasts has been of no prognostic value to date,[147] although the degree of nucleolar differentiation may be of value. In one study patients with mean nucleolar scores of zero from bone marrow lymphoblasts at the time of diagnosis had a median survival of 26 months, whereas those with higher scores had a median survival of 17 months.[188]

Acute lymphoblastic leukemia cells can be classified by the presence or absence of cellular immune markers on lymphoblasts. The blast cells of approximately 75% of patients do not have surface receptors to sheep red blood cells (T cells) nor do they contain IgG, IgA, or IgM on their surface (B cells).[37,168] Approximately 25% of patients with acute lymphocytic leukemia, especially adolescent boys with mediastinal masses and initial white blood counts greater than 25×10^9/liter[387] have T cell blasts in their bone marrow and blood. Less than 1% of acute lymphocyte leukemia in childhood is associated with increased B cell lymphoblasts in the bone marrow.[102] A terminal transferase enzyme found in thymocytes has been identified in 25% of cases of acute lymphocytic leukemia.[204] It seems likely that lymphoblasts that carry immunologic markers and contain enzymes

similar to lymphocytes of thymus or lymph node origin may arise from these sites as lymphosarcomas that go on to invade bone marrow and transform into acute lymphocytic leukemia.

Chronic granulocytic or chronic myelocytic leukemia, in contrast to acute leukemia, is not associated with a hiatus in maturation of myeloid cells but rather results from excessive proliferation of bone marrow myeloid elements. The neutrophil granule alkaline phosphatase is reduced in chronic myelocytic leukemia, whereas it is increased in leukemoid reactions caused by infection or inflammation.[155] In one study of eighteen cases, six were juvenile type, seven were adult type, four were familial, and one was unclassified.[292] Since the juvenile form of chronic myelocytic leukemia is refractory to chemotherapy, it is important to differentiate it from the adult form in children. Table 21-5 (p. 598) lists these differences.

INCIDENCE

The incidence of childhood leukemia is 3.45 cases/100,000 children under age 15 yearly in the United States. Children of all ages are affected; the highest incidence is between 1 and 5 years, and the peak is reached between 3 and 4 years of age.[219] A similar incidence has been noted in England.[196] In 22 cases of leukemia in identical twins the other twin was affected in five instances, usually within weeks to months. Siblings of leukemic children have a slight increased risk, 1/720 within the first 10 years of life. These statistics can be compared to the average for a white child under age 15 years living in the United States, who has an approximate 1/2,880 risk of developing leukemia in the first 10 years of life.

Patients with a group of congenital disorders associated with chromosomal abnormalities have a higher risk of leukemia. Patients with Fanconi's anemia and their unaffected relatives may develop myelomonocytic or monocytic leukemia.[241] Three cases of acute leukemia have occurred in twenty-three patients with Bloom's syndrome before the age of 30 years.[275] Four patients with ataxia telangiectasia (Louis-Bar syndrome),[127,182] and several patients with congenital agranulocytosis (Kostmann's disease)[108] have also contracted leukemia. Children with Down's syndrome have a leukemic risk of 1/95 before the age of 10 years.[149]

Radiation-treated patients with polycythemia vera have an increased incidence (1/6) of leukemia between 10 and 15 years after treatment.[223] Survivors of Hiroshima who were within 1,000 meters of the hypocenter had a 1/60 risk of developing leukemia within 12 years.[220] Radiation-treated patients with ankylosing spondylitis have a 1/270 risk of leukemia within 15 years.[59] The risk of subsequent leukemia for the fetus after in-

Table 21-3. Incidence of leukemia among selected population groups

	Risk
Family member of leukemia patient	
Identical twin	1/5 until age 4 years
Sibling	1/720 until age 10 years
White child younger than 10 years	1/2,880
Persons with diseases with chromosome abnormality	
Down's syndrome, younger than 10 years	1/95
Fanconi's anemia, and unaffected siblings	1/50?
Bloom's syndrome	1/8
Ataxia telangiectasia	
Persons with exposure to excess radiation	
Polycythema vera, treated with ^{32}P or radiation	1/6
Atomic bomb, 1,000 meters	1/60
Ankylosing spondylitis	1/720
Persons with exposure to chemical carcinogens	
Dimethyl benzanthracene	?
Ethyl carbonates	?

trauterine radiation exposure is low (in the relative risk range of 1.5 to 2.0); children of mothers with a previous miscarriage or stillbirth experienced slightly higher leukemic risks[111] (Table 21-3).

Occupational exposure to benzene is generally accepted as incurring a risk of leukemia (especially erythroleukemia), although the incidence is low compared to the incidence of bone marrow hypoplasia from benzene.[90] Although there have been many reports blaming microepidemics of leukemia, the evidence to incriminate "clustering" is still not conclusive in any of them.[169]

PRELEUKEMIC SYNDROME

The hematologic abnormalities that precede development of the acute nonlymphocytic leukemias constitute a recognizable syndrome that may be appropriately labeled preleukemia. The clinical usefulness of such a designation is enhanced if one excludes by definition the high-risk groups of patients just described.[194] Recognition of the preleukemia syndrome is difficult and often is done in retrospect. The incidence of preleukemia is unknown. In one series a preleukemic phase was observed in 21 of 322 cases of acute leukemia; it was more common in adult patients, especially over the age of 50, than in children.[34] The following group of conditions could be considered preleukemic: idiopathic chronic aplastic anemia,

pure red cell aplasia, neutropenia, monocytosis, thrombocytopenia, refractory macrocytic anemias, and sideroblastic anemias.

Laboratory data are nonspecific and include elevated plasma and urine muramidase levels, increased concentrations of Hb F, abnormal chromosome patterns of bone marrow cells, increased cluster:colony ratio on in vitro bone marrow culture, and positive red blood cell tests for paroxysmal nocturnal hemoglobinuria.

ETIOLOGY

Although the cause of acute leukemia is unknown, certain leukemogenic factors are well known. Ionizing radiation and 7,12-dimethyl benzanthracene and the ethyl carbonates (e.g., hydroxyurethane, urethane, hydroxyurea) used alone or as coleukemogens induced leukemia in animals. Recent research has focused on viral relationships in leukemia. Although the interaction of genetic, hormonal, immunologic, and environmental factors are all important determinants in the development of leukemia, leukemia will not develop in experimental animals unless the animal is infected with the appropriate virus. For example, myeloblastosis virus causes leukemia only in chickens, and murine leukemia virus induces a similar disease only in mice.[306] No efficient human cancer-causing virus is known. Although animal cancer-causing viruses do not indicate the etiology of human cancer, they may be relevant to an understanding of human cancer. All of the viruses that are known to cause cancer are believed to form viral DNA integrated with cellular DNA. For DNA viruses such as herpesvirus[257] and Epstein-Barr virus,[132] formation of viral DNA integrated with cellular DNA is a result of recombination of the viral DNA with the cellular DNA. For RNA viruses such as C-type virus,[65] formation of viral DNA integrated with cellular DNA is a result of synthesis of viral DNA using the viral RNA as a template and then apparently recombination of this viral DNA with cell DNA. Viruslike particles in human leukemic cells and body fluids have been described. The question still remains whether virus particles are merely passengers or whether they play a causative role in the development of the leukemic process. It has been established that type-C RNA tumor virus can cause leukemia and lymphoma in birds, mice, and cats. No such proof exists for humans. However, as a result of progress in understanding the biochemistry of RNA tumor viruses, particularly the process of "reverse transcription" of viral genomic RNA, molecular components related to these in RNA tumor viruses have been found in human leukemic cells. These so-called viral footprints consist of two essential replicative components of RNA tumor viruses intact 70S or subunit 35S viral-related RNA, and RNA-directed DNA polymerase, i.e., reverse transcriptase.[104] Recently human leukemias, sarcomas, and lymphomas were found to contain RNA with sequence homology to murine leukemia virus but not to murine mammary tumor virus or avian myeloblastosis virus. Furthermore, the RNA was encapsulated in a particle possessing the density and size of RNA tumor viruses and was associated with similar reverse transcriptase activity. DNA from human leukemia and lymphoma contains particle-related sequences that could not be detected in normal DNA. In studies with identical twins the DNA from a leukemic twin contained particle-related sequences that could not be detected in the leukocytes of the healthy sibling. These findings support the idea that complete copies of information required to produce malignancy are acquired rather than transmitted genetically.[295]

IMMUNOLOGY

In recent years increasing attention has been paid to the possibility that neoplasms arise because clones of cells with abnormal growth characteristics escape destruction by reason of a defect in the normal mechanism for recognizing and eliminating abnormal cells. Normal cells possess a variety of surface antigens, and changes in these antigens may occur when the cells undergo neoplastic transformation. The breakdown in ''recognition'' of these antigens may permit the establishment of malignant clones. Leukemia-specific antigens have been identified,[165,314] and specific antisera have been raised in animals to detect the antigen.[122] Depending on the conditions used to raise the antibody, cytotoxic antibody to both acute and chronic forms of lymphocytic and myelocytic leukemia have been made.[124] Cytotoxic antibody that is specific for the histologic type of leukemia has been found in sera of some leukemic patients and some of their relatives.[29] Although there are no major alterations of serum immunoglobulin levels in acute lymphoblastic leukemia, low levels of IgG have been seen in a group with poor prognosis.[256] On the other hand, recent studies in adult acute leukemia indicate that cellular immune competence as measured by delayed hypersensitivity to a variety of skin test antigens (streptokinase-streptodornase, *Candida,* diphtheria, and tetanus) is associated with improved prognosis[136] and that relapse is associated with a loss of these responses.

The presence or absence of surface receptors on the leukemic cells for sheep red blood cells or for immunoglobin has provided a way to classify lymphoblastic leukemia into T, B, or null cell types; approximately 80% are null, 15% are T, and 5% are B types.[399a] T cell leukemia is frequently

associated with elevated white blood counts and the presence of a mediastinal mass in a teenage male patient.[36] B cell leukemia occurs in association with retroperitoneal lymphomas.[88a]

GENETICS
Acute leukemia

Chromosomal changes are present in bone marrow cells of approximately half of patients with acute leukemia.[273] The predominant abnormality is aneuploidy, and the modal chromosome numbers range from forty-one to fifty-three in acute granulocytic leukemia and from forty-six to ninety in acute lymphocytic leukemia. Although hypodiploidy has been seen occasionally in acute myelocytic leukemia, it was not found in more than 100 cases of acute lymphocytic leukemia studied for chromosomal changes. Although abnormal karyotypes vary greatly from one patient to another, the original chromosome changes are quite stable in the individual patient. Aneuploid cells become less common during remission, but the same cell line reemerges unchanged when the disease relapses.[262]

Familial leukemia

Chromosome studies have been carried out in relatives of affected siblings with familial leukemia. No consistent finding has been noted despite the evidence that in certain families the incidence is as high as 6% with as many as five siblings from the same generation affected. The following observations have been made:

1. Five members of one generation of an Icelandic family had acquired Pelger-Huët anomaly of their neutrophils, aneuploidy of C-group chromosomes, and acute myeloid leukemia.
2. Five cases of acute lymphoblastic leukemia occurred in a New Zealand Maori sibship of nine within 5 years in children between the ages of 10 months and 6 years.[163]
3. Cytogenetic studies were normal in the bone marrow and blood of a patient with familial leukemia and three affected siblings.[119]
4. Skin fibroblasts of certain surviving members of a family that had six cases of acute myelogenous leukemia and two cases of reticuloendothelial malignancy could be transformed by the oncogenic virus SV40.[293] Dermatoglyphic studies are of no real value in patients with acute leukemia.[271]

Chronic myelogenous leukemia

In chronic granulocytic leukemia the chromosomal anomaly involves most or all of the dividing bone marrow cells and is present in remission as well as relapse.[230,297] In the adult form the Philadelphia chromosome (Ph[1]) is usually the result of a translocation of the long arm of chromosome 22 to chromosome 9. In one study sixty of seventy-three consecutive patients with clinical and laboratory features of chronic myelocytic leukemia had the Ph[1] chromosome.[310] The thirteen Ph[1]-negative patients differed from the Ph[1]-positive group as follows: they had lower white blood cell counts (median 133.7×10^9/liter as compared to 41.5), three of thirteen were under 7 years of age while eight out of sixty Ph[1]-positive patients were under age 7; and they had a median survival of 18 months versus 45 months for the Ph[1]-positive group.

Recent evidence suggests that in some cases of adult chronic myelogenous leukemia the Philadelphia chromosome is lacking because the breaking point was quite near the end of the long arm of chromosome 22 or the patients have the juvenile form of the disease.[31] The defect likely arose from a single clone of cells since G-6-PD heterozygotes, which have two distinct populations of cells, each with its own isoenzyme pattern (either A or B), demonstrate only one isoenzyme pattern in their red cells and myelocytes once they acquire Ph[1]-positive chronic myelocytic leukemia.

CLINICAL AND LABORATORY FEATURES
Acute leukemia

The clinical manifestations of acute leukemia are extremely variable and nonspecific, and they usually appear 2 to 6 weeks before the diagnosis. Bone discomfort and arthritis may persist for even longer periods of time.[85] The child with acute leukemia generally experiences one or more of the following symptoms: insidious onset of pallor, easy fatiguability, lethargy, fever, bleeding, easy bruising, infection, lymph node enlargement, abdominal distension, bone pain, arthralgia, and abnormality of gait or inability to walk. Less common symptoms include vomiting, headache, and priapism. The presenting clinical and laboratory findings of more than 1,000 patients with acute lymphocytic leukemia treated by the Southwest Oncology Group are listed in Table 21-4.[83]

Physical examination reveals one or more of the following: irritability, pallor, tachycardia, petechiae, cutaneous bruises, gingival bleeding, epistaxis, melena, fever, evidence of infection including perianal disease, hepatosplenomegaly, adenopathy, leukemic skin infiltrates, periorbital edema, bone pain elicited by pressure. Skin infiltrates and gingival hypertrophy are more common in monocytic leukemia.[64] Skin involvement varies. It is either specific with leukemic infiltration or nonspecific with erythema multiforme–like papulonecrotic and eczematous lesions. More specific are the small, yellow, discrete, elevated, flat-topped plaques that are either dispersed or

Table 21-4. Presenting clinical and laboratory findings in children with acute leukemia*

Characteristic	Per-cent	Characteristic	Per-cent
Age (yr)		Platelets	
<2	14	($\times 10^9$/liter)	
2-10	71	<20	29
≥11	15	20-49	23
White blood cell		50-99	20
count ($\times 10^9$/liter)		≥100	29
<10	34	Sex (male)	57
10-49	47	Race (white)	85
≥50	19	Hemorrhage	48
Hemoglobin (gm/dl)		Liver enlarged	29
<7	44	Spleen enlarged	79
7-11	43	Nodes enlarged	
>11	14	Cervical	62
Blasts (%)		Inguinal	54
<65	25	Axillary	47
65-94	50	Fever	61
≥95	25	Bone pain	23

*Modified from Fernbach, D. J.: In Sutow, W. W., Vietti, T. J., and Fernbach, D. J., eds.: Clinical pediatric oncology, St. Louis, 1972, The C. V. Mosby Co.

confined to localized areas on the abdomen and extremities. Infrequently maculopopular eruptions cover the face initially and spread to the chest and back and eventually to the abdomen and extremities (Fig. 21-1). Each lesion may become hemorrhagic and necrotic and is eventually covered by a grayish membrane. Biopsy reveals extensive leukemic infiltration around blood vessels and adnexa in the epidermis and subcutaneous tissue (Fig. 21-2). A soft tissue granulocytic tumor called chloroma may be seen in acute myelocytic leukemia.[153] Papilledema or evidence of increased intracranial pressure with morning vomiting and headache is an uncommon finding at the time of initial presentation. Testicular leukemia presents as painless swelling of the testes, usually later in the course of the disease, in 5% to 10% of boys. Priapism (Fig. 21-3) has been reported in children with acute and chronic leukemia and marked leukocytosis.[115,149] Among the various mechanisms proposed for this is sludging and mechanical obstruction of the corpora cavernosa and dorsal veins of the penis by leukemic infiltration or coagulation of the platelet-rich leukemic blood within the corpora cavernosa. The more common association of priapism with chronic myelocytic than with acute lymphocytic leukemia may be related to the elevated platelet count and leukocytosis in chronic myelocytic leukemia.

The peripheral blood count and blood smear usually reveal a normocytic normochromic anemia and thrombocytopenia in approximately 90% of

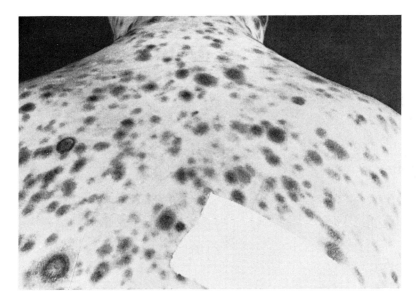

Fig. 21-1. Skin lesions in child with acute lymphoblastic leukemia (leukemia cutis). The lesions, originally discrete, were later confluent and covered the face, trunk, and eventually the entire body. The individual lesions were slightly nodular, erythematous, and purpuric. Many were eventually necrotic.

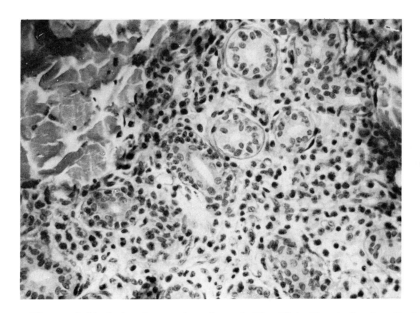

Fig. 21-2. Biopsy of skin lesion from patient shown in Fig. 21-1. Note leukemic cells densely infiltrating corium about sweat glands. (×435.)

cases.[323] The reticulocyte count is normal or low. Approximately two thirds of patients present with white blood cell counts less than 20×10^9/liter. Circulating blast cells generally are noted, but in some cases the differential blood smear is normal. Most often the absolute granulocyte count is less than 1×10^9/liter. Elevated white blood cell counts of 20 to 900×10^9/liter are usually asso-

ciated with prominent lymphadenopathy and hepatosplenomegaly.

Bone marrow aspiration and/or biopsy is almost always necessary to confirm the diagnosis. Bone marrow aspirate may be obtained from the following sites: posterior iliac spine or crest, anterior iliac spine, vertebral spinous process, or tibia. Sternal samples are obtained infrequently in chil-

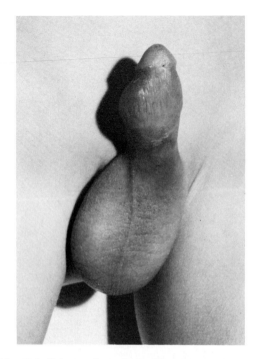

Fig. 21-3. Priapism in patient with acute myeloblastic leukemia. The initial white blood cell count was 125 × 10⁹/liter. Complete response occurred with induction chemotherapy and local radiation therapy.

dren, and the tibia is used frequently in infants. Sites of prior irradiation should be avoided because of local marrow aplasia. Removal of more than 0.5 ml of bone marrow results in dilution from the peripheral blood. Spicules of bone marrow should be quickly identified, isolated with a small pipette, and smeared on glass slides. Some hematologists prefer to use mild sedation, such as with chlorpromazine, and/or local anesthesia (1% to 2% tetracaine [Pontocaine]) administered with a 25-gauge needle, anesthetic patch, or a high-pressure anesthetic gun.* In acute leukemia at time of initial diagnosis the bone marrow is cellular because of replacement by leukemic cells, which generally comprise more than 80% of the marrow; megakaryocytes are decreased to absent in more than 90% of marrow samples at the time of diagnosis. So-called aleukemic leukemia is characterized by pancytopenia and absence of circulating blast cells; bone marrow is required for diagnosis. If marrow tissue is not obtained by aspiration, a bone marrow biopsy must be done. The Jamshidi needle† has facilitated success in obtaining sufficient marrow tissue. Touch preparation of the biopsy tissue to a glass slide for Wright's stain before it is placed in Zenker's fixative for conven-

tional processing, sectioning, and hematoxylin-eosin stain usually gives an immediate diagnosis.

Bleeding abnormalities are almost always a result of thrombocytopenia and/or aspirin-induced defects of platelet aggregation. Leukemic infiltrates of the liver rarely prolong the prothrombin time and partial thromboplastin time and decrease serum fibrinogen level but generally not to the extent to induce bleeding. Marked alteration of these test results occurs in progranulocytic leukemia as a result of diffuse intravascular coagulation, especially when treatment commences. Fibrin split products may be demonstrated by protamine sulfate precipitation or staphylococcal clumping tests.

Uric acid levels may be elevated and, if overlooked, can rapidly result in uric acid nephropathy aggravated by dehydration and acidosis.[5,142] This metabolic dysfunction has been seen with uric acid levels as low as 10 mg/dl. Since food intake may be poor, the serum creatinine level rather than the BUN should be used to gauge renal function. SGOT levels may be moderately increased and serum LDH levels even more elevated, probably reflecting liberation of enzymes from degenerating blast cells in the bone marrow. Tetany caused by hypocalcemia and hyperphosphatemia has been reported as a rare complication as chemotherapy commences, especially in patients with large leukemic cell burdens.[334]

The serum muramidase level and urinary excretion of muramidase are markedly elevated in acute monocytic and myelomonocytic leukemia, slightly elevated in acute myelocytic leukemia,[238,289] and normal in acute lymphoblastic leukemia.[281] Serum transcobalamine I levels are increased in promyelocytic leukemia and in chronic myelocytic leukemia.[254]

Radiographic examination of the chest reveals a mediastinal mass in 8% to 10% of patients, and 25% of these have white blood cell counts greater than 100 × 10⁹/liter.[49] Rarely pulmonary infiltrates can be seen at the time of diagnosis, but this may be a result of infection rather than leukemic cell infiltration. Organomegaly of the liver, spleen, and kidneys as a result of leukemic infiltration is often evident but does not result in dysfunction of these organs. The skeletal survey shows osseous abnormalities in about 50% of cases.[285] The following abnormalities have been noted in a large series[308]: generalized rarefaction of bones (most common) (Fig. 21-4), transverse metaphyseal radiolucent lines adjacent to the zone of provisional calcification at the end of long bones (Fig. 21-5) and beneath the cortex of flat bones, periosteal new bone formation, cortical and trabecular osteolytic lesions, osteosclerosis, leukemic infiltrations and hemorrhage, and pathologic fractures (Fig. 21-6). None of these findings have prognostic significance.

---

*Mizzy Instrument Co., New York, N.Y.
†Kormed Corp., Minneapolis, Minn. 54108.

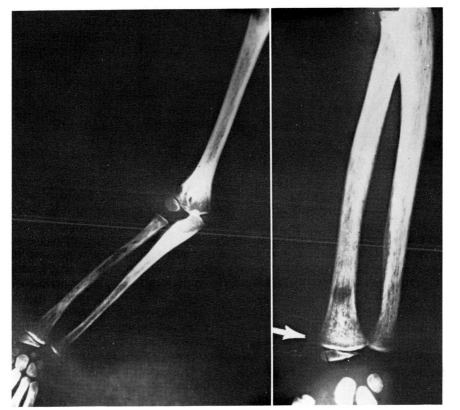

Fig. 21-4

Fig. 21-5

Fig. 21-4. Skeletal lesion of leukemia. Note generalized and local rarefaction and focal areas of bone absorption associated with replacement of bone marrow by leukemic tissue.

Fig. 21-5. Arrow points to a narrow, deep, transverse zone of rarefaction just proximal to the metaphysis of the long bones, usually most marked in the lower end of the radius. Note also multiple areas of rarefaction in medullary portion of bones.

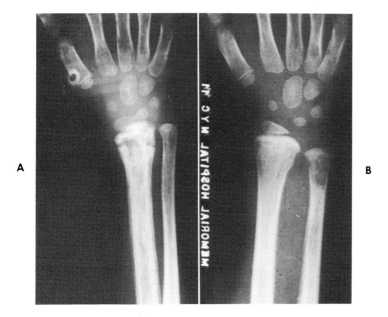

A

B

Fig. 21-6. Skeletal lesions of acute lymphoblastic leukemia. **A,** Pathologic fracture of distal radius with marked destruction by diffuse osteolytic involvement of entire radius and periosteal reaction along shaft of radius. **B,** Four months after treatment with 6-mercaptopurine, steroids, and radiation therapy, residual demineralization with slight deformity at area of fracture is present, but otherwise there is complete restoration. (Courtesy Dr. M. Lois Murphy, New York, N.Y.)

Blood cultures may be positive in 25% of newly diagnosed cases of acute leukemia.[48] Cultures of all body fluids should be obtained if fever is present.

Chronic myelocytic leukemia

The juvenile form of chronic myelocytic leukemia usually appears before the age of 2 years with an eczematoid facial rash, pallor, lymphadenopathy with a tendency to suppuration, moderate but progressive hepatosplenomegaly, respiratory infection, and thrombocytopenic petechiae and bleeding of mucosal surfaces and skin.[123] The adult form is usually seen in children over the age of 2 years with massive splenomegaly, pallor, and moderate lymphadenopathy and hepatomegaly. Laboratory findings in juvenile chronic myelogenous leukemia include leukocytosis with counts in the range of 50×10^9/liter as a result of absolute increases in both granulocytic and monocytic forms at all stages of maturation.[26] Nucleated red blood cells, early myelocytes, and monoblasts are also evident on the blood smear.[26] In vitro culture of the blood produces colonies that are almost exclusively monocytic.[7] Anemia with evidence of ineffective erythropoiesis,[203] such as disparity between bone marrow erythroid hyperplasia and blood reticulocyte counts and elevated red cell and heart-type LDH isoenzyme, is often present. The fetal hemoglobin level is elevated and adult type antigen I is reduced on the red blood cell.[318] Platelet counts are reduced below 100×10^9/liter, often below 25×10^9/liter. Serum and urinary muramidase levels are markedly elevated.[237] Serum immunoglobulin levels are high, and there is a high incidence of antinuclear and anti-IgG antibodies.[43] Bone marrow reveals diminished megakaryocytes, granulocytic and monocytic hyperplasia with no maturation arrest, and disordered erythroid hyperplasia. Spontaneous mitotic figures from bone marrow cells lack the Ph[1] chromosome.[261] Laboratory findings in the adult form of chronic myelogenous leukemia include a leukocyte count usually in excess of 100×10^9/liter. Monocytosis and normoblastemia are not present and there is a more orderly arrangement of all granulocytic forms, including eosinophils and basophils. Thrombocytopenia is uncommon prior to chemotherapy and there is no evidence of ineffective erythropoiesis or elevation of fetal hemoglobin levels. Muramidase is not usually increased in serum or urine, and no alterations of immunoglobulins are recorded. In vitro colony growth from the blood of patients with adult-type

Table 21-5. Differences between adult and juvenile forms of chronic granulocytic leukemia*

	Adult	Juvenile
Age of onset	Usually more than 2 years	Usually less than 2 years[123]
Physician findings		
Facial rash	Absent	Present[123]
Lymphadenopathy	Occasional	Frequent, with tendency to suppuration[123]
Splenomegaly	Marked	Variable[123]
Hemorrhagic manifestations	Absent	Frequent[123]
Hematologic findings*		
White blood cell count at onset	Usually >100×10^9/liter	Usually <100×10^9/liter[123]
Monocytosis of peripheral blood and bone marrow	Absent	Usually present[26]
Eosinophilia and basophilia	Common	Uncommon
Thrombocytopenia	Uncommon at onset	Frequent at onset[26,58]
Red blood cell abnormalities		
Ineffective erythropoiesis	Absent	Present[203]
I antigen on red blood cell	Normal	Reduced[318]
Fetal hemoglobin level	Normal	15%-50%[21,318]
Normoblasts in peripheral blood	Unusual	Frequent
Other laboratory findings		
Chromosome studies	Ph[1] chromosome positive	Ph[1] chromosome negative[261]
Urinary and serum muramidase levels	Slightly elevated	Markedly elevated[43,237]
Immunologic abnormalities	None	Strikingly high immunoglobulin levels, high incidence of antinuclear antibodies (52%) and anti-IgG antibodies (43%)[43]
Nature of colonies produced in vitro from peripheral blood	Predominantly granulocytic	Almost exclusively monocytic[7]
Response to busulfan	Uniformly good[292]	Poor
Median survival	2½ to 3 years[105]	Less than 9 months[123]

*Both forms have low alkaline phosphatase levels in blood neutrophils.

chronic myelogenous leukemia (in contrast to the juvenile form) is predominantly granulocytic. Bone marrow is hypercellular with all stages of granulocytic cells evident. Megakaryocytes and erythroid precursors are present. Ph[1] chromosome is found in spontaneously dividing bone marrow cells but not in blood lymphocytes or skin fibroblast cultures. Leukocytic alkaline phosphatase values are reduced in both forms of chronic myelogenous leukemia (Table 21-5).

Myelofibrosis and myeloid metaplasia

Myeloid metaplasia with or without myelofibrosis is rare in children. Most of the cases are idiopathic. Some have been secondary to acute leukemia, to other causes of myelophthisic anemia, or to toxic destruction of bone marrow elements. In children the primary myeloproliferative form has usually followed an acute course with rapidly progressive anemia and thrombocytopenia. A diagnosis of myeloid metaplasia is based on the following findings:

1. Hepatosplenomegaly
2. Anemia, often with nucleated red cells and teardrop forms in the peripheral blood smear
3. Immature leukocytes in the peripheral blood smear
4. Large misshapen platelets
5. Normal or elevated leukocyte alkaline phosphatase
6. Extramedullary hematopoeisis
7. Variable degrees of myelofibrosis on bone marrow biopsy

Of the twenty-seven reported pediatric cases, idiopathic myelofibrosis occurs twice as frequently in girls as in boys. Some patients with idiopathic myelofibrosis have had radiologic skeletal alterations, including osteosclerotic changes, manifested by metaphyseal striations. Newborn infants with marble bone disease, or osteosclerosis, may have associated myelofibrosis. Corticosteroids, testosterone, and splenectomy have been tried in selected patients without any real benefits.[37a]

Congenital leukemia

Congenital leukemia is a rare disease, of which approximately fifty adequately documented cases have been reported.[239,299] Some infants exhibit signs of leukemia at birth and die shortly thereafter. In another group the infants are normal at birth but develop clinical and hematologic signs later in the newborn period. In a third group the disease is not detected until the third to the sixth week of life[38] with a suggestive history of a hematologic abnormality dating back to the first weeks of life.

The presence of associated cardiac, orthopedic,

skeletal, and other developmental anomalies in patients with congenital leukemia[27] is analogous to the well-documented combination of leukemia and Down's syndrome.[179,180] In addition to trisomy 21, other specific congenital anomalies include isolated malformations such as absence of radii,[299] Klippel-Feil syndrome,[299] patent ductus arteriosus, atrial and ventricular septal defects,[299] the D_1 trisomy syndrome,[276] Bonnevie-Ullrich syndrome,[251] and a variant of the Ellis–van Creveld syndrome.[216]

The leukemia is principally myelogenous and is marked by a hyperleukocytosis and a predominance of promyelocytes and myelocytes.*

Myeloblasts vary from 10% to 80%. Anemia is uncommon but develops soon thereafter, with a rapid progression to pancytopenia. Large numbers of normoblasts may be present in the peripheral blood, regardless of anemia. Platelets are reduced in number. Physical signs include skin, mucous membrane, and umbilical hemorrhage, nodular skin infiltration, and hepatosplenomegaly.

In the newborn period leukemia must be differentiated principally from the leukemoid reaction of sepsis and congenital syphilis, hemolytic disease of the newborn, folate deficiency, and congenital thrombocytopenic purpura. In patients with a leukemoid reaction myelocytes as well as segmented and nonsegmented polynuclear leukocytes are increased, but myeloblasts are usually absent. The essential differentiating feature of leukemia is the extensive organ infiltration by immature myeloid cells and the absence of such infiltration in patients with a leukemoid reaction. Erythroblastosis can be diagnosed by evidence of blood group incompatibility, and in congenital thrombocytopenic purpura hepatosplenomegaly is absent and early myeloid cells do not appear in the peripheral blood. It is of interest that, except for the case reported by Cramblett et al.,[60] congenital leukemia has never been encountered in a newborn infant whose mother had leukemia during pregnancy.

DIFFERENTIAL DIAGNOSIS

The differential diagnosis of acute leukemia depends in part on the initial presenting manifestations.

Pancytopenia

The child with anemia, granulocytopenia, and/or thrombocytopenia may be mistaken to have aplastic anemia. Hepatosplenomegaly and lymphadenopathy are unusual physical findings in aplastic anemia and more common in acute leukemia. Rarely infiltration of the bone marrow by metastatic neuroblastoma cells may produce my-

---

*References 27, 61, 164, 166, 247.

elophthisic anemia or pancytopenia. Retinoblastoma and rhabdomyosarcoma will metastasize to bone marrow. Bone marrow aspirates may reveal clumps of tumor cells most noticeable on a low-power scan; bone marrow biopsy will aid in the search for metastatic tumor in bone marrow tissue. Skeletal survey and bone scan with technetium Tc 99m diphosphonate may reveal a metastatic tumor in bone cortex; 24-hour urine excretion of vanillylmandelic acid, homovanillic acid, metanephrine, and catecholamines is elevated in greater than 80% of patients with metastatic neuroblastoma.

Bone pain

Bone pain in acute leukemia produces arthralgia and occasionally frank arthritis to the extent that it mimics rheumatoid arthritis, rheumatic fever, or other collagen vascular diseases. To ensure that acute leukemia is not present a bone marrow aspiration should be performed when rheumatoid arthritis or collagen vascular disease is considered the most likely diagnosis.

Organomegaly

Viral infection may produce lymphadenopathy, hepatosplenomegaly and lymphocytosis. Infection by Epstein-Barr virus, cytomegalovirus, toxoplasmosis, adenovirus, or herpesvirus produces most of the nonspecific signs and symptoms seen in acute leukemia. Inspection of the peripheral blood smear during the height of the viral infection reveals lymphocytes with morphologic features of the so-called atypical lymphocyte and not those associated with leukemic blast cells. Atypical lymphocytes have abundant basophilic vacuolated cytoplasm and an irregular bean-shaped mature nucleus.

Non-Hodgkin's lymphoma of the diffuse, poorly differentiated, lymphocytic type or of the histiocytic type frequently spreads to bone marrow to produce leukemic transformation that is at times indistinguishable from acute leukemia. Generalized involvement of the reticuloendothelial system in infants and young children is noted in the Letterer-Siwe form of histiocytosis X and at times may simulate acute leukemia. Purpura, fever, lymphadenopathy, hepatosplenomegaly, skin infiltration, and pancytopenia may be seen in both conditions. Biopsy of involved tissue and bone marrow in histiocytosis X reveals histiocytes, eosinophils, and other inflammatory cells rather than leukemic cells.

Purpura

Thrombocytopenic purpura is a relatively common disorder of children generally not associated with alterations in the white blood cell count or with anemia. It most often follows a nonspecific viral infection, the majority of which are suspected to be caused by antiplatelet antibody. The physical examination in idiopathic thrombocytopenic purpura is normal except for petechiae and purpura.

Leukocytosis

Elevation of the white blood count as a result of mature lymphocytes has been associated with pertussis and parapertussis infections and benign infectious lymphocytosis. In each instance no leukemic cells are noted in the peripheral blood or bone marrow. A granulocytic leukemoid reaction caused by infection by *Diplococcus pneumoniae, Staphylococcus aureus, Haemophilus influenzae,* tubercle bacillus, or certain fungi or caused by inflammatory disease such as rheumatoid arthritis may produce white blood counts in excess of 50×10^9/liter with an increased percentage of metamyelocytes, myelocytes, and promyelocytes in the peripheral blood. This so-called shift to the left must be differentiated from chronic myelogenous leukemia; splenomegaly is marked and mature granulocytes lack granule alkaline phosphatase. True leukocyte alkaline phosphatase values are elevated in leukemoid reactions.

Leukocytosis in the newborn

Congenital leukemia is usually a form of acute myelomonocytic leukemia. Symptoms are present in the neonatal period; hepatosplenomegaly and lymphadenopathy are evident. Skin infiltration is a prominent feature.[260] Leukemic cells are evident in the blood, bone marrow, and extramedullary sites. This disease must be differentiated from the transient leukemoid reaction of the newborn, most frequently noted with Down's syndrome[74]; neonatal infections with rubella virus, cytomegalovirus, *Toxoplasma gondii,* herpesvirus; neonatal syphilis; erythroblastosis fetalis; and Letterer-Siwe syndrome.

Increased intracranial pressure

Central nervous system leukemia produces signs and symptoms of increased intracranial pressure, irritability, morning headache, vomiting, papilledema, and facial and ocular nerve palsy. Skull x-ray films show spread suture lines in a child under age 2 years and erosion of the anterior and posterior clinoids in a child over age 2. Similar signs and symptoms also occur with primary brain tumor, metastatic tumor to the brain, hydrocephalus, postinfectious polyneuritis, bacterial or viral meningitis, and meningoencephalitis. The diagnosis of central nervous system leukemia is established by observing leukemic cells in the cerebrospinal fluid. The Cytocentrifuge* provides a sim-

---

*Shandon Scientific, Sawitcky, Penn.

ple, convenient method to concentrate neoplastic cells from body fluids yet retain excellent morphology. Other centers have employed the Millipore filter technique with equal success.

PATHOPHYSIOLOGY
Leukemic cell cycle kinetics

Until rather recently it was generally believed that leukemic blast cells of human acute leukemia (1) proliferated rapidly, (2) were quite homogeneous in their kinetic behavior, and (3) were unable to differentiate. At the present it appears that these are misconceptions. Early observations that the mitotic index, i.e., the fraction of cells in mitosis, was lower in acute leukemia bone marrow cells than in normal granulocytic precursors went unheeded.[22,259] A true reorientation of the concepts concerning leukemic cell proliferation in man did not take place until ^{3}H-labeled thymidine became available to label cells in DNA synthesis.[171] The fraction of cells labeled 1 hour after infusion of ^{3}H-labeled thymidine was very low in leukemic myeloblasts—4% to 14% compared to 40% to 70% in normal myeloblasts.[170] Similar results were obtained in children with acute lymphocytic leukemia.[202] These observations led to the important conclusion that the fraction of proliferating leukemic blast cells in acute leukemia is only between 15% and 35% of all marrow blast cells at the time of diagnosis. The labeled blasts are larger and after division give rise to small blast cells.[201] In contrast to the larger proliferating blasts, the small blast cell is in a "nonproliferative" state. Proof of this stems from results of long-term infusion of ^{3}H-labeled thymidine for 8 to 10 days, which failed to label 7% to 18% of these marrow blasts, and for 21 days, which left 1% to 8% of blast cells unlabeled.[55] The average generation time for proliferating lymphoblasts, i.e., the time to complete one cell division, is prolonged to 40 to 50 hours, compared to the normal 18 to 24 hours. The cell cycle can be divided into four phases:

1. Mitosis (M phase) is increased from 30 minutes in the normal to 1 hour in the leukemic cell.
2. The postmitosis gap phase, termed G_1, is a dormant period of variable duration. The cell may move into a nonproliferative state termed G_0, then return to G_1.
3. The next phase is termed S_1. During this period new DNA, RNA, and protein synthesis occur. S_1 is increased from 8 to 14 hours to 15 to 20 hours in blast cells.
4. A brief second gap phase, termed G_2, lasting approximately 3 hours, occurs before the next mitosis.

Cells in the nonproliferative or slow proliferative compartments represent 65% to 85% of bone marrow blast cells and pose a most serious obstacle to cytostatic chemotherapy, which generally attacks cells in DNA synthesis (S_1) or mitosis (M) phase.

Leukemic cell proliferation in vitro

With time there is an accumulation of blast cells in the bone marrow leading to depletion of normal myeloid, erythroid, and megakaryocyte precursors. Quantitation of the bone marrow pool of stem cells committed to myeloid and monocyte-macrophage lines of differentiation has been facilitated by the development of techniques to culture colonies of the cells in vitro in semisoft and liquid media[235,242] enriched with feeder layers of monocyte-macrophages from blood or other tissues that secrete colony stimulating factor.[225] Cultures of bone marrow from patients with acute myeloblastic and lymphoblastic leukemia in relapse contain fewer colony forming stem cells, numbers of which return when complete remission is obtained.[40,255] The leukemic stem cell in acute myeloblastic leukemia is responsive to colony stimulating factor, but many small clusters of granulocytic cells are usually noted instead of normal colonies.[213] In contrast, no clusters or colonies are grown from the relapsed marrow of children with acute lymphocytic leukemia.[72]

The loss of normal progenitor cells by infiltration of leukemic blast cells produces progressive anemia, granulocytopenia, and thrombocytopenia.

Leukemic cell proliferation in vivo

The experimental L-1210 mouse leukemia model proposed by Skipper et al.[291] cannot be rigorously applied to human leukemia, but it does provide a basis for understanding the pathophysiology of leukemia. Prior to treatment or during severe relapse it is estimated that the patient with acute leukemia has about 10^{12} leukemic cells, i.e., 1 kg of tumor tissue.[96] In a logarithmic sense this figure is quite accurate since 10^{13} cells (10 kg) is obviously too much while 10^{11} cells (100 gm) is clearly an underestimate. Since less than 10^8 total body leukemic cells are undetectable in bone marrow aspiration, treatment programs can produce an apparent remission by a cytoreduction of greater than 4 logs of leukemic cell mass; even a 2 log cytoreduction of leukemic cells can convert bone marrow from 100% blast cells to 1% blast cells, yet 10^{10} leukemic cells remain. The L-1210 model has also shown that the fractional kill of leukemic cells is the same for a given amount of treatment regardless of the actual number of cells present so that, in theory, it should be possible, in humans as well as mice, to destroy all leukemic cells in the body by repeated or long continued treatment. Limiting factors are (1) drug toxicity to normal tissue, (2) resistance of some leukemic cells to drug therapy, (3) isolation of the leukemic cells in body compartments that cannot be reached by leukemic drugs in the circulation, and (4) a high proportion of slowly proliferating or non-proliferating leukemic cells not vulnerable to cell cycle–specific chemotherapy.

PATHOLOGY

Practically every organ has at times been found to be involved in the leukemic process. However, organ dysfunction as a result of leukemic infiltration is rare. The following organs and incidence of involvement have been noted in pathologic postmortem studies of patients who died in relapse.

1. Lymph nodes are always infiltrated with leukemic cells, lose normal architecture, and become matted together because of invasion of the surrounding capsule. It is not possible to differentiate primary involvement with lymphosarcoma from those changes caused by leukemia.

2. The liver is almost always diffusely infiltrated; there may be evidence of portal fibrosis in some cases.

3. The spleen shows diffuse infiltration of the splenic pulp and sinusoids with loss of normal malpighian corpuscles. Splenic infarctions are seen in 35% of cases.

4. Kidneys show diffuse infiltration in greater than 95% of cases, which produces enlargement without loss of renal function.

5. The bone shows attenuation of trabeculae with slender irregular borders lined by giant osteoclasts. Erosion of the cortex is less common. Widening of cortical haversian canals and plugging of them with leukemic cells may lead to bone necrosis and pathologic fractures.

6. The gastrointestinal tract is involved 13% of the time with dense leukemic infiltrates in the mucosa or submucosa that may pierce the muscularis mucosa. The esophagus is the only area of the gastrointestinal tract not involved with leukemic cells but often becomes the site of fungal infection. Lymph nodes, Peyer's patches, and appendix become infiltrated, and the appendix may be the site of perforation.

7. The heart shows silent infiltration of the myocardium in 34% of cases.

8. The lungs are involved in 13% to 27% of cases with parenchymal infiltration in either a diffuse or nodular pattern; at times it is difficult to differentiate from infection or infarction. Nonparenchymal involvement of the lung includes bronchial, peribronchial, pleural, and subpleural areas with pleural effusions common in lymphocytic leukemia.

9. Ocular involvement with hemorrhage and infiltration of the anterior chamber, choroid plexus, or retina occurs in 43% to 65% of cases (Fig. 21-7). Subconjunctival and subsclerosal infiltration can also be noted.

10. Foci of leukemic cells diffusely involve endocrine organs in 18% of cases. The thyroid, testes, ovaries, and adrenal glands may be involved.

11. Central nervous system involvement is found in a high percentage of cases prior to prophylactic treatment of the central nervous system. In an early study by Leidler and Russell,[190] sixty-seven cases had the following anatomic involvement: cerebral hemispheres, 61%; basal ganglia, 46%; brain stem, 31%; cerebellum, 28%; and cerebral and spinal meninges, 18%. Cranial nerves, especially the sixth, seventh, and eighth, were involved more frequently than peripheral nerves (Fig. 21-8). Thirty-two percent of patients died of cerebral hemorrhage secondary to brain infiltration.[278] A recent histopathologic study of 126 brains of children with leukemia noted 70 cases of central nervous system involvement. The earliest evidence of leukemia was seen in the walls of superficial arachnoid veins, whereas in more advanced disease there was extension into the deep arachnoid surrounding blood vessels coursing through the brain. Brain parenchymal involvement appeared to be caused by destruction of the pia-glial membrane or by interference with local per-

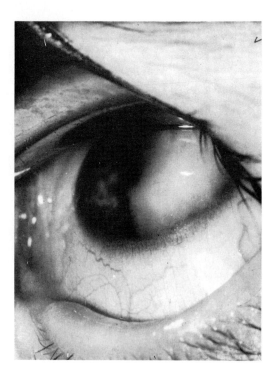

Fig. 21-7. Eye of a child with acute monocytic leukemia. Note the fluffy white leukemic aggregates, conglomerate and more discrete, occupying part of the anterior chamber.

fusion resulting from constriction of blood vessels by perivascular arachnoid leukemia.[250]

TREATMENT AND MANAGEMENT OF ACUTE LEUKEMIA
General principles

A new patient with acute leukemia generally requires hospitalization. Physiologic imbalances should be restored prior to chemotherapy, e.g., correction of anemia, establishment of adequate hydration, transfusion of platelets if bleeding is present, and antibiotic treatment of possible infection. If anemia is present, transfusion of packed red blood cells (10 ml/kg) will help restore normal physiologic function to vital organs. Most patients require red blood cell transfusion early in their course because of suppression of erythroid production by leukemia or chemotherapy. If bleeding is present, a rapid assessment of the cause is made and specific therapy initiated.

A vigorous search for infection is made in the febrile patient with absolute granulocyte counts less than 0.5×10^9/liter. Renal and hepatic function are evaluated with serum creatinine and SGOT, LDH, and prothrombin time, respectively. Serum calcium and phosphorous levels should be determined since hypocalcemic tetany has been reported in patients with a large leukemic cell burden after initiation of chemotherapy.[334] Tuberculin skin testing should be applied prior to initiation of prednisone therapy. Additional skin testing with streptokinase-streptodornase, *Candida,* diphtheria, and tetanus antigens determines the presence or absence of anergy and may have prognostic value.[136]

Specific areas of management of the child with acute leukemia that deserve special emphasis include hyperuricemia, hemorrhage, and infection.

Hyperuricemia. Most children with acute leukemia manifest hyperuricemia at the time of diagnosis. They are asymptomatic and occasionally renal failure caused by uric acid nephropathy may be the presenting complication[328] (Fig. 21-9). It normally is associated with bilateral renal involvement and serum uric acid levels greater than 10 mg/dl. Hyperuricemia results from increased purine turnover as a result of increased proliferation and destruction of leukemic cells by chemotherapy and radiation therapy. Purines are degraded to uric acid by the hypoxanthine-xanthine pathway catalyzed by xanthine oxidase.[258] Regulation of uric acid excretion is controlled by several mechanisms: (1) glomerular filtration, (2) proximal tubular reabsorption and excretion, and (3) distal tubule reabsorption.[67] Initial therapy is directed toward establishing adequate urine flow, alkalinization of the urine, and initiation of allopurinol therapy. Uric acid excretion increases with increased urine flow as fluid volume expansion develops.[67] Intravenous solutions with 5% dextrose should be administered at 3,000 ml/square meter/ 24 hours to ensure good urine flow. Alkalinization of the urine is accomplished by intravenous administration of sodium bicarbonate, 3 to 4 gm/ square meter/24 hours. Dosage adjustments, based on results of pH monitoring of the urine, are aimed to obtain pH values of 7.0 to 7.5. Sodium lactate should not be used since lactate inhibits uric acid excretion. With administration of bicarbonate the possibility of hypocalcemia and hypokalemia must be kept in mind. Allopurinol is given as 10 to 20 mg/kg/24 hours in divided doses three or four times per day. It competitively inhibits xanthine oxidase; the conversion of hypoxanthine to xanthine and xanthine to uric acid is blocked with resultant increase in the urinary excretion of the

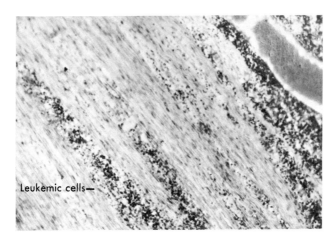

Leukemic cells—

Fig. 21-8. Leukemic cell infiltration in the eighth cranial nerve in a child with acute lymphoblastic leukemia. (×125.) (Courtesy Dr. Ferdinand La Venuta and Dr. James A. Moore, New York, N.Y.)

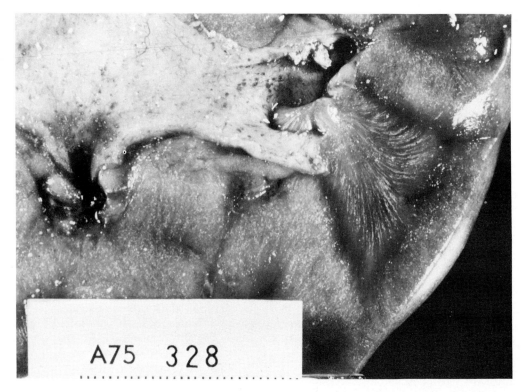

Fig. 21-9. Uric acid crystals in 12-year-old boy with acute myeloblastic leukemia. The initial uric acid level was 81 mg/dl.

oxypurines, hypoxanthine and xanthine. Since oxypurines and uric acid are more soluble in alkaline than acid urine, alkalinization of the urine helps prevent their precipitation in renal tubules.

If anuria from uric acid nephropathy does occur, osmotic diuresis induced by intravenous infusions of mannitol may be lifesaving.[67] Furosemide (Lasix) should be avoided since it produces acid urine; thiazides should be avoided since they decrease urate excretion through competitive inhibition for renal tubular secretion sites. Salicylates inhibit secretion of uric acid and raise serum urate levels.

Chemotherapy is withheld until adequate evaluation and management of these factors have been attained. Chemotherapy is often begun at reduced dosage in leukemic children with high white blood counts, adenopathy, and organomegaly because of their increased risk of developing urate nephropathy. Dosages of 6-mercaptopurine, a purine antagonist, should be reduced by 75% when used with allopurinol since degradation of 6-mercaptopurine is also dependent on xanthine oxidase.

Hypercalcemia and hypocalcemia. The clinical picture of patients with hypercalcemia may vary from no symptoms at all to a full blown hypercalcemic crisis manifested by nausea, vomiting, abdominal pains, lethargy, coma, dehydration,

and renal failure. The most common presenting complaints are anorexia, nausea, constipation, polydypsia, and polyuria. The metabolic basis for hypercalcemia may be either ectopic hyperparathyroidism or enhanced cortical bone resorption because of metastatic involvement with tumor. Ectopic hyperparathyroidism is associated with hypercalcemia, increased serum parathormone activity, and often hypophosphatemia, whereas elevations in urinary metabolites of prostaglandins, PGE_1 and PGE_2, occur in metastatic bone disease. Leukemia or lymphoma is occasionally associated with ectopic hyperparathyroidism, whereas most adult cancers produce hypercalcemia by directly invading the bone.

Treatment of this condition depends on its severity. Mild degrees of hypercalcemia (<13 mg/dl) in an asymptomatic patient require no treatment other than that indicated for the primary malignancy. Patients with more severe forms of hypercalcemia with serum calcium levels between 14 and 20 mg/dl often are water depleted from vomiting, poor intake, and polyuria, resulting in renal azotemia. Replacement of fluids, especially saline, will help correct dehydration and restore intravascular volume. The increased sodium excretion is accompanied by increased calcium excretion and will induce calciuresis. Intravenous administration of furosemide—40 to 80 mg every 4 to 6 hours—may result in significant calcium diuresis by blocking tubular reabsorption, but depletion of sodium, potassium, and magnesium may occur as a side effect if the regimen is administered too vigorously. Thiazide diuretics are contraindicated because they depress urinary calcium excretion. Hemodialysis has been used to control severe hypercalcemia in patients with severe renal disease, and peritoneal dialysis has been employed for long-term management. The oral administration of phosphate effectively controls hypercalcemia but is contraindicated in renal disease. Corticosteroids have been effective in reducing serum calcium levels toward normal. Cytotoxic agents found to inhibit bone marrow absorption at doses lower than antitumor doses include mithramycin and actinomycin D. Mithramycin, 25 μg/kg body weight, given intravenously as a direct injection or as a 4-hour infusion, reverses hypercalcemia in 48 hours. Actinomycin D, 10 μg/kg, has also been useful.

Hypocalcemic tetany results in patients with large leukemic cell burdens who are started immediately on chemotherapy. It has been postulated that there is release of phosphorus from the leukemic cells producing hyperphosphatemia and secondary hypocalcemia. Measures to reduce serum phosphorus levels and the addition of calcium gluconate or other calcium solutions are required to combat the hypocalcemia.[227a]

Hemorrhage. Bleeding is second only to infection as the major cause of death in leukemia and is usually a result of thrombocytopenia.[112,135] Bleeding may occur when platelet counts drop to 50×10^9/liter but becomes more likely when platelet levels reach less than 20×10^9/liter. The presence of high leukemic blast counts or infection tends to increase the risk of bleeding from thrombocytopenia. Transfusion with type-specific platelet concentrates, 1 unit/6 kg/day, should be given to treat bleeding episodes. Platelet concentrates have a volume of 20 to 30 ml/unit, and one unit is the amount of platelets obtained from one unit of fresh whole blood. The development of platelet antibodies is reduced markedly by administering donor platelets compatible with patient's platelets based on HLA typing.[326,327] Cutaneous, mucosal, gingival, retinal, conjunctival, and nares bleeding are common, but gastrointestinal, central nervous system, and pulmonary hemorrhage may be more life threatening. Hematuria is unusual in thrombocytopenia.

Salicylates decrease platelet aggregation through inhibition of release of endogenous ADP, resulting in prolonged bleeding time and a bleeding tendency.[78] They should be avoided in the leukemic patient with or without thrombocytopenia.

Other drugs reported to impair platelet function in vitro include antihistamines (promethazine and diphenhydramine), glyceryl guaiacolate, phenylbutazone, and tranquilizers of the phenothiazine class (chlorpromazine, prochlorperazine, and diazepam).[246] Other causes of bleeding in acute leukemia include hepatic dysfunction caused by leukemic infiltration of the liver with decrease in all factors but factors VIII and XIII and disseminated intravascular coagulation with decreased platelets, fibrinogin, and factors II, V, VIII, IX and increased circulating soluble fibrin monomers.[187] Bleeding manifestations in acute promyelocytic leukemia are a result of disseminated intravascular coagulation and may become worse with chemotherapy.[113] If disseminated intravascular coagulation is present, heparin therapy (50 to 100 units/kg given intravenously every 4 hours) is begun prior to initiation of chemotherapy and is followed by platelet transfusion. This approach has produced a more sustained response of the platelet count to platelet transfusion and has reduced the incidence of serious bleeding.[113]

Infection
Bacterial infection. Approximately 80% of children with leukemia die as a result of infection during either relapse or remission.[144,288] The nature of the infection varies with the phase of the disease and the intensity of chemotherapy. Infection during induction therapy is quite common. Fifty-one percent had documented infection during the first 6 weeks of therapy, resulting in a 3% mortality rate; half of these infections occurred during the first week of treatment.[146] The incidence of infection is related directly to the degree of granulocytopenia.[33] Organisms causing sepsis during induction of remission include *Staphylococcus aureus, Pseudomonas aeruginosa, Candida albicans, Haemophilus influenzae, Proteus mirabilis,* and species of *Klebsiella.* The incidence of pulmonary infection during early phases of remission in a group of 569 children was 29%.[284] The etiology of 157 cases (78%) could not be documented; 32 patients underwent lung biopsy and 9 cases of pneumocystis, 4 of viral pneumonia, and 4 of bacterial pneumonia were documented. Fifty-six patients died as a consequence of their pulmonary disease (10%). In one study 92% of infections occurring during remission were nonbacterial, e.g., caused by *Pneumocystis carinii,* herpesvirus, cytomegalovirus, hepatitis viruses, varicella, respiratory viruses, and fungi.[192] Patients with long-term immunosuppressive chemotherapy are at a high risk for gram-negative bacterial infections. Most oncology centers report that *Pseudomonas aeruginosa, Klebsiella pneumoniae,* and *Escherichia coli* are most frequently isolated, followed by group D *Streptococcus*

and *Serratia marcescens*. A special concern is the development of gram-negative sepsis from the patient's own enteric tract during prolonged periods of drug-induced granulocytopenia and bone marrow hypoplasia. Heat-stable opsonic activity against *Pseudomonas aeruginosa* is decreased in this group of patients.[325] These patients are similar to patients at the time of diagnosis in that severe granulocytopenia renders them more susceptible to pyogenic organisms.[33]

ANTIBIOTIC THERAPY. Patients with granulocytopenia or who have received corticosteroid therapy may not manifest the usual signs of infection or inflammation. Fever and chills in the leukemic patient must be considered to be of bacterial origin until proved otherwise; after appropriate bacterial and fungal cultures are obtained antibiotic therapy is begun promptly.[191,277] Since the etiology of the infection is unknown at the time intravenous administration of gentamicin, 3 to 5 mg/kg for 24 hours; a penicillinase-resistant penicillin such as methicillin, 200 to 400 mg/kg/day (maximum of 12 to 16 gm/24 hours), or oxacillin at the same dosage; and ampicillin, 200 mg/kg/day, should be started. If *Pseudomonas* infection is suspected or documented, carbenicillin, 400 to 500 mg/kg/ 24 hours, should be added. Carbenicillin in combination with cephalosporin, 170 mg/kg/24 hours (maximum of 12 gm/24 hours), also has been suggested in this situation. If a specific organism is isolated, antibiotic therapy should be altered according to in vitro sensitivities in each case. Carbenicillin and gentamicin have a synergistic effect in the treatment of severe *Pseudomonas* infection.[8,174] Carbenicillin and other penicillins inactivate gentamicin in vitro if mixed and allowed to stand for a period of time in the intravenous setup.[266] When a gram-negative organism other than *Pseudomonas* is isolated, carbenicillin should be discontinued and gentamicin continued alone or in combination with cephalosporin based on in vitro sensitivities.

SUPPORTIVE MEASURES. Leukocyte transfusions may aid in the treatment of bacterial infections in granulocytopenic patients. Patients with chronic myelogenous leukemia may serve as donors,[226] but their availability and higher risk to transfer hepatitis, toxoplasmosis, and cytomegalovirus infection mitigates against their common use. Granulocytes obtained from compatible normal donors can be concentrated either with the NCI IBM continuous blood flow cell separator or by filtration leukapheresis techniques. An average 4-hour collection with the NCI machine yields about 10^{10} mature functional granulocytes,[206] whereas the simpler, less expensive filtration leukapheresis yields up to 10^{11} granulocytes,[70] but the side effects and effectiveness of these cells in vivo re-

mains in question.[137] Donors should be screened for VDRL antibody, Australian antigen, and serologic evidence of *Toxoplasma* infection. All donors and recipients should be ABO and HLA compatible for maximum posttransfusion recovery of granulocytes, and recipients should be evaluated, if possible, for antineutrophil antibodies. Repeated transfusions of granulocytes from compatible normal donors seem to reduce mortality in patients with granulocytopenia and gram-negative septicemia.[114] Single transfusions are of no benefit and generally must be repeated daily for 5 days or longer.

Protected environments and prophylactic oral nonabsorbable antibiotics for patients with severe granulocytopenia were shown to decrease the incidence of infectious morbidity but no difference was found in remission rate or duration of remission between investigation and control groups.[193] The practical value of diligent hand washing cannot be overemphasized to the hospital personnel caring for these patients. The most common source of gram-negative infections is from endogenous (usually gastrointestinal) sources. Infections with *Staphylococcus aureus* often arise from superficial skin infections (e.g., paronychia and finger-prick blood sampling). The common practice of gown-and-mask reverse isolation often precludes good medical care and is no substitute for meticulous observation and diagnosis of early infection. The results of several extensive studies to determine the efficacy of heptavalent *Pseudomonas aeruginosa* vaccine in patients with malignant disease have been disappointing.[120,330]

Protozoan infection. Recently *Pneumocystis carinii* has become a common cause of death in leukemic children during remission, presumably secondary to immunosuppression. It accounts for 30% of deaths during remission in one series.[288] The incidence of *Pneumocystis* pneumonia was 4.1% in 1,251 children with malignancies of varied types.[145] Children have fever, nonproductive cough, tachypnea, nasal flaring, intercostal retraction, lack of rales on auscultation, and progressive cyanosis. Arterial blood gases reveal a Po_2 of less than 60 mm Hg with no evidence of CO_2 retention in the early stages. Chest films reveal diffuse bilateral interstitial pneumonitis. The organism cannot be cultured, and serologic confirmation appears to be of limited value.[269] Diagnosis must be made by histochemical identification of the organism on smears from lung tissue or fluid. The Gomori methenamine silver nitrate or Gram-Weigert stain can be used to identify the organism. Open- or closed-needle lung biopsy or lung aspiration is used to obtain fluid or tissue for culture and stains. Open lung biopsies are preferred since more tissue is available for bacterial, viral, and fungal cultures and for histologic study. Simple needle aspiration provided material containing *Pneumocystis* in 87.5% of first aspirations in one series.[145] However, the procedure was accompanied by a 30% incidence of pneumothorax, so thoracotomy tube suction should be available before lung aspiration is performed. Endobronchial brush biopsy has also been used to identify the organisms.[263] *Pneumocystis* infection is treated with pentamidine isethionate (available from the Center for Disease Control, Atlanta, Georgia), 4 mg/kg/day given intramuscularly for 12 to 14 days, with the total dosage not to exceed 56 mg/kg. Forty-eight percent to 81% of patients with documented *Pneumocystis carinii* infection recovered when given this treatment.[144,319] Trimethoprim-sulfamethoxazole, 20 mg/kg/day either by mouth or intravenously, is also effective. Toxic effects of pentamidine isethionate include hypotension, hypoglycemia, hypocalcemia, axotemia, elevated SGOT, neutropenia, and local reactions at the injection sites.[319] Differential diagnosis of interstitial pneumonia includes cytomegalovirus infection, varicella, herpes simplex, *Candida albicans,* aspergillosis, nocardiosis, *Myocoplasma* (Eaton agent) infection, tuberculosis, histoplasmosis, toxoplasmosis, leukemic infiltration of the lung, pulmonary alveolar proteinosis, adenovirus infection, influenza virus infection, parainfluenza virus infection, respiratory syncytial virus infection, pulmonary methotrexate toxicity, and cyclophosphamide lung disease.[144]

Rarely toxoplasmosis complicates the course of a patient with leukemia. Diagnosis may be established by observing rising or high titers using the Sabin-Feldman dye test or the complement fixation test for *Toxoplasma gondii.*[81] Sulfadiazine and pyrimethamine is the therapy of choice for systemic toxoplasmosis.[80]

Fungal infection. Between 28% and 33% of children with leukemia who die have evidence of fungal infection. *Candida albicans* and *Aspergillus fumigatus* were the most common.[270] *Candida* is a normal inhabitant of the oral pharynx, intestinal tract, and vagina, and these areas serve as a source of infection in the patient with altered host defenses.[222] Systemic disease from *Candida* involves the lungs, gastrointestinal tract, kidneys, heart, brain, meninges and blood, and there is a macular nodular skin rash.[222,252] Diagnosis depends on demonstration of the organism in blood or tissue, and this is difficult to achieve because of its invasiveness into deep tissues. Skin testing and serologic testing are not much help.[18]

Aspergillosis with *A. fumigatus* (59%), *A. flavus* (31%), or *A. glaucus* (5%) produces a deep-seated visceral infection. The usual port of entry is the respiratory tract. In some series it has surpassed

Candida albicans as the most common fungal infection in patients with acute leukemia.[109] Lung involvement is most common and is manifested as nodular pneumonia and hemorrhagic infarction. Other organs less frequently involved include the brain, heart, gastrointestinal tract, kidney, and liver. Aspergillosis is often associated with infection by other organisms, including *Candida albicans* and *Pseudomonas aeruginosa.* Antemortem diagnosis is difficult. In one study only 34% of infected patients had positive cultures. Since culture of blood is rarely, if ever, positive, diagnosis must be made by biopsy, such as lung biopsy.[214,331] Skin tests and serologic testing are not reliable. Mucomyosis is almost impossible to diagnose antemortem and has been demonstrated in lung tissue and gastrointestinal tract.[227] Cryptococcosis is an acute or chronic meningeal, pulmonary, or disseminated mycosis caused by *Cryptococcus neoformans.*[317] *Histoplasma capsulatum* produces disseminated disease with involvement of one or more organs of the reticuloendothelial system, lungs, liver, and central nervous system. It is different from many of the other mycoses in that blood and bone marrow cultures are positive in as many as 50% of patients with the disseminated form.[311]

Treatment of these five fungal infections is important since untreated cases have a mortality rate in excess of 80%. Amphotericin B remains a drug of choice despite the many toxicities that it possesses. Among its side effects are fever, chills, anorexia, nausea, headache, phlebitis, anemia, hypocalcemia, hypokalemia, azotemia, renal tubular acidosis, and hypotension.[9] The initial test dose of amphotericin B is 0.1 mg/kg intravenously to be increased to 1 mg/kg/24 hours. It should be infused slowly over a 6- to 8-hour period[41] since rapid infusions cause cardiac arrhythmias, chest pain, or convulsions. The drug should be given for a 10-week period. 5-Fluorocytosine is useful in *Candida* infections, especially cystitis. The dosage is 25 to 150 mg/kg daily in divided doses every 6 hours.[79] Marrow depression and hepatic necrosis are side effects. Potentiation of amphotericin B by 5-fluorocytosine has been described recently for infection with *Candida, Crytococcus,* and *Histoplasma.*[212] It is important to differentiate the infections with *Nocardia asteroides,* an aerobic, partially acid-fast member of the family Actinomycetaceae, because sulfonamides, erythromycin, and ampicillin may be effective.[329] Pulmonary infiltrates in association with peculiar skin abscesses should suggest the diagnosis, and the organism can be cultured from infected tissue.

Viral infection. Viral infection in acute leukemia can be severe and devastating; the infection may be a result of varicella zoster, respiratory viruses, cytomegalovirus, herpes simplex, vaccinia, measles, and viral hepatitis virus. Infection may be expressed as pneumonia, hepatitis, encephalitis, hemorrhagic varicella, or disseminated zoster. Fulminant varicella pneumonia occurs more frequently in children with acute lymphocytic leukemia, and mortality is significant.[82] In a retrospective study there were 10 deaths for 225 cases of varicella zoster in leukemic children during a period from 1971 to 1973, a mortality of 4.4%.[17] Zoster immune globulin (ZIG) prepared from high-titer plasma will prevent or modify the clinical manifestations of varicella in leukemic patients given a dose of 0.2 ml/kg (maximum of 5 ml) intramuscularly within 72 hours of household exposure. Cytosine arabinoside (Ara C) has been given in a dose of 20 to 40 mg/square meter/24 hours by continuous intravenous infusion for 3 days in an attempt to arrest the varicella infection in immunosuppressed patients with varied results.[148,298] Adenine arabinoside (Ara A) has also

been advocated at a dose of 10 mg/kg/day intravenously given continuously for 5 days.[218]

Cytomegalovirus infection produces fever, rash, pneumonia, hepatosplenomegaly, vomiting, and diarrhea,[267] or the infected patient may remain asymptomatic.[10] It appears to be the more common infection in children with leukemia, probably because of the immunosuppression from combined chemotherapy. Diagnosis is made by isolation of the virus. The throat is the most reliable source of virus isolation. Several cultures are necessary, since only 25% of the cytomegalovirus-excreting leukemic children were detected on the first culture attempt in one series.[133] Although some leukemic children excrete virus without a rise in antibody titers, complement fixation and indirect hemagglutination antibody titers may be of diagnostic value if determined in the acute and convalescent phases.[177] A fourfold rise in antibody titer correlates with the clinical syndrome of pneumonia, fever, and rash. Treatment with cytosine arabino-

Table 21-6. Antimicrobial therapy of infections in leukemia

Microorganism	Drug	Dosage	Toxicity
Bacteria			
S. aureus	Methicillin, oxacillin	200-400 mg/kg/day IV q6h	Allergy
P. aeruginosa	Gentamicin	3-5 mg/kg/day IV q6h 3Q 60 min	Renal, inner ear
	Carbenicillin	400-500 mg/kg/day IV q4h for 15 min	Allergy
E. coli, Klebsiella	Gentamicin	3-5 mg/kg/day	Renal, inner ear
Anaerobes—Penicillin-resistant Bacteroides fragilis	Clindamycin	20-40 mg/kg/day IV q6h for 30 min	Diarrhea, allergy
Protozoan			
P. carinii	Pentamidine isethionate	4 mg/kg/day IM for 10 days	Hypotension, hypoglycemia, hypocalcemia, azotemia, hepatitis, local reactions at injection site
	Trimethoprim-sulfamethoxazole	20 mg/kg/day orally or IV	Rash, neutropenia
T. gondii	Pyrimethamine	14.5 mg/M²/day orally for 28 days	Marrow suppression (Add folinic acid 6 mg/day orally.)
	Sulfadiazine	2.4 gm/M²/day q6h for 28 days	
Fungus			
C. albicans A. fumigatus C. neoformans H. capsulatum	Amphotericin B*	0.1-1.0 mg/kg/day IV for 6 hr for 1-3 months	Cardiac arrhythmias, chest pain, fever, chills, headache, nausea, vomiting, azotemia, renal tubular acidosis, hypocalcemia, phlebitis, hypokalemia
	5-Fluorocytosine*	25-150 mg/kg/day orally q6h	Marrow suppression, hepatic necrosis
Viral			
Varicella-zoster, cytomegalovirus	Ara C? Ara A?	20-40 mg/day 6 IV, continuously for 3-5 days	Marrow and immune suppression

*Effects may be additive.

side has been of varied success.[177,205,245] Floxuridine[42] and idoxuridine[19] have also been used in treatment; however, a large control study to evaluate the efficacy of these agents has yet to be reported.

Because of the apparent increased susceptibility of children with acute leukemia to viral infections, live viral vaccines should be avoided, including measles, mumps, rubella, smallpox, and attenuated polio vaccines. A treatment summary is given in Table 21-6.

Chemotherapy

General concepts. The goal of chemotherapy is to induce a complete remission and then to maintain the remission. Relapse can occur in the bone marrow, central nervous system, or extramedullary parenchymal sites, and each may occur independently of the others. Survival is directly related to the length of the first remission.[99] Combinations of two or more drugs are significantly more effective than single agents for induction of remission. This is based on the assumption that each drug acts independently and that the leukemic cell responsiveness or resistance to a drug is unrelated to its responsiveness or resistance to any other drug. For example, using a combination of two drugs, A and B, should in theory produce the following complete remission rate (CRR) by the formula:

$$CRR_{A+B} = CRR_A + CRR_B \times 100 - \frac{CRR_A}{100}$$

For example, if both drugs have a CRR of 50%, half of the patients will respond to drug A, and half the remainder will respond to B. The CRR of the combination will be 75%.[96] Clinical experience is slightly better than the formula predicts. In acute lymphocytic leukemia, prednisone has a complete remission rate of 57% and vincristine 55%. The combination of prednisone and vincristine produces a complete remission rate of 86% to 90%. This theoretical equation applies in some cases of lymphoblastic leukemia; it does not apply in acute myeloblastic leukemia (Tables 21-7 and 21-8).

Since the median duration of bone marrow remission without chemotherapy was 2.2 months, maintenance therapy with sequential and cyclic drug schedules were developed. Sequential ther-

Table 21-7. Remission induction by chemotherapy in children with lymphoblastic leukemia

Treatment	No. patients	Complete remission (%)	Reference
Single drugs			
Methotrexate	48	21	4
Prednisone	72	57	3
Mercaptopurine	43	27	4
Cyclophosphamide	44	18	84
Vincristine	119	55	158
Daunorubicin	32	33	25
Cytosine arabinoside	10	30	143
L-Asparaginase	21	67	231
Drug combinations			
Prednisone + mercaptopurine	154	82	97
Prednisone + vincristine	63	84	280
Prednisone + vincristine + daunorubicin	33	97	25
Prednisone + vincristine + methotrexate + mercaptopurine (POMP)	35	94	128
Prednisone + vincristine + L-asparaginase	582	93	139

Table 21-8. Remission induction by chemotherapy in acute myeloid leukemia*

Treatment	No. patients	Complete remission (%)	Reference
Single drugs			
Methotrexate	44	16	315
Prednisone	39	15	210
Mercaptopurine	31	10	4
Cyclophosphamide	45	4	69
Vincristine	14	36	159
	7	0	56
Daunorubicin	21	43	25
Cytosine arabinoside	31	44	131
5-Azacytidine	14	43	159
L-Asparaginase†			
Drug combinations			
Prednisone + mercaptopurine	77	3	309
Methotrexate + prednisone + mercaptopurine + vincristine	83	29	130
Cytosine arabinoside + thioguanine	36	36	106
Daunorubicin + cytosine arabinoside (± L-asparaginase)	23	60	60
Cytosine arabinoside + cyclophosphamide + vincristine	134	57	294

*Most patients were adults.
†Information inadequate, but response seems rare. Addition of L-asparaginase to the combination prednisone + daunorubicin + cytosine arabinoside apparently does not improve results.

Table 21-9. Cell cycle–specific drugs

Drug	Class	Mechanism of action	Dosage	Side effects and toxicity*
Vincristine	Vinca alkaloid	1. Inhibits flow of cells from G_0 to G_1[207] 2. Arrests cells in mitosis (metaphase) by inhibiting mitotic spindle formation	1.5-2.0 mg/m²/wk IV†	Neurotoxicity (parathesias, jaw pain, loss of deep tendon reflexes, constipation, ileus, hoarseness, sensory loss, muscle weakness, slapping gait), local reactions with injection site extravasation, alopecia, rarely inappropriate ADH secretion
Methotrexate	Folic acid antagonist (inhibits dihydrofolic reductase)	1. Inhibits DNA synthesis[184,185] 2. Synchronizes cells in S phase	15-30 mg/m² once or twice weekly IM or orally†	Bone marrow suppression, megaloblastosis, oral and gastrointestinal tract ulcerations, hepatotoxicity, osteoporosis, pneumonitis, necrotizing enteropathy, anorexia, nausea, vomiting
6-Mercaptopurine‡	Purine antagonist	1. Inhibits DNA and RNA synthesis, probably by interfering with purine synthesis, incorporation into DNA, and coenzyme inhibition[118]	50-90 mg/m²/day orally†	Bone marrow suppression, hepatotoxicity, rarely oral ulcerations, occasionally nausea and vomiting (toxicity accentuated by allopurinol administration)
Thioguanine‡	Purine antagonist	1. Inhibits DNA and RNA synthesis, probably in same manner as 6-mercaptopurine[118]	75 mg/m²/day orally[46a]	Bone marrow suppression, rarely hepatotoxicity, occasionally gastrointestinal upset
Cytosine arabinoside	Pyrimidine antagonist (inhibits DNA polymerase)[14]	1. Inhibits DNA synthesis 2. Synchronizes cells in S phase of mitotic cycle 3. Recruits cells from G_0 to G_1[184,185]	100-150 mg/m²/day IV continuously over 4 hr[110] or 25 mg/m² every 8 hr IV[46a]	Bone marrow suppression, megaloblastic marrow, oral ulcerations, anorexia, nausea, vomiting, fever; rarely diarrhea, abdominal pain, hepatotoxicity, and alopecia
5-Azacytidine	Cytidine analog	1. Interferes with DNA, RNA and protein synthesis[161]	100-150 mg/m²/day IV (dose not well established[161])	Bone marrow suppression, nausea, vomiting, diarrhea, rash, fever

*References 46a, 50, 118, 161, 181, 183, 232, 253, 265, 304, 313.

†References 11, 51, 138a, 141, 244.

‡Cell cycle specificity in humans not yet defined.

Table 21-10. Non–cell cycle–specific drugs

Drug	Class	Mechanism of action	Dosage	Side effects and toxicity*
Prednisone	Steroid	1. Lympholytic agent[75,184,185] 2. Prevents entry into S phase	40-60 mg/m²/day orally in 3 or 4 doses†	Hypertension, increased appetite and weight gain, cushingoid appearance, personality changes, osteoporosis, diabetes mellitus, pancreatitis, increased susceptibility to infection (varicella, fungal, tuberculosis, etc.), gastrointestinal ulceration
L-Asparaginase	Enzyme (deaminates L-asparagine)	1. Lympholytic[184] 2. Prevents entry into S phase[274] 3. Deprives cell of intra- and extracellular L-asparagine[172]	6,000 units/m² IM or IV 3 times/wk[51]	Hypersensitive reactions, hepatotoxicity, fever, coagulation abnormalities, azotemia, weight loss, anorexia, nausea, vomiting, transient hyperglycemia, diabetes mellitus, pancreatitis, EEG changes, hyperammonemia, encephalopathy
Cyclophosphamide	Alkylating agent	1. Inhibits DNA synthesis[184] 2. Arrests cells in mitosis 3. Prevents entry into S phase	2.0-3.0 mg/kg/day orally[118] or 200 mg/m²/wk orally or IV[11,244]	Bone maarow suppression, alopecia, anorexia, nausea, vomiting, hemorrhagic cystitis, bladder fibrosis, sterility
Daunorubicin	Antibiotic	1. Complexes DNA[290] 2. Cytocidal (perhaps more sensitive in S phase)	25-50 mg/m²/wk IV[11,313] (dose not well established); total dose should not exceed 20-30 mg/kg	Bone marrow suppression, oral ulcerations, anorexia, nausea, vomiting, fever, alopecia, cardiac toxicity; rarely abdominal pain, local reactions with injection site extravasation or phlebitis
γ-Radiation		1. Lethal to cells in all phases of cell cycle	150-200 rads/day	Tissue necrosis, bone marrow suppression, alopecia, pneumonitis, hepatitis, nephritis, bone growth arrest, encephalopathy

*References 46a, 50, 118, 161, 181, 183, 232, 253, 265, 304, 313.
†References 11, 138a, 232a, 244.

Table 21-11. Duration of remission and survival in children with lymphoblastic leukemia treated by various regimens

Maintenance therapy	Median duration of remission (months)	Median survival (months)	Reference
None	2.2	11	3
Mercaptopurine	8.2	12.5	
Cyclic prednisone, methotrexate, mercapto-purine	11	17	332
Intermittent parenteral or oral methotrexate (high dose)	10.4	16	2
Vincristine, mercaptopurine, cyclophosphamide, methotrexate sequentially or in cycles	12	24	13
Prednisone, vincristine, mercaptopurine, methotrexate (POMP) daily	13.5	33	129
Methotrexate, cyclophosphamide, vincristine weekly	15	35	243
Radiation (1,200 rads), cerebrospinal axis	15		12
Radiation (2,400 rads), cranial, with intrathecal methotrexate	36		12

apy involved maintenance with one drug such as 6-mercaptopurine or methotrexate until relapse occurred and then reinduction of a second remission and maintenance by a second drug. The sequences were continued until no drugs remained. Cyclic therapy involved maintenance with one of several agents for 6 to 12 weeks and then use of another agent for a similar period of time. The rotation of maintenance drugs was continued until relapse occurred. Individual drugs are not equally effective for prolonging remission in acute lymphocytic leukemia. Intermittent methotrexate and 6-mercaptopurine are better than cyclophosphamide, cytosine arabinoside, and daunomycin; vincristine, L-asparaginase, and prednisone are not useful for long-term maintenance therapy.

Three obstacles impede the goal of obtaining a long-term continuous first remission:

1. Drug resistance may develop so that some leukemic cells survive exposure to drug concentrations that would initially kill them.
2. A small but significant fraction of leukemic cells may persist in an extended G_1 phase of the cell cycle in which they are relatively insensitive to cytotoxic agents.
3. Leukemic cells may be sequestered in sanctuaries, especially the central nervous system, where they escape the effect of lethal concentrations of chemotherapy.

A modern approach to maintenance chemotherapy is based on the following principles posed by these problems.

1. To combat drug resistance combinations of drugs with different mechanisms of action should be used concurrently or in sequence. Since it is possible to have evidence of bone marrow remission and yet have leukemic cells survive, it may be useful to consolidate the remission using the initial induction treatment regimen at intervals.

2. The use of cell cycle–specific drugs and non–cell cycle–specific agents should be used in combination to attack and kill cells both in an active cell cycle and those in an extended G_1 phase. Lists of these agents are found in Tables 21-9 and 21-10.

3. Approximately 50% of patients with acute lymphocytic leukemia who remained in continuous first remission for 12 months developed central nervous system relapse during this time. Prophylactic treatment of the central nervous system with radiation therapy was first utilized with 500 rads, then 1,200 rads, and finally 2,400 rads to the cranium plus multiple intrathecal injections of methotrexate. Although some prophylactic central nervous system programs that have employed intrathecal methotrexate alone have showed a marked decrease in the incidence of central nervous system relapse, regimens that have utilized radiation therapy to the cranium appear somewhat superior unless methotrexate is continued during maintenance. In either case, central nervous system prophylactic treatment with 2,400 rads of cranial irradiation and intrathecal methotrexate (12 mg/square meter/injection, not to exceed 15 mg given at regular intervals) have virtually eliminated this problem and have reduced the incidence to less than 5%. Moreover, as indicated in Table 21-11 and Fig. 21-10, the length of the continuous first remission has been markedly prolonged so that 50% of the patients can be expected to remain in disease-free remission for periods greater than 5 years.

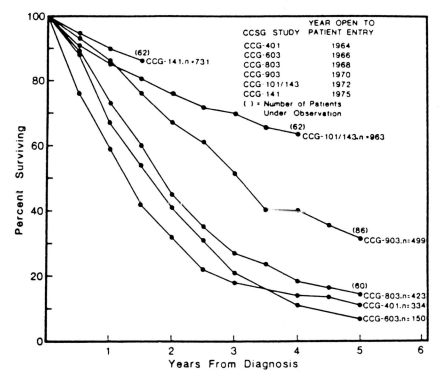

Fig. 21-10. Progressive improvement in survival of children with acute lymphoblastic leukemia treated according to Children's Cancer Study Group protocols during the years 1964 to 1977.

Current treatment of acute lymphocytic leukemia. One example of a modern chemotherapy program for acute lymphocytic leukemia is the following. For induction of remission dosages are prednisone, 40 mg/m²/day for 4 weeks; vincristine, 1.5 mg/m²/week intravenously; and L-asparaginase, 6,000 units/m² intramuscularly three times a week for 3 weeks. On day 28 a bone marrow aspiration is performed; approximately 92% of patients have a complete remission. For those who do not another effort should be made to be certain that the leukemia is truly lymphocytic and not myelocytic or monocytic. Addition of cyclophosphamide may be indicated to induce remission.[84]

Following induction, central nervous system prophylaxis is begun with cranial irradiation, 200 rads/day for a total of 2,400 rads, and six intrathecal injections of methotrexate, 12 mg/m²/week or twice weekly are administered; prednisone and vincristine are continued during this period. Following central nervous system prophylaxis a repeat bone marrow can be done to assure complete bone marrow remission.

Then the patient is placed in a maintenance therapy program with 6-mercaptopurine, 75 mg/m²/day; methotrexate, 20 mg/m² once a week orally; and monthly pulses with vincristine, 1.5 mg/m² intravenously; and 5 days of prednisone,

40 mg/m²/day orally. In those patients who have evidence of larger leukemic cell burden with initial high white blood cell counts or mediastinal masses the addition of cyclophosphamide, daunorubicin, or cytosine arabinoside may be indicated. However, the relative risk of toxicity must be balanced against the benefits. Maintenance therapy is continued and the dosage is adjusted to maintain the absolute granulocyte count between 1.0 and 1.5 × 10⁹/liter. The benefit of maintenance chemotherapy beyond 3 years is questionable, and most programs stop therapy after 3 years.

The issue of how long to treat a patient with chemotherapy in continuous first remission has only become evident in the past few years, reflecting the success of modern therapy. In one study fifteen patients receiving cyclic or sequential chemotherapy were randomly selected after 2½ to 3½ years of complete remission for continuation or cessation of therapy. After more than 5 years relapse had occurred in four of eight in whom therapy was stopped and in four of seven who had continued receiving therapy; relapses in both groups continued at the same exponential rate, suggesting that a point is reached at which chemotherapy ceases to eradicate leukemia cells or prevent proliferation.[178] In another study 103 children who received preventive central nervous system irradiation and were removed from therapy after

2 to 3 years of remission experienced a 12% rate of relapse in the bone marrow or testes, but central nervous system relapse did not occur.[11]

An immunologic rebound occurs within 2 to 3 months after cessation of long-term chemotherapy, with following features: (1) bone marrow lymphocytosis followed by peripheral blood lymphocytosis, (2) a rise in serum immunoglobulin levels and in antibody titers to previously sensitized antigens, and (3) an increase in reactive T lymphocytes in the blood.[35,116]

Treatment of bone marrow and extramedullary relapse. With the initial relapse after induction of complete remission, several alternatives are available. Early relapses are more likely to occur in patients with unfavorable prognostic factors (Table 21-12). Reinduction with the original therapy may be only partially effective, and more intensive programs are indicated, such as the "L-2" intensive chemotherapy program utilized at Memorial-Sloan Kettering Cancer Center[121] or regimens employing moderate-dose intravenous methotrexate therapy.[93,318a] A trial with a non–acute lymphocytic leukemia type of therapy should also be considered in patients who have a relapse within the first few months of treatment. Patients relapsing after chemotherapy has been discontinued usually respond successfully to the initial induction and maintenance therapy, and prolonged second remissions are not unusual. The central

nervous system should be reevaluated and retreated whether or not there is evidence of central nervous system relapse. If the patient had received central nervous system radiation initially, an additional course of cranial radiation (2,400 rads) plus spinal radiation (1,000 rads) can be given if high-dose methotrexate is not used. In a recent trial conducted in Britain the addition of craniospinal irradiation to a course of intrathecal methotrexate greatly prolonged the period of subsequent control of central nervous system leukemia.[321,322] Intrathecal or intraventricular methotrexate via an Ommaya shunt,[296] 12 mg/m^2/week for 6 weeks and then monthly is also recommended for overt central nervous system leukemia at the time of a bone marrow relapse. Patients not responding to intrathecal methotrexate have been treated with monthly intrathecal injections of methotrexate, 10 to 15 mg/m^2; cytosine arabinoside, 30 mg/m^2; and hydrocortisone sodium succinate, 10 to 15 mg/m^2.[303]

Maintenance therapy after the first relapse is usually less successful than initially, and each subsequent remission is shorter. The rates of remission induction with subsequent relapses also diminish. Combinations of agents not used during the first remission are indicated and include cytosine arabinoside, moderate-dose or high-dose methotrexate, cyclophosphamide, adriamycin, and daunomycin. Newer more experimental or phase II agents are reserved for subsequent relapses

Table 21-12. Prognostic factors in acute lymphocytic leukemia of childhood

Factor	Favorable	Unfavorable
Demographic		
Age	3-7 years	<3, >7 years
Race	White	Black
Leukemic burden		
Initial white cell count	<10 × 10^9/liter	>50 × 10^9/liter
Mediastinal mass	Absent	Present (with high white cell count)
Central nervous system disease at diagnosis	Absent	Present
Organomegaly and adenopathy	Absent	Present
Hemoglobin	<7 gm/dl	>11 gm/dl
Platelets	>100 × 10^9/liter	<25 × 10^9/liter
Morphology and histochemistry		
Lymphoblasts	Microlymphoblasts or L1[24]	Sarcomatous,[32] L2, or prolymphoblastic
PAS stain	Positive	Negative
Immunologic factors		
Immunoglobulins	Normal or increased IgG, IgA, IgM[215]	Low IgG, IgA, IgM
Surface markers	Null cell leukemia	B or T cells
Other receptors	Increased glucocorticoid receptors[175]	Decreased glucocorticoid receptors
Response to induction therapy	M$_1$ marrow (<5% blasts) on day 14[215]	M$_3$ marrow (>25% blasts) on day 14

and must be evaluated under the supervision of experienced centers.

Testicular relapse. In a recent large series reported by the Children's Cancer Study Group testicular relapse occurred in approximately 13% of the patients at risk.[229] Although testicular relapse may occur simultaneously with bone marrow relapse, frequently painless unilateral testicular swelling in a patient in complete remission heralds testicular relapse. Invariably bone marrow relapse follows. Diagnostic studies should include a confirmatory testicular biopsy and reevaluation of the bone marrow and central nervous system. Bilateral involvement is the rule rather than the exception despite the presence of unilateral testicular enlargement. The treatment of choice is bilateral testicular irradiation, 2,000 rads, including the inguinal canal. This dosage appears to irradicate leukemic cells but preserves hormonal function. Survivors who reach the age of puberty have secondary sexual changes but are sterile. If patients have bone marrow and central nervous system remission, reinduction therapy should be given in an attempt to prevent frank relapse.

Complications of central nervous system therapy. Recently 39% of children who received central nervous system prophylaxis with either 2,400 rads to the craniospinal axis in 28 days or 2,400 rads to the brain and four weekly injections of methotrexate, 10 mg/m[2], developed a syndrome occurring 3 to 8 weeks following irradiation with all or some of the following: anorexia and irritability leading to somnolence, fever, nausea, vomiting, diarrhea, and upper respiratory infection symptoms. EEG studies show a diffuse, slow, and patchy wave pattern over both hemispheres consistent with encephalopathy. All made a recovery within a few weeks.[95]

The more irreversible lesions ending in progressive neurologic deterioration and death have been associated with methotrexate and irradiation together. A distinctive degenerative change in telencephalic white matter consisting of diffuse reactive astrocytosis and multiple noninflammatory necrotic foci was evident in 13 of 231 brains from leukemic children.[249] The direct neurotoxicity of methotrexate ranges from chemical arachnoiditis (seventeen of twenty patients) to transient paresis (one of twenty) to encephalopathy (two of twenty).[71]

Irradiation depletes lymphocytes from lymph nodes, peripheral blood, and bone marrow. Patients who received craniospinal irradiation between the ninth and eleventh weeks of treatment were compared to those who did not receive irradiation. After 18 months of maintenance therapy with prednisone, vincristine, methotrexate, and 6-mercaptopurine, the irradiation group still had lower total lymphocyte counts, lower lymphocyte responsiveness to phytohemagglutinin, and relatively higher percentages of B cells, indicative of the prolonged depletion and sensitivity of T lymphocytes to irradiation.[209]

Irradiation has an effect on phagocyte function.[16] During craniospinal irradiation, in contrast to cranial irradiation with intrathecal methotrexate, peripheral blood neutrophils phagocytized bacteria normally but did not kill *Staphylococcus aureus, Pseudomonas aeruginosa,* and *Diplococcus pneumoniae.*

Treatment of acute myeloblastic leukemia

General principles. In myeloblastic and related types of acute leukemia, vincristine, prednisone, and L-asparaginase have a negligible combined therapeutic effect. Moreover, other cell cycle–specific and non–cell cycle–specific agents have relatively little selectivity of action for leukemic myeloblasts and usually cause serious suppression of normal hematopoietic stem cells. The rate of movement of leukemic myeloblasts from the resting or slowly proliferating G_1 state into the S phase is so slow that induction usually requires several courses of 5 or more days of treatment in cycles every 2 weeks to obtain remission. Even so, many normal hematopoietic precursors are killed in the process. The risk of the patient dying from infection as a result of granulocytopenia or hemorrhage caused by thrombocytopenia is 10% to 40% depending on the age of the patient. The problem is more evident in adults.[60]

Four drugs are effective inducers of remission in acute myeloblastic and related leukemias: cytosine arabinoside, daunomycin, 6-thioguanine, and 5-azacytidine. Remission induction rates of approximately 60% to 70% have been obtained with one or more of these agents. Remission induction is attended by severe bone marrow suppression from the effect of chemotherapy on normal stem cells as well as on the leukemic myeloblast. Generally induction programs are designed for courses of 5 to 7 days with separation by a treatment-free interval of about 2 weeks to allow normal hematopoiesis to recover and yet prevent leukemic cells from moving from the slow G_1 phase into an active cell cycle. Usually four to six such courses are required before a bone marrow remission can be obtained. It may be impossible to reduce the leukemic cell number to less than 15%. It appears that the length of the remission is not different in patients with less than 5% and those with between 6% and 15% blast cells in their bone marrow at the time that maintenance therapy is initiated.

Maintenance of remission in acute myeloblastic leukemia is generally obtained with the same drugs used to induce the remission but given at 3-week or monthly intervals. It is in this setting that immunotherapy with allogeneic acute myelocytic leukemia cells and BCG has been used in an attempt to produce further reduction of leukemic cell numbers. The immunotherapy consisted of weekly injections of irradiated allogeneic leukemic cells together with BCG delivered by skin multipuncture technique.[63] The median duration of remission was 188 days for those receiving chemotherapy alone but 310 days for those having immunotherapy as well; median survival from the time of complete remission was 303 days for the chemotherapy group and 545 days for the immunotherapy group.[20] Additional studies are needed.

Since the median duration of remission in acute myeloblastic leukemia is short, the problem of central nervous system leukemia has not been a significant one. The incidences of central nervous system involvement in childhood acute lymphocytic and acute myelocytic leukemia when expressed per month at risk are not greatly different.[77] Although central nervous system complications were found in acute lymphocytic and acute myelocytic leukemia with incidences of 32% and 7%, respectively, this was entirely a result of the longer survival in acute lymphocytic leukemia. Thus at 4 months central nervous system involvement had occurred in 3% of patients with acute myelocytic and 4% of those with acute lymphocytic leukemia and at 8 months was 13% for both groups.[236]

Current treatment. An acceptable chemotherapy program for children with acute nonlymphocytic leukemia is the following: for induction 6-thioguanine, 75 mg/m²/day by mouth for 4 days; cytosine arabinoside and cyclophosphamide, 25 mg/m² IV every 8 hours for twelve doses, with or without vincristine, 1.5 mg/m²/week, and prednisone, 40 mg/m²/day. Four to six courses are given at 14-day intervals. Platelet transfusions and leukocyte transfusions with appropriate antibiotics are used as needed to combat bleeding and infection.

Following successful induction the remission is maintained with monthly pulses of cytosine arabinoside and cyclophosphamide, 75 mg/m²/day for 4 days, and thioguanine, 75 mg/m²/day. This treatment program has produced an induction remission rate greater than 60% with a median duration of remission greater than 1 year.[46]

Treatment of chronic myelogenous leukemia. As in adults, the duration of survival in children with chronic myelogenous leukemia has not been altered by chemotherapy. The median duration of survival is still 3 to 4 years, which is similar to that of the group of patients described by Minot et al.[221] in 1924. Treatment seems indicated for patients with white blood counts greater than 200 ×

10^9/liter, in whom the chance for leukothrombosis is great, and in those patients with progressive weight loss as a result of a negative nitrogen balance from excessive myeloproliferation. Observations that DNA synthesis time (S_1) is normal (10 to 15 hours) and that ³H-thymidine labeling of the proliferating bone marrow myeloid cells is also normal (23%) support the idea that the rate of myeloid proliferation is normal.[301] Rather, the clinical observation that immature myeloid cells in the blood increase progressively faster and faster after each course of myelosuppressive therapy suggests a progressive maturation defect of the self-perpetuating precursors with an exponential expansion of the precursor compartment culminating in a blastic crisis or transformation. There is almost no effective treatment of blastic crisis once it occurs. Myelofibrosis, chromosome abnormalities in addition to the Ph¹ chromosome, increased leukocyte alkaline phosphatase in neutrophils, and a short doubling time of blasts in the blood are events that herald the onset of this crisis.[301] The leukocytosis is to a minor degree caused by the prolonged circulation of the neutrophils; the T½ of chronic myelogenous leukemia neutrophils is 26 hours, compared to 7 hours for normal neutrophils.[103]

Drugs active in chronic myelogenous leukemia are nitrogen mustard, uracyl mustard, vinblastine, 6-thioguanine, 6-mercaptopurine, triethylenemelamine (TEM), melphalan, and busulfan. Median survival statistics are available for certain of these agents given over most or all of the duration of the disease (Table 21-13); these drugs can be used to decrease spleen size and white blood count. Since 80% of acute myelogenous leukemia ends with a blastic crisis and the Ph¹ chromosome persists in bone marrow even when remission occurs, new attempts at more vigorous treatment designed to eradicate the leukemic cell and the Ph¹ chromosome seem justified. Regimens of radiotherapy of the spleen followed by splenectomy and an intensive course of chemotherapy with cytosine arabinoside and 6-thioguanine or other drugs used in

Table 21-13. Survival of patients treated for chronic myelogenous leukemia

Treatment	Dose	Median survival (months)	Reference
None		31	221
Busulfan	2-6 mg/day	40-42	125, 211
Splenic irradiation	600-1,000 rads	28	211
		43	68
Dibromomannitol	250 mg daily to twice weekly		
Hydroxyurea		39-50	167, 279

acute myeloblastic leukemia have been proposed.[176] It has been possible to eradicate the Ph[1] chromosome in two of eight patients treated in this manner. Recently a number of reports have documented the occurrence of Ph[1] chromosome–positive chronic myelogenous leukemia in children presenting with lymphoblastic crisis.[320] These patients responded to conventional acute lymphocytic leukemia–type therapy and specifically to combinations including prednisone and vincristine. Morphologic, histochemical, immunologic, and enzyme markers confirmed that the blasts were indeed lymphoblasts.

Psychotherapeutic management

The most difficult, and perhaps most important, aspect of management of the child with leukemia is the approach to the psychotherapeutic problems created by the diagnosis. After the diagnosis of acute leukemia has been established with certainty and verified by an experienced hematologist-oncologist, both parents are requested to meet with the medical personnel involved in the patient's care. This usually includes the hematologist-oncologist, the ward or family physician, the nursing specialist, and the social worker. The initial conference should be held in a quiet room where distractions can be held to a minimum, allowing ample time for discussion. A frank but sympathetic discussion of the diagnosis should be given in a manner that allows the parents time to give each other emotional support and to ask questions of the staff so that misconceptions can be eliminated.[73,76,186] Certain myths such as that leukemia is preventable, highly contagious, or hereditable should be dispelled. Many parents display guilt feelings about their tardiness in seeking medical evaluation; these guilt feelings should be allayed. A realistic prognosis for the patient should be described and important aspects of supportive therapy and chemotherapy outlined. Cautious optimism is indicated for the patient with good prognostic factors. Parents should be cautioned about sensational reports in the news media regarding immediate cures using nonmedical approaches. Emphasis is placed in the idea that their child will be returned to his or her normal life setting as quickly as possible. Overprotection should be avoided, if possible.[1] Repeated conferences are usually necessary to reinforce these points made during the initial conference. During the initial hospitalization and throughout the next few months of the illness ample time is allowed for parents to experience their grief reactions and to meet with the medical personnel to clarify points made in previous discussions. Parents usually progress through a mourning reaction including sadness, anger, and finally rejuvenation of energies to meaningful activities that may take several months to complete.

Parental support requires an understanding of and an ability to deal positively with the initial reactions of shock, guilt, denial, hostility, and anger that frequently occur. The patterns of adjustment and adoptive mechanisms developed by parents (''coping behavior'') will protect them from overwhelming stress and permit them to function more effectively in providing their child with as normal a life as possible.[100]

Green[117] has outlined a number of important principles of management of children with fatal illnesses. These include (1) the competence and availability of the physician, (2) continuity and personalization of care, and (3) preparation of the patient for required medical procedures. The problem of what to tell the child about his disease has led to the appreciation that all children should be permitted to have an active role,[162] ask questions, select the vein for intravenous injection, and maintain lines of communication between their parents and physician about their illness.

Discussions about the disease and its treatment depend on the age and maturity of the child, but it has been suggested that the child who is totally cut off from any meaningful discussion concerning his disease may have anxieties and develop feelings of hopelessness and guilt.[312] An ''open policy'' atmosphere can be sensed by the child, and confidence in the physician and the medical team is generated in this setting. The term ''leukemia'' should be explained to the child. The immediate and long-term commitments of the patient to the treatment program are briefly outlined, and procedures such as blood tests, bone marrow aspirations, and lumbar punctures are always explained in detail before they are performed. A realistic approach to pain and other physical discomforts also eventually instills more confidence and strengthens the relationship.

Total emotional support requires an understanding of the impact of the disease on other family members, including siblings and grandparents. Recent studies have emphasized the relatively high incidence of emotional disturbances during the course or following the death of a child with leukemia.[30] Preparing families for the death of a child,[101] or ''anticipatory grieving,'' may decrease the sudden, overwhelming sense of loss that occurs in parents who were unwilling or unable to accept the implications of the diagnosis. Patients with a relapse or other life-threatening situation require even more time so that the patient and family never feel lost or that ''the doctors have given up.''

Several important principles of management in the care of the dying child should be followed.[100,117] The physician must attend the needs of the child and family in a competent and conscientious manner and be available when needed. The family should have access to telephone numbers so that the responsible physician can be reached when an emergency arises. The physician must exhibit a willingness to answer questions and be sensitive to the child's emotional needs in order to dispel anxieties, fears, anger, or guilt feelings. He or she must be sympathetic, comforting, and supportive to the child and to the family but must avoid loss of control of his or her own feelings without becoming distant or impersonal. An environment of steady, constant support in which the child can receive honest answers should prevail. It is particularly important that the physician continue to comfort and support the child by his or her physical presence until death. Parents should be encouraged, if they wish, to return several months after death to extinguish lingering guilt and feelings of anxiety.[92]

Finally the problems and reactions of the physician should not be overlooked. On the one hand, emotional overinvolvement may compromise medical management and decision making; on the other hand, repulsion of death and the impulse to retreat from the dying child may deny the child and the family vital support. Senior physicians must be prepared to support their students and staff and be willing to communicate openly and continuously with the medical team managing the patient. Conflicts frequently arise regarding experimental therapy with new agents and heroic measures to sustain the life of a terminally ill child. The physician who treats children with leukemia, and whose aim is to provide optimal total care, must find a compromise between the extremes of overinvolvement and detachment.[272]

PROGNOSIS

It is obvious that not all patients with acute leukemia have the same prognosis. Prognostic indicators well substantiated to survival are age at diagnosis, histiologic type of leukemia, and initial peripheral blood leukocyte count in acute lymphocytic leukemia. Children younger than 2 years of age, and to a lesser extent children over 9 years of age, did poorly as compared to patients between ages 2 and 9 years. In terms of survival, age groups can be classified, from best to worst, as follows: 3 to 5 years, 6 to 12 years, 1 to 2 years, older than 10 years, and younger than 1 year.[107]

In a more recent study performed by the Children's Cancer Study Group[57] white blood cell count and age at diagnosis accounted for 75% of

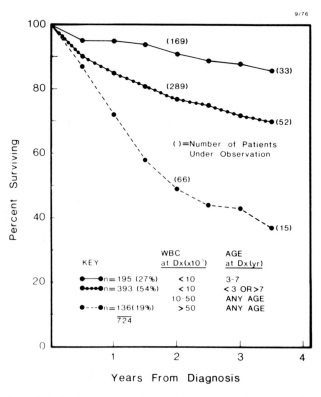

Fig. 21-11. Survival of similarly treated patients with acute lymphocytic leukemia. Three prognostic groups are identified on the basis of initial white blood cell count and age at diagnosis.

the probability of survival. In a group of more than 700 children in whom therapy was not a variable, three prognostic groups emerged:

1. The patients with most favorable prognosis, accounting for 27% of the total, had initial white blood cell counts of less than 10×10^9/liter and were between 3 and 7 years of age. Nearly 80% of the patients are alive 4 years after diagnosis.
2. An average-risk group, accounting for 55% of the total, had initial white blood cell counts between 10 and 50×10^9/liter in all age groups or were less than 3 or greater than 7 years of age with an initial white blood cell count of less than 10×10^9/liter. The median survival of this group is 3 years.
3. A poor-prognosis group had initial white blood cell counts greater than 50×10^9/liter at any age. Their median survival is less than 2 years (Fig. 21-11).

Patients with acute lymphocytic leukemia have a much more favorable prognosis than patients with other types of leukemia. The median length of first remission in acute lymphocytic leukemia is 4 to 5 years but only 1 year in acute myelocytic leukemia. Response to therapy can be predicted on the basis of the prognostic factor of the initial white cell count.[217] Patients with an initial white blood count of less than 10×10^9/liter[107] or 20×10^9/liter[286] have the best survival; those with white blood counts ranging from 10 to 99×10^9/liter in turn have better survival than those with white blood counts of greater than 100×10^9/liter. In acute lymphocytic leukemia, but not acute myeloblastic leukemia, nonwhite children have a poorer prognosis than white children.[107,286] Enlargement of the liver, spleen, and peripheral and mediastinal lymph nodes; the initial platelet count; and any hemorrhagic tendency may be other important prognostic factors for an unfavorable response. A mediastinal mass, however, is not an independent variable but appears to be related to the initial white blood cell count.[47] There is virtually no prognostic significance of the initial percentage of blast cells in bone marrow or of the sex of the patient.[107] However, patients with normal levels of hemoglobin have higher initial white cell counts and a poorer prognosis. It is suggested that the following factors may have prognostic value in acute lymphocytic leukemia: morphologic characteristics of lymphoblasts, i.e., large size, nucleolar prominence, PAS reactivity, and karyotypic pattern[320]; the rate of attaining remission[151]; delayed cutaneous hypersensitivity[134]; HLA type[268]; immunoglobulin levels[256]; the presence or absence of T or B cell markers on lymphoblasts[282,324]; and the presence of central nervous system disease at diagnosis. The characteristics of in vitro clusters and colonies grown in semisoft agar may provide prognostic information in acute myelocytic leukemia.[224] Recent Children's Cancer Study Group studies indicate that, in acute myelocytic leukemia, a favorable outcome occurs in only 20% of cases, especially in the age group between 5 and 10 years and with a white cell count of less than 20×10^9/liter at diagnosis.[15,46]

FUTURE RESEARCH AND NEW METHODS OF TREATMENT

Since the cause or causes of acute leukemia in humans have not been determined, vigorous pursuit of the basic etiology of this disease is required. Molecular biologists and virologists will continue to investigate the viral etiology of human leukemia. Cellular immunologists will try to define further immunologic alterations of the leukemic cell, identifying specific leukemic surface antigens as well as unraveling the interrelationships between the autoimmune processes and the leukemic process. Mathé et al.[197] investigated the efficacy of immune reactions in the control of human leukemia. The demonstration of virus-specific new antigens in murine leukemia induced by a virus and similar findings in the cells of human leukemia prompted the application of active immunotherapy procedures. One direction of research, nonspecific immunotherapy to stimulate the immune defenses, has had mixed and conflicting results. Although Mathé et al.[197] were able to show a significant prolongation of remission and survival in patients treated with BCG vaccinations, irradiated leukemic cells, or a combination of both, controlled studies from Britain,[208] the United States,[137] and Belgium[300] were unable to demonstrate any beneficial effect of immunotherapy in childhood acute lymphocytic leukemia over that provided by conventional chemotherapy. Additional clinical trials of immunotherapy in leukemia will be carried out.

Currently under investigation in childhood acute myelocytic leukemia is the use of BCG,[15] irradiated[247] and nonirradiated leukemic[15] cells, mercaptonal-extractable residue (MER),[23,140] and neuraminidase-treated leukemic cells[23] as adjunctive immunotherapy. Although preliminary results showed a beneficial effect of immunotherapy in adults,[248] the benefit of immunotherapy in children with acute myelocytic leukemia has not been established.[15]

Bone marrow transplantation (Chapter 17) will likely be performed earlier in the course of disease on selected patients determined to have a poor prognosis with conventional therapy. In one major transplant center HLA-identical, MLC-compatible bone marrow transplants have resulted in prolonged survival of more than 1 year in approximately 20% of cases refractory to conventional chemotherapy.[307] Relapse occurred in 40% of cases of acute lymphocytic and myelocytic leukemia; the other patients died of intercurrent infection. In two recipients leukemia developed in the donor leukemic cells, pointing out that environmental and host factors are very important in leukemia.

Clinical research trials will become more difficult to evaluate because of improved long-term survival and the time required to tell whether one treatment program is significantly different from another. For example, elimination of 10% to 20% of poor prognostic groups from a population compared in a treatment protocol can significantly affect survival statistics at the end of 5 and 10 years even though earlier statistics may not appear to be different.[157] Standardized methods to express results of clinical trials and chemotherapy must be used so that different treatment protocols can be compared. At present some investigators believe that the most significant figure is the percentage of all patients started on a treatment program to achieve a complete remission; others believe that the group of patients with inadequate treatment because therapy was stopped for reasons other than treatment failure or because of early death of the patient should be subtracted from the denominator. Since there are good reasons to support both views, all clinical facts must be given in results of these studies.

Hodgkin's disease and non-Hodgkin's lymphoma

HODGKIN'S DISEASE

Hodgkin's disease is a malignant neoplastic process of the lymphoreticular system. The cause is unknown, and it is characterized histologically by infiltration of the involved organ with Reed-Sternberg cells.

Historical perspective[370]

In 1832 Dr. Thomas Hodgkin described clinical histories and postmortem findings for seven patients with a primary disease of the "absorbent" (lymphatic) glands, which he believed was not secondary to obscure inflammatory conditions. Sir Samuel Wilkes in 1856 described ten cases, including Hodgkin's original four cases in the Guys Hospital, and coined the term "Hodgkin's disease" to describe this affliction. He differentiated it from leucocythaemia described by Bennet and Virchow in 1845 by noting that Hodgkin's disease was not associated with superabundant white corpuscles but was a disease primary to the spleen and lymphatic glands.

Dreshveld in 1892 and Kundrat in 1893 independently distinguished lymphosarcoma from the aleukemic leukemias. Follicular nodular lymphomas were not recognized until 1925 when Brill, Baehr, and Rosenthal described the clinical, laboratory, and histopathologic features of 2 cases. Two years later Symmers independently described the same entity, which since has been known as Brill-Symmers disease. Rappaport, Winter, and Hicks in 1956 recognized five types of follicular lymphoma in which the neoplastic cell resembled a lymphocyte, lymphoblast, histiocyte, or mixture thereof. Reticulum cell sarcoma of bone was first distinguished from myelomas in 1928 by Oberling; he considered Ewing's sarcoma of bone to be a variant of this type, which he designated as reticuloendothelial sarcoma. Two years later in 1930 Roulet first separated off the group of primary reticulum cell sarcomas of lymphoid tissue. In 1942 Gall and Mallory suggested that reticulum cell sarcomas should be further subdivided into two major groups: stem cell lymphomas and clasmatocytic lymphomas. The final entrant into the lymphoma family was reported in 1958 by Denis Burkitt, who described the clinical, radiologic, and histologic features of thirty-eight cases of sarcoma involving the jaw in African children, to which the name "Burkitt's lymphoma" has generally been given.

The first descriptive histopathologic study of Hodgkin's disease was performed by Sternberg in 1898 and Reed in 1902 when they clearly illustrated the appearance of the multinucleated giant cell that now bears their names and remains the hallmark of the disease (Fig. 21-12). It is fascinating that Fox in 1926 reexamined microscopic sections of gross specimens, preserved in the Gordon Museum of Guys Hospital Medical School, from three of Hodgkin's original cases and was able to confirm the diagnosis of Hodgkin's disease in two of them. Fox considered the third case to be more likely an example of lymphosarcoma or lymphatic leukemia.

The classification of Hodgkin's disease was begun by Jackson and Parker in 1937. They assigned the name Hodgkin's granuloma to the more typical cases; the pleomorphic, anaplastic tissue type was termed Hodgkin's sarcoma, and that with a relative paucity of Reed-Sternberg cells and a great abundance of lymphocytes was called Hodgkin's paragranuloma. Lukes et al. in 1963 recognized another characteristic subtype within the category of heterogenous Hodgkin's granuloma, to which they assigned the name nodular sclerosis. Whereas lymphosarcoma, reticulum cell sarcoma, and Burkitt's lymphoma were regarded as malignant neoplasms from the beginning, follicular lymphomas were initially regarded as benign.

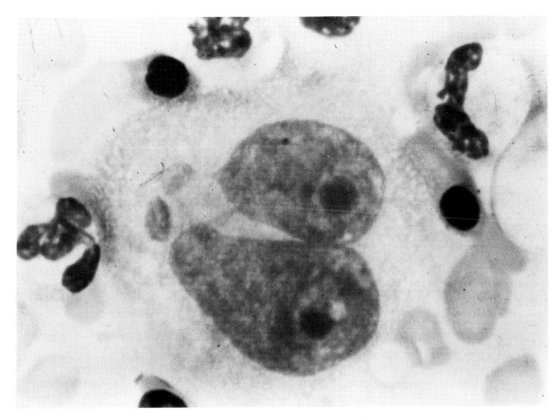

Fig. 21-12. Reed-Sternberg cell in Hodgkin's disease. The cell is binucleated, with a thick nuclear membrane and large regular nucleoli surrounded by a perinucleolar halo.

In 1887 Pell and Epstein first described the peculiar cyclic bouts with fever, and Reed in 1902 observed that her patient was tuberculin negative, despite the fact that he had open and active tuberculosis. Schier et al. in 1956 first demonstrated the relative anergy of patients with Hodgkin's disease, and in 1962 Aisenberg carried out the first systematic study in this series of patients and showed that anergy was closely linked to the activity of the disease.

The introduction by Peters in 1950 of a three-stage clinical classification ushered in a new era of increased emphasis on diagnostic evaluation and systematic analysis of the anatomic extent of involvement. This movement gained impetus in 1952 when Kinmonth showed that lower extremity lymphangiography could be used to identify pelvic and retroperitoneal lymph nodes and pointed out the sensitivity of this procedure for a more accurate definition of clinical disease than could be obtained by clinical palpation, inferior venacavagram, or intravenous urography. Glatstein et al.[358] in 1969 pointed out the importance of surgical laparotomy to document the involvement of spleen, liver, and retroperitoneal nodes in Hodgkin's disease.

Therapy of Hodgkin's disease and lymphomas was far ahead of that of leukemia. In 1902 Pussy treated a 24-year-old man with bilateral cervical lymphadenopathy caused by small cell sarcoma with x-rays and obtained a dramatic decrease in the size of the masses. Radiation remained the primary modality of treatment for the next two decades. Between 1920 and 1950 there was interest in the use of radical surgery for the eradication of localized lymphomas. However, x-ray therapy was also combined in most cases. Chemotherapy became a part of the treatment program only after Farber introduced aminopterin in 1948. The combination of these treatment modalities and an understanding of the relative timing and clinical indications for their use is a recent story that has produced the dramatic improvement in survival in Hodgkin's disease and, to a lesser extent, non-Hodgkin's lymphoma.

Classification

The classification of Hodgkin's disease is based on histopathologic patterns. The early classification by Jackson and Parker into paragranuloma, granuloma, and sarcoma correlated well with prognosis, since Hodgkin's granuloma had a prognosis intermediate between paragranuloma and the sarcoma types. In a series of 377 cases reviewed by Lukes[379] the median survival was 11.2 years for paragranuloma, 3.2 years for granuloma, and 0.6 years for sarcoma. However, the Jackson-Parker classification suffered a major drawback that limited its practical utility since cases were not distributed into roughly comparable numbers in the three categories. In Lukes' review 344, or 91%, were classified as granulomas, whereas 30, or 8%, were paragranulomas, and only 3, or 1% were sarcomas.

The classification of Lukes et al.[380] had six categories: (1) lymphocytic and/or histiocytic, nodular; (2) lymphocytic and/or histiocytic, diffuse; (3) nodular sclerosis; (4) mixed; (5) diffuse fibrosis; and (6) reticular. The distribution of 377 cases among the six categories was considerably more uniform with 6%, 11%, 40%, 25%, 12%, and 5%, respectively, of the cases. There was also a good correlation with prognosis; median survival was 12.4, 7.4, 4.2, 2.5, 0.9, and 2.3 years, respectively. Nonetheless, it was thought that six categories were unacceptably complex, and an effort was made at the Rye conference to simplify this classification. It was decided to combine the nodular and diffuse forms of lymphocytic and/or histiocytic types as well as the diffuse fibrosis and reticular types. This provides the current classification of (1) lymphocyte predominance, (2) nodular sclerosis, (3) mixed cellularity, and (4) lymphocyte depletion.[381]

Incidence

The incidence of Hodgkin's disease is age specific, with two peaks, one at age 20 and another at age 60. Although the incidence varies with geographic distribution, the annual incidence for Hodgkin's disease in the United States is 3.5/100,000 population for white males and 2.6/100,000 population for white females, with annual death rates of 2.3/100,000 and 1.3/100,000, re-

spectively.[385] Thirty percent of cases occur in patients under 20 years of age and more than half of these occur between the ages of 15 and 19. There is a male:female ratio of 1.8 in the group under age 20 and over age 35, but the ratio becomes equal between ages 20 and 34 years.[389] The incidence of childhood Hodgkin's disease in socioeconomically underdeveloped countries is higher than in the more affluent societies. Of African children 38.4% have the lymphocyte-depletion type; this type accounts for less than 2%[409] in the United States, where nodular sclerosis is the most common type and accounts for 50% of the disease in children between 0 and 14 years and for 60% to 80% in the 15 to 19 year age group[389] (Table 21-14).

Etiology

The cause of Hodgkin's disease is unknown, although infection by a wide variety of microorganisms has been proposed. The argument still continues, but observations of aneuploidy and marker chromosomes from cells of Hodgkin's disease tissue support that it is a true neoplasm.[348] Malignant lymphoid tumors have been reported in many species of animals. It is known that viruses, radiation, and genetic factors can be implicated as causal. Kaplan[371] has suggested three possible etiologic mechanisms: (1) release or activation of a latent virus, (2) atrophy of lymphoid tissue followed by compensatory hyperplasia of thymocytes more susceptible to malignant transformation in the proliferative stage, and (3) injury to marrow and thymus with impaired regeneration of the thymus and increased susceptibility of the tissue to neoplastic change.

RNA viruses have been demonstrated to be etiologic factors in lymphomas of chickens, mice, cats, and hamsters. C-type particles with similarity to RNA leukogenic viruses have been observed in electron microscopic study of tissues of dogs, cattle, and humans with lymphomas and

Table 21-14. Hodgkin's disease in Connecticut: histologic subtypes

Age group (yr)	Nodular sclerosis		Lymphocyte predominance		Mixed cellularity		Lymphocyte depletion		Not classified		Total No.
	No.	%	No.	%	No.	%	No.	%	No.	%	
0-14	24	47	11	22	16	31	0	—	0	—	51
15-19	48	68	4	6	14	19	2	3	4	5	72
20-34	41	53	11	14	19	24	5	6	2	3	78
35-49	21	46	8	17	12	26	4	9	1	2	46
50-69	9	15	4	7	29	50	9	16	7	12	58
70+	14	17	10	12	28	34	23	27	8	10	83
Unknown	1	100	0	—	0	—	0	—	0	—	1
TOTAL	158		48		118		43		22		389

leukemia.[343] The Epstein-Barr virus (EBV) has been incriminated as the possible cause of Burkitt's lymphoma. But there is an opposing argument that EBV simply is a passenger residing in proliferating lymphoid tissue. However, certain biologic characteristics such as the ability of the EBV to stimulate lymphocytes grown in vitro, the production of characteristic chromosomal aberrations by EBV, and the ability of EBV to induce membrane antigens in infected cells support the idea that the EBV is oncogenic in this disease.[363]

In one study the sera of 489 patients with Hodgkin's disease were examined for antibodies to EBV capsid antigens (VCA) and to the DNA components of EBV-induced early antigen complex, and results were compared with those obtained in infectious mononucleosis, Burkitt's lymphoma, nasopharyngeal carcinoma, and chronic lymphatic leukemia. In Hodgkin's disease many patients lacked antibodies to VCA and early antigen complex. This serologic evidence and other evidence seem to show a certain etiologic role of EBV in infectious mononucleosis, a probable role in Burkitt's lymphoma, but an unlikely role in Hodgkin's disease and nasopharyngeal carcinoma. It seems more likely that the immunosuppressive effects of Hodgkin's disease activate latent persistent EBV infections, which boost antibody titers in certain patients.[364] The idea that tonsillectomy increases the development of Hodgkin's disease by a factor of 2.9 times has been challenged because no patients with infected tonsils who did not have tonsillectomies were included in the study.[404]

Immunology

The incidence of anergy among patients with Hodgkin's disease is greater than in other lymphatic neoplasms, carcinomas, or controls. This observation was made in 1956 before staging procedures to assess the extent of disease were performed.[396] In one study the incidence of anergy was 53% in Hodgkin's disease, 12% in leukemia, 5% in non-Hodgkin's lymphoma, 0% in carcinoma, and 1.4% in controls.[375] Responsiveness decreased appreciably with increasing anatomic extent of disease. One or more of four different recall antigen intradermal skin tests were positive in seven of eight stage I patients, thirteen of twenty-four stage II patients, three of seven stage III patients, and five of eleven stage IV patients. There was no influence of constitutional symptoms within each stage.[342]

Dinitrochlorobenzene (DNCB) responses, which test both the afferent and the efferent arms of the cellular immune mechanism, parallel the recall skin test responses in advancing disease. For example, 36% of stage I, 17% of stage II, 10% of stage III, and 8% of stage IV patients had positive reactions to 0.1% DNCB challenge on the opposite arm 3 weeks after sensitization to 2% DNCB.[371] Homograph rejection, blastogenic transformation of peripheral blood lymphocytes to specific antigen or nonspecific mitogens, and absolute peripheral blood lymphocyte counts show a similar incidence of defects with advancing disease.[336] On the other hand, except for advanced near-terminal stages of illness, patients with Hodgkin's disease show normal humoral antibody responses to antigens to which they were previously exposed.[374]

Genetics

There appears to be a slightly increased risk (2½ to 3-fold) of Hodgkin's disease and perhaps other lymphomas in close relatives of patients.[393] Both mortality and incidence rates for nonwhites are appreciably lower than those for whites. Some evidence of clustering has been noted, suggesting that this disease, when it occurs in a family, could have an infectious rather than genetic etiology.[376] Although normal lymphocytes both in peripheral blood and in lymph nodes yield cells with a normal karyotype when stimulated by phytohemagglutinin, chromosome studies in lymph nodes in patients with any histologic type of Hodgkin's disease show a uniformity of pattern, a mixture of normal diploid cells together with an abnormal population of polyploid cells.[397] One possible explanation for the finding of two cell populations is that both cancer cells and other benign reacting cells (presumably lymphocytes) can be found in the affected lymph nodes from patients with Hodgkin's disease. Singular aneuploid lines can be found in the lymph nodes of patients with Hodgkin's disease. Changes in benign human cells rarely involve more than one or two chromosomes and never match the degree of abnormality seen in cancer cells, in which counts range from 51 to 154 chromosomes in both Hodgkin's disease and non-Hodgkin's lymphoma.[386]

Clinical and laboratory presentation

Clinical manifestations. The clinical manifestations of Hodgkin's disease in children mostly parallel those observed in adults. Usually the patient has a lump, swelling, or mass caused by an enlarged lymph node. In most instances the enlarged nodes are not painful or tender, and they may grow quite large before they become noticeable. The apparent rate of growth of the lymph node mass exhibits markable variation. Some enlarge rapidly in a few days, and rarely the mass may be present for as long as 2 years. Generally the mass grows larger over a few months. There are cases of waxing and waning of the size

Table 21-15. Sites of initial lymph node involvement in stage I Hodgkin's disease*

	Smithers (children and adults)	Jenkins (children)
Number	115	29
Cervical	73 (64%)	23 (80%)
Mediastinal	21 (18%)	1 (3%)
Axillary	8 (7%)	3 (10%)
Abdominal and pelvic	8 (7%)	2 (7%)

*From Smithers, D.: Hodgkin's disease, Edinburgh, 1973, Churchill Livingstone.

of the lymph node masses, occasionally associated with cycles of tenderness or fever. In 90% to 93% of cases lymph node involvement in Hodgkin's disease is manifested as follows: superficial nodes, 90% to 93% of cases; cervical, 60% to 80%; axillary, 6% to 20%; and inguinal, 6% to 12%. Primary mediastinal involvement is found in 6% to 11%, and retroperitoneal disease in 25% of the cases.[402] The sites of initial lymph node involvement in stage I Hodgkin's disease are presented in Table 21-15. Although mediastinal Hodgkin's disease has an initial incidence of 6% to 11%, it occurs in more than 60% of patients in the course of their illness and is most frequently noted in young women with nodular sclerosis type.[403] The two major complications seen in mediastinal Hodgkin's disease are compression of the major vessels, producing the superior vena cava syndrome, and regional spread from the lymph node to the lung parenchyma. Superior vena cava obstruction is one of the true emergencies encountered in both Hodgkin's disease and non-Hodgkin's lymphoma. Impairment of venous return to the heart results in marked venous distension of the neck veins, plethora, and edema of the face (which may become massive); airway or esophageal obstruction with dyspnea or dysphagia may occur rather suddenly.[401] Although the lungs are involved clinically in about 40% of the cases in which the mediastinum is enlarged, parenchymal involvement usually produces few symptoms. Cardiac involvement, if it does occur, is usually asymptomatic. Congestive heart failure, murmurs, and tachycardia have been described, although usually these are more related to the radiation therapy.

Generally in children the presentation pattern is that of cervical or supraclavicular mass in 75% of the patients; the mediastinum is involved in half of these. Twenty-three of 109 children with Hodgkin's disease who had staging by laparotomy were found to have splenic involvement.

In this series Hodgkin's disease arising primarily at an extranodal site was not encountered; extranodal involvement was only found as a late manifestation of the disease.[367]

Hodgkin's disease in the abdomen and retroperitoneum usually is progressive. Retroperitoneal lymphoma is regularly found at laparotomy in almost all of the 6% to 12% of patients presenting with inguinal adenopathy. Lymphedema of the legs and scrotal edema may develop secondary to large inguinal or abdominal nodes. Mechanical obstruction of the intra-abdominal tract or direct infiltration may occur rarely and it produces obstructive complications. Obstruction of the urinary tract may occur when massive retroperitoneal disease encircles one or both ureters. Malabsorption syndrome as a result of Hodgkin's disease of the bowel has been described. Usually a fullness or discomfort in the abdomen may lead a patient to palpate the abdomen and detect a mass.

Pain in the low back, often radiating down one or both legs, may be a presenting manifestation of a spinal cord compression syndrome produced by infiltration of the extradural space. The occurrence of spinal cord compression is a surgical emergency. The incidence of spinal cord compression in Hodgkin's disease is 3% to 7.5%.[357]

Constitutional nonspecific clinical manifestations of Hodgkin's disease include weakness, fatigability, anorexia, weight loss, cachexia, diaphoresis, fever, and pruritus. Fever occurs in 30% to 50% of patients and is continuous or cyclic.[403] There is a significant association of systemic symptoms with advanced anatomic stages as well as with the more aggressive histologic types of mixed cellularity and lymphocyte depletion.[373] The cause of the fever in the absence of infection is unknown.

Constitutional symptoms of Hodgkin's disease do not appear to be related to the existing splenic disease. Usually splenic involvement is silent but may present with hepatosplenomegaly; occasionally it is associated with sequestration manifested by anemia, leukopenia, thrombocytopenia, or a combination of any of these.[403]

Liver is involved in progressive disease when there is widespread involvement. In contrast to splenic involvement, hepatic Hodgkin's disease commonly causes constitutional symptoms. Jaundice and pruritus occur in 10% to 15% of cases. Usually the jaundice is secondary to intrahepatic obstruction by portal peribiliary infiltration.[341] It may be related to extrahepatic biliary obstruction from portal adenopathy or to an associated secondary hemolytic anemia, rarely Coombs positive in nature.

Pruritus may occur early in the course of the disease. As many as 85% of adult patients have pruritus at certain times in their disease. It may be localized or generalized. Most patients with generalized pruritus are found to have a mediastinal or abdominal mass, although the cause of the pruritus is not known. It is hypothesized that an autoimmune reaction to substances activated by tumor cytolysis produces this symptom.[388]

A variety of nonspecific skin lesions have been described in Hodgkin's disease and resolve with treatment. These are (1) excoriation, pyoderma, and lichenification secondary to pruritus, (2) pigmentation, (3) prurigo-like papular lesions, (4) urticaria and erythematous lesions, (5) erythema multiforme, (6) erythema nodosum–like lesions, (7) eczematous and seborrheaform lesions, (8) erythroderma and exfoliative dermatitis, (9) bullous pemphigoid lesions, (10) edema secondary to lymphatic obstructions, and (11) atrophic lesions of generalized anhidrosis and acquired ichthyosis.

Physical examination. Examination of most young patients with Hodgkin's disease reveals the presence of resilient, rubbery, firm lymph nodes, often in matted groups that may or may not be sufficiently distinct to permit the experienced observer to distinguish them from chronic infectious lymphadenopathy or from other benign conditions. Generally if the adenopathy involves the supraclavicular regions, which are unusual anatomic sites for common drainage from infection, neoplasm is likely. A definitive histologic diagnosis must be established by lymph node biopsy in every case. Careful palpation of all lymph node areas including those in the groin should be done.

Examination may also reveal evidence for compression of the superior vena cava with massive facial edema and engorgement of the veins in the neck and the upper anterior chest. Friction rub from invasion of the pericardium or from pericardial effusion may be accompanied by diminished intensity of the heart sounds and a paradoxical pulse. Small pulmonary parenchymal infiltrates are usually silent, but large infiltration affecting entire segments or lobes of the lung yield typical signs of pulmonary consolidation. Pleural involvement may be detected by a pleural friction rub. Palpation of an enlarged liver and spleen should be attempted with the realization that further laboratory studies are necessary to confirm involvement of these organs by Hodgkin's disease. The liver and spleen are seldom massive, but if they are enlarged, this usually indicates hepatic and splenic involvement. Careful neurologic examination is indicated to detect paresis and paralysis; alteration of normal reflexes may indicate a cord compression syndrome.

Laboratory data. Hematologic data on admission of 100 newly selected previously untreated patients with Hodgkin's disease revealed a hemo-

globin value of less than 10 gm/dl in only one patient who had stage III disease. Leukocyte counts greater than 12×10^9/liter were noted in nine of seventy-two patients with stage I or II disease and in six of twenty-eight patients with stage III or IV disease; monocyte percentages greater than 10% were found in five of seventy-two patients with stages I and II and two of the twenty-eight patients with stage III or IV disease; eosinophil counts greater than 10% were noted in three of seventy-two and in three of twenty-eight, respectively. Absolute lymphocytopenia ($<1 \times 10^9$/liter) was noted in ten of the seventy-two patients and nine of twenty-eight patients, respectively. Sedimentation rate elevations greater than 20 mm/hour were noted in twenty of thirty-seven patients with stage I or II and eleven of seventeen patients with stage III or IV disease.[370] Other acute phase glycoproteins claimed to be useful indicators of active Hodgkin's disease include ceruloplasmin (abnormal in fourteen of twenty-seven patients tested, with no correlation with clinical stage or presence or absence of constitutional symptoms). In addition, orosomucoid, haptoglobin, α_1-antitrypsin, ferritin, fibrinogen, plasminogen, and C-reactive protein concentrations may be elevated. γ-Globulin levels are elevated in 40% of patients. Initially there is a slightly raised IgG level, and IgA and IgM levels are often decreased. Moderate hypogammaglobulinemia occurs in 50% of cases, particularly in patients with more advanced disease.[359,368] Serum copper level elevation parallels the elevation in ceruloplasmin.

Anemia can be present late in the course of the illness in 80% of patients with progressive disease, but hemolytic anemia has been observed in only 2.7% of patients with Hodgkin's disease.[352] The basis for progressive disease anemia is most often ascribed to impaired mobilization of iron tissue stores and defective reutilization of the red blood cell iron, i.e., the anemia of chronic infection. The serum iron level is low, and the total iron-binding capacity is slightly decreased or normal.[356] Infiltration of the bone marrow can be suspected by observing either anemia or leukoerythroblastic changes in the blood smear, i.e., nucleated red cells, teardrop red cells, and a left shift of the granulocytes. Bone marrow biopsy is required to confirm this and may show either granulomas or myelofibrosis.

Roentgenologic study

Radiographs. Chest films identify mediastinal and hilar lymphadenopathy and pulmonary involvement. Although lymphangiography is almost routine, it should not be performed until the chest radiographs have been examined. Since the hazards of pulmonary oil embolization, which are ordinarily trivial, may be quite serious in the patient with diffused chronic pulmonary disease, whether specifically caused by Hodgkin's disease or not, conventional radiographic examination of the chest, including tomograms in selected situations, may be extremely useful. In a smaller child multiple views of the chest may be substituted for tomography.[346]

Lymphangiography. Lymphangiography is a sensitive means to detect retroperitoneal nodes involved in Hodgkin's disease. The technique involves identification and isolation of a lymphatic vessel in the dorsum of both feet for injection of a radiopaque dye through a catheter into the isolated, canulated lymphatic. The dye fills the lymph nodes of the deep inguinal and retroperitoneal areas and outlines gross distortions of their normal architectural patterns. The procedure is technically difficult in the preschool-age child because of the size of the lymphatic vessels. In one study lymphangiography demonstrated a 98% accuracy in predicting histologically normal or abnormal lymph nodes of 107 cases. There were no false negative results for Hodgkin's disease in sixty-nine consecutive untreated patients; however, a high incidence of benign histologic abnormalities caused 26% false positive results when prediction of involvement with tumor was attempted. In 15% of all patients who had relapses roentgenographic detection of changes in opacified retroperitoneal lymph nodes was the first manifestation of the initial relapse. Experience with repeat lymphangiography indicates that approximately 30% of the time a patient with previously normal lymphangiogram has an abnormal one. Yet 10% of these repeat studies showed distinct changes in the opacified lymph nodes caused by recurrent tumor. Lymphangiography serves as an important guide to surgical sampling of the retroperitoneal area and in radiotherapy field planning.

Bone survey and scan. The skeletal survey employs radiographs of the skull, vertebrae, ribs, pelvis, and long bones and is complemented by technetium Tc[99m] diphosphonate bone scan to detect osteoblastic or, less commonly, osteolytic lesions. The lesions are most often first seen in the vertebrae and pelvis.[349]

Total body scanning with radioactive gallium citrate (^{67}Ga) is a useful technique in staging of Hodgkin's disease and histiocytic-type malignant lymphoma. Scans are performed 5 and 7 days after injection of the ^{67}Ga rather than at 24 hours when abscess identification is the main issue. One study of thirty patients indicated an overall accuracy of approximately 80%. Identification of disease in the abdomen, including liver, spleen, periaortic nodes, and periiliac nodes, is sometimes difficult because of interference of ^{67}Ga uptake

in the liver, colon, and marrow. However, identification of disease in lymphatic tissues above the diaphragm is highly accurate.[365] In another study of 108 patients with Hodgkin's and non-Hodgkin's lymphoma who were evaluated with ^{67}Ga scans for staging, diagnosis, determining recurrence, or determining the results of treatment, accuracy was confirmed by comparing the scans with histologic material or roentgenologic and clinical findings and was found to be 83%. Known lymph node involvement was diagnosed correctly in 87%, but accuracy was only 48% for extranodal areas. Bone lesions were diagnosed correctly in 83%, compared to only 48% of lesions in the

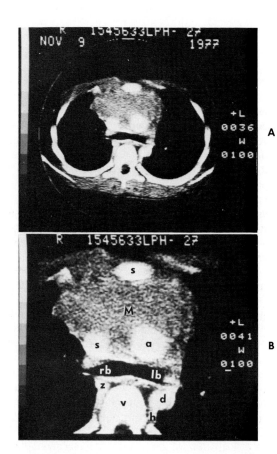

Fig. 21-13. CAT section at level of tracheal bifurcation performed during intravenous infusion of iodinated contrast medium in a 15-year-old boy. Conventional view **(A)** and labeled magnified view **(B)** of the same section show an anterior mediastinal mass *(M)* displacing the ascending aorta *(a)*, the superior vena cava *(s)*, and the trachea posteriorly. The mass is hypovascular and clearly demarcated from the opacified vessels. *rb* = right bronchus; *lb* = left bronchus; *z* = azygos vein; *d* = descending aorta; *h* = hemiazygos vein; *v* = vertebral body; *s* = sternum. Non-Hodgkin's lymphoma was diagnosed at surgery. (Courtesy Dr. Elias Kazam, New York Hospital–Cornell Medical Center.)

lungs and liver. [67]Ga scans were 75% accurate in twenty-eight patients scanned for initial staging. False negative results occurred in 12%; recurrent tumor in an area of prior radiation therapy appeared to be the most common cause of this. There were also 5% false positive results.[335] Liver-spleen scans with technetium ^{99m}Tc sulfur colloid is not a useful procedure because of its lack of specificity in Hodgkin's and non-Hodgkin's lymphoma.

Other noninvasive techniques. Computerized axial tomography (CAT) of the abdomen and chest is an extremely useful new technique that employs a low dose of radiation and has a high degree of resolution. It is particularly useful in the identification of retroperitoneal and mediastinal masses in Hodgkin's disease and non-Hodgkin's lymphoma (Fig. 21-13).

Ultrasound also provides useful information and is entirely noninvasive.

Clinical staging

Surgical laparotomy is now an accepted diagnostic procedure developed for the purpose of documenting involvement of spleen, liver, and retroperitoneal nodes. It supplements the information obtained by indirect means such as lymphangiography and various types of scanning. At the present time the choice between radiation and chemotherapy for treatment rests on the extent and site of involvement. The principle objective of exploratory laparotomy is to delineate the extent of disease. Early Hodgkin's lymphoma may not be grossly evident anywhere among the abdominal lymph nodes or in the spleen, liver, or other viscera. Guided somewhat by the scans and lymphangiogram, a complete surgical exploration of the abdominal contents is made and findings are recorded. Biopsy specimens are taken routinely of the largest and apparently most involved lymph nodes in each of the following groups and metal clips are placed to mark the areas: portal, celiac, splenic, aortic at the level of T12 and L1 and on both sides and below and behind the duodenum at the level of L2 to L4, external iliac on both sides; and the superior mesenteric. Specimens of nodes from other intra-abdominal areas are taken when lymphangiography indicates enlarged nodes or when they are discovered at operation. Biopsy specimens may also be taken from peripheral node groups during the same period of anesthesia when indicated. Splenectomy and biopsy of splenic hilar nodes is done. A wedge biopsy specimen from the anterior edge of the liver and a needle biopsy sample from both lobes of the liver centrally are taken, and the hepatic lymph nodes are also sampled. Even if the bone marrow has been examined and found to be normal preoperatively, a bone marrow biopsy specimen from the iliac crest is taken.[353] In a combined series of Hodgkin's disease in children under 16 years of age involving forty-two patients, there was a change in the staging of seventeen. Generally the staging involved patients with apparent stage I and II disease who were found to have disease below the diaphragm, or stage III (Table 21-16). This was the case in ten of eleven such patients.*

Generally it is unusual to find massive involvement of the liver early in the course of the disease. Abnormalities of liver function tests including sulfobromophthalein (Bromsulphalein [BSP]) excretion, serum alkaline phosphatase levels, SGOT, and moderate hepatomegaly on ^{99m}Tc scan may all

---

*References 358, 362, 377, 392.

Table 21-16. Changes in staging by laparotomy in childhood (<16 years) Hodgkin's disease

Series	No. patients	M:F	Age (years) (mean)	Stage	Staging No. prelaparotomy	Staging No. postlaparotomy	No. with change in status
Stanford	9	6:3	11-15 (13)	I-II	2	4	5/9
				III	4	4	
				IV	3	1	
Baltimore	3	1:2	11-15 (12)	I-II	1	1	0/3
				III	2	2	
Yale	7	4:3	5-15 (12)	I-II	6	5	1/7
				III	1	2	
Los Angeles	23	13:10	2-15 (9)	I-II	22	12	11/23
				III	0	10	
				IV	1	1	
Toronto	34			I-II	25	16	18/34
				III	7	15	
				IV	2	3	

be misleading. These abnormalities occur non-specifically, especially in patients with systemic symptoms, and hepatic involvement must be sought through histologic verification by biopsy. Conversely, liver involvement can be demonstrated rarely with no laboratory abnormalities. There is an excellent correlation between the size of the spleen and probability of liver involvement. This was documented at laparotomy in sixteen patients with Hodgkin's disease with spleens weighing more than 400 gm; thirteen (81%) had documented hepatic tumor. Of twenty-one patients with involved spleens weighing less than 400 gm, six (29%) had involvement of the liver. It is extremely rare to observe involvement of the liver without previous or concurrent splenic involvement.[394]

The Ann Arbor staging classification adapted in 1971 is the current and worldwide accepted method for staging of Hodgkin's disease. Stage I is involvement of a single lymph node region (I) or a single extralymphatic organ or site (Ie); stage II is involvement of two or more lymph node regions on the same side of the diaphragm (II) or localized involvement of an extralymphatic organ or site and of one or more lymph node regions on the same side of the diaphragm (IIe); stage III is involvement of lymph node regions on both sides of the diaphragm (III), which may also be accompanied by involvement of the spleen (IIIs) or by localized involvement of an extralymphatic organ or site (IIIe) or both (IIIse); stage IV is diffuse or disseminated involvement of one or more extralymphatic organs (liver, lung, or marrow) with or without associated lymph node involvement. The absence or presence of fever, night sweats, or unexplained loss of 10% or more of body weight in the 6 months preceding admission is denoted in all cases by the suffix letters A and B, respectively.

Certain recommendations for the diagnostic evaluation of patients with Hodgkin's disease were also adopted at the workshop in Ann Arbor in April 1971:

A. Mandatory procedures
 1. Biopsy of the involved lymph node or organ with interpretation by a qualified pathologist
 2. History with special attention to the presence and duration of fever, night sweats, generalized pruritus, and unexplained loss of 10% or more body weight in the 6 months preceding admission
 3. Physical examination
 4. Laboratory tests
  a. Complete blood cell count and platelet count
  b. Erythrocyte sedimentation rate
  c. Serum alkaline phosphatase

 5. Radiographic examinations
  a. Posteroanterior and lateral chest x-ray films
  b. Lymphangiogram
  c. Intravenous urogram
  d. Skeletal survey including spine and pelvis
B. Additional procedures
 1. Chest tomogram, frontal and lateral, when pulmonary hilar and/or mediastinal involvement is present or suspected
 2. Bone marrow biopsy, needle or open, if disease is clinical stage III, if alkaline phosphatase is elevated, if anemia is present, or at time of laparotomy
 3. Staging laparotomy if decision regarding management is likely to be influenced by staging
 4. Inferior venacavagram if lymphangiogram or urogram is equivocal or unsatisfactory
 5. Liver biopsy if there is a strong indication of hepatic involvement
C. Optional ancillary procedures
 1. Radioisotopic bone scans in selected patients with bone pain and negative unequivocal roentenograms
 2. Radioisotopic liver and spleen scans in selected patients (of limited value)
 3. Tests of immunologic function
 4. Additional blood chemistry determinations
  a. Uric acid
  b. Calcium
D. Promising procedures for clinical investigation: [67]Ga and selenium ^{75}Se scans and tests biologic indicators of disease activity, including ceruloplasmin, serum copper, serum iron, ferritin, and other acute phase reactants

Pathophysiology and pathology

The Reed-Sternberg cell in the appropriate histologic setting is required to establish the diagnosis of Hodgkin's disease. This cell can be identified by the large inclusion-like nucleoli and the double or multiple nuclei of large size (Fig. 21-12). A peculiar clear zone around a huge nucleus is the distinctive feature of this cell. The number and type of Reed-Sternberg cells vary inversely to the intensity of lymphocyte proliferation; when lymphocyte proliferation is prominent, characteristic Reed-Sternberg cells are rare, but when lymphocytes appear depleted, Reed-Sternberg cells predominate. The histopathologic classification of Hodgkin's disease is given in Table 21-17.[372] There are four histopathologic types and all of them cause total disruption of the normal lymph node architecture with characteristic invasion of the lymph node capsule: lymphocyte predominance, nodular sclerosis, mixed cellularity, and lymphocyte depletion. In an analysis of ninety-three children with Hodgkin's disease, the overall percentage distribution was nodular sclerosis, 57%; mixed cellularity, 28%; lymphocyte predominance, 14%; and unclassified, 1%. Lympho-

Table 21-17. Histopathologic (Rye) classification in Hodgkin's disease

Type	Features	Relative prognosis
Lymphocyte predominance (LP)	Abundant lymphocytic stroma; sparse Reed-Sternberg cells*	Most favorable
Nodular sclerosis (NS)	Nodules of lymphoid tissue of varying size separated by bands of collagen and containing "lacunar" cell variants of Reed-Sternberg cells	Favorable
Mixed cellularity (MC)	More numerous Reed-Sternberg cells in pleomorphic stroma rich in eosinophils, plasma cells, fibroblasts, and lymphocytes	Guarded
Lymphocyte depletion (LD)	Paucity of lymphocytes; diffuse, irregular fibrosis in some instances; bizarre, anaplastic Reed-Sternberg cells usually numerous	Least favorable

*Reed-Sternberg cells are essential for diagnosis of Hodgkin's disease but are not pathognomonic; they may be seen in infectious mononucleosis, metastatic breast cancer, etc. It is therefore important to observe them in an appropriate stroma.

cyte depletion was not seen. In stage I disease there was a relative excess of lymphocyte predominance and a decrease in nodular sclerosis.[367]

Fundamental lymphocyte abnormalities in Hodgkin's disease have long been suspected because of the apparent defect in delayed hypersensitivity responsiveness, increased susceptibility to certain infections such as herpes zoster, and tendency for the development of lymphocyte depletion with disease progression. The mediastinal prevalence of nodular sclerosis also suggests evidence of a thymic relationship in Hodgkin's disease. The early focal involvement of lymph node paracortical regions with sparing of sinusoids provides further evidence for thymic-dependent lymphoid tissue affinity with Hodgkin's disease. Recent evidence suggests a close interrelationship between the lymphocyte and the Reed-Sternberg cell. One recent hypothesis suggests that the development of Hodgkin's disease is based on a defective T cell surveillance system promoting development of Reed-Sternberg cells from reticulum cells.[391] Lukes and Collins[383] suggest that Reed-Sternberg cells represent a polypoid expression of transformed lymphocytes rather than traditional malignant reticulum cells. The clinical manifestations then would express the struggle between the host T cell and the Reed-Sternberg cell.

Recent functional and immunologic studies suggest that the abnormal cell in Hodgkin's disease is best classified as a malignant monocyte-macrophage rather than a T or B lymphocyte.[371a]

Treatment and management

During the last decade major progress has been made in the understanding and treatment of Hodgkin's disease. This has resulted in a marked increase in the proportion of patients who survive, both adults and children. A recent report showed a 95% actuarial 5-year survival rate for children in all stages aged 16 years or less at diagnosis.[367]

General principles of treatment applicable to adults pertain to children with Hodgkin's disease. It is obvious that treatment must be based on accurate clinical staging. Major treatment modalities include radiotherapy and chemotherapy alone or in combination. Modern radiotherapy of Hodgkin's disease is designed to totally irradicate the tumor and cure the patient. This requires a tumorcidal dose of 3,500 rads in 3.5 weeks to 4,400 rads in 4 weeks. In addition, a local "boost" to 5,000 rads in 5 to 6 weeks should be given to exceptionally larger, slowly regressing lymph node masses. When large lymph nodes areas are involved, the irradiation field must be shaped to encompass multiple lymph node chains, and this is usually best approached from an anterior and posterior opposed radiation port. The exception is for Waldeyer's ring. Megavoltage beam energies with a linear accelerator or cobalt 60 teletherapy apparatus with a treatment distance capability of 100 to 140 cm should be used. Treatment with small cobalt 60 teletherapy units operating at a treatment distance of 80 cm or less forces the use of multiple small treatment fields rather than one large treatment port and is a source of frequent technical errors. Patients with previously untreated, potentially curable Hodgkin's disease deserve optimal treatment the first time. Radiotherapy fields in Hodgkin's disease are the following:

1. The *mantle* encompasses the mediastinal, hilar, and bilateral supraclavicular infraclavicular, cervical, and axillary node chains with lead shields shaped to the lungs, heart, and spinal cord after 2,000 rads have been delivered.
2. The *inverted* Y encompasses the spleen and splenic pedicle and the periaortic, iliac, inguinal, and femoral node chains. Lead shields are used for the rectum and bladder

and the iliac and upper femoral bone marrow. Careful attention is paid to obtain continuous radiation at the "gap" junction with the mantle field.

3. The *total nodal* field encompasses the lymph node area included in both the mantle and inverted Y fields.

4. The *Waldeyer port* consists of opposed lateral fields encompassing the preauricular nodes and lymphatic tissues of Waldeyer's ring if it is clinically involved or if adenopathy is present in the high cervical nodes.

Radiation therapy is the treatment of choice for stages I, II, and III, whereas chemotherapy is reserved for stage IV; however, supplemental chemotherapy may be added to stages II and III when clinically indicated. In the growing child there is an even more valid reason for a graded sequence of radiation therapy based on stage, symptoms, histopathology, and presenting site. Local involved field, or limited, radiotherapy has a valid place in the management of certain stage IA and IIA presentations and subtotal radiotherapy in others. For example, those cases of lymphocyte predominance or nodular sclerosis that carry a better prognosis on the basis of histology and are confined to one upper cervical region (stage IA) require only ipsilateral local cervical, supraclavicular involved field radiotherapy.

Mantle field radiotherapy is indicated for stage IA nodular sclerosis type limited to the mediastinal region, and an inverted Y is indicated for stage IA lymphocyte predominance or nodular sclerosis limited to one inguinal-femoral region. Subtotal lymphoid radiotherapy involves the mantle field as well as the spleen, spleen pedicle, and para-aortic and iliac nodes and would be indicated for stage IA lymphocyte predominance and nodular sclerosis involving one lower cervical supraclavicular region; Waldeyer's field should also be included when the upper cervical nodes are involved.

For more extensive symptomatic stage II disease or for a case with an unfavorable histologic pattern such as mixed cellularity or lymphocyte depletion, total lymphoid radiotherapy is the treatment of choice, either alone or supplemented by six cycles of MOPP combination chemotherapy (see below).

In stage IIIA of the nodular sclerosis or lymphocyte predominance type disease with splenic involvement, total lymphoid radiotherapy may be supplemented with either hepatic irradiation of 2,200 rads for 4 weeks or six cycles of MOPP chemotherapy; in the presence of constitutional symptoms and/or an unfavorable histologic type, both hepatic irradiation and MOPP therapy are added to the total lymphoid radiotherapy.

Patients with stage IV disease require combination chemotherapy as the mainstay of their management. But those treated with chemotherapy alone have a relatively high rate of relapse in sites of initially bulky lymphadenopathy, so that strategies that incorporate moderate-dose radiotherapy in a split course between the chemotherapy at the end of multiple drug cycles after complete remission has been obtained are now used in many stage IV situations if tolerated. However, such combined therapy is very toxic, producing marked immunologic suppression.

Chemotherapy regimens most used in Hodgkin's disease involve multiple courses of combinations of four drugs. The program proposed by DeVita et al. is called MOPP therapy and is the one program most frequently used. This included nitrogen mustard (Mustard), 6 mg/m^2 intravenously on days 1 and 8; vincristine (Oncovin), 1 to 1.4 mg/m^2 intravenously on days 1 and 8; procarbazine, 100 mg/m^2/day orally on days 1 through 14; and prednisone, 40 mg/m^2/day orally on days 1 through 14. Fourteen-day cycles are separated by 14-day rest periods, and usually six or more cycles are given. Prednisone is included only in cycles 1 and 4. Other drugs found to have activity in Hodgkin's disease are chlorambucil, cyclophosphamide, adriamycin, bleomycin, the nitrosureas (BCNU and CCNU) and dimenthyltriazino imadizole carboxamide (DTIC).

When previously treated patients with Hodgkin's disease have a relapse in multiple extranodal areas or heavily irradiated sites, MOPP or other intensive combinations of chemotherapy are given if hematologic tolerance permits. Local radiotherapy can be given when relapse involves local nodes or extranodal sites if hematologic tolerance is too poor to withstand multiple-agent chemotherapy. Single-drug palliative chemotherapy is indicated when relapse involves multiple node or extranodal heavily irradiated sites and hematologic tolerance is poor.

Prognosis

The dramatic improvement in the prognosis of Hodgkin's disease has resulted from systematic application of modern diagnostic and therapeutic advances. At present the 5-year survival percentage is 81.3%, and the 5-year relapse-free percentage is 61.5%, including all cases and all stages at diagnosis. At 10 years relapse-free survival has persisted at about 50%, suggesting that at least 50% of all patients may now be permanently cured of their once inevitably fatal disease. Of course, this assumes a meticulous diagnostic evaluation including proper staging and judicious selection and skillful administration of radiotherapy and/or multidrug combination chemotherapy.

In a series of 504 consecutive biopsy-proved, previously untreated cases of Hodgkin's disease routinely staged with lymphangiography and laparotomy, including splenectomy, most patients were treated with high-dose total lymph node radiotherapy for stages IA, IB, IIA, IIB, and III SA; total lymph node irradiation supplemented with either hepatic radiotherapy or MOPP chemotherapy in stages IIISB and IV (hepatic A or B); and MOPP chemotherapy with or without supplemental radiotherapy for stage IV bone marrow disease with A or B symptoms. The following statistics were obtained:

Five-year survival: stage IA and IB, 86%; stage IIA and IIB, 93.6%; stage IIIA and IIIB, 81.3%; stage IVA and IVB 39%.

Five-year relapse-free percentage: stage I, 72.5%; stage II, 69%; stage III, 61%; stage IV, 26.9%.

Large series of similarly treated children are lacking at this time, but it is likely that similar results will be obtained. One contrasting difference is the higher incidence of life-threatening septicemia and meningitis in children with Hodgkin's disease who had staging with splenectomy and laparotomy. In more than 200 children and young adults, ages 3 to 18 years, the incidence of sudden pneumococcal, *Haemophilus influenzae,* and/or meningococcal infection was 10%; 50% of patients died suddenly.[347]

DIFFERENTIAL DIAGNOSIS OF LYMPHOMAS

Lymph node enlargement caused by Hodgkin's or non-Hodgkin's lymphoma may be localized or generalized. Regional lymphadenopathy is most commonly secondary to infection with β-hemolytic *Streptococcus, Staphylococcus aureus,* tubercle bacillus including atypical mycobacteria, cat-scratch fever, and typhoid fever. Generalized lymphadenopathy is a more common feature of infections with Epstein-Barr virus, cytomegalovirus, and adenovirus type 6 and acquired toxoplasmosis. Systemic tuberculosis, histoplasmosis, coccidiomycosis, and other deep fungal infections may also produce generalized adenopathy. Chronic granulomatous reactions in the lymph node resulting from bactericidal defects of circulating neutrophils and monocytes often reveal unusual infections with less virulent microorganisms such as *Serratia marcescens.* Generalized lymph node enlargement can be associated with sarcoidosis, serum sickness, and other allergic reactions, particularly eczematoid skin eruptions. Phenytoin (Dilantin) may occasionally produce striking lymphadenopathy.

Lymph nodes that are matted together, nontender, and of a firm consistency should be biopsied immediately. Many errors in diagnosis are attributed to technically unsatisfactory biopsy slides. Many technical pitfalls in histologic processing of lymph node tissue have been stressed by Butler.[344] Differential diagnosis is seldom a problem when classical Reed-Sternberg cells are observed, although cells indistinguishable from them have been found in infectious mononucleosis.[384] In some instances of Hodgkin's disease of the nodular lymphocytic predominant variety, Reed-Sternberg cells may be sufficiently sparse to be missed in the initial section. Such cases are not unlikely to be erroneously diagnosed as follicular nodular lymphocytic lymphoma. Similarly the diffuse lymphocytic predominance type of Reed-Sternberg cells may not be present in every section, leading to the erroneous diagnosis of diffuse lymphocytic lymphoma.

From the pathologic point of view, benign conditions to be differentiated from Hodgkin's disease and other malignant lymphomas include the hydantoin-induced pseudolymphomas, rheumatoid lymphadenitis, herpes zoster, and postvaccinal lymphadenitis.

Chronic lymphadenopathy simulating malignant lymphoma

A symptom complex has been described with the following features: onset of disease between 1 month and 2 years of age, hepatosplenomegaly, generalized lymphadenopathy, decrease in size of nodes during infections, fever, variable lymph node histologic changes but most suggestive of immunoblastic lymphadenopathy, hypercellular bone marrow, deviations in immunologic status with various manifestations of autoimmune disease (weakly to moderately positive Coombs test with hemolytic anemia, neutropenia with leukocyte antibodies, and thrombocytopenia with or without demonstrable platelet antibodies), and a chronic, intermittent course.[345] Variable responses to corticosteroids and to other immunosuppressive agents (azathioprine and 6-mercaptopurine) have been observed, and organomegaly decreased. Splenectomy was performed for hemolytic anemia and pancytopenia with a partial response. Many aspects of this disorder suggest an immunologic disease. Zuelzer et al.[410] have reported cases of chronic lymphadenopathy with intermittent hemolytic anemia associated with the presence of cytomegalovirus in lymphoid cells at the time of active hemolysis. Although the symptom complex simulated lymphoma, no evidence of malignancy has developed in prolonged follow-up.

NON-HODGKIN'S LYMPHOMA

In children malignant lymphoma of the lymphocytic or histiocytic type is markedly different from Hodgkin's disease in regard to the anatomic extent of disease at diagnosis, rate and manner of progression, incidence of leukemic conversion, central nervous system involvement, and response to irradiation and chemotherapy. Compared with lymphocytic or histiocytic lymphoma in adults, in children there is a markedly greater proportion with involvement of the gastrointestinal tract, the abdomen, or the mediastinum. These lymphomas may rapidly spread within a few weeks with a progression rate as high as for any human malignancy. This is reflected in the fact that the majority of children (60% to 80%) already have extensive spread of tumor at diagnosis. There is a small proportion (10% to 20%) in whom the disease is truly localized and who may be cured by surgery, radiation, and chemotherapy. There have been major improvements in survival over the last decade. In one study of childhood non-Hodgkin's lymphoma, fourteen of seventy-two (19%) of children were well at 3 years and nine of fifty-seven (16%) at 5 years from the time of diagnosis. However, the median survival for the entire group was 0.68 years.[366]

Classification

The classification of non-Hodgkin's lymphoma that appears most reasonable is a modification of that originally proposed by Gall and Rappaport.[355] These pathologists classified the disease on the basis of histologic features into (1) lymphoma, lymphocytic type, well differentiated, (2) lymphoma, lymphocytic type, poorly differentiated, (3) lymphoma, histiocytic type (reticulum cell sarcoma), (4) lymphoma, mixed lymphocytic-histiocytic type, (5) lymphoma, undifferentiated, pleomorphic type, and (6) lymphoma, undifferentiated, Burkitt type. Berard[338] modified this classification so that all forms can be either of a nodular or diffuse pattern except the Burkitt type.

Incidence

The incidence of non-Hodgkin's lymphoma is about 6/100,000, and it is responsible for 5% of all cancer deaths. The incidence is highest in the 15- to 34-year-old group, intermediate for those under 15 years of age, and lowest in the 35- to 45-year-old group.[361] Burkitt's tumor is a distinct form of non-Hodgkin's lymphoma seen predominantly in children between the ages of 2 and 14 years with a peak incidence at 7 years in tropical Africa, Papua, and New Guinea; more than 100 cases have been identified in the United States and within a 3½-year period more than 150 cases were found in Uganda.

Immunology

Hypogammaglobulinemia is a common sign in patients with histiocytic and lymphocytic lymphomas.[387] Peripheral lymphopenia and decreased production of antibodies to antigens are common.

Immunologic markers of surface immunoglobulins on peripheral blood lymphocytes and lymph node lymphocytes reveal most lymphomas to be of the B cell type of the IgM subclass. Some are T cell types identified by their capacity to form rosettes with sheep red blood cells spontaneously. In contrast, skin tests reactivity to recall antigens are usually normal.

Certain genetic disorders of immunity predispose to non-Hodgkin's lymphoma. Patients with ataxia telangiectasia, Wiskott-Aldrich syndrome, congenital sex-linked agammaglobulinemia, and Chediak-Higashi syndrome have an apparently increased incidence of lymphoma or a lymphoma-like illness.[354] There is a higher incidence of autoimmune disorders in patients with malignant lymphomas than in patients with various other solid tumors.[387]

Clinical manifestations

The peak distribution of non-Hodgkin's lymphoma is between 3 and 7 years and between 9 and 14 years. Males are affected five to six times more commonly than females.[395] Lymphadenopathy, usually painless, is the most common presenting complaint. In a series of 784 children, 505 presented with lymphocytic lymphosarcoma in the following regions: 132 in cervical lymph nodes; 136 in mediastinal lymph nodes; 107 in other lymph node sites; 63 in the gastrointestinal tract; 28 in bone; and 39 in other non–lymph node sites including paravertebral and paranasal sinuses, orbit, parotid and submaxillary glands, ovary, gingiva, breast, bone marrow, joint space, thyroid, lung, intracranium, spleen, kidney, and vagina. In 75 of these 584 cases the disease was disseminated at time of initial presentation and 4 were unknown. Of 200 reticulum cell sarcomas, 171 were localized as follows: 38 were localized in the cervical area, 12 in mediastinal nodes, and 46 in other lymph nodes; 24 were primary in the gastrointestinal tract; 34 were primary in bone; and 17 were in other non–lymph node sites. Disease was disseminated in 28 of 200 and 1 was unknown.[360]

Skin nodules, tonsil lesions, gastrointestinal or bone pain may occur. Weight loss, fever, anorexia, and malaise are seen in about 10% of patients. Peripheral edema, ascites, and pleural effusion result primarily from central lymphatic obstruction by lymphoma. Rarely in children non-Hodgkin's lymphoma may serve as a lead point for an intussusception.[351] Hepatic involvement may occur in a high percentage of patients although jaundice and alteration of serum bilirubin, SGOT, and alkaline phosphatase may be normal or only slightly altered. Histologic verification of involvement of the liver is obtained in a high number of cases. At autopsy liver involvement with tumor has been noted in more than 50% of patients, and the rate is no doubt higher in children than in adults since they have a higher incidence of diffuse disease.

Renal problems associated with lymphoma may be the result of parenchymal involvement, hydronephrosis, secondary ureteral obstruction, compression of the renal vascular supply, hypercalcemic nephropathy, and complications of therapy, i.e., uric acid nephropathy and radiation nephritis.

Bone lesions occur in 10% of patients. Primary histiocytic lymphoma of bone marrow usually occurs more frequently than the other types of lymphoma. The long bones, pelvis, and scapula are most commonly involved. Neurologic manifestations of lymphoma usually result from extradural compression by direct extension from diseased lymph nodes, by bone involvement, or by interference with the vascular supply to the cord. In more than 50% of the patients the disease may convert to acute leukemia.[369,398]

The most common clinical manifestations relate to the particular area of lymph node involvement. Paratracheal and mediastinal involvement cause symptoms of fatigue, hoarseness, dry hacking cough, and fever. The mass can displace the trachea and compress the mediastinal vascular structures, creating the superior mediastinal syndrome of facial edema, plethora, cyanosis, and distended neck veins. Small bowel and colon involvement may cause obstruction; gastrointestinal obstruction most commonly involves the ileum. Occasionally diffuse lymphosarcoma of the bowel can mimic protein-losing enteropathy, hemorrhage into the bowel wall, malabsorption, or sprue. Retroperitoneal disease may produce complaints of weight loss and back pain, abdominal pain, and a feeling of abdominal fullness.

Two major complications from malignant lymphoma in childhood are leukemic conversion and central nervous system involvement. The frequency of leukemic conversion in lymphocytic and histiocytic lymphoma is dependent on the disease pattern at diagnosis. In one study, when the disease was primary in the abdominal, gastrointestinal, or extranodal head and neck areas, 6% developed leukemia later in the disease compared to 29% of patients with primary mediastinal, lymph node, or mixed patterns.

Involvement of the central nervous system occurred in 30 of 102 children with non-Hodgkin's lymphoma. In six the complication was present at diagnosis but most frequently central nervous system disease occurred later in the course. Only seven of twenty-three developed central nervous system disease at the time after leukemic conversion; the remainder developed it without prior leukemic conversion. Central nervous system complication was common in all patterns of disease; 24% for abdominal, gastrointestinal, and extranodal head and neck disease and 35% for mediastinal, nodal, and mixed patterns.[366]

Laboratory data

Generally the complete blood count is normal, except when leukemic transformation occurs. In that case pancytopenia or frank leukemia may be present with circulating lymphoblasts. Bone marrow biopsy is indicated in addition to the bone marrow aspiration, and a higher incidence of leukemic transformation is revealed by testing in this manner. The conversion of poorly differentiated lymphocytic lymphoma resembles acute lymphocytic leukemia, whereas histiocytic lymphoma generally resembles monohistiocytic leukemia. Lumbar puncture reveals an elevation of spinal fluid pressure, an increase in malignant blast cells, and occasionally a slight elevation in protein levels when central nervous system involvement occurs. Generally results of liver function studies are normal and often the serum LDH is proportionally higher than the SGOT because of a release of this enzyme from the malignant cells themselves. This is especially the case with leukemic transformation. Serum creatinine and BUN should be monitored as indicators of renal function. Uric acid elevations may occur and can produce nephropathy, if unrecognized.

Radiologic studies include chest x-ray films to exclude an anterior mediastinal mass or other nodal masses and pleural effusion. A skeletal survey is done to exclude gross areas of osteolytic bone destruction. Soft tissue views of the nasopharynx are obtained for evidence of involvement of Waldeyer's ring. An intravenous pyelogram after initial assessment of renal function and hydration may be done to exclude renal parenchymal disease, retroperitoneal disease, or obstruction of the ureters, particularly by lymphomatous masses in the pelvis.

In selected cases examination of the upper and lower gastrointestinal tract is indicated to exclude or evaluate primary or secondary involvement of the gastrointestinal tract. Sonography and CAT scans are also helpful in evaluating suspected masses. Lymphangiography may be of particular value in evaluation of a child presenting with apparent localized disease. In the majority of cases with evidence of widespread non-Hodgkin's lymphoma this is not necessary, since the required systemic therapy is not influenced by knowledge of the state of the limited number of retroperitoneal nodes. A ^{99m}Tc liver-spleen scan may be useful, although nonspecific, to gauge the size of organs in response to therapy. Inferior venacavagrams are helpful in selected cases. A ^{67}Ga citrate scan is useful in defining lymph node and bone involvement but is less accurate in defining extranodal sites of involvement such as the lungs and liver.[335]

Quantitative evaluation of immunoglobulins may reveal alterations in one or more of the immunoglobulin subclasses. Generally the degree of hypogammaglobulinemia is mild and does not produce symptoms. Surface marker studies on biopsied nodes should be performed as well.

Staging procedures

Since the pattern of spread of non-Hodgkin's lymphoma is unpredictable and does not follow the more orderly movement from one contiguous lymph node site to the next as is the case in Hodgkin's disease, no generally accepted staging method has emerged for lymphosarcoma of childhood. The value of diagnostic laparotomy in the staging of Hodgkin's disease is clearly proved, but this procedure cannot be logically extended to non-Hodgkin's lymphoma since the dissemination is often to the bone marrow or central nervous system or to undetectable lymph node sites not reached by laparotomy.

Pathophysiology and pathology

The classification of non-Hodgkin's lymphoma depends on the predominant cell type, either lymphocyte or histiocyte, the differentiation of the lymphocyte or histocyte, and the histology of the involved lymph node either in a diffuse or nodular pattern. The classification is given on p. 632.

In children virtually all lymphomas are diffuse and all of the lymphocytic types are poorly differentiated. The predominant type and histopathologic subtypes appear to be (1) diffuse, poorly differentiated lymphocytic, (2) diffuse histiocytic, (3) diffuse undifferentiated, Burkitt's type, and (4) diffuse undifferentiated pleomorphic or stem cell type.

A new functional classification of lymphomas has been proposed on the basis of techniques for identification of T and B lymphocytes and histiocytes, quantitation of lymphocyte transformation, and certain morphologic observations.[372] More than 70% of non-Hodgkin's lymphomas studied in this way revealed evidence of B cell involvement. Furthermore, lymphomas of the true histiocytic variety appeared rare. Redefinition with functional studies may be needed since those previously recorded as histiocytic lymphomas are undistinguishable morphologically from transformed lymphocytes. Lymphomas of large transformed lymphocytes called immunoblastic sarcomas of the B and T cell types have been observed to develop in

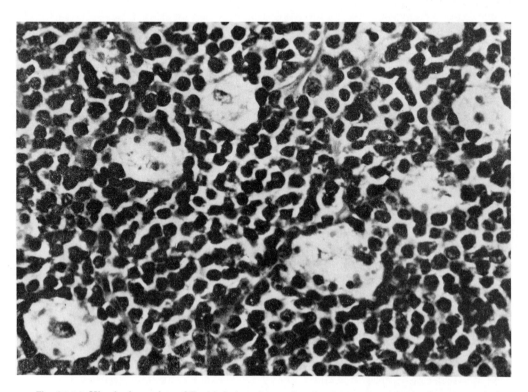

Fig. 21-14. Histologic section of Burkitt's lymphoma showing large, clear histiocytes set between undifferentiated lymphoid cells, giving the so-called starry sky pattern. (From Ziegler, J. L., Wright, D. H., and Kyalwazi, S. K., Cancer **27:**503, 1971.)

abnormal immune states. Further information in this area is required for better interpretation of histology.

Burkitt's lymphoma. The only lymphoid neoplasm that has been closely linked to viral etiology is Burkitt's tumor. This distinct clinical pathologic syndrome was originally described by Burkitt in 1958 and is classified as a malignant lymphoma composed of uniformly undifferentiated lymphoblasts with a characteristic histologic and cytologic feature. It is predominantly seen in children between the ages of 2 and 14 with a peak incidence at 7 years. Males are slightly more affected than females. The incidence is highest in tropical Africa, Papua, and New Guinea, although sporadic cases have been reported throughout many different countries of the world. More than 100 cases have been confirmed in the United States. The Epstein-Barr virus, a herpeslike DNA virus, has been cultured from Burkitt's lymphoblasts and can be identified by electron microscopy from these cells. The pathologic features include a uniformity of small undifferentiated lymphoreticular cells with little variation in size and shape interspersed with phagocytic histiocytes, producing a so-called starry sky pattern (Fig. 21-14). In Africa 60% of the patients present with a jaw tumor. These are painless, appear to originate from the marrow of the maxilla or mandible, grow rapidly, and distort the face and gingivae with loosening of the teeth.

The second most common presenting feature is abdominal involvement. Bilateral renal tumors, mesenteric retroperitoneal tumors, and ascites occur. In decreasing order of incidence, kidneys, ovaries, mesenteries, retroperitoneal tissue, liver, and spleen may be involved. Patients with abdominal tumors may or may not have associated jaw tumors. Other sites less frequently involved include the thyroid, salivary glands, pelvis, long bones, grafts, bone marrow, heart, and skin. The peripheral and mediastinal lymph nodes in Waldeyer's ring are conspicuously spared since only 5% of patients, even in the late stages of their disease, demonstrate peripheral lymph node involvement.

Central nervous system involvement is the third most common presenting manifestation. Paraplegia occurs in 15% of patients. Spinal cord involvement reflected by paresis, lower extremity sensory defect, and loss of sphincter control does occur. Growth of these tumors is rapid within 2 to 4 weeks. A recent study suggests that one form of childhood leukemia represents a malignant transformation of a Burkitt's lymphoma, American type, with B cell involvement.[406] These patients have a poor prognosis. In African Burkitt's lymphoma, although delayed hypersensitivity response is normal, there is impaired production of IgM antibodies.[408]

Treatment and management

The initial treatment of non-Hodgkin's lymphoma is dependent on the anatomic site involved.

Nonlymphoid sites

Gastrointestinal tract. Patients with gastrointestinal tract involvement present with a short history of abdominal pain, abdominal mass, acute or recurrent intussusception, and rarely perforation with peritonitis. When possible, the diagnosis is established during laparotomy by frozen section, but often it is not suspected. The tumor is excised if possible, but most often a right hemicolectomy is necessary, and occasionally a segmental excision of ileum is adequate; appropriate mesentery is also removed. The surgeon should carefully inspect the abdomen to determine the extent of lymphomatous disease with particular regard to the liver, spleen, retroperitoneal space, and ovaries. A through-and-through liver biopsy is indicated for adequate staging, since this organ is so frequently involved. The entire abdomen is irradiated postoperatively for a total of 2,500 rads in 28 days. The kidneys should be shielded appropriately so that they do not receive greater than 1,500 rads.

In one study eight of ten children treated by this combined approach have apparently been cured of their disease, compared with the approximately 10% chance for cure generally reported with surgery alone.[339,366] On the other hand, patients with massive abdominal disease outside of the gastrointestinal have a very poor prognosis. Median survival of 11 weeks was noted in one study. These patients should be treated with total irradiation followed by chemotherapy. Chemotherapy most useful in non-Hodgkin's lymphoma included combinations of prednisone, vincristine, cyclophosphamide, methotrexate, and 6-mercaptopurine.

Bone. Malignant lymphoma ("reticulum cell sarcoma") of the bone usually involves the diaphysis of the long bones. Affected sites in order of frequency are the femur, humerus, pelvis, skull, tibia, ribs, scapula, and vertebra. Histologically these tumors resemble Ewing's sarcoma; the latter tumor cells are often PAS-positive and form clusters around vascular lakes, findings not seen in bone lymphomas. Arising within the medullary cavity, the tumor spreads in both directions. Outward infiltration and destruction of cortical bone, periosteal penetration, and soft tissue invasion cause the presenting symptoms of pain and swelling and radiographic changes.[405] Metastases to other bones and distant lymph nodes also occur late in the disease. The later occurrence of chronic granulocytic leukemia has been observed.[378]

Localized disease can be controlled with radiation therapy.[340] Doses of 4,000 to 4,500 rads are required but, because of the risk of late local recurrence and/or distant metastases, additional intensive multiagent chemotherapy as proposed by

Wollner et al.[407] is recommended. Late amputation has been recommended if the site of the primary mass makes this feasible 6 to 12 months after the local primary mass has been controlled with radiotherapy and chemotherapy.[399]

Lymphosarcoma of the bone carries the poorest prognosis of the lymphomas, particularly when there is generalized dissemination or involvement of relatively inaccessible sites (pelvis and vertebrae). In a review of forty-three cases a 5-year disease free-survival of 40% and a 10-year survival of 30% were reported.[399] Amputation had been performed in 25% of the cases.

Head and neck. Adults who present with primary lymphoma of Waldeyer's ring including tonsil and nasopharynx, mandible, or maxilla usually have localized disease with no evidence of spread, and a 5-year survival rate of 40% to 50% may be expected with adequate wide field irradiation following excisional biopsy.[337,350] Although this may be the case for adults, the results obtained in children treated this way are uniformly poor. Therefore in childhood lymphoma of extranodal origin in the head and neck, even with completely negative results of investigation for distant disease, should always be considered an indication for systemic disease. Management must include aggressive chemotherapy combined with local irradiation of 4,500 rads over 4 to 5 weeks as the main hope for long survival.

Central nervous system. Involvement of the central nervous system is common in non-Hodgkin's lymphomas; it occurs in more than 30% of the cases. It is common with all patterns of disease including abdominal, gastrointestinal, and extranodal head and neck disease, as well as mediastinal, nodal, and mixed patterns. Presenting manifestations include headache, vomiting, facial palsy, convulsions, deteriorating vision or blindness, behavioral disturbances, and photophobia. Papilledema and cranial nerve palsies are frequently observed. Management of these patients is designed to relieve the increased pressure and irradicate the lymphoma from the brain and spinal fluid. Cranial-spinal irradiation (2,400 rads over 3 weeks) or cranial radiation (2,400 rads) and intrathecal injections of methotrexate (12 mg/m²/injection) are used. Prospective studies designed to obtain better results with combinations of chemotherapy and radiation therapy, including central nervous system prophylaxis and/or total body irradiation, are now in progress for this disease, which currently carries such a poor prognosis.

Lymphoid sites

Mediastinal lymphoma. Tracheal obstruction by compression from mediastinal lymphoma is truly a medical emergency. Intravenous hydro-cortisone, 200 mg/m², should be given immediately and repeated for every 6 hours; in addition, emergency irradiation of 400 rads/day for several days is required to relieve the respiratory distress. Most patients with mediastinal involvement do not demonstrate symptoms of airway or superior vena cava obstruction. In one study 24 of 100 children had a large anterior mediastinal mass as the prominent site of disease; however, in only nine was this site the only area of involvement. Those who did have a single involvement without evidence of blast cells in the blood smear did well and obtained a complete remission with local irradiation of the mediastinum. First relapse in the other group of patients with more generalized disease included seven with leukemia (usually T cell type), three with bone marrow infiltration without evidence of leukemia in the blood, and three with central nervous system disease. Thus vigorous attempts to properly stage these patients is indicated, especially if systemic chemotherapy is to be withheld. Patients with nonlocalized disease should be treated with a combination of irradiation of the mediastinum, 2,500 rads in 28 days, plus multiple-agent chemotherapy similar to that given patients with acute lymphocytic leukemia. Long-term maintenance therapy is required as in acute leukemia.

Abdominal lymphoma. Retroperitoneal lymphoma is a rapidly progressive disease, usually of the B cell type, IgM subclass, which frequently is associated with bone marrow and other extranodal sites of infiltration by lymphoma cells.[57a]

Primary peripheral lymph node lymphoma. Crude vital statistics show a poor response to therapy in patients who present with peripheral lymph node non-Hodgkin's lymphoma. Detailed investigation of the extent of disease is required, including complete blood count, bone marrow biopsy, liver biopsy, lumbar puncture, and ^{67}Ga scan. If these procedures fail to demonstrate disseminated disease, a lymphangiogram and/or elective exploratory laparotomy can be justified. Since greater than 80% of these patients eventually demonstrate disseminated disease, it is most reasonable to consider systemic involvement in all these patients and treat them accordingly. Local irradiation of the grossly involved region should not be less than 3,500 rads in 4 weeks. Chemotherapy is the main method of management. Those patients with poorly differentiated lymphocytic lymphoma who already have leukemic conversion at the time of initial presentation are managed similarly to patients with acute lymphocytic leukemia. Those patients with histiocytic lymphoma may have a conversion to histiocytic, monocytic leukemia; if so, appropriate treatment for that type of leukemic process is given.

Prognosis

Prior to 1967 the survival of children with non-Hodgkin's lymphoma was extremely poor; less than 10% survived more than 40 months.[400] Survival has improved somewhat with more aggressive treatment of localized lymph node diseases as well as systemic chemotherapy for long periods of time similar to treatment given to patients with leukemia. The duration of survival since 1967 has been improved to 30% beyond 40 months for both poorly differentiated lymphocytic and histiocytic lymphoma.[400] The best results to date have been recorded in a group of forty-three children, 76% with advanced disease and 86% with diffuse histology at initial presentation, who were treated with multiple-agent therapy designed to (1) rapidly and maximally decrease bulky lymph node disease with high-dose cyclophosphamide given in a single intravenous push with adjunctive radiation therapy for any tumor greater than 5 cm; (2) immediately initiate intensive induction, consolidation, and maintenance chemotherapy as for leukemia, even in those without marrow metastases; and (3) provide maximum protection of the central nervous system throughout all phases of treatment. In contrast to all previous studies, 76% of these patients are surviving free of disease with a median observation beyond 25 months, and 51% of the survivors are not now receiving therapy and are without evidence of disease.[407]

FUTURE RESEARCH AND NEW TREATMENT METHODS

The etiology of these disorders is yet to be determined. More and more attention will be turned toward the idea that Hodgkin's disease is a progressive disorganization involving the immune system with disturbances of immunologically competent cells. Impaired host reaction may set the scene for primary immune deficiency, autoimmune disease, or therapeutic immunosuppression. On the other hand, aberrant immunocompetent cells may arise from several causes, the most likely of which is lymphoproliferation induced by Epstein-Barr virus. In such situations a graft-versus-host reaction or a host-versus-graft response may lead to tumor formation. This idea has been proposed in Hodgkin's disease.[390]

Newer methods of classification based on functional lymphocyte studies and immunologic surface markers of lymphocytes will be obtained. Diagnostic evaluation in Hodgkin's disease will continue to show improvement in newer methods of scanning and more refinement in the assessment of individual risk and need for specific therapy.

The progress that must be made in non-Hodgkin's lymphoma is more considerable because of the poor prognosis in these children. Clear methods to identify the patient at risk as well as more aggressive combinations of radiation, chemotherapy, and perhaps immunotherapy remain challenges for the future.

REFERENCES
Leukemia

1. Ablin, A. R., Binger, C. M., Stein, R. C., et al.: A conference with the family of a leukemic child, Am. J. Dis. Child. **122:**362, 1971.
2. Acute Leukemia Group B: Acute lymphocytic leukemia in children, J.A.M.A. **207:**923, 1969.
3. Acute Leukemia Group B: The effect of 6-mercaptopurine on the duration of steroid-induced remissions in acute leukemia: a model for evaluation of other potentially useful therapy, Blood **21:**699, 1963.
4. Acute Leukemia Group B: Studies of sequential and combination antimetabolite therapy in acute leukemia: 6-mercaptopurine and methotrexate, Blood **18:**431, 1961.
5. Alsarraf, D., and Reese, L.: Management of acute renal failure due to marked hyperuricemia, Can. Med. Assoc. J. **106:**352, 1972.
6. Altman, A. J., and Baehner, R. L.: In vitro colony-forming characteristics of chronic granulocytic leukemia in childhood, J. Pediatr. **86:**221, 1975.
7. Altman, A. J., Palmer, C. G., and Baehner, R. L.: Juvenile "chronic granulocytic" leukemia: a panmyelopathy with prominent monocytic involvement and circulating monocyte colony-forming cells, Blood **43:**341, 1974.
8. Andriole, A. T.: Synergy of carbenicillin and gentamycin in experimental infection with *Pseudomonas*, J. Infect. Dis. **124:**46, 1971.
9. Andriole, V. T., and Dravetz, H. M.: The use of amphotericin B in man, J.A.M.A. **180:**269, 1962.
10. Armstrong, D., Haghbin, M., Balakrishnan, S. L., and Murphey, M. L.: Asymptomatic cytomegalovirus infection in children with leukemia, Am. J. Dis. Child. **122:**404, 1971.
11. Aur, R. J. A., Simone, J. V., Histu, H. O., et al.: Cessation of therapy during complete remission of childhood acute lymphocytic leukemia, N. Engl. J. Med. **291:**1230, 1974.
12. Aur, R. J. A., Simone, J. V., Hustu, H. O., et al.: Central nervous system therapy and combination chemotherapy of childhood lymphocytic leukemia, Blood **37:**272, 1971.
13. Australian Cancer Society's Childhood Leukaemia Study Group L: Cyclic drug regimen for acute childhood leukaemia, Lancet **2:**313, 1968.
14. Bach, M. K.: Biochemical and genetic studies of a mutant strain of mouse leukemia L 1210 resistant to 1-B-D-ara binofuranosylcytosine (Cytarabine), Cancer Res. **29:**1036, 1969.
15. Baehner, R., Bernstein, T., Higgins, G., McCreadie, S., Chard, R., and Hammond, D.: Improved induction in children with acute nonlymphocytic leukemia treated with daunomycin 5-azacytidine (D-ZAPO), Proc. Am. Soc. Clin. Oncol. **18:**349, 1977. (Abstract.)
16. Baehner, R. L., Neiburger, R. G., Johnson, D. E., and Murrman, S. M.: Transient bactericidal defect of peripheral blood phagocytes from children with acute lymphoblastic leukemia receiving cranio-spinal irradiation, N. Engl. J. Med. **289:**1209, 1973.
17. Baehner, R. L., et al.: The incidence of varicella zoster infection in children with leukemia and solid tumors, Minutes of meeting of Children's Cancer Study Group, September 30, 1974, p. 41.
18. Baladran, L., Rothschild, H., Pugh, N., and Seabury, J.: A cutaneous manifestation of systemic candidiasis, Ann. Intern. Med. **78:**400, 1973.

19. Bartow, B. W., and Tobin, J.: The effect of iodoxuridine on the excretion of cytomegalovirus on congenital infection, Ann. N.Y. Acad. Sci. **173:**90, 1970.

20. Beard, M. E., and Fairley, G. H.: Acute leukemia in adults, Semin. Hematol. **11:**5, 1974.

21. Beaven, G. H., Ellis, M. J., and White, J. C.: Studies on human fetal hemoglobin. II. Fetal hemoglobin levels in healthy children and adults and in certain hematological disorders, Br. J. Haematol. **6:**201, 1960.

22. Begeman, H., and Hemmerle, W.: Die Mitosetätigkeit des menschlichen Knochenmarks und ihre Beeinflussfung durch cytostatische Substanzen, Klin. Wochenschr. **27:** 530, 1949.

23. Bekesi, J. G., Holland, J. F., Cuttner, J., et al.: Chemoimmunotherapy in acute myelocytic leukemia, Proc. Am. Assoc. Cancer Res. **18:**198, 1977.

24. Bennett, J. M., Catovsky, D., Daniel, M. T., et al.: Proposals for the classification of the acute leukemias, Br. J. Haematol. **33:**451, 1976.

25. Bernard, J., Boiron, M., Jacquillat, C., and Weil, M.: Rubidomycin in 400 patients with leukemia and other malignancies. In Abstracts of the simultaneous sessions, Twelfth congress of International Society of Hematology, 1968.

26. Bernard, J., Seligmann, M., and Acar, J.: La leucémie myeloide chronique de l'enfant (étude de vingt observations), Arch. Fr. Pediatr. **19:**881, 1962.

27. Bernard, W. G., Gore, I., and Kilby, R. A.: Congenital leukemia, Blood **6:**990, 1951.

28. Bessis, M.: Cytologic diagnosis of leukemias by electron microscopy. In Mathé, G., Pouillart, P., and Schwarzenberg, L., eds.: Recent results in cancer research: nomenclature, methodology, and results of clinical trials in acute leukemia, New York, 1973, Springer-Verlag New York, Inc.

29. Bias, W. B., Santos, G. W., Burke, P. J., et al.: Cytotoxic antibody in normal human serums reactive with tumor cells from acute lymphocytic leukemias, Science **178:**304, 1972.

30. Binger, C. M., Ablin, A. R., Feuerstein, R. C., et al.: Childhood leukemia: emotional impact on patients and family, N. Engl. J. Med. **280:**414, 1969.

31. Bloom, G. E., Gerald, P. S., and Diamond, L. K.: Chronic myelogenous leukemia in an infant: serial cytogenetic and fetal hemoglobin studies, Pediatrics **38:**295, 1966.

32. Bloomfield, C. D., and Brunning, R. D.: Prognostic implications of cytology in acute leukemia in the adult, Hum. Pathol. **5:**641, 1974.

33. Bodey, G. P., Buckley, M., Sathe, Y. S., and Freireich, E. J.: Quantitative relationships between circulating leukocytes and infection in patients with acute leukemia, Ann. Intern. Med. **64:**328, 1966.

34. Boggs, D. R., Wintrobe, M. N., and Cartwright, G. E.: The acute leukemias: analysis of 322 cases and a review of the literature, Medicine **41:**163, 1962.

35. Borella, L., Green, A. A., and Webster, R. G.: Immunologic rebound after cessation of long-term chemotherapy in acute leukemia, Blood **40:**42, 1972.

36. Borella, L., and Sen, L.: Clinical importance of lymphoblasts with T-markers in childhood leukemia. N. Engl. J. Med. **292:**828, 1975.

37. Borella, L., and Sen, L.: T- and B-lymphocytes and lymphoblasts in untreated acute lymphocytic leukemia, Cancer **34:**646, 1974.

37a. Boxes, L. A., Camitta, B. M., Berenberg, W., and Fanning, J. P.: Myelofibrosis-myeloid metaplasia in childhood, Pediatrics **55:**861, 1975.

38. Brescia, M. A., Santora, E., and Sarnatora, V. F.: Congenital leukemia, J. Pediatr. **55:**35, 1959.

39. Bruce, W. R., Meeker, B. E., and Valeriote, F. A.: Comparison of the sensitivity of normal hematopoietic and transplanted lymphoma colony-forming cells to chemotherapeutic agents administered in vivo, J. Natl. Cancer. Inst. **37:**233, 1966.

40. Bull, J. M., Duttera, M. J., Stashick, E. D., et al.: Serial in vitro marrow culture in acute myelocytic leukemia, Blood **42:**679, 1973.

41. Butler, W. T.: Pharmacology, toxicity, and therapeutic usefulness of amphotericin B, J.A.M.A. **195:**371, 1966.

42. Cangir, A., Sullivan, M. P., Sutow, W. W., and Taylor, G.: Cytomegalovirus syndrome in children with acute leukemia, J.A.M.A. **201:**612, 1967.

43. Cannat, A., and Seligmann, M.: Immunological abnormalities in juvenile myelomonocytic leukemia, Br. Med. J. **1:**71, 1973.

44. Carey, R. W.: Comparative study for cytosine-arabinoside therapy alone and combined with thioguanine, mercaptopurine, or daunomycin in acute myelocytic leukemia, Proc. Am. Assoc. Cancer Res. **11:**15, 1970.

45. Carter, S. K.: Introduction to methodology of clinical trials and the varieties of acute leukemias: defining the numerator and denominator in leukemic trials. In Mathé, G., Pouillart, P., and Schwarzenberg, L., eds.: Recent results in cancer research: nomenclature, methodology, and results of clinical trials in acute leukemias, New York, 1973, Springer-Verlag New York, Inc.

45a. Chard, R., Finkelstein, J., Sonley, M., and Hammond, D.: Improved survival in childhood acute non-lymphocytic leukemia. Proc. Am. Soc. Clin. Oncol. **18:**354, 1977. (Abstract.)

46. Chard, R. L., Finkelstein, J. Z., Sonley, M. J., et al.: Increased survival in childhood acute non-lymphocytic leukemia after treatment with prednisone, cytosine arabinoside, 6-thioguanine, cyclophosphamide, and oncovin (PATCO) combination chemotherapy — 163 patients. In preparation.

47. Chilcote, R., Coccia, P., Sather, H., et al.: Mediastinal mass and prognosis in acute lymphocytic leukemia (ALL), Proc. Am. Soc. Clin. Oncol. **17:**292, 1976. (Abstract.)

48. Chilcote, R. R., and Baehner, R. L.: Infection in childhood cancer: Experience in management of infection in acute leukemia. In Pochedly, C., ed.: Clinical management of cancer in children, Action, Mass., 1975, Science Group, Inc.

49. Chilcote, R. R., and Coccia, P.: Personal communication.

50. Choice of therapy in the treatment of malignancy, Med. Lett. **15:**3, 1973.

51. Reference deleted in proofs.

52. Reference deleted in proofs.

53. Reference deleted in proofs.

54. Reference deleted in proofs.

55. Clarkson, B.: Review of recent studies of cellular proliferation in acute leukemia, Nat. Cancer Inst. Monogr. **30:**81, 1969.

56. Cline, M. J., and Rosenbaum, E.: Prediction of in vivo cytotoxicity of chemotherapeutic agents by their in vitro effect on leukocytes from patients with acute leukemia, Cancer Res. **28:**2516, 1968.

57. Coccia, P., Sather, H., Nesbit, M., et al.: Interrelationship of initial WBC, age, and sex in predicting prognosis in childhood acute lymphoblastic leukemia, Presented to American Society of Hematology December, 1976. (Abstract 214.)

57a. Coccia, P. F., Kersey, J. H., Karamiera, J., et al.: Prognostic significance of surface marker analysis in childhood non-Hodgkin's lymphoproliferative malignancies, Am. J. Hematol. **1:**405, 1976.

58. Cooke, J. V.: Chronic myelogenous leukemia in children, J. Pediatr. **42:**537, 1953.

59. Court-Bronw, W. M., and Abbatt, J. D.: The incidence of leukaemia in ankylosing spondylitis treated with x-ray, Lancet **1:**1283, 1955.

60. Cramblett, H. J., Friedman, J. L., and Najjar, S.: Leukemia in an infant born of a mother with leukemia, N. Engl. J. Med. **259:**727, 1958.

61. Cross, F. S.: Congenital leukemia: report of 2 cases, J. Pediatr. **24:**191, 1944.

62. Crowther, D., Bateman, C. J. T., Vartan, C. P., et al.: Combination chemotherapy using L-asparaginase, daunorubicin, and cytosine arabinoside in adults with acute myelogenous leukaemia, Br. Med. J. **4:**513, 1970.

63. Crowther, D., Powles, R. L., Bateman, C. J. T., et al.: Management of adult acute myelogenous leukaemia, Br. Med. J. **1:**131, 1973.

64. Dameshek, W., and Gunz, F.: Leukemia, New York, 1964, Grune & Stratton, Inc.

65. Deinhardt, F.: Introduction to virus-caused cancer: type C virus, Cancer **34:**1363, 1974.

66. DeVita, V. T., and Schein, P. S.: The use of drugs in combination for the treatment of cancer: rationale and results, N. Engl. J. Med. **288:**998, 1973.

67. Diamond, H. S., Lazarus, R., Kaplan, D., and Halverstam, D.: Effect of urine flow rate on uric acid excretion in man, Arthritis Rheum. **15:**338, 1972.

68. Dibromomannitol Cooperative Study Group: Survival of chronic myeloid leukemia patients treated by dibromommannitol, Eur. J. Cancer **9:**583, 1973.

69. Dick, D. A. L.: The response to cyclophosphamide: a review of a sample of the literature. In Fairley, G. H., and Simister, J. M. P., eds.: Cyclophosphamide, Bristol, 1964, John Wright & Sons, Ltd.

70. Djerassi, I., Kim, J. S., Mitrakul, C., et al.: Filtration of leukopoiesis for separation and concentration of transfusible amounts of normal human granulocytes, J. Exp. Clin. Med. **1:**368, 1970.

71. Duttera, M. J., Bleyer, W. A., Pomeroy, T. C., et al.: Irradiation, methotrexate toxicity, and the treatment of leukemia, Lancet **2:**703, 1973.

72. Duttera, M. J., Whang-Peng, J., Bull, J. M. C., and Carbone, P. P.: Cytogenically abnormal cells in vitro in acute leukaemia, Lancet **1:**715, 1972.

73. Easson, W. M.: The family of the dying child, Pediatr. Clin. North Am. **19:**1157, 1972.

74. Engel, R. R., Hammond, D., Eitzman, D. V., et al.: Transient congenital leukemia in seven children with mongolism, J. Pediatr. **65:**303, 1964.

75. Ernst, P., and Killmann, S.: Perturbation of generation cycle of human leukemic blast cells by cytostatic therapy in vivo: effect of corticosteroids, Blood **26:**689, 1970.

76. Evans, A. E., and Edin, S.: If a child must die . . . , N. Engl. J. Med. **278:**138, 1968.

77. Evans, A. E., Gilbert, E. S., and Zandstra, R.: The increasing incidence of central nervous system leukemia in children (Children's Cancer Study Group A), Cancer **26:**404, 1970.

78. Evans, G., Packham, M. A., Nishizawa, E. E., et al.: The effect of acetyl salicyclic acid on platelet function, J. Exp. Med. **128:**877, 1968.

79. Fass, R. J., and Perkins, R. L.: 5-fluorocytosine in the treatment of cryptococcal and candida mycoses, Ann. Intern. Med. **74:**535, 1971.

80. Feldman, H. A.: Toxoplasmosis, N. Engl. J. Med. **279:**1370, 1968.

81. Feldman, H. A., and Lamb, G. A.: A micromodification of the toxoplasma dye test, J. Parasitol. **52:**415, 1966.

82. Feldman, S., Hughes, W. T., and Kim, H. Y.: Herpes zoster in children with cancer, Am. J. Dis. Child. **126:**178, 1973.

83. Fernbach, D.: The natural history of leukemia. In Sutow, W., Vietti, T., and Fernbach, D., eds.: Clinical pediatric oncology, St. Louis, 1972, The C. V. Mosby Co.

84. Fernbach, D. J., Sutow, W. W., Thurman, W. G., Vietti, T. J.: Clinical evaluation of cyclophosphamide: a new agent for the treatment of children with acute leukemia, J.A.M.A. **182:**30, 1962.

85. Fink, C. W., Windmiller, J., and Sartain, P.: Arthritis as the presenting feature of childhood leukemia, Arthritis Rheum. **15:**347, 1972.

86. Fischer, R., and Schmalzl, F.: Über die Hemmearkeit der Esterase aktivität in Blutmonocyten durch Natriumfluorid, Klin. Wochenschr. **42:**751, 1964.

87. Flandrin, G., and Bernard, J.: Cytological classification of acute leukemias: a survey of 1400 cases, Blood Cells **1:**7, 1975.

88. Flandrin, G., and Daniel, M. T.: Practical value of cytochemical studies for the classification of acute leukemias. In Mathé, G., Pouillart, P., and Schwarzenberg, L., eds.: Recent results in cancer research: nomenclature, methodology, and results of clinical trials in acute leukemias, New York, 1973, Springer-Verlag New York, Inc.

88a. Flandrin, G., Brovet, J. C., Daniel, M. T., and Preud'homme, J. L.: Acute leukemia with Burkitt's tumor cells: a study of six cases with special reference to lymphocyte surface markers, Blood **45:**183, 1975.

89. Forman, E. N., Padre-Mendoza, T., Smith, P. S., et al.: Ph[1]-positive childhood leukemias: spectrum of lymphoid-myeloid expressions, Blood **49:**549, 1977.

90. Forni, A., and Moreo, L.: Chromosome studies in a case of benzene-induced erythroleukemia, Eur. J. Cancer **5:**459, 1969.

91. Fraumeni, J. F., Jr., and Miller, R. W.: Leukemia mortality: downward rates in the United States, Science **155:**1126, 1967.

92. Freedman, A. R.: Interview the parents of dead child? Absolutely! Clin. Pediatr. **8:**564, 1969.

93. Freedman, A. R., Wang, J., and Sinks, L.: High dose methotrexate in acute lymphocytic leukemia, Blood **46:**1040, 1975. (Abstract.)

94. Freeman, J. A.: Origin of Auer bodies, Blood **27:**499, 1966.

95. Freeman, J. E., Johnston, P. G. B., and Voke, J. M.: Somnolence after prophylactic cranial irradiation in children with acute lymphoblastic leukaemia, Br. Med. J. **4:**523, 1973.

96. Frei, E., and Freireich, E. J., III: Progress and perspectives in the chemotherapy of acute leukemia. In Goldin, A., Hawking, F., and Schnitzer, R. J., eds.: Advances in chemotherapy, New York, 1965, Academic Press, Inc.

97. Frei, E., III, Karon, M., Levin, R. H., et al.: The effectiveness of combinations of antileukemic agents in inducing and maintaining remission in children with acute leukemia, Blood **26:**642, 1965.

98. Freireich, E. J., Bodey, G. P., Rodriques, V., et al.: Remission-induction in adults with AML. In Mathé, G., ed.: Advances in acute blastic leukemias, Berlin, 1973, Springer-Verlag.

99. Freireich, E. J., Gehan, E. A., Sulman, D., et al.: The effect of chemotherapy on acute leukemia in the human, J. Chronic Dis. **14:**593, 1961.

100. Friedman, S. B.: Care of the family of the child with cancer, Pediatrics **40:**498, 1967.

101. Friedman, S. B., Chodoff, P., Mason, J. W., et al.: Behavioral observation on parents anticipating the death of a child, Pediatrics **32:**610, 1963.

102. Gajl-Peczalaska, K. J., Bloomfield, C. D., Nesbit, M. E., and Kersey, J. H.: B-cell markers on lymphoblasts in acute lymphoblastic leukemia, Clin. Exp. Immunol. **17:**561, 1974.

103. Galbraith, P. R., and Abu-Zahra, H. T.: Granulopoiesis in chronic granulocytic leukaemia, Br. J. Haematol. **22:**135, 1972.

104. Gallo, R. C., Gallagher, R. E., Sarngadharan, M. G.,

et al.: The evidence for involvement of type C RNA tumor viruses in human acute leukemia, Cancer **34:**1398, 1974.

105. Galton, D. A. G.: Chemotherapy of chronic myelogenous leukemia, Semin. Hematol. **6:**323, 1969.

106. Gee, T. S., Yu, K. P., and Clarkson, B. D.: Treatment of adult acute leukemia with arabinosylcytosine and thioguanine, Cancer **23:**1019, 1969.

107. George, S. I., Fernbach, D. J., Vietti, T. J., et al.: Factors influencing survival in pediatric acute leukemia: The SWCCSG experience, 1958-1970, Cancer **32:**1542, 1973.

108. Gilman, P. A., Jackson, D. P., and Guild, H. G.: Congenital agranulocytosis: prolonged survival and terminal acute leukemia, Blood **36:**576, 1970.

109. Goldstein, E., and Hoeprich, P. D.: Problems in the diagnosis and treatment of systemic candidiasis, J. Infect. Dis. **125:**190, 1972.

110. Goodell, B., Leventhal, B., and Henderson, E.: Cytosine arabinoside in acute granulocytic leukemia, Clin. Pharmacol. Ther. **12:**599, 1971.

111. Graham, S., Levin, M. L., Lilinfeld, A. M., et al.: Preconception intrauterine and post natal irradiation is related to leukemia, Nat. Cancer Inst. Monogr. **19:**347, 1965.

112. Gralnick, H. R., and Henderson, E.: Acquired coagulation factor deficiencies in leukemia, Cancer **26:**1097, 1970.

113. Gralnick, H. R., and Sultan, C.: Acute promyelocytic leukaemia: hemorrhagic manifestation and morphologic criteria, Br. J. Haematol. **29:**373, 1975.

114. Graw, R. G., Jr., Herzig, G. P., Perry, S., and Henderson, E. S.: Normal granulocyte transfusion therapy: treatment of septicemia due to gram-negative bacteria, N. Engl. J. Med. **287:**367, 1972.

115. Graw, R. J., Jr., Skeel, R. T., and Carbone, P. P.: Priapism in a child with chronic granulocytic leukemia, J. Pediatr. **74:**788, 1969.

116. Green, A. A., and Borella, L.: Immunologic rebound after cessation of long-term chemotherapy in acute leukemia. II. In vitro response to phytohemagglutinin and antigens by peripheral blood and bone marrow lymphocytes, Blood **42:**99, 1973.

117. Green, M.: Care of the dying child, Pediatrics **40:**492, 1967.

118. Greenwald, E. S.: Cancer chemotherapy, ed. 2, Flushing, N.Y., 1973, Medical Examination Publishing Co., Inc.

119. Gunz, F. W., Fitzgerald, P. H., Crossen, P. E., et al.: Multiple cases of leukemia in a sibship, Blood **27:**482, 1966.

120. Haghbin, M., Armstrong, D., and Murphy, M. L.: Controlled prospective trial of *Pseudomonas aeruginosa* vaccine in children with acute leukemia, Cancer **32:**761, 1973.

121. Haghbin, M., Ian, C., Clarkson, B. D., et al.: Intensive chemotherapy in children with acute lymphoblastic leukemia (L-2 protocol), Cancer **33:**1491, 1974.

122. Halterman, R. W., Leventhal, B. G., and Mann, D. L.: An acute-leukemia antigen: with clinical status, N. Engl. J. Med. **287:**1272, 1972.

123. Hardisty, R. M., Speed, D. R., and Till, M.: Granulocytic leukemia in childhood, Br. J. Haematol. **10:**551, 1964.

124. Harris, R.: Leukaemia antigens and immunity in man, Nature **241:**95, 1973.

125. Haut, A., Abbott, W. S., and Wintrobe, M. M.: Busulfan in the treatment of chronic myelocytic leukemia: the effects of long-term intermittent therapy, Blood **17:**1, 1961.

126. Hayhoe, F. G., Quaglino, D., and Flemans, R. J.: Consecutive use of Romanowsky and periodic-acid-Schiff techniques in the study of blood and bone-marrow cells, Br. J. Haematol. **6:**23, 1960.

127. Hecht, F., Koler, R. D., Rigas, D. A., et al.: Leukaemia and lymphocytes in ataxia-telangiectasia, Lancet **2:**1193, 1966.

128. Henderson, E. S.: Combination chemotherapy of acute lymphocytic leukemia of childhood, Cancer Res. **27:** 2570, 1967.

129. Henderson, E. S., and Samaha, R. J.: Evidence that drugs in multiple combinations have materially advanced the treatment of human malignancies, Cancer Res. **29:**2272, 1969.

130. Henderson, E. S., and Serpick, A.: The effect of combination drug therapy and prophylactic oral antibiotic treatment in adult acute leukemia, Clin. Res. **15:**336, 1967.

131. Henderson, E., Serpick, A., Leventhal, B., and Henry, P.: Cytosine arabinoside infusions in adult and childhood acute myelocytic leukemia, Proc. Am. Assoc. Cancer Res. **9:**29, 1968.

132. Henle, W., and Henle, G.: Epstein-Barr virus and human malignancies, Cancer **34:**1368, 1974.

133. Henson, D., Siegel, S. E., Fuccillio, D. A., et al.: Cytomegalovirus infections during acute childhood leukemia, J. Infect. Dis. **126:**469, 1972.

134. Hersh, E.: Serial studies of immunocompetence in patients undergoing chemotherapy for acute leukemia, Proceedings of American Society of Clinical Oncology, Houston, March, 1974.

135. Hersh, E. M., Bodey, G. P., Nies, B. A., and Freireich, E. J.: Causes of death in acute leukemia, J.A.M.A. **193:** 105, 1965.

136. Hersh, E. M., Whitecar, J. P., Jr., McCredie, K. B., et al.: Chemotherapy, immunocompetence, immunosuppression, and prognosis in acute leukemia, N. Engl. J. Med. **285:**1211, 1971.

137. Herzig, G. P., Root, R. K., and Graw, R. G., Jr.: Granulocyte collection by continuous-flow filtration leukapheresis, Blood **39:**554, 1972.

138. Heyn, R., Joo, P., Karon, M., et al.: BCG in the treatment of acute lymphocytic leukemia, Blood **46:**431, 1975.

138a. Heyn, R., Joo, P., Karon, M., et al.: BCG in the treatment of acute lymphoblastic leukemia, Immunotherapy of Cancer, 1976. (Abstract.)

139. Hittle, R., Ortega, J., Donaldson, M., et al.: Effectiveness of presymptomatic treatment (preRx) on the occurrence of central nervous system (CNS) disease in childhood lymphoblastic leukemia (ALL), Submitted to sixty-sixth annual meeting of American Society of Clinical Oncology, San Diego, May, 1975. (Abstract.)

140. Holland, J. F.: Cancer and leukemia group B protocol, 1977.

141. Holland, J. F., and Glidelwell, O.: Oncologists' reply: Survival expectancy in acute lymphocytic leukemia, N. Engl. J. Med. **287:**769, 1972.

142. Holland, P., and Holland, N. H.: Prevention and management of acute hyperuricemia in childhood leukemia, J. Pediatr. **72:**358, 1968.

143. Howard, J. P., Albo, V., and Newton, W. A.: Cytosine arabinoside: results of a cooperative study in acute childhood leukemia, Cancer **21:**341, 1968.

144. Hughes, W. T.: Fatal infections in childhood leukemia, Am. J. Dis. Child. **122:**283, 1971.

145. Hughes, W. T., Price, R. A., Kin, H., et al.: Pneumocystis carinii pneumonitis in children with malignancies, J. Pediatr. **82:**404, 1973.

146. Hughes, W. T., and Smith, D. R.: Infection during induction of remission in acute lymphocytic leukemia, Cancer **31:**1008, 1973.

147. Humphrey, G. B., Nesbit, M. E., and Brunning, R. D.: Prognostic value of the periodic acid-Schiff (PAS) reaction in acute lymphoblastic leukemia, Am. J. Clin. Pathol. **61:**393, 1974.

148. Hyrniuk, W., Foerster, J., and Shojania, M.: Cytoarabine for herpes virus infection, J.A.M.A. **219:**750, 1972.

149. Jackson, E. W., Turner, J. H., Klauber, M. R., and Norris, F. D.: Down's syndrome: variation of leukemia occurrence in institutionalized population, J. Chronic Dis. **21:**247, 1968.

150. Jacquillat, C., Flandin, G., Weil, M., et al.: Correlation between cytological varieties and prognosis in acute lymphocytic leukemia, Proc. Am. Assoc. Cancer Res. **14:**2, 1972.

151. Jacquillat, C., Weil, M., and German, M. F.: Combination therapy in 130 patients with acute lymphocytic leukemia, Cancer Res. **33:**3278, 1973.

152. Jaffe, N., and Kim, B. S.: Priapism in acute granulocytic leukemia, Am. J. Dis. Child. **118:**619, 1969.

153. Kandel, E. V.: Chloroma, Arch. Intern. Med. **59:**691, 1937.

154. Kaplow, L. S.: Simplified myeloperoxidase stain using benzidine, dihydrochloride, Blood **26:**215, 1965.

155. Kaplow, L. S.: Cytochemistry of leukocyte alkaline phosphatase, Am. J. Clin. Pathol. **39:**439, 1963.

156. Karnovsky, M. L.: Metabolic basis of phagocytic activity, Physiol. Rev. **42:**143, 1962.

157. Karon, M.: Problems in evaluation of long-term results. In Mathé, G., Pouillart, P., and Schwarzenberg, L., eds.: Recent results in cancer research: nomenclature, methodology, and results of clinical trials in acute leukemia, New York, 1973, Springer-Verlag New York, Inc.

158. Karon, M.: Preliminary report on vincristine (Oncovin) from Acute Leukemia Group B, Proc. Am. Assoc. Cancer Res. **4:**33, 1963.

159. Karon, M., Freireich, E. J., Frei, E., III, et al.: The role of vincristine in the treatment of childhood acute leukemia, Clin. Pharmacol. Ther. **7:**332, 1966.

160. Karon, M., Sieger, L., Leimbrock, S., et al.: 5-Azacytidine: a new active agent for the treatment of acute leukemia, Blood **42:**359, 1973.

161. Karon, M., Sieger, L., Leimbrock, S., et al.: 5-Azacytidine: effective treatment for acute leukemia in children, Proc. Am. Assoc. Cancer Res. **14:**94, 1973.

162. Karon, M., and Vernick, J.: An approach to the emotional support of fatally ill children, Clin. Pediatr. **7:**274, 1968.

163. Kaur, J., Catovsky, D., Valdimarsson, H., et al.: Familial acute myeloid leukaemia with acquired Pelger-Huet anomaly and aneuploidy of C group, Br. Med. J. **4:**327, 1972.

164. Keith, H. M.: Chronic myelogenous leukemia in infancy: report of a case, Am. J. Dis. Child. **69:**366, 1945.

165. Kelin, G.: Tumor antigens, Annu. Rev. Microbiol. **20:**223, 1966.

166. Kelsey, N. M., and Anderson, D. H.: Congenital leukemia, Am. J. Dis. Child. **58:**1268, 1939.

167. Kennedy, B. J.: Hydroxyurea therapy in chronic myelogenous leukemia, Cancer **29:**1052, 1972.

168. Kersey, J. H., Sabad, A., Gajl-Peczalaska, K., et al.: Acute lymphoblastic leukemic cells with T (thymus-derived) lymphocyte markers, Science **182:**1355, 1973.

169. Kessler, I. I., and Kilienfeld, A. M.: Perspectives in the epidemiology of leukemia, Adv. Cancer Res. **12:**225, 1969.

170. Killmann, S. A.: Acute leukemia: the kinetics of leukemic blast cells in man: an analytical review, Ser. Hematol. **1:**38, 1968.

171. Killmann, S. A., Cronkiet, E. P., Robertson, J. S., et al.: Estimation of phases of the life cycle of leukemic cells from labeling in human beings in vivo with tritiated thymidine, Lab. Invest. **12:**671, 1963.

172. Killman, S. A., and Ernst, P.: An analysis of the relationship of leukemia cell kinetics to chemotherapy. In Proceedings of the fifth international symposium on comparative leukemia research, Padua, Italy, 1971.

173. Kirby, H. B., Kenamore, B., and Guckian, J. C.: *Pneumocystis carinii* pneumonia treated with pyrimethamine and sulfadizaine, Ann. Intern. Med. **73:**695, 1970.

174. Klastersky, J., Cappel, R., and Danau, D.: Therapy with carbenicillin and gentamycin for patients with cancer and severe infections caused by gram-negative rods, Cancer **31:**331, 1973.

175. Konior, G. S., Lippman, M. E., Johnson, G. E., et al.: Correlation of glucocorticoid receptor levels and complete remission duration in "poor prognosis" acute lymphatic leukemia, Proc. Am. Assoc. Cancer Res. **18:**353, 1977. (Abstract.)

176. Krakff, I. H., Downling, M. D., and Gee, T.: A perspective of intensive treatment aiming at prolonged control and/or eradication of chronic granulocytic leukemia, In Proceedings of the second Padua seminar on clinical oncology, October, 1972, Padua, 1973, Piccin Medical Books.

177. Kraybill, E. N., Sever, J. L., Avery, G. B., and Movassagi, N.: Experimental use of cytosine-arabinoside in congenital cytomegalovirus infections, J. Pediatr. **80:**485, 1972.

178. Krivit, W., Gilchrist, G., and Beatty, E. C., Jr.: The need for chemotherapy after prolonged complete remission in acute leukemia of childhood, J. Pediatr. **76:**138, 1970.

179. Krivit, W., and Good, R. A.: Simultaneous occurrence of mongolism and leukemia: report of a nationwide survey, Am. J. Dis. Child. **94:**289, 1957.

180. Krivit, W., and Good, R. A.: The simultaneous occurrence of leukemia and mongolism; report of 4 cases, Am. J. Dis. Child. **91:**218, 1956.

181. Kumar, R., Biggart, J. D., McEvoy, J., and McGeown, M. G.: Cyclophosphamide and reproductive function, Lancet **1:**1212, 1972.

182. Lambert, F.: Akute lymphoblastische Leukaemie bei Geschwistern mit progressiver Kleinhirnataxie (Louis-Barr Syndrom), Dtsch. Med. Wochenschr. **94:**217, 1969.

183. Lampkin, B. C., McWilliams, N. B., and Mauer, A. M.: Treatment of acute leukemia: symposium on pediatric hematology, Pediatr. Clin. North Am. **19:**1123, 1972.

184. Lampkin, B. C., Niagao, T., and Mauer, A. M.: Synchronization and recruitment in acute leukemia, J. Clin. Invest. **50:**2204, 1971.

185. Lampkin, B. C., Niagao, T., and Mauer, A. M.: Drug effect in acute leukemia, J. Clin. Invest. **48:**1124, 1969.

186. Lascari, A. D.: The family and the dying child: a compassionate approach, Med. Times **97:**207, 1969.

187. Leavey, R. A., Kahn, S. B., and Brodsky, I.: Disseminated intravascular coagulation: a complication of chemotherapy in acute myelomonocytic leukemia, Cancer **26:**142, 1970.

188. Lee, S. L., and Glidwell, O.: Cytology and survival in acute lymphatic leukemia of children. In Mathé, G., Pouillart, P., and Schwarzenberg, L., eds.: Recent results in cancer research: nomenclature, methodology, and results of clinical trials in acute leukemia, New York, 1973, Springer-Verlag New York, Inc.

189. Lee, S. L., Vopel, S., and Glidwell, O.: Cytology and survival in acute lymphoblastic leukemia of children, Semin. Oncol. **3:**209, 1976.

190. Leidler, F., and Russell, W. O.: The brain in leukemia, Arch. Pathol. **40:**14, 1945.

191. Levine, A. S., Graw, R. G., Jr., and Young, R. C.: Management of infections in patients with leukemia and lymphoma: current concepts and experimental approaches, Semin. Hematol. **9:**141, 1972.

192. Levine, A. S., Schimpff, S. C., Graw, R. G., Jr., and Young, R. C.: Hematologic malignancies and other marrow failure states: progress in the management of complicating infections, Semin. Hematol. **11:**141, 1974.

193. Levine, A. S., Siegel, S. E., Schreiber, A. D., et al.:

Protected environments in prophylactic antibiotics: a prospective controlled study of their utility and the therapy of acute leukemia, N. Engl. J. Med. **288:**477, 1973.

194. Linman, J. W., and Saarni, M. I.: The preleukemia syndrome, Semin. Hematol. **11:**93, 1974.

195. Loffler, H.: Indications and limits of cytochemistry, In Mathé, G., Pouillart, P., and Schwarzenberg, L., eds.: Recent results in cancer research: nomenclature, methodology, and results of clinical trials in acute leukemia, New York, 1973, Springer-Verlag New York, Inc.

196. Marsden, H. B., and Steward, J. K.: Tumors in children. In Recent results in cancer research, New York, 1968, Springer-Verlag New York, Inc.

197. Mathé, G., Amiel, J. L., Schwarzenberg, L., et al.: Active immunotherapy for acute lymphoblastic leukaemia, Lancet **1:**697, 1969.

198. Mathé, G., Belpomme, D., Dantchev, D., et al.: Search for correlations between cytological types and therapeutic sensitivity of acute leukemia, Blood Cells **1:**37, 1975.

199. Mathé, G., Pouillart, P., Sterescu, M., et al.: Subdivision of classical varieties of acute leukemia: correlations with prognosis, cure expectancy, Eur. J. Clin. Biol. Res. **16:**554, 1971.

200. Mathé, G., Pouillart, P., Weiner, R., et al.: Classification and subclassification of acute leukemias correlated with clinical expression, therapeutic sensitivity, and prognosis. In Mathé, G., Pouillart, P., and Schwarzenberg, L., eds.: Recent results in cancer research: nomenclature, methodology, and results of clinical trials in acute leukemias, New York, 1973, Springer-Verlag New York, Inc.

201. Mauer, A. M., and Fisher, V.: Characteristics of cell proliferation in four patients with untreated acute leukemia, Blood **28:**428, 1966.

202. Mauer, A. M., and Fisher, V.: In vivo studies of cell kinetics in acute leukemia, Nature **197:**574, 1963.

203. Mauer, A. M., Vida, L. N., and Honig, G. R.: Similarities of the erythrocytes in juvenile chronic myelogenous leukemia to fetal erythrocytes, Blood **39:**778, 1972.

204. McCaffrey, R., Harrison, T. A., Parkman, R., and Baltimore, D.: Terminal transferase activity in leukemic cells and normal thymocytes, N. Engl. J. Med. **292:**761, 1975.

205. McCracken, G. H., Jr., and Luby, J. P.: Cytosine arabinoside in the treatment of congenital cytomegalic inclusion disease, J. Pediatr. **80:**488, 1972.

206. McCredie, K. B., and Freireich, E. J.: Increased granulocyte collection from normal donors with increased granulocyte recovery following transfusion, Proc. Am. Assoc. Cancer Res. **12:**58, 1971.

207. McWilliams, N. B., Mauer, A. M., and Lampkin, B. C.: Dose dependent vincristine effects, Clin. Res. **19:**494, 1971.

208. Medical Research Council: Treatment of acute lymphoblastic leukemia: comparison of immunotherapy (BCG), intermittent methotrexate, and no therapy after a five-month intensive cytotoxic regimen Concord trial, Br. Med. J. **4:**189, 1971.

209. Medical Research Council: Treatment of acute lymphoblastic leukemia: effect of "prophylactic" radiotherapy against central nervous system leukaemia, Br. Med. J. **2:**381, 1973.

210. Medical Research Council Working Party on the Evaluation of Different Methods of Therapy in Leukaemia: Treatment of acute leukaemia in adults: comparison of steroid and mercaptopurine therapy alone and in conjunction, Br. Med. J. **1:**1383, 1966.

211. Medical Research Council Working Party for Therapeutic Trials in Leukemia: Chronic granulocytic leukaemia: comparison of radiotherapy and busulfan therapy, Br. Med. J. **1:**201, 1968.

212. Medoff, G., Kobayashi, G. S., Kwan, C. N., et al.: On potentiation of Rifampicin and 5-fluorocytosine as antifungal antibiotics by amphotericin B, Proc. Natl. Acad. Sci. **69:**196, 1972.

213. Metcalf, D., Moore, M. A., Sheridan, J. W., and Spitzer, G.: Responsiveness of human granulocytic leukemic cells to colony-stimulating factor, Blood **43:**847, 1974.

214. Meyer, R. D., Young, L. S., Armstrong, D., and Yu, B.: Aspergillosis complicating neoplastic disease, Am. J. Med. **54:**6, 1973.

215. Miller, D. R.: Children's Cancer Study Group Protocol 141, 1977.

216. Miller, D. R., Newstead, G. J., and Young, L. W.: Perinatal leukemia with a possible variant of the Ellis van-Creveld syndrome, J. Pediatr. **74:**300, 1969.

217. Miller, D., Sonley, M., Karon, M., et al.: Additive therapy in the maintenance of remission in acute lymphoblastic leukemia of childhood: the effect of prognostic factors, Cancer **33:**508, 1974.

218. Miller, F. A., Dixon, G. J., Ehrlich, J., Sloan, B. J., and McLean, I. W.: Antiviral activity of 9-beta-D-arabinosuranosyladenine, Antimicrob. Agents Chemother. p. 136, 1968.

219. Miller, R. W.: Fifty-two forms of childhood cancer: United States mortality experience, 1969-1966, J. Pediatr. **75:**685, 1969.

220. Miller, R. W.: Genetics of leukemia: epidemiological aspects, Jpn. J. Hum. Genet. **13:**100, 1968.

221. Minot, G. R., Buckman, J. E., and Isaacs, R.: Chronic myelogenous leukemia: age incidence, duration and benefit derived, J.A.M.A. **82:**1486, 1924.

222. Mirsky, H. S., and Kuttner, J.: Fungal infection in acute leukemia, Cancer **30:**348, 1972.

223. Modan, B., and Lilienfeld, A. M.: Polycythemia vera and leukemia: the role of radiation treatment. Medicine **44:**305, 1965.

224. Moore, M. A. S., Spitzer, G., Williams, N., et al.: Agar culture studies in 127 cases of untreated acute leukemia: the prognostic value of reclassification of leukemia according to in vitro growth characteristics, Blood **44:**1, 1974.

225. Moore, M. A. S., Williams, N., and Metcalf, D.: In vitro colony formation by normal and leukemic human hematopoietic cells: interaction between colony-forming and colony-stimulating cells, J. Natl. Cancer Inst. **50:**591, 1973.

226. Morse, E. E., Freireich, E. J., Carbone, P. P., et al.: The transfusions of leukocytes from donors with chronic myelocytic leukemia to patients with leukopenia, Transfusion **6:**183, 1966.

227. Myer, R. D., Rosen, P., and Armstrong, D.: Phycomycosis complicating leukemia and lymphoma, Ann. Intern. Med. **77:**871, 1972.

227a. Myers, W. P. L.: Differential diagnosis of hypercalcemia and cancer, Cancer J. Clin. **27:**258, 1977.

228. Naegeli, O.: Blutkankheiten und Blutdiagnostik, Leipzig, 1908, Verlag von Veit.

229. Nesbit, M., Ortega, J., Donaldson, M., et al.: Prevention of testicular relapse by prophylactic radiation in childhood acute lymphoblastic leukemia, Proc. Am. Assoc. Cancer Res. **18:**317, 1977.

230. Nowell, P. C., and Hungerford, D. A.: Chromosome studies on normal and leukemic human leukocytes, J. Natl. Cancer Inst. **25:**85, 1960.

231. Oettgen, H. F., Old, L. J., Boyse, E. A., et al.: Inhibition of leukemias in man by L-asparaginase, Cancer Res. **27:**2619, 1967.

232. Oettgen, H. F., Stephenson, P. A., Schwartz, M. K., et al.: Toxicity of E. coli L-asparaginase in man, Cancer **25:**253, 1970.

232a. Ortega, J., Nesbit, M., Donaldson, M., et al.: L-asparaginase, vincristine, and prednisone for induction of first remission in acute lymphocytic leukemia, Cancer Res. **37:**535, 1977.

233. Paintrand, M., Dantchev, D., and Mathé, G.: Electron microscopic aspects of cells in the four subvarieties of acute lymphoid leukemia. In Mathé, G., Pouillart, P., and Schwarzenberg, L., eds.: Recent results in cancer research: nomenclature, methodology, and results of clinical trials of acute leukemias, New York, 1973, Springer-Verlag New York, Inc.

234. Pantazopoulos, N., and Sinks, L. F.: Morphologic criteria for prognostication of acute lymphoblastic leukemia, Br. J. Haematol. **27:**25, 1974.

235. Paran, M., Sachs, L., Barak, Y., and Resnitsky, P.: In vitro induction of granulocyte differentiation in hematopoietic cells from leukemic and non-leukemic patients, Proc. Natl. Acad. Sci. **67:**1542, 1970.

236. Pavlovsky, S., Eppinger-Helft, M., and Muriel, F. S.: Factors that influence the appearance of central nervous system leukemia, Blood **42:**935, 1973.

237. Perillie, P. E., and Finch, S. C.: Muramidase studies in Philadelphia chromosome positive and chromosome negative chronic granulocytic leukemia, N. Engl. J. Med. **283:**456, 1970.

238. Perillie, P. E., Kaplan, S. S., Lefkowitz, E., et al.: Studies of muramidase (lysosyme) in leukemia, J.A.M.A. **203:**317, 1968.

239. Pierce, M. I.: Leukemia in the newborn infant, J. Pediatr. **54:**691, 1959.

240. Pierce, M. I., Borges, W. H., Heyn, R., et al.: Epidemiological factors and survival experience in 1770 children with acute leukemia: treated by members of Children's Study Group A between 1946 and 1964, Cancer **23:**1296, 1969.

241. Pierre, R. V.: Preleukemia states, Semin. Hematol. **11:** 73, 1974.

242. Pike, B. L., and Robinson, W. A.: Human bone marrow colony growth in agar-gel, J. Cell. Physiol. **75:**77, 1970.

243. Pinkel, D.: Five-year follow-up of "total therapy" of childhood lymphocytic leukemia, J.A.M.A. **216:**648, 1971.

244. Pinkel, D., Hernandez, K., Borella, L., et al.: Drug dosage and remission duration in childhood lymphocytic leukemia, Cancer **27:**247, 1971.

245. Plotkin, S. A., and Stetler, H.: Treatment of congenital cytomegalic inclusion disease with antiviral agents, Antimicrob. Agents Chemother. p. 372, 1969.

246. Pochedly, C., and Ente, G.: Adverse hematologic effects of drugs, Pediatr. Clin. North Am. **19:**1095, 1972.

247. Poncher, H. G., Weir, H. F., and Limarzi, L. R.: Chronic myelogenous leukemia in early infancy: case report, J. Pediatr. **21:**73, 1942.

248. Powles, R. L., Crowther, D., Bateman, C. J. T., et al.: Immunotherapy for acute myelogenous leukemia, Br. J. Cancer **28:**365, 1975.

249. Price, J. A., and Jamiesin, P. A.: The central nervous system in childhood leukemia. II. Subacute leukoencephalopathy, Cancer **35:**306, 1975.

250. Price, R. A., and Johnson, W. W.: The central nervous system in childhood leukemia. I. The arachnoid, Cancer **31:**520, 1973.

251. Pridie, G., and Dumitriscu-Pirvu, D.: Laucemie acuta sindrom Bonnevie-Ullrich la un non rascat, Pediatria **10:**345, 1961.

252. Quie, P. G., and Children, R. A.: Acute disseminated and chronic mucocutaneous candidiasis, Semin. Hematol. **8:**227, 1971.

253. Qureshi, M. S. A., Goldsmith, H. J., Pennington, J. H., and Cox, P. E.: Cyclophosphamide therapy and sterility, Lancet **2:**1290, 1972.

254. Rachmilewitz, B., Rachmilewitz, M., and Moshkowitz,

B.: Serum transcobalamin in myeloid leukemia, J. Lab. Clin. Med. **78:**275, 1971.

255. Ragab, A. H., Gilkerson, E. S., and Myers, M. L.: Granulopoiesis in childhood leukemia, Cancer **33:**791, 1974.

256. Ragab, A. H., Lindquist, K. J., Vietti, T. J., et al.: Immunoglobulin pattern in childhood leukemia, Cancer **26:**890, 1970.

257. Rapp, F., and Duff, R.: Oncogenic conversion of normal cells by inactivated herpes simplex viruses, Cancer **34:** 1353, 1974.

258. Rasteger, A., and Thier, S. O.: The physiologic approach to hyperuricemia, N. Engl. J. Med. **286:**470, 1972.

259. Ravatta, M.: Studio and anatomo-funzionlie dell midollo osso nella leucemia acuta, Haematologica **24:**657, 1942.

260. Reimann, D. L., Clemmens, R. L., and Pillsbury, W. A.: Congenital acute leukemia: skin nodules, a first sign, J. Pediatr. **46:**415, 1955.

261. Reisman, L. E., and Trujillo, J. M.: Chronic granulocytic leukemia of childhood: clinical and cytogenetic studies, J. Pediatr. **62:**710, 1963.

262. Reisman, L. E., Zuelzer, W. W., and Thompson, R. I.: Further observations on the role of aneuploidy in acute leukemia, Cancer Res. **24:**1448, 1964.

263. Repsher, L. H., Schröeter, G., and Hammond, W. S.: Diagnosis of *Pneumocystis carinii* pneumonitis by means of endobronchial brush biopsy, N. Engl. J. Med. **287:** 340, 1972.

264. Reschad, H., and Schilling-Torgau, V.: Ueber eine neue Leukämie durch echote Uebergangsformen (Splenozytenleukämie) und ihre Bedeutung für die Selbständigkeit dieser Zellen, Munch. Med. Wochenschr. 60, 1913.

265. Riemenschneider, T. A., Wilson, J. F., and Vernier, R. L.: Glucocorticoid-induced pancreatitis in children, Pediatrics **41:**428, 1968.

266. Riff, L. J., and Jackson, G. G.: Laboratory and clinical conditions for Gentamicin inactivation by carbenicillin, Arch. Intern. Med. **130:**887, 1972.

267. Rinker, C. T., and McGraw, J. P.: Cytomegalic inclusion disease in childhood leukemia, Cancer **20:**36, 1967.

268. Rogentine, G. N., Yankee, R., Gart, J., et al.: HLA antigens in disease (acute lymphocytic leukemia), J. Natl. Cancer Inst. **51:**2420, 1972.

269. Rosen, P., Armstrong, D., and Ramos, C.: *Pneumocystis carinii* pneumonia, Am. J. Med. **53:**428, 1972.

270. Rosenow, E. C.: The spectrum of drug induced pulmonary disease, Ann. Intern. Med. **77:**977, 1972.

271. Rosner, F.: Dermatoglyphics in leukaemic children, Lancet **2:**272, 1969.

272. Rothenberg, M. G.: Reactions of those who treat children with cancer, Pediatrics **40**(part II):507, 1967.

273. Sandberg, A. A., Takagi, N., Sofuni, T., and Crosswhite, L. H.: Chromosomes and causation of human cancer and leukemia. V. Karyotypic aspects of acute leukemia, Cancer **22:**1268, 1968.

274. Saunders, E. F.: The effect of L-asparaginase on the nucleic acid metabolism and cell cycle of human leukemia cells, Blood **29:**575, 1972.

275. Sawitsky, A., Bloom, D., and German, J.: Chromosomal breakage and acute leukemia and congenital talangiectatic erythema and stunted growth, Ann. Intern. Med. **65:**487, 1966.

276. Schade, H., Schoeller, L., and Schultze, K. W. D.: D-trisomie (Patau) mit kongenitaler myeloischer leukaemie, Med. Welt. **50:**2690, 1962.

277. Schimpff, S. C., Satterlee, W., Young, V. M., and Serpick, A.: Empiric therapy with carbenicillin and gentamycin for febrile patients with cancer and granulocytopenia, N. Engl. J. Med. **284:**1061, 1971.

278. Schwab, R. S., and Weiss, S.: The neurologic aspect of leukemia, Am. J. Med. Sci. **189:**755, 1935.

279. Schwarzenberg, L., Mathé, G., and Pouillart, P.: Hydroxurea, leucophoresis and splenectomy in chronic myelogenous leukemia at the problast phase, Br. Med. J. **1:**700, 1973.
280. Selawry, O. S.: New treatment schedule with improved survival in childhood leukemia: intermittent parenteral vs. daily oral administration of methotrexate for maintenance of induced remission, J.A.M.A. **194:**75, 1965.
281. Seligman, B. R., Rosner, F., Parise, F., and Lee, S. L.: Serum muramidase levels in acute leukemia, Am. J. Med. Sci. **264:**69, 1972.
282. Sen, L., and Borella, L.: Clinical importance of lymphoblasts with T markers in childhood leukemia, N. Engl. J. Med. **292:**828, 1975.
283. Sheehan, H. L.: The staining of leucocyte granules by Sudan black, Br. J. Pathol. Bacteriol. **49:**580, 1939.
284. Siegel, S. E., Baehner, R. L., and Nesbit, M.: Pulmonary complications during the therapy of childhood acute lymphocytic leukemia, Presented to American Society of Hematology, Atlanta, December 9, 1974. (Abstract.)
285. Simmons, C. R., Harle, T. S., and Singleton, E. B.: The osseous manifestations of leukemia in children, Radiol. Clin. North Am. **6:**115, 1968.
286. Simone, J.: Acute lymphocytic leukemia in childhood, Semin. Hematol. **11:**25, 1974.
287. Simone, J. V.: Treatment of children with acute lymphocytic leukemia, Adv. Pediatr. **19:**13, 1972.
288. Simone, J. V., Holland, E., and Johnson, W.: Fatalities during remission of childhood leukemia, Blood **39:**759, 1972.
289. Skarin, A. T., Matsuo, Y., and Maloney, W. C.: Muramidase in myeloproliferative disorders terminating in acute leukemia, Cancer **29:**1336, 1972.
290. Skipper, H. E.: Leucocyte kinetics in leukemia and lymphoma. In Leukemia-Lymphoma, Chicago, 1970, Year Book Medical Publishers, Inc.
291. Skipper, H. E., Schabel, F. M., Jr., and Wilcox, W. S.: Experimental evaluation of potential anti-cancer agents. XIII. On the criteria and kinetics associated with "curability" of experimental leukemia, Cancer Chemotherapy Reports 35, U.S. Department of Health, Education, and Welfare, Public Health Service, 1964.
292. Smith, K. L., and Johnson, W.: Classification of chronic myelocytic leukemia in children, Cancer **34:**670, 1974.
293. Snyder, A. L., Li, F. P., Henderson, E. S., and Todaro, G. T.: Possible inherited leukaemogenic factors in familial acute myelogenous leukemia, Lancet **1:**586, 1970.
294. Sonley, M. J., Nesbit, M., Pearce, M., et al.: Cytosine arabinoside, cyclophosphamide, and vincristine for the treatment of children with acute myelogenous leukemia (acute non-lymphatic leukemia). (In press.)
295. Speigelman, S., Axel, R., Baxt, W., et al.: Human cancer and animal viral oncology, Cancer **34:**1406, 1974.
296. Spiers, A. S. O.: Chemotherapy of acute leukemia, Clin. Haematol. **1:**127, 1972.
297. Stemple, R. M.: The Philadelphia chromosome and leukemia research: bibliography, ORNL:TM 2103, U.S. Atomic Energy Commission, 1968.
298. Stevens, D. A., Jordan, G. W., Waddell, T. F., and Merigan, T. C.: Adverse effect of cytosine-arabinoside on disseminated zoster in a controlled trial, N. Engl. J. Med. **289:**873, 1973.
299. Stransky, E.: Perinatal leukemia, Acta Paediatr. Acad. Sci. Hung. **8:**121, 1967.
300. Stryckmans, P. A.: Immuno-versus chemotherapy during complete remission (CR) of acute lymphoblastic leukemia (ALL), Int. Soc. Haematol. Eur. Afr. Soc. Div. **21:**6, 1975. (Abstract.)
301. Stryckmans, P. A.: Current concepts in chronic myelogenous leukemia, Semin. Hematol. **11:**101, 1974.
302. Sullivan, M. P., Hanshaw, J. B., Cangir, A., and Butler, J. J.: Cytomegalovirus complement-fixation antibody levels of leukemic children, J.A.M.A. **206:**569, 1968.
303. Sullivan, M. P., Sutow, W. W., Taylor, H. G., et al.: Intrathecal (IT) combination chemotherapy for meningeal leukemia using methotrexate (MTX), cytosine arabinoside (CA) and hydrocortisone (HDC), Proc. Am. Assoc. Cancer Res. **12:**45, 1971.
304. Suskind, R. M., Brusilow, S. W., and Zehr, J.: Syndrome of inappropriate secretion of antidiuretic hormone produced by vincristine toxicity (with bioassay of ADH level), J. Pediatr. **81:**90, 1972.
305. Sutow, W. W., Vietti, T. J., and Fernback, D. J., eds.: Clinical pediatric oncology, St. Louis, 1972, The C. V. Mosby Co.
306. Temin, H. M.: Introduction to virus-caused cancers, Cancer **34:**1347, 1974.
307. Thomas, E. D.: Marrow transplantation in acute leukemia, Presented at sixty-sixth American Association for Cancer Research Meeting, San Diego, May, 1975.
308. Thomas, L. B., Forkner, C. E., Jr., Frei, E., III, et al.: The skeletal lesions of acute leukemia, Cancer **14:**608, 1961.
309. Thompson, I., Hall, T. C., and Moloney, W. C.: Combination therapy of adult acute myelogenous leukemia, N. Engl. J. Med. **273:**1302, 1965.
310. Tjio, G. H., Carbone, P. P., Whang, J., and Frei, E., III: The Philadelphia chromosome and chronic myelogenous leukemia, J. Natl. Cancer Inst. **36:**567, 1966.
311. Utz, J. P.: The spectrum of opportunistic fungus infections, Lab. Invest. **11:**1018, 1963.
312. Vernick, J., and Karon, M.: Who's afraid of death on a leukemia ward? Am. J. Dis. Child. **109:**393, 1965.
313. Vietti, T. J., Starling, K., Wilbur, J. R., et al.: Vincristine, prednisone, and daunomycin in acute leukemia of childhood, Cancer **27:**602, 1971.
314. Viza, D., Davies, D. A. L., and Harris, R.: Solubilization and partial purification of human leukaemic specific antigens, Nature **227:**1249, 1970.
315. Vogler, W. R., Huguley, C. M., and Rundles, R. W.: Comparison of methotrexate with 6-mercaptopurine-prednisone in treatment of acute leukemia in adults, Cancer **20:**1221, 1967.
316. Volkman, A.: The origin of macrophages from bone marrow in the rat, Br. J. Exp. Pathol. **46:**62, 1966.
317. Warr, W., Bates, J. H., and Stone, A.: The spectrum of pulmonary cryptolcoccis, Ann. Intern. Med. **69:**1109, 1968.
318. Weatherall, D. J., Edwards, J. A., and Donohue, W. T. A.: Hemoglobin and red cell enzyme changes in juvenile myeloid leukemia, Br. Med. J. **1:**679, 1968.
318a. Weetman, R. M.: Relapsing CGG—141, 101 and 143 (open), Minutes of the meeting of the Children's Cancer Study Group, Feb. 8-10, 1978, Park City, Utah.
319. Western, K. A., Perera, D. R., and Schultz, M. G.: Pentamidine isathionate in the treatment of *Pneumocystis carinii* pneumonia, Ann. Intern. Med. **73:**695, 1970.
320. Whang-Peng, J., Knutsen, T., Ziegler, J. et al.: Cytogenetic studies in acute lymphocytic leukemia: special emphasis in long-term survival, Med. Ped. Oncol. **2:**333, 1976.
321. Willoughby, M. L. N.: Treatment of overt meningeal leukemia, Br. Med. J. **1:**864, 1976.
322. Willoughby, M. L. N.: Treatment of overt meningeal leukemia, Lancet **1:**363, 1974.
323. Wolff, J. A.: Acute leukaemia in children, Clin. Haematol. **1:**189, 1972.
324. Wolff, L. J., Irwin, D., Richardson, S., et al.: Poor prognosis in childhood acute lymphocytic leukemia of B cell type, Presented to Society for Pediatric Research, October, 1975. (Abstract.)
325. Wollman, M. R., Young, L. S., Armstrong, D., and

Haghbin, M.: Anti-*Pseudomonas* heat-stabile opsonins in acute lymphoblastic leukemia of childhood, J. Pediatr. **86:**376, 1975.

326. Yankee, R. A., Graff, K. S., Dowling, R., and Henderson, E. S.: Selection of unrelated compatible platelet donors by lymphocyte HL-A matching, N. Engl. J. Med. **288:**760, 1973.

327. Yankee, R. A., Grumet, F. C., and Rogentine, G. N.: Platelet transfusion therapy: the selection of compatible platelet donors for refractory patients by lymphocyte HL-A typing, N. Engl. J. Med. **281:**1208, 1969.

328. Yolken, R. H., Wanless, I., and Miller, D. R.: Hyperuricemia and renal failure-presenting manifestations of occult hematologic malignancies, J. Pediatr. **89:**775, 1977.

329. Young, L. S., Armstrong, D., Blevins, D., and Lieberman, P.: *Nocardia asteroides* infection complicating neoplastic disease, Am. J. Med. **50:**356, 1971.

330. Young, L. S., Meyer, R. D., and Armstrong, D.: *Pseudomonas aeruginosa* vaccine in cancer patients, Ann. Intern. Med. **79:**518, 1973.

331. Young, R. C., Bennett, J. E., Vogel, C. L., et al.: Aspergillosis: the spectrum of the disease in 98 patients, Medicine **79:**147, 1970.

332. Zuelzer, W. W.: Implications of long-term survival in acute stem cell leukemia of childhood treated with composite cyclic therapy, Blood **24:**477, 1964.

333. Zuelzer, W. W., and Cox, D. E.: Genetic aspects of leukemia, Semin. Hematol. **6:**228, 1969.

334. Zusman, J., Brown, D. M., and Nesbit, M. E.: Hyperphosphatemia, hyperphosphaturia, and hypocalcemia in acute leukemia, N. Engl. J. Med. **289:**1335, 1973.

Hodgkin's disease and non-Hodgkin's lymphoma

335. Adler, S., Parthasarathy, K. L., Bakshi, S. P., and Stutzman, L.: Gallium 67 citrate scanning for the localization and staging of lymphomas, J. Nuclear Med. **16:**255, 1975.

336. Aisenberg, A. C.: Quantitative estimation of the reactivity of normal and Hodgkin's disease lymphocytes with thymadine-2-C_{14}, Nature **205:**1233, 1965.

337. Banfi, A., Bonadonna, G., Ricci, S. B., et al.: Malignant lymphomas of Waldeyer's ring: natural history and survival after radiotherapy, Br. Med. J. **3:**140, 1972.

338. Berard, C. W.: Histopathology of lymphoreticular disorders: Conditions with malignant proliferative response: lymphoma. In Williams, W. J., Butler, E., Erslev, A. J., and Rundles, R. W., eds.: Hematology, New York, 1972, McGraw-Hill Book Co.

339. Berry, C. L., and Keeling, J. W.: Gastrointestinal lymphoma in childhood, J. Clin. Pathol. **23:**459, 1970.

340. Boston, A. C., Dahler, D. C., Ivins, J. C., et al.: Malignant lymphoma (so called reticular cell sarcoma) of bone, Cancer **33:**1131, 1974.

341. Bouroncle, B. A., Old, J. W., and Vazques, A. G.: Pathogenesis of jaundice in Hodgkin's disease, Arch. Intern. Med. **110:**872, 1962.

342. Brown, R. S., Haynes, H. A., Foley, H. T., et al.: Hodgkin's disease: immunological clinical and histologic features of 50 untreated patients, Ann. Intern. Med. **67:**291, 1967.

343. Bryan, R. H.: Rationale for virus research in human leukemia. In Zarafonetis, C. J. D., ed.: Proceedings of the international conference on leukemia-lymphoma, Philadelphia, 1968, Lea & Febiger.

344. Butler, J. J.: Non-neoplastic lesions of lymph nodes of man to be differentiated from lymphomas, Natl. Cancer Inst. Monogr. **32:**233, 1969.

345. Canale, V. C., and Smith, C. H.: Chronic lymphadenopathy simulating malignant lymphoma, J. Pediatr. **70:**891, 1967.

346. Castellino, R. A., and Blank, N.: 1. Current role of

347. Chilcote, R. R., Baehner, R. L., et al.: The incidence of overwhelming infection in children staged for Hodgkin's disease, Presented at American Society of Clinical Oncology, San Diego, 1974. (Abstract.)

348. Cif, G. F. S., and Spriggs, A. I.: Chromosome changes in Hodgkin's disease, J. Natl. Cancer Inst. **39:**557, 1967.

349. Davidson, J. W., and Clarke, E. A.: Influence of modern radiologic techniques in clinical staging of malignant lymphoma, Can. Med. Assoc. J. **99:**1196, 1968.

350. Derz, J. J., and Warr, H. G.: Primary lymphosarcoma of the tonsil, Surgery **65:**772, 1969.

351. Ehrlich, A. N., Stalder, G., Geeler, W., and Sherlock, T.: Gastrointestinal manifestations of malignant lymphoma, Gastroenterology **54:**1115, 1968.

352. Eisner, E., Ley, A. B., and Mayer, K.: Coombs positive hemolytic anemia in Hodgkin's disease, Ann. Intern. Med. **66:**258, 1967.

353. Ferguson, D. J., Allen, L. W., Griem, M. L., et al.: Surgical experience for staging laparotomy in 125 patients with lymphoma, Arch. of Intern. Med. **131:**356, 1973.

354. Fraumeni, J. F.: Constitutional disorders of man predisposing to leukemia-lymphoma. In Lingeman, C. H., and Garner, F. M., eds.: Hematopoietic neoplasms, Natl. Cancer Inst. Monogr. **32:**221, 1969.

355. Gall, E. A., and Mallory, T. B.: Malignant lymphoma; clinicopathologic survey of 618 cases, Am. J. Pathol. **18:**381, 1942.

356. Giannopoulos, B. P., and Bergsagel, D. E.: Mechanism of the anemias associated with Hodgkin's Disease, Blood **14:**856, 1959.

357. Ginsberg, S.: Hodgkin's disease with predominant localization in the nervous system: early diagnosis and radiotherapy, Arch. Intern. Med. **39:**571, 1927.

358. Glatstein, E., Guernsey, J. M., Rosenberg, S. A., and Kaplan, H. S.: The value of laparotomy in splenic staging of Hodgkin's disease, Cancer **24:**709, 1969.

359. Goldman, J. M., and Hobbs, J. R.: The immunoglobulins in Hodgkin's disease, Immunology **13:**421, 1967.

360. Grundy, G. W., Creagan, E. T., and Fraumeni, J. F.: Non-Hodgkin's lymphoma in childhood: epidemiologic features, J. Natl. Cancer Inst. **14:**767, 1973.

361. Gunz, F. M.: The leukemia lymphoma problem. In Zarofonetis, C. J. D., ed.: Proceedings of the international conference on leukemia-lymphoma, Philadelphia, 1968, Lea & Febiger.

362. Hays, D. M., Karon, M., Isaacs, H., and Hittle, R. E.: Hodgkin's disease: technique and results of staging laparotomy in childhood, Arch. Surg. **106:**507, 1973.

363. Henle, G., Clifford, P., Diehle, V., et al.: Antibodies of Epstein-Barr virus in Burkitt's Lymphoma in control groups, J. Natl. Cancer Inst. **43:**1147, 1969.

364. Henle, W., and Henle, G.: Epstein-Barr virus related serology in Hodgkin's disease, Natl. Cancer Inst. Monogr. **36:**79, 1973.

365. Hoffer, P. B., Turner, D., Gottschalk, A., et al.: Whole body radiogallium scanning for staging of Hodgkin's disease and other lymphomas, Natl. Cancer Inst. Monogr. **36:**277, 1973.

366. Jenkin, R. D.: The management of malignant lymphomas in childhood: modern radiotherapy. In Thomas, J., and Deeley, A., eds.: Malignant diseases in children, London, 1974, Butterworth & Co., Ltd.

367. Jenkin, R. D., Brown, T. C., Peters, M. V., and Sonley, M. J.: Hodgkin's disease in children: a retrospective analysis, 1958-1973, Cancer **35:**979, 1975.

368. Jensen, K. B., Thorling, E. G., and Andersen, C. J.: Serum copper in Hodgkin's disease, Scand. J. Hematol. **1:**63, 1964.

lymphangiography, Natl. Cancer Inst. Monogr. **36:**271, 1973.

369. Jones, B., and Klingbart, W. G.: Lymphosarcoma in children, J. Clin. Pathol. **45:**653, 1966.
370. Kaplan, H. S.: Hodgkin's disease, Cambridge, Mass., 1972, Harvard University Press.
371. Kaplan, H. S.: The role of radiation in experimental leukomogenesis. Natl. Cancer Inst. Monogr. **14:**207, 1964.
371a. Kaplan, H. S., and Gartner, S.: "Sternberg-Reed" giant cells of Hodgkin's disease: cultivation in vitro, heterotransplantation, and characterization as neoplastic macrophages, Int. J. Cancer **19:**511, 1977.
372. Kaplan, H. S., and Rosenberg, S. A.: Management of Hodgkin's disease, Cancer **36:**797, 1975.
373. Keller, A. R., Kaplan, H. S., Lukes, R. J., and Rappaport, H.: Collation of histopathology with other prognostic indicators in Hodgkin's disease, Cancer **22:**487, 1968.
374. Kelly, W. D., Good, R. A., Varco, R. L., and Levitt, M.: The altered response to skin hemografts in delayed allergens in Hodgkin's disease, Surg. Forum **9:**785, 1958.
375. Lamb, D., Pilney, F., Kelly, W. D., and Good, R. A.: Comparative study of the incidence of anergy in patients with carcinoma, leukemia, Hodgkin's disease, and other lymphomas, J. Immunol. **89:**555, 1962.
376. Londin, F. E., Jr., Fraumeni, F. J., Lloyd, J. W., and Smith, E. M.: Temporal relationships with leukemia and lymphoma deaths and neighborhoods, J. Natl. Cancer Inst. **37:**123, 1966.
377. Lowenbreum, S., Ramsey, H., Sutherland, J., and Serpick, A. A.: Diagnostic laparotomy and splenectomy for staging Hodgkin's disease, Ann. of Intern. Med. **72:**655, 1970.
378. Luban, N. C., and Miller, D. R.: Unpublished observations.
379. Lukes, R. J.: Relationship of histologic features to clinical stages in Hodgkin's disease, Am. J. Roentgenol. **90:**944, 1963.
380. Lukes, R. J., Butler, J. J., and Hicks, E. D.: Natural history of Hodgkin's disease as related to its pathologic picture, Cancer **19:**317, 1966.
381. Lukes, R. J., Carver, L. F., Hall, T. C., et al.: Report of the nomenclature committee, Cancer Res. **26:**1311, 1966.
382. Lukes, R. J., and Collins, R. D.: A functional post to the classification of malignant lymphoma, Recent Results Cancer Res. **46:**18, 1974.
383. Lukes, R. J., and Collins, R. D.: Immunologic characterization of human malignant lymphomas, Cancer **34:**1488, 1974.
384. Lukes, R. J., Tindle, B. H., and Parker, J. W.: Reed-Sternberg-like cells in infectious mononucleosis, Lancet **2:**1003, 1969.
385. MacMahon, B.: Epidemiology of Hodgkin's disease, Cancer Res. **26:**1189, 1966.
386. Miles, C. P.: Chromosome changes in Hodgkin's disease, Natl. Cancer Inst. Monogr. **36:**197, 1973.
387. Miller, D. G.: Patterns of immunologic deficiency and lymphomas and leukemias, Ann. Intern. Med. **57:**703, 1962.
388. Newbold, P. C. H.: Skin markers of malignancies, Arch. Dermatol. **102:**680, 1970.
389. O'Connor, G. T., Correa, P., Christine, B., et al.: Hodgkin's disease in Connecticut: histology and age distribution, Natl. Cancer Inst. Monogr. **36:**3, 1973.
390. Order, S. E., Chism, S. E., and Hellman, S.: Hodgkin's disease associated with antigens: studies on segregation and specificity, Natl. Cancer Inst. Monogr. **36:**139, 1973.
391. Order, S. E., and Hellman, S.: Pathogenesis of Hodgkin's disease, Lancet **1:**571, 1972.
392. Prosnitz, L. R., Neuland, S. P., and Klingerman, M. N.: Role of laparotomy and splenectomy in the management of Hodgkin's disease, Cancer **29:**44, 1972.
393. Rigby, P., Pratt, P., Rosenlof, R., and Lemon, H.: Genetic relationship in familial leukemia and lymphoma, Arch. Intern. Med. **121:**67, 1968.
394. Rosenburg, S. A.: Hodgkin's disease. In Holland, J. F., and Frei, E., III, eds.: Cancer medicine, Philadelphia, 1974, Lea & Febiger.
395. Schey, W. L., White, H., Conway, J. J., and Kidd, J. M.: Lymphosarcoma in children: a roentgenologic and clinical evaluation of 60 children, Am. J. Roentgen. Radiat. Ther. Nucl. Med. **117:**59, 1973.
396. Schier, W. W., Roth, A., Ostroff, G., and Schrift, M. H.: Hodgkin's disease in immunity, Am. J. Med. **20:**94, 1956.
397. Seif, G. F., and Spriggs, A. I.: Chromosome changes in Hodgkin's disease, J. Natl. Cancer Inst. **39:**557, 1967.
398. Sherman, R. S., and Wolfson, S. L.: Roentgen diagnosis of lymphosarcoma and reticulum cell sarcoma in infancy and childhood, Am. J. Roentgenol., Radiat. Ther. Nucl. Med. **986:**693, 1961.
399. Shoji, H., and Miller, T. R.: Primary reticular cell sarcoma of bone: significance of clinical features upon the prognosis, Cancer **28:**1234, 1971.
399a. Siegal, F. P., Filippa, D. A., and Koziner, B.: Surface markers in leukemia and lymphomas, Am. J. Pathol. **90:**461, 1978.
400. Sullivan, M. P.: Treatment of lymphoma, Cancer **35:**991, 1975.
401. Ultmann, J. E.: Current status in the management of lymphoma, Semin. Hematol. **7:**441, 1970.
402. Ultmann, J. E.: Clinical features in diagnosis of Hodgkin's disease, Cancer **19:**297, 1966.
403. Ultmann, J. E., Cunningham, J. E., and Gellhorn, A.: The clinical picture of Hodgkin's disease, Cancer Res. **26:**1047, 1966.
404. Vianna, N. J., Greenwald, P., and Davies, J. N. P.: Tonsillectomy in Hodgkin's disease: the lymphoid tissue barrier, Lancet **1:**431, 1971.
405. Wilson, T. W., and Pugh, D.: Primary reticular cell sarcoma of bone with emphasis on roentgen aspects, Radiology **65:**343, 1955.
406. Wolff, L. J., Irwin, D., Richardson, S., et al.: Poor prognosis in childhood acute lymphocytic leukemia of B cell type, Presented at Midwest Society for Pediatric Research, October, 1975, Madison, Wisc. (Abstract.)
407. Wollner, N., Burchenal, J. H., Lieberman, P. H., et al.: Non-Hodgkin's lymphoma in children: a comparative study of two modalities of therapy, Proceedings of the Symposium on Conflicts in Childhood Cancer, 1975.
408. Ziegler, J. L.: Burkitt's tumor. In Holland, J. E., and Frei, E., eds.: Cancer medicine, Philadelphia, 1974, Lea & Febiger.
409. Ziegler, J. L., Morrow, R. H., and Fass, L.: Childhood Hodgkin's disease in Uganda, East Afr. Med. J. **47:**191, 1970.
410. Zuelzer, W. W., Mastrangelo, R., Stulberg, C. S., et al.: Autoimmune hemolytic anemia: natural history and viral-immunologic interactions in childhood, Am. J. Med. **49:**80, 1970.

22 □ The spleen and disorders of the reticuloendothelial system

Robert L. Baehner
Denis R. Miller

THE SPLEEN
Role of the spleen in blood disorders

The spleen plays an essential part in the pathogenesis of so many blood disorders that a review of its structure and function serves as a frame of reference for appraising deviations from the normal.

Structure of the spleen

The spleen is structurally organized to perform its main physiologic functions of blood formation, sequestration and destruction of blood cells (principally the erythrocytic series), and protection against infection. It possesses a smooth muscle capsule and trabeculae permitting its contraction, a vascular system with connecting sinusoids allowing withdrawal of cells from the circulation, a lymphoid system (malpighian corpuscles) corresponding to similar tissue elsewhere in the body, and a rich supply of reticuloendothelial tissue.[22]

The spleen is the largest mass of lymphatic tissue in the body, but, unlike other similar collections of this tissue, it is integrally associated with the bloodstream.[49] Splenic tissue fills the spaces between the capsule and trabeculae and is composed of white pulp and red pulp. The white pulp is made up of diffuse and nodular or cylindrical masses of lymphoid tissue, forming a sheath about small arterial branches. The red pulp consists of venous sinuses, while the tissue filling the spaces between them contains the splenic cords. The splenic artery subdivides into arterioles and capillaries, the majority terminating in venous sinuses. The veins of the spleen begin as networks of venous sinuses. The sinuses are lined by long narrow cells and fixed macrophages, which are identical in properties with those in surrounding splenic cords.

Arterioles and venules in the spleen connect by two pathways. In the closed circulation system[44] the blood in the spleen follows endothelial-lined pathways throughout so that arterial capillaries communicate directly with venous sinuses without initial sidetracking through the splenic cords. In a second, or open, circulation pathway, the arterial capillaries pour the blood directly into the pulp cords and then filter it into venous sinuses.

It is now known that the sinus wall is a fenestrated membrane perforated by numerous slits through which the sinuses communicate with the surrounding pulp cords. Through a system of sphincters it is possible for the red cells to be sequestered in the venous sinuses for considerable periods of time, during which the plasma filters through the slits in the sinus wall into the cords.[7] Red cells discharged into the cords of Billroth must traverse the fenestrations, which measure 2.5 to 3 μ in diameter, to gain entry into the sinuses[96] (Fig. 22-1). Inspissated blood is eventually discharged from the sinuses into veins. However, during the process of deplasmatization the entrapped red corpuscles are made more spheroidal and their membranes are weakened and thus rendered susceptible to hemolysis in the trauma of the circulation.

Elements of the reticuloendothelial system are either scattered through the pulp or line the vascular and lymphatic sinusoids. Whether free or fixed, these cells exert a phagocytic action. Mesenchymal cells and lymphoid tissue serve as a source of monocytes and lymphocytes. The sequestration of blood into pulp spaces and venous sinuses exposes bacteria and particulate matter to phagocytosis by the reticuloendothelial tissue and at the same time promotes the stasis and destruction of red blood cells.

Normal functions of the spleen

The normal functions of the spleen include the production, storage, and destruction of blood and protection against infection.

Blood production. The spleen is one of the principal sites of blood formation from the second to the fifth month of fetal life. After passing through the hemocytoblast stage, mesenchymal

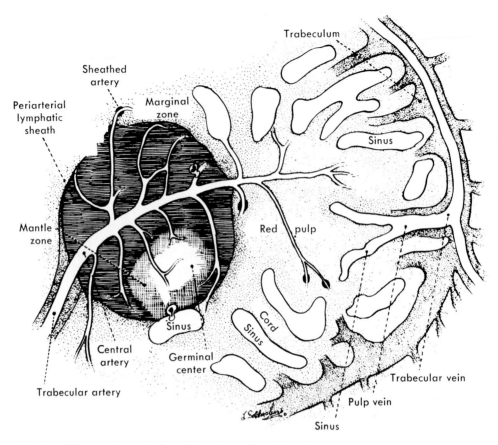

Fig. 22-1. Schema of organization of the spleen. The white pulp consists primarily of a periarterial lymphatic sheath of large and small lymphocytes surrounding the central trabecular artery and is separated from the red pulp by a marginal zone of large, oval reticular cells. The red pulp consists of patent venous sinuses with discontinuous basement membranes alternating with the cords, which are partially collapsed, narrow passages without true walls. (From Weiss, L.: In Greep, R., ed.: Histology, New York, 1965, McGraw-Hill Book Co. Used with permission of McGraw-Hill Book Co.)

cells in the fifth month give rise to erythroblasts. After the fifth month red cell production diminishes and it is absent by the sixth month.[13] Lymphocytes are produced in the spleen mainly in the white pulp (lymphatic tissue and malpighian bodies). According to the unitarian theory, monocytes are derived from lymphocytes on migrating into the red pulp. In stress situations such as hemorrhage, hemolysis, and leukoblastic infiltration in infants and children, fetal blood foci are reactivated with the resumption of hematopoiesis. This function, by which the spleen, liver, and lymph nodes revert to their fetal function of hematopoiesis, is known as extramedullary hematopoiesis and applies equally to the production of red blood cells, granulocytes, and platelets. The relationship of the spleen to blood formation is further confirmed by the observation that in adult mice recovery of blood-forming tissues after total irradiation is accelerated by previously shielding the surgically exteriorized spleen with lead.[38]

Blood storage. Although the spleen serves as a reservoir of red blood cells in the dog, cat, and horse, evidence indicates that blood reservoirs of this nature do not exist in humans.[24,62] In the average-sized adult the spleen holds 20 to 30 ml of red blood cells.[13] During the passage through the spleen even normal red blood cells are rendered more fragile, and a mild degree of spherocytosis is attained. It has been estimated that of the 120-day life cycle of the human red blood cell, about 2 days are spent in the spleen.[13] However, in in patients with pathologic conditions, significant withdrawal of red blood cells from the circulation may take place, producing sudden severe anemia.[54]

In many enlarged spleens a stasis compartment exists in which blood slowly exchanges with the main arteriovenous stream. This "pool" of closely packed cells is especially prominent in patients with splenomegaly.[87] During repeated circuits through this compartment the red cells become progressively more susceptible to splenic destruction. In patients with red cell abnormalities splenic pooling is greater in relation to spleen size than in those patients in whom normal cells are circulating. In sickle cell anemia in young children sudden pooling of the blood into the spleen results in increased size of the organ, accompanied by severe anemia (Chapter 13).

It has been demonstrated that circulation of ^{51}Cr-labeled red cells is slowed in patients with splenomegaly, leading to increased erythrostasis.[33] Whereas in normal subjects labeled red cell mixing in the spleen is completed within less than 1 minute, in patients with splenomegaly complete red cell mixing may require 45 minutes. The resulting erythrostasis may be associated with destruction of red cells within the spleen or the movement of altered cells through the circulation. The detention of red cells in an enlarged spleen and their resulting spheroidicity may be responsible for transient hemolytic anemias encountered in a variety of systemic infections such as bacterial endocarditis, infectious hepatitis, and infectious mononucleosis.[40]

Postsplenectomy thrombocytosis. Approximately 30% of the circulating platelets are stored in the spleen. In any patient who has undergone splenectomy the number of platelets may rise excessively. Although hemorrhagic and thromboembolic complications have been reported with postsplenectomy thrombocytosis in adults,[34] these have not occurred in our patients or in the experience of others dealing with splenectomized children.[19] Accordingly the need for instituting anticoagulant therapy is minimal.

Blood maturation and destruction. Splenic control of normal maturation of the red cell surface is indicated by the loss of stickiness of the reticulocytes during maturation, the loss of reticulum, and shrinkage of diameter and volume from loss of water.[13] This function is lost after splenectomy. Evidence of splenic control over the bone marrow is also suggested by the peripheral blood changes occurring after splenectomy, i.e., prompt increase in the number of white blood cells, platelets, nucleated red cells, and target cells; tendency toward thinness of the red cells; decreased osmotic fragility; and appearance of siderocytes, Heinz bodies, and red cells containing nuclear fragments (Howell-Jolly bodies).[79] On the other hand, erythrocytes containing Heinz bodies are removed and destroyed primarily in the spleen.[70] In a study in which such damaged cells were injected intravenously, the rate of their disappearance was slower in splenectomized patients than in control subjects.[1]

The "culling" function of the spleen describes the ability of this organ to scrutinize passing cells and to remove from the circulation those that do not meet certain minimum requirements.[13] The "pitting" function refers to its ability to remove a solid particle from the cytoplasm of a red cell without destroying the cell itself.[13] The increase in normoblasts following splenectomy may result from the loss of an organ that is able to remove the nucleus of these red cells. Although the spleen may remove nucleated red cells from the circulation, some, at least, are normally pitted and returned to the circulation. The pitting function may extend to siderin granules and other intraerythrocytic inclusions.

Through the reticuloendothelial system the spleen removes worn out and fragmented cells and red cells sensitized by agglutination, resulting in degradation of hemoglobin and formation of bile pigment. Abnormally shaped red cells are trapped and destroyed by the normal spleen, as illustrated by the fate of the spherocytes in patients with hereditary spherocytosis.

The activity of the enzymes of the red cell gradually diminishes[4]; the aging cell grows thinner,[80] becoming brittle and mechanically fragile,[84] and hence more susceptible to fragmentation. The fragments of the old red cells are finally destroyed in the spleen. ATP is a known determinant of erythrocyte deformability, i.e., the ability of the erythrocyte to traverse the restrictive passages of the microcirculation of the spleen and other reticuloendothelial structures.[96] The intracellular content of ATP decreases with aging, and a significant difference in the concentration of ATP between young and old erythrocytes has been detected.[64] Thus with ATP depletion spheroidicity and membrane rigidity increase, deformability decreases, and erythrocyte fragmentation occurs, leading to splenic entrapment and destruction of aged erythrocytes.[46]

Protection against infection. The spleen with its abundant content of macrophages, plasma cells, and lymphocytes is strategically located in the direct stream of the circulating blood for effective phagocytosis and antibody production.[64] The extent to which the spleen participates in antibody response is estimated by comparing the normal with the splenectomized animal and human being after the injection of microorganisms and other antigens. It has been shown in the rabbit that abolition of antibody formation by roentgen rays may be prevented by shielding the surgically mobilized spleen.[39] A comparison of the antibody response to different types of agents in splenectomized and nonsplenectomized animals and human beings has led to divergent results.* These differences may be due to the need for intravenous[72,73] rather than

---

*References 53, 60, 65, 72-74, 81.

subcutaneous[74] injections to demonstrate the depression of antibody response following splenectomy. There is satisfactory evidence that filtration of organisms or other particulate material takes place from the bloodstream by the local phagocytic action of the macrophages in the spleen. Evidence for such a protective mechanism is suggested by experiments[6] in which intravenously injected bacteria cleared from the blood were recovered in the macrophages of the reticuloendothelial tissues of the liver and spleen. Trapping of organisms by removal mechanisms of the liver and spleen have been demonstrated for staphylococci and *Escherichia coli*.[66,67]

Properdin, a natural serum protein that (in association with magnesium and complement) is involved in the destruction of selected bacteria and viruses, has been found to be in lower concentration in splenectomized persons than in normal persons.[9] The activation of the alternate pathway of complement activation (the properdin system) may be defective in asplenic persons as well.[41]

Several studies have recently reemphasized that under certain circumstances the splenectomized child may show increased susceptibility to infection, particularly in the form of septicemia and meningitis.* The least susceptible is the child who has sustained a traumatic rupture of the spleen. An increased incidence, 10% or more, is found in children with portal hypertension and thalassemia major. The splenectomized infant younger than 1 year of age is most susceptible, with an incidence of infection of 20%.[38] The risk of overwhelming infection after splenectomy for hereditary spherocytosis is 2.3% and for thrombocytopenic purpura, 4.8%.

The basis of this increased susceptibility is not known. Perhaps it results from removal of a substantial part of the monocyte-macrophage system lodged in the spleen or from the fact that this organ provides an important site of antibody synthesis.[30] Recently Shinefield et al.[78] found that splenectomized mice are strikingly susceptible to *Diplococcus pneumoniae* type 6. By using small numbers of organisms, in contrast to previous investigators who had experimented with large numbers, they were able to show that earlier and increased death rates were observed in splenectomized mice, that diminished resistance persisted for a prolonged period after splenectomy, and that factors other than a deficiency of blood clearance of these organisms by the spleen were responsible for increased susceptibility.

It has been suggested that the high transferrin level appearing after splenectomy supports the concept of an immunologic function for this protein in addition to iron-binding capacity.[76]

The growth of microorganisms in vitro is greater in the presence of saturated transferrin and a high serum iron concentration than it is in media containing a low concentration of iron and decreased transferrin saturation, supporting the concept of "nutritional immunology."[94]

Since serious infections occur most frequently in the first 2 years after splenectomy, oral therapy with antibiotics, usually penicillin, has been prescribed as a continuous prophylactic measure during this period. Recent clinical trials have shown the prophylactic benefit of vaccination of susceptible groups with pneumococcal antisera.[4a] Infections have also occured 5 to 10 years after splenectomy. Although the incidence of postsplenectomy infection is avowedly small in comparison with the ever-increasing number of splenectomies, close supervision of the splenectomized child is necessary for several years postoperatively until further information is obtained. Such patients should receive immediate and energetic treatment in the event of sudden and severe illness.[81]

DISORDERS OF THE SPLEEN
Splenomegaly

The causes for enlargement of the spleen are listed in the following outline. As shown, splenomegaly accompanies both hematologic and nonhematologic disorders.

A. Blood dyscrasias
  1. Hemolytic anemias
    a. Acquired hemolytic anemia
    b. Hereditary spherocytosis (other membrane defects)
    c. Thalassemia syndromes
    d. Sickle cell anemia (other hemoglobinopathies)
    e. Enzymopathies
  2. Leukemias
B. Storage diseases
  1. Lipid
    a. Gaucher's disease
    b. Niemann-Pick disease
    c. GM gangliosidoses
    d. Wolman's disease
  2. Mucopolysaccharidoses
  3. Amyloidosis
C. Reticuloendothelioses
D. Vascular diseases
  1. Chronic congestive splenomegaly (Banti's syndrome)
  2. Chronic passive congestion
E. Infectious diseases
  1. Acute
    a. Septicemia
    b. *Salmonella* infection
    c. Brucellosis
    d. Infectious mononucleosis

---

*References 20, 27, 35, 45, 50, 82, 83.

2. Chronic
   a. Malaria
   b. Kala-azar
   c. Trypanosomiasis and other parasitic infections
3. Subacute bacterial endocarditis
4. Tuberculosis
5. Sarcoidosis
6. Syphilis
F. Neoplasms and cysts
   1. Hodgkin's disease
   2. Non-Hodgkin's lymphoma
   3. Hemangioma and lymphangioma
   4. Dermoids
G. Miscellaneous
   1. Lupus erythematosus
   2. Rheumatoid arthritis

In interpreting the pathologic significance of an enlarged spleen, it is important to remember that the spleen may be palpable in normal infants and children and at times does not recede in size until puberty. At birth the weight of the spleen is approximately 10 gm; at 1 year of age, approximately 30 gm; at 6 years of age, about 55 gm; at puberty, approximately 95 gm; and in adulthood, about 155 gm.[92] It is estimated that spleens must be enlarged two and one-half to three times the normal size to be palpable.

In a group of 2,200 entering college students 2.86% had palpable spleens.[51] Of the sixty-three students studied, approximately 30% persisted with this finding for at least 3 years after the initial detection. The finding of a palpable spleen could not be explained on the basis of body habitus or infectious mononucleosis or other blood dyscrasias.

The soft edge of the spleen tip can be palpated in many normal children and even in young adults.

Hypersplenism

The spleen exerts a regulatory influence on the control of blood formation and in the delivery of cellular elements from the bone marrow. This function is greatly exaggerated when the spleen becomes hyperactive, a condition that is termed hypersplenism and implies an exaggeration of inhibitory and destructive activities of the spleen. Hypersplenism represents a functional and not an anatomic change. Inherent in this concept is the reduction of one or more cellular elements in the peripheral blood with compensatory hyperplasia in the bone marrow of the corresponding cells, the presence of an enlarged spleen, and the expectation that the peripheral blood picture will be returned to normal, or nearly normal, by splenectomy. The blood disturbances dependent on hypersplenism have been attributed to either selective sequestration and increased destruction

of formed cell elements in the enlarged spleen[23] or to an inhibitory influence on a normal or hyperactive bone marrow by a hormonal mechanism.[16,17] By inhibitory action it is understood that the growth and maturation of various cells are prevented or their delivery from the marrow to the blood is blocked. There is increasing evidence favoring the concept of hypersplenic sequestration, but it does not exclude the possibility that other splenic mechanisms may cause cytopenic diseases. In reviewing the data on which the two concepts of hypersplenism are based, Crosby[14] concludes that "although the evidence in favor of inhibitory hypersplenism is fragile and loopholed, there is still reason to suspect the existence of splenic humoral factors." In either case, whether by increased destruction or inhibition, the removal of an abnormally functioning spleen has been shown to restore normal blood levels with varying degrees of success. Hypersplenism therefore is associated with neutropenia, thrombocytopenia, or anemia either singly or in combination, by splenomegaly and a normal or hypercellular marrow.

Hypersplenism may be primary when there is no obvious cause for the depletion of blood cell types, as in patients with splenic neutropenia, splenic panhematopenia or pancytopenia, and idiopathic thrombocytopenic purpura. It is secondary in patients with splenomegaly in combination with well-defined disorders such as Banti's syndrome, Hodgkin's disease, chronic leukemia, Gaucher's disease, lymphosarcoma, or Boeck's sarcoid. Splenectomy frequently restores a normal peripheral blood picture without affecting the underlying disorder.

Experimental hypersplenism has been produced by a variety of methods. The most consistent of these is the intraperitoneal injection into rats of macromolecular inert polymers such as methyl cellulose.[58] Splenomegaly of up to eight times its normal weight can be produced by this method in the rat. The histology of such spleens reveals packing of splenic phagocytes with methyl cellulose particles and congestion of the pulp with blood. The rats develop anemia, leukopenia, and thrombocytopenia with hyperplastic bone marrow. The spleen, liver, and kidneys are infiltrated with "storage cell" macrophages. The administration of methyl cellulose to previously splenectomized rats produced similar histologic lesions but failed to produce the hematologic abnormalities. In experimental hypersplenism of this type a humoral factor is responsible for the thrombopenia, which is eliminated in the urine. When such urine is given to normal rats, it is responsible for the thrombopenia and partially for the anemia.[59]

Tests for diagnosis of hypersplenism. Various hypersplenic states are associated with a depletion of one or more classes of cells in the peripheral blood.[23] Neutrophils transiently marginate along vessel walls[42] or circulate, the two aggregations of the blood neutrophil population being about equal in size and in constant equilibrium. *Epinephrine* effects a redistribution of granulocytes of the blood by causing a shift from the marginating to the circulating compartment. Although the objective of the epinephrine stimulation tests is to determine the extent of granulocyte sequestration in the spleen, the results are not always constant. In splenomegalic conditions[10] there was no correlation between the degree of splenic contraction and the degree of epinephrine-induced leukocytosis.

The liver-spleen scan with ^{99m}Tc, measurement of survival of ^{51}Cr-labeled red cells combined with surface counting for organ sequestration, and an exact quantification of increased transfusion requirements all provide additional useful information.

Splenic aspiration[11,93] is no longer used in children. Other noninvasive or less invasive diagnostic tests have supplanted splenic aspiration.

Primary splenic neutropenia

Primary splenic neutropenia,[98] is characterized by neutropenia with normal erythrocytes and platelets and often a palpable spleen but without evidence of an underlying disease. Primary splenic neutropenia is a rare disease in childhood and should be differentiated from chronic or periodic neutropenia. The symptoms and signs in both conditions overlap. There are frequent bouts of fever, sore throat, and ulcerative lesions of the gums, mouth, tonsils, vulva, and vagina. The leukocyte count varies between 1 and 3×10^9/liter with granulocytes varying from 0% to 20%.[16] In the typical patient symptoms are completely relieved by splenectomy.

Primary splenic panhematopenia

Although splenic panhematopenia occurs frequently in children with splenomegaly as a manifestation of secondary hypersplenism, the primary disease is rare. The case of a 14-year-old girl with the primary disease was described by Doan and Wright[23]; she had weakness, pallor, unexplained fever, skin disorders, and anorexia, accompanied by pancytopenia, a hyperplastic marrow, a slightly palpable nontender spleen, and no adenopathy. Splenectomy was followed by a hematologic as well as clinical recovery. As contrasted with aplastic anemia, in which pancytopenia also exists, the bone marrow in patients with primary splenic panhematopenia is hyperplastic, and each cellular element is present in normal or increased numbers.

Felty's syndrome

Felty's syndrome occurs in adults. It consists of neutropenia, splenomegaly, and chronic rheumatoid arthritis and usually responds to splenectomy.[68]

Chronic congestive splenomegaly (Banti's syndrome, portal hypertension, splenic anemia)

Definition. Chronic congestive splenomegaly is characterized by enlargement of the spleen, progressive anemia, leukopenia, often thrombocytopenia, gastrointestinal hemorrhage caused by portal hypertension, and, in later stages, cirrhosis of the liver and ascites.

Clinical features. The onset is insidious, usually with an unexplained enlargement of the spleen. The most common manifestations are fatigability, pallor, splenomegaly, hematemesis, and melena. Portal hypertension should be suspected in children of any age, even in the first year of life, when hematemesis or melena is associated with an enlarged spleen. In an infant who had had melena and hematemesis from 3 months of age, splenoportography at 14 months revealed anomalies of the portal system. In patients with fully developed chronic congestive splenomegaly the liver is palpable and the spleen is massive, and in more than one half of the patients hematemesis has occurred. Less often, hemorrhoids are a source of bleeding. The majority of these features are attributable to the rupture of varices in strategic locations. Epistaxis and early bruising are noted in a small number of patients.

Laboratory data. Normochromic and hypochromic anemia and leukopenia, with or without thrombocytopenia, are usually noted. With increasing size of the spleen, marked reduction in the number of leukocytes occurs, ranging usually between 1.5 and 4×10^9 white blood cells/liter, with a predominance of lymphocytes. Leukocytosis accompanies severe hemorrhage, and when blood loss is repeated a hypochromic microcytic anemia results. In the presence of portal cirrhosis the red blood cell survival may be shortened and indirect serum bilirubin may be elevated.[3] The mechanism postulated for hemolysis is a high portal venous pressure and probably a major degree of congestive splenomegaly with red cell stasis. Macrocytosis,[99] target cells, teardrop poikilocytes, and an increase in the MCH have been noted in patients with long-standing disease and cirrhosis of the liver.[69] In patients with marked thrombocytopenia, prolonged bleeding time and occasionally increased bruising follow, but this association is inconstant. The coagulation time is usually normal. The bone marrow reveals either a normal pattern, despite leukopenia and anemia, or a hyperplasia involving megakaryocytes and myeloid and erythroid elements.

Etiology and pathogenesis. As originally described by Banti in 1894,[5] the disease progresses in three stages. The first is that of splenic enlargement and increasing anemia; the second, enlargement of the liver and jaundice; and, terminally, cirrhosis of the liver, gastrointestinal hemorrhage, and ascites. The sequence according to this concept is initiated by a toxin elaborated by an enlarged spleen that acts locally and is also carried to the liver and other tissues and organs. The causative agent, being lodged primarily in the arteriole of the malpighian corpuscle, produces a thickening of the surrounding reticulum while maintaining a glandlike structure. Banti designated this pathologic picture as fibroadenie. It has since been shown[52] that fibroadenie is indeed a peripheral fibrosis representing a nonspecific manifestation of passive congestion and the end result of hemorrhage around the splenic arterioles. More recently the concept of Banti's disease has been changed from a homogeneous entity originating in the spleen to one of congestion and enlargement of the spleen resulting from high portal venous pressure.[97] Congestive splenomegaly has therefore replaced the term "Banti's disease."

The portal system is formed by the portal, the superior and inferior mesenteric, and the splenic veins and their tributaries. The portal vein itself is formed by the union of the superior mesenteric and splenic veins. Unlike other veins, the portal vein ends like an artery, breaking up into numerous small channels that ultimately terminate in capillaries in the substance of the liver. The portal vein has no valves and carries about 75% of the circulation of the liver, whereas the hepatic artery carries oxygen and supplies the other 25% of the circulation.[2] Both vessels have a common outlet in the hepatic vein, which empties into the inferior vena cava. It is important to bear in mind that back pressure in the valveless portal system does not possess the anatomic barriers found in the peripheral veins.[95]

The location of the obstruction in the portal system determines the type of portal hypertension. If obstruction is within the liver, it is classified as intrahepatic; if outside the liver parenchyma, it is classified as extrahepatic. Normally the venous pressure in the portal system ranges from 140 to 220 mm of saline solution or from 60 to 140 mm of water.[95] In the adult the portal pressure is normally below 225 mm of water; readings above 250 mm can be regarded as abnormally high.[32]

The commonest cause of portal obstruction is cirrhosis of the liver resulting from congenital diseases, infiltrations, hepatitis, schistosomiasis, Wilson's disease, and neoplasms. Fibrocystic disease of the pancreas is one of the more important causes of biliary cirrhosis and portal hypertension in childhood. It stems from mechanical obstruction of the bile ductules by inspissated secretions.[21] Cirrhosis of the liver, which accounts for 70% of cases of portal hypertension in the adult, is rare in children. In children extrahepatic lesions are more common and are caused by congenital malformations such as congenital stenosis or atresia, aneurysm of the splenic artery, and distortions of the portal vein extending into the liver. Other causes are thrombosis resulting from thrombophlebitis caused by omphalitis or generalized infection in early life involving splenic or portal veins or both, cavernomatous transformation of the portal vein, hepatic fibrosis secondary to irradiation in Wilms' tumor, and compression from pancreatic fibrosis and tumors, especially of the pancreas.

Extrahepatic portal vein obstruction and portal hypertension may result from umbilical vein catheterization in the course of exchange transfusion.[57,77] To avoid the potential hazard of portal vein thrombosis as a consequence of catheterization, it has been recommended that fluids should not be administered parenterally via an indwelling umbilical vein catheter, that catheters should not be left in the umbilical vein between exchange transfusions, and if clinical evidence of umbilical sepsis exists or difficulty is encountered during insertion of the catheter, another site for catheterization should be chosen.[57]

Pathology. The long-standing back pressure on the venous sinuses of the spleen eventually results in hemorrhage, with fibrotic and regenerative changes within this organ resulting in a characteristic fibrotic spleen.[97] The pathologic histology of the spleen has been described as consisting of periarterial hemorrhages developing into areas of periarterial fibrosis, siderotic nodules, and dilated venous sinuses with thickening of the reticulum of the wall, giving a collagen-staining reaction.[52]

Collateral circulation. In the patient with chronic portal hypertension a collateral circulation that tends to lower the pressure in the portal system develops between the portal and systemic veins. These collaterals are located at the lower end of the esophagus and the upper end of the stomach, in the umbilicus, and in the rectum. Collateral vascular channels are sometimes seen in the abdominal wall. Of the greatest clinical significance are the collateral routes beneath the mucous membranes at the cardioesophageal junction, which give rise to esophageal varices. The latter are thin walled and are likely to rupture when exposed to trauma, resulting in massive and at times fatal hemorrhage. The hemorrhoidal varices represent connections between the portal system and systemic veins through the middle hemorrhoidal vessels and constitute a source of hemorrhage.[95] Although it is known that bleeding from ruptured esophageal varices can occasionally occur in the absence of associated portal hypertension, patients with a high portal venous pressure and massive bleeding from esophageal varices have been described in whom neither intrahepatic nor extrahepatic portal vein obstruction was found.[86] Esophageal varices have been observed also in patients with extensive intrahepatic Hodgkin's disease.[47]

Diagnosis. The combination of massive enlargement of the spleen, a palpable liver, and pancytopenia often presents a difficult diagnostic problem. Before a definite diagnosis can be made, other conditions associated with splenomegaly, leukopenia, and pancytopenia must be eliminated. These include Gaucher's disease, Niemann-Pick disease, reticuloendotheliosis (Letterer-Siwe disease), and infiltrations of the bone marrow with leukemic or neoplastic cells.

A history of hematemesis or melena is, of course, highly suggestive of portal hypersplenism. After barium is swallowed esophageal varices can be seen in only about 40% of patients.[18] Esophagoscopy with the flexible esophagoscope is utilized to visualize varices at the site of the lesion. In patients suspected to have chronic congestive splenomegaly, the use of percutaneous splenoportal venography has been helpful in diagnosis. With this method roentgenographic visualization of the portal vein and its branches is achieved by percutaneous intrasplenic injection of contrast material.[28]

Extrahepatic portal hypertension may be differentiated from that which is secondary to liver cirrhosis[36] and is suggested by the following: a history of omphalitis or severe bacterial infection during early infancy that is followed by an uneventful course until signs of portal hypertension appear; an essentially negative and benign history prior to the onset of signs of portal hypertension, such as hematemesis and/or splenomegaly; an absence of jaundice or other signs of liver disease prior to the onset of symptoms; and normal liver function tests. In contrast, portal hypertension secondary to cirrhosis of the liver is suggested by positive liver function tests, evidence of a previous history of jaundice or liver enlargement, hepatomegaly, and tenderness of the liver, which is prominent. Hepatic enlargement, ascites, and other evidences of liver failure tend to appear prior to portal hypertension.

Newer techniques have led to an elucidation of the pathogenetic factors of portal hypertension and the possible identification of the site of obstruction. Appraisal of liver function, manometric measurement of portal pressures, and the use of portal venography and celiac axis arteriography contribute to the accuracy of diagnosis and facilitate surgical intervention for decompression of the portal area.[75] In portal venography the portal venous system is rendered opaque by contrast medium and then visualized by serial x-ray studies. At present percutaneous splenoportography and anteriography of the celiac axis are in common use. The latter may aid diagnosis by delineating abnormalities of the hepatic circulation during the arterial phase; during the venous phase it shows the condition of the splenic and portal veins. Anteriography also confirms the presence of esophageal varices and provides important data with regard to size and conformation of the vessels; this aids in the selection of the optimal type of shunt.[100]

Treatment. Adequate treatment depends on the discovery of the site and nature of the portal obstruction. Splenorenal, mesocaval, and portacaval anastomoses are the three types of shunts in common use, and the choice of one of these depends primarily on the patency and caliber of the vessels available for the procedure. Splenectomy might be considered preferable in children with moderate or marked enlargement of the spleen, especially when pancytopenia exists. Although blood values would be restored to normal or nearly normal, it is now realized that once the spleen is removed the splenic vein is no longer available for anastomosis should it later become necessary. Splenectomy without a venovenous shunt is indicated only in patients with lesions obstructing the splenic hilum.[71] The prognosis is best in those children with a normal liver and with obstruction located in the splenic vein.

Splenectomy with a splenorenal shunt is usually recommended in patients with marked splenomegaly, hypersplenism, large caliber splenic veins, or an obliterated portal vein resulting from cavernomatous transformation or aplasia of the portal vein. A portacaval shunt is advocated with small caliber splenic veins or cirrhosis of the liver. Because of the progressive nature of the disease and the likelihood that a fair percentage of splenorenal shunts will tend to close spontaneously, there has been a tendency to decompress the portal system by an immediate portacaval shunt, especially in the small child. Should the latter procedure eventually prove ineffective, the now larger splenic vein will be available for anastomosis.

In general the most effective relief of portal hypertension in children with intrahepatic obstruction is obtained from portacaval anastomosis, a procedure normally successful in children older than 5 years.[88] For children with extrahepatic portal obstruction the most effective remedy is to bypass the obstruction by means of a portal-system venous shunt. Since the portal vein is usually occluded by the obstructive process, a splenorenal or mesocaval shunt may be used. The former procedure has rarely been found successful in children less than 10 years of age.[88] When a shunt is inadvisable or impossible and control of bleeding cannot otherwise be achieved, the mesocaval shunt devised by Marion and Clatworthy[12,89] may prove useful. This shunt is worthwhile in patients whose portal and splenic veins have been rendered useless for shunting. The mesocaval shunt represents an anastomosis of the proximal end of the divided inferior vena cava into the root or side of the superior mesenteric vein in an end-to-side fashion. There is no definite way, unfortunately, to visualize the superior mesenteric vein preoperatively to determine its patency. Celiac and superior mesenteric arteriograms may be utilized to demonstrate the venous phase of the superior mesenteric vein, but this method is not sufficiently trustworthy.

It is of interest that a salutary effect on the hematologic features of hypersplenism has been observed after a portacaval shunt, with a reversal of the pancytopenia and without splenectomy.[25] Once portal hypertension is relieved, esophagogastric varices recede, the hazard of hemorrhage diminishes, and the spleen shrinks in size.[90,91] Transthoracic ligation and endoscopic injection of esophageal varices have also proved of value for the temporary control of esophageal bleeding.

Anemia due to hemorrhage responds to iron therapy. Blood transfusions are given for values of 8 gm/dl or less, but the hemoglobin concentration need not be elevated to maximal levels. Esophageal bleeding remains a constant source of concern, and methods for its control by tamponade with esophageal balloons have proved of questionable value.

Course and prognosis. The course depends on the degree and site of obstruction and the effectiveness of a remedial operation in relieving the excessive portal venous pressure and retarding liver damage. The control of gastrointestinal hemorrhage from ruptured varices and eradication of the obstruction are important factors in projecting the outcome. The presence of ascites and persistent anorexia are of serious prognostic importance.

The site of portal venous obstruction is the most significant single factor in the management and prognosis of patients with portal hypertension in childhood. Intrahepatic portal obstruction carries a much poorer outlook than extrahepatic obstruction because of the serious and progressive nature of the primary hepatic disease. Posthepatic obstruction of the hepatic veins rarely leads to the development of esophageal varices and bleeding.[88]

Congenital absence of the spleen

Agenesis of the spleen usually occurs in combination with malformation of the heart, most often atrioventricular communis, and partial transposition of the abdominal viscera.[8,61,63] Rarely is there an absence of an associated anomaly.[37,55,56] In either case a presumptive diagnosis of agenesis of the spleen can be made from the peripheral blood by the presence of normoblastemia and Howell-Jolly bodies and Heinz bodies in the erythrocytes. The diagnostic value of Heinz bodies (particles of denatured hemoglobin) has been emphasized by their presence in 10% of the red cells in the peripheral blood of mature newborn infants with agenesis of the spleen.[120]

Hereditary splenic hypoplasia has been described in three siblings in whom the use of radioactive scanning techniques helped to establish the diagnosis.[43]

Indications for splenectomy

Splenectomy is most successful in patients with hereditary spherocytosis and, to a lesser extent, in those with thrombocytopenic purpura. By removing the inhibitory or destructive influence in patients with secondary hypersplenism, it frequently restores the blood count to normal either in part or completely. As mentioned in Chapter 14, in patients with thalassemia major the beneficial effects of splenectomy result in the elimination of a hemolytic factor and in a material decrease in transfusion requirements. Splenectomy is discussed in connection with management of the specific disorder in other sections of this text.

A. Hemolytic disorders
  1. Hereditary spherocytosis
  2. Acquired hemolytic anemia
  3. In selected cases
    a. Thalassemia major
    b. Sickle cell anemia
    c. Certain enzymopathic hemolytic anemias
B. Hypersplenic syndromes
  1. Without splenomegaly: chronic idiopathic thrombocytopenic purpura
  2. With splenomegaly
    a. Banti's syndrome
    b. Splenic neutropenia
    c. Splenic pancytopenia
    d. Gaucher's disease
    e. Other lipid storage diseases
C. Miscellaenous
  1. Rupture of spleen
  2. Cysts
  3. Tumors (i.e., staging in Hodgkin's disease)

DISEASES OF THE MONOCYTE-MACROPHAGE (RETICULOENDOTHELIAL) SYSTEM

The reticuloendothelioses constitute a group of disorders of unknown etiology, having in common hyperplasia of cellular elements of the reticuloendothelial system. Reticulum cells and histiocytes undergo proliferation principally in the spleen, liver, bone marrow, lymph nodes, and, to some extent, other tissues and organs. These disorders have been subject to varied classifications but are now separated on the basis of presence or absence of distinctive intracellular lipids. Gaucher's disease and Niemann-Pick disease are the prominent members of the storage disease group, and Letterer-Siwe disease (nonlipid reticuloendotheliosis), Hand-Schüller-Christian disease, and eosinophilic granuloma constitute the group designated histiocytosis X. The difficulty of classification is exemplified by Hand-Schüller-Christian disease, in which the proliferating histiocytes initially contain little cholesterol but later accumulate enough to give the appearance of foam cells.

Gaucher's disease

Definition. Gaucher's disease is an uncommon hereditary metabolic disorder characterized by the storage of kerasin and other cerebrosides in the reticuloendothelial system. It has been most often observed in Jewish families, but cases have been described in many nationalities over the world. The disease occurs as an acute infantile type and a chronic or adult type. Gaucher first described this entity in 1882, regarding it as a primary epithelioma of the spleen.

Genetics. The disease has been noted in siblings, in a parent and child both with the full clinical picture of Gaucher's disease,[126] and in asymptomatic parents of typically affected children.[122,149] In this respect the parent can be regarded as a carrier. The mode of inheritance varies with different groups, the majority of cases being caused

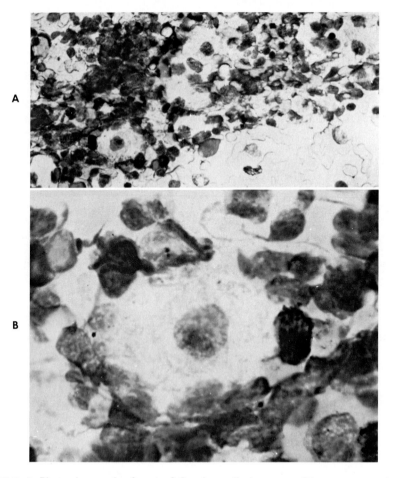

Fig. 22-2. A, Photomicrograph of nest of Gaucher cells in smear of bone marrow. (×900.) **B,** A single Gaucher cell from the smear shown in **A.** Note crinkled, fibrillar appearance of cytoplasm and relatively small, slightly eccentric nucleus. (×1,500.)

by an autosomal recessive gene.[126] Zoltnick and Groen[157] in an analysis of cases of Gaucher's disease found that the disease tends to become more severe in successive generations. The authors noted that not a single patient with Gaucher's disease was born of a father or mother with manifest disease, indicating that death in utero results from the severe metabolic disturbance. They concluded that "patients with manifest Gaucher's disease can at least be freed from worry about their offspring." The patients can expect either healthy children or none at all. More extensive observations are required in confirmation of this principle.

Clinical and laboratory features. The clinical features of the acute infantile and chronic forms of Gaucher's disease are discussed separately.

Acute infantile form. The infant may appear normal at birth and for the first weeks and months of life but soon undergoes mental and physical retardation and deterioration. Splenomegaly followed by enlargement of the liver contributes to prominence of the abdomen, which is further exaggerated by wasting of the extremities. Severe neurologic symptoms and signs characterize the infantile form of the disease. Generalized hypertonia, opisthotonus and rigidity, dysphagia, laryngeal spasm, cyanosis, severe cough due in part to pulmonary infiltration with Gaucher cells,[142] (Fig. 22-2) and fever dominate the clinical picture. Death occurs before the age of 2 years.[121] The cerebral changes observed at postmortem examination indicate chronic disease of the ganglion cells progressing to sclerosis and complete destruction. Rarely typical Gaucher cells are found in the intracerebral vascular spaces.[155]

Lipid analysis of liver and spleen in young patients reveals a consistent increase in the level of water-insoluble glycolipid (cerebroside).[148] Acid phosphatase is increased in these tissues. The elevations of cerebroside and acid phosphatase usually are not of the magnitude characteristic of children with the chronic disease. Alteration in the metabolism of certain large neurons results in an accumulation of glycolipid within their cytoplasm, which is then apparently followed by cell death and neuronophagia. A patchy loss of nerve cells is especially marked in layers three and five of cortex, as well as a prominence of microglia and Gaucher cells in the same location.[102] Neuronophagia is a conspicuous finding in the nuclei of the basal ganglia and brainstem. In contrast, it is rare in Tay-Sachs, Hurler's, and Niemann-Pick diseases.

Chronic form. The chronic form has an insidious onset (starting in childhood or at any age thereafter), most commonly with splenomegaly followed soon after by liver enlargement. Lymph-adenopathy is not a conspicuous feature. The skin reveals a yellow or patchy brown pigmentation that is particularly prominent on exposed parts of body — face, neck, hands, and legs. Pingueculae of the conjunctiva are rare in children and common in adults. They consist of a brownish yellow wedge-shaped thickening of the subconjunctival tissue with bases situated close to the corneal margins and apices pointed to the inner and outer canthi. Infiltration with Gaucher cells causes pulmonary and bone involvement. Pulmonary infiltration is uncommon in the chronic form although common in the acute form of the disease. Pain in the legs, occasionally accompanied by swelling of adjacent joints, is caused by bony infiltration by Gaucher cells. The roentgenogram shows diffuse or localized destructive and productive changes often producing a characteristic deformity in the lower femora. This consists of a widening of the lower halves and thinning and flaring of the cortices, giving a trumpet or an Erlenmeyer flask appearance.[105,140] This feature is reminiscent of the swollen appearance in similar areas in patients with thalassemia major. Pathologic fractures caused by marked osteoporosis and replacement by Gaucher cells may occur[124] (Figs. 22-3 and 22-4).

In some cases osteosclerosis is a major feature of the disease. New bone may be laid down around and between areas of bone destruction, or it may be found along the inner aspect of the cortex in the affected areas.[135] A periosteal reaction is produced by elevation of the periosteum by Gaucher cells, resulting in new bone formation.[150] The clinical picture of osteomyelitis may be simulated. Gaucher's disease may also exhibit the roentgenographic features of Legg-Perthes disease.[112] Proliferation of Gaucher cells in the femoral heads, leading to their subsequent collapse, creates a picture indistinguishable from aseptic necrosis.[135,152] Gaucher cell infiltration of the vertebrae may lead to their collapse.

The clinical differentiation between osteomyelitis and the condition produced by extensive infiltration of the bone marrow by Gaucher cells may be extremely difficult. It has been emphasized that an intractable sinus may result when patients with Gaucher's disease are subjected to operation under the mistaken diagnosis of osteomyelitis.[150]

Blood. The anemia is usually of a mild or moderate normochromic and normocytic type. Leukopenia with relative lymphocytosis and slight to marked thrombocytopenia may be present. Thrombocytopenia with hemorrhage may be sufficiently severe to require splenectomy. The complete pancytopenic blood picture of hypersplenic disorders may ultimately develop. Serum lipid and choles-

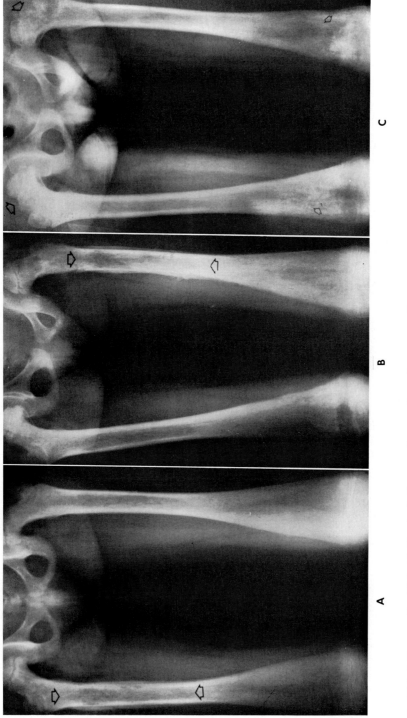

Fig. 22-3. A, Femurs of a child with Gaucher's disease at 7 years of age. Large area of bone destruction associated with subperiosteal new bone formation in the proximal half of the right femur (between arrows). The process was preceded by fever, swelling, and local pain of several days' duration. Subsequently, the patient was asymptomatic. The bone changes cleared completely in 4 months without residuum. **B,** Six months after the onset of the previous episode the patient developed a similar lesion in the left femur (between arrows) with identical clinical history, findings, course, and duration. **C,** Seven months later; complete clearing of the destructive process in the left femur. Note undertubulation of the distal segment of the femoral shafts (Erlenmeyer flask appearance) characteristic of Gaucher's disease (arrows). Note also in **B** and **C** signs (more marked in **C**) of aseptic necrosis of the femoral heads and necks (arrows)—not uncommon complications of Gaucher's disease. Radiolucent defects in distal femoral metaphysis are presumably a result of infiltration of bone by Gaucher cells.

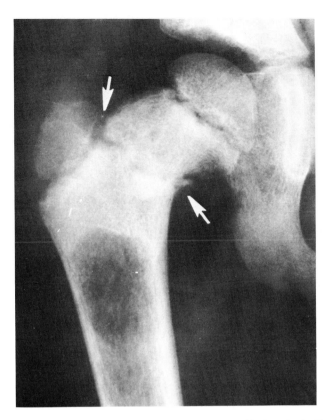

Fig. 22-4. Pathologic fracture of right hip in a 9-year-old girl with Gaucher's disease of 4 years' duration. Fracture and mild subluxation of right femoral neck indicated by arrows.

terol levels are normal. With phenylphosphate substrate the serum acid phosphatase level is elevated in Gaucher's disease, perhaps by spillage from tissue accumulations.[106,115] Gaucher cells have been found infrequently in smears of the peripheral blood. They should be sought along the edges of the slide. In one case in which this finding was reported a leukoerythroblastic reaction was observed many years after splenectomy.[157]

Pathology and pathogenesis. At least three substances have been isolated from tissues containing Gaucher cells: a galactocerebroside (kerasin), a glucocerebroside, and a water-soluble glycolipid polycerebroside.[153,154] The pathogenesis of the disease has been ascribed to a primary deficiency of the enzyme causing an accumulation of cerebrosides and glucocerebrosidase[104] in reticuloendothelial cells. The site of the biochemical error in the disease is at the conversion of the glucocerebroside to the galactocerebroside so that the abnormal glucose form accumulates.

Postmortem examination reveals Gaucher cells in the spleen, liver, lymph nodes, bone marrow, lungs, and other organs (Fig. 22-2). The disease is diagnosed by the proliferation of cells in these areas, the most accessible of which is the bone marrow. Gaucher cells are large and distinctive, 20 to 80 μ in diameter, round or oval, and possess one or more small dense nuclei eccentrically located. The cytoplasm has an opaque wrinkled tissue paper appearance caused by the presence of fine wavy fibrils running parallel to the long axis of the cell. The cytoplasm occupies the major part of the Gaucher cell and stains slightly gray or bluish. It exhibits an intense PAS reaction for glycogen and a positive reaction for acid phosphatase.[116] Electron microscopy indicates that the cytoplasmic striations, pathognomonic of the Gaucher cell, correspond to tubule-containing bodies. Mitochondria could be identified within such bodies. These round or ovoid bodies may be derived from transformations of the mitochondria.[116]

Course and treatment. There is no cure for Gaucher's disease, and in children beyond infancy the disease may either progress or remain chronic. Pregnancy does not aggravate the course of Gaucher's disease, nor is there any effect on the fetus.[125] Those patients who survive to adolescence live for many years. Most adults die of intercurrent diseases rather than of Gaucher's disease. Steroids are sometimes of value in relieving bone pains and joint swelling without altering the progress of the disease. Splenectomy is usually effective in relieving the development of a massive spleen and in reversing the severe pancytopenia.[132] Acceleration of bone involvement by splenectomy has been a controversial issue because the spleen is the main storage place for glucocerebrosides. However, based on wide experience, the theory that splenectomy hastens the onset of bone lesions finds no support from most authors on this subject.[140] Splenectomy induces improvement in symptoms, particularly if there are signs of hypersplenism such as bleeding from thrombocytopenia. Occasionally massive enlargement of the liver follows splenectomy. In these cases microscopic examination reveals diffuse infiltration by Gaucher cells, some arranged in tumorlike nodules. Experience with a new form of therapy, enzyme replacement,[114] is too preliminary at this time but provides hope for the future.

Sea-blue histiocyte syndrome

Cases of hepatosplenomegaly have been described in which abnormal cells, probably of reticuloendothelial origin, containing large blue cytoplasmic granules have been found in bone marrow and other organs.[131,145] Cells similar to those initially described by Sawitsky et al.[145] have been observed in the bone marrow by Silverstein et al.[146] in a black girl who had been followed from the age of 16 months until her death at 10 years of age. This disorder, termed the syndrome of the sea-blue histiocyte, is characterized by the presence of this destructive, blue, granulated histiocyte and an associated splenomegaly. Clinically patients with the disease may have a relatively benign course with mild purpura secondary to thrombocytopenia or may have progressive hepatic cirrhosis, hepatic failure, and death. Two biochemical events appear to accompany this disease: storage of specific phospholipids and glycosphingolipids, and abnormal urinary excretion and perhaps hepatic storage of mucopolysaccharide-type substances. All patients had numerous sea-blue histiocytes in aspirated specimens of bone marrow demonstrated by either Wright's or Giemsa stain. This histiocyte is a large cell, up to 20 μ in diameter, containing a varying number of blue-staining granules. The cells are differentiated from those of Gaucher's disease, Niemann-Pick disease, and other storage diseases.

Two siblings 10 and 12 years of age with the sea-blue histiocyte syndrome have been reported.[127] The 10-year-old child had an enlarged spleen, and chest x-ray films showed diffuse nodular densities in both lung fields with bilateral hilar adenopathy. He had varying degrees of hypersplenism as manifested by mild anemia, leukopenia, and thrombocytopenia. Bone marrow aspiration showed numerous large histiocytes whose cytoplasm contained varying numbers of granules staining light blue with Wright's or May-Grünwald-Giemsa stain. A 12-year-old sister had bone

marrow containing numerous sea-blue histiocytes identical in number and morphology to those found in the patient's bone marrow. Her spleen was not palpable. It was postulated that this is a hereditary disorder of lipid metabolism transmitted as an autosomal recessive trait.

Objection has been made that the sea-blue histiocyte is not a specific cell. Kattlove et al.[128] regard this cell as a normal reticuloendothelial cell that contains partially digested cells, which become apparent when there is increased destruction of blood or bone marrow cells. They think that the inclusions are the remnants of partially phagocytosed cells and are responsible for the appearance of these histiocytes on light microscopy.

Gaucher-like cells bearing a resemblance to the sea-blue histiocyte have been reported in congenital dyserythropoietic anemia, chronic granulocytic leukemia, and idiopathic thrombocytopenic purpura.

Niemann-Pick disease

Definition. Niemann-Pick disease is a rare hereditary disease, clinically resembling the infantile type of Gaucher's disease.[139] It is characterized by the widespread storage of sphingomyelin in the reticuloendothelial system, the nervous system, and some other tissues. At least four types or variants have been described.[118]

Genetics. There is a striking predilection for Jews, which is more marked than in Gaucher's disease. The occurrence among siblings is well known. Tay-Sachs disease has been noted among relatives of patients with Niemann-Pick disease. All four variants are inherited as autosomal recessive disorders. The homozygous form of the disease can be detected antenatally.[113]

Clinical and laboratory features. The onset may date from birth or may occur after the first 6 months of life. Progressive physical and mental deterioration is accompanied by massive and equal enlargement of the liver and spleen. In contrast, in patients with Gaucher's disease the spleen is larger than the liver. A brownish yellow pigmentation occurs, especially in the parts exposed to light. In an appreciable number of patients (estimated as high as 60%)[155] a cherry-red spot appears in the macula, corresponding to that seen in patients with Tay-Sachs disease. Nervous system involvement is manifested by spasticity, blindness, and deafness; the patient finally lapses into a state of apathy and idiocy. With the patient profoundly emaciated, death usually occurs before the third year of life. Although the bone marrow is infiltrated with foam cells, survival is not sufficiently prolonged for changes to be conspicuously apparent on x-ray examination.

Chronic forms of the disease are described extending to adolescence,[106,117,130] and in cases reported in two brothers death occurred at 29 and 33 years of age, respectively.[151] In patients who have survived beyond infancy extensive pulmonary infiltrations are observed on roentgenographic examination. In a 19-year-old boy under observation from early childhood with the typical Niemann-Pick cells in the bone marrow, marked hepatosplenomegaly, and pulmonary infiltration, normal mental and physical growth took place.

Hematologic findings. Vacuoles appear in the cytoplasm of the circulating lymphocytes and monocytes, but no definite histochemical studies on such cells are known. The vacuoles are discrete, unstained, and round and vary in number from 1 or 2 to 15 or 20.[106]

In the older patient anisocytosis and poikilocytosis with many oval cells are noted. A mild or moderate microcytic anemia is found. White blood cells vary between slight leukocytosis and moderate leukopenia. Blood cholesterol either is not increased or is slightly elevated.

Pathology and pathogenesis. The striking features at autopsy are involvement of the liver, spleen, lungs, bone marrow, and lymph nodes and the replacement of reticular cells and histiocytes by the foam or Niemann-Pick cells. The nervous system is almost invariably affected. Degenerative changes take place in the ganglion cells. The large neurons are distended or ballooned with loss of their usual triangular or pyramidal shape. Usually there are lipid deposits in the ganglion and neuroglia cells.[155] Often there is a paucity of nerve cells as if many had disintegrated.[106]

The storage material in the foam cells that accumulates in the viscera of patients with Niemann-Pick disease consists largely of phospholipids, sphingomyelin, and cholesterol. The foam cells that characterize the disease are readily available for examination by bone marrow aspiration. These are large, more or less rounded, occasionally oval or polyhedral cells averaging 15 to 90 μ in diameter[106] and containing one or two nuclei often eccentrically placed with loosely arranged chromatin material. The abundant cytoplasm is filled with highly refractile lipid droplets that give a weblike, honeycombed, or foamy appearance. Unlike the Gaucher cells, the foam cells of the disease are readily detected in the counting chamber and can be separated from the megakaryocytes (Fig. 22-5). Electron microscopy revealed in one case that the lipid inclusions were made up of lamellated muliple membranes.[130]

Assays of sphingolipid-cleaving enzymes in the leukocytes and other tissues of patients with Niemann-Pick disease are of diagnostic value and have provided much useful information concerning the abnormal lipid metabolism in these diseases. Decreased activity of sphingomyelinase has been found in type A and type B Niemann-Pick disease,[147] respectively. The spleen and skin fibroblasts also demonstrate these enzymatic lesions.[103]

Treatment and prognosis. There is no effective treatment. Splenectomy may be carried out, but except for the relief of anemia and mild evidences of hypersplenism this procedure does not alter the course of the disease.[106] In patients with type A or type C disease death occurs before 4 years

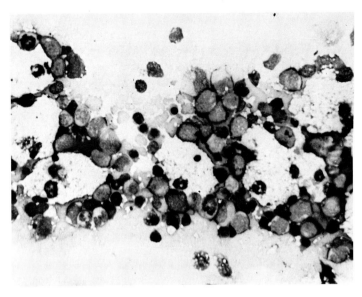

Fig. 22-5. Photomicrograph of bone marrow smear of patient with Niemann-Pick disease. Note group of typical cells—their large size, relatively small, round, or oval nucleus, and foam droplets giving a honeycomb appearance of cytoplasm.

of age or in later childhood, respectively. Children with type B Niemann-Pick disease have visceral but no central nervous system involvement, are intellectually normal, and attain adulthood. Death is usually associated with progressive neurologic deterioration and superimposed pulmonary infections.

Generalized gangliosidosis

In patients with generalized gangliosidosis[129] (GM$_1$ gangliosidosis, familial neurovisceral lipidosis, pseudo-Hurler disease, Hurler variant, Tay-Sachs disease with visceral involvement), abnormal gargoyle-like facies, macroglossia, peripheral edema, hepatosplenomegaly, and infrequently cherry-red spots in the macula have been described. The clinical and radiologic features resemble Hurler's disease. Vacuoles in the lymphocytes and monocytes, Reilly bodies in the polymorphonuclear leukocytes, and foam cells in the bone marrow are prominent hematolgoic characteristics. Pathologically there is lipid histiocytosis of the reticuloendothelial system, neural lipidosis, and ballooning of the glomerular epithelium. The metabolic abnormality present in the brain, liver, skin, leukocytes, and other tissues results from a deficiency of β-galactosidase, with progressive accumulation of ganglioside.[137] Death usually occurs before the second or third year of life.

Wolman's disease

Wolman's disease, or primary familial xanthomatosis with involvement and calcification of the adrenals, was originally described in Israeli children[152] and has been reported in children from New Zealand,[101] Austria,[110] and the United States.[108] Clinically patients have failure to thrive, gastrointestinal complaints, and hepatosplenomegaly. Death usually occurs by 2 to 4 months of age. Vacuolated lymphocytes in the peripheral blood and foam cells in the bone marrow, similar to those seen in Neimann-Pick disease, have been described. Markedly increased amounts of structurally normal cholesterol have been identified in the liver, spleen, and, to a lesser extent, brain of these patients, suggesting that the biochemical defect may be an abnormality in the regulation of the rate of production or disposal of cholesterol.[140]

Mucopolysaccharidoses

The mucopolysaccharidoses are a group of rare diseases of early childhood characterized by dull, coarse, cretinoid facies, dwarfism, skeletal deformities, clouding of the corneas, and mental retardation. Fine and coarse blue granules have been described by Reilly in some 60% to 90% of the granulocytes and their precursors in the bone marrow and occasionally in the lymphocytes and monocytes.[138] These granules are the same as

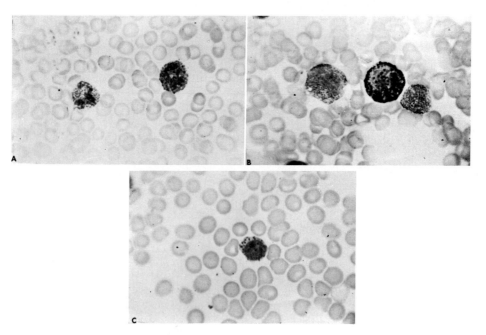

Fig. 22-6. Blood and bone marrow smears from a 3½-year-old boy with gargoylism (Hurler's syndrome). Heavy granulation (Reilly bodies) present in polymorphonuclear leukocytes of the peripheral blood, **A;** myelocytes of the bone marrow, **B;** and lymphocytes (Mittwoch bodies), **C,** are characteristic of this disease. These granules differ from toxic granulation and those found in the basophilic leukocytes. Although coarse granules are common, fine and medium granules may also be present. (Courtesy Dr. Ralph L. Engle, Jr., New York, N.Y.)

those noted by Alder as a hereditary anomaly (Fig. 22-6, *A* and *B*). Patients with mucopolysaccharidoses have been described in whom the abnormal inclusions were confined to the lymphocytes ("Mittwoch bodies"), the granulocytes being unaffected[133,134] (Fig. 22-6, *C*).

In the lymphocytes of gargoylism the cytoplasmic inclusions also stain with May-Grünwald-Giemsa stain and metachromatically with toludine blue.[134] These inclusions are described as distinct from those in polynuclear cells (Reilly bodies) and appear typically as deeply stained granules in the center of vacuoles, sharply defined against the surrounding cytoplasm. These staining reactions indicate that the inclusions consist of acid mucopolysaccharides and are correlated with the excessive excretion of this substance in the urine of many clinically diagnosed cases of mucopolysaccharidosis.[136]

In addition, basophilic granules have also been described in the bone marrow, both extracellular and intracellular within large mononuclear cells, resembling histiocytes. In a few patients the granules are largely intracellular. However, in most cases they are dispersed throughout the particles of bone marrow, perhaps resulting from rupture of cells during preparation. The basophilic granules were described originally by Gasser[119] and more recently by Pearson and Lorincz[138] in the bone marrow of seventeen of eighteen patients with documented gargoylism. Thus the coarse granulations once thought to be present solely in the circulating granulocytes of the mucopolysaccharidoses have now also been found in lymphocytes as well as in bone marrow aspirates.

Several different variants of the mucopolysaccharidoses have been described and are listed in Table 22-1. Some have lymphocyte and/or granulocyte inclusions.[123] Mucopolysaccharides have now been identified by several investigators as chondroitin sulfuric acid B (Dermatan sulfate) and in smaller amounts, heparitin sulfate (heparin sulfate).

The nature of the metabolic defect underlying the mucopolysaccharidoses is most likely related to a hereditary deficiency of a different enzyme resulting in the intracellular storage of a specific metabolite.[111]

In vitro studies have demonstrated intracellular deposition of mucopolysaccharides in fibroblasts of patients with Hurler's and Hunter's disease[109] and have initiated research of the metabolic defect[114] and the antenatal diagnosis of the disease.

Histiocytosis X and other monocyte-macrophage disorders

Definition. Histiocytosis X is a disorder of the reticuloendothelial system with proliferation of normal-appearing macrophages with or without an associated inflammatory reaction of eosinophils, neutrophils, and mononuclear cells involving integument, bone, and viscera. The cause is unknown. Three recognized clinical syndromes of eosinophilic granuloma of bone, Hand-Schüller-Christian syndrome and Letterer-Siwe syndrome share a similar pathology. Severity varies from benign in patients with solitary or multifocal bone lesions to progressive deterioration and death in young infants with visceral involvement.

Historic perspective. The first patient to be described was a 3-year-old boy with hepatosplenomegaly, generalized lymphadenopathy, exophthalmos, polyuria, and an osteolytic lesion of the skull; he was originally thought to have tuberculosis. However, when the case was reconsidered 28 years later in 1921 by the boy's physician, Dr. Hand, it was clear that his signs and symptoms mimicked those of the patients previously described by Christian and Schüller.*

In 1924 Letterer[196] reported the case of a 6-month-old boy with fever, purulent bilateral otitis media, lymphadenopathy, hepatosplenomegaly, and generalized purpura. At autopsy, collections of abnormal histiocytes characterized by large indented nuclei surrounded by abundant eosinophilic cells were found principally in the spleen, lymph

---

*References 169, 182, 183, 189, 212.

Table 22-1. Classification of the mucopolysaccharidoses

		Inclusions in	
Type	**Syndrome**	**Granulocytes**	**Lymphocytes**
I	Hurler's	Present	Diffuse
II	Hunter's	Present	Diffuse
III	Sanfilippo's	Present	Localized
IV	Morquio's	Present in 90%	Rare or absent
V	Scheie's	Absent	Variable (10%)
VI	Maroteaux-Lamy	Packed (EOS also)	Absent
VII	Thompson-Nelson-Grobelney	Absent	Rare

nodes, tonsils, bone marrow, and skin. Intracellular fatty material present in many histiocytes was first noted then by Rowland in 1928.[211] In 1933 Siwe[214] described a 16-month-old girl with hepatosplenomegaly, lymphadenopathy, and large bone lesions in the left fibula. At autopsy the organs were infiltrated by a cell thought to be reticular endothelial or histiocytic in origin; the bone lesions contained lipid-laden mononuclear cells and occasional giant cells.

Subsequently Abt and Denholz[158] reviewed nine cases, including one of their own, and described an entity of unknown etiology that they called Letterer-Siwe disease. Otani and Ehrlich[208] as well as Lichtenstein and Jaffe[197] described five cases of eosinophilic granuloma of bone occurring in older children and adults with solitary lesions in the long bones or the axial skeleton. The granulomas were composed of mixtures of histiocytes with vesicular nuclei surrounded by polymorphonuclear cells and eosinophils. The growth of many of the lesions appeared self-limited. The presence of proliferative histiocytes in patients with Hand-Schüller-Christian syndrome, Letterer-Siwe syndrome, and eosinophilic granuloma offered histologic evidence that these entities were part of a single disease process. In particular the bony lesions in all three disease categories were indistinguishable by both pathologic description and x-ray studies. Furthermore, hepatosplenomegaly, anemia, thrombocytopenia, and skin eruptions were noted in patients and termed by some physicians as clinical manifestations of Hand-Schüller-Christian syndrome and by others as Letterer-Siwe syndrome. Lichtenstein[197] formulated the term "histiocytosis X" as a means of grouping the three clinical types: (1) disease localized in bone similar to eosinophilic granuloma, (2) disseminated chronic histiocytosis X similar to Hand-Schüller-Christian syndrome, and (3) disseminated acute and subacute histiocytosis X similar to Letterer-Siwe syndrome. It remains to be determined whether these three clinical syndromes are related.

Classification. Histiocytosis X and other related disorders can be classified on the basis of whether the disorder is hereditary, by the distribution and histopathology of the affected organs, or by the clinical signs and symptoms.

Heredity

FAMILIAL. Cases of familial histiocytic disorders have been associated with a rapidly fatal, progressive disease characterized by fever, hepatosplenomegaly, lymphadenopathy, purpura, jaundice, and hypergammaglobulinemia. Affected tissue reveals reticuloendothelial hyperplasia with widespread infiltration by bizarre mononuclear cells and plasma cells.[174,200,202]

NONFAMILIAL. Letterer-Siwe syndrome is usually encountered in infants or very young children as a progressive and frequently fatal disease. It involves the skin, liver, lymph nodes, lungs, bones, and hematopoietic system. In fact, the number of systems involved in any given case seems to have prognostic significance.[194]

Hand-Schüller-Christian disease occurs in young children more frequently than in infants. The classic triad of osteolytic defects in membrane bones, exophthalmos, and diabetes insipidus is present in only a small percentage of cases; however, it is diagnostic when it occurs. The disease usually is not fatal, but it is chronic and sometimes progressive.

Eosinophilic granuloma of bone may involve long bones in adults and more typically the skull, vertebrae, ribs, and pubic bones in children.[219]

Systemic distribution. There are a number of pathologic entities in the broad category of reticuloendotheliosis distinct from histiocytosis X. These diseases can be best divided into those with local or systemic distributions. These diseases involve the histiocytic cell capable of ingesting foreign particles. In some instances the cells accumulate lipid material demonstrating xanthomatous characteristics. Although these diseases are similar to histiocytosis X, there is no association with any qualitative or quantitative lipid abnormalities.

LOCALIZED RETICULOENDOTHELIOSIS

HISTIOCYTOMA. Histiocytoma (fibroma simplex, dermatofibroma, sclerosing hemangioma) is a well-defined, circumscribed, painless, freely movable, reddish brown skin lesion varying from 1 to 10 mm found principally over the extensor surfaces of the tibia, forearms, and shoulders.[160]

JUVENILE XANTHOGRANULOMA. Juvenile xanthogranuloma (juvenile xanthoma, endothelioma, nevoxanthoma endothelioma, multiple eruptive xanthoma) consists of sharply demarcated, painless, yellow, usually multiple, pinhead lesions with a predilection for the face and scalp. It is common before 6 months of age and tends to regress spontaneously within several months or years, leaving an atrophic, scarlike area. The tumor is composed of dense infiltration of histiocytes. Most have foamy cytoplasm; no treatment is required.[172]

GRANULOMA FACIALE. Granuloma faciale (facial granuloma with eosinophilia) is a purplish, slowly developing, nodular or placquelike eruption found almost exclusively on the face in a patchlike distribution. Histologic findings consist of a granulomatous infiltration composed of polymorphonuclear leukocytes with a high but variable proportion of eosinophils. There are no areas of necrosis. The corium of the skin is involved with complete sparing of the epidermis. It differs from the lesions of idiopathic histiocytosis X in which the epidermis is often infiltrated and skin ulcerations may occur. This asymptomatic benign lesion does not respond to radiation therapy.[171]

EOSINOPHILIC GRANULOMA OF GASTROINTESTINAL AND GENITOURINARY TRACTS. Eosinophilic granulomas of the gastrointestinal and genitourinary tract are lesions that may be caused by a wide range of allergic reactions or parasitic infestations including *Toxocara;* in contrast to histiocytosis X, they are commonly associated with peripheral blood eosinophilia.[166,221]

SYSTEMIC RETICULOENDOTHELIOSIS

HISTIOCYTIC MEDULLARY RETICULOSIS. Histiocytic medullary reticulosis is a rapidly fatal disease seen most often in adults, but it has been reported in children younger than 14 years of age.[167] This rare disorder was described originally by Scott and Robb-Smith[213] in 1939. Diffuse proliferation of malignant-appearing histiocytes and their precursors destroy normal lymph node architecture. The liver, spleen, and bone marrow may also be involved by histiocytes showing striking erythrophagocytosis (Fig. 22-7). Patients are febrile and often jaundiced; lymphadenopathy, hepatosplenomegaly, anemia, and pancytopenia are all present with or without skin involvement.

Electron microscopy of the neoplastic histiocytes and ferrokinetic studies support the hypothesis that the anemia in patients with this disorder is caused by the unavailability of iron stores, resulting from excessive erythrophagocytosis.[222] The entity has been thought by some to be the adult expression of the progressive and disseminated acute histiocytosis X of the Letterer-Siwe variant in children, but erythrophagocytosis is not prominent in the latter disease. Histiocytic medullary reticulosis is unresponsive to radiation or chemotherapy. The course of histiocytic medullary reticulosis is fulminant with death occurring in a matter of weeks to a few months. Malignant histiocytes in the peripheral blood may simulate a leukemic picture initially. Protein-losing enteropathy attributed to histiocytic infiltration of the lamina propria of the small intestine has also been reported.[170] The disease may represent a form of malignant lymphoma rather than reticuloendotheliosis. This and similar reticuloendothelial disorders must be distinguished from drug-induced (e.g., phenobarbital) bone marrow aplasia with pancytopenia and a histiomonocytic proliferation in the marrow. Hepatosplenomegaly and adenopathy are usually absent in drug-induced histiocytic reactions.

FAMILIAL HEMOPHAGOCYTIC RETICULOSIS. Patients with familial hemophagocytic reticulosis (lymphohistiocytic erythrophagocytosis), in contrast to patients with histiocytosis X, show no skin changes or infiltrates and frequently have prominent clinical involvement of the central nervous system, which on microscopic examination demonstrates infiltration of the reticuloendothelial system and meninges by histiocytes with prominent erythrophagocytosis and leukophagocytosis.[164,176]

DISSEMINATED LIPOGRANULOMATOSIS. Disseminated lipogranulomatosis, a fatal disease similar to acute histiocytosis X with involvement of pleura, pericardium, and abdominal viscera by granulomas was described in three infants by Farber[175] in 1952. The histiocytes, on closer inspection, contained mucopolysaccharide rather than lipid, but the material could not be biochemically identified at the time.

RETICULOHISTIOCYTOMA. Reticulohistiocytoma (reticuloendothelial granuloma, giant cell histiocytoma, lipid dermatoarthritis) describes firm multiple nodules derived from reticuloendothelial ele-

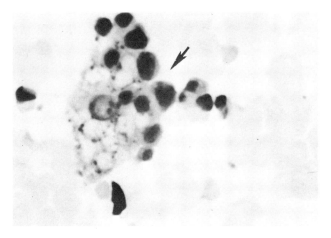

Fig. 22-7. Histiocytic medullary reticulosis. Bone marrow aspirate from a 10-year-old boy who had fever and adenopathy shows erythroid hyperplasia and marked erythrophagocytosis.

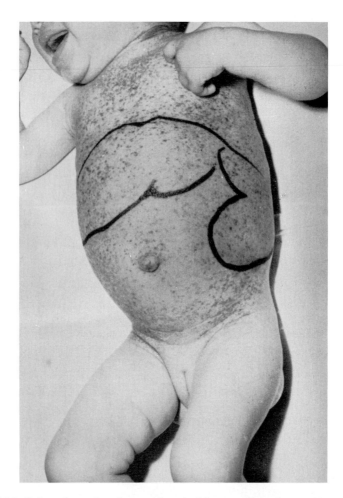

Fig. 22-8. Child of about 6 months of age with typical Letterer-Siwe disease. Note diffuse seborrheic eruption over the body in combination with petechiae and purpura. The enlarged liver and spleen are outlined. (Courtesy Dr. Philip Lanzkowsky, New York, N.Y.)

ments in the dermis. The lesions are composed of irregularly shaped histiocytes accompanied by an infiltration of inflammatory cells and supported by a stroma of spindle-shaped fibroblasts; multinucleated giant cells are quite prominent. The lesions are flesh-colored, yellow, or reddish brown, and located most commonly on the dorsum of the hands, wrist, and elbows, on the extensor surfaces of the extremities and scalp, and behind the ears (Fig. 22-8). It is considered systemic because of its association with progressive, often mutilating, arthritis.[162]

FAMILIAL LIPOCHROME HISTIOCYTOSIS. Familial lipochrome histiocytosis was described in three sisters with susceptibility to bacterial infection, splenomegaly, pulmonary infiltration, and arthritis. The symptoms were similar in some respects to those of patients with chronic granulomatous disease of childhood. However, affected tissue contained lipochromic granules with histiocytes.

Langerhans granules similar to those seen in patients with idiopathic histiocytosis X were found in the histiocytes.[177,209]

LIPOGRANULOMA OF BONE. Five patients with cysts of the medullary cavity of bone filled with brown liquid and surrounded by lipid foamy histiocytes in a fibrotic capsule have been described.[176] This could be merely a type of solitary histiocytosis X.

LYMPHADENOPATHY AND SINUS HISTIOCYTOSIS. Lymphadenopathy and sinus histiocytosis, a benign condition, has been described in thirty-six patients. These patients had protracted course of fever, leukocytosis, and prominent cervical lymph node enlargement on histologic examination, showing dilation of the subcapsulary and medullary sinuses and proliferation of histiocytes within them. More than half the patients were black. Although a transient immune defect was observed in one infant, cultured histiocytes phagocytize normally.[163,188] Although the histologic findings are quite similar to those of the Letterer-Siwe variant of idiopathic histiocytosis X, the course is always benign and does not involve bone, skin, liver, spleen, or lung; it is restricted to lymph nodes.[210] Sinus histiocytosis also occurs in acquired toxoplasmosis and other types of infections.

Incidence. The exact incidence of histiocytosis X is unknown, but it is probably greater than the estimated 1/100,000/year in children less than 1 year of age or the 0.2/100,000 in children less than 15 years of age. The data used for the estimate did not include children with solitary or disseminated eosinophilic granuloma or those with Hand-Schüller-Christian syndrome.[179] In a recent survey of 162 black children with cancer in the United States, histiocytosis X had the same relative frequency in blacks as in whites (i.e., about 3%); however, it was found to be rare in African blacks.[206]

Etiology. The cause of histiocytosis X is unknown. The identification of a cytoplasmic organelle, the Langerhans granule, in the histiocytes[178] stimulated speculation as to their origin. Theories have ranged from interpretation of virus particles to possible derivation from the Golgi apparatus or plasma membrane of the cell.[184] These Langerhans granules have also been identified in at least one case of malignant histiocytosis. One can speculate as to whether the disease process is principally neoplastic, infectious, a consequence of a hereditary abnormality, or the result of a tissue immunologic disorder. However, this presumes that there is a single etiology, a point contested by a number of authors who think that eosinophilic granuloma and diffuse histiocytosis X of the Letterer-Siwe variant reflect different initiating causes.[198] They consider the latter to be a neoplastic process but are uncertain as to the cause of the granuloma.

Immunology. A study of thirteen infants and children with histiocytosis X at various phases of activity and/or treatment generally showed normal skin test reactivity and lymphocyte blastogenesis to mitogens and allogeneic cells and normal neutrophil nitroblue tetrazolium dye reduction and bactericidal killing. Immunoglobulin levels were decreased in two infants, but others exhibited elevated levels. In general the immunologic alterations improved following chemotherapy. No evidence of a combined immunodeficiency disorder was found.[195] Infants with fulminant, fatal Letterer-Siwe syndrome may have some of the clinical, laboratory, and pathologic characteristics of combined immunodeficiency, but in most cases the findings can be ascribed to the immunosuppressant therapy or the histiocytic infiltration of lymph nodes.[168]

Genetics. Although histiocytosis X is considered a nonhereditary disorder, males are affected twice as frequently as females.[159] A number of cases have occurred in more than one member of the same family. The usual pattern has been for siblings to develop disseminated life-threatening or fatal forms of the disease. Of at least five sets of twins, three in which monozygosity was fairly certain, both children have developed disseminated histiocytosis. Chromosome analysis and more sophisticated genetic studies have been lacking in most familial cases.[187,202,207]

Clinical and laboratory features

Clinical manifestations. Clinical manifestations usually appear within the first decade with the highest incidence in the 2- to 6-year-old age group. Since histiocytosis X may affect almost any organ, the clinical findings are extremely variable. In one series of thirty-nine patients 16 years old and younger the initial presenting manifestations were as follows[159,173,205]:

Symptoms	Number
Bone lesions	38
Skull	14
Femur	9
Scapula	6
Mandible	4
Ribs	5
Pelvis	5
Vertebrae	3
Humerus	2
Maxilla	1
Sternum	1
Otitis	18
Dermatitis	15
Hepatomegaly	16
Lymphadenopathy	12
Anemia	14
Diabetes insipidus	10
Splenomegaly	11
Exophthalmos	10

The infant with the Letterer-Siwe syndrome often presents with hepatosplenomegaly, diffuse scalp or skin lesions with a papular, purpuric, or seborrheic appearance (Fig. 22-8), fever, pallor, and/or otitis media. The otitis media, often bilateral, is frequently a direct result of invasion of the mastoids and petrous portions of the temporal bones. Occasionally the lymphadenopathy may predominate. The classic triad of exophthalmos, diabetes insipidus, and skeletal bone lesions rarely exists separate from some of the other clinical manifestations although it tends to occur between 2 and 4 years of age. The exophthalmos, which may be unilateral or bilateral, can produce visual disturbances and is often associated with destructive skeletal lesions of the orbit. Bone lesions may or may not produce symptoms, depending on the site of bone involvement. Those lesions involving the long bones of the lower extremities may cause a limp or pain. One or more of the vertebrae may collapse. Maxillary or mandibular involvement often produces loose teeth, prompting the parents to first seek dental attention. Skull lesions may produce local areas of swelling and are the most common site of bone involvement in histiocytosis X.

Pulmonary involvement occurs in approximately 25% of cases. However, respiratory distress and pneumothorax are rare manifestations more frequently associated with other systemic manifestations of the disease. Four infants younger than 1 year of age and a 10- and 16-year-old were among eleven cases of symptomatic pulmonary histiocytosis X proved by lung biopsy in which no other clinical features of the disease occurred.[216] The gums may become hypertrophic from direct tissue invasion, producing gingivitis. Liver dysfunction may cause edema, jaundice, and ascites. Occasionally weight loss is also a feature. Diarrhea and malabsorption have been associated with histiocytic infiltration of the small bowel.[190]

The long-term consequences of so-called burned out or healed histiocytosis X may produce pulmonary insufficiency and cor pulmonale caused by lung fibrosis or portal hypertension caused by hepatic fibrosis.[181,191] Diabetes inspidus may also be a later sequela but usually occurs within 18 months after onset of bone involvement. Other central nervous system manifestations associated with histiocytosis X include seizures, increased intracranial pressure, focal neurologic deficits, mental retardation, hearing loss, intention tremor, and optic atrophy.[199] Growth retardation has been noted in one third of patients[159] and is often associated with retardation of bone age, delay in epiphyseal closure, and hypogonadism with lack of sexual development, indicating involvement of the hypothalamus or pituitary. Diabetes insipidus and retardation of linear growth are often associated findings.[161]

Laboratory data. Anemia may be the result of decreased red blood cell formation, blood loss secondary to thrombocytopenia, or enlargement of the spleen with trapping of red blood cells. Reticulocytosis of more than 1.5% occurs in 30% of the cases with soft tissue and visceral involvement.[199] Moderate thrombocytopenia with platelet counts of less than 100×10^9/liter occurs in half the patients with visceral involvement who have splenomegaly. Sometimes thrombocytopenia is associated with decreased megakaryocytes in the bone marrow. A leukocyte count of more than 10×10^9/liter occurs in approximately half of those with soft tissue involvement, but eosinophilia is not a feature. The bone marrow aspiration usually shows erythroid or myeloid hyperplasia and decreased megakaryocytes occasionally. Although histiocytic infiltration of the marrow is observed in 10% to 15% of patients, it is difficult to establish the diagnosis from the marrow aspirate alone.

Serum levels of calcium, phosphorous, and alkaline phosphatase are normal. Serum cholesterol and phospholipids values, once thought to be related to the basic disease process, are not helpful.[207] The extent of liver dysfunction can be determined by the total serum protein content. Values of less than 5.5 gm/dl for total protein, less than 2.5 gm/dl for albumin, and more than 1.5 gm/dl total serum bilirubin in the absence of hemolysis; a prothrombin time 50% or more longer than the control values; and an elevated LDH level more than two times that of normal adult values are indicative of liver dysfunction. Arterial blood gas measurements and pulmonary function studies are useful to assess lung dysfunction. The diagnosis of antidiuretic hormone deficiency is usually made clinically and confirmed by the urine specific gravity and/or osmolarity. The defect in urinary concentrating ability may be incomplete; however, spontaneous remissions are rare.

Abnormalities of chest x-ray films occur in 14% to 30% of cases.[159,199] The usual pattern is the presence of prominent, coarse pulmonary markings and small, well-defined, nonconfluent pulmonary nodular densities often giving a honeycomb pattern. These changes may be present at diagnosis or may develop later in the course of the disease, and half the affected patients die.[199] Unilateral or bilateral pneumothorax occurs rarely in those patients. Bacterial pneumonia has been noted with equal frequency in this group and in those with previously normal chest x-ray films.

Skeletal involvement may manifest itself as either solitary or multiple circumscribed areas of osteolytic destruction within bone. These may develop rapidly and if multiple lesions do occur, they may be in various stages of healing. ^{99m}Tc bone scans may be positive in lesions with osteoblastic activity. The skull is the most common site of bone involvement in which lesions appear as sharply punched-out areas of destruction with well-defined regular margins. In long bones both medullary and cortical destruction as well as periosteal new bone formation is common. When the mandible is involved, destruction of the lamina dura of the tooth socket and the supporting alveolar bone often gives the appearance that the teeth are floating in air. If the base of the skull is affected, destruction is often seen in the mastoid and petrous portions of the temporal bone. Vertebral body involvement usually begins as a purely osteolytic area that progresses to collapse of the involved body to a uniformly thin and dense disc (vertebra plana). The collapse may be asymmetric with anterior wedging common at some stage in the process. An important feature to differentiate these lesions from infections of the vertebral bodies is the preservation in the height of the disc space.[173]

Differential diagnosis

Skeletal system. The radiologic changes of irregular medullary destruction, soft tissue swelling, sclerosis, and periosteal reaction are also common in osteomyelitis, Ewing's sarcoma, osteogenic sarcoma, giant cell tumor of bone, metastatic neuroblastoma, epidermoid of the skull, and fibrous dysplasia. Osteolytic skull lesions and proptosis and ecchymosis of the upper eyelid are one initial manifestation of metastatic neuroblastoma.

Lymphoreticular system. Hepatosplenomegaly and lymphadenopathy, especially in the cervical region, suggest diffuse granulomatous diseases such as tuberculosis, histoplasmosis, brucellosis, Hodgkin's disease, non-Hodgkin's lymphoma, leukemia, or an underlying immune defect such as chronic granulomatous disease of childhood or Wiskott-Aldrich syndrome.

Skin. The scalp involvement closely resembles seborrheic dermatitis. Atopic eczema, pyoderma, petechiae caused by thrombocytopenia or vasculitis, and cutaneous moniliasis at times may be confused with the so-called flea-bitten scaly lesions of histiocytosis X. Healed lesions form small craters in the skin because of fibrosis in the dermal areas. Skin scrapings touched onto glass slides and Wright's-stained smears show the accumulation of clumps of mature histiocytes[203] (Fig. 22-9). Chronic draining otitis media and gingivitis also occur in neutropenia with or without immunoglobulin deficiency.

Pathophysiology and pathology. The basic tissue abnormality is a proliferation of histiocytes with moderate pale cytoplasm often occurring in sheets with fused histiocytes occasionally forming multinucleated giant cells. Mitotic figures are absent. Although less prominent in infants with widespread disease, eosinophils and a few lymphocytes, plasma cells, and neutrophils are superimposed on the sheets of histiocytes. The increased sudanophilic material found in vacuolated histiocytes reflects the increased tissue cholesterol and phospholipids. In the same areas of healing, fibroblastic proliferation is evident. All of these clinical findings can be explained by direct tissue infiltration. A uniform histiocytic proliferation and lack of eosinophilic infiltrate and necrosis have been associated more often with a fatal outcome.[205] Bone lesions almost always show eosinophilia, fibrosis, and necrosis.

Biopsy of lymph nodes, liver, lung, and soft tissues may be useful not only to establish the diagnosis but also to provide prognostic information, whereas biopsy of bone and skin lesions is helpful to establish the diagnosis. Benign lesions are characterized by a mixture of eosinophils and histiocytes in varying degrees. In most lesions the histiocyte predominates, appearing in sheets. These cells are usually polygonal with indistinct cell membranes, and they form an almost syncytial appearance. Areas of fibrosis, focal necrosis, hemorrhage, and hemosiderin granules in macrophages as well as multinucleated giant cells complete the picture.

Malignant lesions are characterized by diffuse

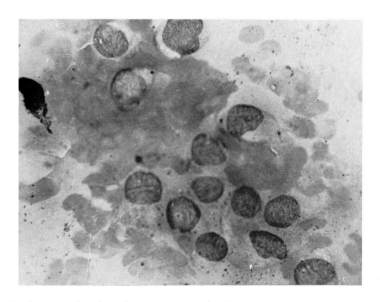

Fig. 22-9. Touch preparation from the skin lesions of a 20-month-old patient with nonlipid histiocytosis (Letterer-Siwe disease). The large mononuclear cells resemble those seen in affected lymph nodes. (×725.) (From Moore, T. D.: Pediatrics **19:**438, 1957.)

infiltration of individual histiocytes throughout the reticuloendothelial system with preservation of tissue architecture. The histiocytes are large with abundant, weakly basophilic cytoplasm and relatively distinct cell membranes. Their nuclei are folded with invaginated nuclear membranes and dark basophilic clumped chromatin. Multinucleated giant cells, eosinophils, necrosis, and fibrosis are rarely seen.[204] Biopsy of skull lesions should be performed with caution since both the outer and inner tables of the skull have usually eroded, exposing the dura mater.

Treatment. Localized eosinophilic granuloma of a single bone can be successfully treated with curettage, surgery, or radiation. The location of disease and ease of surgical approach are often the deciding factors as to whether radiotherapy is utilized in preference to surgery. Radiotherapy is preferred to surgery in the treatment of periorbital, mandibular, mastoid, or vertebral disease or for recurrence after simple surgical procedure and for producing rapid suppression of lesions in weight-bearing bones in which pathologic fracture may result. It is recommended that the dose level be less than 1,000 rads and preferably in the range of 550 to 600 rads for a typical lesion.[211] There is general agreement that no improvement in urinary concentrating ability follows irradiation of the pituitary region.[161,186] The cutaneous manifestations are also insensitive to irradiation.

The evaluation of chemotherapy in histiocytosis X is difficult because of (1) diversity of clinical manifestations and organ system involvement, (2) lack of clear-cut diagnostic criteria, and (3) occasional spontaneous remission. Survival was compared in untreated patients and those receiving various forms of chemotherapy (singly or in combination, antimetabolites, antibiotics, steroids, or alkylating agents) matched for age (mean of 10.5 and 15 months for untreated and treated patients, respectively) and number of organ systems involved (4.8 and 5.0, respectively). The 50% survival time in the untreated patients was 4 months, compared with 18 months in the treated group[194] (Fig. 22-10). A variety of drug combinations offers approximately the same benefit. Vinblastine alone given intravenously once weekly in an initial dose of 0.15 mg/kg and increased by 0.05 mg/kg until the white cell count falls lower than 3×10^9/liter; prednisone, 2 mg/kg/day; and vinblastine or prednisone and oral 6-mercaptopurine, 2.5 mg/kg/day, are about equally efficacious in inducing complete and parital remissions (60%, 60%, and 44%, respectively).[189]

Recent data from the Southwest Cancer Chemotherapy Study Group suggests that vincristine, 1.5 to 2 mg/m²/week intravenously; vinblastine, 5 to 6.5 mg/m²/week intravenously; and oral

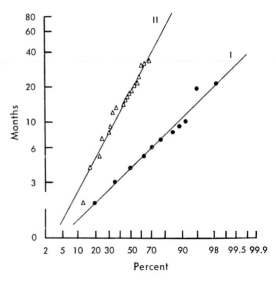

Fig. 22-10. Survival in months of treated (II) and untreated (I) patients with histiocytosis X. Group I, twenty-seven patients; group II, sixty-four patients. (From Lahey, M. E.: J. Pediatr. **60:**664, 1962.)

cyclophosphamide, 2.5 to 5.0 mg/kg/day, used singly are equivalent in effectiveness in the treatment of histiocytosis X. The complete and partial remission rates for the three drugs were 50%, 65%, and 59%, respectively.[217] Methotrexate has also been shown to be an effective therapeutic agent in this disorder. A study recently conducted in twenty-eight children by members of Cancer and Acute Leukemia Group B indicates that the response is essentially equal in patients receiving either oral prednisone, 40 mg/m²/day, and methotrexate, 30 mg/m² twice a week (50%), or oral prednisone and intravenous vincristine, 2 mg/m² once weekly (64%); however, the completeness of the response to prednisone and methotrexate was much better than to prednisone and vincristine.[181] Furthermore, in the same study patients who did respond were subsequently randomized into two groups: one receiving long-term maintenance with methotrexate and the other receiving nothing. The former group remained in remission 315 days, the latter for only 70 days, which suggests that long-term maintenance is valuable. Oral chlorambucil, 0.1 to 0.2 mg/kg/day, has also produced complete remissions in some cases.[218]

Diabetes insipidus can be controlled with intramuscular vasopressin tannate in oil (Pitressin) or with vasopressin nasal spray. The oil preparation must be shaken vigorously before injection to ensure homogenous distribution of the drug. The dose and frequency of administration varies with each patient but generally 0.3 to 1.0 ml intramuscularly every day or every other day or two to three nasal applications per day are required.[201]

Prognosis. On the basis of four large series of 223 cases the overall survival rate in histiocytosis X in children is 70%.* Several factors have been documented to be important as "front end" prognostic indicators: (1) age of patient at onset of disease, (2) extent of clinical disease as determined by physical examination and laboratory evaluation, (3) specific organ site of involvement, and (4) likelihood of a good response to therapy based on retention of normal function of the involved organ as well as the specific pathologic picture of the biopsy specimen from the involved organ. Seventy-five percent of all children become symptomatic during the first 3 years of life (40% during the first year, 25% during the second year, and 10% during the period between ages 2 and 3 years); the survival rate during this period is approximately 50%. There is a close relationship between age and extent of disease; 60% of children younger than age 3 and less than 5% of those older than age 3 have three or more organ systems involved, based on a scoring system to objectively evaluate the presence or absence of disease in each organ. Patients with disease involving the lung, liver, spleen, or hematopoietic system manifested by anemia, leukopenia, and/or thrombocytopenia with or without hemorrhagic cutaneous lesions have a poor outlook, whereas those with skeletal involvement or diabetes insipidus more often have a favorable outcome. The incidence of multiple skeletal lesions as the sole manifestation of disease is much higher in those over age 3 years.[194,199]

Consideration should be given to the so-called benign and malignant lesions of biopsies from suitable organs (skin excluded) and the presence or absence of dysfunction of liver (total protein <5.5 gm/dl, albumin <2.5 gm/dl, bilirubin >1.5 mg/dl, not attributable to hemolysis, edema, or ascites); lung (tachypnea and/or dyspnea, cyanosis, cough, pneumothorax, or pleural effusion not attributable to infection, excluding the more frequently occurring isolated radiographic densities or infiltrates); and bone marrow (hemoglobin <10.0 gm/dl, not attributable to iron deficiency or infection, white count $<4 \times 10^9$/liter or absolute granulocyte count $<1.5 \times 10^9$/liter, platelet count $<100 \times 10^9$/liter, excluding histiocytes in the bone marrow aspirate). Thirty-two of thirty-three children with organ dysfunction were less than 3 years of age, most had malignant histology, and only one third responded to therapy; 66% died. On the other hand, forty of fifty children without organ dysfunction were also less than age 3, almost all had benign pathology, two thirds responded to therapy, and only 4% are dead. The real prognostic value for evaluating organ function

appears to be in children with five or more organ systems involved. In a recent retrospective study, fourteen of forty of this group without organ dysfunction had an excellent response to therapy and only one death occurred (7% mortality rate); whereas the twenty-six with organ dysfunction had poor responses to therapy, and nineteen of this group died (73% mortality).[188]

REFERENCES
The spleen and disorders of the spleen

1. Acevedo, G., and Mauer, A. M.: The capacity for the removal of erythrocytes containing Heinz bodies in premature infants and patients following splenectomy, J. Pediatr. **63:**61, 1963.
2. Ackerman, J.V.: Surgical pathology, ed. 4, St. Louis, 1968, The C. V. Mosby Co.
3. Allen, F. A., Carr, M. H., and Klotz, A. P.: Decreased red blood cell-survival time in patients with portal cirrhosis: correlation of laboratory and clinical findings, J.A.M.A. **164:**955, 1957.
4. Allison, A. C., and Burn, G. P.: Enzyme activity as a function of age in the human erythrocyte, Br. J. Haematol. **1:**291, 1955.
4a. Ammann, C. J., Addiego, J., Wara, D. W., et al.: Polyvalent pneumococcal polysaccharide immunization of patients with sickle cell anemia and patients with splenectomy, N. Engl. J. Med. **297:**897, 1977.
5. Banti, G.: La splenomegalia con cirrose del fegato, Sperimentale (sez biol.) **48:**407, 1894.
6. Bennett, I. L., Jr., and Beeson, P. B.: Bacteremia; a consideration of some experimental and clinical aspects, Yale J. Biol. Med. **26:**241, 1954.
7. Bjorkman, S. E.: The splenic circulation with special reference to the function of the spleen sinus wall, Acta Med. Scand. Suppl. 191, 1947.
8. Bush, J. A., and Ainger, L. E.: Congenital absence of spleen with congenital heart disease, Pediatrics **15:**93, 1955.
9. Carlisle, H. N., and Saslaw, S.: Properdin levels in splenectomized persons, Proc. Soc. Exp. Biol. Med. **102:**150, 1959.
10. Chatterjea, J. B., Dameshek, W., and Stefanini, M.: The adrenalin (epinephrine) test as applied to hematologic disorders, Blood **8:**211, 1953.
11. Chatterjea, J. B., Mesa Arrau, C., and Dameshek, W.: Splenic puncture, Br. Med. J. **1:**987, 1952.
12. Child, C. G., III: The liver and portal hypertension. In Dunphy, J. E., consulting editor: Major problems in clinical surgery, vol. I, Philadelphia, 1964, W. B. Saunders Co.
13. Crosby, W. H.: Normal functions of the spleen relative to red blood cells: a review, Blood **14:**399, 1959.
14. Crosby, W. H.: Is hypersplenism a dead issue? Blood **20:**91, 1962.
15. Dale, O. C., Fauci, A. S., DuPont, J., et al.: Comparison of agents producing a neutrophilic leukocytosis in man: hydrocortisone, prednisone, endotrin, and etiocholanolone, J. Clin. Invest. **56:**808, 1975.
16. Dameshek, W.: Hypersplenism, Bull. N.Y. Acad. Med. **31:**113, 1955.
17. Dameshek, W., and Estren, S.: Hypersplenism, Med. Clin. North Am. **34:**1271, 1950.
18. DeGrucny, C. C.: Clinical haematology in medical practice, ed. 2, Springfield, Ill., 1964, Charles C Thomas, Publisher.
19. Diamond, L. K.: Indications for splenectomy in childhood, Am. J. Surg. **39:**400, 1938.

---

*References 192-194, 199, 218.

20. Diamond, L. K.: Splenectomy in childhood and the hazard of overwhelming infection, Pediatrics **43**:886, 1969.

21. Di Sant'Agnese, P. A., and Blane, W. A.: A distinctive type of biliary cirrhosis of the liver associated with disease of the pancreas: recognition through signs of portal hypertension, Pediatrics **18**:387, 1956.

22. Doan, C. A.: The spleen and reticuloendothelial system. In Sodeman, W. A., editor: Pathologic physiology, Philadelphia, 1956, W. B. Saunders Co.

23. Doan, C. A., and Wright, C. S.: Primary congenital and secondarily acquired splenic panhematopenia, Blood **1**: 10, 1946.

24. Ebert, R. V., and Stead, E. A., Jr.: Demonstration that in normal man no reserves of blood are mobilized by exercise, epinephrine, and hemorrhage, Am. J. Med. Sci. **201**:655, 1941.

25. Ekman, C. A.: Portal hypertension; diagnosis and surgical treatment, Acta Chir. Scand. **1**(suppl. 222): 143, 1957.

26. Ellis, E. F., and Smith, R. T.: The role of the spleen in immunity: with special reference to the post-splenectomy problem in infants, Pediatrics **37**:111, 1966.

27. Erickson, W. D., Burgert, E. O., Jr., and Lynn, H. B.: The hazards of infection following splenectomy in children, Am. J. Dis. Child. **116**:1, 1968.

28. Figley, M. M.: Splenoportography: some advantages and disadvantages, Am. J. Roentgen. **80**:313, 1958.

29. Gasser, C., and Willi, H.: Spontane Innenköperbildung bei Milzagenesie, Helvet. Paediatr. Acta **7**:369, 1952.

30. Gitlin, D., Rosen, F. S., and Janeway, C. A.: Undue susceptibility to infection, Pediatr. Clin. North Am. **9**: 405, 1962.

31. Godwin, H. A., Zimmerman, T. S., Kimball, H. R., Wolff, S. M., and Perry, S.: The effect of etiocholanolone on the entry of granulocytes into the peripheral blood, Blood **31**:461, 1968.

32. Gross, R. E.: The surgery of infancy and childhood: its principles and techniques, Philadelphia, 1953, W. B. Saunders Co.

33. Harris, I. M., McAlister, J. M., and Prankerd, T. A. J.: Splenomegaly and the circulating red cell, Br. J. Haematol. **4**:97, 1958.

34. Hayes, D. M., Spurr, C. L., Hutaff, R. J., and Sheets, J. A.: Postsplenectomy thrombocytosis, Ann. Intern. Med. **58**:259, 1963.

35. Horan, M., and Colebatch, J. H.: Relation between splenectomy and subsequent infection, Arch. Dis. Child. **37**:398, 1962.

36. Hsia, D. Y-Y., and Gellis, S. S.: Portal hypertension in infants and children, Am. J. Dis. Child. **90**:290, 1955.

37. Ivemark, B. I.: Implications of agenesis of the spleen on the pathogenesis of cono-truncus anomalies in childhood, Acta Paediatr. **44**(suppl. 104):1, 1955.

38. Jacobson, L. O., Marks, E. K., Gaston, E. O., Simons, E. L., and Robson, M. J.: Modification of radiation, Bull. N.Y. Acad. Med. **30**:675, 1954.

39. Jacobson, L. O., Robson, M. E., Marks, E. K., and Goldman, M. C.: The effect of x-radiation on antibody formation, J. Lab. Clin. Med. **34**:1612, 1949.

40. Jandl, J. H., Jacob, H. S., and Daland, G. E.: Hypersplenism due to infection: a study of 5 cases manifesting hemolytic anemia, N. Engl. J. Med. **264**:1063, 1961.

41. Johnston, R. B., Jr., and Newman, S. L.: Serum opsonine and the alternate pathway in sickle cell disease, N. Engl. J. Med. **288**:803, 1973.

42. Kauder, E., and Mauer, A. M.: Neutropenias of childhood, J. Pediatr. **69**:147, 1966.

43. Kevy, S. V., Tefft, M., Vawter, G. F., and Rosen, F. S.: Hereditary splenic hypoplasia, Pediatrics **42**:752, 1968.

44. Knisely, M. H.: Microscopic observations of the circulatory system of living unstimulated mammalian spleens, Anat. Rec. **65**:23, 131, 1936.

45. Krivit, W.: Overwhelming postsplenectomy infection, Am. J. Hematol. **2**:193, 1977.

46. La Celle, P. L., and Weed, R. I.: The contribution of normal and pathologic erythrocytes to blood rheology. In Brown, E. B., and Moore, C. V., eds.: Progress in hematology, vol. VII, New York, 1971, Grune & Stratton, Inc.

47. Levitan, R., Diamond, H. D., and Craver, I. F.: Esophageal varices in Hodgkin's disease involving the liver, Am. J. Med. **27**:137, 1959.

48. Marsh, J. C., and Perry, S.: The granulocyte response to endotoxin in patients with hematologic disorders, Blood **23**:581, 1964.

49. Maximow, A. A., and Bloom, W.: A text book of histiology, ed. 6, Philadelphia, 1953, W. B. Saunders Co.

50. McCracken, G. H., and Dickerman, J. D.: Septicemia and disseminated intravascular coagulation: occurrence in four asplenic children, Am. J. Dis. Child. **118**:431, 1969.

51. McIntyre, O. R., and Ebaugh, F. G.: Palpable spleens in college freshmen, Ann. Intern. Med. **66**:301, 1967.

52. McMichael, J.: Pathology of hepatolienal fibrosis, J. Pathol. Bacteriol. **39**:481, 1934.

53. Meyerson, R. M., Stout, R., and Havens, W. P.: Production of antibody by splenectomized persons, Am. J. Med. Sci. **234**:297, 1957.

54. Motulsky, A. G., Casserd, F., Giblett, E. R., Broun, G. O., Jr., and Finch, C. A.: Anemia and the spleen, N. Engl. J. Med. **259**:1164, 1958.

55. Muir, C. S.: Splenic agenesis and multilobulate spleen, Arch. Dis. Child. **34**:431, 1959.

56. Murphy, J. W., and Mitchell, W. A.: Congenital absence of the spleen, Pediatrics **20**:253, 1957.

57. Oski, F. A., Allen, D. M., and Diamond, L. K.: Portal hypertension: a complication of umbilical vein catheterization, Pediatrics **31**:297, 1963.

58. Palmer, J. G., Eichwald, E. J., Cartwright, G. E., and Wintrobe, M. M.: The experimental production of splenomegaly, anemia, and leukopenia in albino rats, Blood **8**:72, 1953.

59. Perez-Tamayo, R., Mora, J., and Montfort, J.: Humoral factor(s) in experimental hypersplenism, Blood **16**:1145, 1960.

60. Perla, D., and Marmorston, J.: The spleen and resistance, Baltimore, 1935, Williams & Wilkins Co.

61. Polhemus, D. W., and Schafer, W. B.: Absent spleen syndrome: hematologic findings as an aid to diagnosis, Pediatrics **24**:254, 1959.

62. Prankerd, T. A. J.: The spleen and anaemia, Br. J. Med. **2**:517, 1963.

63. Putschar, W. G. J., and Manion, W. C.: Congenital absence of the spleen and associated anomalies, Am. J. Clin. Pathol. **26**:429, 1956.

64. Ramot, B., Brok, F., and Ben-Bassat, I.: Alterations in the metabolism of human erythrocytes with aging, Plenary Session Papers, XII Cong. Int. Soc. Hematol., New York, 1968.

65. Robinson, T. W., and Sturgeon, P.: Postsplenectomy infection in infants and children, Pediatrics **25**:941, 1960.

66. Rogers, D. E.: Studies on bacteremia: mechanisms relating to the persistence of bacteremia in rabbits following the intravenous injection of staphylococci, J. Exp. Med. **103**:713, 1956.

67. Rogers, D. E., and Melly, M. A.: Studies on bacteremia: the blood stream clearance of *Escherichia coli* in rabbits, J. Exp. Med. **105**:113, 1957.

68. Rogers, H. M., and Langley, F. H.: Neutropenia associated with splenomegaly and atrophic arthritis (Felty's syndrome): report of a case in which splenectomy was performed, Ann. Intern. Med. **32**:745, 1950.

69. Rosenberg, D. H.: Macrocytic anemia in liver disease, particularly cirrhosis, Am. J. Med. Sci. **192**:86, 1936.

70. Rothberg, H., Corallo, L. A., and Crosby, W. H.: Observations on Heinz bodies in normal and splenectomized rabbits, Blood **14:**1180, 1959.

71. Rousselot, L. M.: The present status of surgery for portal hypertension, Am. J. Med. **16:**874, 1954.

72. Rowley, D. A.: The effect of splenectomy on the formation of circulating antibody in the adult male albino rat, J. Immunol. **64:**289, 1950.

73. Rowley, D. A.: The formation of circulating antibody in the splenectomized human being following intravenous injection of heterologous erythrocytes, J. Immunol. **65:**515, 1950.

74. Saslow, S., Bouroncle, B. A., Wall, R. L., and Doan, C. A.: Studies on the antibody response in splenectomized persons, N. Engl. J. Med. **261:**120, 1959.

75. Schuckmell, N., Grove, W. J., and Remenchik, A. P.: The diagnosis of operable portal obstruction in children, Am. J. Dis. Child. **90:**692, 1955.

76. Schumacher, J. J.: Serum immunoglobulins and transferrin levels after childhood splenectomy, Arch. Dis. Child. **45:**114, 1970.

77. Shaldon, S., and Sherlock, S.: Obstruction to the extrahepatic portal circulation in childhood, Lancet **1:**63, 1962.

78. Shinefield, H. R., Kaye, D., and Eichenwald, H. F.: The effect of splenectomy on the mortality of mice inoculated with *Diplococcus pneumoniae,* J. Pediatr. **65:**1104, 1964.

79. Singer, K., Miller, E. B., and Dameshek, W.: Hematologic changes following splenectomy in man with particular reference to target cells, hemolytic index and lysolecithin, Am. J. Med. Sci. **202:**171, 1941.

80. Singer, K., and Weisz, L.: The life cycle of the erythrocyte after splenectomy and the problems of splenic hemolysis and target cell formation, Am. J. Med. Sci. **210:**301, 1945.

81. Smith, C. H., Erlandson, M. E., Schulman, I., and Stern, G.: Hazard of severe infections in splenectomized infants and children, Am. J. Med. **22:**390, 1957.

82. Smith, C. H., Erlandson, M. E., Stern, G., and Hilgartner, M. W.: Postsplenectomy infection in Cooley's anemia: an appraisal of the problems in this and other blood disorders, with a consideration of prophylaxis, N. Engl. J. Med. **266:**737, 1962.

83. Smith, C. H., Erlandson, M. E., Stern, G., and Hilgartner, M. W.: Postsplenectomy infection in Cooley's anemia, Ann. N.Y. Acad. Sci. **119:**748, 1964.

84. Stewart, W. B., Stewart, J. M., Izzo, M. J., and Young, L. E.: Age as affecting the osmotic and mechanical fragility of dog erythrocytes tagged with radioactive iron, J. Exp. Med. **91:**147, 1950.

85. Thatcher, L. G., and Smith, N. J.: Granulocyte responses of children to bacterial endotoxin, J. Pediatr. **62:**484, 1963.

86. Tisdale, W. A., Klatskin, G., and Glenn, W. W. L.: Portal hypertension and bleeding esophageal varices, their occurrence in the absence of both intrahepatic and extrahepatic obstruction of the portal vein, N. Engl. J. Med. **261:**209, 1959.

87. Reference omitted.

88. Trusler, G. A., Morris, F. R., and Mustard, W. T.: Portal hypertension in childhood, Surgery **52:**664, 1962.

89. Vorhees, A. B., Jr., and Blaksmore, A. H.: Clinical experience with superior mesenteric vein, inferior vena cava shunt in the treatment of portal hypertension, Surgery **51:**35, 1962.

90. Walker, R. M., Shaldon, C., and Vowles, K. D. J.: Late results of portacaval anastamoses, Lancet **2:**727, 1961.

91. Wantz, G. E., and Payne, M. A.: Experience with portacaval shunt for portacaval hypertension, N. Engl. J. Med. **265:**721, 1961.

92. Watson, E. H., and Lowrey, G. H.: Growth and development of children, Chicago, 1951, Year Book Medical Publishers, Inc.

93. Watson, R. J., Shapiro, H. D., Ellison, R. R., and Lichtman, H. C.: Splenic aspiration in clinical and experimental hematology, Blood **10:**259, 1955.

94. Weinberg, E. D.: Infectious diseases influenced by trace element environment, Ann. N.Y. Acad. Sci. **199:**274, 1972.

95. Welch, C. S.: Portal hypertension, N. Engl. J. Med. **243:**598, 1950.

96. Wennberg, E., and Weiss, L.: The structure of the spleen and hemolysis, Ann. Rev. Med. **20:**29, 1969.

97. Whipple, A. O.: Problems of portal hypertension in relation to hepatosplenopathies, Ann. Surg. **122:**449, 1945.

98. Wiseman, B. K., and Doan, C. A.: Primary splenic neutropenia; a newly recognized syndrome, closely related to congenital hemolytic icterus and essential thrombocytopenic purpura, Ann. Intern. Med. **16:**1097, 1942.

99. Wright, D. O.: Macrocytic anemia in Banti's disease, Ann. Intern. Med. **8:**814, 1935.

100. Zeid, S. S., Felson, B., and Schiff, L.: Percutaneous splenoportal venography, with additional comments on transhepatic venography, Ann. Intern. Med. **52:**782, 1960.

Diseases of the monocyte-macrophage (reticuloendothelial) system

101. Alexander, S.: Niemann-Pick's disease showing calcification in the adrenal glands, New Zealand Med. J. **45:**43, 1946.

102. Banker, B. Q., Miller, J. Q., and Crocker, A. C.: The neurological disorder in infantile Gancher's disease, Trans. Am. Neurol. Assoc. **86:**43, 1961.

103. Brady, R. O.: Genetics and the sphingolipidosis, Med. Clin. North Am. **53:**827, 1969.

104. Brady, R. O., Kanfer, J. N., Bradley, R. M., et al.: Demonstration of a deficiency of glucocerebrosidase clearing enzyme in Gaucher's disease, J. Clin. Invest. **45:**1112, 1966.

105. Caffey, J.: Pediatric x-ray diagnosis, Chicago, 1956, Year Book Medical Publishers, Inc.

106. Crocker, A. C., and Farber, S.: Niemann-Pick disease; a review of eighteen patients, Medicine **37:**1, 1958.

107. Crocker, A. C., and Landing, B. H.: Phosphatase studies in Gaucher's disease, Metabolism **9:**341, 1960.

108. Crocker, A. C., Vawter, G. F., Neuhauser, E. B. O., and Rosowsky, A.: Wolman's disease: three new patients with a recently described lysidosis, Pediatrics **35:**627, 1965.

109. Danes, B. S., and Bearn, A. G.: Hurler's syndrome: demonstration of an inherited disorder of connective tissues in cell culture, J. Exp. Med. **123:**1, 1966.

110. Dienet, G., and Hamperl, H.: Lipoid splenohepatomegalie (typus Niemann-Pick), Wien Klin. Wochenschr. **40:**1432, 1927.

111. Dorfman, A., and Matalon, R.: The Hurler and Hunter syndromes, Am. J. Med. **47:**691, 1969.

112. Draznin, S. Z., and Singer, K.: Legg-Perthes disease; a syndrome of many etiologies with clinical and roentgenographic findings in a case of Gaucher's disease, Am. J. Roentgen. **60:**490, 1948.

113. Epstein, C. J., and Brady, R. O.: In utero diagnosis of Niemann-Pick disease, Am. J. Hum. Gen. **24:**533, 1971.

114. Erbe, R. W.: Therapy in genetic disease, N. Engl. J. Med. **291:**1028, 1974.

115. Estborn, B., and Hillborg, P. O.: On the increased serum acid phosphatase in Gaucher's disease, Scand. J. Clin. Lab. Invest. **12:**504, 1960.

116. Fisher, E. R., and Reidbord, H.: Gaucher's disease; pathogenetic considerations based on electron micro-

scopic and histochemical observations, Am. J. Pathol. **41:**679, 1962.

117. Forsythe, W. I., McKeown, E. F., and Neill, D. W.: Three cases of Niemann-Pick's disease in children, Arch. Dis. Child. **34:**406, 1959.

118. Fredrickson, D. S., and Sloan, H. R.: Sphengomyelin lepidoses: Niemann-Pick disease. In Stanburg, J. B., Wyn-gaarden, J. B., and Fredrickson, D. S., eds.: Metabolic basis of inherited disease, ed. 3, New York, 1972, McGraw-Hill Book Co.

119. Gasser, G.: In discussion of paper by Alder, A.: Konstitutionellbedingte Granulationsveränderungen der Leükocyten und Knochenveränderungen, Schweiz, Med. Wochenschr. **80:**1095, 1950.

120. Gaucher, E.: De l'épithelima primitit de la rate, Theśe de Paris, 1882.

121. Geddes, A. K., and Moore, S.: Acute (infantile) Gaucher's disease, J. Pediatr. **43:**61, 1953.

122. Groen, J.: The hereditary mechanism of Gaucher's disease, Blood **2:**1328, 1948.

123. Hansen, H. G.: Hematologic studies in mucopolysaccharidoses and mucolipidoses, Birth Defects **8:**115, 1972.

124. Harrison, W. E., Jr., and Louis, H. S.: Osseous Gaucher's disease in early childhood; report of a case with extensive bone changes and pathological fractures with splenomegaly, J.A.M.A. **187:**107, 1964.

125. Hoja, W. A.: Gaucher's disease in pregnancy, Am. J. Obstet. Gynecol. **79:**286, 1960.

126. Hsia, D. Y.-Y., Naylor, J., and Bigler, J. A.: Gaucher's disease, report of two cases in father and son and review of the literature, N. Engl. J. Med. **261:**164, 1959.

127. Jones, B., Gilbert, E. F., Zugibe, F. T., and Thompson, H.: Sea-blue histiocyte disease in siblings, Lancet **2:**73, 1970.

128. Kattlove, H. E., Gaynor, E., Spivack, M., and Gottfried, E. L.: Sea-blue indigestion, N. Engl. J. Med. **282:**630, 1970.

129. Landing, B. H., Silverman, F. N., Craig, J. M., et al.: Familial neurovisceral lipidosis, Am. J. Dis. Child. **108:**503, 1964.

130. Lynn, R., and Terry, R. D.: Lipid histochemistry and electron microscopy in adult Niemann-Pick disease, Am. J. Med. **37:**987, 1964.

131. Malinin, T. I.: Unidentified reticuloendothelial cell storage disease, Blood **17:**675, 1961.

132. Medoff, A. S., and Bayrd, E. D.: Gaucher's disease in 29 cases; hematologic complications and effects of splenectomy, Ann. Intern. Med. **40:**481, 1954.

133. Mittwoch, U.: Abnormal lymphocytes in gargoylism, Br. J. Haematol. **5:**365, 1959.

134. Mittwoch, U.: Inclusions of mucopolysaccharides in the lymphocytes of patients with gargoylism, Nature **191:**1315, 1961.

135. Moseley, J. E.: Bone changes in hematologic disorders, New York, 1963, Grune & Stratton, Inc.

136. Muir, H., Mittwoch, U., and Bitter, T.: The diagnostic value of isolated urinary polysaccharides and the lymphocyte inclusions in gargoylism, Arch. Dis. Child. **38:**358, 1963.

137. Okada, S., and O'Brien, J. S.: Generalized gangliosidosis; beta galactosidase deficiency, Science **160:**1002, 1968.

138. Pearson, H. A., and Lorincz, A. E.: A characteristic bone marrow finding in the Hurler syndrome, Pediatrics **34:**280, 1964.

139. Pick, L.: Niemann-Pick disease and other forms of so-called xanthomatosis, Am. J. Med. Sci. **185:**601, 1933.

140. Reich, C., Seife, M., and Kessler, B. J.: Gaucher's disease; a review and discussion of 20 cases, Medicine **30:**1, 1951.

141. Reilly, W. A.: The granules in the leukocytes in gargoylism, Am. J. Dis. Child. **62:**489, 1941.

142. Rodgers, C. L., and Jackson, S. H.: Acute infantile Gaucher's disease, Pediatrics **7:**53, 1951.

143. Rosowsky, A., Crocker, A. C., Tritis, D. H., and Modest, E. J.: Gas-liquid chromatographic analysis of the tissue sterol fraction in Wolman's disease and related lipidosis, Biophys. Acta **98:**617, 1965.

144. Rowland, R. S.: Constitutional disturbances of lipid metabolism and the reticuloendothelial system, constitutional disturbances of the lipid metabolism. In McQuarrie, I., and Kelley, V. C., eds.: Brennemann's practice of pediatrics, vol. 3, Hagerstown, Md., W. F. Prior Co., Inc.

145. Sawitsky, A., Hyman, G. A., and Hyman, J. B.: An unidentified reticuloendothelial cell in bone marrow and spleen, Blood **9:**977, 1954.

146. Silverstein, M. N., Ellefson, R. D., and Ahern, E. J.: The syndrome of the sea-blue histiocyte, N. Engl. J. Med. **228:**1, 1970.

147. Snyder, R. A., and Brady, R. O.: The use of white cells as a source of diagnostic material for lipid storage diseases, Clin. Chem. Acta **25:**331, 1969.

148. Stein, M., and Gardner, L. J.: Acute infantile Gaucher's disease, Pediatrics **27:**491, 1961.

149. Stransky, E., and Conchu, T. L.: Heredity in the infantile type of Gaucher's disease, Ann. Paediatr. **177:**319, 1951.

150. Strickland, B.: Skeletal manifestations of Gaucher's disease with some unusual findings, Br. J. Radiol. **31:**246, 1958.

151. Thannhauser, S. J.: Lipoidoses diseases of the cellular lipid metabolism, ed. 2, Oxford, 1950, Oxford University Press.

152. Todd, R., and Keidan, S. E.: Changes in the head of the femur in children suffering from Gaucher's disease, J. Bone Joint Surg. **34B:**454, 1952.

153. Uzman, L. L.: The lipoprotein of Gaucher's disease, Arch. Pathol. **51:**329, 1951.

154. Uzman, L. L.: Polycerebrosides in Gaucher's disease, Arch. Pathol. **55:**181, 1953.

155. van Creveld, S.: The lipoidoses. In Levine, S. Z., ed.: Advances in pediatrics, vol. 6, Chicago, 1953, Year Book Medical Publishers, Inc.

156. Wolman, M., Sterle, V. V., Gatt, S., and Frenkel, M.: Primary familial xanthomatosis with involvement and calcification of the adrenals, Pediatrics **28:**742, 1961.

157. Zlotnick, A., and Groen, J. J.: Observations on a patient with Gaucher's disease, Am. J. Med. **30:**637, 1961.

Histiocytosis X and other monocyte-macrophage disorders

158. Abt, A. F., and Denholz, E. J.: Letterer-Siwe disease: splenohepatomegaly associated with widespread hypoplasia of nonlipoid storing macrophages: discussion of the so-called reticuloendotheliosis, Am. J. Dis. Child. **51:**499, 1936.

159. Alvioli, L. V., Lasersohn, J. T., and Lopresti, J. M.: Histiocytosis X (Schuller-Christian disease): a clinicopathological survey: review of ten patients and the results of prednisone therapy, Medicine **42:**119, 1963.

160. Arnold, H. L., Jr., and Tilden, I. L.: Histiocytoma cutis: variant of xanthema: histologic and clinical studies of 27 lesions in 23 cases, Arch. Dermatol. Syphil. **49:**498, 1943.

161. Avery, M. E., McAfee, J. C., and Guild, H. G.: The course and prognosis of reticuloendotheliosis: a study of 40 cases, Am. J. Med. **12:**636, 1957.

162. Barrow, M. V., and Holubar, K.: Multicentric reticulohistiocytosis, Medicine **43:**287, 1969.

163. Becroft, D. M. O., Dix, M. R., Gillman, J. C., MacGregor, B. J. L., and Shaw, R. L.: Benign sinus histio-

cytosis with massive lymphadenopathy: transient immunological defects in a child with mediastinal involvement, J. Clin. Pathol. **26:**463, 1973.

164. Bell, R. J. M., Brafield, A. J. E., Barnes, N. D., and France, N. E.: Familial haemophagocytic reticulosis, Arch. Dis. Child. **43:**601, 1968.

165. Bodley-Scott, R., and Robb-Smith, A. H. T.: Histiocytic medullary reticulosis, Lancet **2:**194, 1939.

166. Brown, E. W.: Eosinophilic granuloma of the bladder. J. Urol. **83:**665, 1960.

167. Castleman, B., and McNealey, B. U.: Case report of the Massachusetts general hospital, N. Engl. J. Med. **282:**917, 1970.

168. Cederbaum, S. D., Niwayama, G., Stiehm, E. R., et al.: Combined immunodeficiency presenting as the Letterer-Siwe syndrome, J. Pediatr. **85:**466, 1974.

169. Christian, H. A.: Defects of membranous bones, exophthalmos, and diabetes insipidus: an unusual syndrome of dyspituitarism: a clinical study, Med. Clin. North Am. **3:**849, 1920.

170. Clarke, B. S., and Dawson, P. J.: Histiocytic medullary reticulocytosis presenting with a leukemic blood picture, Am. J. Med. **45:**314, 1969.

171. Cobane, J. H., Straith, C. O., and Pinkus, H.: Facial granulomas with eosinophilia: their relations to other eosinophilic granulomas of skin and to reticulogranuloma, Arch. Dermatol. Syphil. **61:**442, 1950.

172. Crocker, A. C.: Skin xanthomas in childhood, Pediatrics **8:**573, 1951.

173. Ennis, J. T., Whitehouse, G., Ross, F. G. M., and Middlemiss, J. H.: The radiology of the bone changes in Histiocytosis X, Clin. Radiol. **24:**212, 1973.

174. Falletta, J. M., Fernbach, D. J., Singer, D. M., South, M. A., Landing, B. H., Heath, C. W., Jr., Shore, N. A., and Barrett, F. F.: A fatal x-linked recessive reticuloendotheliosis, J. Pediatr. **83:**549, 1973.

175. Farber, S.: A lipid metabolic disorder: disseminated "kipogranulomatosis": a syndrome with similarity to and important differences from Niemann-Pick and Hand-Schuller-Christian disease, Am. J. Dis. Child. **84:**499, 1952.

176. Farquhar, J. W., and Claireaux, A. E.: Familial haemophagocytis reticulosis, Arch. Dis. Child. **27:**519, 1952.

177. Ford, D. K., Price, C. E., Culling, C. F., and Vassar, P. S.: Familial lipochrome pigmentation of histiocytes with hyperglobulinemia, pulmonary infiltration, splenomegaly, arthritis, and susceptibility to infections, Am. J. Med. **33:**478, 1962.

178. Friedmen, B., and Hanaoka, H.: Langerhans cell granules in eosinophilic granuloma of bone, J. Bone Joint Surg. **51A:**378, 1969.

179. Glass, A. G., and Miller, R. W.: U.S. Mortality from Letterer-Siwe disease in 1960-1964, Pediatrics **42:**364, 1968.

180. Gresham, G. A., Melcher, D. H., and Whitelaw, A. J.: Lipogranuloma of bone, J. Clin. Pathol. **19:**65, 1966.

181. Grosfeld, J. L., Fitzgerald, J. F., Wagner, V. M., Newton, W. A., and Baehner, R. L.: Portal hypertension in infants and children with Histiocytosis X, Am. J. Surg. **131:**108, 1976.

182. Hand, A.: Defects of membranous bone, exophthalmos, and polyuria in childhood: is it dyspituitarism? Am. J. Med. Science **162:**509, 1921.

183. Hand, A.: Polyuria and tuberculosis, Arch. Pediatr. **10:**673, 1893.

184. Hashimoto, K.: Langerhans cell granule: an endocytotic organelle, Arch. Dermatol. **104:**148, 1971.

185. Jones, B.: Chemotherapy of reticuloendotheliosis, Cancer Chemother. Rep. **57:**110, 1973.

186. Jorhsholm, B.: Roentgen therapy in Hand-Schüller-Christian and related disease, Acta Radiologica **50:**468, 1958.

187. Juberg, R. C., Kloepfer, H. W., and Oberman, H. A.: Genetic determination of acute disseminated histiocytosis X (Letterer-Siwe syndrome), Pediatrics **45:**753, 1970.

188. Karpas, A., Arno, J., and Crawley, J.: Sinus histiocytosis with massive lymphadenopathy: properties of cultures histiocytes, Eur. J. Cancer **9:**729, 1973.

189. Kaye, T. W.: Acquired hydrocephalus with atropic bone changes, exophthalmos and polyuria, Pa. Med. **9:**520, 1905-1906.

190. Keeling, J. W., and Harris, J. T.: Intestinal malabsorption in infants with histiocytosis X, Arch. Dis. Child. **48:**350, 1973.

191. Komp, D., El-Mahdi, A., Easley, J., Vietti, T., Berry, D., George, S.: Quality of survival in histiocytosis X, Pediatr. Res. **10:**455, 1976. (Abstract No. 921.)

192. Lahey, M. E.: Histiocytosis X: an analysis of prognostic factors, J. Pediatr. **87:**184, 1975.

193. Lahey, M. E.: Histiocytosis X: comparison of three treatment regimens, J. Pediatr. **87:**179, 1975.

194. Lahey, M. E.: Prognosis in reticuloendotheliosis in children, J. Pediatr. **60:**664, 1962.

195. Leikin, S., Puruganan, G., Frankel, A., Steerman, R., and Chandra, R.: Immunologic parameters in histiocytosis X, Cancer **32:**796, 1973.

196. Letterer, E.: Aleukaemische Retikulse (ein Beitrag zu den proliferatvan Erkrenkungendes Retikuloendothelial partas, Z. Pathol. **30:**377, 1924.

197. Lichtenstein, L.: Histiocytosis X: integration of eosinophilic granuloma of bone "Letterer-Siwe" disease and "Schüller-Christian disease" as related manifestations of a single nosologic, Arch. Pathol. **56:**84, 1953.

198. Lieberman, P. H., Jones, C. R., Dargeon, H. W. K., and Begg, C. F.: A reappraisal of eosinophilic granuloma of bone, Hand-Schuller-Christian syndrome, and Letterer-Siwe syndrome, Medicine **48:**375, 1969.

199. Lucaya, J.: Histiocytosis X, Am. J. Dis. Child. **121:**289, 1971.

200. MacMahon, H. E., Bedizel, M., and Ellis, C. A.: Familial erythrophagocytic lymphohistiocytosis, Pediatrics **32:**868, 1963.

201. Mermann, A. C., and Dargeon, H. W.: The management of certain nonlipid reticuloendotheliosis: 28 cases treated over a 22-year period, Cancer **8:**112, 1955.

202. Miller, D. R.: Familial reticuloendotheliosis: concurrence of disease in five siblings, Pediatrics **38:**896, 1966.

203. Moore, T. D.: A simple technique for the diagnosis of nonlipid histiocytosis, Pediatrics **19:**438, 1957.

204. Newton, W. A., Jr., and Hamoudi, A. B.: Histiocytosis: a histologic classification with clinical correlation, Perspect. Pediatr. Pathol. **1:**251, 1973.

205. Oberman, H. A.: Idiopathic histiocytosis: A clinico-pathologic study of 40 cases and review of the literature on eosinophilic granuloma of bone, Hand-Schuller-Christian disease, and Letterer-Siwe disease, Pediatrics **28:**307, 1961.

206. Olisa, E. G., Chandra, R., Jackson, M. A., Kennedy, J., and Williams, A. O.: Malignant tumors in American black and Nigerian children: a comparative study, J. Natl. Cancer Inst. **55:**281, 1975.

207. Omern, G.: Familial reticuloendoteliosis with eosinophilia, N. Engl. J. Med. **273:**427, 1965.

208. Otani, S., and Ehrlich, J. C.: Solitary granuloma of bone stimulating primary neoplasm, Am. J. Pathol. **16:**479, 1940.

209. Quasson, C. C., Roddy, G. E., and Good, R. E.: Altered structure of familial lipochrome histiocytosis, Lab. Invest. **22:**294, 1970.

210. Rosai, J., and Dorfman, R. F.: Sinus histiocytosis with

massive lymphadenopathy: a pseudolymphomatous benign disorder: analysis of 34 cases, Cancer **30:**1174, 1972.

211. Rowland, R. S.: Xanthomatosus and reticuloendothelial system, Arch. Int. Med. **42:**611, 1928.

212. Schuller, A.: Uber eingenareig Schadeldefekte im Jugendalter, Forstschur. Roentgenstr **23:**12, 1915-1916.

213. Scott, R. B., and Robb-Smith, A. H. T.: Histiocytic medullary reticulosis, Lancet **2:**194, 1939.

214. Siwe, S. A.: Die Reticuloendotheliose ein neuses Krankheitsbild unter den Hepatosblvnome galien, J. Z. Kinderheilk **55:**212, 1933.

215. Smith, D. G., Nesbit, M. E., D'Angio, G. J., and Levitt, S. H.: Histiocytosis X: role of radiation therapy in management with special references to dose levels employed, Therap. Radiol. **106:**419, 1973.

216. Smith, M., McCormack, L. J., Van Ordstrand, H. S., and Mercer, R. D.: "Primary" pulmonary histiocytosis X, Chest **65:**776, 1974.

217. Starling, K. A., Donaldson, M. H., Haggard, M. E., et al.: Therapy of histiocytosis X with vincristine, vinblastine, and cyclophosphamide, Am. J. Dis. Child. **123:**105, 1972.

218. Starling, K. A., and Fernbach, B. J.: Histiocytosis. In Sutow, W. W., Vietti, T. J., and Ferbbach, D. J., eds.: Clinical pediatric oncology, St. Louis, 1972, The C. V. Mosby Co.

219. Talbot, M. L.: Histiocytosis X, Am. Surg. **40:**89, 1974.

220. Vaith, I. A., Nathan, T., Fishkin, S., and Gruhn, J. G.: Histiocytic medullary reticulosis, Am. J. Clin. Pathol. **47:**160, 1967.

221. Virshup, M., and Mandelberg, G. A.: Eosinophilic granuloma of the gastrointestinal tract: report of a case involving the ileum, Ann. Surg. **139:**236, 1954.

222. Zawadzki, Z. A., Pena, C. E., and Fisher, E. R.: Histiocytic medullary reticulosis, case report with electron microscopic study, Acta Haematol. **42:**50, 1969.

PART FOUR **HEMOSTASIS**

edited by
CAMPBELL W. McMILLAN

23 □ Hemostasis: general considerations

Campbell W. McMillan

The purpose of this chapter is twofold: (1) to provide a foundation for subsequent discussion of platelet and vascular disorders in Chapter 24 and coagulation disorders in Chapter 25 and (2) to suggest general principles for a clinical approach to disorders of hemostasis.

Hemostasis may be defined as the sum total of those specialized functions within the circulating blood and its vessels that are designed to stop hemorrhage. These functions are delicately balanced so that although the blood may circulate freely within intact vessels, sites of bleeding can be efficiently sealed by formation and subsequent disposition of blood clots. Hemostasis is principally mediated by the blood vessel walls, platelets, and specialized plasma factors. Plasma factors, in turn, consist of coagulation factors directly involved in clot formation, fibrinolytic factors involved in clot removal, and natural inhibitors of coagulation and fibrinolysis that help to harness these powerful forces. Hemostasis is a highly integrated set of functions, but it is conceptually helpful to divide the overall process into components according to their approximate sequence: (1) vascular phase, (2) platelet phase, and (3) plasma phase.

HISTORICAL PERSPECTIVE

Current concepts of hemostasis are largely the product of an explosion of new knowledge that began at the end of World War II and is still continuing. However, prior to 1945 a relatively limited but critically important body of knowledge about hemostasis had gradually evolved. A summary of the essential components of this knowledge follows.

In the event of blood vessel injury platelets adhere to the exposed vessel surfaces and to each other, thus forming an initial hemostatic plug, including admixed red and white blood cells.[45,132] In accordance with the classic coagulation scheme proposed by Morawitz[81] in 1905, this plug is converted into a blood clot by deposition within it of insoluble strands of *fibrin,* derived from a soluble plasma protein precursor, *fibrinogen,* through the action of a potent enzyme, *thrombin;* this enzyme is derived from an inert plasma precursor, *prothrombin.* The conversion of prothrombin to

thrombin is dependent on trace amounts of ionized *calcium* and is accelerated by tissue extracts broadly termed *thromboplastin.* (The important distinction between complete and partial thromboplastins was not made until 1953.) At the turn of the twentieth century evidence had begun to suggest that plasma also contains substances leading to the formation of an enzyme capable of dissolving fibrin clots[87] and other substances that inhibit thrombin and fibrinolytic activity.[24,81,96] This information is schematically summarized in Fig. 23-1.

The coagulation component of this sequence was neatly unified in a classical and now standard laboratory test by Quick[94] in 1935, known as the prothrombin time (PT). This one-stage test consists of measuring the clotting time of plasma decalcified by sodium citrate or oxalate after calcium is replaced and a saline suspension of dried rabbit brain is added. Assuming optimal concentrations of calcium, tissue extract, and plasma fibrinogen to be in the system, the result was thought to indicate the plasma prothrombin content. A more specific test for prothrombin was introduced in 1936 by Warner et al.[121] These researchers utilized a standard fibrinogen substrate in a two-stage method instead of the fibrinogen in the test plasma itself.

By means of these tests hypoprothrombinemia was identified in hemorrhagic disease of the newborn and obstructive jaundice in humans[22,94] and in hemorrhagic disease of chicks on highly purified diets and of Canadian cattle fed spoiled sweet clover.[28,29,102] The hypoprothrombinemia in these diverse states proved to be caused by a simple lack of vitamin K in the case of human newborns and chicks, decreased absorption of vitamin K in obstructive jaundice, and a coumarin anticoagulant in cattle.[23,30,95,119]

These exciting discoveries of the 1930s established certain basic principles of hemostasis in addition to yielding major practical results. However, in keeping with consistent effects of progress in basic research, some gaps in the existing knowledge of hemostasis became even more apparent. As a prime example, no explanation emerged for the prolonged whole blood clotting time characteristic of the bleeding disorder in males known as

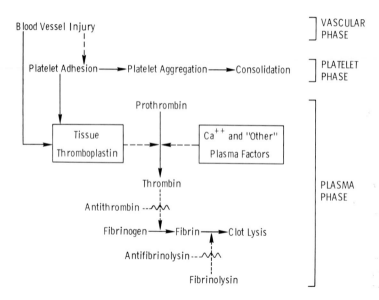

Fig. 23-1. Concept of hemostasis in 1945. Solid lines represent transformation; broken lines, action.

hemophilia. Specifically the prothrombin time was found to be entirely normal in patients with hemophilia.[94] However, by the end of the 1940s evidence suggested that abnormal clotting in hemophilia might result from the lack of a plasma antihemophilic factor that was somehow required, along with platelets, for normal conversion of prothrombin to thrombin.[3,19,20,89,97] The possibility of more than one such antihemophilic factor was suggested in 1947 by Pavlovsky,[90] who reported that the clotting time of one hemophiliac was transiently corrected by transfusion with blood from another hemophiliac.

Another major gap in the existing knowledge of hemostasis was identified and solved through a series of brilliant studies by Owren[88] in 1947. He found that a prolonged prothrombin time in a 29-year-old woman with a lifelong bleeding disorder was clearly *not* the result of a deficiency of prothrombin. Rather, Owren showed that her disorder, termed parahemophilia, was caused by deficiency of a plasma factor required for the *conversion* of prothrombin to thrombin in addition to calcium and tissue thromboplastin. Owren named the new clotting element "factor V" because it constituted the fifth established clotting factor as of 1947—the other four being fibrinogen, prothrombin, tissue thromboplastin, and calcium. He also suggested that factor V is changed to an activated substance during the process of clotting and designated the active principle "factor VI." Subsequently it has been shown that factor V probably acts as a single entity in the conversion of prothrombin to thrombin[108]; therefore both the term "factor VI" and its concept have been set aside.

Owren's epochal work spurred an intensive search for other clotting principles involved in the conversion of prothrombin to thrombin. His studies also emphasized the decisive role that clinical investigation might play in the identification of hemostatic mechanisms. Appropriately the discovery and ultimate acceptance of seven new coagulation factors between 1948 and 1960 were critically linked to studies of patients with a variety of bleeding problems.

The terminology of these new factors by different investigators had become so confusing by 1960 that an International Nomenclature Committee was formed to recommend standard terms. In 1962 a Roman numeral nomenclature system was formally introduced.[131] Owren's factor V served as an anchor point, and subsequent numerals were assigned to coagulation factors in the order of their discovery, with the omission of factor VI. These factors are shown in Table 23-1. This nomenclature system has been well accepted by investigators and clinicians alike. However, in this and succeeding chapters factors I, II, III, and IV are generally referred to as fibrinogen, prothrombin, tissue thromboplastin, and calcium, respectively.

The roles of fibrinogen, prothrombin, and factor XIII in hemostasis have been rather precisely defined. Although it is known that tissue thromboplastin, calcium, and factors V through XII are all involved in the conversion of prothrombin to thrombin, the interactions and single roles of these factors have been the subject of continuing investigation and changing interpretation. Certain major ideas about prothrombin conversion have emerged over the years, largely initiated with the

Table 23-1. Nomenclature of coagulation factors in plasma

Coagula-tion factor	Descriptive names (synonyms and abbreviations)
I	Fibrinogen
II	Prothrombin
III	Tissue thromboplastin
IV	Calcium
V	Plasma Ac globulin, proaccelerin, labile factor
VII	Proconvertin, serum prothrombin conversion accelerator (SPCA), stable factor
VIII	Antihemophilic globulin (AHG), antihemophilic factor (AHF)
IX	Christmas factor, plasma thromboplastin component (PTC)
X	Stuart-Prower factor
XI	Plasma thromboplastin antecedent (PTA)
XII	Hageman factor
XIII	Fibrin-stabilizing factor (FSF)

discovery of factor V and accelerated by a series of critical developments in 1952.

In 1952 clarification of prothrombin conversion and hemophilia took a giant step forward through definitive and independent studies by Aggeler et al.,[4] Schulman and Smith,[107] and Biggs et al.[14] These researchers showed conclusively that so-called hemophilia is not a single disease but two clinically identical disorders resulting from a lack of either of two clotting factors, each with markedly different laboratory properties. The more common disorder, which came to be known as classic hemophilia, is caused by lack of plasma factor VIII activity. The less common form of hemophilia, caused by lack of plasma factor IX activity, is most familiarly known as Christmas disease, based on the surname of the propositus in the report by Biggs et al.[14] published in the December 27, 1952, issue of the *British Medical Journal*. A major common denominator of all these reports was the finding that plasma from patients with different deficiencies is mutually corrective while plasma from patients with the same deficiency is not. This simple but basic observation has become a cornerstone of the clinical and laboratory identification of hemostatic disorders. Likewise it was shown that Christmas disease was the proper diagnosis of Pavlovsky's hemophilic patient whose clotting time was transiently corrected after transfusion with blood from another hemophiliac; the donor had classic hemophilia.[91]

A definitive contribution to understanding the relationship of the coagulation defect in hemophilia to the problem of prothrombin conversion was included in the report by Biggs et al.[14] The two forms of hemophilia were differentiated by a new test, the thromboplastin generation test (TGT). A more formal report on the TGT was published by Biggs and Douglas[13] in 1953. These researchers showed through this complex two-stage test that a prothrombin-deficient mixture of platelets, barium sulfate–adsorbed plasma, aged serum, and calcium generated a prothrombin-converting principle *in the absence of tissue thromboplastin*. They termed the principle plasma thromboplastin in contradistinction to tissue thromboplastin. Specific results were that patients with either form of hemophilia do not generate normal amounts of plasma thromboplastin, the factor lacking in classic hemophilia is normally present in the adsorbed plasma fraction, and the factor lacking in Christmas disease is normally present in the serum fraction. It should be noted here that adsorption of plasma with barium sulfate removes most of the prothrombin and factors VII, IX, and X; serum harvested from clotted blood lacks fibrinogen, prothrombin, and factors V and VIII.

In 1953 Langdell et al.[60] introduced a test of the partial thromboplastin time (PTT)—a landmark laboratory test that, like the TGT, has proved to be critical to studies of coagulation in general and prothrombin conversion in particular. The remarkably simple PTT differs from the PT of Quick[94] only in that the lipid part of tissue thromboplastin obtained by ether extraction of dried brain tissue is used in a one-stage system instead of a saline suspension of whole brain tissue. Langdell et al.[60] showed that the use of such a "partial" thromboplastin in the PTT uncovers prolonged clotting in hemophilic plasma whereas the use of a "complete" thromboplastin in Quick's PT clearly does not. Furthermore, they showed that the use of substrate plasma deficient in a given hemophilic factor could be applied to an assay of that factor in test plasma. Despite modifications since its introduction in 1953, the PTT has become a definitive screening test of coagulation and the method of choice for many factor assays as well.

By the early 1960s it was widely held that the conversion of prothrombin to thrombin is mediated by an active product generated in plasma and derived from two sources: (1) an extrinsic pathway, reflected in the PT and resulting from the interaction of certain clotting factors with tissue thromboplastin, normally extrinsic to the circulating blood, and (2) an intrinsic pathway, reflected in the PTT and TGT and resulting from the interaction of certain clotting factors with platelet phospholipids, all intrinsic to the circulating blood.

However, it was not at all clear how the several pieces of the prothrombin conversion puzzle actually fitted together. Two different but not necessarily mutually exclusive schools of thought domi-

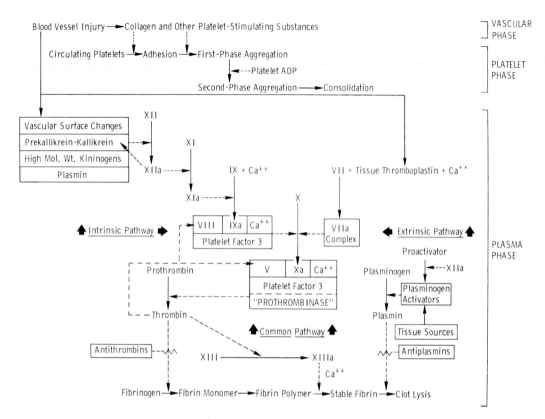

Fig. 23-2. Concept of hemostasis in 1978. Solid lines represent transformation; broken lines, action.

nated the scene during the 1960s. Seegers et al.[108] proposed that thrombin is derived from prethrombin, which in turn is derived from the parent prothrombin molecule along with autoprothrombin I (factor VII), autoprothrombin II (factor IX), and autoprothrombin III (factor X). Davie and Ratnoff[31] and Macfarlane[68] suggested a "waterfall" or "cascade" model in which conversion of prothrombin to thrombin is the last step in sequential activation of a series of distinct procoagulants.

By the early 1970s a substantial resolution of these divergent views[70] had produced a relatively unified concept of prothrombin conversion: A prothrombin-converting principle, or prothrombinase, is generated in plasma through the interaction of activated factor X, calcium, factor V, and platelet phospholipids; factor X is activated both by an extrinsic pathway dependent on the interaction of complete tissue thromboplastin (factor III) with factor VII and calcium and by an intrinsic pathway dependent on interactions of certain clotting factors, namely, factors XII, XI, IX, and VIII, calcium, and partial thromboplastin derived from platelet phospholipids (platelet factor 3).

During the evolution of a consensus on prothrombin conversion after Owren's discovery of factor V, enormous progress was also being made

in virtually all other aspects of hemostasis. An updated concept of hemostasis is broadly depicted in Fig. 23-2. It should be emphasized that this scheme will undoubtedly prove to be as incomplete 70 years from now as the 1905 version of Morawitz looks today.

CLINICAL APPROACH TO DISORDERS OF HEMOSTASIS

Subsequent sections of this chapter are designed to provide not only a continuing overview of hemostasis but also ingredients for a clinical approach to its disorders, including (1) a workable knowledge of hemostasis, (2) a scheme for classification of its clinical disorders, (3) components of a data base, and (4) familiarity with specific therapeutic agents and principles for their use. These topics are discussed in the order listed and should be regarded as general guidelines only; there is by no means a universal clinical approach to problems of hemostasis.

HEMOSTATIC MECHANISMS AND METHODS OF MEASUREMENT
Vascular phase

Although blood vessel injury triggers the hemostatic process, the role of the vessel itself is relatively difficult to define since it does not lend itself to direct study. The vascular phase is largely understood in terms of its known interactions with platelets and plasma factors. Thus vasoconstriction is mediated by serotonin released from platelets and by vasoactive peptides related to the activation of factor XII.[99] Also it is known that the vessel makes the following major contributions to platelet and plasma phases of hemostasis: (1) exposed vascular collagen is the major site of platelet adhesion and plays a major role in stimulating platelet aggregation,[10] (2) injury-induced vascular surface changes induce activation of the intrinsic pathway of coagulation beginning with factor XII,[85] and (3) tissue thromboplastin released by vascular injury interacts with factor VII and calcium to activate the extrinsic pathway of coagulation.[55]

There is no test that specifically measures the vascular phase of hemostasis. The bleeding time and tests that measure the effects of either positive pressure on vessel walls (tourniquet test) or negative pressure (suction devices such as the petechiometer) undoubtedly reflect platelet function much more than vascular integrity. Indeed, the diagnosis of vascular hemostatic defects depends on the clinical recognition of known vascular disorders such as Ehlers-Danlos syndrome and on the absence of platelet and coagulation abnormalities.

Platelet phase

The platelet phase of coagulation may be divided into three approximately sequential components: (1) adhesion of platelets to exposed subintimal vascular elements, particularly collagen, (2) aggregation of platelets to each other, largely mediated by the release of endogenous ADP, and (3) consolidation of the "platelet plug" by deposition of fibrin within it.[112] Platelet aggregation may be subdivided into a first phase that is reversible and a second phase that is irreversible: The first phase is induced by low concentrations of ADP and by the direct effect of certain substances, notably epinephrine and thrombin; the second phase is mediated by endogenous platelet ADP released in response to a large number of pathologic and physiologic substances, including ADP itself.[124,125] A discussion of the complex participation of platelets in the plasma phase of hemostasis is beyond the scope of this overview and is discussed in Chapter 24. However, it should be noted that certain platelet factors involved in coagulation have been designated by Arabic numerals, principally platelet factor 3, or platelet phospholipid; these are listed in Table 23-2.

Major screening tests of platelets include the platelet count, inspection of platelets on a good blood smear, and a standardized bleeding time

Table 23-2. Nomenclature of platelet factors

Platelet factors*	Descriptive characteristics
1	Adsorbed factor V
2	Accelerator of conversion of fibrinogen to fibrin monomer by thrombin
3	Platelet phospholipids, derived from lipoproteins of the membranes and granules
4	Heparin-neutralizing activity
5	Platelet fibrinogen
6	Antiplasmin activity
7	Tissue thromboplastin cofactor
8	Tissue thromboplastin inhibitor
9	Factor V stabilizing activity
10	Platelet serotonin

*Only platelet factors 2, 3, and 4 are generally recognized at the present time and referred to as such.

measurement—preferably by the forearm method of Ivy et al.[52] In measuring the bleeding time the template method of Mielke et al.[79] is preferred by many workers to the use of separate stabs. The ear lobe puncture method for the bleeding time, originally introduced in 1910 by Duke,[34] tends to be more cumbersome and more susceptible to hemorrhagic complications than tests performed on the forearm. The Duke bleeding time is generally inappropriate for children. By whatever method used, a standardized bleeding time is a powerful tool for overall assessment of platelet function. This test combined with determination of numbers of platelets by appropriate counting and observation of the characteristics and distribution of platelets on a blood smear constitute a highly comprehensive screen for platelets. If these three tests reveal no abnormalities in a given patient, a significant platelet disorder at that time is unlikely.

Most specific tests of platelets are comprised of a wide variety of measurements of platelet function. Such tests are particularly indicated in children in whom a platelet count within the normal range of 150 to 400 × 10^9/liter is combined with an Ivy bleeding time beyond the normal range of about 2 to 10 minutes, which suggests a qualitative platelet defect. Representative tests include quantitative measurement of clot retraction; measurement of platelet factor 3 activity in PTT, TGT, or prothrombin consumption systems; measurement of platelet retention (reflecting both adhesiveness and aggregation) in a standardized glass bead device; and differential assessment of first-phase and second-phase platelet aggregation in response to a variety of inducing agents, utilizing an instrument called an aggregometer.[9] The clinical application of these methods is discussed in Chapter 24.

Tests of platelet function are generally not indicated when the platelet count is below 50 × 10^9/liter; this count may be taken as the minimal hemostatic level of functionally intact platelets. If platelet counts are above this level, particularly above 150×10^9 platelets/liter, evaluation of platelet function by carefully selected specific tests becomes increasingly appropriate.

Plasma phase

In general the plasma phase of hemostasis is comprised of those mechanisms involved in the maintenance of an equilibrium between the formation and dissolution of fibrin within the blood clot. As noted previously, these mechanisms may be broadly divided into coagulation, fibrinolysis, and natural inhibitors of coagulation and fibrinolysis.

Coagulation. The coagulation component of the plasma phase of hemostasis may be subdivided into the following sequential stages: (1) generation of plasma prothrombinase, (2) conversion of plasma prothrombin to thrombin by prothrombinase, (3) conversion of plasma fibrinogen to fibrin monomer, leading to formation of fibrin polymer, and (4) stabilization of fibrin polymer by factor XIII, resulting in a firm clot.

The major features of plasma prothrombinase generation are (1) tissue thromboplastin released from injured tissues interacts with factor VII and calcium in a relatively rapid extrinsic pathway for activation of factor X; (2) vascular surface changes lead to sequential activation of factors XII, XI, and IX, and activated factor IX interacts with factor VIII, platelet factor 3, and calcium in the intrinsic pathway for activation of factor X; and (3) activated factor X interacts with factor V, platelet factor 3, and calcium in the common pathway for generation in plasma of an active product that converts prothrombin to thrombin, generally termed prothrombinase.[46,70]

Prothrombinase divides each prothrombin molecule into smaller functional pieces including a molecule of thrombin.[69] Thrombin in turn enzymatically cleaves four peptide groups from the fibrinogen molecule, thereby converting it to fibrin monomer.[17] Monomeric forms aggregate both end-to-end and side-to-side to form fibrin polymer. Fibrin polymer is stabilized by specific peptide cross-links in the presence of calcium, a process catalyzed by thrombin-activated factor XIII.[58,67,101,118] Without stabilization by factor XIII, fibrin polymer is abnormally soluble in solutions of urea and monochloracetic acid.[58]

The entire coagulation system is effectively screened by PTT,[60] the PT,[94,100] and a fibrin solubility test with 5M urea or 1% monochloracetic acid.[5,58] Pertinent details of these and other screening tests are summarized in Table 23-3.

Both the PTT and PT are one-stage tests that reflect activities of factors V and X in the common pathway of prothrombin conversion as well as prothrombin and fibrinogen. However, the PTT reflects the intrinsic pathway and is therefore insensitive to deficiency of factor VII. Conversely the PT reflects the extrinsic pathway and is therefore insensitive to deficiencies of factors VIII, IX, XI, and XII. In instances in which the PTT and PT are both prolonged, defective conversion of fibrinogen to fibrin may be specifically screened by adding dilute thrombin to plasma under standard conditions in the so-called thrombin clotting time or TCT.[116] Deficiency of factor XIII is uncommon but should be assessed by appropriate tests of clot solubility in any case in which a clinically significant bleeding disorder is characterized by normal platelets and by a normal PTT and PT.

The TGT, like the PTT, reflects the intrinsic

Table 23-3. Major screening tests of hemostasis

Test	Hemostatic functions measured
Platelet count and examination of blood smear	Platelet quantity and morphology
Standard bleeding time	Platelet quality
Plasma PT	Extrinsic and common pathways of coagulation: factors VII, X, and V, prothrombin, and fibrinogen
Plasma PTT	Intrinsic and common pathways of coagulation: factors XII, XI, IX, VIII, X, and V, prothrombin, and fibrinogen
Whole blood clotting time	Intrinsic and common pathways of coagulation
Plasma recalcification time	Intrinsic and common pathways of coagulation
Plasma TCT	Plasma fibrinogen concentration and antithrombin activity
TGT	Adsorbed plasma fraction: factors XII, XI, VIII, and V Serum fraction: factors XII, XI, IX, and X
Prothrombin consumption of whole blood	Factors XII, XI, IX, VIII, X, and V and platelet factor 3
Clot solubility in 5M urea or 1% monochloracetic acid	Factor XIII

and common pathways of prothrombin conversion but, unlike the PTT, is independent of deficiencies of prothrombin or fibrinogen. It is a two-stage test in which an aliquot of a prothrombin-deficient mixture (containing adsorbed plasma, aged serum, a source of phospholipids, and calcium) is added to normal plasma with additional calcium at specified intervals. In this system the normal plasma provides a constant source of prothrombin and fibrinogen. The resulting clotting time of the normal substrate plasma reflects plasma thromboplastin or intrinsic prothrombinase generated in the incubation mixture.[13] Because of the relative complexity of the TGT, it is now less frequently used for screening purposes than the much simpler and equally sensitive PTT.

Indirect estimation of intrinsic prothrombinase may be done by measuring the change in prothrombin activity during the coagulation of whole blood or platelet-rich plasma. Normally about 90% of the starting prothrombin activity in such a sample is consumed at the end of 1 hour as a result of the generation and subsequent rapid clearance of thrombin. Such prothrombin consumption reflects proper functioning of the several ingredients of the intrinsic and common pathways of prothrombin conversion, including platelet factor 3 activity. Representative methods for estimating prothrombin consumption include sequential measurements of specific prothrombin activity during clotting to determine the rate of prothrombin utilization and measurements of specific prothrombin activity in serum from blood allowed to clot for 1 hour and in plasma to determine 1-hour prothrombin consumption.[111] It should be emphasized that it is inappropriate to use the PT test for these procedures because, despite its name, it is not specific for prothrombin. Prothrombin consumption tests remain useful for assessment of platelet factor 3 activity but are not nearly as sensitive as the PTT to clotting factors in the intrinsic and common pathways.[111]

Both the whole blood clotting time and the plasma recalcification time reflect activities of factors in the intrinsic and common pathways of prothrombin conversion, prothrombin itself, and fibrinogen; thus these tests are entirely analogous to the PTT. Although these relatively insensitive screening tests of clotting function[61] have been superseded almost entirely by the PTT, they are cornerstones of all tests of clotting activity and deserve brief discussion.

The time-honored test of whole blood clotting time was introduced by Lee and White[62] in 1913. As originally described by these workers, the test is performed under standard conditions using three untreated glass tubes. In recent decades several modifications have been introduced: e.g., the

use of siliconized glass tubes to decrease contact activation of clotting and thereby to increase sensitivity of the test and the use of capillary tubes to increase the clinical convenience of the test.[11] By whatever method it is performed, the whole blood clotting time is highly susceptible to technical variables and at best is less sensitive than the PTT. Nonetheless, it remains a useful means for direct observation of clot formation, can be directly incorporated into tests of prothrombin consumption and clot retraction, and is still preferred by some clinicians for bedside monitoring of heparin therapy.

The plasma recalcification time was introduced by Howell[50] in 1916. This test simply measures the clotting time of decalcified plasma to which an optimal quantity of calcium is added under standard conditions. It is now recognized that a given result will vary, depending on the concentration of platelets remaining in the plasma after centrifugation of the whole blood sample. Thus the recalcification time of platelet-free plasma is longer than that of platelet-rich plasma, which of course contains partial thromboplastin. Indeed, it should be recognized that the PT and PTT are both plasma recalcification times modified by the addition of specific clot-promoting agents: a suspension of dried brain in the PT, a lipid fraction of whole brain (or its equivalent) in PTT, and a contact-activating substance such as kaolin[93] as well as lipid in the so-called activated PTT. Furthermore, the second stage of the TGT is a plasma recalcification time with the addition of intrinsic prothrombinase generated in the incubation mixture. The thrombin clotting time and fibrin solubility tests for factor XIII activity are the only major screening tests of plasma clot formation that are not directly accompanied by recalcification of the test sample.

Patients with evidence of a coagulation disorder by history or any of the screening tests may be checked for one or more specific deficiencies by a variety of quantitative assays. In general clotting factors may be quantitated either in functional terms by appropriate assays or in structural terms by biochemical or immunologic techniques. Fibrinogen is relatively unique among clotting factors because it is readily measurable in both regards; it may be functionally assayed by means of thrombin clotting time, and the plasma fibrinogen level may be measured immunologically or by a variety of biochemical methods.[41,51] The average plasma fibrinogen level is about 250 mg/dl with a range of 150 to 400 mg/dl.

Measurement of specific clotting factors other than fibrinogen is generally limited at the present time to functional assays utilizing a selected deficient substrate plasma and a method appropriate for the factor in question. For example, factors

VIII, IX, XI, and XII may be assayed in a PTT system, factor VII in a PT system; and factors V and X in either a PTT or PT system. Specific prothrombin activity may be measured either by the two-stage method of Warner et al.[121] or in a PT system using artificially prepared prothrombin-deficient substrate plasma.[6]

Deficiency of a specific clotting factor may be screened by testing a 1:1 mixture of abnormal test plasma and plasma with a known deficiency, either artificially prepared or obtained from an appropriate patient. If the clotting time of the mixture is prolonged, the test plasma may be assumed to lack the same factor as the known plasma and a presumptive diagnosis is established. However, if the clotting time of the mixture is normal, mutual correction of different deficiencies has occurred and the diagnostic search must continue. In any case a precise diagnosis ultimately demands a quantitative assay of the deficient factor with results expressed as a percentage of the activity in average normal plasma, arbitrarily taken to be 100%; the normal range for factors is within 50% to 200%.

During the past decade research in the molecular properties of the clotting factors, in contrast to their functional properties, has been accelerated. With the exception of certain findings regarding factor VIII, the results of these studies are not yet generally applicable to clinical practice. In the case of factor VIII the finding of normal factor VIII–associated antigen in classic hemophilia and relatively low antigen levels in von Willebrand's disease[133] has introduced important new dimensions to the differential diagnosis and fundamental nature of these disorders. In addition, it has been found that patients with von Willebrand's disease lack a factor required for ristocetin-induced platelet aggregation, a deficiency not shared by patients with classic hemophilia.[49]

Fibrinolysis. The fibrinolytic component of the plasma phase of hemostasis may be broadly subdivided into two stages: (1) conversion of plasminogen to plasmin by plasminogen activators and (2) proteolysis of fibrin and other substrates of plasmin.

Current concepts of fibrinolysis have been summarized in a review by Astrup and Thorsen[7] and recent findings on relationships between factor XII and fibrinolysis have been outlined by Kaplan et al.[54] Plasminogen, formerly termed profibrinolysin, is the inert plasma precursor of the active proteolytic enzyme plasmin, formerly termed fibrinolysin. Sherry[110] has suggested that plasminogen exists in a two-phase system: (1) in a *soluble* plasma phase and (2) in a *gel* phase through its incorporation into any fibrin clots that may be formed. The effects of conversion of plasminogen to plas-

min differ among these phases; plasmin formed in plasma is readily accessible to inhibition by naturally occurring antiplasmins, whereas plasmin formed within clots is less susceptible to such inhibition. This useful concept accounts for physiologic fibrinolysis within formed clots, in which plasmin is needed, as opposed to the circulating blood, in which plasmin (like thrombin) most assuredly is not needed. If the formation of circulating plasmin should exceed its inhibition, pathologic proteolysis of fibrinogen and other plasmin substrates may occur, constituting so-called primary fibrinolysis. Such a disorder should be distinguished from widespread pathologic proteolysis of formed fibrin, representing secondary fibrinolysis typically associated with disseminated intravascular coagulation.

Activators that convert plasminogen to plasmin are widely distributed among body tissues and fluids and in urine, where such activators are called urokinase.[57,122,128] For many years there was uncertainty about the existence of a plasminogen proactivator in plasma leading to an intrinsic plasminogen activator in addition to activators of tissue or extrinsic origin. Within recent years Kaplan and Austen[53] have described a plasma proactivator that is converted to plasminogen activator by activated factor XII or its fragments. Existing evidence points to interdependence of the early steps of the coagulation and fibrinolytic systems and to the existence of intrinsic and extrinsic pathways for activation of fibrinolysis as well as coagulation.

Once formed, plasmin is a potent enzyme with broader proteolytic specificity than thrombin. The major natural substrates for plasmin are fibrin, fibrinogen, and factors V, VIII, and XII. The digestion of the fibrinogen molecule by plasmin has been extensively studied[72] and is summarized in Fig. 23-3. The pieces into which fibrinogen or fibrin divides are commonly referred to as fibrin or fibrinogen degradation products (FDPs).

Neither heritable nor acquired primary deficiencies of fibrinolytic factors have been clearly defined. In addition, clinical disorders of increased fibrinolysis are usually secondary to other hemostatic abnormalities. Finally, clinically useful tests of fibrinolysis are limited in number. Thus the laboratory investigation of abnormal fibrinolysis is generally less extensive than that of coagulation disorders.

Fibrinolytic activity may be evaluated directly by specific assays of plasminogen and activator levels in plasma and by the relatively nonspecific euglobulin lysis time or indirectly by measurement of FDPs. In clinical practice the latter approach is utilized in most cases. The thrombin clotting time is a useful screening test for FDPs if the

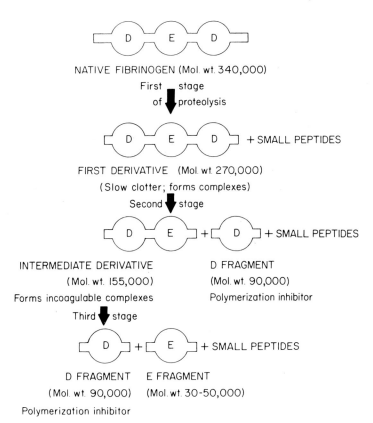

NATIVE FIBRINOGEN (Mol. wt. 340,000)

First stage of proteolysis

FIRST DERIVATIVE (Mol. wt. 270,000)
(Slow clotter; forms complexes)

Second stage

INTERMEDIATE DERIVATIVE
(Mol. wt. 155,000)
Forms incoagulable complexes

D FRAGMENT
(Mol. wt. 90,000)
Polymerization inhibitor

Third stage

+ SMALL PEPTIDES

D FRAGMENT   E FRAGMENT
(Mol. wt. 90,000)   (Mol. wt. 30-50,000)
Polymerization inhibitor

Fig. 23-3. Marder's concept of stepwise digestion of the fibrinogen molecule by plasmin. The first derivative is frequently referred to as fragment X and the intermediate derivative as fragment Y.[72] (From Sherry, S.: In Williams, W. J., Beutler, E., Erslev, A. J., and Rundles, R. W., eds.: Hematology, New York, 1972, McGraw-Hill Book Co. Used with permission of McGraw-Hill Book Co. Originally proposed by Marder, V. J., et al.: Trans. Assoc. Am. Phys. **80:**156, 1967.)

fibrinogen level is not markedly decreased; high concentrations of these products are known to interfere with polymerization of fibrin monomer.[86,115]

Numerous methods have been described for quantitating FDPs, including direct titration with specific antisera,[59] inhibition of hemagglutination utilizing tanned red cells,[73] and assay of antithrombin activity.[116] In most instances tests for FDPs are carried out on serum obtained from a sample of fresh whole blood to which standard amounts of thrombin and ε-aminocaproic acid (EACA) are added; thrombin ensures maximal conversion of clottable protein to fibrin, and EACA, an inhibitor of plasminogen activator activity, prevents in vitro fibrinolysis. Although all current methods for measurement of FDPs have certain limitations, techniques for rapid titration of FDPs by specific antisera are particularly convenient and therefore widely utilized.

Normally fibrin monomer derived from the action of thrombin on fibrinogen undergoes polymerization to form insoluble fibrin as noted previous-

ly. However, if the formation of fibrin monomer is associated with pathologic fibrinolysis, soluble complexes of fibrin monomer with FDPs and fibrinogen that are not clotted by added thrombin may be formed.[56] Such fibrin monomer complexes may be converted to insoluble fibrin by so-called paracoagulants, including certain strains of staphylococci,[65] protamine sulfate,[66] and ethanol.[42] Furthermore, if these complexes are present in plasma in excessive amounts, they may be precipitated as cryofibrinogen by cooling the plasma to 4° C.[65] Since these complexes include fibrin monomer, their presence in serum is theoretically diagnostic of secondary fibrinolysis in contrast to primary fibrinolysis. A variety of standard paracoagulation tests have been developed, such as the ethanol gelation test.[18] Although the detection of FDPs is unquestionably useful in the overall diagnosis of pathologic fibrinolysis, the usefulness of paracoagulation tests in the separation of secondary from primary fibrinolysis is not yet established.

Natural inhibitors of coagulation and fibrinolysis. The potent products generated by the forces

Table 23-4. Major antiproteases controlling coagulation and fibrinolysis

Natural inhibitors	Properties	Functions
Antithrombin III*	α_2-globulin; mol. wt., 63,000 daltons; range, 20-35 mg/dl	Heparin cofactor; inhibitor of thrombin and XIIa, XIa, IXa, and Xa; inhibitor of plasmin
α_2-Macroglobulin*	α_2-globulin; 19s; mol. wt., 725,000 daltons; range, 200-400 mg/dl	Inhibitor of plasmin and plasminogen activator; inhibitor of thrombin, XIIa, and kallikrein; neutrophil chemotaxis
α_1-Antitrypsin	α_1-globulin; mol. wt., 65,000 daltons; 275 mg/dl	Inhibitor of plasmin and XIa
CT inhibitor (C$\bar{1}$ INH)	α_2-globulin; mol. wt., 100,000 daltons; 20 mg/dl	Inhibitor of XIIa, kallikrein, and plasmin

*Antithrombin III is the major natural inhibitor of thrombin, and α_2-macroglobulin is the major inhibitor of plasmin.

of coagulation and fibrinolysis are essential for the speedy arrest and orderly disposition of hemorrhage. However, if these forces were not properly controlled, their effects would be lethal. For example, the thrombin that can be generated by 1 ml of normal plasma would, if unchecked, convert the fibrinogen in 250 ml of normal plasma to fibrin in a matter of seconds.

Within recent years there has been increasing recognition of the importance of the control of coagulation and fibrinolysis, both by certain physiologic processes and by natural inhibitors. Physiologic processes include rapid blood flow itself; the clearance of activated clotting and fibrinolytic factors by the liver; the selective incorporation of these factors into formed clots as opposed to their free circulation in the blood; and the reciprocal checks and balances between coagulation and fibrinolysis, notably the inhibition of thrombin activity by plasmin-induced FDPs.[33] In addition to these physiologic processes, certain natural inhibitors of coagulant and fibrinolytic enzymes are known to play critical roles in the control of hemostasis. Major antiproteases of this group include antithrombin III, α_2-macroglobulin, α_1-antitrypsin, and the inhibitor of activated C1 (C$\bar{1}$ INH).[106] Principal properties and functions of these inhibitors are summarized in Table 23-4; all members of this group have overlapping roles in the control of coagulation and fibrinolysis.

Recent advances in knowledge of control mechanisms require readjustment of former concepts and nomenclature. This is particularly well illustrated in the case of antithrombins, which were previously designated by a series of Roman numerals, each representing a broadly characterized activity: antithrombin I, inhibition of thrombin by its adsorption onto fibrin; antithrombin II, plasma heparin cofactor; antithrombin III, true plasma antithrombin; antithrombin IV, an inhibitor of the conversion of prothrombin to thrombin; antithrombin V, antithrombin activity associated with hy-

pergammaglobulinemia; and antithrombin VI, plasmin-induced FDP.[71] In general this system of nomenclature is obsolete with the exception of antithrombin III, which now designates a well-characterized antiprotease that encompasses activities formerly attributed to antithrombins II, III, and IV and participates in the control of fibrinolysis as well.

Major contributions to the understanding of antithrombin III have been recently provided by the studies of Rosenberg[103] and Rosenberg et al.[104] They have shown that arginine in the antithrombin molecule is the reactive site for its stoichiometric combination with serine in the thrombin molecule and that heparin produces a conformational change in antithrombin that vastly enhances its attachment to thrombin. Furthermore, it has been shown that inhibition of serine esterase activity by antithrombin III accounts for its effects not only on thrombin but also on other enzymes in the coagulation mechanism, i.e., activated forms of factors XII, XI, IX, and X.[105,113]

So far there has been rather limited adaptation to clinical practice of recent progress in the understanding of mechanisms that control coagulation and fibrinolysis. The diagnosis and management of certain disorders of hemostasis will undoubtedly be improved when the clinical effects of abnormal antithrombins and antiplasmins are more fully identified. It is already recognized that inherited deficiency of antithrombin III may be associated with thrombotic disorders[35] and that acquired deficiency of this antiprotease is typically observed in disseminated intravascular coagulation.[12]

Neonatal hemostasis

There is substantial evidence that hemostatic mechanisms in newborn infants are not uniformly developed in comparison to those of older children and adults. A grasp of relative hemostatic deficits that may be observed in healthy full-term and premature newborns is essential for appropriate interpretation of hemorrhagic disorders as well as diagnostic tests in this special age group. A summary of major features of neonatal hemostasis may be helpful. Also, the reader should consult excellent reviews by Bleyer et al.[16] and Hathaway.[44]

There is no convincing evidence of deficiency in the vascular phase of neonatal hemostasis, except possibly in small premature infants.[16] However, there is clear evidence of deficits in the platelet phase of hemostasis. Although platelet counts in healthy newborns do not differ significantly from those in adults, a variety of platelet functions are relatively deficient. Also, platelets of the newborn are significantly more susceptible than those of adults to drug-induced inhibition of platelet aggregation.[16,26,82] However, the bleeding time is usually within normal limits, both in full-term and premature newborns.[44]

By far the most thoroughly studied of all the components of neonatal hemostasis is the coagulation mechanism. Activities of the prothrombin complex (prothrombin and factors VII, IX, and X) may be depressed during the first week of life; dangerous progression of this combined deficiency is effectively prevented by prophylactic administration of vitamin K at birth.[1] Activities of factors XI, XII, and possibly XIII are moderately low at birth.[43,47] For the most part, factor VIII activity is within the normal range for adults although the mean for newborns may be lower than the adult mean, and factor VIII activity lower than 50% unassociated with any clinical coagulation disorder may rarely be observed.[76] Fibrinogen concentration and factor V activity are both usually normal by adult standards. These generalizations are intended to reflect coagulation factor profiles in full-term newborns; exaggeration of deficiencies tends to be correlated with the degree of prematurity. Physiologic depressions, particularly of the prothrombin complex factors, may not become fully corrected for months. In general the coagulation mechanism of a 1-year-old infant is equivalent to that of an adult.

In view of the multiple physiologic deficiencies of coagulation factors that may exist in a healthy newborn, it is not surprising that the PT and PTT may be significantly prolonged beyond the control times. The PT may be about 5 seconds longer than the control; the activated PTT may be 10 seconds longer and the nonactivated PTT 20 seconds longer than corresponding controls. Prolongation of the thrombin clotting time (TCT), which may be 5 seconds longer than the control, is not so readily explained since concomitant fibrinogen levels are usually normal and FDP are not increased. This finding may be related to unique molecular characteristics of fibrinogen in the newborn, i.e., a fetal fibrinogen analogous to fetal hemoglobin, a

possibility for which there is some evidence.[129,130]

Studies of fibrinolysis in healthy newborns have shown evidence for increased activity, characterized by increased activity of plasminogen activator expressed in shortened euglobulin lysis times and by decreased levels of plasminogen.[36,37] As noted above, FDPs are usually not significantly increased.

Despite a spectrum of measurable hemostatic deficits in comparison to adults, healthy newborns do not have a bleeding tendency. A possible expression of the overall efficiency of neonatal hemostasis is the impressively short whole blood clotting time characteristic of both full-term and premature newborns.[82] Decreased activity of natural inhibitors of coagulation and fibrinolysis may contribute to the enhancement of neonatal hemostasis. Decreased activity as well as molecular concentration of antithrombin III in newborn infants has been described.[84,127] Intensified studies of neonatal hemostasis at the molecular level in all its phases will undoubtedly explain much that is presently unclear on the basis of screening tests and functional assays.

A note is in order on the procurement of blood for studies of hemostasis in newborns. Frequently it is extremely difficult to obtain a properly drawn and properly citrated sample of venous blood for such studies. If a suitable blood sample is to be obtained, at least two major conditions must be met: (1) the time from onset of venipuncture to completed mixing of blood with citrate should be no more than 1 minute, and (2) the amount of citrate to be used for a given blood sample must be adjusted for hematocrits of more than 50% to avoid excessive citration and plasma dilution that will certainly prolong times of screening tests and decrease activities of assayed factors.

As tests of hemostasis are improved, both in scientific and technologic respects, it should be possible in due course to carry out comprehensive tests on newborns with capillary blood samples only. To some extent this is already possible.[78]

CLASSIFICATION OF DISORDERS OF HEMOSTASIS

The following outline is a general framework for classification of bleeding and clotting disorders that is developed in considerably more detail in Chapters 24 and 25. This scheme is designed to emphasize the use of simple clinical data readily obtained from the history, physical examination, and routine tests of hemostasis.

A. Purpuras without major coagulation disorders (Chapter 24)
1. With low platelet count
   a. Acquired thrombocytopenias (e.g., idiopathic thrombocytopenic purpura)

b. Heritable thrombocytopenias (e.g., Fanconi's anemia)
c. Neonatal thrombocytopenias (e.g., isoimmune purpura)
2. With normal platelet count
  a. Qualitative platelet disorders
    (1) Acquired thrombocytopathies (e.g., effects of aspirin)
    (2) Heritable thrombocytopathies (e.g., Glanzmann's disease)
  b. Vascular disorders
    (1) Acquired vascular disorders (e.g., Henoch-Schönlein purpura)
    (2) Heritable vascular disorders (e.g., Ehlers-Danlos syndrome)
3. With high platelet count
B. Major coagulation disorders (Chapter 25)
  1. With decreased activity of one or more coagulation factors
    a. Heritable coagulation disorders (e.g., classic hemophilia)
    b. Acquired coagulation disorders (e.g., disseminated intravascular coagulation)
    c. Neonatal coagulation disorders (e.g., hemorrhagic disease of the newborn)
  2. With normal or increased coagulation factors
    a. Heritable thrombotic disorders (e.g., effects of congenital deficiency of antithrombin III)
    b. Acquired thrombotic disorders (e.g., effects of oral contraceptive drugs)

GUIDELINES FOR DATA BASE

The child with a problem in hemostasis should be evaluated by an orderly series of steps with highest priority for the history, followed by a careful physical examination and a selective approach to laboratory testing. Although diseases of hemostasis include both thrombosis and hemorrhage, the following discussion emphasizes bleeding problems, which comprise the overwhelming majority of clinical disorders of hemostasis seen in the pediatric age group.

It should be emphasized that attempts to solve a child's bleeding problem by ordering every test of hemostasis that a given hospital can offer is not only poor medical practice but also potentially misleading to a physician unfamiliar with the "territory." Moreover, the best way to acquire the necessary familiarity is in the management of affected children; the medical literature, including chapters in textbooks, simply does not fully suffice. Specifically, wide-ranging knowledge about disorders of hemostasis should be a by-product of the continuing care of children with idiopathic thrombocytopenic purpura and classic hemophilia. The pathologic physiology, differential diagnosis, and principles of management of these two relatively common diseases constitute a highly comprehensive core curriculum in hemostasis and its disorders.

History

Ideally the written history of the present illness should consist of three parts: (1) a succinct summary of the patient's bleeding problem, analogous to the leading sentence in a newspaper article, (2) a narrative summary of the present illness in which the time and nature of onset should be carefully identified, and (3) positive and negative information pertinent to possible causes of the problem. Etiologic considerations may be probed by keeping in mind the following questions: (1) Is the bleeding problem caused by defective hemostasis or is it an appropriate response to vascular injury? (2) Assuming defective hemostasis, does expression of the problem suggest an isolated vascular, platelet, or coagulation defect or rather a combination of defects? (3) Does available evidence suggest that the problem is inherited or acquired? These are important but by no means exclusive questions that should guide effective history taking. The following general comments are related to these questions.

Recurrent bleeding from a single site without other evidence of a bleeding tendency is usually seen with vascular disruption without hemostatic dysfunction. For example, recurrent, painless hematuria in an otherwise well preschool child should primarily raise questions about renal disease, notably Wilms' tumor. However, epistaxis constitutes a special problem. In most cases nosebleeds are probably caused by little fingers and perhaps are aggravated by effects of aspirin given for colds and minor ailments. However, recurrent epistaxes may be the only manifestation of platelet dysfunction, including von Willebrand's disease. Finally, mechanisms may be mixed, as in a 7-month-old male infant with a skull fracture and subarachnoid hemorrhage who was shown to be a victim of child abuse and also to have mild classic hemophilia.

Close questioning should yield valuable clues as to which one or more components of the hemostatic mechanism may be involved in the expression of defective hemostasis. Isolated vascular defects may be associated with diagnostic clinical expression, notably Henoch-Schönlein purpura with its constellation of cutaneous and visceral signs and symptoms. Thrombocytopenia and platelet dysfunction are characterized by superficial hemorrhage into the skin and mucous membranes. Plasma defects, of which the overwhelming majority are coagulation disorders, are usually manifested by a chronic bruising tendency, the occurrence of deep-seated hematomas including hemorrhage into muscles, a tendency for surface wounds to exhibit troublesome recurrent hemorrhage that may extend for days or weeks, and bleeding into joints, which is the hallmark of severe classic hemophilia and Christmas disease. The history should include close questioning about any accidental or surgical wounds. Healing of scalp lacerations and after dental extractions, tonsillectomy, or adenoidectomy should be carefully observed since normal healing of wounds in these instances is critically dependent on efficient coagulation; appendectomy and herniorrhaphy are relatively less demanding as far as hemostasis is concerned. However, a young man with mild classic hemophilia (factor VIII level of 22%) had had a tonsillectomy at 6 years of age without recollected problems; his diagnosis was established at 16 years of age when an alert orthopedist initiated a clotting workup after the boy developed an acute hemarthrosis of the right knee after a hard tackle in a high school football game. Circumcision in newborns may provide misleading evidence; Baehner and Strauss[8] have pointed out that this procedure may be uneventful in about 50% of infants subsequently shown to have severe hemophilia. However, a history of prolonged bleeding from the umbilical cord is highly suggestive of congenital deficiency of either fibrinogen or factor XIII.

There are at least three major sources of clues as to whether a bleeding problem is inherited or acquired. First, inherited diseases usually emerge during infancy, are chronic or recurrent in nature, and are expressed in rather specific ways; acquired diseases are variable in time of onset, are usually acute, and are typically associated with other identifiable conditions including infections, immunologic disorders, malignancies, and drug reactions. Second, the nature of the bleeding problem may constitute an important clue. For example, hemarthrosis is a sign typical of hemophilia rather than acquired disease; the same is true of delayed, recurrent bleeding after such procedures as dental extraction. Third, and of paramount importance, is the family history. The family history may be entirely negative in many cases of heritable disease, but the identification of similarly affected family members is of critical value in establishing both the existence of inherited disease and the mode of its inheritance. The history of the present illness should include a notation about the family history, and a detailed summary along with an appropriate diagram should be recorded in the subsequent family history section of the workup.

The past medical history, social history, and review of systems should include supplements to the essentials of the bleeding history described in the present illness as well as routine information.

Physical examination

The physician should move from history taking to the physical examination with a strong sense of direction as to what the bleeding problem might be, if any. A careful examination should then add

a major dimension to the problem-solving process. In addition to the general examination including assessment of the overall state of health of the child, particular attention should be paid to the skin, mucous membranes, and joints.

The skin is a major target for expression of disorders of hemostasis. If purpura is present, its distribution and the character of individual lesions should be closely examined. Random bruises with petechiae are characteristic of thrombocytopenia and platelet dysfunction. Deep hematomas including intramuscular hematomas without petechiae are typical of coagulation disorders. Severe bruises about the buttocks and head, particularly if associated with evidence of fractures, may signal child abuse. Peculiar ecchymotic lesions with bizarre distribution are seen in factitious purpura. Symmetrical purpura of the lower extremities in children with abdominal and joint complaints is diagnostic of Henoch-Schönlein purpura. In an acutely ill child symmetrical purpura accompanied with evidence of ischemia, if not necrosis, suggests purpura fulminans and is a major emergency. Mushy skin with marked elasticity, confluent patches of purpura, especially on the shins; broad scar formation; and hypermobile joints are diagnostic of Ehler-Danlos syndrome. Broad scar formation is also characteristic of factor XIII deficiency. In the case of active surface wounds, recurrent bleeding around large, very dark, friable clots is seen in coagulation disorders, particularly hemophilia; minor scratches in hemophilia are usually not as troublesome as they may be in states of platelet lack or dysfunction.

The mucous membranes of the mouth and nose should be closely examined. Petechiae in these regions and a tendency to gum bleeding are typical of platelet disorders. The mucous membranes of the mouth and particularly the nose and major sites of telangiectases, lesions that are more likely to be identified by the astute internist than by a pediatrician.

Acute hemarthroses and chronic joint deformities are particularly characteristic of classical hemophilia and Christmas disease. In chronic arthropathy of the knees there is not only limited extension of these joints but also frequently evidence of associated atrophy of the quadriceps muscle. Acute unilateral hip flexion contracture in a person with hemophilia is usually a sign of hemorrhage into the corresponding psoas muscle rather than into the hip itself. Extreme mobility of the joints, as noted above, is typical of Ehlers-Danlos syndrome.

Laboratory tests

If the vast diagnostic resources of the history and physical examination are properly utilized, selected laboratory tests should extend established impressions rather than initiate a diagnosis. Four screening tests constitute the first step: (1) a platelet count, combined with examination of the blood smear for platelets and other formed elements, (2) a standard Ivy bleeding time to assess platelet function, (3) a test of the PT to assess the extrinsic and common pathways of coagulation, and (4) a test of the PTT to assess the intrinsic and common pathways of coagulation. In a child with a significant hemorrhagic disorder in whom these tests are all negative, a test of clot solubility in 5M urea of 1% monochloracetic acid should be carried out to assess factor XIII deficiency, but this heritable disorder is vanishingly rare.

Normality of the four screening tests is potent evidence for lack of a significant hemostatic defect, but caution must be used if the history strongly suggests the possible presence of a platelet or coagulation defect. Specifically, the PTT is not reliable in detecting factor levels higher than 20% of normal and it may therefore be normal in cases of von Willebrand's disease or very mild classic hemophilia or Christmas disease. Likewise, a single Ivy bleeding time is not capable of screening out every case of platelet dysfunction and von Willebrand's disease.

Conversely, abnormality of these tests does not establish without question the presence of a clinically significant hemorrhagic disorder. Inappropriate collection and citration of blood samples, as well as clerical and technical errors in the laboratory, must first be ruled out if the history and examination simply do not suggest a bleeding problem. Also, marked isolated abnormality of the PTT may reflect factor XII deficiency, which is typically not associated with a clinically expressed hemorrhagic tendency.[98]

In most cases the data generated by the history, physical examination, and screening tests of hemostasis should provide a firm base on which further specific diagnostic measures can be added rationally. Screening test results and appropriate additional tests for representative disorders of hemostasis are summarized in Table 23-5.

Conventional tests of hemostatic function are of little or no value in the diagnosis of thrombotic disease unassociated with coagulation deficiency. Although inherited deficiency of antithrombin III activity is a rare cause of such disorders in any age group, this antiprotease should be measured in affected patients.

Table 23-5. Screening test profiles and diagnostic procedures in selected disorders of hemostasis

Disorder	PC	BT	PT	PTT	Diagnostic procedures
Vascular disorders					
Henoch-Schönlein purpura	N	N	N	N	Clinical diagnosis only
Ehlers-Danlos syndrome	N	N†	N	N	Clinical diagnosis only
Platelet disorders					
Idiopathic thrombocytopenic purpura (ITP)	L	P	N	N	Clinical diagnosis supported by bone marrow examination and, if available, tests for platelet antibodies (positive)
Glanzmann's disease (thrombasthenia)	N	P	N	N	Clot retraction (abnormal) and platelet aggregation studies (defective first-phase aggregation)
Aspirin effect	N	P	N	N	Platelet aggregation studies (defective second-phase aggregation)
Coagulation disorders					
Classic hemophilia	N	N	N	P	Factor VIII assay (deficient activity)
Christmas disease	N	N	N	P	Factor IX assay (deficient activity)
von Willebrand's disease	N	P	N	P	Assays of factor VIII activity, VIII antigen, and ristocetin cofactor activity (all low in typical cases)
Factor VII deficiency	N	N	P	N	Factor VII assay (deficient activity)
Factor X deficiency	N	N	P	P	Factor X assay (deficient activity)
Vitamin K deficiency	N	N†	P	P	Assays of factors II, VII, IX, X (specific deficiencies with other factors normal)
Disseminated intravascular coagulation	L	P	P	P	Assays of factors I, II, V, and VIII (deficient activities) and FDP titer (increased)

*PC = platelet count, BT = standard bleeding time, PT = prothrombin time, PTT = partial thromboplastin time; N = normal result, L = low, P = prolonged.
†Bleeding time may be prolonged.

GUIDELINES FOR MANAGEMENT

Management of specific disorders of hemostasis is discussed in Chapters 24 and 25. Some general principles of management and a survey of specific therapeutic agents are outlined in the following discussion. The comments emphasize issues related to hemorrhage as opposed to thrombosis.

General management

Childhood hemorrhagic disorders may be divided into at least four broad groups with respect to overall modes of management. First, isolated vascular disorders, including transient acquired disorders such as Henoch-Schönlein purpura as well as lifelong heritable disorders such as Ehlers-Danlos syndrome, are not specifically treatable at this time and management therefore is limited to variable supportive care only. Second, isolated platelet disorders are variably responsive to platelet replacement therapy, but overall management overwhelmingly consists of a variety of supportive measures. This group includes both quantitative and qualitative platelet disorders, either heritable or acquired. Third, heritable deficiency of a single coagulation factor, notably classic hemophilia and Christmas disease, is effectively treated as needed by specific replacement therapy; appropriate blood components or commercially available concentrates may be used for this purpose. Fourth, a wide-ranging group of hemorrhagic disorders may be secondary to an underlying disease process; in these instances the management of choice usually emphasizes treatment of the primary disease. Disorders of hemostasis in this group are generally characterized by complex combinations of defects, illustrated by disseminated intravascular coagulation, or rare isolated defects such as acquired inhibitors of specific coagulation factors. These disorders may be easy to treat, such as vitamin K deficiency complicating cystic fibrosis in early infancy, or difficult to treat, such as parenchymal liver disease producing multiple defects of hemostasis.

Two other quite distinct groups include traumatic purpura and nonhemorrhagic thrombotic disorders. Traumatic purpura is not the result of a defect in hemostasis, for example, bruising caused by child abuse or self-inflicted injury (so-called factitious purpura). Management of acquired or heritable thrombotic disorders generally includes treatment with anticoagulant agents.

The management of children with disorders of hemostasis may require specialized knowledge of diagnosis and treatment that is beyond the scope of the generalist. It is therefore not surprising that such children are referred to hematologists who provide not only specialized care but also makeshift primary care as well. This is a mistake. The overall management of these children should be provided by a primary care physician, particularly when their disorder is classified in one of the first three groups just described. A firm commitment to the continuing care of children with disorders of hemostasis, including diagnosis and treatment, is a satisfying professional investment for the generalist.

Principles of replacement therapy

The principles of replacing deficient clotting factors are ideally illustrated in the use of appropriate factor concentrates in the management of classic hemophilia and Christmas disease. Specific details are fully discussed in Chapter 25.

When instituting replacement therapy for a patient with a given factor deficiency, a physician should have appropriate information in the following categories: (1) the meaning and application of the unit in which activity of the factor is expressed, (2) available sources of the appropriate concentrate, (3) the effects of replacement on the initial

Table 23-6. Materials used for replacement therapy of disorders of hemostasis

Replacement product	Contents and concentration
Blood components	
Platelet concentrate	5.5×10^{10} platelets in 50 ml plasma/bag
Cryoprecipitate	About 100 units factor VIII, 75 units factor XIII, 100 units ristocetin cofactor activity, and 150 mg fibrinogen in 25 ml plasma/bag
Cryoprecipitate-poor plasma	About 225 units of factors V, VII, IX, X, XI, and XII in about 225 ml plasma/bag
Commercially available factor concentrates	
Factor VIII concentrates: Factorate (Armour), Hemofil (Hyland), Humafac (Parke-Davis), Koate (Cutter), Profilate (Abbott)	250 to 1,000 units factor VIII/lyophilized vial, reconstituted with 4 to 30 ml accompanying sterile water
Prothrombin complex concentrates: Konyne (Cutter), Proplex (Hyland)	About 500 units/lyophilized vial, reconstituted with 20 to 30 ml accompanying sterile water
Fibrinogen concentrates: Fibrinogen, human (Merck, Sharp and Dohme), Parenogen (Cutter)	1.0 to 2.0 gm fibrinogen/lyophilized vial, reconstituted with 50 to 200 ml accompanying sterile water

plasma level of the factor and the rate of its subsequent disappearance, and (4) the relationship between a given plasma level of the factor and resulting hemostasis.

Unit of activity. The biologic activity of coagulation factors, excluding fibrinogen, tissue thromboplastin, and calcium, is currently expressed in two ways: as a percentage of average normal activity in reference to hemostasis and in arbitrary units in reference to content and dosage. One unit of a given factor is simply defined as its activity in 1 ml of average normal plasma. Thus 1 factor unit/ml plasma equals 100% activity. This remarkably simple terminology is useful in identifying the total activity of a factor in a bottle of concentrate, in calculating a dosage for a patient, and in estimating the expected percent of activity in the patient after infusion.

Fibrinogen is readily measurable in quantitative terms and therefore packaged in gram quantities; the plasma concentration is expressed in milligrams per deciliter.

Source of factor replacement. Blood components and commercially available factor concentrates variously appropriate for replacement therapy are given in Table 23-6.

Behavior of infused factor in plasma. The initial plasma level of a given factor after its infusion and its half-time of disappearance are generally characteristic for each factor. For example, 1 unit of factor VIII/kg body weight produces an increment in plasma of about 0.02 unit/ml, followed by exponential disappearance with a half-time of about 12 hours. The same dose of factor IX produces an increment in plasma of only 0.01 unit/ml or even less with a disappearance half-time of about 24 hours.

Relationship of the plasma factor level to hemostasis. Although the minimum hemostatic level for each coagulation factor is unknown, sufficient empirical information is available to guide replacement therapy in most clinical situations. For example, a factor VII level of about 10% for only 1 day is probably adequate coverage for appendectomy in a child with inherited deficiency of factor VII. In contrast, a factor VIII level of no less than 25% for 8 days should probably be maintained for the same operation in a child with classic hemophilia.

Specific therapeutic agents

The large number of agents currently available for specific treatment of disorders of hemostasis may be grouped as blood components, coagulation factor concentrates, vitamin K, agents affecting fibrinolysis, and antithrombotic agents.

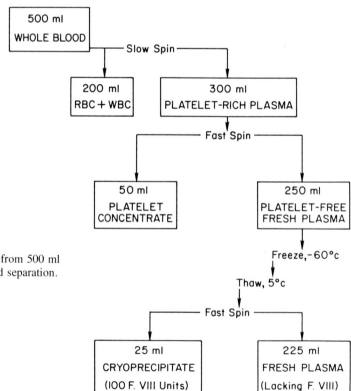

Fig. 23-4. Components obtained from 500 ml of whole blood by nonautomated separation.

Blood components. Whole blood and all its components prepared in the blood bank are applicable to overall treatment of bleeding and clotting disorders. However, those components principally used for replacement of platelet and coagulation factor deficiencies are platelet concentrates, cryoprecipitate from fresh plasma, and fresh plasma from which cryoprecipitate has been removed (cryoprecipitate-poor plasma). Steps for manual separation of components from 500 ml whole blood are outlined in Fig. 23-4. Such manual methods will probably become obsolete shortly, being increasingly superseded by automated blood component separators.

Platelet concentrates are available in individual bags, each representing the harvest from 500 ml fresh whole blood. Assuming appropriate recovery of platelets infused into a recipient, such a bag of platelets should produce an increment in the platelet count of about 10×10^9/liter/m^2 body surface.[83] This increment is not achieved in a variety of conditions, notably states in which the recipient has platelet antibodies that are directed against donor platelet antigens or that become nonspecifically adsorbed to donor platelets.

As shown in Fig. 23-4, a cryoprecipitated fraction of plasma is derived from platelet-free plasma that is first frozen at $-60°$ C (rapidly) and then thawed at $5°$ C. The discovery of important practical applications of cryoprecipitate by Pool and Shannon[89] in 1965 is one of the major developments in plasma fractionation during the past three decades. Cryoprecipitate is primarily a concentrate of factor VIII and the plasma cofactor of ristocetin-induced platelet aggregation (factor lacking in typical cases of von Willebrand's disease); one bag of standard cryoprecipitate contains, on the average, activities of factor VIII and ristocetin cofactor equivalent in to that normally contained in about 100 ml of fresh plasma.[83] Thus an average bag of cryoprecipitate should contain 100 factor VIII units. Fibrinogen and factor XIII are also modestly concentrated in cryoprecipitate, each present in amounts equivalent to that in about 60 ml and 75 ml of fresh plasma, respectively.[83] No other known coagulation factors are substantially concentrated in cryoprecipitate.

After removal of formed elements and cryoprecipitate from the initial 500 ml fresh whole blood, about 225 ml of plasma remains. This cryoprecipitate-poor plasma may serve as an agent for expansion of blood volume or for nonconcentrated replacement of prothrombin and factors V, VII, IX, X, and XI. The plasma also contains factor XII, but factor XII deficiency is not clinically expressed and thus does not require replacement therapy. The amount of whole plasma that can be infused is limited by the volume that can be safely tolerated without producing congestive heart failure. In states of normal blood volume the maximum for total infusion of plasma is 30 ml/kg/24 hours.

Coagulation factor concentrates. During the past three decades replacement therapy for deficiencies of coagulation factors has undergone spectacular improvement through progress in plasma fractionation. At the present time a variety of clinically effective fractions are commercially available, each containing variously concentrated fibrinogen, factors II, VII, IX, and X of the prothrombin complex, and factor VIII. These concentrates are clearly superior to whole plasma for aggressive replacement therapy of appropriate deficiencies, notably factor VIII deficiency, because desired levels of activity can be readily achieved without attendant danger of volume overload. As a result successful major surgery and home therapy program have become commonplace for children with heritable coagulation disorders. Concentrates for treatment of deficiencies of factors V, XI, and XIII are not commercially available, primarily because the factor levels produced by whole plasma therapy (or cryoprecipitate in the case of factor XIII) are sufficient even for major bleeding and surgical episodes.

The modern era of coagulation factor concentrates largely began as a by-product of plasma fractionation programs for development of blood transfusion substitutes during World War II, notably in the laboratory of Dr. Edwin J. Cohn and his colleagues at Harvard. The immediate problem-solving product of Cohn's group was albumin, but the first fraction (fraction I) of his low-temperature ethanol fractionation system was found to contain fibrinogen and factor VIII (then known only as antihemophilic globulin or antihemophilic factor) in amounts significantly more concentrated than in whole plasma.[25] Thereafter progress in development of a variety of concentrated fractions was closely linked to overall progress through discoveries about hemostasis. During the late 1950s clinical trials with the relatively crude fractions than available began to proliferate.[74,75,77,117] A quantum leap in factor VIII fractionation occurred in 1965 when Pool and Shannon[92] reported their discovery that this factor is concentrated in cryoprecipitate of plasma. Further purification of factor VIII in cryoprecipitate, such as by glycine extraction,[21,120] produced the potent factor VIII concentrates now available.

Despite the tremendous benefits that concentrated plasma fractions have provided for patients with coagulation deficiencies, it should be pointed out that certain problems remain. First, some patients with heritable deficiencies, notably those with classic hemophilia, spontaneously acquire antibodies to the factor replaced and thereby become variably resistant to such therapy.[109] Second, despite elimination of donors with hepatitis-associated antigen, the occurrence of hepatitis in recipients of plasma fractions persists.[63] Third, a variety of adverse reactions may complicate the use of plasma fractions, such as potentially serious thrombotic episodes in patients receiving prothrombin complex concentrates.[15]

Vitamin K. Vitamin K, notably in its natural form as vitamin K_1, is specific and highly effective therapy for depression of the prothrombin complex (factors II, VII, IX, and X) by vitamin K deficiency of any cause. A major recent discovery is that vitamin K is responsible for formation of calcium-binding sites on factors of the prothrombin complex rather than for their overall molecular synthesis as was formerly thought.[114] It should be emphasized that vitamin K is of no value in the treatment of prothrombin complex deficiency caused by parenchymal liver disease *not* associated with vitamin K deficiency.

Agents affecting fibrinolysis. Agents affecting fibrinolysis may be divided into fibrinolytic and antifibrinolytic agents. Major examples of the first group are streptokinase and urokinase, both of which are plasminogen activators. These agents have been extensively evaluated in clinical trials for their effects, along with standard anticoagulation, on thromboembolic disease; so far results have not established their additive usefulness in this regard.[2,80]

Major examples of the second group are epsilon aminocaproic acid and tranexamic acid, both of which are primarily inhibitors of plasminogen activation. These agents, notably EACA, have been evaluated for hemostatic effects in a variety of bleeding disorders in which excessive fibrinolysis may play a real or presumed role. Clinical indications for the use of these agents are not uniformly established, but there is clear evidence that EACA decreases the need for replacement therapy after dental extractions in patients with classical hemophilia and Christmas disease.[48,123]

Antithrombotic agents. Antithrombotic agents consist of anticoagulants for control of venous thrombosis and, of more recent vintage, antiplatelet agents for possible control of arterial thrombosis. The two standard anticoagulants are heparin and warfarin. As noted previously, heparin potentiates the inhibition of thrombin and other serine esterases in the coagulation cascade by antithrombin III.[103] Warfarin is a vitamin K antagonist. Since thrombotic disease is much less common in children than in adults, anticoagulant therapy is rarely indicated in pediatric practice and uniform guidelines for such therapy have not been established. As to syndromes of disseminated intra-vascular coagulation, heparin therapy has been shown to be of definite value in purpura fulminans and promyelocytic leukemia but its usefulness in other instances is not certain.[27]

Since Weiss and Aledort[126] discovered in 1967 that aspirin inhibits platelet function there has been tremendous interest in the pharmacology of platelet inhibition. Some of this concern has to do with the possible benefits of drugs such as aspirin in the prevention of arterial thrombosis, a problem that is not controlled as well by heparin and warfarin as is venous thrombosis. The principal agents being investigated in addition to aspirin are sulfinpyrazone and dipyridamole; final conclusions regarding their effectiveness as antithrombotic agents are not yet available.[38-40]

Finally, the agent ancrod, the official term for the venom of the Malayan pit viper, has been used clinically. This interesting agent causes rapid conversion of fibrinogen to unstable fibrin polymer, which is then rapidly cleared from the circulation. Thrombocytopenia does not accompany the defibrination process and overall mechanisms of coagulation and fibrinolysis are not significantly affected. The obvious antithrombotic potential of this agent has been evaluated in limited clinical trials in adults, and so far evidence for its definite usefulness is lacking.[32]

REFERENCES

1. Aballi, A. J.: The action of vitamin K in the neonatal period, S. Med. J. **58:**48, 1965.
2. Adar, R., and Salzman, E. W.: Treatment of thrombosis of veins of the lower extremities, N. Engl. J. Med. **292:** 348, 1975.
3. Addis, T.: The pathogenesis of hereditary haemophilia, J. Pathol. Bacteriol. **15:**427, 1911.
4. Aggeler, P. M., White, S. G., Glendening, M. B., et al.: Plasma thromboplastin component (PTC) deficiency: a new disease resembling hemophilia, Proc. Soc. Exp. Biol. Med. **79:**692, 1952.
5. Alami, S. Y., Hampton, J. W., Race, G. J., et al.: Fibrin stabilizing factor (factor XIII), Am. J. Med. **44:**1, 1968.
6. Alexander, B.: One-stage method for specific prothrombin (in plasma or serum). In Tocantins, L. M., ed.: The coagulation of blood: methods of study, New York, 1955, Grune & Stratton, Inc.
7. Astrup, T., and Thorsen, S.: The physiology of fibrinolysis, Med. Clin. North Am. **56:**153, 1972.
8. Baehner, R. L., and Strauss, H. S.: Hemophilia in the first year of life, N. Engl. J. Med. **275:**524, 1966.
9. Bang, N. U., Beller, F. K., Deutsch, E., et al.: Thrombosis and bleeding disorders, New York, 1971, Academic Press, Inc.
10. Baumgartner, H. R.: Platelet interaction with vascular structures, Thromb. Diath. Haemorrh. **51**(suppl.):161, 1972.
11. Beller, F. K., and Graeff, H.: Clotting time techniques. In Bang, N. U., Beller, F. K., Deutsch, E., and Mammen, E. F., eds.: Thrombosis and bleeding disorders, New York, 1971, Academic Press, Inc.
12. Bick, R., Kovacs, I., and Fekete, L. F.: A new two stage functional assay for antithrombin III (heparin cofactor):

clinical and laboratory evaluation, Thromb. Res. **8:**745, 1976.

13. Biggs, R., and Douglas, A. S.: The thromboplastin generation test, J. Clin. Pathol. **6:**32, 1953.
14. Biggs, R., Douglas, A. S., Macfarlane, R. G., et al.: Christmas disease: a condition previously mistaken for haemophilia, Br. Med. J. **2:**1378, 1952.
15. Blatt, P. M., Lundblad, R. L., Kingdon, H. S., et al.: Thrombogenic materials in prothrombin complex concentrates, Ann. Intern. Med. **81:**734, 1974.
16. Bleyer, W. A., Wakami, N., and Shepard, T. H.: The development of hemostasis in the human fetus and the newborn infant, J. Pediatr. **79:**838, 1971.
17. Blombäck, B., Blombäck, M., Grondahl, N. J., et al.: Structure of fibrinopeptides: its relation to enzyme specificity and phylogeny and classification of species, Acta Chem. Scand. **25:**411, 1966.
18. Breen, F. A., and Tullis, J. L.: Ethanol gelation: a rapid screening test for intravascular coagulation, Ann. Intern. Med. **69:**1197, 1968.
19. Brinkhous, K. M.: A study of the clotting time in hemophilia: the delayed formation of thrombin, Am. J. Med. Sci. **189:**509, 1939.
20. Brinkhous, K. M.: Clotting defect in hemophilia: deficiency in a plasma factor required for platelet utilization, Proc. Soc. Exp. Biol. Med. **66:**117, 1947.
21. Brinkhous, K. M., Shanbrom, E., Roberts, H. R., et al.: A new high-potency glycine-precipitated antihemophilia factor (AHF) concentrate, J.A.M.A. **205:**613, 1968.
22. Brinkhous, K. M., Smith, H. P., and Warner, E. D.: Plasma prothrombin level in normal infancy and in hemorrhagic disease of the newborn, Am. J. Med. Sci. **193:**475, 1937.
23. Campbell, H. A., and Link, P. K.: Studies on the hemorrhagic sweet clover disease. IV. The isolation and crystalization of the hemorrhagic agent, J. Biol. Chem. **138:**21, 1941.
24. Christensen, L. R., and MacLeod, C. M.: A proteolytic enzyme of serum: characterization, activation, and reaction with inhibitors, J. Gen. Physiol. **28:**559, 1945.
25. Cohn, E. J., Strong, L. E., Hughes, W. L., Jr., et al.: Preparation and properties of serum and plasma proteins. IV. A system for the separation into fractions of the protein and lipoprotein components of biological tissues and fluids, J. Am. Chem. Soc. **68:**459, 1946.
26. Corby, D. G., and Schulman, I.: The effects of antenatal drug administration on aggregation of platelets of newborn infants, J. Pediatr. **79:**307, 1971.
27. Corrigan, J. J.: Heparin should be used cautiously and selectively. In Inglefinger, F. J., Ebert, R., Finland, M., and Relman, A. S.: Controversies in internal medicine, Philadelphia, 1974, W. B. Saunders Co.
28. Dam, H.: Haemorrhages in chicks reared on artificial diets: a new deficiency disease, Nature **133:**909, 1934.
29. Dam, H.: The anti-haemorrhagic vitamin of the chick, Nature **135:**652, 1935.
30. Dam, H., Schonheyder, F., and Tage-Hensen, E.: Studies on the mode of action of vitamin K, Biochem. J. **30:**1075, 1936.
31. Davie, E. W., and Ratnoff, O. D.: Waterfall sequence for intrinsic blood clotting, Science **145:**1310, 1964.
32. Davies, J. A., Merrick, M. V., Sharp, A. A., et al.: Controlled trial of ancrod and heparin in treatment of deep-vein thrombosis of lower limb, Lancet **1:**113, 1972.
33. Deykin, D.: Thrombogenesis, N. Engl. J. Med. **276:**622, 1967.
34. Duke, W. S.: The relation of blood platelets to hemorrhagic disease: description of a method for determining the bleeding time and coagulation time, J. Am. Med. Assoc. **55:**1185, 1910.
35. Egeberg, O.: Inherited antithrombin deficiency causing thrombophilia, Thromb. Diath. Haemorrh. **13:**516, 1965.
36. Ekelund, H., Hedner, U., and Nilsson, I. M.: Fibrinolysis in newborns, Acta Paediatr. Scand. **59:**33, 1970.
37. Ekelund, H.: Fibrinolysis in the first year of life, Acta Paediatr. Scand. **61:**5, 1972.
38. Genton, E., Gent, M., Hirsch, J., et al.: Platelet-inhibiting drugs in the prevention of clinical thrombotic disease, Part I, N. Engl. J. Med. **293:**1174, 1975.
39. Genton, E., Gent, M., Hirsch, J., et al.: Platelet-inhibiting drugs in the prevention of clinical thrombotic disease. Part 2, N. Engl. J. Med. **293:**1236, 1975.
40. Genton, E., Gent, M., Hirsch, J., et al.: Platelet-inhibiting drugs in the prevention of clinical thrombotic disease. Part 3, N. Engl. J. Med. **293:**1296, 1975.
41. Gitlin, D., and Borges, W. H., Studies on the metabolism of fibrinogen in two patients with congenital afibrinogenemia, Blood **8:**679, 1953.
42. Godal, H. C., and Abildgaard, U.: Gelation of soluble fibrin in plasma by ethanol, Scand. J. Haematol. **3:**342, 1966.
43. Hathaway, W. E.: Coagulation problems in the newborn infant, Pediatr. Clin. North Am. **17:**929, 1970.
44. Hathaway, W. E.: The bleeding newborn. In Oski, F. A., Jaffe, E. R., and Miescher, P. A., eds.: Current problems in pediatric hematology New York, 1975, Grune & Stratton, Inc.
45. Hayem, G.: Recherches sur l'évolution des hématies dans le sang de l'homme et des vertébrés, Arch. Phys. Norm. Pathol. **5:**692, 1878.
46. Hemker, H. C.: Interaction of coagulation factors. In Brinkhous, K. M., and Hemker, H. C., eds.: Handbook of hemophilia. Part 1, Amsterdam, 1975, Excerpta Medica.
47. Henriksson, P., Hedner, Nilsson, I. M., et al.: Fibrin-stabilizing factor (factor XIII) in the fetus and newborn infant, Pediatr. Res. **8:**789, 1974.
48. Hilgartner, M. W.: Use of antifibrinolytic agents in hemophilia. In Brinkhous, K. M., and Hemker, H. C., eds.: Handbook of hemophilia. Part 2, Amsterdam, 1975, Excerpta Medica
49. Howard, M. A., and Firkin, B. G.: Ristocetin—a new tool in the investigation of platelet aggregation, Thromb. Diath. Haemorrh. **26:**362, 1971.
50. Howell, W. H.: Structure of the fibrin-gel and theories of gel-formation, Am. J. Physiol. **40:**526, 1916.
51. Huseby, R. M., and Bang, N. U.: Fibrinogen. In Bang, N. U., Beller, F. K., Deutsch, E., and Mammen, E. F., eds.: Thrombosis and bleeding disorders, New York, 1971, Academic Press, Inc.
52. Ivy, A. C., Shapiro, P. R., and Melnick, P.: Bleeding tendency in jaundice, Surg. Gynecol. Obstet. **60:**781, 1935.
53. Kaplan, A. P., and Austen, K. F.: The fibrinolytic pathway of human plasma: isolation and characterization of the plasminogen proactivator, J. Exp. Med. **136:**1378, 1972.
54. Kaplan, A. P., Meier, H. L., and Mandle, R., Jr.: The Hageman factor dependent pathways of coagulation, fibrinolysis, and kinin-generation, Semin. Thromb. Hemost. **3:**1, 1976.
55. Kirk, J. E.: Thromboplastin activities of human arterial and venous tissues, Proc. Soc. Exp. Biol. Med. **109:**890, 1962.
56. Kowalski, E.: Fibrinogen derivatives and their biologic activities, Semin. Hematol. **5:**45, 1968.
57. Lack, C. H.: Proteolytic activity and connective tissue, Br. Med. Bull. **20:**217, 1964.
58. Laki, K., and Lorand, L.: On the solubility of fibrin clots, Science **108:**280, 1948.
59. Lambert, C. J., Marengo-Rowe, A. J., Leveson, J. E., et al.: The tri-F-titer: a rapid test for the estimation of

plasma fibrinogen and the detection of fibrinolysis, fibrin(ogen) split products and heparin, Ann. Thoracic Surg. **18:**357, 1974.

60. Langdell, R. D., Wahner, R. H., and Brinkhous, K. M.: Effect of anti-hemophilic factor in one-stage clotting tests, J. Lab. Clin. Med. **41:**637, 1953.

61. Langdell, R. D., Wagner, R. H., and Brinkhous, K. M.: Antihemophilic factor (AHF) levels following transfusions of blood, plasma, and plasma fractions, Proc. Soc. Exper. Biol. Med. **88:**212, 1955.

62. Lee, R. I., and White, P. D.: A clinical study of the coagulation time of blood, Am. J. Med. Sci. **145:**495, 1913.

63. Lewis, J. H., Hasiba, U., Maxwell, N. G., et al.: Jaundice and hepatitis B antigen/antibody in hemophilia. In Brinkhous, K. M., and Hemker, H. C., eds.: Handbook of hemophilia. Part II, Amsterdam, 1975, Excerpta Medica.

64. Lipinski, B., Hawiger, J., and Jeljaszewicz, J.: Staphylococcal clumping with soluble fibrin monomer complexes, J. Exp. Med. **126:**979, 1967.

65. Lipinski, B., Wegrzynowicz, Z., and Budzynski, A. Z.: Soluble unclottable complexes formed in the presence of fibrinogen degradation products (FDP) during the fibrinogen-fibrin conversion and their potential significance in pathology, Thromb. Diath. Haemorrh. **17:**65, 1967.

66. Lipinski, B., and Worowski, K.: Detection of soluble fibrin monomer complexes in blood by means of protamine sulfate test, Thromb. Diath. Haemorrh. **20:**44, 1968.

67. Lorand, L., and Jacobsen, A.: Studies on the polymerization of fibrin. The role of globulin: fibrin-stabilizing factor, J. Biol. Chem. **230:**420, 1958.

68. Macfarlane, R. G.: An enzyme cascade in the blood clotting mechanism, and its function as a biological amplifier, Nature **202:**498, 1964.

69. Magnusson, S., Sottrup-Jensen, L., Ellebaek-Petersen, T., et al.: The primary structure of prothrombin, the role of vitamin K in blood coagulation, and a thrombin-catalyzed "negative feedback" control mechanism for limiting the activation of prothrombin. In Hemker, H. C., and Veltkamp, J. J., eds.: Prothrombin and related coagulation factors, Leiden, The Netherlands, 1975, Leiden University Press.

70. Mammen, E. F.: Physiology and biochemistry of blood coagulation. In Bang, N. U., Beller, F. K., Deutsch, E., and Mammen, E. F., eds.: Thrombosis and bleeding disorders, New York, 1971, Academic Press, Inc.

71. Mammen, E. F.: Determination of antithrombin. In Bang, N. U., Beller, F. K., Deutsch, E., and Mammen, E. F., eds.: Thrombosis and bleeding disorders, New York, 1971, Academic Press, Inc.

72. Marder, V. J., and Budzynski, A. Z.: The structure of fibrinogen degradation products, Progr. Hemost. Thromb. **2:**141, 1974.

73. Merskey, C., Lalezari, P., and Johnson, A. J.: A rapid, simple method for measuring fibrinolytic split products in human serum, Proc. Soc. Exp. Biol. Med. **131:**871, 1969.

74. McMillan, C. W., Diamond, L. K., and Surgenor, D. M.: Treatment of classic hemophilia: the use of fibrinogen rich in factor VIII for hemorrhage and for surgery. Part 1, N. Engl. J. Med. **265:**224, 1961.

75. McMillan, C. W., Diamond, L. K., and Surgenor, D. M.: Treatment of classic hemophilia: the use of fibrinogen rich in factor VIII for hemorrhage and for surgery. Part 2, N. Engl. J. Med. **265:**277, 1961.

76. McMillan, C. W., and Elston, R. C.: Plasma factor VIII activity in capillary and venous blood samples, J. Lab. Clin. Med. **71:**412, 1968.

77. McMillan, C. W., Tullis, J. L., and Diamond, L. K.:

Preliminary clinical trials with barium sulfate eluate, Vox Sang. **5:**78, 1960.

78. McMillan, C. W., Weiss, A. F., and Johnson, A. M.: Acquired coagulation disorders in children, Pediatr. Clin. North Am. **19:**1029, 1972.

79. Mielke, C. H., Kaneshiro, M. M., Maher, I. A., et al.: The standardized normal Ivy bleeding time and its prolongation by aspirin, Blood **34:**204, 1969.

80. Miller, G. A. H., Sutton, G. C., Kerr, I. H., et al.: Comparison of streptokinase and heparin in treatment of isolated acute massive pulmonary embolism, Br. Heart J. **33:**616, 1971.

81. Morawitz, P.: Die Chemie der Blutgerinnung, Ergebn. Physiol. **4:**307, 1905.

82. Mull, M. M., and Hathaway, W. E.: Altered platelet function in newborns, Pediatr. Res. **4:**229, 1970.

83. Myhre, B. A.: Blood component therapy, ed. 2, Washington, D.C., 1975, American Association of Blood Banks.

84. Neumann, L. L., Hathaway, W. E., Clarke, S., et al.: Antithrombin III levels in term and preterm newborn infants, Clin. Res. **22:**226A, 1974.

85. Niewiarowski, S., Bankowski, E., and Rogowicka, I.: Studies on the adsorption and activation of Hageman factor (factor XII) by collagen and elastin, Thromb. Diath. Haemmorh. **16:**387, 1965.

86. Niewiaroski, S., and Kowalski, E.: Un nouvel enticoagulant dérivé du fibrinogène, Rev. Hématol. **13:**320, 1958.

87. Nolf, P.: Contribution à l'étude de la coagulation du sang. La fibrinolyse, Arch. Int. Physiol. Biochim. **6:**306, 1908.

88. Owren, P. A.: The coagulation of blood, investigations on a new clotting factor, Acta Med. Scand. **194**(suppl.): 1, 1947.

89. Patek, A. J., and Taylor, F. H. L.: Hemophilia. II. Some properties of a substance obtained from normal human plasma effective in accelerating the coagulation of hemophilic boood, J. Clin. Invest. **16:**113, 1937.

90. Pavlovsky, A.: Contribution to the pathogenesis of hemophilia, Blood **2:**185, 1947.

91. Pavlovsky, A., 1959, cited by Brinkhous, K. M.: A short history of hemophilia with some comments on the word "hemophilia". In Brinkhous, K. M., and Hemker, H. C., eds.: Handbook of hemophilia, Amsterdam, 1975, Excerpta Medica.

92. Pool, J. G., and Shannon, A. E.: Production of high-potency concentrates of antihemophilic globulin in a closed-bag system: assay in vitro and in vivo, N. Engl. J. Med. **273:**1443, 1965.

93. Proctor, R., and Rapaport, S.: The partial thromboplastin time with kaolin, Am. J. Clin. Pathol. **36:**212, 1961.

94. Quick, A. J.: The prothrombin in hemophilia and obstructive jaundice, J. Biol. Chem. **109:**lxxiii, 1935.

95. Quick, A. J.: Coagulation defect in sweet clover disease and in the hemorrhagic chick disease of dietary origin, Am. J. Physiol. **118:**260, 1937.

96. Quick, A. J.: The normal antithrombin of the blood and its relation to heparin, Am. J. Physiol. **123:**712, 1938.

97. Quick, A. J.: Studies on the enigma of the hemostatic dysfunction of hemophilia, Am. J. Med. Sci. **214:**272, 1947.

98. Ratnoff, O. D., and Colopy, J. E.: A familial hemorrhagic trait associated with a deficiency of a clot-promoting fraction of plasma, J. Clin. Invest. **34:**602, 1955.

99. Ratnoff, O. D., and Miles, A. A.: The induction of permeability-increasing activity in human plasma by activated Hageman factor, Br. J. Exp. Path, **45:**328, 1964.

100. Rizza, C. R., and Walker, W.: One-stage prothrombin time techniques. In Bang, N. U., Beller, F. K., Deutsch, E., and Mammen, E. F., eds.: Thrombosis and bleeding disorders, New York, 1971, Academic Press, Inc.

101. Robbins, K. C.: A Study on the conversion of fibrinogen to fibrin, Am. J. Physiol. **142**:581, 1944.
102. Roderick, L. M.: A problem in the coagulation of the blood "sweet clover disease of cattle", Am. J. Physiol. **96**:413, 1931.
103. Rosenberg, R. D.: Actions and interactions of antithrombin and heparin, N. Engl. J. Med. **292**:146, 1975.
104. Rosenberg, R. D., and Damus, P. S.: The purification and mechanism of human antithrombin heparin cofactor, J. Biol. Chem. **248**:6490, 1973.
105. Rosenberg, J. S., McKenna, P. W., and Rosenberg, R. D.: Inhibition of human factor IXa by human antithrombin, J. Biol. Chem. **250**:883, 1975.
106. Schreiber, A. D.: Plasma inhibitors of the Hageman factor dependent pathways, Semin. Thromb. Hemost. **3**:43, 1976.
107. Schulman, I., and Smith, C. H.: Hemorrhagic disease in an infant due to deficiency of a previously undescribed clotting factor, Blood **7**:794, 1952.
108. Seegers, W. H., Schröer, H., and Marciniak, E.: Activation of prothrombin. In Seegers, W. H., ed.: Blood clotting enzymology, New York, 1967, Academic Press, Inc.
109. Shapiro, S. S., and Hultin, M.: Acquired inhibitors to the blood coagulation factors, Semin. Thromb. Hemost. **1**:336, 1975.
110. Sherry, S.: Fibrinolysis, Ann. Rev. Int. Med. **19**:247, 1968.
111. Shulman, N. R.: Prothrombin consumption tests. In Bang, N. U., Beller, F. K., Deutsch, E., and Mammen, E. F., eds.: Thrombosis and bleeding disorders, New York, 1971, Academic Press, Inc.
112. Spaet, T. H., and Zucker, M. G.: Mechanism of platelet plug formation and role of adenosine diphosphate, Am. J. Physiol. **206**:1267, 1964.
113. Stead, N., Kaplan, A. P., and Rosenberg, R. D.: Inhibition of activated factor XII by antithrombin-heparin cofactor, J. Biol. Chem. **251**:6481, 1976.
114. Stenflo, J.: Vitamin K, prothrombin, and gammacarboxyglutamic acid, N. Engl. J. Med. **296**:624, 1977.
115. Triantaphyllopoulos, D. C.: Anticoagulant effect of incubated fibrinogen, Canad. J. Biochem. Physiol. **36**:294, 1958.
116. Triantaphyllopoulos, D. C., and Triantaphyllopoulos, E.: Fibrinogen and fibrinogen derivatives. In Bang, N. U., Beller, F. K., Deutsch, E., and Mammen, E. F., eds.: Thrombosis and bleeding disorders, New York, 1971, Academic Press, Inc.
117. Tullis, J. L., and Breen, F. A., Jr.: Christmas Factor concentrates. The clinical use of several preparations, Bibl. Haematol. **34**:40, 1970.
118. Tyler, H. M.: Studies of the activation of purified factor XIII, Biochem. Biophys. Acta **222**:396, 1970.
119. Waddell, W. W., Guerry, D. P., Bray, W. E., et al.: Possible effects of vitamin K on prothrombin and clotting time in newly-born infants, Proc. Soc. Exp. Biol. Med. **40**:432, 1939.
120. Wagner, R. H., McLester, W. D., Smith, M., et al.: Purification of antihemophilic factor (factor VIII) by amino acid precipitation, Thromb. Diath. Haemorrh. **11**:64, 1964.
121. Warner, E. D., Brinkhous, K. M., and Smith, H. P.: A quantitative study on blood clotting: prothrombin fluctuations under experimental conditions, Am. J. Physiol. **114**:667, 1936.
122. Warren, B. A.: Fibrinolytic activity of vascular endothelium, Br. Med. Bull. **20**:213, 1964.
123. Webster, W. P., McMillan, C. W., Lucas, O. N., et al.: Dental management of the bleeder patient. In Haemophilia, Proceedings of the eighth congress of the World Federation of Haemophilia) International Congress Series No. 252, Amsterdam, 1971, Excerpta Medica.
124. Weiss, H. J.: Platelet physiology and abnormalities of platelet function, Part 1, N. Engl. J. Med. **293**:531, 1975.
125. Weiss, H. J.: Platelet physiology and abnormalities of platelet function. Part 2, N. Engl. J. Med. **293**:580, 1975.
126. Weiss, H. J., and Aledort, L. M.: Impaired platelet connective tissue reaction in man after aspirin ingestion, Lancet **2**:495, 1967.
127. Weissbach, G., Domula, M., and Lenk, H.: The progressive antithrombin activity and its relation to other factors of the coagulation system, Acta Paediatr. Scand. **67**:555, 1974.
128. White, W. F., Barlow, G. H., and Mozen, M. M.: The isolation and characterization of plasminogen activators (urokinase) from human urine, Biochem. **5**:2160, 1966.
129. Witt, I., and Muller, H.: Phosphorus and hexose content of human foetal fibrinogen, Biochem. Biophys. Acta **221**:402, 1970.
130. Witt, I., Muller, H., and Kunzer, W.: Evidence for the existence of foetal fibrinogen, Thromb. Diath. Haemorrh. **22**:101, 1969.
131. Wright, I. S.: The nomenclature of blood clotting factors, Thromb. Diath. Haemorrh. **7**:381, 1962.
132. Wright, J. H., and Minot, G. R.: The viscous metamorphosis of the blood platelets, J. Exp. Med. **26**:395, 1917.
133. Zimmerman, T. S., Ratnoff, O. D., and Powell, A. E.: Immunologic differentiation of classic hemophilia (factor VIII deficiency) and von Willebrand's disease, J. Clin. Invest. **50**:244, 1971.

24 □ Platelet and vascular disorders

Campbell W. McMillan

PURPURA

The word "purpura" is a Latin derivative of the Greek word "porphyra," the designation for the purple fish *(Purpura lapillus)* from whose gills a purple dye was obtained. Although the term was used for many centuries to designate the color purple, it did not come into use in disease until about the sixteenth century. At that time epidermoid spotted fevers—plague, typhus, or cerebrospinal fever—were called purpura fevers. Thereafter the term was used to designate any eruption of a purple color. With the discovery that the purple spots often were independent of fever, purpura acquired a narrower meaning within the context of abnormal hemostasis.[208]

Purpura may be defined as any hemostatic disorder presumed to be caused by one or more underlying defects of the circulating blood or its vessels and clinically characterized by purplish discoloration of the skin by leakage of blood from blood vessels. The purpuras have come to embrace a large group of bleeding disorders in which abnormal bruising is a prominent feature, with or without bleeding elsewhere. Extravasations of blood may vary from small pinpoint petechiae characteristic of thrombocytopenic purpura to large ecchymotic areas seen in Ehlers-Danlos syndrome.

If purpura is defined as any hemostatic disorder characterized by abnormal bruising, its application to the classification of bleeding problems obviously is too broad to be useful unless it is restricted. This chapter will deal only with those purpuras associated with platelet and vascular defects but *not* with major plasma coagulation abnormalities.

A basis for understanding the purpuras can be provided by a summary of: (1) the steps in the evolution of current concepts of the roles of the platelet and blood vessel in hemostasis; (2) current knowledge of the normal platelet and blood vessel; and (3) characteristics of these structures and their functions in the normal newborn.

HISTORICAL PERSPECTIVE

One of the earliest definitive observations about the initial phase of hemostasis was made by Hayem.[168] He showed that, in the event of vascular injury, platelets adhered to each other and to the injured site. The term "viscous metamorphosis" was introduced by Eberth and Schimmelbusch[112] to describe the transformation of aggregated platelets into a homogeneous gelatinous mass, an observation that was refined by Wright and Minot.[454] With the explosion of new knowledge about coagulation in the 1950s the participation of platelets in the plasma coagulation process was emphasized. No less than ten platelet factors related to coagulation were subsequently described, designated by Arabic instead of Roman numerals to distinguish them from the plasma coagulation factors.[448] This approach to the role of platelets in hemostasis proved unsatisfactory, for both laboratory investigation and clinical application. In fact, all these factors have sunk into oblivion except for platelet factors 2, 3, and 4.[101]

The current era of knowledge about platelets began in 1960 when Hellem[170] observed that (1) if citrated whole blood were passed through a column of glass beads, 46% of the blood platelets were retained by the beads, and (2) if platelet-rich plasma, free of red cells, were passed through such a column, only 4% of the platelets were retained by the beads. He determined that this difference was the result of a factor derived from red cell stroma, termed R factor, which was responsible for increased platelet adhesiveness and aggregation around the glass beads.[170] The following year Gaarder et al.[128] showed convincingly that R factor was, in fact, ADP.

Thereafter ensued a tremendous proliferation of laboratory and clinical studies, which have continued to the present. Laboratory highlights have included development of a clinically applicable glass bead test of platelet retention[346] and the introduction by Born[51] and O'Brien[306] of the aggregometer, a machine that measures platelet aggregation in vitro by detecting decreasing optical density of platelet-rich plasma to which an aggregation-inducing agent is added.

From a clinical viewpoint, critical breakthroughs occurred in 1967. In that year five important reports appeared describing separate groups of patients who shared in common a functional platelet disorder characterized by defective platelet aggregation caused by deficient release (or content) of endogenous ADP.* The article by Weiss and Aledort[431] describes such a disorder in normal subjects after ingestion of aspirin. The other reports describe the disorder as congenital and include the Portsmouth syndrome[307] and what is now known as ADP storage pool disease.[427,430,430a]

These studies established the central importance of ADP-induced platelet aggregation, particularly the ADP release from the platelets themselves, in contrast to the exogenous erythrocytic ADP that Hellem[170] encountered. These studies also established the clinical relevance of investigating platelet aggregation and relegated to lower priority the platelet factor approach to platelet problems.

More recent developments include the discovery that ristocetin, an antibiotic agent that proved to be unsuitable for clinical use, is an important tool for study of platelet aggregation.[131,191] Platelets suspended in plasma from a person with von Willebrand's disease are not normally aggregated by ristocetin because there is lack of factor VIII–associated protein on which ristocetin-induced aggregation is dependent.[192] In the rare Bernard-Soulier (giant platelet) syndrome, platelets taken from affected persons and suspended in normal plasma are not normally aggregated by ristocetin,[193] presumably because of lack of a proper platelet receptor site for human factor VIII–associated protein.[203,422]

In summary, in 1960 ADP was discovered to be involved in platelet aggregation; ADP has subsequently been shown to be the critical ingredient in a complex assembly line culminating in the formation of a platelet plug; and the search for an explanation of the role of ADP has been going on furiously since 1960 and is by no means complete.[102]

THE NORMAL PLATELET

The platelet is a small, disc-shaped cell without a nucleus, normally measuring 1 to 2 μm in diameter and 0.5 to 1 μm in thickness with volume of about 6 μl.[190,347] The mean platelet count in normal children and adults is about 250×10^9/liter, usually ranging from 150 to 400×10^9/liter. The platelet is derived from the cytoplasm of megakaryocytes, primarily located in the bone marrow. After its formation the platelet is released to the bloodstream, where it circulates for about 10 days before its removal, largely by the spleen. If a platelet is not required to perform a task, it circulates freely without adhesion to the vessel wall or aggregation with other platelets. If a task is required

—its major task is to seal holes in blood vessels— the stimulated platelet turns into a bloated sphere, develops thornlike pseudopodia, and becomes very sticky as it participates with the blood vessel, coagulation factors, and other platelets in the initiation of hemostasis.

Platelet production

The megakaryocyte, parent cell of the platelet, is presumed to be derived from pleuripotential stem cells in the bone marrow, which are capable of differentiating into myeloid or erythroid elements as well as megakaryocytes. Maturation of the megakaryocyte is characterized by enlargement up to 160 μ in diameter, endomitotic nuclear maturation followed by nuclear lobulation, and cytoplasmic maturation. Mature cytoplasm is then fragmented by platelet formation and release. The platelet is literally a "pinch" of megakaryocytic cytoplasm, created by invaginations of the surface of the megakaryocyte around previously processed cytoplasmic organelles.[38] The cytoplasm of the megakaryocyte thereby becomes an aggregate of platelets, which are released to the bloodstream, mainly from cytoplasmic pseudopodia extending into adjacent marrow sinusoids,[37] just as Wright[453] surmised many years ago. Eventually the entire cytoplasm is dissipated in platelet formation and the remaining nucleus degenerates and is removed by bone marrow phagocytes. The life span of the megakaryocyte in man has been estimated to be about 5 days.[86]

The regulation of thrombopoiesis is not yet fully understood, but there is evidence for a humoral thrombopoietin that may have a role analogous to that of erythropoietin in red cell production.[2,319,358] In any event, the normal platelet count reflects a well-regulated balance between production of platelets in the bone marrow and their subsequent destruction.[159]

Structure and content

Ultrastructural studies have shown that the platelet is composed of three principal components: (1) membrane structures, (2) granules, and (3) microtubules.[430,430a] (Fig. 24-1). The platelet has a three-layered *membrane* and an overlying *amorphous coat*. There are numerous invaginations of the surface, forming a system of underlying channels that provide a direct connection between the interior and the surface of the platelet. Interspersed among these structures is another set of narrower channels termed the *dense tubular system*. The platelet membrane is composed of specific proteins that mediate the response to platelet stimulation. Major examples of such proteins are thrombosthenin, probably identical to muscle actomyosin, critically involved in platelet contractility

---

*References 158, 181, 307, 427, 431.

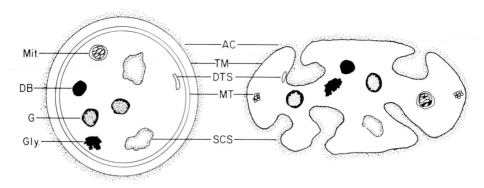

Fig. 24-1. Schematic view of platelet ultrastructure. Latitudinal (left) and longitudinal (right) cross-sections of the platelet are shown. *AC,* amorphous coat; *TM,* trilaminar membrane; *DTS,* dense tubular system; *MT,* microtubules; *SCS,* surface-connecting system; *Mit,* mitochondria; *DB,* dense bodies (storage-pool ADP and ATP, serotonin, and calcium); *G,* α-granule (acid hydrolases); *Gly,* glycogen. (From Weiss, H. J.: N. Engl. J. Med. **293:**533, 1975. Reprinted by permission.)

and aggregation[50]; glucosyl transferases, probably involved in the adhesion of platelets to collagen[52]; adenyl cyclase, the catalyst for synthesis of cyclic AMP, which inhibits platelet aggregation[60]; and lipoproteins, the source of platelet factor 3, involved in the activation of prothrombin and factor X.[255] Also contained in the membrane are platelet-specific antigens and antigens shared with other formed elements. Antigens of the Pl^A system[371] are platelet specific. ABO antigens are shared with red cells, and transplantation antigens (HLA system) are shared with granulocytes and lymphocytes.[129] (See Chapter 4.) The amorphous coat of the platelet may serve as the site for attachment of certain plasma proteins, including fibrinogen and factors V, VIII and XI.[430,430a] The term ''platelet factor 1'' denotes an entity now known to be adsorbed factor V.[101]

Platelet granules are characterized by two degrees of electron density: *α-granules* with moderate density and *dense bodies* with higher density. α-Granules principally contain lysosomal enzymes. They may also be the site of heparin-neutralizing material, termed platelet factor 4.[247] Dense bodies are less numerous than α-granules but are particularly critical to platelet function because they are the storage depot for ADP involved in the second phase of platelet aggregation.[432] In addition, dense bodies contain ATP, serotonin, and calcium.[323]

Microtubules are arranged in the form of an inner ring beneath the surface of the platelet, distinct from the surface-connecting and dense tubular systems of the membrane. Available evidence suggests that the microtubules provide structural support of the platelet and influence the character of its contractile functions.[441,464]

In addition to these structures, the platelet contains glycogen granules, occasional ribosomal particles, and small amounts of RNA and mitochondria. Important intracellular platelet constituents that have not been precisely localized include thrombosthenin, fibrinogen,[296] factor XIII,[262] fibrinogen-activating factor termed (platelet factor 2),[303] and platelet factor 3. Finally, although most of the intracellular calcium is stored in the dense bodies, a critical fraction directly related to platelet contractility is probably located elsewhere, perhaps in the dense tubular system.[442]

Metabolism

The source of energy for platelet function is ATP generated within the platelet from plasma glucose and a limited, nonrenewable supply of adenine nucleotides, presumably acquired from the megakaryocyte at the time of platelet formation.[185] Approximately 85% of the glucose is metabolized in the Embden-Meyerhof glycolytic pathway; 15% is oxidized in the Krebs cycle and hexose monophosphate shunt.[213,423] However, the glycolytic and oxidative pathways each generate approximately the same amount of ATP because of the greater efficiency of the oxidative pathways, particularly the Krebs cycle.[107] A critical level of ATP in the platelet is required for all of its functions, and the platelet responds to stimulation with increased glucose metabolism and ATP renewal.[185] ATP consumption primarily occurs with change in platelet shape.[186] Platelet adhesion to collagen is not energy dependent,[249] and first-phase platelet aggregation, although dependent on a high basal ATP level, is not associated with ATP consumption.[280]

The platelet is also equipped to carry out limited protein and fatty acid synthesis.[253,424] However, these capabilities appear to have little or no

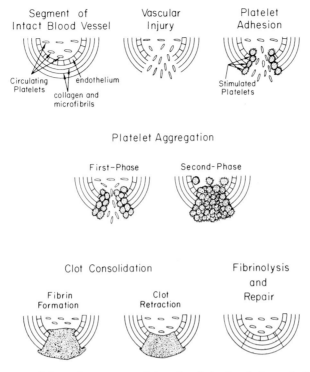

Segment of Intact Blood Vessel — Vascular Injury — Platelet Adhesion

Circulating Platelets, endothelium, collagen and microfibrils, Stimulated Platelets

Platelet Aggregation

First-Phase — Second-Phase

Clot Consolidation — Fibrinolysis and Repair

Fibrin Formation — Clot Retraction

Fig. 24-2. Schematic summary of the role of platelets in hemostasis.

significance in relation to the major functions of the platelet.

Functions

The platelet is able to carry out the following specialized functions: (1) hemostasis, (2) phagocytosis, (3) inflammatory response, and (4) endothelial support, particularly in the microvasculature. The reader should consult other sources for information on topics of phagocytosis,[76] inflammatory response,[297,438] and endothelial support.[140,207] Clearly the critical work of the platelet is its contribution to hemostasis, particularly in the initial phases. This function is highly integrated but may be divided into the following components, in order of their approximate sequence: (1) adhesion, (2) aggregation, and (3) consolidation[389] (Fig. 24-2).

Adhesion. The platelet is sensitive to any disturbance in the integrity of the blood vessel wall and adheres to a variety of vascular components that may be exposed. By far the most important of these is collagen.[34] The adhesion of platelets to collagen is not calcium dependent and may be effected through enzyme-substrate links involving glucosyl transferases on the platelet membrane.[201] Other vascular components to which platelets are known to adhere include microfibrils associated with elastin (but not elastin itself) and basement membrane; adhesion to these noncollagenous sub-

stances is calcium dependent. These biologic phenomena must be clearly differentiated from the retention of platelets by glass beads, which is now known to reflect both adhesion and aggregation.[430,430a]

Aggregation. Current knowledge of platelet aggregation is largely based on in vitro studies utilizing a platelet aggregometer. In addition, studies more nearly reproducing in vivo conditions have also been carried out, such as those by Baumgartner[35] in which segments of rabbit aorta denuded of endothelium are perfused with citrated whole blood. Representative aggregation patterns produced by collagen, epinephrine, thrombin, and various concentrations of ADP are shown in Fig. 24-3.

Concomitant with their adhesion to disturbed endothelium or exposure to aggregation-inducing agents, platelets change in shape from smooth discs to spiny, sticky spheres and begin to aggregate with each other. This process may be divided into first and second phases, bridged by accelerating release by platelets of their granular contents, particularly ADP.

First-phase (or primary) aggregation is reversible and is largely mediated by low concentrations of exogenous ADP, presumably derived from release of ADP from the first platelets to arrive at the injured vessel and to a lesser extent from red cells and other tissues.[292] The initiation of aggregation is dependent on the presence of calcium and fibrinogen.

Second-phase (or secondary) aggregation is mediated by high concentrations of ADP derived from the explosive release of endogenous ADP from platelets rapidly added to the enlarging platelet mass. This phase of aggregation is irreversible.

The release of ADP and other ingredients contained within platelets is critical to the orderly progression of aggregation through its two phases.[96] Release is induced by a variety of agents, presumably acting on contractile protein of the platelet membrane. Expulsion of the contents of dense bodies and α-granules has been termed release I and release II, respectively.[96] Release I is particularly critical to platelet aggregation because dense bodies contain most of the endogenous ADP as noted above. The following outline summarizes the agents causing platelet aggregation and release. All induce release I, and the enzymes and particulate substances induce release II.

A. Low molecular weight compounds
   1. ADP
   2. Epinephrine
   3. Norepinephrine
   4. Serotonin
   5. Vasopressin
   6. Endoperoxide precursors of prostaglandins E_2 and F_{2a}
B. Proteolytic enzymes
   1. Thrombin
   2. Trypsin
   3. Snake venoms
   4. Papain
C. Particulate substances
   1. Collagen (high concentration)
   2. Latex particles
   3. Fatty acid micelles
   4. Thorium dioxide
   5. Viruses
   6. Antigen-antibody complexes

These considerations raise the question of whether platelet-aggregating agents and release-inducing agents are performing separate tasks or really the single task of mobilizing endogenous ADP, which is ultimately responsible for all platelet aggregation. The latter concept is probably correct in general, but some substances — notably thrombin — appear to aggregate platelets directly in addition to inducing the release reaction.[188]

Substances that inhibit platelet aggregation appear to interfere largely with effects of ADP on the platelet rather than with ADP itself. Physiologic inhibition of aggregation appears to be largely mediated through any process that raises the platelet concentration of cyclic AMP.[348] Prostaglandins are of particular interest in this regard: PGE_1 inhib-

its platelet aggregation by stimulation of membrane adenyl cyclase, the catalyst of cyclic AMP[457]; PGE_2 promotes platelet aggregation by potentiating ADP release induced by endoperoxide precursors of PGE_2 and PGF_{2a}.[446] Chemical agents, notably mercurials, that combine with sulfhydryl groups on the platelet membrane also inhibit platelet aggregation.[163] The following agents inhibit platelet aggregation.

A. Compounds related to stimulation of platelet adenyl cyclase
   1. Cyclic AMP
   2. Prostaglandin E_1 (PGE_1)
B. Compounds that inhibit degradation of cAMP
   1. Papaverine
   2. Methyl xanthines
   3. Adenosine
C. Sulfhydryl-binding compounds
   1. Mercurials
   2. Arsenicals
D. Pharmacologic agents that inhibit platelet release reactions (p. 736)

In summary, it is now very clear that ADP is the principal substance mediating platelet aggregation. However, despite exhaustive studies and many theories, the precise mode of its action and inhibition are not yet known.

Consolidation. Platelets interact with plasma coagulation mechanisms in three major respects to promote consolidation of the platelet plug by fibrin. First, platelets contribute to the surface changes that activate factors XII and XI[421] and provide the initial framework on which fibrin formation occurs. Second, the platelet is a direct contributor of coagulation factors. Intracellular factors are calcium, fibrinogen, and factor XIII. Factors tightly adsorbed to the surface of the platelet include fibrinogen and factors V, VIII, and XI; others may be loosely adsorbed.[182] Third, the platelet furnishes three recognized factors of its own to the coagulation mechanism: platelet factors 2, 3, and 4. The most significant of these is platelet factor 3, derived from platelet lipoproteins associated with both membranous and granular components of the platelet.[256] It primarily acts as a surface catalyst for the activation of prothrombin and factor X and thus participates in the generation of thrombin through two steps of the intrinsic pathway. Lesser roles in coagulation are played by platelet factor 2 (fibrinogen-activating factor) and platelet factor 4 (antiheparin factor).

The complex steps in the fibrin consolidation of the platelet plug may be usefully integrated by considering the interacting roles of the platelet and thrombin in fibrin formation. Thrombin causes platelet aggregation directly and participates with other substances in the induction of ADP release; aggregated platelets provide coagulation factors

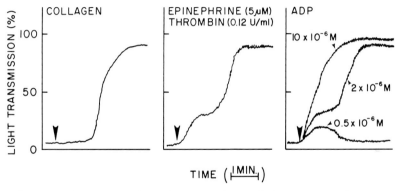

Fig. 24-3. Representative patterns of platelet aggregation. *Left,* Response to collagen, in which a lag period is followed by monophasic aggregation; this response is mediated by release of endogenous platelet ADP. *Middle,* Typical diphasic response to epinephrine and thrombin; these agents produce first-phase aggregation directly and second-phase aggregation by mediating platelet ADP release. *Right,* Three patterns of response to ADP, depending on its concentration: immediate and monophasic aggregation in response to a relatively high ADP concentration (e.g., 10 μM); a diphasic response to an intermediate ADP concentration (e.g., 2 μM); and a first-phase response only to a low concentration of ADP (e.g., 0.5 μM).

and platelet-specific factors that promote thrombin generation; thrombin catalyzes the conversion of fibrinogen to fibrin, and aggregated platelets provide the initial surface on which fibrin deposition takes place.

The final event in the evolution of the hemostatic plug is shrinkage of the mass, presumably mediated by thrombosthenin.[246] Although clot retraction is teleologically attractive as a last step to ''wrap it all up,'' its hemostatic significance is not entirely clear.

THE NORMAL BLOOD VESSEL

Although vascular injury initiates the hemostatic process, current knowledge of the contribution of the blood vessel to this process is largely a by-product of intensive research efforts directed at coagulation and platelets. Thus our understanding of the vessel itself is relatively limited. This deficiency, which may or may not prove to be significant with respect to an overall grasp of hemostasis, is an obvious target for future research. However, for the moment it does not seem to be a major shortcoming. The known vascular contributions to hemostasis will be briefly summarized here.

In the event of vascular injury, platelets adhere to exposed collagen and noncollagenous vascular components, including elastin-associated microfibrils and basement membrane. The role of collagen is particularly significant in that it appears to stimulate adherent platelets more than any other substance in the vessel wall.[34] Exposed collagen, along with aggregating platelets, also promotes surfaces changes that activate factor XII to trigger the intrinsic pathway of thrombin generation.[302] Injured vascular endothelium furnishes tissue

thromboplastin (factor III), which interacts with factor VII and calcium in the extrinsic pathway to activate factor X.[221] Plasminogen activator derived from the intimal layer of blood vessels[184] presumably helps to control fibrin deposition in the hemostatic plug and works with phagocytes to remove the plug as vascular integrity is restored by healing.

In blood vessels with smooth muscle elements vasoconstriction is a prominent characteristic of the vascular response to injury. Apart from its purely reflex nature, vasoconstriction is mediated by substances related to the hemostatic process. These include serotonin released from platelets and vasoactive peptides (kinins) released in connection with catalytic effects of activated factor XII.[333]

PLATELETS AND BLOOD VESSELS OF THE NEWBORN

The subject of platelets and blood vessels of newborns has not been studied as vigorously as coagulation in the newborn, but available data suggest certain differences between the neonatal period and later life, particularly in regard to platelets.

The platelet count in the neonate has been extensively surveyed, most results showing means for full-term infants that approximate the norm for adults and children. The mean pooled from five surveys of full-term infants reported by Bleyer et al.[47] is 249×10^9/liter. On the other hand, the mean pooled from three surveys of healthy premature infants is 216×10^9/liter. Aballi et al.[1] found the incidence of platelet counts below 100×10^9/liter during the first month of life in the premature infant to be less than 3.6%. In consideration of all available data, thrombocytopenia in the newborn period may be defined as a platelet count below 100×10^9/liter.

Platelet function in premature and full-term newborns has been shown by several investigators to be less efficient than that in adults.[47,82,176,290] These differences are expressed in two respects. First, platelets of the newborn do not aggregate as well as those of adults in response to thrombin, collagen, and ADP at equivalent platelet concentrations of 100×10^9/liter. However, this disparity may be decreased or corrected by using a relatively higher concentration of platelets from the newborn. For example, Bleyer et al.[47] showed that maximum collagen-induced platelet aggregation required a newborn platelet concentration of 700×10^9/liter, whereas the equivalent response for the infant's mother was achieved with a platelet concentration of 250×10^9/liter. Second, the platelets of the newborn are more susceptible than those of adults to inhibition of aggregation by certain drugs. For example, Corby and Schulman[82] have shown clear maternal-neonatal differences in the inhibition of collagen-induced platelet aggregation by given in vitro concentrations of aspirin and promethazine.

In the absence of significant contributing factors such as drugs, it appears unlikely that these functional platelet deficits in the newborn are capable of producing clinical problems. This conclusion is strongly supported by surveys showing normal bleeding times in all but severely premature newborns.[47]

As in the case of adults and children, little information is available about the role of the blood vessel in neonatal hemostasis. Furthermore, this information is largely derived from results of highly inconclusive tests of vascular function, i.e., the bleeding time and capillary fragility tests. Although such measurements are imprecise, suction-type measurements of capillary fragility have been shown to be abnormal to a degree that is roughly proportional to the degree of prematurity, whereas full-term newborns have normal capillary fragility.[290,458]

The platelet and blood vessel of the newborn may not be as well equipped for hemostatic functions as these structures become later in life, but there is no evidence that these relative deficits are clinically significant in the healthy newborn, full-term or premature.

CLASSIFICATION OF PURPURAS WITHOUT MAJOR COAGULATION DISORDERS

Purpuras without major coagulation disorders are arbitrarily divided into three major categories: (1) thrombocytopenic purpuras with a platelet count of less than 100×10^9/liter; (2) purpuras with a normal platelet count, including qualitative platelet disorders and vascular disorders; and (3) purpuras with thrombocytosis, i.e., a platelet count greater than $1,000 \times 10^9$/liter. The following classification should be regarded as a continuation of the overall scheme introduced in Chapter 23.

A. Purpuras with low platelet counts
 1. Acquired thrombocytopenic purpuras
  a. Increased destruction or loss of platelets
   (1) Idiopathic thrombocytopenic purpura
   (2) Identifiable immunologic disorders
    (a) Specific autoimmune diseases
    (b) Immunologic drug sensitivity
    (c) Posttransfusion purpura
   (3) Massive transfusion
   (4) Infections
   (5) Microangiopathic diseases
    (a) Hemolytic uremic syndrome
    (b) Thrombotic thrombocytopenic purpura
  b. Decreased or ineffective production of platelets
   (1) Idiopathic aplastic anemia
   (2) Neoplastic replacement of bone marrow
   (3) Myelosuppressive disorders
    (a) Marrow damage by radiation, chemical agents, and drugs
    (b) Infections
   (4) Diseases with ineffective platelet production
   (5) Hypoplastic thrombocytopenia
   (6) Cyclic thrombocytopenia
  c. Abnormal distribution of platelets
   (1) Diseases associated with splenomegaly
   (2) Liver disease
 2. Inherited thrombocytopenic purpuras
  a. Decreased production of platelets
   (1) Fanconi's anemia
   (2) Thrombocytopenia with absent radius syndrome
   (3) Other hypomegakaryocytic purpuras
   (4) Congenital deficiency of thrombopoietin
  b. Increased destruction of defective platelets
   (1) Wiskott-Aldrich syndrome
   (2) Disorders with giant platelets
    (a) May-Hegglin anomaly
    (b) Bernard-Soulier syndrome
    (c) Other giant platelet disorders
   (3) Disorders with morphologically normal platelets
 3. Neonatal thrombocytopenic purpuras
  a. Neonatal purpuras without hepatosplenomegaly
   (1) Immunologic disorders
    (a) Isoimmune neonatal thrombocytopenic purpura
    (b) Thrombocytopenias caused by maternal autoantibodies
   (2) Nonimmunologic disorders
    (a) Infections

(b) Congenital malformations
(c) Thrombotic disorders
(d) Other disorders
b. Neonatal purpuras with hepatosplenomegaly
  (1) Infectious diseases
    (a) Congenital rubella
    (b) Other infections
  (2) Non-infectious diseases
    (a) Congenital leukemia
    (b) Isoimmune hemolytic disease
    (c) Other diseases
B. Purpuras with normal platelet counts
  1. Qualitative platelet disorders
    a. Acquired thrombocytopathies
      (1) Drug-induced thrombocytopathies
        (a) Aspirin
        (b) Other drugs
      (2) Thrombocytopathies associated with systemic diseases
        (a) Uremia
        (b) Other diseases
    b. Inherited thrombocytopathies
      (1) Isolated thrombcytopathies
        (a) Glanzmann's disease
        (b) ADP storage pool disease
        (c) ADP-release disease
        (d) Considerations on von Willebrand's disease and Bernard-Soulier syndrome
      (2) Associated with inherited systemic disease
    c. Neonatal thrombocytopathies
  2. Vascular disorders
    a. Acquired vascular disorders
      (1) Traumatic purpuras
        (a) Battered-child syndrome
        (b) Factitious purpura
      (2) Inflammatory disorders
        (a) Henoch-Schönlein purpura
        (b) Other inflammatory disorders
      (3) Other acquired vascular disorders
    b. Inherited vascular disorders
      (1) Ehlers-Danlos syndrome
      (2) Hereditary hemorrhagic telangiectasia
      (3) Other inherited vascular disorders
    c. Neonatal vascular disorders
C. Purpuras with high platelet counts

Purpuras with low platelet counts

ACQUIRED THROMBOCYTOPENIC PURPURAS

Increased destruction or loss of platelets

Idiopathic thrombocytopenic purpura. Idiopathic thrombocytopenic purpura (ITP, Werlhof's disease, purpura hemorrhagica) is an acquired hemorrhagic disorder characterized by (1) thrombocytopenia that may be acute, recurrent, or chronic in clinical presentation, (2) purpura that is typically petechial in nature, occurring to an extent

usually correlated with the degree of thrombocytopenia, and (3) absence of otherwise identifiable thrombocytopenic disorders. Major negative findings should include absence of significant hepatosplenomegaly on physical examination and the presence of abundant megakaryotytes in a bone marrow aspirate.

Historical perspective. The history of ITP is described in an article on this subject by Jones and Tocantins.[208] Hippocrates may have been the first to describe ITP, but this disease was not separated from the larger body of purpuras until Werlhof identified it as a distinct entity in 1735, naming it morbus maculosus hemorrhagicus. His observations were extended in 1808 by Willan,[445] who included ITP in a classification of purpuras under the term "purpura hemorrhagica," separating it from other conditions including "purpura urticans" — Henoch-Schönlein or anaphylactoid purpura. The existence of thrombocytopenia in ITP was not known until Krauss observed decreased numbers of platelets in affected patients in 1883. The first actual platelet count documenting thrombocytopenia in ITP was performed by Hayem in 1890.

The treatment of ITP by splenectomy was inaugurated by Kasnelson[217] in 1916. As a medical student in Prague, he decided that the thrombocytopenia of ITP was a result of removal of platelets by the spleen and induced one of his instructors, a Professor Schloffer, to perform a splenectomy on an affected woman. The operation was a total success, followed by a rise in the patient's platelet count from a preoperative level of 0.2×10^9/liter to a postoperative level of 500×10^9/liter and, as would be expected, clearance of the purpura. The idea that the spleen might have something to do with purpura was considered as early as the days of Hippocrates, but Kasnelson was the first to act on this idea. Splenectomy thereby became the mainstay of treatment of ITP, but the role of the spleen in this disorder, many theories notwithstanding, was not determined until more than 30 years later.

The current era of ITP was launched by three major developments beginning in 1949: a provocative observation by Evans and Duane[117] a dramatic clinical experiment by Harrington et al.,[160,161] and the first measurement of platelet survival in ITP by Hirsch and Gardner.[179] Evans and Duane[117] described the association of thrombocytopenia with acquired (Coombs-positive) hemolytic anemia and suggested that an immunologic disorder, already established with respect to the red cell, might be affecting the platelet as well. A subsequent report by Evans et al.[118] presented evidence to support an immunologic basis for ITP itself, apart from its association with Coombs-positive hemolytic anemia. Then Harrington et al.[161] transfused ten normal persons (including Harrington) with blood from patients with ITP and demonstrated that eight of the recipients promptly developed thrombocytopenia and in some cases purpura as well. One of the recipients was a patient with cancer whose spleen had been previously removed. These observations established conclusively the primary role of a "humoral factor" in ITP and a relatively secondary role of the spleen. The reverse clinical experiment was performed by Hirsch and Gardner[179] who transfused fresh normal blood into patients with ITP and thereby demonstrated decreased platelet survival in this disorder.

Thereafter many pieces of the puzzle began to fall rapidly into place. In the case of adults with chronic ITP, it was convincingly shown that this disorder could be largely explained by attachment to platelets of IgG antibody, resulting in increased destruction of sensitized platelets by the reticuloendothelial system.[374] Contributing significantly to this concept of ITP was the recognition that neonatal thrombocytopenic purpura, first described by Dohrn[108] in 1873, could be related in certain instances to placental transfer of maternal antibodies associated either with isoimmunization* or maternal ITP.[162,372]

The immunologic basis for ITP has become sufficiently well established that as long ago as 1966 Baldini suggested that the "I" of ITP should stand for "immunologic" instead of "idiopathic" in appropriate instances. That this has not yet occurred is a reflection of two salient problems: (1) incomplete knowledge of the pathogenesis of the acute type of ITP, largely occurring in children after infections, and (2) profound and persisting technical problems with methods for detecting antibodies on platelets, caused by difficulties in separating antibody-mediated platelet agglutination from the natural aggregation of stimulated platelets. Thus a final note on the history of ITP is that an ideal test for antibodies on platelets, analogous to the Coombs test for red cells, has not yet been devised. Until such a test arrives, the "I" of ITP will probably continue to stand for "idiopathic."

Classification. The most objective method of classifying ITP is to divide it into acute and chronic types on the basis of duration rather than the nature of its clinical presentation. This approach is widely utilized but is modified as follows to integrate various classifications by others:

1. Acute ITP: complete and sustained remission within 6 months from onset
   a. Single episode, variable severity
   b. Recurrent, largely biphasic

2. Chronic ITP: sustained remission not achieved within 6 months from onset
   a. Continuous episode, variable severity
   b. Recurrent, multiphasic

In subsequent discussions the acute and chronic types of ITP will each be considered in a general sense. Recurrent ITP, which is at the interface of acute and chronic types, does not lend itself to separate consideration. However, its very existence tends to suggest that *all* forms of ITP may consist of variations on a single theme.

Incidence. Taken as a whole, ITP occurs more frequently in all age groups than any other thrombocytopenic disease.[106] Although ITP may appear at any age, it largely affects children and young adults, approximately half of all cases occurring in children under 15 years of age according to one large survey.[245] The disease appears to be more common in whites than in blacks.[197]

Acute and chronic ITP differ rather sharply from each other in regard to incidence and to age and sex predilection. Acute ITP is approximately twice as common as chronic ITP, its peak incidence is from 2 to 6 years of age, and it is rather evenly distributed among boys and girls.[234,248] Chronic ITP affects older children and adults for the most part, occurring principally in persons between 10 and 30 years of age,[178,380] and is about three times as common in females as in males.[245]

Etiology. Although the cause of ITP is unknown, there has been significant progress in determining its pathogenesis. In a classical sense ITP is an autoimmune disorder specifically affecting platelets, caused by an abnormal response of the human host to disease-related or indeterminate antigenic agents.

Genetics. Since ITP is an acquired disorder, genetic considerations do not strictly apply. However, the appearance of ITP is undoubtedly conditioned by certain poorly understood constitutional factors, including age, sex, and race. Genetic factors may also be operational in some cases of bona fide ITP. Roberts and Smith[339] described a family with presumed autosomal recessive inheritance in which four children of both sexes developed severe ITP-like disease between 3 and 7 years of age and died of hemorrhage. Bithell et al.[45] reported mild thrombocytopenia inherited as an autosomal dominant trait in eleven of fifty-one members of four generations of an affected kindred. Further, several workers have described thrombocytopenic purpura associated with sex-linked recessive inheritance.[71,351,413] Canales and Mauer[66] have also described a kindred with sex-linked recessive inheritance of thrombocytopenic purpura, but they regarded this disorder as a variant of Wiskott-Aldrich syndrome, although increased infections and

*Forms of immunization are designated as follows: *auto,* antibodies against "self" antigens; *iso,* IgG maternal antibodies against antigens of the fetus; *allo,* antibodies against "nonself" antigens.

eczema typical of this syndrome were not evident. Finally, Ata et al.[24] have described a thrombocytopenic disorder presumably inherited as a sex-linked dominant trait with incomplete penetrance in females, occurring in ten of forty-seven members of five generations of an affected kindred.

At the present time it is difficult to know exactly what to make of reports such as these. They do suggest the existence of genetic determinants of this disorder, but particular care in diagnostic evaluation needs to be carried out in such instances. The ultimate understanding of the role of inheritance in ITP will, of course, be obtained only when ITP becomes less "idiopathic."

Clinical features. The hallmark of ITP, regardless of type, is purpura with an otherwise normal physical examination. Purpuric lesions vary from pinpoint petechiae—the classic expression of thrombocytopenia—to large ecchymoses. Depending on the time the patient is seen in relation to the onset of purpura, lesions vary in color from the blue of fresh extravasation to the greenish yellow of older hemorrhage undergoing resolution. Random distribution of purpura is absolutely essential for a diagnosis of any type of ITP. Any suggestion of symmetry should alert the clinician to the possibility of diseases other than ITP.

Purpura is frequently associated with variable bleeding elsewhere. By far the most dangerous complication of ITP is intracranial hemorrhage. Fortunately this problem is uncommon, its incidence ranging between 2% and 4%[132] with a mortality of 1% or less.[234,380] Unfortunately it does not have a predictable association with any particular mode of presentation of ITP; intracranial hemorrhage may occur early in the course of fulminating acute ITP or at any time in the course of chronic ITP. Aside from neurologic abnormalities suggesting central nervous system hemorrhage, the clinician should be alerted by a history of significant headaches and by the finding of retinal hemorrhages. There is no evidence that subconjunctival hemorrhages or petechiae of the soft palate have any significance in relation to intracranial hemorrhage.

Other sites of hemorrhage rarely if ever constitute dangerous complications. Epistaxes are common, especially in acute ITP, and are probably largely responsible for the melena that may be associated with ITP, although substantial gastrointestinal bleeding may also occur. Menorrhagia is not a common problem in acute ITP simply because menses have not occurred in the majority of girls who develop acute ITP. It is a significant problem in chronic ITP, which largely occurs in females older than 10 years. Hematuria may occur in any type of ITP but is uncommon.

Types of bleeding that are *not* appropriate for a diagnosis of ITP also should be emphasized. Purpura that is largely ecchymotic rather than petechial should raise questions. Symmetrical, as opposed to random, purpura has been mentioned. Hemarthroses are totally inappropriate for thrombocytopenia of any variety but are characteristic of certain plasma coagulation disorders, particularly classical hemophilia and Christmas disease. Brisk capillary oozing from a fresh surface wound is characteristic of thrombocytopenic hemorrhage, but delayed or recurrent hemorrhage from such a wound is more suggestive of a plasma coagulation disorder.

It cannot be overemphasized that, aside from purpura, the physical examination of a patient with ITP should reveal nothing of significance. For example, a young child with fulminating acute ITP may be frightened, but he or she should not "look sick" in the manner typical of patients with sepsis or meningitis. More specifically the presence of significant lymphadenopathy or hepatosplenomegaly should raise serious doubts about a diagnosis of ITP, although a palpable spleen tip or liver edge may occur.

ACUTE ITP. Although acute ITP is most objectively defined in terms of its overall duration, it is also typically characterized by the sudden and spontaneous onset of generalized purpura, usually associated with variable bleeding elsewhere. Epistaxes are particularly common, as are petechiae and hemorrhagic bullae involving the mucous membranes of the mouth and pharynx. Florid purpura usually subsides naturally within a week or two, while the platelet count returns to normal more slowly. There is no certain way to predict the duration of a specific case of ITP, but 60% to 90% of all patients recover completely within 6 months,[248,380] the vast majority having only a single episode of purpura. Indeed, sustained remission in such cases usually occurs within 6 weeks.[300]

Approximately 80% of acute-onset cases of ITP are preceded by an illness occurring within 3 weeks of the appearance of purpura.[132,248] The majority of such antecedent illnesses are nonspecific upper respiratory infections during the winter and spring months, but about 20% may be specific infectious diseases, particularly exanthems: rubeola,[125,194] rubella,[3,124,392,420] and varicella.[439] Other associated conditions include mumps,[223] infectious mononucleosis,[17,75,331] cat-scratch disease,[39,44,205] Colorado tick fever,[257] smallpox vaccination,[273] and rubeola vaccination.[14]

The temporal relation between the onset of thrombocytopenic purpura and associated infections is highly variable. Cases of exanthem-associated ITP may be most objectively examined in this regard. For example, development of thrombocytopenia with rubella has variously occurred anywhere from the same time as the exanthem to 11 days later[124] with a mean interval of 4 days from the onset of the rash to the onset of purpura.[287]

The association of an antecedent illness with the acute onset of ITP may be of some help in predicting an early remission from a single episode of thrombocytopenia, thereby fulfilling in a total sense the diagnosis of acute ITP. Lammi and Lovric[234] have reported that patients developing ITP without a history of an antecedent illness tended to have a more protracted course, including development of chronic ITP.

CHRONIC ITP. In addition to its extended duration, chronic ITP is typically characterized by an insidious onset and a mild course. There is usually no history of a preceding illness. Menorrhagia may be a presenting complaint in female patients of an appropriate age. Petechial purpura is characteristic of chronic ITP but is typically mild and may be expressed only as an increased bruising tendency, unlike the relatively florid, spontaneous purpura seen in acute ITP. Indeed, depending on the platelet count, there may even be no bleeding problems.

Unlike affected adults, a significant number of children with chronic ITP may recover spontaneously in time. For example, in a study of ITP in 152 children up to 13 years of age, Lammi and Lovric[234] found that twenty-three of thirty-six patients who did not recover within 6 months ultimately recovered naturally within a period of 3½ years, a remission rate of 64%.

Laboratory evaluation. At the present time there is no specific test that establishes a diagnosis of ITP. Therefore the role of laboratory evaluation largely consists of excluding otherwise identifiable causes of thrombocytopenia. Three categories of testing should be carried out: (1) examination of the blood counts and smear, (2) examination of a bone marrow aspirate, and (3) selected tests of venous blood to exclude certain diseases, notably identifiable autoimmune diseases and plasma coagulation disorders.

In general blood counts in ITP should reveal no abnormalities of any of the formed elements, except a deficiency of platelets. Anemia or white cell changes may be present also, but such findings should be readily explainable by associated blood loss or expected effects of an associated infection, respectively. Typically the degrees of thrombocytopenia and purpura are proportional to each other. Purpura usually does not become significant until the platelet count drops below 50×10^9/liter, and severe purpura with associated spontaneous bleeding elsewhere usually occurs when the platelet

count is below 25×10^9/liter. Examination of the blood smear is an important adjunct to the platelet count. Platelets on a good smear of fresh blood are readily seen and tend to clump together when the count is above 50×10^9/liter. When the count is below this level, platelets on the smear are increasingly isolated, large, and scarce.

A variety of simple tests of overall platelet function also reflect the effects of thrombocytopenia. These include the bleeding time (the Ivy method is recommended), clot retraction, capillary fragility testing by tourniquet or petechiometer, and the prothrombin consumption test for platelet factor 3 activity. In the absence of an associated qualitative platelet defect, results of these tests should be within normal limits or nearly so, with platelet counts as low as 50×10^9/liter. Indeed, results may not become clearly abnormal until the platelet count falls below 25×10^9/liter. These tests add virtually nothing to the diagnostic assessment of acute-onset ITP; the clinical data, the platelet count, and inspection of the blood smear suffice.

However, these tests, particularly the Ivy bleeding time, may be helpful in screening for a qualitative platelet defect that may occur in some cases of chronic ITP.[73] Such a defect should be suspected in any patient with impressive purpura associated with a platelet count above 50×10^9/liter.

The bone marrow in ITP is generally easy to aspirate, and the smear should show abundant megakaryocytes along with normal myeloid and erythroid elements and absence of any abnormal cells. Although megakaryocytes may frequently appear immature by virtue of decreased size, absence of nuclear lobulation, and scanty cytoplasm, this finding should not be regarded as having any special diagnostic or prognostic significance. Likewise, the association of marrow eosinophilia and greater likelihood of spontaneous recovery from ITP[364] has not been confirmed. Representative megakaryocytes are shown in Figs. 24-4 and 24-5.

Finally, to exclude certain immunologic and plasma coagulation disorders that may be associated with thrombocytopenia, the following tests should be performed: an antinuclear antibody test for systemic lupus erythematosus; direct and indirect Coombs tests for Coombs-positive acquired hemolytic anemia; and tests of PT and PTT, which are typically prolonged in plasma coagulation disorders but entirely normal in ITP.

Differential diagnosis. In one sense the differential diagnosis of ITP is hopelessly complex. That is, a complete list of possibly similar disorders would properly include *all* purpuras, both with and without associated plasma coagulation abnormalities. However, if one adheres to a strict definition of ITP and obtains appropriate data from the history, physical examination, and laboratory eval-

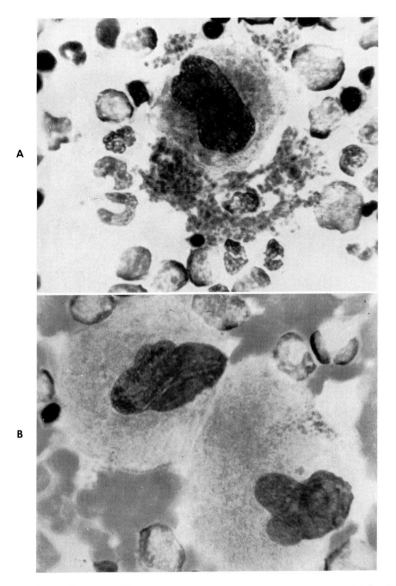

Fig. 24-4. A, Smear from normal bone marrow. Note mature megakaryocyte containing large lobulated nucleus. Cytoplasm is granular with platelets in the process of formation. Masses of platelets are chiefly grouped about the periphery of the cell. **B,** Intermediate megakaryocytes. These are usually found in increased numbers in the bone marrow of patients with idiopathic thrombocytopenic purpura. Cytoplasm is more abundant and less granular than that shown in **A,** and platelet differentiation is either absent (upper cell) or slight (lower cell). (Courtesy Dr. Robert L. Rosenthal, New York, N.Y.)

uation, the diagnosis of ITP is usually not at all difficult to establish.

The entire group of nonthrombocytopenic purpuras is excluded by a significantly low platelet count. Acquired thrombocytopenia caused by impaired production of platelets, notably leukemia and aplastic anemia, should be definitively excluded by the bone marrow aspiration. Absence of significant enlargement of the liver and spleen should exclude abnormal sequestration of platelets as seen in portal hypertension associated with splenomegaly. The clinical picture of the patient and the blood smear should rule out microangiopathic disorders, notably hemolytic-uremic syndrome in children. Appropriate laboratory tests usually rule out specifically identifiable immunologic diseases such as systemic lupus erythematosus and also generalized coagulation disorders such as purpura fulminans.

Perhaps the most important entry in the differential diagnosis of ITP is infection, particularly treatable life-threatening septicemia, such as me-

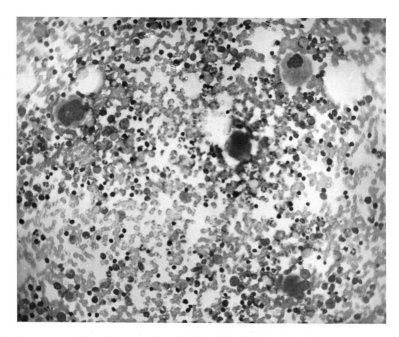

Fig. 24-5. Low-power view of bone marrow in idiopathic thrombocytopenic purpura. Typically the megakaryocytes are not only relatively increased but also frequently appear immature like those shown above. (×150.)

ningococcemia. Such an infection may mimic ITP completely, notably in its early stages, and should always be considered in a child who "looks sick."

Pathogenesis and pathophysiology. Numerous theories have been advanced in the past to explain the pathogenesis of ITP. Representative ideas since the turn of the century have included the following: deficient production of platelets by megakaryocytes,[127] increased attraction of platelets to defective blood vessels,[404] elaboration by the spleen of abnormal humoral factors that suppress platelet production by megakaryocytes,[91] and selective sequestration of platelets by the spleen.[105] Probably the most decisive of the events establishing the immunologic nature of ITP were the clinical experiments of Harrington et al.[161] in which normal volunteers developed thrombocytopenia when transfused with plasma from subjects with ITP. These experiments firmly established the existence of a circulating "factor" in ITP capable of causing thrombocytopenia, at least in adults with chronic ITP such as the subjects whose plasma was tested. This "factor" was conclusively shown by Shulman et al.[374] to be a 7S γ-globulin (IgG) by virtue of the following characteristics: localization in the IgG fraction of serum, adsorption onto normal platelets, and association with platelet destruction in direct proportion to the quantity of plasma infused. Further confirmation of the role of IgG was provided by the discovery that this is the only immunoglobulin that crosses the placenta,[141] coupled with the long-recognized association of neonatal thrombocytopenic purpura and maternal ITP.[162]

Thus the pathogenesis of chronic ITP can now be largely attributed to IgG autoantibodies directed against platelet antigens. Chronic ITP is therefore analogous to Coombs-positive hemolytic anemia, as Evans and Duane[117] first suggested in 1949. On the other hand, it is not yet known whether this immunologic error in "self" recognition is the result of a normal immunologic response to an altered profile of platelet antigens, an abnormal immunologic response to normal platelets, or perhaps some combination of these two mechanisms. This dilemma is largely unresolved with respect to immunologic disorders in general.

The pathogenesis of acute ITP usually seen after infectious diseases in young children has not been as well determined as that of chronic ITP. Acute ITP is also widely regarded as immunologic in nature. However, decreased platelet survival in acute ITP may be caused by relatively nonspecific adsorption onto platelets of antigen-antibody complexes derived from associated disease processes[295] rather than by autoantibodies directed against platelet antigens, as in chronic ITP. In any case, it does not appear that the pathogenesis of acute ITP is significantly related to direct suppression of platelet production by viruses or other infectious agents. A model probably illustrating such suppression has been provided by the studies of Oski and Naiman,[312] who documented mild and transitory thrombocytopenia in normal children over a 3-week period after they received live measles vaccine. Decreased numbers of megakaryocytes as well as increased vacuolization suggested direct inhibitory effects of the virus on platelet production. This mechanism of thrombocytopenia can usually be excluded in acute ITP, even without conclusive studies such as measurement of platelet survival, on at least two clinical grounds: (1) although acute ITP may coincide with appearance of an exanthem, viral inoculation of the host will have preceded the exanthem by several weeks, depending on its incubation time, and (2) the explosive purpura characteristic of acute ITP is quite different from the largely subclinical thrombocytopenia that may be associated with the early phases of viral illnesses.

With the assumption of an immunologic pathogenesis for all types of ITP, the pathophysiology of this disorder may be summarized as follows: Antibody-coated platelets have an abnormally short survival time because they are rapidly filtered from the blood by the reticuloendothelial system, particularly the spleen; the bone marrow responds to thrombocytopenia by formation of increased numbers of megakaryocytes and thus increased production of platelets but, even with maximal effort, is not able to provide sufficient platelets to offset the effects of their shortened survival.

Many methods for studying platelet survival are now available, largely utilizing appropriate radioisotopes for platelet labeling: ^{32}P as sodium phosphate or diisopropyl fluorophosphate (DFP), ^{75}Se as selenomethionine, and ^{51}Cr as sodium chromate.[132] Of these methods ^{51}Cr labeling of platelets has probably been the most widely used. Platelets normally survive about 10 days.[28,159] By whatever method studied, it has been consistently shown that survival of homologous (donor) platelets is short in patients with ITP and that this finding is unrelated to alloimmunization. Furthermore, in accord with the pioneering experiments of Harrington et al.,[161] autologous (self) platelets of normal persons have shortened survival if they are reinfused along with ITP plasma. Finally, there is evidence that the degree of shortened survival is directly proportional to the degree of thrombocytopenia, presumably a reflection of the similar relationship between thrombocytopenia and the amount of circulating platelet antibodies. Indeed, the essentially universal agreement on increased platelet destruction in ITP makes this finding a particularly firm cornerstone of the pathophysiology of this disorder.

As a general rule in clinical practice, measurement of platelet survival is not necessary to establish a diagnosis of ITP. However, if the diagnosis is uncertain, the finding of a normal life span of autologous or homologous platelets in the patient effectively removes ITP from further consideration.

Platelets sensitized by specific antibodies are removed by the reticuloendothelial system, particularly the spleen.[23] In the event of marked sensitization, typically correlated with severe thrombocytopenia and short platelet survival, hepatic sequestration of platelets may also occur.[374] Surface scanning of the spleen and liver for ^{51}Cr uptake after injection of ^{51}Cr-labeled platelets in ITP has been helpful in defining the relative roles of these organs in platelet destruction.[23] Theoretically this technique should be useful in predicting effects of splenectomy in a given case of ITP. However, results tend to be sufficiently variable that this technique has not yet gained a firm place in clinical practice.

There is increasing evidence that the spleen also may play a major role in ITP by producing platelet-binding IgG antibodies, both in chronic and acute forms of the disease.[242,269] Synthesis rates of IgG by cultured splenic leukocytes in ITP have been shown to be increased up to seven times normal.

The bone marrow plays a secondary role in the pathophysiology of ITP. Although the antibodies that sensitize platelets may conceivably impair platelet production by direct effects on megakaryocytes, available evidence suggests that thrombopoiesis in ITP is effectively increased beyond normal rates.[159] Thus the thrombocytopenia of ITP may be largely regarded as the result of platelet destruction uncompensated for even by maximal production.

There is preliminary evidence that the bone marrow may also be a site for production of platelet-binding IgG antibodies, suggested in a 10-year-old boy whose ITP was not controlled by splenectomy.[242] His disease was subsequently controlled in association with aggressive immunosuppressive therapy. The effect on platelet production of bone marrow synthesis of platelet-binding IgG antibodies was not investigated. Further studies on such cases surely will be forthcoming.

Despite many speculations regarding the possible role of a vascular disorder in the pathophysiology of ITP,[251] there is no substantive evidence for such a role. The beneficial effects of corticosteroids that may be observed in ITP are largely related to decreased platelet phagocytosis rather than to improved vascular integrity. This issue will be considered in the discussion of treatment of ITP.

Pathology. The prinicpal pathologic manifestation of ITP is nonspecific gross and microscopic cutaneous extravasation corresponding to the clinical appearance of purpura. The extent of extracutaneous hemorrhage that occurs in ITP obviously cannot be fully known aside from clinically evident signs or autopsy in the rare event of death. It is rather distressing to speculate on possible events within the brain of a child who has fulminating purpura and numerous bleeding sites elsewhere. Fortunately lethal intracranial hemorrhage in ITP is extremely rare in children.

The most extensively studied organs in ITP are the bone marrow and the spleen because they are critically important from diagnostic and therapeutic standpoints, respectively. Bone marrow findings have been discussed previously. Splenic pathology is largely nonspecific, consisting of enlargement of germinal centers, dilation of the sinusoids of the red pulp, variable presence of extramedullary elements (including megakaryocytes), and presence of lipid-laden histiocytes.[58,174] In rare instances the spleen may show changes diagnostic of specific diseases, thereby excluding ITP.

Management. The therapeutic approach to ITP may be divided into two broad categories: (1) supportive care only and (2) specific treatment, variously consisting of corticosteroids and other drugs, splenectomy, and platelet infusions.

ACUTE ITP. In acute ITP supportive care alone is the cornerstone of management against which all other approaches must be judged. This is so because acute ITP is rarely associated with serious complications, and by definition it undergoes a natural and permanent remission within 6 months. The principal adjunct to supportive care is watchful waiting, carefully explained to the parents and also to the child if he or she is 6 years of age or older. Particular ingredients of supportive care include the following: replacement of acute hypovolemic blood loss with stored bank blood, replacement of subacute isovolemic blood loss with packed red cells if the hematocrit falls below approximately 20%, treatment of chronic blood loss anemia with ferrous sulfate orally as needed, and commonsense restriction of the child's activities until purpura has begun to subside with concomitant rise in the platelet count.

The main problem in carrying out supportive care alone undoubtedly lies with the physician rather than with the disease. It is extremely difficult to restrain oneself from "doing something" when confronted with a child suddenly covered with purpura and usually bleeding elsewhere as well. Furthermore, in a given case the ultimate course of ITP cannot be precisely predicted, and the urge to influence the course favorably may not be adequately relieved by chapters in textbooks suggesting that the course is probably going to be favorable anyway. At the point of this classical dilemma, specific measures for management of ITP, notably corticosteroids, come into the picture.

A summary of the principal corticosteroids is shown in Table 24-1. Over the past three decades these agents and adrenocorticotrophic hormone (ACTH) have been used in a variety of pharmacologic regimens. The agent most widely administered is probably prednisone. ACTH offers no advantages over corticosteroids, is rarely used, and need not be discussed.

Corticosteroids are usually administered during the first month of acute-onset ITP when the risk of death is greatest.* In individual instances corticosteroid therapy unquestionably seems to be causally related to a rise in platelet counts and clearance of purpura. These benefits have been variously attributed to hemostatic effects of corticosteroids on the vascular wall[119] and to immunosuppression.[92] More recent studies suggest that clinical improvement with corticosteroids is largely related to their inhibition of platelet phagocytosis by the reticuloendothelial system, especially the spleen,[374] although immunosuppression may also play a significant role.[104]

In a disease with as inherently good a prognosis as acute ITP, it is not surprising that it has been difficult to demonstrate statistically significant benefits from corticosteroid therapy on platelet counts, the incidence of complications, or the

*References 224, 261, 355, 419.

Table 24-1. Relative potency and dosages of corticosteroids commonly used in clinical practice

	Approximate relative potency	Representative pharmacologic dose (mg/m²/day)	Approximate physiologic dose (mg/m²/day)
Cortisone	0.8	300	25
Hydrocortisone	1	240	20
Prednisone	4	60	5
Prednisolone	4	60	5
Methylprednisolone	5	48	4
Triamcinolone	5	48	4
Dexamethasone	40	6	0.5

duration of illness. Lusher and Zuelzer[248] and Lammi and Lovric[234] found no such benefits. On the other hand, the host of believers in steroid therapy of ITP have undoubtedly derived great comfort from the report of Simons et al.,[380] who found statistically higher platelet counts during the second week of illness in treated as compared with untreated patients. These workers administered the equivalent of approximately 60 mg prednisone/m^2/day for 3 to 4 weeks. They did not find significant differences between treated and untreated patients during the first and most of the third weeks of therapy. Clinicians still await the results of a well-designed, controlled clinical trial in this disease.

Splenectomy, immunosuppressive therapy other than corticosteroids, and platelet infusions generally have limited application in the management of acute ITP. However, life-threatening hemorrhage (particularly intracranial hemorrhage) or intercurrent surgical emergencies[352] may constitute exceptions to this generalization. In such instances emergency splenectomy may be indicated, followed by additional surgical or medical treatment as needed.

Immunosuppressive agents other than corticosteroids are generally not used within 6 months of onset of ITP unless uncontrolled and dangerous complications persist beyond splenectomy. Variable success in treatment of ITP has been reported with azathioprine[177] and cyclophosphamide,[236] but the overall value of these agents in ITP has not yet been conclusively determined. The same is true for vincristine.[9] The mechanism whereby vincristine tends to raise the platelet count is uncertain, but this effect does not appear to be related to immunosuppression.[340]

There are unfortunately no rational guidelines for the use of platelet infusions in ITP. Even massive platelet infusions are generally not capable of raising the platelet count significantly in fulminating ITP. On the other hand, platelets quantitatively bind platelet antibodies, and at least a few platelets may conceivably reach critical bleeding sites before they are removed by the spleen. In any case, in the event of life-threatening hemorrhage it is entirely appropriate to administer platelet concentrates, preferably HLA matched,[456] along with supportive transfusions, corticosteroids, and preparations for emergency splenectomy. It can be shown that 1 unit of platelets derived from 500 ml whole blood produces an increment of about 10×10^9 platelets/liter/m^2 body surface area in the absence of excessive platelet destruction.[293] With this assumption, 5 to 10 units of platelet concentrate/m^2 every 12 hours constitutes reasonable therapy for ITP, depending, of course, on local blood bank resources.

In summary, the mainstays of management should be supportive care and nonfrantic watchful waiting. After completion of diagnostic studies *but never before* prednisone may be given in a single daily oral dose of 60 mg/m^2. This treatment should be terminated completely within 1 month, regardless of the platelet count; abrupt cessation of therapy (no tapering) after 2 weeks is quite appropriate. By 1 month any one of three outcomes may be observed: (1) the platelet count may be normal and remain so for life; (2) thrombocytopenic purpura may be completely corrected during therapy but recur on its discontinuation; or (3) thrombocytopenic purpura may show partial correction or no improvement at all. In the event of the latter two outcomes, further prednisone therapy should be strongly resisted because it frequently happens that an otherwise normal child with ITP is transformed into a cushingoid child with ITP. Side effects of corticosteroids are minimal or absent if a single daily dose (rather than divided doses) is combined with complete termination of therapy within a month. Recurrent or continuing thrombocytopenic purpura is usually not a major problem and the child should remain in school but avoid contact sports. On the other hand, if purpura is rather marked, particularly if previous prednisone therapy was objectively helpful, it may be appropriate to prescribe the lowest possible dose of this agent that will control the purpura, preferably administered every other day. Such a program must be developed empirically. Finally, if ITP extends beyond 6 months in a continuous or recurrent fashion, the disorder then shifts by definition from acute to chronic ITP and a new set of therapeutic considerations begin to apply.

CHRONIC ITP. In chronic ITP watchful waiting and supportive care should continue to be mainstays of management, whereas long-term corticosteroid treatment should be avoided insofar as possible.[77] Indeed, if a child maintains a platelet count above 50×10^9/liter and is largely free of purpura, watchful waiting without treatment should probably be continued indefinitely. This is especially true for children under 10 years of age, whose chances of eventual recovery remain rather good as long as approximately 4 years from the onset of ITP.[234] On the other hand, for children over 10 years of age, whose chances of recovery become increasingly slight, consideration of elective splenectomy is appropriate, preferably after 1 year from onset of ITP. Menorrhagia in teenage girls is a particularly clear indication for splenectomy in chronic ITP.

Splenectomy is followed by sustained remission in about 70% of otherwise refractory cases of ITP.[380] The benefits of this operation cannot be accurately predicted in advance, but return of platelet counts to normal limits at least within 1 week of surgery seems to be associated with sustained remission.[311] The benefits of splenectomy can be rationally attributed to removal of a major site, if not *the* major site, for destruction of sensitized platelets and for production of platelet-binding antibodies. Elective splenectomy has been sufficiently tested that it should probably be regarded as the first choice for management of chronic ITP in those instances in which conservative support and time have not sufficed.

Most patients with ITP undergoing splenectomy or any other surgical procedure will have received corticosteroids previously. Such patients *must* be carefully supported during the stress of surgery to prevent potentially lethal adrenal insufficiency, even if steroids have not been administered for more than a year. The anesthesiologist should be thoroughly apprised of the circumstances, and baseline electrolyte levels along with serum creatinine and blood glucose levels should be obtained. Recommendations for the management of corticosteroid therapy of patients with ITP undergoing surgery are outlined below.

  A. Patients currently treated with corticosteroids
    1. Minor surgical procedure requiring general anesthesia: 50 mg/m² hydrocortisone intravenously before the procedure and 50 mg/m² intravenously on completion of the procedure
    2. Major surgical procedure: 100 mg/m² hydrocortisone intravenously during induction of anesthesia and 100 mg/m² intravenously in a slow drip of 5% dextrose in water throughout surgery
    3. Postoperative management: resumption of regular dosage, temporarily substituting parenteral equivalent of the dose as needed until oral intake is resumed
  B. Patients previously treated with corticosteroids
    1. Preoperative management
      a. Twelve hours before surgery: 50 mg/m² hydrocortisone intravenously
      b. One hour before surgery: 100 mg/m² hydrocortisone intravenously
    2. During the operation: 100 mg/m² hydrocortisone in a slow drip of 5% dextrose in water throughout surgery
    3. Postoperative management
      a. In recovery room: 100 mg/m² hydrocortisone intravenously
      b. First and second postoperative days: 50 mg/m² hydrocortisone intravenously every 12 hours
      c. Third and fourth postoperative days: 10 mg/m² prednisone orally every 12 hours or its equivalent parenterally until oral intake is resumed
      d. Corticosteroid discontinued abruptly (no need to taper)

Following splenectomy a reactive thrombocytosis may be observed with the platelet count some-

times rising to levels of 200×10^9/liter or more. Indeed, such a rise has been thought by some observers to be indicative of a favorable prognosis.[61] Anticoagulation has been recommended for postsplenectomy platelet counts above $1,000 \times 10^9$/liter,[149] but this is generally unnecessary in children because of the virtual absence of thrombotic complications. Although high platelet counts may persist for several months, they usually return to normal limits within a month.

Patients on a given dose of corticosteroids at the time of splenectomy should be maintained on this same dose during the first postoperative week. Thereafter dosage may be empirically tapered over a 1- to 3-week period. Indeed, a test of the patient's clinical response to cessation of corticosteroid therapy probably should be carried out even in those instances in which the platelet count remains low after splenectomy.

Persistent or recurrent thrombocytopenia usually reflects uncontrolled ITP. However, on rare occasions this problem may be related to one or more accessory spleens missed at the time of original surgery.[19] Evaluation of this possibility should consist of a careful examination of both routine and specially stained blood smears and a ^{99m}Tc spleen scan. Red cells of a truly asplenic person usually contain some identifiable particles of rubbish that are normally extracted by the pitting mechanism of the spleen. Such particles include nuclear remnants (Howell-Jolly bodies), siderotic granules (Pappenheimer bodies), and denatured hemoglobin (Heinz bodies). The absence of such findings combined with evidence of an accessory spleen by a ^{99m}Tc scan warrant another splenectomy in a persistently thrombocytopenic patient.

Until recent years splenectomy was largely regarded as a harmless procedure, although as early as 1919 Morris and Bullock[285] suggested a connection between splenectomy and an increased risk of infection. The present era of concern with this problem probably began in 1952 when King and Shumaker[220] reported five infants with overwhelming sepsis following splenectomy for hereditary spherocytosis. The current status of postsplenectomy sepsis has been carefully reviewed by Singer.[381] (See Chapter 22.)

Splenectomy for ITP has been shown to be associated with a low but nonetheless significant risk of sepsis, particularly pneumococcal. In reviewing 489 reported splenectomies for ITP up to 1973, Singer[381] identified sepsis in ten patients (2.05%) of whom seven died (1.43%). The overall risk of sepsis for such patients was estimated to be about 100 times that for the general population. Children under 5 years of age, especially infants less than 1 year of age, appear to be at particular risk. The interval between splenectomy and sepsis varied from 13 days to 14 years.

These findings add a new and rather disturbing dimension to the management of ITP as well as other conditions in which splenectomy may be indicated. A 1% chance of fatal postsplenectomy sepsis must be weighed against an overall 1% chance of fatal intracranial hemorrhage in ITP. Definitive recommendations cannot be made at this time, but the following principles of management are suggested: (1) there should be no hurry about splenectomy for ITP in children except in cases of life-threatening hemorrhage; (2) in the case of infants and preschool children splenectomy should be deferred insofar as possible until the child is more than 5 years old; (3) in the event of splenectomy in children under 5 years of age prophylaxis against pneumococcal infection probably should be instituted (e.g., 400,000 units of penicillin G twice daily and polyvalent pneumococcal vaccine); (4) even in older children the risk of postsplenectomy sepsis needs to be recognized and explained to the patient and family in obtaining informed consent for splenectomy.

Finally, if splenectomy fails to relieve ITP, immunosuppressive agents and vincristine may be tried. In chronic as well as in acute ITP definitive guidelines for their use have not yet been established and their value in treatment of otherwise refractory ITP is uncertain. Indeed, if judicious corticosteroid therapy, watchful waiting, and splenectomy have all failed, it may be in the best interests of the child with ITP to stop further active therapeutic efforts and return to watchful waiting. Fortunately for pediatric practice this impasse is uncommon.

Prognosis. In a given patient under 16 years of age with ITP there is about a 70% chance that the child will entirely recover within 6 months (acute ITP). This chance is increased to approximately 90% if the child is less than 10 years of age and has had a clearly defined onset of purpura associated with a preceding infection.

There is about a 30% chance that ITP in a given patient will persist or recur beyond 6 months (chronic ITP). Of such patients recoveries of approximately 70% have been separately reported for natural remission[234] and response to splenectomy[380]; whether these outcomes are somehow additive or variations on a single theme is totally unclear at this time.

In any case, an overall 90% chance for ultimately complete recovery from ITP is a solid and probably conservative estimate for any patient younger than 16 years. Of the remaining 10% or less of cases a mortality rate of 1% may be assigned to intracranial hemorrhage and an additional 1% to sepsis following splenectomy. A small and indeterminate percentage of children initially presenting with ITP may have other identifiable diseases, notably immunologic disorders such as systemic lupus erythematosus.[92] A subsequent diagnosis of aplastic anemia or leukemia may be made, but these diagnoses should not be missed initially if careful examination of the bone marrow is carried out. Finally, it appears that about 5% or less of all children with ITP simply have to continue to live with persistent but usually rather tolerable thrombocytopenic purpura. Such children tend to have exacerbations of ITP with intercurrent infections and need specially attentive medical care and overall support at these times.

Future perspectives. The overriding need in the immediate future is the development of reliable laboratory methods for identifying conclusively those cases that are truly "immunologic" rather than "idiopathic." Such methods must be capable of direct, rather than indirect, detection of antibodies on platelets, which are causally related to platelet destruction. A representative step in this direction has been taken by Dixon et al.,[104] who described a quantitative complement lysis-inhibition assay of platelet-bound IgG. With this sensitive but complex test they detected increased levels of platelet IgG in all adults with chronic ITP and also in a child with varicella-associated acute ITP. They also found that the amount of platelet-bound IgG could be usefully correlated with the clinical response to corticosteroid therapy.

It may be hoped that the near future will yield answers to the following questions about ITP: (1) Is all chronic ITP characterized by platelet-specific IgG autoantibodies? (2) Is all acute ITP characterized by adsorption onto platelets of antigen-antibody complexes—and therefore fundamentally different from chronic ITP? (3) How does recurrent ITP fit into the picture? (4) What is the role of cellular immunity in ITP? (5) How far away is a truly rational basis for the use of corticosteroids, immunosuppressive agents, platelet infusions, and splenectomy in the clinical management of ITP? (6) What are the prospects for vaccines capable of preventing postsplenectomy sepsis? These are only a few questions; there are many more.

Specific autoimmune diseases. Instead of being an isolated finding, as in ITP, thrombocytopenia may be associated with a variety of diseases regarded as autoimmune in nature. The clinical expression of thrombocytopenia in such diseases is largely similar to chronic ITP. Likewise, the pathophysiology of thrombocytopenia in these instances is presumably mediated by platelet-specific autoantibodies. The factors that determine differences in cellular specificity and clinical effects of autoantibodies in this group of diseases, as well as in ITP, are not clearly understood. Indeed, the strict requirements for "autoimmune disease" prescribed by Witebsky[450] are not uniformly met by most of the clinical disorders currently so designated.

McClure[261] has reported the association of thrombocytopenia with the following diseases: systemic lupus erythematosus (five cases); acquired hemolytic anemia (three cases); hyperthyroidism (two cases); and Raynaud's phenomenon with a positive antinuclear antibody test, rheumatoid arthritis associated with Coombs-positive hemolytic anemia, isolated rheumatoid arthritis, and immune leukopenia (one case each). These fourteen patients were evaluated with 399 children with isolated thrombocytopenia ("true" ITP by our definition); thus they constituted 3.4% of an overall group with presumed immunologic thrombocytopenias. Such thrombocytopenia has also been described in certain neoplastic disorders, notably Hodgkin's disease and non-Hodgkin's lymphoma,[106] but this association appears to be considerably more common in adults than in children.

Immunologic drug sensitivity. It has been thoroughly established that severe thrombocytopenic purpura following ingestion of a given drug by certain sensitive persons may be mediated by antibodies against the drug. Many agents have been implicated in immunologic thrombocytopenia,[154] but conclusive evidence for this mechanism is limited to the following: quinine, quinidine, digitoxin, stibophen, novobiocin, and allylisopropylacetylurea—more familiarly known by the trade name "Sedormid"—a now-defunct sedative.[22]

Although the association of acute thrombocytopenic purpura and quinine was described by Vipan[415] in 1865, an immunologic basis for certain drug-related thrombocytopenias was not identified for more than 80 years. In 1948 Grandjean[147] showed that normal platelets were destroyed by a mixture of quinine and serum from a quinine-sensitive person but not by either ingredient alone. Ackroyd[4] obtained similar results in classical investigations of Sedormid purpura and suggested that drug-dependent antibodies are responsible both for thrombocytopenia and for vascular damage in sensitive persons. He further proposed that drug-related immunologic thrombocytopenia is mediated by antibodies formed against an antigenic platelet-drug complex, where the drug acts as a hapten.[6] However, in their studies on Sedormid sensitivity, Miescher et al.[278,279] concluded that the platelet does not participate with the drug in antigenic stimulation but rather adsorbs drug-antibody complexes in a relatively nonspecific fashion. These conclusions were supported and extended by Shulman[368,369] in a series of important studies on quinidine sensitivity.

The clinical picture of drug-related immunologic thrombocytopenic purpura is largely analogous to acute ITP. The disorder usually begins within 24 hours of exposure to the offending drug and is self-limited, clearing on riddance of the drug. Once sensitivity has been established, it is generally assumed to be permanent.

The key to management of a patient whose platelets may be affected by a given drug is to identify the problem by a careful history supported by in vitro testing insofar as possible[7] and to avoid the drug in question thereafter. As to treatment of the episode itself, there is virtually nothing that will predictably alter the natural course, which usually lasts less than 2 weeks. In general the principles for management of acute ITP are quite applicable, including consideration of corticosteroids and avoidance of splenectomy except in the event of life-threatening hemorrhage. As in acute ITP, platelet infusions offer little or nothing as long as the offending drug is circulating, because in its presence antibodies attach equally to homologous and autologous platelets.

The mechanism by which drug-related antibodies destroy platelets has not been unequivocally established. However, the consensus seems to be aligned with the concept that the platelet is sensitized by innocent adsorption of immune complexes rather than by attachment of a specific antibody. If this were proved to be so, the role of viruses and the like in acute ITP and the role of drugs in the disorder in question might be neatly unified.

Posttransfusion purpura. Posttransfusion purpura is a rare hemorrhagic disorder characterized by the onset of severe thrombocytopenic purpura in patients about 1 week after uneventful transfusion of routinely cross-matched whole blood. Of seventeen cases reported from 1959 to 1975 all but two have shown the following: (1) The patients have been adult women who have been pregnant in the past; (2) platelets of donors have contained the Pl^{A1} antigen; and (3) platelets of recipients have lacked this antigen, but their sera have contained anti-Pl^{A1} antibodies.* The recent report of posttransfusion purpura in a nulliparous female *with* the Pl^{A1} antigen and also in a male suggests that the profile of this disorder may be less constant than previously thought.[461] Although posttransfusion purpura is a rare disease apparently limited to adults, it should claim the attention of pediatricians because it is clinically similar to acute ITP and it is relevant to the broad question of immunization against platelet antigens.

Cross-matching procedures for transfusion of whole blood or its components are generally restricted to compatibility tests of the red cells only. Therefore repeated transfusions of whole blood or platelet concentrates from random donors will sooner or later result in the alloimmunization of

---

*References 144, 371, 373, 408, 461.

most recipients against foreign platelet antigens. Indeed, Shulman[370] has estimated that approximately 5% of such recipients may become so immunized after only a single unit of blood. Clinically the most important antigens are those of the transplantation, or human leukocytes, locus A (HLA) system,[457] *not* the Pl^A system. In any case, alloimmunization caused by transfusion of antigenically incompatible platelets usually causes only shortened survival of such platelets without additional effects on the patient's own platelets.

Since the Pl^{A1} antigen is present in about 98% of the population,[371] women lacking this antigen who developed posttransfusion purpura may well have been isoimmunized during their previous pregnancies. But even so, why did their reexposure to this antigen result in severe, delayed destruction of their *own* platelets instead of the harmless, orderly removal of donor platelets that would normally be expected?

The answer to this question is not yet known, but the studies of Shulman et al.[371] suggest that posttransfusion purpura may be pathogenically as well as clinically similar to drug-related immunologic thrombocytopenia. That is, soluble complexes of persisting Pl^{A1} antigen from the donor and antibody of the patient may be nonspecifically absorbed onto the patient's platelets, thereby causing their paradoxical destruction. However, without "appropriate adjustments" this explanation fails to account for the apparent absence of posttransfusion purpura in the 2% of children and adults lacking the Pl^{A1} antigen who are even now receiving whole blood and platelets without crossmatching to exclude this antigen. The further clarification of posttransfusion purpura will undoubtedly add much to our understanding of acute thrombocytopenic purpura as an overall syndrome consisting of acute ITP and drug purpura as well as posttransfusion purpura.

Massive transfusion. Thrombocytopenia has been observed in patients receiving large amounts of compatible banked blood, usually for treatment of simple blood loss[227] and also for multiple exchange transfusions in newborn infants.[100] Thrombocytopenia in these instances appears to be largely the result of the interaction of the following factors: dilution of the recipient's platelet pool, deficiencies in quality and quantity of donor platelets, and inability of megakaryocytes to compensate for rapid platelet depletion. Significant purpura is rarely associated with thrombocytopenia in these circumstances, and the problem is usually quite manageable by appropriate platelet replacement therapy. Such therapy may consist of giving platelet concentrates or interspersing banked blood with fresh whole blood.

Infections. Thrombocytopenia presumed to be a result of increased destruction of platelets may be associated with infectious diseases caused by virtually the entire spectrum of etiologic agents. The two most investigated mechanisms of such thrombocytopenia are discussed elsewhere: immunologic thrombocytopenia as seen in acute ITP and DIC (discussed in Chapter 25). Actually in most instances thrombocytopenia associated with infection may be unrelated to these two mechanisms. For example, in a study of forty-six infants and children with proved bacterial sepsis, Corrigan[83] discovered no specific reason for thrombocytopenia other than sepsis itself in twenty-one of twenty-eight patients who had platelet counts less than 150×10^9/liter. Since platelets have phagocytic functions[76] and participate in inflammatory reactions,[438] increased consumption of platelets in certain infectious processes is not difficult to presume, particularly when such a process is severe.

It should be emphasized that in cases in which a decreased platelet count is associated with a serious infection, the central issue in both diagnosis and treatment is the infection, not the thrombocytopenia. However, appropriate component therapy should be used for support of the patient, and serial platelet counts may provide a useful "weather vane" for assessing overall clinical progress. To help differentiate the thrombocytopenia of increased platelet destruction from that of decreased production, a bone marrow aspirate should be examined. As in ITP, megakaryocytes should be abundant if the platelet lack is largely a result of increased destruction. Unfortunately, aside from evaluation of the bone marrow, there is little that the laboratory can offer in the resolution of this problem. Platelet survival studies, for example, have limited usefulness in the absence of a "steady state," and a severe infection is hardly that. Thrombocytopenia associated with infection in most instances may well be related *both* to decreased production and to increased destruction of platelets. Intensive efforts to separate these mechanisms generally add little or nothing to appropriate clinical management.

Microangiopathic diseases
Hemolytic-uremic syndrome. Hemolytic-uremic syndrome (HUS) is an acquired disorder largely affecting infants and young children and is characterized by the triad of microangiopathic hemolytic anemia, acute renal failure, and thrombocytopenia.

HISTORICAL PERSPECTIVE. In 1955 Gasser et al.[134] introduced the term "hemolytic-uremic syndrome" to describe a constellation of clinical and pathologic findings in a group of children from 2 months to 7 years of age. These authors particularly emphasized the renal failure, which clinically resembled acute glomerulonephritis with hematuria and proteinuria, and the finding of bilateral renal cortical necrosis at autopsy. In time it was noted that schistocytes (fragmented red cells), previously described in such conditions as uremia and disseminated carcinoma,[89,365] were an integral part of this syndrome.

There has been relatively little progress in the understanding and specific management of this disorder since it was first described. Fibrin deposition within diseased microvasculature of the renal cortex appears to be the basic lesion, and this in turn presumably mediates the associated abnormalities of the red cells and platelets. Brain[54] pointed out the clinical and pathologic similarities of HUS and thrombotic thrombocytopenic purpura (TTP) and applied the term "microangiopathy" to both these diseases. However, the pathologic mechanisms underlying the observed changes are not yet clear. A lively debate has occurred over the years regarding the occurrence of disseminated as well as localized intravascular coagulation in HUS.[216,241,350] At the present time the bulk of evidence does not support the concept that HUS is a manifestation of DIC.

CLASSIFICATION. The clinical and pathologic findings that have been observed in HUS do not lend themselves to meaningful classification. Furthermore, there may be unpredictable shifts in the clinical expression of recurrent microangiopathic disease. For example, one of the earliest reported patients with HUS[375] was a child who had many exacerbations of the disease and finally died at 13½ years of age with a clinical and pathologic picture best fitting TTP.[252]

INCIDENCE. In accord with the original description of HUS by Gasser et al.,[134] subsequent reports have confirmed that this syndrome usually occurs in infants and young children. For example, in a recent study of 212 cases of HUS, van Wieringen et al.[409] found that 84% of the patients were 4 years old or younger, with a peak incidence at about 1 year of age. However, this disease may rarely affect teenagers and even young adults.[366] No predilection for sex or race has been observed.

HUS is a relatively uncommon disorder occurring in isolated instances. However, the appearance of this disease in geographically limited outbreaks resembling an epidemic has also been described. For example, Gianantonio et al.[139] reported the occurrence of fifty-eight cases among children younger than 3 years in Buenos Aires. Similarly McLean et al.[268] reported an outbreak of HUS in ten patients over a short period of time in a small area of North Wales.

ETIOLOGY. The etiology of HUS is unknown. However, its occurrence has been associated with a wide variety of infectious agents, both in iso-

lated and epidemic settings. In the series of Gianantonio et al.[139] a viral agent was isolated from the blood of patients during the acute phase of the disease but was not specifically identified. Mettler[275] isolated from two patients with HUS and one with TTP a rickettsia. The same organism was recovered from mites collected in the bedroom of one of the children. Bacteria have also been implicated,[121,367] but in the studies of HUS by van Wieringen et al.[409] no evidence for a bacterial etiology could be found. In a few instances HUS has appeared following immunizations.[111,202]

It seems plausible to believe that HUS may be triggered in susceptible patients by one or more specific infectious agents to be identified in due course. Such an etiology is suggested by the occasional epidemic character of its appearance and its tendency to occur at certain times of the year, notably during the spring months.[409]

GENETICS. Although the occurrence of HUS in young children underscores important constitutional factors in this disease, there is so far no evidence that genetic factors are also involved. The disease has been reported in siblings[18] but, as in outbreaks, such occurrence may be related to environmental rather than hereditary factors.

CLINICAL FEATURES. The onset of HUS is typically preceded by a prodromal illness of about 1 week's duration, ranging from 1 to 15 days.[409] Signs of gastroenteritis with vomiting and diarrhea, particularly bloody diarrhea, are most frequently observed. Fever and nonspecific upper respiratory illness may also occur during this period. The actual onset of HUS is characterized by anemia and thrombocytopenia as well as effects of acute renal disease, notably hematuria and oliguria or even anuria. On physical examination the child with HUS is usually subacutely ill and shows findings appropriate for the disease, particularly pallor, petechial purpura, and variable edema. Other findings that may be encountered include jaundice, enlargement of the liver and to a lesser extent the spleen, hypertension, and a spectrum of central nervous system signs ranging from mild changes in the sensorium to coma or convulsions, which are largely caused by effects of renal failure.

LABORATORY EVALUATION. In most cases the diagnosis of HUS can be readily established by clinical findings and the following laboratory studies: (1) blood counts and inspection of the blood smear, showing a normocytic normochromic anemia with a high reticulocyte count, a platelet count usually well below 100×10^9/liter, and evidence on the blood smear of typical red cell fragmentation (Fig. 24-6) along with polychromatophilia and decreased platelets; (2) urinalysis, showing protein and abundant red cells, including red cell casts on occasion; (3) assessment of renal function, show-

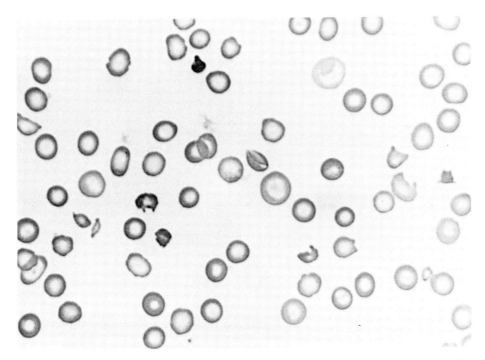

Fig. 24-6. Blood smear of a child with hemolytic-uremic syndrome, showing red cell fragmentation (schistocytosis) and marked deficiency of platelets. (×450.)

ing marked elevation of blood urea nitrogen and serum creatinine levels and variable abnormalities of serum electrolytes, notably hyperkalemia; (4) selected negative test results, including results of direct and indirect Coombs tests and serum antinuclear antibody tests; and (5) a bone marrow examination, confirming expected normal megakaryocytes and erythroid hyperplasia.

Although HUS is not associated with consistent plasma coagulation abnormalities, the three standard one-stage clotting tests should be carried out to determine TCT, PT, and PTT. If these tests are within acceptable limits, as they typically are in HUS, continued pursuit of coagulation problems is hardly indicated. However, significant abnormalities shown by these tests should be followed up with specific assays of fibrinogen, prothrombin, factor V, and factor VIII and appropriate measurement of fibrinogen degradation products in serum. If these further tests establish the presence of DIC, additional considerations for its management are of course in order.

DIFFERENTIAL DIAGNOSIS. In classic cases of HUS differential diagnosis does not pose a major problem if appropriate laboratory evaluation is carried out. Difficulties arise in those instances in which HUS may not have completely evolved or there are other hemolytic, thrombocytopenic, or renal disorders presenting signs overlapping with HUS. In older children particular care must be taken to differentiate HUS from TTP and from immunologic disorders, notably systemic lupus erythematosus.

PATHOGENESIS AND PATHOPHYSIOLOGY. The mechanisms that underlie the clinical expression of HUS are at best poorly understood. Within this limitation the following partial concept of the pathogenesis and pathophysiology of HUS is offered, largely assembled from reports by Brain[54], Katz et al.,[215,216] and Kisker and Rush.[222]

First, a constitutionally susceptible subject is challenged by a foreign antigen. Second, an abnormal immunologic reaction occurs that for unknown reasons is largely limited to glomerular capillaries and adjacent arterioles. Brain[54] has suggested that soluble immune complexes may be involved. Katz et al.[216] have compared the process to that of renal allograft rejection. Third, reactive inflammation of the affected renal blood vessels occurs with intense but transient *localized* intravascular coagulation and deposition of fibrin, ranging from fine intraluminal strands to complete vascular occlusion with necrosis. Fourth, both red blood cells and platelets are damaged in their passage through the partially obstructed renal microvasculature, resulting in their early demise within the general circulation or their prompt removal by the reticuloendothelial system. Fifth, renal failure is mediated by the ischemic process that is pathologically characterized by widespread fibrin deposition within renal arterioles and glomerular capillaries and by variable cortical necrosis.

There is particular agreement among most workers on two parts of this concept. First, DIC is no longer believed to account for the overall clinical picture of HUS. Even studies carried out in the prodromal period of this disease have failed to show evidence for DIC.[222] Thus the suggestive similarities between HUS in humans and the Sanarelli-Shwartzman reaction in rabbits, particularly the occurrence of bilateral renal cortical necrosis,[349,377] may not represent a meaningful similarity in their pathogenesis, as has been postulated.[235,376]

There is also general agreement that the hemolytic anemia of HUS is the result of damage to red cells in transit through diseased small blood vessels. The cells are thought to be sliced by intraluminal fibrin strands (Fig. 24-7). The concept was first advanced by Monroe and Strauss,[282] and the pathologic process was termed microangiopathic

hemolytic anemia by Brain et al.[55] in 1962. There is more uncertainty about the pathophysiology of the thrombocytopenia in HUS. Brain[54] suggested that the same mechanism affecting red cells might affect platelets as well but implied that platelets might be trapped within the kidneys. Katz et al.[215] found no evidence for intrarenal sequestration of platelets in HUS and suggested that they are damaged in their passage through the renal vessels and then removed by the reticuloendothelial system, particularly the spleen.

PATHOLOGY. Although the pathology of HUS is by no means unique, certain consistent features have been described.* Foremost among these are histologic changes of the glomerular capillaries and adjacent arterioles, characterized by widespread deposition of fibrin with formation of hyaline thrombi and variable endothelial changes associated with parietal thickening. These lesions tend to be focal, and their severity as well as dis-

---

*References 54, 137, 202, 416.

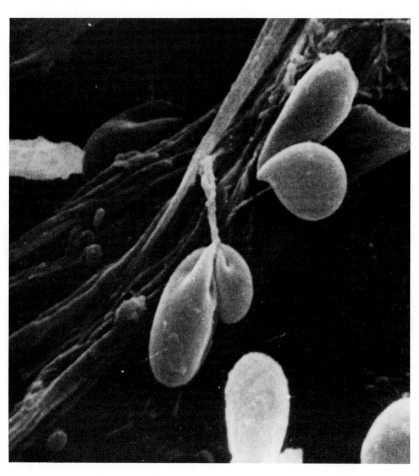

Fig. 24-7. Scanning electron micrograph of formation of fragmented erythrocytes by fibrin strands in an in vitro model. (×2,100.) (From Bull, B. S., and Kuhn, I. N.: Blood **35:**104, 1970.)

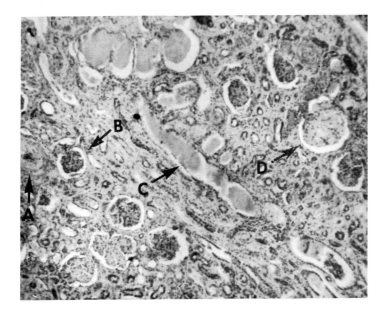

Fig. 24-8. Photomicrograph of section of kidney of child with hemolytic-uremic syndrome. Child was almost 5 years of age at time of death. Illness lasted 3 months with periods of marked anuria and oliguria. *A,* Small artery with markedly thickened wall; *B,* shrunken hypercellular glomerulus with two similar glomeruli nearby; *C,* cast of proteinaceous precipitate in a dilated tubule; *D,* necrotic glomerulus with disappearance of all cellular elements. (×120.)

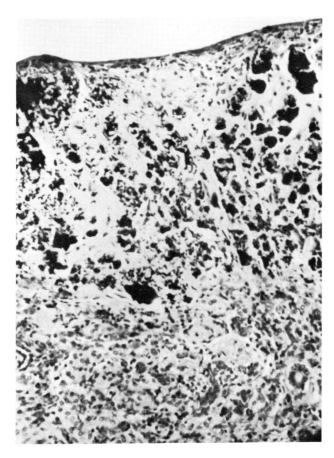

Fig. 24-9. Photomicrograph of kidney of 20-month-old child with hemolytic-uremic syndrome. Note widespread necrosis of outer three fourths of renal cortex with degenerative calcification. Heavily pigmented masses of finely granular basophilic material staining as calcium are scattered through the cortex. A zone of less severely affected cortex is observed in the lower portion of the section. Illness was progressive, lasting 3 months.

tribution determine the extent of bilateral renal cortical necrosis. Although Brain[54] has suggested that soluble immune complexes may mediate these changes in HUS, it should be noted that Gervais et al.[137] were unable to demonstrate immunoglobulin or complement at the site of vascular lesions. Photomicrographs of representative renal lesions in HUS are shown in Figs. 24-8 and 24-9.

MANAGEMENT. The major principles for management of HUS are early diagnosis and supportive treatment of renal failure. Peritoneal dialysis has enabled children to recover renal function after periods of 2 or more weeks of anuria[54] and should be undertaken as early as possible to control azotemia.[202] Other useful supportive measures include treatment of hypertension and control of anemia with transfusion of whole blood or packed red cells as indicated. Transfusion of platelet concentrates may be administered in the event of marked thrombocytopenic hemorrhage but is seldom required.

Other reported modes of treatment and their rationales are as follows: corticosteroids, for improving platelet survival; aspirin and dipyridamole, for inhibition of platelet aggregation; heparin, for inhibition of thrombin activity; and streptokinase, for promotion of thrombolysis.[210,322,326] With the exception of corticosteriod therapy, these measures are based on the premise that control of intravascular coagulation should be useful in the management of HUS. So far there is no convincing evidence that any of these measures, alone or in combination, offers any benefits beyond supportive management alone.

PROGNOSIS. In the large series described by Gianantonio et al.[139] the most significant prognostic factor in HUS was the severity of renal failure in the acute phase of the disease, based on renal function and the degree of glomerular damage on renal biopsy. These workers found an overall mortality of 29% among fifty-eight affected infants and children. Later in a series of 250 cases Gianantonio et al.[138] found that a mortality of 23% in the first 150 patients fell to 5% in the last 100 patients. They pointed out that, although part of this decreased mortality could be attributed to inclusion of milder cases of HUS, a major role was also played by improvements in the supportive management of acute renal failure. In a more recent series of 212 cases of HUS reported by van Wieringen et al.[409] the overall mortality was 16%, but all deaths occurred before management included systematic peritoneal dialysis.

In survivors thrombocytopenia and anemia generally clear within 1 month of diuresis. Renal function is substantially improved by this time but complete return to normal, particularly renal concentrating function, may require as long as a year. Recurrence of HUS is uncommon but has been de-scribed up to 4 years after complete remission.[202] Transition of HUS into TTP has also been reported.

FUTURE PERSPECTIVES. Although there is increasing agreement that DIC does not play a definable role in the overall picture of HUS, there is need to clarify both the pathogenesis and the timing of the renal deposition of fibrin that is at the heart of the disease. The respective roles of possible etiologic agents and response of the host remain to be defined. It must be determined whether renal deposition of fibrin represents the residual of a transient burst of intravascular coagulation, either localized or disseminated: a sustained but self-limited process of localized intravascular coagulation, a sustained but self-limited state of partially compensated DIC, some combination of these, or none of these. The clarification of these issues would contribute to greater understanding and more specific management not only of HUS but of many other diseases as well. In the meantime the results of supportive care are quite impressive.

Thrombotic thrombocytopenic purpura. Thrombotic thrombocytopenic purpura (TTP, Moschcowitz's syndrome) is an acquired disorder largely affecting young adults and typically characterized by (1) thrombocytopenic purpura, (2) severe microangiopathic hemolytic anemia, (3) variable neurologic abnormalities, (4) renal disease, and (5) fever.

This disorder was first described by Moschcowitz[288] in 1925. His observation of widespread hyaline thrombi in capillaries and arterioles has

Table 24-2. Differences between HUS and TTP*

	Hemolytic-uremic syndrome (HUS)	Thrombotic thrombocytopenic purpura (TTP)
Peak age incidence	1-4 years	20-25 years
Male:female ratio	1:1	1:2
Prodromal illness	Usual	Variable
Fever	Rare	Usual
Neurologic abnormalities	Variably related to renal failure	Usual
Renal disease	Usual	Usual
Renal failure	Common	Rare
Hypertension	Common	Rare
Major organs affected	Kidneys	Kidneys, brain, heart, pancreas, and adrenals
Prognosis	Relatively good	Poor

*Modified from Berman, N., and Finklestein, J. Z.: Scand. J. Haematol. **14:**286, 1975.

been thoroughly confirmed since that time, and this finding is now established as the pathologic hallmark of TTP. Moschcowitz regarded these lesions as the result of a circulating toxin affecting platelets and red cells. However, Altschule[15] suggested almost two decades later that the primary defect lay in the blood vessels themselves rather than in the formed elements of the blood. His concept is now accepted. A later major contribution was the demonstration by Craig and Gitlin[84] in 1957 that the hyaline microthrombi of TTP are largely composed of fibrin instead of aggregated platelets as previously thought. In 1962 Brain et al.[55] introduced the term "microangiopathic hemolytic anemia" to describe the damaging effect of diseased small blood vessels on red cells. This concept was experimentally supported by Brain and Hourihane[56] in the same year and is now accepted as the basis of the hemolytic anemia in TTP. As previously noted, Brain[54] underscored the similarities between TTP and HUS. These two disorders are now generally regarded as widely varying expressions of a unitary pathologic process involving small blood vessels in both cases. A summary of their major differences is shown in Table 24-2.

There is no specific treatment for TTP. As in HUS, supportive care should be a cornerstone of any scheme of management with particular emphasis on support of those organ systems most critically affected. There is also some evidence suggesting that aggressive corticosteroid therapy combined with early, if not emergency, splenectomy may be effective in the treatment of TTP.[283,362] Many other approaches similar to those discussed in connection with HUS have been tried, but conclusive evidence of their benefit is lacking so far. Thus unfortunately there is no true consensus at present on the most effective mode of treatment for TTP, many findings and claims notwithstanding. A useful survey of the "state of the art" on TTP in childhood has recently been reported by Berman and Finklestein.[42]

TTP tends to be a rather grim disease. In the series of 271 cases reported by Amorosi and Ultmann[16] the majority of patients died within 3 months, and the mortality 1 year from onset was approximately 95%. However, despite lack of agreement on optimal treatment, the current prognosis of TTP may be considerably better. For example, in their survey of childhood TTP in a large number of institutions in the United States and Canada Berman and Finklestein[42] reported seven of twelve children surviving 3 to 32 months from onset of TTP. Treatment variously consisted of supportive care alone, corticosteriods alone, and combinations of corticosteriods, splenectomy, heparin, aspirin, and dipyridamole.

Other microangiopathic hemolytic diseases.
Although HUS and TTP represent classical examples of microangiopathy, similar platelet and red cell changes may be observed in a variety of other disorders. These include immunologic diseases, disseminated malignancy, and DIC. Various types of surgical cardiac repair may also cause red cell fragmentation similar to that seen in microangiopathy ("Waring blender" syndrome).

Decreased or ineffective production of platelets

The following disorders are discussed elsewhere in this book and are primarily listed here for the sake of completeness. Thrombocytopenia is a variably significant component of these disorders and may or may not be associated with purpura, depending on the platelet count in a given instance.

1. Idiopathic aplastic anemia (Chapter 17)
2. Neoplastic replacement of marrow: Leukemia (all types) and metastatic tumors (Chapter 21)
3. Myelosuppressive disorders: infections and chemical or physical agents (Chapter 16)
4. Ineffective thrombopoiesis: megaloblastic anemia and iron-deficiency anemia (Chapters 6 and 7)

Certain aspects of these disorders warrant further brief comments. First, although most myelotoxic agents produce generalized marrow depression with pancytopenia, specific depression of platelet production has been attributed to derivatives of thiazide diuretics,[231] diethylstilbestrol,[79] and alcohol.[325] Second, although thrombocytopenia may be associated with iron-deficiency anemia, the platelet count in this disorder is more commonly normal or elevated. Whether such thrombocytopenia is a result of iron lack itself or of associated folic acid deficiency is not entirely clear, but it is clear that the platelet count normalizes with correction of the anemia. Third, although specific mechanisms may be difficult to identify in thrombocytopenia associated with certain infections, decreased thrombopoiesis may well be interwoven with decreased platelet survival in most instances. Above all, the primary emphasis should be directed at management of the infection rather than the mechanism of the thrombocytopenia.

Hypoplastic thrombocytopenia. Acquired hypoplastic thrombocytopenia is an uncommon disorder characterized by chronic hypomegakaryocytic thrombocytopenia without associated erythroid or myeloid marrow defects or congenital anomalies. In most if not all instances these findings do not constitute a distinct entity such as hypoplastic anemia (Diamond-Blackfan anemia) but rather a phase in the evolution of aplastic anemia with ultimate pancytopenia.[308] Treatment should be limited to supportive measures insofar as possible and an emphasis placed on watchful waiting.

Cyclic thrombocytopenia. Physiologic variation in the platelet count has been documented in a majority of normal women[324] and in some normal men.[284] In premenopausal women the count begins to fall 2 weeks before menstruation, reaches its lowest point at the onset of menstruation, and rises to its highest level 2 weeks thereafter. Occasionally a similar variation in platelet counts in men has been recorded with cycles of 3 to 7 weeks.

Pathologic cyclic thrombocytopenia with purpura has been observed in women at the time of menstruation[281] and at midcycle.[383] In these instances megakaryocytic hypoplasia was not noted. On the other hand, cyclic thrombocytopenia has been described in a few men in whom corresponding cyclic hypoplasia of megakaryocytes was also observed.[114,444]

Cyclic thrombocytopenia may be sharply differentiated from recurrent ITP by the finding of normal platelet survival, measurement of which should be carried out if differentiation of these disorders is required. However, possible overlapping of cyclic thrombocytopenia and ITP is suggested by the report by Pepper et al.[320] of highest and lowest platelet counts occurring at ovulation and at menstruation, respectively, in women with ITP.

The existence of physiologic variation in the platelet count underscores the probable operation of factors regulating thrombopoiesis. These factors are poorly understood at the present time. Thus it is not yet clear whether pathologic cyclic thrombocytopenia represents an amplified ''norm'' in certain persons or specific derangement of one or more regulatory factors. So far descriptions of cyclic thrombocytopenia have been limited to adults.

Abnormal distribution of platelets

Diseases associated with splenomegaly. Aster[20] has shown that the spleen normally contains about one third of the total platelet mass. In conditions associated with splenic enlargement the spleen may sequester as much as 90% of the body's platelets. The resulting platelet count varies, presumably in accord with the degree of compensatory platelet production. In typical cases the count ranges from 50 to 150×10^9/liter and purpura is rarely evident. In these instances thrombocytopenia is not associated with qualitative platelet defects, megakaryocytes in marrow aspirates range from normal to increased, and platelet survival is either normal or slightly decreased.[78,159]

Aside from liver disease producing portal hypertension, thalassemia major (Cooley's anemia), congenital dyserythropoietic anemia, and Gau-

cher's disease are examples of disorders in children in which thrombocytopenia may result from splenic sequestration of platelets. Such thrombocytopenia should be clearly distinguished from sequestration of antibody-coated platelets by the normal-sized spleen in ITP and related disorders.

Thrombocytopenia directly related to splenomegaly is generally relieved by splenectomy. However, the decision regarding splenectomy should be based on overall indications pertinent to the underlying disease and not necessarily on the thrombocytopenia alone.

Liver disease. Hepatic disorders, both inflammatory and degenerative, should be specifically identified as a major childhood cause of portal hypertension leading to splenomegaly with thrombocytopenia caused by platelet sequestration. In some instances an abnormal liver may conceivably sequester platelets itself, but such a role, if it exists, is minor compared to that of an enlarged spleen. Above all, it should be emphasized that the indirect contribution of liver disease to platelet sequestration is only one of several mechanisms by which a deranged liver may produce hemostatic defects. Indeed, these other defects, such as decreased hepatic production of coagulation factors, are generally far more critical than platelet sequestration.

INHERITED THROMBOCYTOPENIC PURPURA
Decreased production of platelets

Fanconi's anemia. Although Fanconi's anemia is discussed in detail in Chapter 17, this disorder should be firmly identified as a major cause of heritable thrombocytopenic purpura resulting from decreased production of platelets. Fanconi's anemia is an uncommon autosomal recessive disease that occurs twice as often in males as in females.[155] In its fully expressed form and in accord with the original description of the disorder by Fanconi[120] in 1927, it is characterized by the association of bone marrow failure and pancytopenia with variable congenital anomalies, most commonly affecting the musculoskeletal and genitourinary systems. Although the congenital anomalies are evident at birth, pancytopenia typically is delayed for 5 or more years. Thrombocytopenic purpura may be the first expression of progressive bone marrow failure. Combined therapy with androgens and corticosteroids is widely used in Fanconi's anemia, but this treatment generally affects erythropoiesis more favorably than thrombopoiesis. Indeed, thrombocytopenic hemorrhage, particularly intracranial, is a major cause of death in Fanconi's anemia.

Thrombocytopenia with absent radius syndrome. In 1969 Hall et al.[155] presented a detailed

Table 24-3. Comparison of Fanconi's anemia and TAR syndrome*

	Fanconi's anemia	Thrombocytopenia with absent radius (TAR) syndrome
Inheritance	Autosomal recessive	Autosomal recessive
Male:female ratio	2:1	1:2
Absence of both radii with fingers and thumbs present	0%	100%
Nonmusculoskeletal congenital anomalies	Frequent	Rare
Chromosome breaks in leukocytes	Increased	None
Onset of hematologic signs (usual)	5-10 years	Birth or early infancy
Blood findings	Pancytopenia	Thrombocytopenia and leukemoid reactions, with or without blood-loss anemia
Marrow findings	Panmyelopathy	Decreased or defective megakaryocytes
Prognosis	Poor	Relatively good after first year of life

*Modified from Hall, J. G., Levin, J., Kuhn, J. P., et al.: Medicine **48:**411, 1969.

analysis of forty cases of a syndrome consistently characterized by thrombocytopenia and *bilateral* absence of the radii. These cases were drawn both from the literature and the authors' own experience. In most instances megakaryocytes were decreased or absent in bone marrow aspirates. The authors carefully distinguished this syndrome, designated by the abbreviation "TAR syndrome," from other superficially similar hypomegakaryocytic thrombocytopenias, including Fanconi's anemia, trisomy 18, and congenital defects induced by teratogenic drugs and infections. Particularly important differences as well as similarities between TAR syndrome and Fanconi's anemia are summarized in Table 24-3.

In general the finding of thrombocytopenic purpura and bilateral absence of the radii in an infant, with or without other congenital anomalies, establishes the diagnosis of TAR syndrome. However, a bone marrow aspirate should be obtained to assess megakaryocytes, which are typically decreased in number. Although it may be appropriate to classify TAR syndrome as a disorder of decreased thrombopoiesis, it should be noted that functional defects caused by a lack of platelet ADP content (storage pool disease) have been described in at least two cases.[97,398]

Myeloid hyperplasia of the marrow is not unusual, and impressive peripheral leukocytosis may be observed, especially in the early months of life. Indeed, the white cell count may fluctuate over a wide range, at times suggesting leukemia with levels of 100×10^9/liter or more as well as increased numbers of immature forms.

It should be emphasized that the prognosis of TAR syndrome may be rather favorable with respect to thrombocytopenic purpura if the affected infant survives the first year of life. There is no evidence that corticosteroids are beneficial, and splenectomy should be avoided. However, supportive component therapy with red cells for blood-loss anemia and platelet concentrates for thrombocytopenic hemorrhage are helpful and should be vigorously instituted as needed.

Other hypomegakaryocytic purpuras. Of the several disorders in which thrombocytopenia may be attributed to hypoplasia of megakaryocytes, Fanconi's anemia and TAR syndrome appear to be the best established as to a genetic origin. Other such disorders associated with congenital anomalies largely represent specific chromosomal defects or fetal insults from certain drugs and infections. However, Estren and Dameshek[116] reported familial aplastic anemia and pancytopenia without congenital anomalies. These issues will be further considered in the discussion of neonatal thrombocytopenia.

Congenital deficiency of thrombopoietin. In 1959 Schulman et al.[357] reported a truly remarkable and so far unique female subject with onset in infancy of chronic thrombocytopenia consistently responding to infusions of whole plasma. Continuing studies of this patient showed that her disorder, as well as the response to plasma, persisted into adulthood.[2] Her megakaryocytes were normal in quantity although suggestively immature at times of thrombocytopenia. Plasma infusions were predictably associated with a return of her platelet count to normal for about 2 weeks, along with corresponding maturation of megakaryocytes. Laboratory investigations suggested that the patient lacked an α_2-globulin required for megakaryocytic maturation and platelet production.[356,359] It was postulated that her response might represent replacement of a thrombopoietin-like substance.

A possible hereditary basis for such a disorder was tenuously supported by an anecdotal report of "several" members of a Chilean family with chronic thrombocytopenia similarly responsive to plasma infusions.[414]

Increased destruction of defective platelets

Wiskott-Aldrich syndrome. Wiskott-Aldrich syndrome is a rare sex-linked recessive disorder characterized by (1) chronic thrombocytopenic purpura, (2) eczema, and (3) increased incidence of recurrent infections.

The syndrome was first described by Wiskott in 1937 and independently by Aldrich, et al.[10] in 1954. The sex-linked mode of its inheritance was first identified by Aldrich et al.,[10] and this is now fully established.[81,145,452] The names of Wiskott and Aldrich have been jointly linked to this syndrome since the early 1960s.[135] Wiskott-Aldrich syndrome is now known to be an immunodeficiency disorder with thrombocytopenia as well as humoral and cellular abnormalities, but there is not yet a hypothesis that satisfactorily explains both its immunologic and hematologic components.[228,343]

Clinical features. Wiskott-Aldrich syndrome becomes clinically evident in affected boys during early infancy with onset of thrombocytopenic purpura, atopic dermatitis, and frequent viral and bacterial infections ranging from minor upper respiratory illnesses to sepsis and meningitis. Specific problems often observed include bloody diarrhea, epistaxis, recurrent otitis media (often with chronic tympanic perforation and drainage), and anemia related both to blood loss and to effects of frequent infections.* An increased incidence of malignancy in Wiskott-Aldrich syndrome is recognized, particularly lymphoma.[402] (See p. 569.)

Physical examination of affected patients typically reveals petechial purpura, generalized eczema, variable enlargement of the liver and spleen, and evidence of infection, particularly draining otitis media. In addition, any complication of thrombocytopenic hemorrhage or infection may be encountered.[27,338] The significance of the association of Wiskott-Aldrich syndrome and infantile cortical hyperostosis in two cases remains to be determined.[263]

Laboratory evaluation. Major laboratory findings are as follows: (1) blood counts usually reveal significant thrombocytopenia with small infrequent platelets on the smear, relative lymphopenia, and, depending on blood loss and characteristics of infection, a variable normocytic normochromic anemia with little or no reticulocytosis; (2) bone mar-

row examination should reveal adequate numbers of megakaryocytes, which may show a variety of bizarre nuclear abnormalities[318]; and (3) levels of IgG and IgA are normal or increased, but IgM levels are low, specifically the titers of antibodies (isohemagglutinins) against A and B blood groups.

Differential diagnosis. Major disorders from which Wiskott-Aldrich syndrome should be differentiated include disseminated histiocytosis X of infancy (Letterer-Siwe disease) and other heritable purpuras and immunodeficiency syndromes. A biopsy of affected skin showing no characteristic histiocytic infiltration should generally separate Wiskott-Aldrich syndrome from Letterer-Siwe disease. Other immunodeficiencies and purpuras may be differentiated from Wiskott-Aldrich syndrome in most cases by absence of key components of the diagnostic triad.

Immunology. Although a detailed discussion of the immunologic defects in Wiskott-Aldrich syndrome is beyond the scope of this chapter (see Chapter 20), major characteristics should be cited. These include (1) inability to form antibodies against polysaccharide antigens, e.g., A and B blood group and Forssman antigens, and (2) progressive deterioration of thymus-dependent cellular immunity manifested by increasing relative lymphopenia and depletion of lymphocytes in the paracortical areas of lymph nodes.[46,81]

Pathogenesis. The thrombocytopenia of Wiskott-Aldrich syndrome may be largely ascribed to increased destruction of qualitatively abnormal platelets. The intrinsic defect has been shown to be the result of a lack of ADP and ATP in the dense granules of platelets and is characterized by deficient energy release and by impaired second-phase platelet aggregation in response to ADP, collagen, and epinephrine.[29,152,229] Survival of autologous platelets is significantly shortened as a result of their excessive removal by the reticuloendothelial system, whereas survival of homologous platelets is normal.[152,318] Pearson et al.[318] have shown striking morphologic changes in numerous megakaryocytes of persons with Wiskott-Aldrich syndrome and suggested that impaired thrombopoiesis may contribute to the thrombocytopenia of this disorder. Indeed, the small platelets characteristic of Wiskott-Aldrich syndrome, in contrast to the larger platelets seen in thrombocytopenic states with effective thrombopoiesis (e.g., ITP), may possibly reflect abnormal platelet production.

Management. Treatment of Wiskott-Aldrich syndrome is limited to supportive care with appropriate management of recurrent infections and blood component therapy. A graft-versus-host reaction has been observed as a presumed result of infusion of viable lymphocytes in blood prod-

---

*References 196, 219, 342, 391.

ucts into a patient with Wiskott-Aldrich syndrome.[110] Irradiation of blood products should be considered before their use, particularly in older children with severely compromised cellular immunity.

Topical corticosteroids may be used judiciously to control eczema, but systemic use of these agents should be avoided, both because there is no real evidence that they are useful and because existing immunodeficiency may be aggravated. Likewise, splenectomy should be avoided because whatever benefits it may offer in terms of platelet survival appear to be offset by increased risks of postsplenectomy sepsis.[196,318] Stiehm et al.[395] found that periodic infusions of fresh plasma designed to replace deficient IgM in patients with Wiskott-Aldrich syndrome appeared to decrease the incidence of recurrent infection.

In recent years two new avenues of treatment have been explored: infusion of "transfer factor" derived from dialysis of normal lymphocytes[390] and bone marrow transplantation.[26,276] Although a final assessment of the value of these approaches is not yet possible, it appears that they are helpful for immunologic but not for thrombocytopenic components of Wiskott-Aldrich syndrome.

Prognosis. The prognosis of Wiskott-Aldrich syndrome is poor. Most affected children die of infection or hemorrhage in the early years of life, but rarely patients may survive into adulthood.[271] Canales and Mauer[66] have described a relatively mild sex-linked form of thrombocytopenic purpura that they suggested might be a variant of Wiskott-Aldrich syndrome on the basis of increased IgA levels and decreased isohemagglutinin titers. It is not yet clear whether Wiskott-Aldrich syndrome is, after all, a consistently severe disease or whether it actually encompasses cases with a spectrum of severity.

Disorders with giant platelets

May-Hegglin anomaly. May-Hegglin anomaly is a rare autosomal dominant disorder characterized by giant platelets, leukocytic inclusions resembling Döhle bodies, and a variable bleeding tendency.[169,313] About one third of affected persons are thrombocytopenic, but a prolonged bleeding time is typical. Survival of autologous platelets was found to be decreased in two cases.[95] The platelet defect in this disorder has not been fully characterized.

Bernard-Soulier syndrome. Bernard-Soulier syndrome is a rare autosomal and incompletely recessive hemorrhagic disorder of considerable severity, characterized by large platelets that superficially resemble lymphocytes.[43] The majority of affected patients are thrombocytopenic and in these decreased platelet survival has been noted.[298] The bleeding disorder is not benefited by cortico-

steroid therapy or splenectomy and should be controlled by appropriate blood component therapy as indicated. The Bernard-Soulier "giant platelet" syndrome, though rare, is of great importance among qualitative platelet disorders because it has yielded greatly to recent investigations.

Conventional laboratory studies reveal, in addition to giant platelets on the smear and a mild to moderate thrombocytopenia, a consistently prolonged bleeding time and decreased platelet adhesiveness but normal clot retraction. A critical discovery was made in 1973 by Howard et al.,[193] who observed that platelets in Bernard-Soulier syndrome were not aggregated in response to ristocetin or a fraction of bovine fibrinogen containing factor VIII. First- and second-phase aggregation induced by other agents was largely normal. Howard and Firkin[192] had previously shown that ristocetin-induced platelet aggregation is dependent on factor VIII–associated protein. The presence of normal concentrations of this protein in the plasma of patients with Bernard-Soulier syndrome as well as the lack of response to bovine factor VIII[109] clearly separate the platelet defect in this syndrome from the plasma defect in von Willebrand's disease. More recent studies have indicated that the platelets in Bernard-Soulier syndrome lack a critical receptor site for factor VIII–associated protein.[203]

Other giant platelet disorders. A variety of less familiar inherited disorders characterized by giant platelets and thrombocytopenia have also been described. Most of these are autosomal dominant or sporadic,* but autosomal recessive disorders have also been reported.[87,294] Furthermore, the following disorders characterized by rather specific findings have been described: "gray platelet" syndrome,[330] "Swiss cheese" platelets,[387] and hereditary syndrome of giant platelets, nephritis, and deafness.[115] In general the underlying defects in these disorders, as in the May-Hegglin anomaly, have not yet been fully characterized or classified.

Disorders with morphologically normal platelets.

In the discussion of possible factors in ITP, a variety of hereditary disorders resembling ITP were cited. Proof that these are in fact ITP clearly depends on demonstration of decreased survival of intrinsically normal platelets, as well as an immunologic basis for their increased destruction. The future application of appropriate laboratory techniques will clearly help sort out this group of thrombocytopenias. An autosomal dominant disorder with thrombocytopenia caused by an intrinsic defect with decreased survival of autologous plate-

---

*References 25, 153, 230, 304.

lets appears to be well established in the cases reported by Murphy et al.[291]

NEONATAL THROMBOCYTOPENIC PURPURAS

Neonatal thrombocytopenia, like that at any age, may either be acquired or inherited and may be primarily the result of either increased platelet destruction or impaired production. However, it seems more appropriate to consider neonatal thrombocytopenia in a separate category because of the unique role of maternal factors in two major types of disease: (1) immunologic thrombocytopenia caused by maternal isoantibodies or autoantibodies and (2) congenital infections, exemplified by rubella. Furthermore, neonatal thrombocytopenias may be usefully, if not perfectly, divided on clinical grounds into disorders that usually *are not* associated with hepatosplenomegaly (notably immunologic disorders) and those that usually *are* associated with hepatosplenomegaly (notably infectious disorders). This classification will be used in the discussion to follow, but it must be remembered that an unyielding commitment to rigid diagnostic categories is unwise in dealing with any age group, perhaps newborns most of all.

Given a newborn with thrombocytopenic purpura without significant plasma coagulation abnormalities, the following general elements must always be considered: (1) *the infant*—presence or absence of hepatosplenomegaly, congenital anomalies, and signs of systemic illness, notably sepsis; (2) *the mother*—platelet count and appearance of her blood smear, past and current history of hematologic and infectious disease, complete drug history, and physical evidence of infection transmissible to the infant; and (3) *family history*—presence or absence of parental consanguinity and hematologic disease in family members. Finally, it should be emphasized that absence of significant plasma coagulation abnormalities on a single blood sample never precludes the appearance of such an abnormality in due course. This issue is discussed in the section on coagulation disorders of the newborn in Chapter 25.

Neonatal purpuras without hepatosplenomegaly

Immunologic disorders

Isoimmune neonatal thrombocytopenic purpura. Isoimmune purpura is an acquired hemorrhagic disorder in an otherwise normal newborn infant characterized by thrombocytopenic purpura in the infant, a normal maternal platelet count, and evidence for maternal IgG isoantibodies against a fetal platelet antigen not present in maternal platelets. Isoimmune purpura is thus analogous to neonatal isoimmune hemolytic anemia caused by fetal-maternal incompatibility of red cell antigens.

HISTORICAL PERSPECTIVE. Purpura in the newborn was apparently first recognized as a distinct entity by Dohrn[108] in 1873. Investigative interest in this disorder was largely dormant until an immunologic basis for neonatal purpura in certain instances was demonstrated 80 years later through the pioneering work of Harrington et al.[162] and Schulman et al.[359] Thereafter Schulman et al.[358] used sensitive techniques to apply maternal isoantibodies to the definition of certain platelet antigens. In a comprehensive report in 1964 Pearson et al.[317] described the diagnosis and management of isoimmune purpura involving three platelet antigens: a specific platelet antigen (Pl[A1]) in four families and two antigens shared with leukocytes (PlGrLy[B1] and PlGrLy[C1], now known to be transplantation antigens) in one family each. Additional specific platelet antigens that have been discovered through maternal isoimmunization include DUZO[a], the first platelet antigen to be discovered,[289] and Pl[E2].[373] Although the ABO antigens of the red cell may be present on platelets as well,[21] thrombocytopenia is not a recognized component of isoimmune disease caused by ABO incompatibility.

Of all the currently known platelet antigens, Pl[A1] appears to be the most important in relation to frequency and severity of isoimmune purpura.[265] This is the same platelet antigen implicated in most of the reported cases of posttransfusion purpura in adults.

CLASSIFICATION. In those specialized centers where typing of the platelet antigens and quantitative measurement of platelet antibodies can be performed, isoimmune purpura may be classified according to the specific fetal-maternal incompatibility involved. Classification of this disorder according to its clinical expression is not helpful.

INCIDENCE. Pearson et al.[317] have pointed out that isoimmune purpura occurs in about 1/5,000 births, although the overall chance of fetal-maternal incompatibility is about 1/3 births on the basis of the frequency of the several platelet antigens in the general population. Furthermore, they estimated that absence of maternal hematologic disease occurs only in about 20% of cases of neonatal purpura. It is, of course, in this group that isoimmune thrombocytopenia may be suspected.

In the general population the estimated frequencies of platelet antigens that have been associated with maternal isoimmunization are as follows[369]: Pl[A1], 98%; PlGrLy[B1] (HLA-A2), 46%; PlGrLy[C1], 30%; DUZO[a], 22%; and Pl[E2], 5%.

Like red cell isoimmunization caused by ABO incompatibility but unlike that caused by Rh incompatibility, isoimmune purpura occurs with the first pregnancy in about 50% of cases, even without previous sensitization by blood products. In general, once this disease has appeared in a particular family, it is appropriate to be prepared for its recurrence. However, subsequent newborns may not be thrombocytopenic despite fetal-maternal platelet incompatibility and persistence of maternal isoantibodies.[317] This inconsistency, as well as the discrepancy between the potential and observed incidence of isoimmune purpura, underscores the importance of poorly understood factors in the etiology of this disease.

ETIOLOGY. Isoimmune purpura is caused by maternal isoantibodies of the IgG variety that cross the placenta and attach to specific platelet antigens of the fetus, resulting in their increased destruction, as in ITP. Isoimmune purpura is therefore a classical example of an acquired disease with genetic determinants.

GENETICS. Platelet antigens, like red cell antigens, are inherited as autosomal dominant characteristics. Maternal isoimmunization resulting from fetal-maternal incompatibility may occur only when fetal platelets possess an antigen inherited from the father that is not present on maternal platelets. If a father is homozygous for a given platelet antigen that the mother lacks, all children would be heterozygous for this gene and the chance for maternal isoimmunization would be 100% with each pregnancy. On the other hand, if the father is heterozygous, the chance for maternal isoimmunization with each pregnancy would be 50%.

Again, it should be emphasized that the genetic determination of fetal-maternal platelet incompatibility is only one step, and a relatively small one at that, toward the development of isoimmune purpura in a given infant.

CLINICAL FEATURES. The typical newborn with isoimmune purpura, like the child with ITP, is healthy and shows no abnormalities on physical examination except for randomly distributed and variable petechial purpura. Depending on the circumstances of delivery, there may be exaggerated purpura in areas subjected to trauma, including rapid development of a cephalhematoma, neck and facial petechiae, and large ecchymoses. Purpura is usually evident at birth but may be slightly delayed. In any case, it should be strongly emphasized that purpura that does not appear within the first 24 hours of life should generally never be attributed to an immunologic disorder without first considering other causes, notably infection.

As in the case of ITP, the newborn with isoimmune purpura may show signs of bleeding other than purpura. These include hematuria, upper and lower gastrointestinal tract hemorrhage, prolonged bleeding from the umbilical stump or from heel sticks and venipunctures, and signs of intracranial hemorrhage.

Within 48 hours of life significant, unexplainable jaundice may be observed in affected newborns. Pearson et al.[317] have suggested that such jaundice may be related to an increased bilirubin load from the natural disposition of interstitial blood, as reported by Rausen and Diamond.[334]

Isoimmune purpura tends to be a benign disease, clearing spontaneously within a few weeks and surely within the first 3 months of life. However, as in ITP, intracranial hemorrhage constitutes the one clearly dangerous complication of this disease and is associated with a mortality of about 12%.[317] The clinician should be immediately alerted by an indication of central nervous system disease, ranging from subtle changes in vital signs to jitteriness and convulsions.

LABORATORY EVALUATION. Studies should be carried out first of the infant and then the mother. Minimum initial investigations in each case should include a platelet count, inspection of the blood smear, routine blood counts, and measurement of the one-stage clottings tests—TCT, PT, and PTT. Typically all of these tests are within normal limits except for a platelet count below $50 \times 10^9/$liter in the infant, confirmed by decreased platelets on smear.

Examination of the bone marrow may be less helpful for the diagnosis of isoimmune purpura in newborns than it is for ITP in older children. In general the marrow should show normal megakaryocytes and reactive erythroid hyperplasia. However, marrow aspiration is technically difficult in newborns and findings in isoimmune purpura may be confusing. For example, even in competent hands, marrow aspirates in this disorder may on occasion show no megakaryocytes at all.[317]

Although isoimmune purpura may be suspected in a thrombocytopenic but otherwise normal newborn whose mother has a normal platelet count and no history of hematologic disease, confirmation ultimately rests on appropriate serologic findings. These findings, utilizing serum and whole blood samples from the mother and infant and preferably the father as well, should show the following: (1) presence in the infant's and father's platelets of an antigen lacking in maternal platelets; (2) presence in maternal serum of an IgG antibody specifically directed against this antigen; and (3) ideally the direct demonstration of IgG antibody on the infant's platelets. Over the past three decades analogous testing for neonatal isoimmune hemolytic anemia has become routinely available in blood banks of most community hospitals. However, serologic testing of platelets is an extremely demanding art as well as a science and is available only at certain centers with specific commitments to such work, largely on a research basis. Such a center should be identified by the clinician faced with a case of possible isoimmune purpura and an appropriate workup negotiated. Settlement of the diagnosis will be retrospectively useful for the infant in question, but of more importance is that it provides objective information for parental counseling.

Shulman et al.[372,373] have described their definitive investigations on serologic characteristics of isoimmune purpura. They utilized sensitive complement fixation techniques and reviewed other methods as well as overall problems in serologic studies of platelets. More recently introduced techniques for measuring platelet antibodies include direct assay of platelet-bound IgG,[104] estimation of platelet-associated IgG,[270] and measurement of antibody-induced release of platelet serotonin,[180] release of platelet factor 3,[214] and stimulation of lymphocytes by platelet antigen-antibody complexes.[455]

DIFFERENTIAL DIAGNOSIS. In the most obvious sense neonatal isoimmune purpura must be differentiated from immunologic purpura caused by maternal autoantibodies, most frequently related to maternal ITP. Most neonatal purpuras caused by impaired platelet production are associated with obvious congenital anomalies, notably TAR syndrome. However, it is particularly important not to overlook other causes of thrombocytopenia, such as incompletely evolved DIC and treatable infections such as bacterial sepsis. Indeed, at the same time that blood is being obtained for a platelet count and clotting studies, a sample for blood culture should be obtained.

PATHOGENESIS AND PATHOPHYSIOLOGY. Desai et al.[99] have shown that fetal platelets may enter the maternal circulation during pregnancy. When these fetal platelets are incompatible with maternal platelets, isoimmunization may occur. If the resulting maternal isoantibodies are of the incomplete IgG variety, the fetal platelets may become bound by these antibodies, which are known to cross the placenta.[141] There is particularly clear evidence for the IgG character of anti-Pl[A1] associated with isoimmune purpura. In all of seventeen maternal samples obtained in instances of this disorder, Shulman[373] found that the isoantibodies did not fix complement themselves but instead blocked the effects of complement-fixing antibodies known to have the same antigen specificity. Such interference with complement fixation is a characteristic of IgG.

Once maternal IgG isoantibodies cross the placenta and attach to the platelets of the fetus, the subsequent pathophysiology of isoimmune purpura is identical to that of ITP. However, the termination of the disease is of course much more predictable. Since isoimmune purpura is the result of a given load of maternal IgG with a half-time of no more than a month, there is no such thing as "chronic" or even "recurrent" isoimmune purpura. Within 3 months the disease should be gone forever.

PATHOLOGY. In those infants who die of isoimmune purpura, the principal pathologic finding is intracranial hemorrhage along with generalized and variable extravasations. As in ITP, there are no specific characteristics of such hemorrhage.

MANAGEMENT. Usually neonatal isoimmune purpura is an uncomplicated disorder requiring only routine newborn care. Even so, discharge of an affected infant should be deferred until overall clinical stability and absence of significant complications have been clearly established over a period of about 1 week. Unfortunately a disturbing number of infants suffer from major hemorrhagic complications, of which intracranial hemorrhage is by far the most serious. Indeed, the ultimate intent of all specific measures for treatment of isoimmune purpura should be to prevent or control intracranial hemorrhage. There is no uniform agreement on management in this regard. The following suggestions, assembled from limited published data and personal preferences, are offered for consideration.

In cases in which impending delivery is combined with a history of proved or strongly suspected isoimmune purpura in a previous newborn, it is wisest to assume that the disease will recur and prepare accordingly. Major ingredients of such preparations should include the following: (1) if it has not already been done, maternal and paternal platelets should be typed and maternal serum tested for isoantibodies in an appropriate center; (2) potential donors who have the same platelet type as the mother should be identified if possible; (3) the willingness as well as the fitness of the mother to donate platelets herself in the postnatal period should be established; (4) in accord with the findings of Pearson et al.,[317] prednisone may be administered to the mother beginning 48 hours before delivery in a dose of 60 mg/m^2/day.

On delivery the infant may prove to be normal, to have very mild thrombocytopenia, or to be severely purpuric with or without signs of intracranial hemorrhage. If the infant is not thrombocytopenic, no problem exists. If the infant is mildly affected, prednisone may be administered for 2 weeks in a dose of 60 mg/m^2/day and then stopped. If the infant is severely affected, the most feasible of the following steps may be considered. The ideal course would be to perform an exchange transfusion with fresh whole blood from a type O donor whose platelets are known by previous cross matching not to react with the maternal isoantibody. On the other hand, a more realistic first move would be to give transfusion with a unit of washed platelets obtained from the mother by plasmapheresis. The finding of normal platelet recovery and survival thereafter would serve a diagnostic as well as a therapeutic purpose.[8,265] As a final option, if maternal platelets are unavailable, an exchange transfusion may be performed with whole blood from a random donor cross matched for red cell compatibility only. Obviously, the options are determined by the availability of blood products.

Following platelet transfusion or exchange transfusion prednisone may be administered to the infant according to the schedule noted above. If continuing or new bleeding is a problem in mildly or severely affected infants, support with platelet concentrates, preferably from the mother, may be instituted as needed. Assuming that 1 unit of compatible platelets/m² body surface should produce a platelet increment of about 10×10^9/liter then 1 unit of maternal platelets should raise the average infant's platelet count to about 50×10^9/liter. Such an increment would not be expected, of course, from the platelets obtained from a random donor.

If isoimmune purpura is suspected in a newborn in whom it was not expected, these suggestions may be considered if the infant is severely affected, particularly if there are signs suggesting intracranial hemorrhage. However, if the child is mildly affected, it may be wiser not to institute corticosteroid therapy and to observe the infant closely instead. In such an instance the possibility of infection should never be overlooked, even if the infant does not appear sick.

Although splenectomy has been performed in treatment of neonatal purpura,[48] this should be avoided at all costs in view of the marked risk of postsplenectomy sepsis at this age.[381] Cyclophosphamide, azathioprine, and vincristine sulfate are generally tried in immunologic thrombocytopenias well after other measures have failed and probably have no place in the treatment of isoimmune purpura.

Finally the occurrence of nonspecific hyperbilirubinemia in some infants with isoimmune purpura has already been cited. Usually this complication is not sufficient to warrant exchange transfusion. Jaundice is distinct from the immediate problems of thrombocytopenia and should be approached in a conventional fashion.

PROGNOSIS. As previously noted, intracranial hemorrhage is largely responsible for a mortality of about 12% in isoimmune purpura.[317] This estimate contrasts strikingly with a mortality of about 1% in ITP. Furthermore, there may be a significant incidence of variable brain damage in those infants who survive.[382]

FUTURE PERSPECTIVES. Reliable diagnosis and prompt treatment of isoimmune purpura are severely handicapped by the major problems that beset serologic studies of platelets. Not the least of these problems is the scarcity of centers properly qualified to perform and interpret the rather complex techniques now available. The prospects for substantial remedies are not entirely clear at this time.

Thrombocytopenias caused by maternal autoantibodies. Although substantial discussion has been devoted to isoimmune purpura in the newborn, it should be emphasized that maternal disease associated with circulating IgG autoantibodies is a more common cause of neonatal purpura. The major disease in this group is maternal chronic ITP, which has been estimated to be responsible for about 80% of all cases of neonatal immunologic purpura.[48] Furthermore, about 80% of thrombocytopenic mothers deliver thrombocytopenic newborns[400]; about 20% of mothers with a normal platelet count but a past history of ITP relieved by splenectomy may even be expected to deliver thrombocytopenic newborns.[175] Another possible cause of neonatal thrombocytopenia is maternal systemic lupus erythematosus.[299] Maternal immunologic thrombocytopenia related to certain drugs, notably quinine, may be associated with neonatal purpura,[259] but this appears to be extremely rare.

Although laboratory identification of maternal autoantibodies may be difficult, a clinical diagnosis of neonatal thrombocytopenia caused by such antibodies is relatively simple. In contrast to isoimmune purpura, in which there is no maternal thrombocytopenia, the mother's platelet count is low or there should be a history of ITP or some other disease known to be associated with immunologic thrombocytopenia. In rare cases neonatal thrombocytopenia may actually antedate the clinical and laboratory appearance of maternal thrombocytopenia.

The discussion of the clinical picture and management of isoimmune purpura is largely applicable to neonatal purpura caused by maternal autoantibodies with one major exception. Platelet autoantibodies will attach to *all* platelets and therefore a search for "compatible" platelets is out of order. Indeed, in contrast to the situation in isoimmune purpura, the mother would be the most unsuitable donor of all. Thus, if signs of intracranial hemorrhage develop in an affected infant, whole blood for exchange transfusion or platelet concentrates should be obtained from random donors.

Nonimmunologic disorders
Infections. Neonatal thrombocytopenia as a re-

sult of infections is most typically associated with hepatosplenomegaly or plasma coagulation abnormalities. However, it should be emphasized that any infection, bacterial or otherwise, may be characterized by thrombocytopenia without any other abnormalities. For example, I have recently seen mild and transient thrombocytopenic purpura in an otherwise healthy newborn delivered by a healthy mother, in both of whom a diagnosis of cytomegalovirus infection was established.

Congenital malformations. Evaluation of thrombocytopenia in the newborn must include a careful search for congenital malformations, although usually they are rather obvious. The major examples of these are TAR syndrome and rubella syndrome. As previously noted, Fanconi's anemia may include neonatal thrombocytopenic purpura as well as characteristic anomalies, but hematologic defects usually do not appear until about 5 or more years of age. Thrombocytopenia has been described in newborns with trisomy 18[72,256a,329] and trisomy 13[272] syndromes.

Thrombotic disorders. Thrombosis of both large and small blood vessels may be associated with neonatal thrombocytopenia without significant plasma coagulation abnormalities. A representative example of large vessel disease is renal vein thrombosis.[209] Although HUS is the classical microangiopathic disease of childhood, it is rare in newborns. A more frequently encountered neonatal disease affecting the microvasculature is the syndrome of necrotizing enterocolitis, which is frequently associated with thrombocytopenia, sometimes severe.[394] The syndrome of disseminated intravascular and vegetative cardiac thrombosis in newborns has recently been described by Favara et al.[122] This interesting disorder, rather like TTP, is generally characterized by marked thrombocytopenia without the coagulation abnormalities diagnostic of DIC. The etiology of this disorder is unknown. Severe idiopathic respiratory distress syndrome in newborns may be also associated with thrombocytopenia, presumably related to diffuse microvascular thrombosis.[165]

Other disorders. In the absence of congenital anomalies a diagnosis of "congenital hypoplastic thrombocytopenia" based on isolated deficiency of megakaryocytes in a marrow aspirate is probably unacceptable, both because the apparent deficiency may be a result of technical difficulties and because, even with a good sample, such a deficiency may be associated with mechanisms of increased platelet destruction such as isoimmune purpura. In such instances it may be best to label the disorder ITP in its truest sense, support the infant in a general manner, and wait to see what happens. Such thrombocytopenia may clear up without explanation or may evolve into aplastic ane-

mia, either acquired[308] or familial[116] type. Authentic congenital hypoplastic thrombocytopenia without other abnormalities is vanishingly rare, if indeed it exists at all.

Maternal ingestion of tolbutamide[353] and thiazide diuretics[341] has been implicated in neonatal thrombocytopenia. However, recent studies suggest that thiazides may not play a causal role in this regard.[204,274] In general maternal drug ingestion appears to play a minor role in neonatal thrombocytopenias but may be more important in relation to functional platelet defects in the newborn.

Neonatal thrombocytopenia may occur in association with several other heterogeneous conditions. These include inherited metabolic diseases, i.e., methylmalonic acidemia[286] and isovaleric acidemia,[13] and hyperviscosity syndromes associated with abnormally high hematocrits in certain newborns.[165]

Neonatal purpuras with hepatosplenomegaly

Infectious diseases

Congenital rubella. Rubella is a classical example of an infection that may produce a constellation of disastrous effects in the fetus when transmitted by maternal infection in the first trimester of pregnancy. These effects are variable in surviving newborns but frequently comprise a syndrome with the following components: (1) congenital malformations, including cataracts, congenital heart disease, and deafness; (2) low birth weight reflecting intrauterine growth retardation; (3) signs of active infection, including pneumonitis and hepatitis with hepatosplenomegaly and jaundice; and (4) hematologic abnormalities, notably thrombocytopenic purpura.[80,345] Thrombocytopenic purpura may be an isolated manifestation of congenital rubella,[36] the so-called blueberry muffin baby syndrome.

The rubella virus may be recovered from the amniotic fluid and from placental and fetal tissues well after maternal infection has subsided.[11] Furthermore, the virus may persist in affected infants for several months after birth.[321]

The hematologic effects of congenital rubella have been summarized by Rausen et al.[335] and Zinkman et al.[462] Variable thrombocytopenia, often with purpura, is usually present in at least 50% of affected newborns.[80,345] Leukopenia and anemia with intermittent normoblastemia and reticulocytosis are frequently encountered as well. Examination of the bone marrow usually reveals decreased megakaryocytes and may show impressive phagocytosis of red cells and neutrophils by reticulum cells.[462] Recovery of rubella virus from marrow aspirates tends to correlate with severity of the infection.

The thrombocytopenia of congenital rubella is

self-limited, rarely persisting beyond 1 month. Life-threatening complications of thrombocytopenia such as intracranial hemorrhage are uncommon in congenital rubella, in contrast to neonatal immunologic purpuras. Supportive treatment with platelet concentrates or whole blood as needed is appropriate. However, corticosteroid therapy should be avoided since there is no evidence that it is helpful for the thrombocytopenia or for coping with the infection.

The mechanism of thrombocytopenia in congenital rubella is not well understood. The finding of megakaryocytic hypoplasia would suggest impaired platelet production, but increased destruction of platelets may well coexist or even predominate. Zinkham et al.[462] have pointed out that apparent absence of megakaryocytes may reflect technical problems in sampling rather than true absence of these cells.

Other infections. Aside from rubella, other congenital infections that may be characterized by thrombocytopenia and hepatosplenomegaly include cytomegalovirus disease, toxoplasmosis, and syphilis. Disseminated herpesvirus infection differs from these in that, instead of being an intrauterine infection, it is acquired by the infant by direct exposure to maternal herpetic vulvovaginitis during delivery. As for postnatal infections, thrombocytopenia and enlargement of the liver and spleen may be prominent features of bacterial sepsis.

All congenital infections, including rubella, may be associated with plasma coagulation abnormalities as well as thrombocytopenia, but, except for disseminated herpesvirus infection, this is not the rule. In the case of herpesvirus infection, which is frequently a lethal disease, isolated thrombocytopenia is not as common as a generalized coagulation disorder. (See Chapter 25.)

Noninfectious diseases

Congenital leukemia. In cases of congenital leukemia thrombocytopenic purpura and hepatosplenomegaly are usually present, but these findings are typically far overshadowed by direct evidence of leukemia. The total white cell count tends to be high, frequently over 50×10^9/liter, and blast cells generally make up the majority of the leukocytes seen on the blood smear. The bone marrow examination will confirm the diagnosis of leukemia in these instances, and megakaryocytes are usually markedly reduced or absent.

Isoimmune hemolytic disease. In addition to dilutional thrombocytopenia secondary to exchange transfusions, isoimmune hemolytic anemia may be characterized by thrombocytopenic purpura prior to exchange transfusion in severely affected newborns. This complication is usually seen in infants with disease in which the direct Coombs test is strongly positive, exemplified by Rh incompatibility, rather than weakly positive as is customary in ABO incompatibility. The mechanism of thrombocytopenia in these instances is not clear.[70,113] Since the liver and spleen are usually enlarged when thrombocytopenia is present, platelet sequestration may well play a role. Thrombocytopenia generally does not require treatment beyond that for the isoimmune hemolytic anemia itself.

Other diseases. Any disease characterized by hepatosplenomegaly in a newborn infant may be associated with thrombocytopenia in the absence of plasma coagulation abnormalities. Examples include congenital osteopetrosis[388] and congenital thyrotoxicosis.[460]

Purpuras with normal platelet counts

QUALITATIVE PLATELET DISORDERS

The objectives of this section are twofold: (1) to identify hemorrhagic disorders typically characterized by a normal platelet count and a prolonged Ivy bleeding time reflecting a thrombocytopathy; and (2) to specify the major defects of these disorders according to current concepts of platelet function. Major obstacles to these objectives include incomplete definition of many disorders and frequent overlapping between thrombocytopenia and thrombocytopathy as seen in Bernard-Soulier and Wiskott-Aldrich syndromes. The term "thrombocytopathy" will be used in a general sense to connote any qualitative platelet disorder.

The "state of the art" for classification of thrombocytopathies in the mid-1970s has been lucidly summarized in reviews by Deykin[102] and Weiss.[430] Thrombocytopathies may be classified as

Table 24-4. Classification and major examples of qualitative platelet disorders

Source of defect	Representative clinical disorder
Adhesion	Bernard-Soulier syndrome, von Willebrand's disease
First-phase aggregation	Glanzmann's disease (thrombasthenia)
Second-phase aggregation	
Decreased ADP content	Inherited or acquired storage pool disease
Impaired ADP release	Drug-induced or inherited "aspirin-like" defect

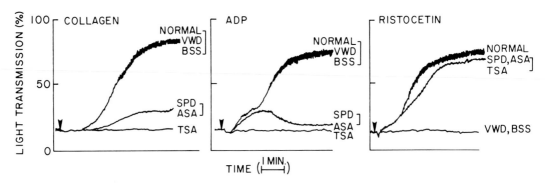

Fig. 24-10. Typical platelet aggregation patterns in representative qualitative platelet disorders. *BSS*, Bernard-Soulier syndrome; *VWD*, von Willebrand's disease; *TSA*, Glanzmann's disease (thrombasthenia); *SPD*, storage pool disease; *ASA*, "aspirin-like" disorders. (From Weiss, H. J.: N. Engl. J. Med. **293:**581, 1975. Reprinted by permission.)

defects of adhesion, first-phase aggregation, or second-phase aggregation. Application of this approach to representative clinical disorders is shown in Table 24-4, and platelet aggregation patterns typical of these disorders are shown in Fig. 24-10.

Acquired thrombocytopathies

Drug-induced thrombocytopathies

Aspirin. The relationship between ingestion of aspirin and prolongation of the bleeding time without change in the platelet count was first emphasized by Quick.[327] In 1967 Weiss and Aledort[431] reported defective collagen-induced platelet aggregation in normal subjects following ingestion of aspirin. Since that time the effects of aspirin on platelets have been exhaustively studied. It has been conclusively established that this drug causes a defect in second-phase platelet aggregation by inhibition of the release of ADP and other contents of the dense granules.[430]

Platelets normally respond to stimulation by synthesizing from membrane phospholipids a cyclic endoperoxide that directly induces release of ADP from dense bodies.[385] This peroxide compound, which Willis et al.[446] have termed labile aggregating-stimulating substance (LASS), is a precursor of PGE_2 and PGF_{2a} and its action is in turn potentiated by PGE_2. Aspirin has been shown to inhibit the cyclo-oxygenase that converts arachidonic acid derived from hydrolysis of membrane phospholipids to LASS.[156,385,446] This effect of aspirin may account, at least in part, for its inhibition of the platelet release reaction. Of particular clinical importance is that a conventional 600 mg dose of aspirin produces a measurable defect in platelets that begins at the time of ingestion and persists for the life span of affected platelets, normally about 10 days. This property of aspirin has been applied to nonradioisotopic methods for estimating platelet survival by Schwartz,[360] who

measured serial changes in platelet aggregation, and by Stuart et al.,[396] who measured inhibition of platelet lipid peroxidation.

Although the major dangers of aspirin intoxication are clearly caused by its metabolic effects, there are certain practical points that should be emphasized regarding its platelet-inhibiting effects. First, a patient with an existing hemorrhagic disorder such as any type of hemophilia should avoid aspirin entirely and take acetaminophen compounds instead. Second, a person scheduled for surgery on an elective basis should avoid aspirin for at least 2 weeks before the operation. Third, the history taken from a child being evaluated for a bleeding tendency should include careful questioning about drugs, especially aspirin.

On the other hand, aspirin should continue to be regarded as a useful drug for treatment of certain disorders such as rheumatoid arthritis. If an unacceptable bleeding tendency develops, a change to sodium salicylate may be helpful, since the acetyl component of aspirin may be critical in its effect.[327] Furthermore, there is much interest in the application of drugs such as aspirin to the possible control of thrombotic disorders.[103]

Other drugs. Aside from aspirin, a large number of pharmacologic agents may cause variable functional platelet defects,[292,429,430] including the following commonly used agents:

A. Anti-inflammatory agents
  1. Aspirin
  2. Phenylbutazone
  3. Sulfinpyrazone
  4. Indomethacin
B. Antihistaminic agents
  1. Diphenhydramine
  2. Promethazine (Phenergan)
C. Psychotropic agents
  1. Phenothiazines
  2. Dibenzazepines

D. Antibiotics
1. Carbenicillin
2. Nitrofurantoin
E. Anticoagulants
1. Coumarins
2. Heparin
F. Miscellaneous
1. Dipyridamole
2. Glyceryl guaiacolate
3. Glyceryl trinitrate
4. Alcohol
4. Dextran

In general, the effects of these drugs on platelets have not been nearly so extensively studied as those of aspirin. However, most of these drugs cause decreased platelet aggregation, particularly in the second phase, by inhibiting ADP release through mechanisms that are largely unknown. In some instances decreased platelet adhesion may play a major role, as in dextran, dipyridamole, sulfinpyrazone, heparin, and glyceryl guaiacolate.[171,344,429] Inhibition of platelet function by these agents is not generally associated with a clinically significant bleeding tendency. Dextran, dipyridamole, and sulfinpyrazone, along with aspirin, have been widely utilized for their antiplatelet effects in the management of various thrombotic disorders.[136]

Thrombocytopathies associated with systemic diseases

Uremia. Patients with uremia not infrequently have a hemorrhagic disorder related to thrombocytopathy rather than thrombocytopenia. The platelet defect in uremia has been thoroughly studied and is characterized by two particularly consistent findings: (1) decreased retention of platelets in a standard glass bead filter, which does not differentiate decreased platelet adhesion and aggregation, and (2) decreased release of platelet factor 3.[430] Direct measurement of platelet aggregation in response to collagen, ADP, and epinephrine has variously yielded normal and abnormal results.[32,430]

Uremic thrombocytopathy appears to be related in some way to effects of abnormal metabolites, since dialysis is associated with improvement in platelet function. Guanidinosuccinic acid and phenolic esters may be major offenders in this regard,[189,328] but the mechanism of their effects is unclear.[94]

Other diseases. As noted previously, patients with chronic ITP may develop thrombocytopathy that is clinically manifested by purpura inappropriate for their platelet counts. Clancy et al.[73] have documented decreased platelet aggregation in chronic ITP, and Regan et al.[336] have described similar findings in systemic lupus erythematosus. Zahavi and Marder[459] have recently reported a pa-

tient with immunologic thrombocytopenia whose platelets showed decreased second-phase aggregation associated with decreased platelet ADP content. This finding may prove to have relevance to other cases of thrombocytopathy complicating chronic ITP.

Thrombocytopathy has also been documented in the following diseases: leukemia and preleukemic states,[397] myeloproliferative disorders,[430] pernicious anemia, scurvy,[447] hepatic cirrhosis,[403] congenital heart disease (notably of the cyanotic type),[260] glycogen storage disease,[88] and macroglobulinemia.[430] The functional platelet abnormalities in these disorders are variably defined and thrombocytopenia is a major feature in some instances. Although congenital heart disease and glycogen storage are not acquired diseases, associated platelet defects are probably acquired, since these defects may disappear with correction of cardiac and metabolic abnormalities respectively. The management of thrombocytopathy associated with systemic disease is not nearly as critical as overall management of the systemic disease itself.

Inherited thrombocytopathies

Isolated thrombocytopathies

Glanzmann's disease. Glanzmann's disease (thrombasthenia) is a rare autosomal recessive hemorrhagic disorder characterized by chronic nonthrombocytopenic purpura, a prolonged bleeding time, and deficient or absent clot retraction. The major underlying abnormality in this disease is grossly defective first-phase aggregation of platelets, which are unresponsive to ADP in any concentration (Fig. 24-10).

In 1918 Glanzmann[142] applied the term "thrombasthenia" to a group of patients with a life-long bleeding disorder in which the principal common denominator was impared clot retraction. It is unlikely that the subjects of his report constituted a homogeneous group since he included patients with a low platelet count and a normal bleeding time, which are not characteristic of Glanzmann's disease as it is now recognized. Furthermore, recent findings suggest that Glanzmann's disease as just defined probably is not a homogeneous disorder either.

Clinically Glanzmann's disease is a chronic generalized purpura of variable severity superficially resembling chronic ITP. Purpura usually begins in early infancy and is unremitting, but hemorrhagic manifestations are generally mild to moderate, although serious or even fatal complications have been described.[64] In affected females menorrhagia is a particular problem, and hormonal suppression of menses is generally required.

With appropriate laboratory evaluation, expected results are as follows: (1) routine blood counts including platelet count should be normal, with the possible exception of blood-loss anemia, and platelets on a smear of fresh nonanticoagulated blood appear normal in number but may not show normal "clumping"; (2) results of screening tests of coagulation (PT, PTT, and TCT) should be normal; (3) results of screening tests of platelet function should be abnormal, i.e., an Ivy bleeding time of more than 10 minutes, markedly reduced clot retraction, and a relatively prolonged kaolin-activated recalcification time of platelet-rich plasma, reflecting decreased platelet factor 3 activity; (4) platelet aggregation studies should show defective aggregation in response to collagen, epinephrine, thrombin, and all concentrations of ADP but normal aggregation in response to ristocetin (Fig. 24-10). Because of the rarity of Glanzmann's disease and its importance to further understanding of platelet function, patients who may have this disease probably should be referred to a center where detailed studies of platelets can be carried out.

The separation of Glanzmann's disease from other platelet disorders is usually not difficult. Its inborn character may be deduced from the lifelong history of purpura, the normal platelet count separates this disease from the thrombocytopenias, and deficient clot retraction largely distinguishes it from other nonthrombocytopenic thrombocytopathies. However, platelet aggregation studies are ultimately required for a definitive diagnosis.

Certain important platelet functions are known to be normal in Glanzmann's disease. These include adhesion to collagen, release of endogenous ADP and platelet factor 4 in response to collagen and thrombin, and ristocetin-induced aggregation.* Although absence of first-phase aggregation as a result of unresponsiveness of platelets to ADP is the major defect in Glanzmann's disease, the precise reason for this defect is unknown. However, recent studies suggest that deficiencies of certain membrane components may be critical in this regard, notably actomyosin[49] and platelet membrane-specific glycoproteins.[305] Other findings in Glanzmann's disease include deficiency of intracellular and adsorbed platelet fibrinogen[434] and variable ATP content, activity of certain glycolytic enzymes, and magnesium-dependence of clot retraction.† The significance of these findings in Glanzmann's disease cannot be fully assessed at the present time, but they suggest that this disease may be subdivided in due course according to specific biochemical defects.

There is no treatment beyond support with appropriate blood components. Insofar as possible,

HLA-compatible persons to serve as platelet donors should be identified, particularly for patients with a clinically significant bleeding tendency. Surgical procedures may be specifically hazardous in patients who have become alloimmunized against random platelet donors and are thus refractory to such replacement therapy. Splenectomy and corticosteroids have no place in the management of this disease.

ADP storage pool disease. ADP storage pool disease is a rare autosomal dominant hemorrhagic disorder typically characterized by mild nonthrombocytopenic purpura and by defective second-phase aggregation of platelets as a result of lack of endogenous stores of ADP (Fig. 24-10). In 1970 Holmsen and Weiss[187] showed that thrombocytopathies characterized by deficient ADP release could be related to a lack of storage ADP as well as to failure of the ADP release mechanism with normal stores. In 1972 they introduced the term "storage pool disease" to designate the former category.[188]

Storage pool disease may exist either as an isolated entity or in association with certain systemic diseases. There are no clinical features that distinguish it from other heritable thrombocytopathies. The diagnosis depends entirely on appropriate laboratory studies. In comparison with Glanzmann's disease, the platelet count in storage pool disease also is typically normal, the bleeding time is prolonged but less impressively so, and the kaolin-activated recalcification time of platelet-rich plasma is less consistently prolonged. Storage pool disease may be sharply differentiated from Glanzmann's disease by the finding of normal clot retraction and defective second-phase but normal first-phase platelet aggregation. The secondary wave of aggregation is lacking in response to those agents that induce first-phase aggregation and trigger the release of endogenous ADP causing second-phase aggregation, notably ADP in an intermediate concentration, e.g., 2 μM. However, platelet aggregation is normal in response to a relatively high concentration of ADP, e.g., 10 μM.

Since the platelet aggregation patterns of storage pool disease and ADP-release disease are identical, the diagnosis of storage pool disease ultimately rests on the demonstration of decreased or absent ADP stores. Functionally this may be shown by isotopic techniques that differentiate the metabolic pool of adenine nucleotides from the storage pool; in storage pool disease the metabolic pool is normal whereas the storage pool is decreased.[187,188] Electron microscopy has shown that the dense granules of platelets, the site of ADP storage, are markedly decreased in number, and the α-granules are normal.[432] Since ATP, serotonin, and calcium are also stored in the dense granules, it is appropriate that platelets of patients with storage pool

---

*References 406, 430, 436, 463.
†References 150, 199, 434, 463.

disease have been found to lack normal content of these substances as well as ADP.[188,233,437]

In accord with these findings the basic abnormality in storage pool disease appears to be defective formation of the platelet dense granules, possibly originating in the cytoplasm of the megakaryocyte.[405] However, the mechanisms underlying this abnormality are unknown at this time.

Storage pool disease appears to be far less demanding as a clinical hemorrhagic disorder than as a means of learning more about the platelet. There is no specific treatment, but this is hardly a major issue since affected persons usually show little more than an increased tendency toward bruising and perhaps epistaxes. Drugs such as aspirin that inhibit the platelet release reaction should be avoided since the function of whatever marginal stores of ADP may exist would be further compromised. In the unlikely event of excessive bleeding, as in surgery, supportive blood component therapy should be instituted as needed.

As storage pool disease is increasingly identified and studied, the overall clinical character of this relative newcomer will surely become more clear, including its true incidence, genetic variants, requirements for treatment, and prognosis.

ADP-release disease. ADP-release disease may be defined as a heterogeneous genetically determined hemorrhagic disorder characterized by clinical and laboratory effects approximating those produced in normal persons following the ingestion of aspirin. As with aspirin effects and storage pool disease, congenital ADP-release disease is characterized by a mild bleeding tendency, a normal platelet count, a variably prolonged bleeding time and defective second-phase platelet aggregation (Fig. 24-10). A reliable diagnosis of this disorder requires the following: (1) a history of a lifelong, mild bleeding tendency; (2) no ingestion of any drugs for at least 2 weeks before laboratory testing; and (3) evidence for defective second-phase platelet aggregation combined with evidence for normal ADP stores.

It was pointed out previously that five separate reports of ADP-release disease in 1967 collectively represented a major development in the evolution of knowledge about the platelet. Furthermore, the discovery of storage pool disease by Holmsen and Weiss[187] in 1970 now demands the finding of normal ADP stores for a diagnosis of "true" ADP-release disease. To date the sorting-out process is far from complete. For instance, the autosomal dominant "Portsmouth syndrome" of platelet dysfunction, described by O'Brien[307] in 1967, has not yet been conclusively identified in these regards. On the other hand, autosomal dominant ADP-release disease with normal ADP storage, as well as sporadic cases, have been reported by Weiss and Rogers[436] and Weiss et al.[433] It has been

suggested that congenital release defects may be relatively common, while storage pool disease is rare.[102,428]

This whole area of investigation is in a tremendous state of ferment at the present time, which is reflected by a bewildering jargon reminiscent of the terms for clotting factors in the bygone era before Roman numeral nomenclature was adopted. In the meantime, it may be helpful to those who have no stake in platelet investigation to point out that a person with storage pool disease, another person with congenital platelet-release disease, and a medical student who has just taken two aspirin tablets for a headache are all rather similarly handicapped with respect to formation of a "platelet plug."

Considerations on von Willebrand's disease and the Bernard-Soulier syndrome. Details of von Willebrand's disease are discussed in Chapter 25 and the Bernard-Soulier syndrome on p. 729. They are cited at this time to emphasize the difference between ristocetin-induced platelet aggregation, which is defective in both conditions, and ADP-related platelet aggregation, which is normal in both (Fig. 24-10).

Platelet aggregation induced by ristocetin reflects the interaction of plasma factors and platelet receptors involved in platelet adhesion to sites of blood vessel injury. The effects of ristocetin on platelets in vitro are not dependent either on the content or the release of platelet ADP.

Defective ristocetin-induced platelet aggregation in von Willebrand's disease appears to be the result of a lack of a factor VIII–related protein in plasma rather than a defect in the platelet itself.[297] In Bernard-Soulier syndrome the defect clearly resides in the platelet receptor apparatus rather than the plasma.

Thrombocytopathies associated with inherited systemic disease. Storage-pool defects have been described in the Wiskott-Aldrich syndrome,[29] the TAR syndrome,[97] and the Hermansky-Pudlak syndrome of oculocutaneous albinism.[443]

Variable and incompletely defined thrombocytopathies have been described in congenital afibrinogenemia,[435] other heritable coagulation disorders,[407] Ehlers-Danlos syndrome,[310] osteogenesis imperfecta,[166] homocystinuria,[465] and G-6-PD deficiency.[361]

As previously noted, thrombocytopathies associated with congenital heart disease[260] and type I glycogen storage disease[88] are probably acquired rather than intrinsic.

Neonatal thrombocytopathies

The platelets of newborns normally do not aggregate as well as adult platelets in response to most inducing agents and are more susceptible to drugs that interfere with platelet function. This physiologic deficit generally clears within 2 weeks after birth.[250] In addition, the newborn may have any of the acquired or inherited thrombocytopathies that have been described.

The major step in diagnosing significant non-thrombocytopenic purpura in an otherwise normal newborn infant without coagulation abnormalities should be a close examination of the maternal drug history and all drugs given to the infant. If an offending drug is identified, discontinuation of drug administration to the infant, or to the mother if she is breast-feeding, and watchful waiting generally suffice. In the event that significant purpura persists well beyond 2 weeks, an inherited thrombocytopathy should be considered, particularly Glanzmann's disease. To avoid confusing overlap between physiologic and pathologic platelet deficits, definitive studies probably should be deferred until the infant is at least 1 month old.

In general neither physiologic nor pathologic thrombocytopathy in the newborn appears to be a clinically significant problem. Neonatal thrombocytopenia and plasma coagulation disorders are vastly more important, in terms of both incidence and demands for precise diagnosis and prompt treatment.

VASCULAR DISORDERS

One category of purpuras includes those that are primarily related to vascular defects and are typically characterized by normal values for the platelet count, bleeding time, and plasma coagulation functions. However, the reader should understand that in this, as in all other categories, a certain amount of overlapping is inevitable. Examples of this include Ehlers-Danlos syndrome, in which the basic vascular disorder may be associated with thrombocytopathy, and certain infectious purpuras such as Rocky Mountain spotted fever, in which abnormalities of the blood vessel, platelet, and coagulation function may be intermingled.

The term "vascular disorder" implies a fundamental pathologic process affecting blood vessels. Purpura caused by injury of normal blood vessels is not strictly consistent with such a process. Nonetheless, traumatic purpura is discussed because the distinction between pathology and trauma may not be at all clear when a patient is initially seen.

Acquired vascular disorders

Traumatic purpuras

Battered-child syndrome. In 1962 Kempe et al.[218] introduced the term "battered-child syndrome" to encompass a complex psychosocial disorder characterized by traumatic lesions in children as a result of physical abuse. The stage for the description of this disorder had been set by certain preceding reports. In 1946 Caffey[65] described the association of multiple fractures with chronic subdural hematoma and in 1953 Silverman[379] convincingly established trauma as a major cause of such lesions. Battered-child syndrome is now fully recognized as a leading cause of morbidity and mortality, especially among infants. Purpura may be a major feature of the syndrome, and affected children are frequently referred for hematologic evaluation in those many instances in which underlying abuse is not initially suspected by the physician.

Salient clinical hallmarks of purpura caused by child abuse are as follows: (1) the purpura is largely nonspecific in character and distribution; (2) screening tests of hemostasis—platelet count and inspection of the blood smear, standard bleeding time, PT, and PTT—are normal; (3) purpura may be associated with other findings compatible with trauma, notably fractures of bones otherwise normal on radiologic examination.

Purpura caused by an underlying hemostatic disorder rather than trauma usually is uncovered by these screening tests. If the test results are normal, judicious consideration of abuse may be far more helpful than extensive tests of specific hemostatic functions. It should also be recognized that the presence of abuse and a hemostatic disorder are by no means mutually exclusive.

Factitious purpura. In addition to purpura caused by physical abuse by others, traumatic extravasations may be self-inflicted, so-called factitious purpura. Such purpura has been largely reported in teenage girls and is usually characterized by bizarre ecchymotic lesions that tend to be quite baffling initially.[167,239,266] Representative causes of factitious purpura include biting, blunt trauma, scarification of skin with broken glass or other sharp instruments, and production of localized petechiae by sustained negative pressure through oral suction or application of a syringe tip. This disorder may overlap with purpura related to possible autosensitivity to blood components. Results of screening tests of hemostatic function are typically normal, although previous ingestion of drugs causing platelet dysfunction, notably aspirin, may confuse the picture.

The key to a diagnosis of factitious purpura is a high index of suspicion of this disorder in those instances in which the physician is faced with variable purpuric lesions that simply do not fit the pattern of any disorder. Above all, it should be emphasized that factitious purpura is a psychiatric and not a hemostatic disorder. The lesions are a cry for help, and management of affected children should be instituted with compassion and professional skill of the highest order.

Inflammatory disorders

Henoch-Schönlein purpura. Henoch-Schönlein purpura (HSP, anaphylactoid purpura, allergic purpura, Henoch's purpura, Schönlein's purpura, peliosis rheumatica) is an acquired disorder of unknown etiology characterized clinically by nonthrombocytopenic purpura with variable joint and visceral abnormalities and pathologically by generalized and diffuse inflammation of small blood vessels.

HISTORICAL PERSPECTIVE. As noted previously, first classification of purpura was probably provided by Willan in 1808. In 1837 Schönlein[354] described several cases in which purpura was associated with acute arthritis, which he termed peliosis rheumatica. In 1868 Henoch[172] pointed out that the term "peliosis rheumatica" was inappropriately restrictive because patients with urticarial purpura and acute arthritis also presented at times with gastrointestinal manifestations including vomiting, abdominal pain, and melena. Henoch[173] also suggested that a single underlying condition might produce these diverse clinical expressions.

The purpuric disorder variously described by Willan, Schönlein, and Henoch was established as a distinct clinical entity by Osler[314,316] at the turn of the century. He regarded Henoch-Schönlein purpura as an expression of anaphylaxis and thus analogous to serum sickness. Osler's concept was extended by Glanzmann,[143] who applied to this disorder the term "anaphylactoid purpura."[127]

Over the past 50 years there have been numerous clinical reports describing specific cases and reviews of experience with Henoch-Schönlein purpura. These reports have contributed to the development of a useful body of knowledge about this disease, particularly its visceral manifestations, but there has been no significant progress in understanding its pathogenesis.

CLASSIFICATION. Despite the diverse anatomic sites affected by Henoch-Schönlein purpura and its occurrence in singly episodic, recurrent, and chronic forms, there is no generally accepted scheme for classification of this disease. This will probably continue to be the case as long as possible approaches to classification continue to have little or no relevance either to mechanisms of pathogenesis or to methods of treatment.

INCIDENCE. The overwhelming majority of persons affected range in age from 6 months to 16 years with a median age of 4 years in the large series reported by Allen et al.[12] About 75% of patients are under 7 years of age, and occurrence in adults is rare. The male:female ratio is approximately 3:1. Although Henoch-Schönlein purpura has been mainly reported in whites, there is no conclusive evidence for racial predilection.[401] The disease tends to occur primarily in the spring and fall.[12,63] Although the true incidence has not been determined, it seems reasonable to presume that it is, aside from traumatic purpura, the most common of all nonthrombocytopenic purpuras.

ETIOLOGY. Although the etiology of Henoch-Schönlein purpura is unknown, it is generally thought that this disease represents an expression in small blood vessels of an abnormal immunologic response to any one of several antigens, in basic accord with the concept of Osler. Such an etiology is suggested by a high incidence of upper respiratory infections 1 to 3 weeks before onset of Henoch-Schönlein purpura, 72% in the study of Bywaters et al.[63] In this study one fourth of the preceding infections were shown to be caused by group A β-hemolytic streptococci, a substantial incidence of this specific agent but clearly insufficient to establish its firm connection in the etiology of Henoch-Schönlein purpura. Other agents that have been implicated by association include vaccines, including smallpox[206] and influenza[394]; insect bites[62]; drugs, including penicillin,[68] quinine[85], and chlorothiazide[126]; and a wide variety of foods, notably milk, eggs, chocolate, wheat, nuts, and beans.[5]

GENETICS. Although age and sex determinants clearly indicate the operation of constitutional factors in Henoch-Schönlein purpura, there is no evidence of genetic factors in the disease at the present time.

CLINICAL FEATURES. The hallmark of Henoch-Schönlein purpura is highly symmetrical purpura, most often involving the buttocks and lower extremities (Fig. 24-11) and typically associated with a maculopapular rash including variable elements of urticaria, erythema, and edema in addition to purpura. The purpuric rash is not a fixed lesion but ranges in color from dark red initially through purple to brown as old lesions regress and new lesions appear in the active phase of cutaneous involvement. Although gastrointestinal involvement may precede skin involvement[12] and the occurrence of renal disease without purpura has been postulated,[440] a definitive diagnosis of Henoch-Schönlein purpura requires identification by inspection of the characteristic purpura.

In addition to involvement of the buttocks and lower extremities, the purpuric rash may be observed on the extensor surfaces of the upper extremities in a symmetrical fashion and less frequently on the palms and soles and external genitalia. The rash impressively spares the trunk above the waist. The mucous membranes are usually not involved, although scattered nonpurpuric erythematous lesions may be observed in the mouth and pharynx.

Although symmetrical maculopapular purpura is the major cutaneous manifestation of Henoch-

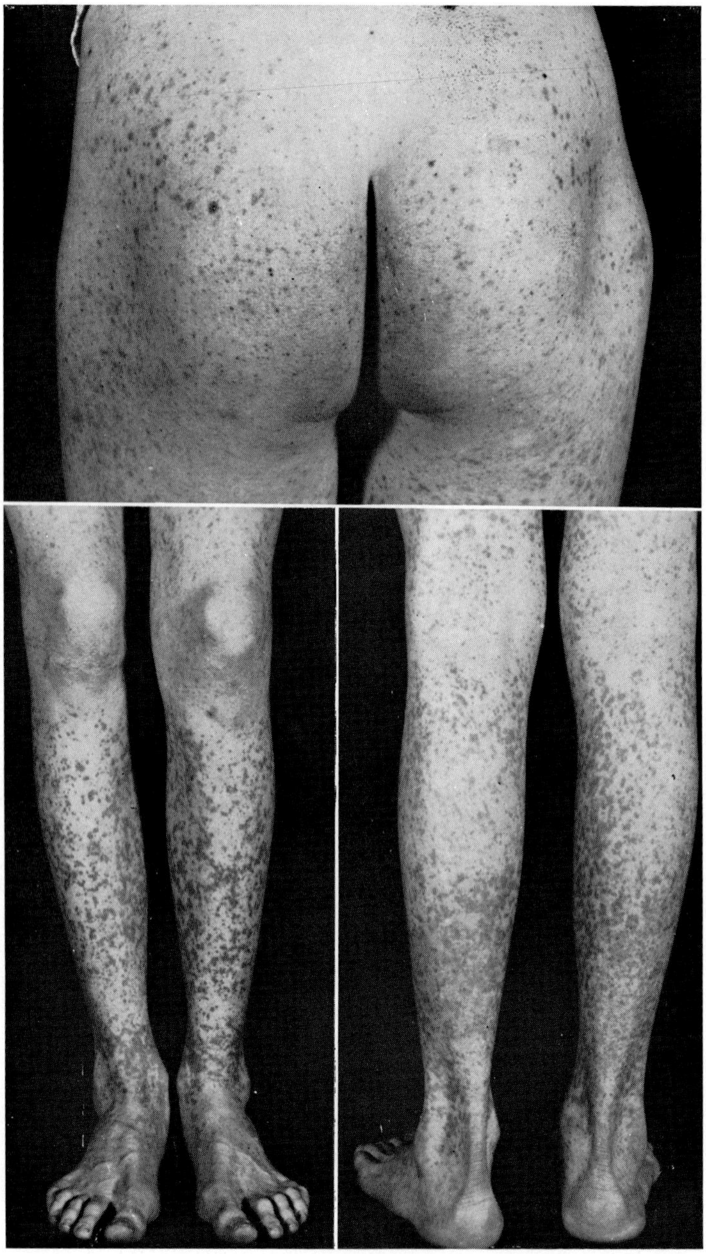

Fig. 24-11. Henoch-Schönlein purpura in a 13-year-old boy, occurring 2 weeks after an acute upper respiratory infection. The hemorrhagic and erythematous lesions are characteristically shown on some of the most commonly affected sites—buttocks and lower extremities.

Schönlein purpura, variable localized edema may also be a prominent feature in many instances, particularly in infants. Such edema is most frequently seen on the dorsum of the hands and feet but may be impressive and sometimes painful in other sites, including the scalp, lips, ears, face, and periorbital areas[12,93] (Fig. 24-12).

Aside from whatever pain may accompany edema, the degree of illness associated with active Henoch-Schönlein purpura is determined not so much by cutaneous manifestations of the disease as by joint and particularly visceral involvement.

Arthritic effects range from asymptomatic swelling around a single joint to painful involvement of one or more joints with significant limitation of function. The knees and ankles are most commonly affected. Regardless of severity, the joint involvement is periarticular rather than intra-

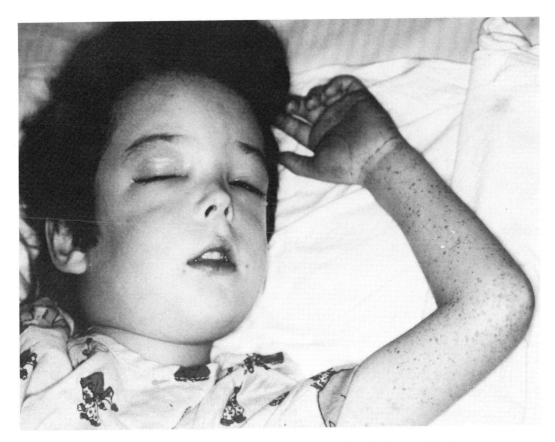

Fig. 24-12. Profound facial and scalp edema in a 4-year-old child with Henoch-Schönlein purpura.

articular. Thus permanent damage to joints does not occur. The synovial structures appear to be spared, and therefore hemarthrosis and other changes characteristic of hemophilic arthropathy are not observed.

Major sites of visceral involvement in Henoch-Schönlein purpura are the gastrointestinal tract and kidneys. Rarely the central nervous system may also be involved.

The major clinical manifestation of gastrointestinal disease is recurrent colicky midabdominal pain in which the attacks are frequently associated with nausea and vomiting and sometimes with passage of blood and mucus in stools as well. The small intestine, particularly the ileum, appears to be the most common site of involvement (Figs. 24-13 and 24-14). Severe colic and associated signs may suggest a surgical condition, notably acute appendicitis or intussusception. Indeed, bowel perforation has been described but is fortunately rare.[33] Abdominal signs may precede or accompany the typical purpura of Henoch-Schönlein purpura. The gastrointestinal lesions have been compared to the cutaneous purpura, but abdominal pain has been attributed to possible epi-

sodic ischemia related to diseased arterioles.[30] In any case, marked abnormalities of the small bowel caused by hemorrhage and edema involving the bowel wall and mesentery, with or without vasospasm, probably account for the severe abdominal pain that may accompany Henoch-Schönlein purpura.

If colicky abdominal pain, vomiting, blood and mucus in the stool, and a palpable abdominal mass occur in a febrile child with Henoch-Schönlein purpura, the occurrence of intussusception should be assumed. In such instances, steps toward immediate surgery should be initiated, with or without preceding barium enema depending on clinical circumstances. In one series nine children had surgical exploration, and intussusception was found in four cases.[123]

Renal involvement has been estimated to occur in as many as 50% of children with Henoch-Schönlein purpura.[309] Although it does not tend to be as stormy a complication as gastrointestinal or joint involvement may be, renal disease potentially appears to be the most serious long-term complication of Henoch-Schönlein purpura. Initially the nephritis of this disease is manifest by variable

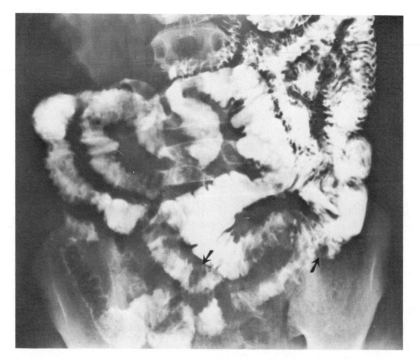

Fig. 24-13. Small intestinal series in Henoch-Schönlein purpura. The small bowel, filled with non-flocculating barium, shows separation of loops, coarse mucosal folds, and polyploid ileal filling defects (arrows). The pattern resembles nonstenotic diffuse ileitis. (From Grossman, H., Berdon, W. E., and Baker, D. H.: Am. J. Dis. Child. **108**:67, 1964.)

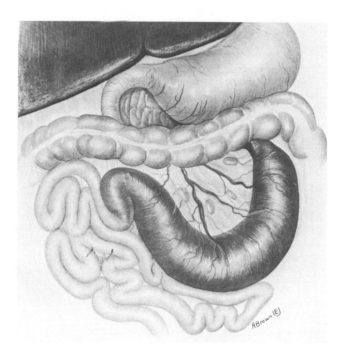

Fig. 24-14. Artist's rendition of edematous, distended, purpuric segment of small intestine in a patient with Henoch-Schönlein purpura. (From Balf, C. L.: Arch. Dist. Child. **26**:20, 1951. Reprinted from Archives of Disease in Childhood, 1951, Volume 26, Page 20, by permission of the Publishers.)

hematuria, casts, and proteinuria. Although the majority of affected children recover completely, some may develop chronic glomerulonephritis with eventual renal failure.[98,426]

Although central nervous system complications are uncommon, it should be noted that fatal subarachnoid hemorrhage has been described in connection with fulminating Henoch-Schönlein purpura.[240]

LABORATORY EVALUATION. A diagnosis of Henoch-Schönlein purpura is made on clinical grounds, particularly recognition of the characteristic purpuric rash by inspection, and does not depend on laboratory studies. Rather, laboratory evaluation serves a twofold supportive purpose: (1) to determine normal hemostatic function by screening tests, including a platelet count, inspection of the blood smear, a standard bleeding time, PT, and PTT, and (2) to determine the existence and degree of visceral involvement, particularly gastrointestinal and renal disease. Tests of gastrointestinal involvement should include the following: hemoglobin determination, hematocrit, reticulocyte count, and guaiac testing of the stool to assess blood loss; white blood cell and differential count to assess the possibility of severe bowel inflammation and necrosis warranting surgical intervention; and serum electrolyte testing to assess metabolic effects of simple vomiting or structural bowel changes. Tests of renal involvement should include a complete urinalysis and careful examination of the urine sediment with particular attention to microscopic hematuria and testing of serum creatinine or blood urea nitrogen to assess renal function. A baseline creatinine clearance test, particularly in severely affected children, is recommended as a sensitive test of renal status with which subsequent clearance tests may be usefully compared to assess recovery, lack of change, or progression of renal disease.

Laboratory studies should also include evaluation of any identifiable illness or other insult that may have preceded the onset of Henoch-Schönlein purpura. For example, although β-hemolytic streptococcal disease does not have a predictable relationship to Henoch-Schönlein purpura a throat culture and testing of anti-streptolysin of O titer may well be in order.

DIFFERENTIAL DIAGNOSIS. In the vast majority of cases the rash combined with appropriate joint and visceral manifestations are sufficiently indicative of Henoch-Schönlein purpura that differential diagnosis simply is not a problem. The whole spectrum of purpuras caused by thrombocytopenic and coagulation disorders are not only usually excluded on clinical grounds but also by tests of hemostasis. Purpura caused by serious infectious diseases such as Rocky Mountain spotted fever and meningococcemia are typically seen in children who "look sick." In contrast, unless Henoch-Schönlein purpura is complicated by a surgical abdominal condition, affected children may be quite uncomfortable from joint and abdominal pains but usually are not seriously ill. A variety of drugs may cause nonthrombocytopenic purpura,[401] but the distribution of such purpura is generalized in most instances and therefore readily differentiated from the symmetrical lesions of HSP.

PATHOGENESIS AND PATHOPHYSIOLOGY. The pathogenesis of Henoch-Schönlein purpura, like its etiology, is unknown. However, the concensus is that this disorder may be the result within a susceptible host of an abnormal immunologic process that somehow produces aseptic inflammation of small blood vessels. Investigations have suggested an autoimmune mechanism[74,225] and effects of phagocytosis within capillary endothelium of antigen-antibody complexes.[412] The latter concept is supported by the occurrence of Henoch-Schönlein purpura following exposure to a variety of antigenic agents.

The pathophysiology of Henoch-Schönlein purpura is characterized by a spectrum of effects of vasculitis: erythema caused by vasodilation, urticarial edema caused by increased vascular permeability, purpura caused by extravasation of blood, and occasionally localized hemorrhagic necrosis caused by thrombosis.[401] The striking symmetry that is characteristic of Henoch-Schönlein purpura is both fascinating and, so far, unexplained.

PATHOLOGY. The basic pathologic lesion of Henoch-Schönlein purpura is a generalized vasculitis affecting capillaries adjacent to arterioles, predominantly characterized by perivascular infiltration of granulocytes and by variable thrombosis and endothelial changes.* In the skin these lesions are limited to dermal vessels, but extravasated red cells may extend to the epidermis. In the gastrointestinal tract there may be marked focal edema and submucosal hemorrhage. In severe cases vascular lesions may be associated with mucosal ulcerations and intussusception. The joint lesions have not been definitively studied but, as previously noted, involvement is periarticular rather than intra-articular; the synovium is spared and progressive arthropathy does not occur.[401] Significant central nervous system involvement is uncommon, but subarachnoid hemorrhage has been described as well as encephalopathy secondary to severe renal disease and renal failure.[240]

Except for the cutaneous manifestations, the pathology of renal disease in Henoch-Schönlein

---

*References 12, 130, 195, 412.

purpura has been perhaps the most fully studied.* On the basis of renal biopsies it appears that a clear majority of children with Henoch-Schönlein purpura have renal involvement, although clinical evidence of such involvement is much less. The acute renal lesion is principally characterized by segmental glomerulitis and occlusion of capillaries by fibrinoid material; older lesions show segmental deposition of hyaline material within glomeruli or fibrous scarring.[411,412] The focal nature of the renal disease is thus similar to that seen in systemic lupus erythematosus, unlike the diffuse involvement characteristic of acute glomerulonephritis. Indeed, West et al.[440] found evidence of focal glomerulonephritis in eleven children without evidence of other systemic manifestations and suggested that these findings might represent Henoch-Schönlein purpura limited to the kidneys. This provocative interpretation will remain unsettled as long as the diagnosis of Henoch-Schönlein purpura hinges on the presence of characteristic skin involvement, as it does now.

MANAGEMENT. The cornerstone of management of Henoch-Schönlein purpura is supportive therapy with watchful waiting, particularly directed at continuing assessment of gastrointestinal and renal manifestations. Every effort should be made to identify and treat as indicated any infection that may be present, but in general the primary institution of antibiotic therapy has no place in the management of Henoch-Schönlein purpura. Along the same line, if there is any suspicious association between a drug or foodstuff and the onset of Henoch-Schönlein purpura, the associated agent should be eliminated even if a cause-and-effect relationship cannot be proved. Painful edema of the skin and arthralgia should be managed with appropriate analgesia and gentle sedation. For analgesia acetaminophen is probably preferable to aspirin because the superimposition of a qualitative platelet defect onto already leaky blood vessels is not desirable. Diphenhydramine or an equivalent antihistamine generally has little or no effect on the urticarial edema, but such compounds are useful sedatives.

Prednisone or an equivalent corticosteroid is the one specific agent that deserves consideration in the management of Henoch-Schönlein purpura. The most definitive guidelines for its use were provided by Allen et al.[12] in 1960, and no substantive basis for changes has emerged since that time. They found that corticosteroids were not associated with beneficial effects on purpura or renal manifestations but were associated with impressive relief of skin edema, arthralgia, and colicky abdominal pain. Indeed, they suggested that timely

*References 31, 40, 41, 410, 412.

institution of such therapy in a child with progressive gastrointestinal signs and symptoms may help prevent the ultimate development of a surgical abdominal condition, notably intussusception.

Available evidence does not warrant the recommendation of corticosteroid therapy in all cases. Indeed, most children with mild or even moderate gastrointestinal manifestations will spontaneously recover without such therapy. However, such manifestations demand careful clinical judgment with close watching. At some indefinable point between mild recurrent abdominal pain and a frank surgical abdominal condition, corticosteroids are probably useful. Prednisone should be instituted without hesitation if there is evidence of severe or increasing gastrointestinal disease. A single daily dose of 60 mg prednisone/m^2 is appropriate and should be continued 2 or 3 days after subsidence of the signs and symptoms; it should be stopped abruptly within 2 weeks in any case. Although such therapy may produce rather dramatic benefits, it should never invoke a false sense of security since continued progression of gastrointestinal disease is not uniformly prevented. The child's primary physician and a consulting surgeon should work together closely in these regards. If a child with Henoch-Schönlein purpura has a surgical abdominal condition, surgery should be instituted without delay and a decision about steroid therapy should be made on the basis of operative findings and overall manifestations of the disease. In typical cases in which impressive edema and hemorrhage of the bowel wall are combined with purpura and arthralgia, postoperative institution of corticosteroid therapy may be quite appropriate. However, if prednisone has already been administered for 2 or 3 days before surgery is needed, further benefit from this agent is unlikely and it may as well be discontinued in favor of supportive measures alone.

Unfortunately there is no evidence that any specific therapeutic approach controls the renal expression of Henoch-Schönlein purpura. However, a close watch on the urinalysis and renal function should begin with the onset of the disease and continue through its initial and recurrent phases, if any, and for at least a year after its complete subsidence. Severe complications, including isolated hypertension, hypertensive encephalopathy, and renal failure, should be managed supportively.

The majority of children with Henoch-Schönlein purpura have, in addition to the characteristic rash, rather tolerable arthritic and visceral manifestations that may be managed with simple supportive measures on an ambulatory basis. Those occasional patients with impressive gastrointestinal or renal disease should generally be hospitalized and watched carefully, with or without prednisone therapy.

PROGNOSIS. Despite its marked clinical variability, the overall prognosis of the disease is good. In approximately 60% of cases it is limited to a single acute episode that spontaneously clears up within an average of 1 month.[12] The remainder may have recurrence or variable chronic persistence of the disease.

Recurrence is typically noted about 6 weeks from the onset of the first attack, follows a period of apparent recovery, and is characterized by purpura without major joint or visceral manifestations. Such recurrence tends to be seasonal, particularly in the spring, and may be observed for as many as 2 to 3 years before permanent remission from purpura.[12]

The most common chronic manifestation of Henoch-Schönlein purpura is renal involvement. In patients with such involvement at the onset, the routine urinalysis will usually become normal within a year. However, by means of 12-hour Addis counts Allen et al.[12] found renal abnormalities persisting from 6 months to 10 years from the onset of Henoch-Schönlein purpura in 21 of 131 patients (28.5%). The significance of these findings in terms of the ultimate development of major renal complications could not be precisely assessed. Certainly in the vast majority of patients such renal abnormalities did not indicate significant renal disease in the face of normal linear growth, normal renal function, and absence of anemia. Vernier et al.[412] showed by renal biopsies that the renal lesions of Henoch-Schönlein purpura are capable of healing and do not necessarily progress to irreversible glomerular damage.

The age of the patient and the degree of renal involvement at the onset of the disease appear to be correlated with the likelihood of subsequent renal abnormalities. In the study of Allen et al.[12] the frequency of such abnormalities was directly proportional to increasing age and the severity of initial renal manifestations. Indeed, Mauer[258] has suggested that, if renal involvement is not detectable within the first week of the disease, it probably will not occur at all.

In summary, a particular case of Henoch-Schönlein purpura has about a 50% chance of complete recovery within a month and about a 95% chance of ultimate recovery that may require years, assuming that minor abnormalities of the urinary sediment that may persist do not constitute disease. A mortality of less than 5% may be attributed to acute visceral complications at the onset of Henoch-Schönlein purpura and to chronic glomerulonephritis with eventual renal failure in those rare instances of progressive renal involvement.

FUTURE PERSPECTIVES. Although Henoch-Schönlein purpura has not been as intensively examined during recent years as other presumed immunologic purpuras, better understanding of this disorder will surely be derived from continued progress in immunologic research. As in all vascular disorders, a major obstacle to basic research is simply that the blood vessel does not readily lend itself to study, in marked contrast to the relative ease of obtaining blood.

Furthermore, even with limited understanding of the pathogenesis of Henoch-Schönlein purpura, it is clear that this disease has a tremendous tendency to resolve spontaneously, especially in infants and preschool children with initially mild disease. Virtually nothing of importance has been added to the management of those children with serious gastrointestinal and renal complications since the development of highly definitive guidelines for these problems by Allen et al.[12] in 1960. Although their findings probably are not the last word, no major resurgence of interest in new clinical approaches to this interesting disease is apparent at this time.

Other inflammatory disorders

INFECTIONS. Although purpura occurring concomitantly with infectious disease generally tends to be characterized by multiple hemostatic defects, lesions presumably caused by isolated vascular changes may be observed. For example, meningococcal purpura is usually associated with thrombocytopenia, if not coagulation abnormalities as well, but it may occur without these findings in relatively milder cases. Such purpura may be caused by septic emboli, as in subacute bacterial endocarditis, or by variable mechanisms of direct vascular damage by virtually any infectious agent. A diagnosis of vascular purpura resulting from an infection hinges on the presence of nonspecific purpura directly correlated with an infectious disease and absence of measurable hemostatic abnormalities in serial screening tests. No treatment of the purpura is needed beyond that for the underlying disease.

AUTOERYTHROCYTE SENSITIVITY. A syndrome of episodic painful bruising in women was first described by Gardner and Diamond,[133] who attributed the disorder to autoerythrocyte sensitization. They found that typical lesions could be reproduced in affected patients by the intradermal injection of autologous intact red cells or stroma but not by injection of autologous leukocytes or plasma. Apparent sensitivity to red cell membrane lipid[148] and to hemoglobin[226] has been subsequently reported. Bruises in affected persons may be associated with bleeding elsewhere. The pathogenesis of autoerythrocyte sensitivity is unknown, there is no typical histologic pattern of the lesions, and a variety of therapeutic approaches have had little or no effect on the bruising tendency. This disorder is largely limited to adolescent girls and adult women.

Ratnoff and Agle[332] have described considerable overlapping of autoerythrocyte sensitivity with factitious purpura in certain persons and have suggested that psychogenic factors may at times play a role in both these disorders. Autoerythrocyte sensitivity has also been documented in the apparent absence of factitious purpura.[146,332]

DNA SENSITIVITY. A syndrome of episodic painful purpura in women has also been attributed to DNA sensitivity. This disorder, unlike autoerythrocyte sensitivity, typically is not associated with trauma.[69,238] Persons affected with this extremely rare disorder have been shown to be sensitive to the intradermal injection of trace amounts of DNA with negative controls.[363] The pathogenesis of DNA sensitivity is unknown at this time. Interestingly, chloroquine has been shown to be effective in the temporary control of this disorder; its mode of action in this regard is unclear.

Other acquired vascular disorders

Drug-induced vascular purpuras. When a drug is associated with the appearance of purpura and measurable hemostatic functions are normal, it is appropriate to assume that the blood vessel itself is directly affected. This assumption is strongly reinforced, of course, if the purpura clears on discontinuation of the drug. A variety of agents have been thereby suspected, including iodides, belladonna, bismuth, mercury, penicillin, phenacetin, chloral hydrate, and notably sulfonamides.[401]

Scurvy. Although scurvy from dietary lack of ascorbic acid is a rare disease in the United States, the purpura of this disease is a classical expression of an acquired vascular defect. Lesions may range from scattered perifollicular petechiae to substantial ecchymoses, particularly on the lower extremities. In affected infants subperiosteal hemorrhages and their effects are usually much more clinically impressive than purpura. Extravasation in scurvy is presumably related to defective synthesis of collagen and other substances that contribute to vascular support, particularly affecting small blood vessels. Oral administration of ascorbic acid rapidly corrects the purpura and promotes steady healing of bony lesions.

Corticosteroid-related purpura. Benign purpuric lesions, including symmetrical striae typically located just above the buttocks, are frequently observed in children with increased levels of corticosteroids: endogenous, as in Cushing's disease, or exogenous, as in prolonged treatment with pharmacologic doses of prednisone. Purpuric lesions usually resolve spontaneously in time if cor-

ticosteroid levels are restored to physiologic levels by appropriate therapeutic means. The mechanism of such purpura is unknown.

Benign hypergammaglobulinemic purpura. A unique form of chronic episodic purpura of the lower extremities associated with hypergammaglobulinemia was first described by Waldenström[417] in 1943. Although about 90% of all affected patients are adult women, benign hypergammaglobulinemic purpura (Waldenström's purpura) has been described in a few children.[200]

This disorder is acquired; its etiology has not been determined. It may occur either in isolated form or in association with a heterogenous group of diseases, including immunologic and neoplastic disorders.[232] The major clinical feature is recurrent purpura progressing to permanent brownish mottling, symmetrically affecting the lower extremities. The principal laboratory finding of this disorder is an increased concentration of IgG, typically found in complexes with intermediate sedimentation coefficients (approximately 12S) as well as in its isolated 7S form.[67] In accord with a vascular basis for this purpura, there is usually no thrombocytopenia or coagulation abnormality, and biopsies of affected skin show vasculitis. No drug has been shown to be effective in management of BHP but plasmapheresis has been shown to produce temporary symptomatic benefit.[200]

Waldenström's purpura should be sharply differentiated from Waldenström's macroglobulinemia. The latter is characterized by high levels of a predominantly monoclonal abnormal protein, usually occurs in adult males, and is rarely associated with purpura.[418] Coagulation abnormalities that may be associated with macroglobulinemia and other dysproteinemias are considered in Chapter 25.

Inherited vascular disorders

Ehlers-Danlos syndrome. Ehler-Danlos syndrome (EDS, cutis hyperelastica) is an autosomal dominant disorder characterized clinically by hyperelasticity of the skin, hyperlaxity of the joints, a generalized bruising tendency with purpura especially evident on the shins, and a tendency to formation of broad scars.[267,384,399] Joint and skin involvement are particularly consistent features (Figs. 24-15 and 24-16). Hemorrhagic manifestations range from mild purpura usually associated with identifiable trauma to life-threatening lesions of major arteries and veins, such as dissecting aneurysm of the aorta.[198,264,267]

The diagnosis of Ehlers-Danlos syndrome is made purely on clinical grounds, usually in a patient with purpura whose joint mobility and skin consistency are carefully examined by an alert physician. Results of screening tests of hemostatic

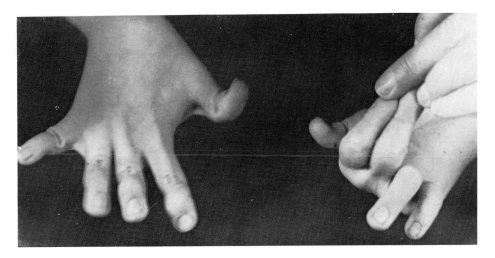

Fig. 24-15. Ehlers-Danlos syndrome. Hyperlaxity of the joints is especially prominent in the fingers. (From Smith, C. H.: J. Pediatr. **14:**632, 1939.)

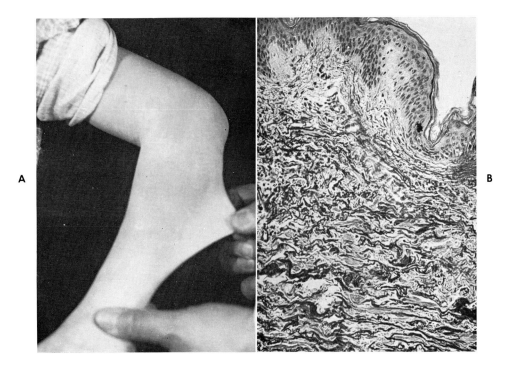

Fig. 24-16. Ehlers-Danlos syndrome. **A,** Loose and hyperelastic skin, stretched beyond normal limits, returns to normal position when released. **B,** High-power photomicrograph of skin. Note that the malpighian layer of the epidermis is reduced in cellular content. The dense reticulum of coarse elastic elements in the corium and the diminution of collagen fibers are important factors in the production of the gaping incised wounds characteristic of the syndrome. (×260.) (From Smith, C. H.: J. Pediatr. **14:**632, 1939.)

function are usually normal, although thrombocytopathy associated with Ehlers-Danlos syndrome has been described,[310] as well as factor IX deficiency.[244] Affected patients generally show no evidence of abnormal bleeding from surface wounds, and surgical procedures are normally tolerated.

The clinical signs of Ehlers-Danlos syndrome are an expression of faulty supportive soft tissue, primarily a result of defective synthesis and structure of collagen.[267] There is also evidence for an abnormal platelet-collagen reaction in this disease.[211] No specific therapy is currently available, but the majority of affected persons do not have serious disability, and commonsense avoidance of trauma suffices.

Hereditary hemorrhagic telangiectasia. Hereditary hemorrhagic telangiectasia (Rendu-Osler-Weber disease) is an autosomal dominant disorder characterized by variably distributed telangiectases involving small veins and by hemorrhage from these lesions. The term "hereditary hemorrhagic telangiectasia" was introduced by Hanes[157] in 1909 following separate definitive reports of this disorder by Rendu,[337] Osler,[315] and Weber.[425]

Rupture of telangiectases is associated with surface bleeding, not purpura. The diagnosis is made by the detection of characteristic macular lesions, which are 1 to 4 mm in diameter, have a reddish purple color, and blanch on pressure. Typically these lesions occur about the face and plantar surfaces of the hands and feet, the nasal mucosa, and less commonly the buccal mucosa and tongue; the trunk is usually spared. Epistaxes should always prompt a careful search for nasal telangiectases. Likewise the finding of such a lesion in an accessible site may provide an important clue to the cause of obscure visceral bleeding.

Laboratory studies, including tests of hemostasis, reveal no specific abnormalities although iron-deficiency anemia caused by chronic gastrointestinal blood loss is a classical finding. Pathologically telangiectases are characterized by marked deficiency of the subendothelial framework of affected veins. The lesions may be widespread, leading to formation of arteriovenous fistulas within major organs, particularly the lungs.[183] There is no specific treatment for this disorder, but the majority of patients may be successfully managed by standard supportive measures, notably treatment of associated iron-deficiency anemia. Lesions progress with age so that adults usually suffer more from hemorrhagic complications of this disease than do children.[386]

Other inherited vascular disorders. Although Ehlers-Danlos syndrome is perhaps the clearest example of a heritable connective tissue disorder associated with vascular purpura, other such disorders may show similar hemorrhagic manifestations. These include pseudoxanthoma elasticum, Marfan's syndrome,[267] and osteogenesis imperfecta.[378] Likewise, certain heritable telangiectatic disorders should be cited in addition to hereditary hemorrhagic telangiectasia: ataxia telangiectasia,[212] Fabry's disease (angiokeratoma corporis diffusum universale),[53] and Majocchi-Schamberg's disease (annular telangiectatic purpura).[301]

Neonatal vascular disorders

In general it is rarely possible to attribute hemorrhage in a newborn to an isolated vascular defect. However, such a defect may play a significant role in the pathogenesis of idiopathic bleeding in certain hypoxic or otherwise sick newborns. Sites in which such hemorrhage may occur with or without associated purpura include the brain, lungs, and gastrointestinal tract. Hathaway[165] has pointed out that a specific hemostatic defect cannot be identified in most cases of neonatal intracranial hemorrhage. Although the absence of measurable platelet or coagulation abnormalities in a bleeding newborn does not necessarily indicate the presence of faulty blood vessels, there is no doubt that mechanisms of such bleeding would be clarified by more knowledge of the neonatal vasculature.

Hemangioma and thrombocytopenia (Kasabach-Merritt syndrome). Hemangioma and thrombocytopenia (Kasabach-Merritt syndrome) are discussed in Chapter 25.

Purpuras with high platelet counts

Thrombocytosis may be defined as a platelet count above the upper limits of the normal range, i.e., approximately 400×10^9/liter.[57] Platelet counts exceeding $1,000 \times 10^9$/liter may be associated with variable hemostatic dysfunction, characterized by hemorrhagic or thrombotic complications. Thrombocytosis largely occurs in two groups of acquired disorders: (1) defective, if not frankly neoplastic, overproduction of platelets by the bone marrow in a group of diseases that Dameshek[90] termed myeloproliferative syndromes and (2) reactive or secondary thrombocytosis associated with a heterogeneous group of pathologic states, including inflammatory diseases,[254] neoplasms,[237] iron-deficiency anemia,[151] and the state following splenectomy and other surgical procedures.[59,243]

The issue of postsplenectomy thrombocytosis has been considered in the discussion of treatment for chronic ITP. In general abnormally high platelet counts in children, regardless of cause, are rarely associated with hemorrhagic or thrombotic complications. Thus the physician who finds thrombocytosis in a child should place a clear priority on diagnosis and management of a possible underlying disorder rather than on management of the thrombocytosis itself.

REFERENCES

1. Aballi, A. J., Puapondh, Y., and Desposito, F.: Platelet counts in thriving premature infants, Pediatrics **42:**685, 1968.
2. Abildgaard, C. F., and Simone, J. V.: Thrombopoiesis, Sem. Hematol. **4:**424, 1967.
3. Ackroyd, J. F.: Three cases of thrombocytopenic purpura occurring after rubella; with a review of purpura associated with infections, Q. J. Med. **18:**299, 1949.
4. Ackroyd, J. F.: The pathogenesis of thrombocytopenic purpura due to hypersensitivity to Sedormid, Clin. Sci. **7:**249, 1949.
5. Ackroyd, J. F.: Allergic purpura, including purpura due to foods, drugs, and infections, Am. J. Med. **14:**605, 1953.
6. Ackroyd, J. F.: The immunologic basis of purpura due to drug hypersensitivity, Proc. R. Soc. Med. **55:**30, 1962.
7. Ackroyd, J. F.: The diagnosis of disorders of the blood due to drug hypersensitivity caused by an immune mechanism. In Immunological methods, Philadelphia, 1964, F. A. Davis Co.
8. Adner, M. M., Fisch, G. R., Starobin, S. G., et al.: Use of "compatible" platelet transfusions in treatment of congenital isoimmune thrombocytopenic purpura, N. Engl. J. Med. **280:**244, 1969.
9. Ahn, Y. S., Harrington, W. J., Seelman, R., et al.: Vincristine therapy of idiopathic and secondary thrombocytopenias, N. Engl. J. Med. **291:**376, 1974.
10. Aldrich, R. A., Steinberg, A. G., and Campbell, D. C.: Pedigree demonstrated a sex-linked recessive condition characterized by draining ears, eczematoid dermatitis, and bloody diarrhea, Pediatrics **13:**133, 1954.
11. Alford, C. A., Jr., Neva, F. A., and Weller, T. H.: Virologic and serologic studies on human products of conception after maternal rubella, N. Engl. J. Med. **271:**1275, 1964.
12. Allen, D. M., Diamond, L. K., and Howell, D. A.: Anaphylactoid purpura in children (Schönlein-Henoch syndrome): review with a follow-up of the renal complications, Am. J. Dis. Child. **99:**833, 1960.
13. Allen, D. M., Necheles, T. F., Reiker, R., et al.: Reversible neonatal pancytopenia due to isovaleric acidemia, Presented to Society for Pediatric Research, Atlantic City, May, 1969.
14. Alter, H. J., Scanlon, R. T., and Schechter, G. P.: Thrombocytopenic purpura following vaccination with attenuated measles virus, Am. J. Dis. Child. **115:**111, 1968.
15. Altschule, M. D.: A rare type of acute thrombocytopenic purpura: widespread formation of platelet thrombi in capillaries, N. Engl. J. Med. **227:**477, 1942.
16. Amorosi, E. L., and Ultmann, J. E.: Thrombotic thrombocytopenic purpura: report of 16 cases and review of the literature, Medicine **45:**139, 1966.
17. Angle, R. M., and Alt, H. L.: Thrombocytopenic purpura complicating infectious mononucleosis: report of a case and serial platelet counts during the course of infectious mononucleosis, Blood **5:**449, 1950.
18. Anthony, P. P., and Kaplan, A. B.: Haemolytic-uraemic syndrome in two sibs, Arch. Dis. Child. **43:**316, 1968.
19. Aspnes, G. T., Pearson, H. A., Spencer, R. P., et al: Recurrent idiopathic thrombocytopenic purpura with "accessory" splenic tissue, Pediatrics **55:**131, 1975.
20. Aster, R. H.: Pooling of platelets in the spleen: role in the pathogenesis of "hypersplenic" thrombocytopenia, J. Clin. Invest. **45:**645, 1955.
21. Aster, R. H.: Effect of anticoagulant and ABO incompatibility on recovery of transfused human platelets, Blood **26:**732, 1965.
22. Aster, R. H.: Drug-induced immunologic thrombocytopenic purpura. In Williams, W. J., Beutler, E., Erslev, A. J., et al. eds.: Hematology, New York, 1972, McGraw-Hill Book Co.
23. Aster, R. H., and Keene, W. R.: Sites of platelet destruction in idiopathic thrombocytopenic purpura, Br. J. Haematol. **16:**61, 1969.
24. Ata, M., Fisher, O. D., and Holman, C. A.: Inherited thrombocytopenia, Lancet **1:**119, 1965.
25. Baadenhuijsen, H., Hirschhauser, C., Kurstjens, R., et al.: Metabolic observations on platelets from patients with familial thrombopathic thrombocytopenia, Br. J. Haematol. **20:**417, 1971.
26. Bach, F. H., Albertini, R. J., Joo, P., et al.: Bone marrow transplantation in a patient with Wiskott-Aldrich syndrome, Lancet **2:**1364, 1968.
27. Baker, D. H., Parmer, E. A., and Wolff, J. A.: Roentgen manifestations of the Aldrich syndrome, Am. J. Roentgenol. **88:**458, 1962.
28. Baldini, M.: Idiopathic thrombocytopenic purpura, N. Engl. J. Med. **274:**1245, 1966.
29. Baldini, M. G.: Nature of the platelet defect in the Wiskott-Aldrich syndrome, Ann. N.Y. Acad. Sci. **201:**437, 1972.
30. Balf, C. L.: The alimentary lesion in anaphylactoid purpura, Arch. Dis. Child. **26:**20, 1951.
31. Ballard, H. S., Eisinger, R. P., and Gallo, G.: Renal manifestations of the Henoch-Schoenlein syndrome in adults, Am. J. Med. **49:**328, 1970.
32. Ballard, H. S., and Marcus, A. J.: Primary and secondary platelet aggregation in uraemia, Scand. J. Haematol. **9:**198, 1972.
33. Basu, R.: Perforation of the bowel in Henoch-Schönlein purpura, Arch. Dis. Child. **34:**342, 1959.
34. Baumgartner, H. R.: Platelet interaction with vascular structures, Thromb. Diath. Haemorrh. **51**(suppl.):161, 1972.
35. Baumgartner, H. R.: The role of blood flow in platelet adhesion, fibrin deposition, and formation of nural thrombi, Microvasc. Res. **5:**167, 1973.
36. Bayer, W. L., Sherman, F. E., Michaels, R. H., et al.: Purpura in congenital and acquired rubella, N. Engl. J. Med. **273:**1362, 1965.
37. Behnke, O.: An electron microscopic study of the rat megakaryocyte: some aspects of platelet release and microtubules, J. Ultrastruc. Res. **26:**111, 1969.
38. Behnke, O.: The morphology of blood platelet membrane systems, Ser. Haematol. **3:**3, 1970.
39. Belber, J. P., Davis, A. E., and Epstein, E. A.: Thrombocytopenic purpura associated with cat-scratch disease, Arch. Intern. Med. **94:**321, 1954.
40. Bergstrand, A., Bergstrand, C. G., and Bucht, H.: Kidney lesions associated with anaphylactoid purpura in children, Acta Pediatr. **49:**57, 1960.
41. Bergstrand, C. G., and Bucht, H.: Renal biopsy in children, Acta Pediatr. **48**(suppl. 117):126, 1959.
42. Berman, N., and Finklestein, J. Z.: Thrombotic thrombocytopenic purpura in childhood, Scand. J. Haematol. **14:**286, 1975.
43. Bernard, J., and Soulier, J. P.: Sur une nouvelle variété de dystrophie thrombocytaire hémorragipare congénitale, Sem. Hop. Paris **24:**3217, 1948.

44. Billo, O. E., and Wolff, J. A.: Thrombocytopenic purpura due to cat-scratch disease, J.A.M.A. **174:**1824, 1960.
45. Bithell, T. C., Didisheim, G. E., and Wintrobe, M. M.: Thrombocytopenia inherited as an autosomal dominant trait, Blood **25:**231, 1965.
46. Blaese, R. M., Strober, W., Brown, R. S., et al.: The Wiskott-Aldrich syndrome: a disorder with a possible defect in antigen processing or recognition, Lancet **1:**1056, 1968.
47. Bleyer, W. A., Hakami, N., and Shepard, T. H.: The development of hemostasis in the human fetus and the newborn infant, J. Pediatr. **79:**838, 1971.
48. Bluestone, S. S., and Maslow, H. L.: Essential thrombocytopenic purpura in the newborn infant. Report of first case treated by splenectomy, Pediatrics **4:**620, 1949.
49. Booyse, F., Kisieleski, D., Seeler, R., et al.: Possible thrombosthenin defect in Glanzmann's thrombasthenia, Blood **39:**377, 1972.
50. Booyse, R. M., and Rafelson, M. E., Jr.: Human platelet contractile proteins: location, properties, and function, Ser. Haematol. **4:**152, 1971.
51. Born, G. V. R.: Aggregation of blood platelets by adenosine diphosphate and its reversal, Nature **194:**927, 1962.
52. Bosmann, H. B.: Platelet adhesiveness and aggregation: the collagen: glycosyl, polypeptide: N-acetylgalactosaminyl and glycoprotein: galactosyl transferases of human platelets, Biochem. Biophys. Res. Commun. **43:**1118, 1971.
53. Brady, R. O., Tallman, J. F., Johnson, W. G., et al.: Replacement therapy for inherited enzyme deficiency: use of purified ceramide trihexosidase in Fabry's disease, N. Engl. J. Med. **289:**9, 1973.
54. Brain, M. C.: The haemolytic uraemic syndrome, Sem. Haematol. **6:**162, 1969.
55. Brain, M. C., Dacie, J. V., and Hourihane, D. O.: Microangiopathic haemolytic anemia; the possible role of vascular lesions in pathogenesis, Br. J. Haematol. **8:**358, 1962.
56. Brain, M. C., and Hourihane, D. O.: Microangiopathic haemolytic anemia; the occurrence of haemolysis in experimentally produced vascular disease, Br. J. Haemat. **13:**135, 1967.
57. Brecher, G., and Cronkite, E. P.: Morphology and enumeration of human blood platelets, J. Appl. Physiol. **3:**365, 1958.
58. Breckenridge, R. T., Moore, R. D., and Ratnoff, O. D.: A study of thrombocytopenia: new histologic criteria for the differentiation of idiopathic thrombocytopenia and thrombocytopenia associated with disseminated lupus erythematosus, Blood **30:**39, 1967.
59. Breslow, A., Kaufman, R. M., and Lawsky, A. R.: The effects of surgery on the concentration of circulating megakaryocytes and platelets, Blood **32:**393, 1968.
60. Brodie, G. N., Baenziger, N. L., Chase, L. R., et al.: The effects of thrombin on adenyl cyclase activity and a membrane protein from human platelets, J. Clin. Invest. **51:**81, 1972.
61. Brooks, P., O'Shea, M., and Pryor, J.: Splenectomy in the treatment of idiopathic thrombocytopenic purpura, Br. J. Surg. **56:**861, 1969.
62. Burke, D. M., and Jellinek, H. L.: Nearly fatal case of Schönlein-Henoch syndrome following insect bite, Am. J. Dis. Child. **88:**772, 1954.
63. Bywaters, E. G. L., Isdale, I., and Kempton, J. J.: Schönlein-Henoch purpura: evidence for a group A beta haemolytic streptococcal aetiology, Q. J. Med. **26:**161, 1957.
64. Caen, J. P., Castaldi, P. A., Leclerc, J. C., et al.: Congenital bleeding disorders with long bleeding time and normal platelet count. I. Glanzmann's thrombasthenia (report of 15 patients), Am. J. Med. **41:**4, 1966.
65. Caffey, J.: Multiple fractures in long bones of infants suffering from chronic subdural hematoma, Am. J. Roentgenol. **56:**163, 1946.
66. Canales, M. L., and Mauer, A. M.: Sex-linked hereditary thrombocytopenia as a variant of the Wiskott-Aldrich syndrome, N. Engl. J. Med. **277:**899, 1967.
67. Capra, J. D., Winchester, R. J., and Kunkel, H. G.: Hypergammaglobulinemic purpura, Medicine **50:**125, 1971.
68. Casser, L.: Anaphylactoid purpura following penicillin therapy, J. Med. Soc. N.J. **53:**133, 1956.
69. Chandler, D., and Nalbandian, R. M.: DNA autosensitivity, Am. J. Med. Sci. **251:**145, 1966.
70. Chessells, J. M., and Wigglesworth, J. S.: Haemostatic failure in babies with Rhesus isoimmunization, Arch. Dis. Child. **46:**38, 1971.
71. Chiaro, J. J., Ayut, D., and Bloom, G. E.: X-linked thrombocytopenic purpura. I. Clinical and genetic studies of a kindred, Am. J. Dis. Child. **123:**565, 1972.
72. Christodoulou, C., and Werner, B.: A girl with 18-trisomy and thrombocytopenia, Acta Genet. **17:**77, 1967.
73. Clancy, R., Jenkins, E., and Firkin, B.: Qualitative platelet abnormalities in idiopathic thrombocytopenic purpura, N. Engl. J. Med. **286:**622, 1972.
74. Clark, W. G., and Jacobs, E.: Experimental non-thrombocytopenic vascular purpura: a review of the Japanese literature with preliminary confirmatory report, Blood **5:**320, 1950.
75. Clarke, B. F., and Davies, S. H.: Severe thrombocytopenia in infectious mononucleosis, Am. J. Med. Sci. **248:**703, 1964.
76. Clawson, C. C., and White, J. G.: Platelet interaction with bacteria. II. Fate of the bacteria, Am. J. Pathol. **65:**381, 1971.
77. Cohen, P., and Gardner, F. H.: The thrombocytopenic effect of sustained high-dose prednisone therapy in thrombocytopenic purpura, N. Engl. J. Med. **265:**613, 1961.
78. Cohen, P., Gardner, F. H., and Barnett, G. O.: Reclassification of the thrombocytopenias by the ^{51}Cr-labeling method for measuring platelet lifespan, N. Engl. J. Med. **264:**1294, 1961.
79. Cooper, B. A., and Bigelow, F. S.: Thrombocytopenia associated with the administration of diethylstilbesterol in man, Ann. Intern. Med. **52:**907, 1960.
80. Cooper, L. Z., Green, K. H., Krugman, S., et al.: Neonatal thrombocytopenic purpura and other manifestations of rubella contracted in utero, Am. J. Dis. Child. **110:**416, 1965.
81. Cooper, M. D., Chase, H. P., Lowman, J. T., et al.: Wiskott-Aldrich syndrome, an immunologic deficiency disease involving the afferent limb of immunity, Am. J. Med. **44:**499, 1968.
82. Corby, D. G., and Schulman, I.: The effects of antenatal drug administration on aggregation of platelets of newborn infants, J. Pediatr. **79:**307, 1971.
83. Corrigan, J. J.: Thrombocytopenia: laboratory sign of septicemia in infants and children, J. Pediatr. **85:**219, 1974.
84. Craig, J. M., and Gitlin, D.: The nature of the hyaline thrombi and thrombotic thrombocytopenic purpura, Am. J. Pathol. **33:**251, 1957.
85. Creger, W. P., and Houseworth, J. H.: Erythrophagocytosis and thrombocytopathy occurring during the course of a Henoch-Schönlein syndrome due to quinine, Am. J. Med. **17:**423, 1954.
86. Cronkite, E. P., Bond, V. P., Fliedner, T. M., et al.: Studies on the origin, production, and destruction of platelets. In Johnson, S. A., ed.: Blood platelets, Boston, 1961, Little, Brown & Co.
87. Cullum, C., Cooney, D. P., and Schrier, S. L.: Familial

thrombocytopenic thrombocytopathy, Br. J. Haematol. **13**:147, 1967.

88. Czapek, E. E., Deykin, D., and Salzman, E. W.: Platelet dysfunction in glycogen storage disease Type I, Blood **41**:325, 1973.

89. Dacie, J. V.: The haemolytic anaemias, New York, 1954, Grune & Stratton, Inc.

90. Dameshek, W.: Some speculations on the myeloproliferative syndromes, Blood **6**:372, 1951.

91. Dameshek, W., and Miller, E. B.: The megakaryocytes in idiopathic thrombocytopenic purpura, a form of hypersplenism, Blood **1**:27, 1946.

92. Dameshek, W., Rubio, F., Jr., Mahoney, J. P., et al.: Treatment of idiopathic thrombocytopenic purpura (ITP) with prednisone, J.A.M.A. **166**:1805, 1958.

93. Davis, E.: The Schönlein-Henoch syndrome of vascular purpura, Blood **3**:129, 1948.

94. Davis, J. W., McField, J. R., Phillips, P. E., et al.: Guanidinosuccinic acid on human platelet effects of exogenous urea, creatinine, and aggregation in vitro, Blood **39**:388, 1972.

95. Davis, J. W., and Wilson, S. J.: Platelet survival in the May-Hegglin anomaly, Br. J. Haematol. **12**:61, 1968.

96. Day, H. J., and Holmsen, H.: Concepts of the platelet release reaction, Ser. Haematol. **4**:3, 1971.

97. Day, H. J., and Holmsen, H.: Platelet adenine nucleotide "storage pool deficiency" in thrombocytopenic absent radii syndrome, J.A.M.A. **221**:1053, 1972.

98. Derham, R. J., and Rogerson, M. M.: The Schönlein-Henoch syndrome with particular reference to renal sequelae, Arch. Dis. Child. **31**:364, 1956.

99. Desai, R. G., McCutcheon, E., Little, B., et al.: Fetomaternal passage of leukocytes and platelets in erythroblastosis fetalis, Blood **27**:858, 1966.

100. Desforges, J. F., and O'Connell, L. G.: Hematologic observations of the course of erythroblastosis fetalis, Blood **10**:302, 1955.

101. Deutsch, E.: Assays for platelet factors. In Bang, N. U., et al.: Thrombosis and bleeding disorders: theory and methods, Stuttgart, 1971, Georg Thieme Verlag.

102. Deykin, D.: Emerging concepts of platelet function, N. Engl. J. Med. **290**:144, 1974.

103. Didisheim, P., Kazmier, F. J., and Fuster, V.: Platelet inhibition in the management of thrombosis, Thromb. Diath. Haemorrh. **32**:21, 1974.

104. Dixon, R., Rosse, W., and Ebbert, L.: Quantitative determination of antibody in idiopathic thrombocytopenic purpura, N. Engl. J. Med. **292**:230, 1975.

105. Doan, C. A.: Hypersplenism, Bull. N.Y. Acad. Med. **25**:625, 1949.

106. Doan, C. A., Bouroncle, B. A., and Wiseman, B. K.: Idiopathic and secondary thrombocytopenic purpura; clinical study and evaluation of 381 cases over a period of 28 years, Ann. Intern. Med. **53**:861, 1960.

107. Doery, J. C. G., Hirsh, J., and Cooper, I.: Energy metabolism in human platelets: interrelationship between glycolysis and oxidative metabolism, Blood **36**:159, 1970.

108. Dohrn, E.: Ein Fall von Morbus maculosus Werlhofi übertragen von der Mutter auf die Frucht, Arch. Gynaekol. **6**:486, 1873.

109. Donati, M. B., de Gaetano, G., and Vermylen, J.: Evidence that bovine factor VIII, not bovine fibrinogen, aggregates human platelets, Throm. Res. **2**:97, 1973.

110. Douglas, S. D., and Fudenberg, H. H.: Graft versus host reaction in Wiskott-Aldrich syndrome: antemortem diagnosis of human GVH in an immunologic deficiency disease, Vox Sang. **16**:172, 1969.

111. Dubilier, L. D., Chadwick, J. A., and Leddy, J. P.: Thymic alymphoplasia with the hemolytic uremic syndrome, J. Pediatr. **73**:714, 1968.

112. Eberth, J. C., and Schimmelbusch, C.: Experimentelle Untersuchungen uber Thrombose, Virchows Arch. Pathol. Anat. **103**:39, 1886.

113. Ekert, H., and Mathew, R. Y.: Platelet counts and plasma fibrinogen levels in erythroblastosis foetalis, Med. J. Aust. **2**:844, 1967.

114. Engstrom, K., Linkquist, A., and Soderstrom, N.: Periodic thrombocytopenia or tidal platelet dysgenesis in a man, Scand. J. Haematol. **3**:290, 1966.

115. Epstein, C. J., Sahud, M. A., Piel, C. F., et al.: Hereditary macrothrombocytopathia, nephritis, and deafness, Am. J. Med. **52**:299, 1972.

116. Estren, S., and Dameshek, W.: Familial hypoplastic anemia of childhood, Am. J. Dis. Child. **73**:671, 1947.

117. Evans, R. S., and Duane, R. T.: Acquired hemolytic anemia: the relation of erythrocyte antibody production to activity of the disease: the significance of thrombocytopenia and leucopenia, Blood **4**:1196, 1949.

118. Evans, R. S., Takahashi, K., Duane, A. B., et al.: Primary thrombocytopenic purpura and acquired hemolytic anemia; evidence for a common etiology, Arch. Intern. Med. **87**:48, 1951.

119. Faloon, W. W., Greene, R. W., and Lozner, E. L.: Hemostatic defect in thrombocytopenia as studied by use of ACTH and cortisone, Am. J. Med. **13**:12, 1952.

120. Fanconi, G.: Familiare infantile perniziosa: artige Anamie (Pernizioses Blutbild und Konstitution), Jahrb. Kinderheilkd. **117**:257, 1927.

121. Farber, S., and Craig, J. M.: Clinicopathological conference: Children's Medical Center, Boston, Mass., J. Pediatr. **51**:85, 1957.

122. Favara, B. E., Franciosi, R. A., and Butterfield, L. J.: Disseminated intravascular and cardiac thrombosis of the neonate, Am. J. Dis. Child **127**:197, 1974.

123. Feldt, R. H., and Stickler, G. B.: The gastrointestinal manifestations of anaphylactoid purpura in children, Proc. Staff Meet. Mayo Clin. **37**:465, 1962.

124. Ferguson, A. W.: Rubella as a cause of thrombocytopenic purpura, Pediatrics **25**:400, 1960.

125. Fisher, O. D., and Kraszewski, T. M.: Thrombocytopenic purpura following measles, Arch. Dis. Child. **27**:144, 1952.

126. Fitzgerald, E. W., Jr.: Fatal glomerulonephritis complicating allergic purpura due to chlorothiazide, Arch. Intern. Med. **105**:305, 1960.

127. Frank, E.: Die Essentielle thrombopenie, Berlin Klin. Wochenschr. **52**:454, 1915.

128. Gaarder, A., Jonsen, J., Laland, S., et al.: Adenosine diphosphate in red cells as a factor in the adhesiveness of human blood platelets, Nature **192**:531, 1961.

129. Gabb, B. W., and Bodmer, W. F.: A micro-complement-fixation test for platelet antibodies. In Teraski, P., ed.: Histocompatibility testing, Baltimore, 1970, The Williams & Wilkins Co.

130. Gairdner, D.: The Schönlein-Henoch syndrome (anaphylactoid purpura), Q. J. Med. **17**:95, 1948.

131. Gangarosa, E. J., Johnson, T. R., and Ramos, H. S.: Ristocetin-induced thrombocytopenia: site and mechanism of action, Arch. Intern. Med. **105**:83, 1960.

132. Gardner, F. H.: Idiopathic thrombocytopenic purpura. In Samter, M., ed.: Immunological diseases, Boston, 1971, Little, Brown & Co.

133. Gardner, F. H., and Diamond, L. K.: Autoerythrocyte sensitization: a form of purpura producing painful bruising following auto-sensitization to red blood cells in certain women, Blood **10**:675, 1955.

134. Gasser, C., Gautier, E., Steck, A., et al.: Hämolytisch-urämische syndrome: bilateral Nierenrindennekrosen bei akuten erwobenen hämolytisehen Anämien, Schweiz. Med. Wochenschr. **85**:905, 1955.

135. Gelzer, J., and Gasser, C.: Wiskott-Aldrich syndrome, Helv. Paediatr. Acta **16**:17, 1961.

136. Genton, E., Hirsch, J., Gent, M., et al.: Platelet-inhibiting drugs in thrombotic disease, N. Engl. J. Med. **293:** 1174, 1975.

137. Gervais, M., Richardson, J. B., Chiu, J., et al.: Immunofluorescent and histologic findings in the hemolytic uremic syndrome, Pediatrics **47:**352, 1971.

138. Gianantonio, C. A., Vitacco, M., Fernando, M., et al.: The hemolytic-uremic syndrome: renal status of 76 patients at long-term followup, J. Pediatr. **72:**757, 1968.

139. Gianantonio, C., Vitacco, M., Mendilaharzu, F., et al.: The hemolytic uremic syndrome, J. Pediatr. **64:**478, 1964.

140. Gimbrone, M. A., Jr., Aster, R. H., Cotran, R. S., et al.: Preservation of vascular integrity in organs perfused in vitro with a platelet-rich medium, Nature **221:**33, 1969.

141. Gitlin, D.: The differentiation and maturation of specific immune mechanisms, Acta Pediatr. Scand. **172**(suppl.): 60, 1967.

142. Glanzmann, E.: Hereditäre haemorrhagische Thrombasthenie, Ein Beitrag zur Pathologie der Blutplättchen, Jahrb. Kinderheilkd. **88:**1, 1918.

143. Glanzmann, E.: Die Konzeption der anaphylaktoiden Purpura, Jahrb. Kinderheilkd. **91:**391, 1920.

144. Gockermann, J. P., and Shulman, N. R.: Isoantibody specificity in posttransfusion purpura, Blood **41:**817, 1973.

145. Gordon, R. R.: Aldrich's syndrome: familial thrombocytopenia, eczema, and infection, Arch. Dis. Child. **35:** 259, 1960.

146. Gottlieb, P. M., Stupniker, S., Sandberg, H., et al.: Erythrocyte autosensitization, Am. J. Med. Sci. **233:** 196, 1957.

147. Grandjean, L. C.: A case of purpura hemorrhagica after administration of quinine with specific thrombocytolysis demonstrated in vitro, Acta Med. Scand. **131**(suppl. 213):165, 1948.

148. Groch, G. S., Finch, S. C., Rogoway, W., et al.: Studies in the pathogenesis of autoerythrocyte sensitization syndrome, Blood **28:**19, 1966.

149. Gross, R. E.: The surgery of infancy and childhood: its principles and techniques, Philadelphia, 1953, W. B. Saunders Co.

150. Gross, R., Gerok, W., Lohr, G. W., et al.: Uber die Natur de Thrombasthenia; Thrombopathie Glanzmann-Naegeli, Klin. Wochenschr. **38:**193, 1960.

151. Gross, S., Keefer, V., and Newman, P. J.: The platelets in iron-deficiency anemia. I. The response to oral and parenteral iron, Pediatrics **34:**315, 1964.

152. Gröttum, K. A., Hovig, T., Holmsen, H., et al.: Wiskott-Aldrich syndrome; qualitative platelet defects and short platelet survival, Br. J. Haematol. **17:**373, 1969.

153. Gröttum, K. A., and Solum, N. O.: Congenital thrombocytopenia with giant platelets; a defect in the platelet membrane, Br. J. Haematol. **16:**277, 1969.

154. Gynn, T. N., Messmore, H. L., and Friedman, I. A.: Drug-induced thrombocytopenia, Med. Clin. North Am. **56:**65, 1972.

155. Hall, J. G., Levin, J., Kuhn, J. P., et al.: Thrombocytopenia with absent radius (TAR), Medicine **48:**411, 1969.

156. Hamberg, M., Svensson, J., Wakabayshi, T., et al.: Isolation and structure of two prostaglandin endoperoxides that cause platelet aggregation, Proc. Natl. Acad. Sci. **71:**345, 1974.

157. Hanes, F. M.: Multiple hereditary telangiectases causing hemorrhage (hereditary hemorrhagic telangiectasia), Bull. Johns Hopkins Hosp. **20:**63, 1909.

158. Hardisty, R. M., and Hutton, R. A.: Bleeding tendency associated with new abnormalities of platelet behavior, Lancet **1:**983, 1967.

159. Harker, L. A., and Finch, C. A.: Thrombokinetics in man, J. Clin. Invest. **48:**963, 1969.

160. Harrington, W. J., Hollingsworth, J. W., Minnich, V., et al.: Demonstration of thrombocytopenic factor in blood of patients with idiopathic thrombocytopenic purpura, J. Clin. Invest. **30:**646, 1951.

161. Harrington, W. J., Minnich, V., Hollingsworth, J. W., et al.: Demonstration of a thrombocytopenic factor in the blood of patients with thrombocytopenic purpura, J. Lab. Clin. Med. **38:**1, 1951.

162. Harrington, W. J., Sprague, C. C., Minnich, V., et al.: Immunologic mechanisms in idiopathic and neonatal thrombocytopenic purpura, Ann. Intern. Med. **38:**433, 1953.

163. Harrison, M. J. G., Emmons, P. R., and Mitchell, J. R. A.: The effect of sulfhydryl and enzyme inhibitors on platelet aggregation in vitro, Thromb. Diath. Haemorrh. **16:**122, 1966.

164. Hathaway, W. E.: Coagulation problems in the newborn infant, Pediatr. Clin. North Am. **17:**929, 1970.

165. Hathaway, W. E.: The bleeding newborn. In Oski, F. A., Jaffe, E. R., and Miescher, P. A., eds.: Hematology, New York, 1975, Grune & Stratton, Inc.

166. Hathaway, W. E., Solomons, C. C., and Ott, J. E.: Platelet function and pyrophosphates in osteogenesis imperfecta, Blood **39:**500, 1972.

167. Hawkings, J. R., Jones, K. S., Sim, M., et al.: Deliberate disability, Br. Med. J. **1:**361, 1956.

168. Hayem, G.: Recherches sur l'évolution des hématies dans le sang de l'homme et des vertébrés, Arch. Phys. Norm. Pathol. **5:**692, 1878.

169. Hegglin, V. R.: Gleichzeitige konstitutionelle Veranderungen a Neutrophilen und Thrombozyten, Helv. Med. Acta **4:**439, 1945.

170. Hellem, A. J.: The adhesiveness of human blood platelets in vitro, Scand. J. Clin. Lab. Invest. **12**(suppl. 51):1, 1960.

171. Hellem, A. J.: Platelet adhesiveness, Ser. Haematol. **1:** 99, 1968.

172. Henoch, E.: Zusammenghang von Purpura und Intestinalstorungen, Berlin Klin. Wochenschr. **5:**517, 1868.

173. Henoch, E.: Ueber eine eigenthumliche Form von Purpura, Berl. Klin. Wochenschr. **11:**641, 1874.

174. Hertzog, A. J.: Essential thrombocytopenic purpura; autopsy findings in thirty-six cases, J. Lab. Clin. Med. **32:**618, 1947.

175. Heys, R. F.: Child bearing and idiopathic thrombocytopenic purpura, J. Obstet. Gynaecol. Br. Comm. **73:** 205, 1966.

176. Hilgartner, M. W.: Transient functional thrombasthenia in the newborn, Presented to Society for Pediatric Research, 1968.

177. Hilgartner, M. W., Lanzkowsky, P., and Smith, C. H.: The use of azathioprine in refractory idiopathic thrombocytopenic purpura in children, Acta Paediatr. Scand. **59:**409, 1970.

178. Hirsch, E. O., and Dameshek, W.: Idiopathic thrombocytopenia, Arch. Intern. Med. **88:**701, 1951.

179. Hirsch, E. O., and Gardner, F. H.: Transfusion of human blood platelets: with note on transfusion of granulocytes, J. Lab. Clin. Med. **39:**556, 1952.

180. Hirschman, R. J., and Shulman, N. R.: The use of platelet serotonin release as a sensitive method for detecting anti-platelet antibodies and a plasma antiplatelet factor in patients with idiopathic thrombocytopenic purpura, Br. J. Haematol. **24:**793, 1973.

181. Hirsh, J., Castelan, D. J., and Yoder, P. B.: Spontaneous bruising associated with defect in interaction of platelets with connective tissue, Lancet **2:**18, 1967.

182. Hirsh, J., and Doery, J. C. G.: Platelet function in health and disease, Prog. Hematol. **7:**185, 1972.

183. Hodgson, C. H., and Kaye, R. L.: Pulmonary arteriovenous fistula and hereditary hemorrhagic telangiectasia;

a review and report of 35 cases of fistula, Dis. Chest **43**:449, 1963.

184. Holemans, R., Johnston, J. G., and McConnell, D. G.: Origin and stability of blood plasminogen activator. In Proceedings of the tenth congress of the European Society of Haematology (Strasbourg, 1965), Basel, 1967, S. Karger.

185. Holmsen, H.: The platelet: its membrane, physiology, and biochemistry, Clin. Haematol. **1**:235, 1972.

186. Holmsen, H., Setkowsky, C. A., and Day, H. J.: Effects of antimycin and 2-deoxyglucose on adenine mucleotides in human platelets: role of metabolic adenine triphosphate in primary aggregation, secondary aggregation, and shape change of platelets, Biochem. J. **144**:385, 1974.

187. Holmsen, H., and Weiss, H. J.: Hereditary defect in the platelet release reaction caused by a deficiency in the storage pool of platelet adenine nucleotides, Br. J. Haematol. **19**:642, 1970.

188. Holmsen, H., and Weiss, H. J.: Further evidence for a deficient storage pool of adenine nucleotides in platelets from some patients with thrombocytopathia—"storage pool disease," Blood **39**:197, 1972.

189. Horowitz, H. I., Stein, I. M., Cohen, B. D., et al.: Further studies on the platelet-inhibiting effect of guanidinosuccinic acid and its role in uremic bleeding, Am. J. Med. **49**:336, 1970.

190. Hovig, T.: The ultrastructure of blood platelets in normal and abnormal states, Ser. Haematol. **1**:3, 1968.

191. Howard, M. A., and Firkin, B. G.: The effect of ristocetin on platelet-rich plasma, J. Aust. Soc. Med. Res. **2**:195, 1968.

192. Howard, M. A., and Firkin, B. G.: Ristocetin: a new tool in the investigation of platelet aggregation, Thromb. Diath. Haemorrh. **26**:362, 1971.

193. Howard, M. A., Hutton, R. A., and Hardisty, R. M.: Hereditary giant platelet syndrome: a disorder of a new aspect of platelet function, Br. Med. J. **2**:586, 1973.

194. Hudson, J. B., Weinstein, L., and Chang, T. W.: Thrombocytopenic purpura in measles, J. Pediatr. **48**:48, 1956.

195. Humble, J. G.: The mechanism of petechial hemorrhage formation, Blood **4**:69, 1949.

196. Huntley, C. C., and Dees, S. C.: Eczema associated with thrombocytopenic purpura and purulent otitis media, Pediatrics **19**:351, 1957.

197. Hyatt, H. W., Jr.: Fatal recurrent of acute thrombocytopenic purpura in an 8-year-old Negro child, J. Pediatr. **65**:456, 1964.

198. Imahori, S., Bannerman, R. M., Graf, C. J., et al.: Ehlers-Danlos syndrome with multiple arterial lesions, Am. J. Med. **47**:967, 1969.

199. Jackson, D. P., Morse, E. E., Zieve, P. D., et al.: Thrombocytopathic purpura associated with defective clot retraction and absence of platelet fibrinogen, Blood **12**:827, 1963.

200. Jacobs, J. C.: Hypergammaglobulinemic purpura in a child, J. Pediatr. **87**:91, 1975.

201. Jamieson, G. A.: Glycosyltransferases in platelet adhesion, Throm. Diath. Haemorrh. **60**(suppl.):111, 1974.

202. Janssen, F., Potvliege, P. R., Vainsel, M., et al.: Le pronostic a court et a long terme du syndrome hemolytique et uremique, Arch. Fr. Pediatr. **31**:59, 1974.

203. Jenkins, C. S. P., Phillips, D. R., Clemetson, K. J., et al.: Platelet membrane glycoproteins implicated in ristocetin-induced aggregation: studies of the proteins on platelets from patients with Bernard-Soulier syndrome and von Willebrand's disease, J. Clin. Invest. **57**:112, 1976.

204. Jerkner, K., Jutti, J., and Victorin, L.: Platelet counts in mothers and their newborn infants with respect to antepartum administration of oral diuretics, Acta Med. Scand. **194**:473, 1973.

205. Jim, R. T. S.: Thrombocytopenic purpura in cat-scratch disease, J.A.M.A. **176**:1036, 1961.

206. Jimenez, E. L., and Dorrington, H. S.: Vaccination and Henoch-Schönlein purpura; correspondence, N. Engl. J. Med. **279**:1171, 1968.

207. Johnson, S. A.: The endothelial supporting function of platelets. In Johnson, S. A., ed.: The circulating platelet, New York, 1971, Academic Press, Inc.

208. Jones, H. W., and Tocantins, L. M.: The history of purpura hemorrhagica, Ann. Med. Hist. **5**:349, 1933.

209. Jones, J. E., and Reed, J. F.: Renal vein thrombosis and thrombocytopenia in a newborn infant, J. Pediatr. **67**:681, 1965.

210. Kaplan, B. S., Katz, J., Krawitz, S., et al.: An analysis of the results of therapy in 67 cases of the hemolytic-uremic syndrome, J. Pediatr. **78**:420, 1971.

211. Karaca, M., Cronberg, L., and Nilsson, I. M.: Abnormal platelet-collagen reaction in Ehlers-Danlos syndrome, Scand. J. Haematol. **9**:465, 1972.

212. Karpati, G., Eissen, A. H., Andermann, F., et al.: Ataxia telangiectasia; further observations and report of eight cases, Am. J. Dis. Child. **110**:51, 1965.

213. Karpatkin, S., and Langer, R. M.: Biochemical energetics of simulated platelet plug formation: effect of thrombin, adenosine diphosphate and epinephrine on intra- and extracellular adenine nucleotide kinetics, J. Clin. Invest. **47**:2158, 1968.

214. Karpatkin, S., and Siskind, G. W.: In vitro detection of antiplatelet antibody in patients with idiopathic thrombocytopenic purpura and systemic lupus erythematosus, Blood **33**:795, 1969.

215. Katz, J., Krawitz, S., Sacks, P. V., et al.: Platelet, erythrocyte, and fibrinogen kinetics in the hemolytic-uremic syndrome of infancy, J. Pediatr. **83**:739, 1973.

216. Katz, J., Lurie, A., Kaplan, B. S., et al.: Coagulation findings in the hemolytic-uremic syndrome of infancy: similarity to hyperacute renal allograft rejection, J. Pediatr. **78**:426, 1971.

217. Kasnelson, P.: Verschwinden der hämorrhagischen Diathese bei einem Falle von essentieller Thrombopenie (Frank) nach Milzextirpation, Wein. Klin. Wochenschr. **29**:1451, 1916.

218. Kempe, C. H., Silverman, F. N., Steele, B. F., et al.: The battered-child syndrome, J.A.M.A. **181**:17, 1962.

219. Kildeberg, P.: The Aldrich syndrome: report of a case and discussion of pathogenesis, Pediatrics **27**:362, 1961.

220. King, H., and Shumaker, H. B., Jr.: Splenic studies: 1. Susceptibility to infection after splenectomy performed in infancy, Ann. Surg. **136**:329, 1952.

221. Kirk, J. E.: Thromboplastin activities of human arterial and venous tissues, Proc. Soc. Exp. Biol. Med. **109**:890, 1962.

222. Kisker, C. T., and Rush, R. A.: Absence of intravascular coagulation in the hemolytic-uremic syndrome, Am. J. Dis. Child. **129**:223, 1975.

223. Kolars, C. P., and Spink, W. W.: Thrombopenic purpura as a complication of mumps, J.A.M.A. **168**:2213, 1958.

224. Komrower, G. M., and Watson, G. H.: Prognosis in idiopathic thrombocytopenic purpura of childhood, Arch. Dis. Child. **29**:502, 1954.

225. Kreidberg, M. B., Dameshek, W., and Latorraca, R.: Acute vascular (Schönlein-Henoch) purpura, an immunologic disorder? N. Engl. J. Med. **253**:1014, 1955.

226. Kremer, W. B., Mengel, C. E., Nowlin, J. B., et al.: Recurrent ecchymoses and cutaneous hyperreactivity to hemoglobin: a form of autoerythrocyte sensitization, Blood **30**:62, 1967.

227. Krevans, J. R., and Jackson, D. P.: Hemorrhagic disorder following massive whole blood transfusions, J.A.M.A. **159**:171, 1955.

228. Krivit, W., and Good, R. A.: Aldrich's syndrome (thrombocytopenia, eczema, and infection in infants): studies of the defense mechanisms, Am. J. Dis. Child. **97:**137, 1959.

229. Kuramoto, A., Steiner, M., and Baldini, M.: Lack of platelet response to stimulation in the Wiskott-Aldrich syndrome, N. Engl. J. Med. **282:**475, 1970.

230. Kurstjens, R., Bolt, C., Vossen, M., et al.: Familial thrombopathic thrombocytopenia, Br. J. Haematol. **15:**305, 1968.

231. Kutti, J., and Weinfeld, A.: The frequency of thrombocytopenia in patients with heart disease treated with oral diuretics, Acta J. Scand. **183:**245, 1968.

232. Kyle, R. A., Gleich, G. J., Bayrd, E. D., et al.: Benign hypergammaglobulinemic purpura of Waldenstrom, Medicine **50:**113, 1971.

233. Lages, B., Scrutton, H. C., Holmsen, H., et al.: Metal ion content of gel-filtered platelets from patients with storage pool disease, Blood **45:**119, 1975.

234. Lammi, A. T., and Lovric, V. A.: Idiopathic thrombocytopenic purpura: an epiodemiologic study, J. Pediatr. **83:**31, 1973.

235. Lanzkowsky, P., and McCrory, W. W.: Disseminated intravascular coagulation as a possible factor in the pathogenesis of thrombotic microangiopathy (hemolytic-uremic syndrome), J. Pediatr. **70:**460, 1967.

236. Laros, R. K., Jr., and Penner, J. A.: "Refractory" thrombocytopenic purpura treated successfully with cyclophosphamide, J.A.M.A. **215:**445, 1971.

237. Levin, J., and Conley, C. L.: Thrombocytosis associated with malignant disease, Arch. Intern. Med. **114:**497, 1964.

238. Levin, M. B., and Pinkus, H.: Autosensitivity to deoxyribonucleic acid (DNA), N. Engl. J. Med. **264:**533, 1961.

239. Levin, R. M., Chodosh, R., and Sherman, J. D.: Factitious purpura simulating autoerythrocyte sensitization, Ann. Intern. Med. **70:**1201, 1969.

240. Lewis, I. C., and Philpott, M. G.: Neurological complications in the Schonlein-Henoch syndrome, Arch. Dis. Child. **31:**369, 1956.

241. Lieberman, E.: Hemolytic-uremic syndrome, J. Pediatr. **80:**1, 1972.

242. Lightsey, A. L., McMillan, R., Koenig, H. M., et al.: In vitro production of platelet-binding IgG in childhood idiopathic thrombocytopenic purpura, J. Pediatr. **88:**414, 1976.

243. Lipson, R. L., Bayrd, E. D., and Watkins, C. H.: The post-splenectomy blood picture, Am. J. Clin. Pathol. **35:**526, 1959.

244. Lisker, R., Nogueron, A., and Sanchez-Medal, L.: Plasma thromboplastin component deficiency in the Ehlers-Danlos syndrome, Ann. Intern. Med. **53:**388, 1960.

245. Lozner, E. L.: The thrombocytopenic purpuras, Bull. N.Y. Acad. Med. **30:**184, 1954.

246. Luscher, E. F., and Bettex-Galland, M.: Thrombosthenin, the contractile protein of blood platelets: new facts and problems, Pathol. Biol. **20**(suppl.):89, 1972.

247. Luscher, E. F., and Kaser-Glanzmann, R.: Platelet heparin-neutralizing factor (platelet factor 4), Thromb. Diath. Haemorrh. **33:**66, 1974.

248. Lusher, J. M., and Zuelzer, W. W.: Idiopathic thrombocytopenic purpura in childhood, J. Pediatr. **68:**971, 1966.

249. Lyman, B., Rosenberg, L., and Karpatkin, S.: Biochemical and biophysical aspects of human platelet adhesion to collagen fibers, J. Clin. Invest. **50:**1854, 1971.

250. Maak, B., Frenzel, J., and Rogner, G.: Aggregation of blood platelets and clot retraction in mature and premature infants, Z. Kinderheilkd. **111:**325, 1972.

251. MacFarlane, R. G.: The mechanism of haemostasis, Q. J. Med. **10:**1, 1941.

252. MacWhinney, J. B., Packer, J. T., Miller, G., et al.: Thrombotic thrombocytopenic purpura in childhood, Blood **19:**181, 1962.

253. Majerus, P. W., Smith, M. B., and Clamos, G. H.: Lipid metabolism in human platelets. I. Evidence for a complete fatty acid synthesizing system, J. Clin. Invest. **48:**156, 1965.

254. Marchasin, S., Wallerstein, R. D., and Aggeler, P. M.: Variation of the platelet count in disease, Calif. Med. **101:**95, 1964.

255. Marcus, A. J.: Platelet function, N. Engl. J. Med. **280:**1213, 1969.

256. Marcus, A. J., Safier, L. B., and Ullman, H. L.: Present concepts of the plasma membrane. In Brinkhous, K. M., Shermer, R. W., and Mostofi, F. K.: eds.: The platelet, Baltimore, 1971, The Williams & Wilkins Co.

256a. Markenson, A. L., Hilgartner, M. W., and Miller, D. R.: Transient thrombocytopenia in 18-trisomy, J. Pediatr. **87:**834, 1975.

257. Markovitz, A.: Thrombocytopenia in Colorado tick fever, Arch. Intern. Med. **111:**307, 1963.

258. Mauer, A. M.: Purpura in childhood, DM **1966:**1, October 1966.

259. Mauer, A. M., DeVaux, L. O., and Lahey, M. E.: Neonatal and maternal thrombocytopenic purpura due to quinine, Pediatrics **19:**84, 1957.

260. Maurer, H. M., McCue, C. M., Caul, J., et al.: Impairment in platelet aggregation in congenital heart disease, Blood **40:**207, 1972.

261. McClure, P. D.: Idiopathic thrombocytopenic purpura in children: diagnosis and management, Pediatrics **55:**68, 1975.

262. McDonagh, J., McDonagh, R. P., Delage, J. M., et al.: Factor XIII in human plasma and platelets, J. Clin. Invest. **48:**940, 1969.

263. McEnery, G., and Nash, F. W.: Wiskott-Aldrich syndrome associated with idiopathic infantile cortical hyperostosis (Caffey's disease), Arch. Dis. Child. **48:**818, 1973.

264. McFarland, W., and Fuller, D. E.: Mortality in Ehlers-Danlos syndrome due to spontaneous rupture of large arteries, N. Engl. J. Med. **271:**1309, 1964.

265. McIntosh, S., O'Brien, R. T., Schwartz, A. D., et al.: Neonatal isoimmune purpura: response to platelet infusions, J. Pediatr. **82:**1020, 1973.

266. McKeown, K. M.: A case of purpura factitia, Lancet **2:**555, 1920.

267. McKusick, V. A.: Heritable disorders of connective tissue, ed. 4, St. Louis, 1972, The C. V. Mosby Co.

268. McLean, M. M., Jones, C. H., and Sutherland, D. A.: Haemolytic-uraemic syndrome: a report of an outbreak, Arch. Dis. Scand. **41:**76, 1966.

269. McMillan, R., Longmire, R. L., Yelenosky, R., et al.: Quantitation of platelet-binding IgG produced in vitro by spleens from patients with idiopathic thrombocytopenic purpura, N. Engl. J. Med. **291:**812, 1974.

270. McMillan, R., Smith, R. S., Longmire, R. L., et al.: Immunoglobulins associated with human platelets, Blood **37:**316, 1971.

271. Meadl, M. A., Walston, J. I., and Rose, B.: The Wiskott-Aldrich syndrome: immunopathologic mechanisms and a long-term survival, Ann. Intern. Med. **68:**1050, 1968.

272. Mehes, K., and Bata, G.: Congenital thrombocytopenia in 13-15 trisomy, Lancet **1:**1279, 1965.

273. Meindersma, T. C., and deVries, S. I.: Thrombocytopenic purpura after small pox vaccination, Br. Med. J. **1:**226, 1962.

274. Merenstein, G. B., O'Loughlin, E. P., and Plunkett, D. C.: Effects of maternal thiazides on platelet counts of newborn infants, J. Pediatr. **76:**766, 1970.

275. Mettler, N. E.: Isolation of a microtatobiote from patients with hemolytic-uremic syndrome and thrombotic thrombocytopenic purpura and from mites in the United States, N. Engl. J. Med. **281:**1023, 1969.

276. Meuwissen, H. J., Gatti, R. A., Terasaki, P. I., et al.: Treatment of lymphopenic hypogammaglobulinemia and bone marrow aplasia by transplantation of allogeneic marrow, N. Engl. J. Med. **281:**691, 1969.

277. Meyer, D., Jenkins, C. S. P., Dreyfus, D., et al.: Willebrand factor and ristocetin. II. Relationship between Willebrand factor, Willebrand antigen and factor VIII activity, Br. J. Haematol. **28:**579, 1974.

278. Miescher, P., and Meischer, R.: Die Sedormid-Anaphylaxie, Schweiz. Med. Wochenschr. **82:**1279, 1952.

279. Miescher, P., and Straessle, R.: Experimentelle Studien uber den Mechanismus der Thrombocyten Schadigung durch antigen-antikorper Reacktionen, Vox Sang. **1:**83, 1956.

280. Mills, D. C. B.: Changes in the adenylate energy charge in human blood platelets induced by adenine diphosphate, Nature **243:**220, 1973.

281. Minot, G. R.: Purpura hemorrhagica with lymphocytosis; acute type and intermittent menstrual type, Am. J. Med. Sci. **192:**445, 1936.

282. Monroe, W. M., and Strauss, A. F.: Intravascular hemolysis: morphologic study of schizocytes in thrombotic purpura and other diseases, South. Med. J. **46:**837, 1953.

283. Moorhead, J. F.: Thrombotic thrombocytopenic purpura: recovery after splenectomy, Arch. Intern. Med. **117:**284, 1966.

284. Morley, A.: A platelet cycle in normal individuals, Aust. Ann. Med. **18:**127, 1969.

285. Morris, D. H., and Bullock, F. D.: The importance of the spleen in resistance to infection, Ann. Surg. **70:**513, 1919.

286. Morrow, G., III, Barness, L. A., Auerbach, V. H., et al.: Observations on the coexistence of methylmalonic acidemia and glycinemia, J. Pediatr. **74:**680, 1969.

287. Morse, E. E., Zinkhaus, W. H., and Jackson, D. P.: Thrombocytopenic purpura following rubella infection in children and adults, Arch. Intern. Med. **117:**573, 1966.

288. Moschcowitz, E.: An acute febrile pleiochromic anemia with hyaline thrombosis of the terminal arterioles and capillaries, Arch. Intern. Med. **36:**89, 1925.

289. Moulinier, J.: Iso-immunisation maternelle antiplaquettaire et purpura neonatal: le systeme de group plaquettair "duzo." In Proceedings of the sixth Congress of the European Society of Haematology, Basel, 1957, S. Karger.

290. Mull, M. M., and Hathaway, W. E.: Altered platelet function in newborns, Pediatr. Res. **4:**229, 1970.

291. Murphy, S., Oski, F. A., and Gardner, F. H.: Hereditary thrombocytopenia with an intrinsic platelet defect, N. Engl. J. Med. **281:**857, 1969.

292. Mustard, J. F., and Packham, M. A.: Factors influencing platelet adhesion, release, and aggregation, Pharmacol. Rev. **22:**97, 1970.

293. Myhre, B. A., ed.: Blood component therapy, Washington, D.C., 1975, American Association of Blood Banks.

294. Myllylä, G., Pelkonen, R., Ikkala, E., et al.: Hereditary thrombocytopenia: report of three families, Scand. J. Haematol. **4:**441, 1967.

295. Myllylä, G., Vaheri, A., Vesikari, T., et al.: Interaction between human blood platelets, viruses, and antibodies. IV. Post-rubella thrombocytopenic purpura and platelet aggregation by rubella antigen-antibody interaction, Clin. Exp. Immunol. **4:**323, 1969.

296. Nachman, R. L., Marcus, A. J., and Zucker-Franklin, D.: Immunologic studies of proteins associated with subcellular fractions of normal human platelets, J. Lab. Clin. Med. **69:**651, 1967.

297. Nachman, R. L., Weksler, B. B., and Ferris, B.: Increased vascular permeability produced by human platelet granule cationic extract, J. Clin. Invest. **49:**274, 1970.

298. Najean, Y.: Survival of radio chromium-labeled platelets in thrombocytopenias, Blood **22:**718, 1963.

299. Nathan, D. J., and Snapper, I.: Simultaneous placental transfer of factors responsible for LE cell formation and thrombocytopenia, Am. J. Med. **25:**647, 1958.

300. Newton, W. A., Jr., and Zuelzer, W. W.: Idiopathic thrombopenic purpura in childhood, N. Engl. J. Med. **245:**879, 1951.

301. Nichamin, S. J., and Brough, A. J.: Chronic progressive pigmentary purpura: purpura annulares telangiectodes of Majocchi-Schamberg, Am. J. Dis. Child. **116:**429, 1968.

302. Niewarowski, S., Bankowski, E., and Rogowicka, I.: Studies on the adsorption and activation of Hageman factor (factor XII) by collagen and elastin, Thromb. Diath. Haemmorh. **16:**387, 1965.

303. Niewiarowski, S., Farbiszewski, R., and Poplawski, A.: Studies on platelet factor 2 (PF2—fibrinogen activating factor) and platelet factor 4 (PF4—antiheparin factor). In Kowalski, E., and Kowalski, S., eds.: Biochemistry of blood platelets, New York, 1967, Academic Press, Inc.

304. Niewiarowski, S., Poplawski, A., Prokopwicz, J., et al.: Abnormalities of platelet function and ultrastructure in macrothrombocytic thrombopathia, Scand. J. Haematol. **6:**377, 1969.

305. Nurden, A. T., and Caen, J. P.: An abnormal platelet glycoprotein pattern in three cases of Glanzmann's thrombasthenia, Br. J. Haematol. **28:**253, 1974.

306. O'Brien, J. R.: Platelet aggregation, J. Clin. Pathol. **15:**446, 1962.

307. O'Brien, J. R.: Platelets: Portsmouth syndrome? Lancet **2:**258, 1967.

308. O'Gorman-Hughes, D. W.: Neonatal thrombocytopenia: assessment of aetiology and prognosis, Aust. Paediatr. **3:**226, 1967.

309. Oliver, T. K., Jr., and Barnett, H. L.: The incidence and prognosis of nephritis associated with anaphylactoid (Schönlein-Henoch) purpura in children, Am. J. Dis. Child. **90:**544, 1955.

310. Onel, D., Ulutin, S. B., and Ulutin, O. N.: Platelet defect in a case of Ehlers-Danlos syndrome, Acta Haematol. **50:**238, 1973.

311. Orringer, E., Lewis, M., Silverberg, J., et al.: Splenectomy in chronic idiopathic thrombocytopenic purpura, J. Chronic Dis. **23:**117, 1970.

312. Oski, F. A., and Naiman, J. L.: Effect of live measles vaccine on the platelet count, N. Engl. J. Med. **275:**352, 1966.

313. Oski, F. A., Naiman, J. L., Allen, D. M., et al.: Leukocytic inclusions—Döhle bodies—associated with platelet abnormality (the May-Hegglin anomaly): report of a family and review of the literature, Blood **20:**657, 1962.

314. Osler, W.: Visceral lesions of the erythema group, Br. J. Dermatol. **12:**227, 1900.

315. Osler, W.: On a family form of recurring epistaxis associated with multiple telangiectases of the skin and mucous membranes, Bull. Johns Hopkins Hosp. **12:**333, 1901.

316. Osler, W.: Visceral lesions of purpura and allied conditions, Br. Med. J. **1:**517, 1914.

317. Pearson, H. A., Shulman, N. R., Marder, V., et al.: Isoimmune neonatal thrombocytopenic purpura; clinical and therapeutic consideration, Blood **23:**154, 1964.

318. Pearson, H. A., Shulman, N. R., Oski, F. A., et al.: Platelet survival in Wiskott-Aldrich syndrome, J. Pediatr. **68:**754, 1966.

319. Pennington, D. G.: Isotope bioassay for "thrombopoietin," Br. J. Med. **1:**606, 1970.

320. Pepper, H., Liebowitz, D., and Lindsay, S.: Cyclical

thrombocytopenic purpura related to the menstrual cycle, Arch. Pathol. **61:**1, 1956.

321. Phillips, C. A., Melnick, J. L., Yow, M. D., et al.: Persistence of virus in infants with congenital rubella and in normal infants with a history of maternal rubella, J.A.M.A. **193:**1027, 1965.

322. Piel, C. F., and Phibbs, R. H.: The hemolytic-uremic syndrome, Pediatr. Clin. North Am. **13:**295, 1966.

323. Pletscher, A., Da Prada, M., Berneis, K. H., et al.: New aspects on the storage of 5-hydroxytryptamine in blood platelets, Experimentia **27:**993, 1971.

324. Pohle, F. J.: Blood platelet count in relation to menstrual cycle in normal women, Am. J. Med. Sci. **197:**40, 1939.

325. Post, R. M., and DesForges, J. F.: Thrombocytopenia and alcoholism, Ann. Intern. Med. **68:**1230, 1968.

326. Powell, H. R., and Ekert, H.: Streptokinase and antithrombotic therapy in the hemolytic-uremic syndrome, J. Pediatr. **84:**345, 1974.

327. Quick, A. J.: Salicylates and bleeding: the aspirin tolerance test, Am. J. Med. Sci. **252:**265, 1966.

328. Rabiner, S. F., and Molinas, F.: The role of phenol and phenolic acids on the thrombocytopathy and defective platelet aggregation of patients with renal failure, Am. J. Med. **49:**346, 1970.

329. Rabinowitz, J. G., Moseley, J. E., Mitty, H. A., et al.: Trisomy 18, esophageal atresia, anomalies of the radius, and congenital hypoplastic thrombocytopenia, Radiology **89:**488, 1967.

330. Raccuglia, G.: Gray platelet syndrome: a variety of qualitative platelet disorder, Am. J. Med. **51:**818, 1971.

331. Radel, E. G., and Schorr, J. B.: Thrombocytopenic purpura with infectious mononucleosis, J. Pediatr. **63:**46, 1963.

332. Ratnoff, O. D., and Agle, D. P.: Psychogenic purpura: a re-evaluation of the syndrome of autoerythrocyte sensitization, Medicine **47:**475, 1968.

333. Ratnoff, O. D., and Miles, A. A.: The induction of permeability-increasing activity in human plasma by activated Hageman factor, Br. J. Exp. Pathol. **45:**328, 1964.

334. Rausen, A. R., and Diamond, L. K.: Enclosed hemorrhage and neonatal jaundice, Am. J. Dis. Child. **101:**164, 1961.

335. Rausen, A. R., Richter, P., Tallal, L., et al.: Hematologic effect of intrauterine rubella, J.A.M.A. **199:**75, 1967.

336. Regan, M. G., Lackner, H., and Karpatkin, S.: Platelet function and coagulation profile in lupus erythematosus: studies in 50 patients, Ann. Intern. Med. **81:**462, 1974.

337. Rendu, M.: Épistaxes répétées chez un sujet porteur de petits angiomes cutanés et maqueux, Bull. Soc. Med. Hop. Paris **13:**731, 1896.

338. Rivera, A. M., and Brehusen, F. C.: Aldrich's syndrome: a report of a case with subperiosteal hemorrhage, J. Pediatr. **57:**86, 1960.

339. Roberts, M. H., and Smith, M. H.: Thrombocytopenic purpura: a report of four cases in one family, Am. J. Dis. Child. **79:**820, 1950.

340. Robertson, J. H., Crozier, E. H., and Woodend, B. E.: The effect of vincristine on the platelet count in rats, Br. J. Haematol. **19:**331, 1970.

341. Rodriguez, S. U., Leikin, S. L., and Hiller, M. C.: Neonatal thrombocytopenia associated with antepartum administration of thiazide drugs, N. Engl. J. Med. **270:**881, 1964.

342. Root, A. W., and Speicher, C. E.: The triad of thrombocytopenia, eczema, and recurrent infections (Wiskott-Aldrich syndrome) associated with milk antibodies, giant-cell pneumonia, and cytomegalic inclusion disease, Pediatrics **31:**444, 1963.

343. Rosen, F. S.: The thymus gland and the immune deficiency syndrome. In Samter, M., ed.: Immunological diseases, Boston, 1971, Little, Brown & Co.

344. Rothman, S., Adelson, E., Schwebel, A., et al.: Adsorption of carbon-14 dextran to human blood platelets and red blood cells, in vitro, Vox Sang. **2:**104, 1957.

345. Rudolph, A. J., Yow, M. D., Phillips, C. A., et al.: Transplacental rubella infection in newly born infants, J.A.M.A. **191:**843, 1965.

346. Salzman, E. W.: Measurement of platelet adhesiveness: a simple in vitro technique demonstrating an abnormality in von Willebrand's disease, J. Lab. Clin. Med. **62:**724, 1963.

347. Salzman, E. W., Ashford, T. P., Chambers, D. A., et al.: Platelet volume: effect of temperature and agents affecting platelet aggregation, Am. J. Physiol. **217:**1330, 1969.

348. Salzman, E. W., and Levine, L.: Cyclic 3', 5'-adenosine monophosphate in human blood platelets. II. Effect of N^6-2'-O-dibutyryl cyclic 3', 5'-adenosine monophosphate on platelet function, J. Clin. Invest. **50:**131, 1971.

349. Sanarelli, G.: De la pathogénie du choléra expérimental, Ann. Inst. Pasteur **38:**11, 1924.

350. Sanchez-Avalos, J., Vitacco, M., Molinas, F., et al.: Coagulation studies in the hemolytic-uremic syndrome, J. Pediatr. **76:**538, 1970.

351. Schaar, F. E.: Familial idiopathic thrombocytopenic purpura, J. Pediatr. **62:**546, 1963.

352. Scharfman, W. A., Tartaglia, A. P., and Propp, S.: Splenectomy preceding surgical intervention in idiopathic thrombocytopenic purpura, Arch. Intern. Med. **116:**406, 1965.

353. Schiff, D., Aranda, J. V., and Stern, L.: Neonatal thrombocytopenia and congenital malformations associated with administration of tolbutamide to the mother, J. Pediatr. **77:**457, 1970.

354. Schönlein, J. L.: Allegemeine und specielle Pathologie und Therapie, St. Gallen, Vol. 2, 1837.

355. Schulman, I.: Diagnosis and treatment; management of idiopathic thrombocytopenic purpura, Pediatrics **33:**979, 1964.

356. Schulman, I., Abildgaard, C. F., Cornet, J., et al.: Studies on thrombopoiesis. II. Assay of human plasma thrombopoietic activity, J. Pediatr. **66:**604, 1965.

357. Schulman, I., Pierce, M., Lukens, A., et al.: A factor in normal plasma which stimulates platelet production; chronic thrombocytopenic purpura due to its deficiency, Am. J. Dis. Child. **98:**633, 1959.

358. Schulman, I., Pierce, M., Lukens, A., et al.: Studies on thrombopoiesis. I. A factor in normal human plasma required for platelet production; chronic thrombocytopenia due to its deficiency, Blood **16:**943, 1960.

359. Schulman, I., Smith, C. H., and Ando, R. E.: Congenital thrombocytopenic purpura: observations on three infants born of a nonaffected mother; demonstration of platelet agglutinins and evidence for platelet isoimmunization, Am. J. Dis. Child. **88:**785, 1954.

360. Schwartz, A. D.: A method for demonstrating shortened platelet survival utilizing recovery from aspirin effect, J. Pediatr. **84:**350, 1974.

361. Schwartz, J. P., Cooperberg, A. A., and Rosenberg, A.: Platelet function studies in patients with glucose-6-phosphate dehydrogenase deficiency, Br. J. Haematol. **27:**273, 1974.

362. Schwartz, J. P., Rosenberg, A., and Cooperberg, A. A.: Thrombotic thrombocytopenic purpura: successful treatment of two cases, Can. Med. Assoc. J. **106:**1200, 1972.

363. Schwartz, R. S., Lewis, B., and Dameshek, W.: Hemorrhagic cutaneous anaphylaxis due to autosensitization to deoxyribonucleic acid, N. Engl. J. Med. **267:**1105, 1962.

364. Schwartz, S. O., and Kaplan, S. R.: Thrombocytopenic purpura; the prognostic and therapeutic value of the eosinophil index; an analysis of 100 cases, Am. J. Med. Sci. **219:**528, 1950.

365. Schwartz, S. O., and Motto, S. A.: The diagnostic sig-

nificance of "burr red cells," Am. J. Med. Sci. **218:**563, 1949.

366. Shapiro, C. M., Kanter, A., Lopas, H., et al.: Hemolytic-uremic syndrome in adults, J.A.M.A. **213:**567, 1970.

367. Sharpstone, P., Evans, R. G., O'Shea, M., et al.: Haemolytic uraemic syndrome: survival after prolonged oliguria, Arch. Dis. Child. **43:**711, 1968.

368. Shulman, N. R.: Immunoreactions involving platelets. I. A steric and kinetic model for formation of a complex from a human antibody, quinidine as a hapten, and platelets, and for fixation of complement by the complex, J. Exp. Med. **107:**667, 1958.

369. Shulman, N. R.: A mechanism of cell destruction in individuals sensitized to foreign antigens and its implications in autoimmunity, Ann. Intern. Med. **60:**507, 1964.

370. Shulman, N. R.: Immunological considerations attending platelet transfusion, Transfusion **6:**39, 1966.

371. Shulman, N. R., Aster, R. H., Leitner, A., et al.: Immunoreactions involving platelets; post-transfusion purpura due to a complement-fixing antibody against a genetically-controlled platelet antigen; a proposed mechanism for thrombocytopenia and its relevance in "autoimmunity," J. Clin. Invest. **40:**1597, 1961.

372. Shulman, N. R., Aster, R. H., Pearson, H. A., et al.: Immunoreactions involving platelets. VI. Reactions of maternal isoantibodies responsible for neonatal purpura. Differentiation of a second platelet antigen system, J. Clin. Invest. **41:**1059, 1962.

373. Shulman, N. R., Marder, V. J., Hiller, M. C., et al.: Platelet and leukocyte isoantigens and their antibodies: Serologic, physiologic, and clinical studies, Prog. Hematol. **4:**222, 1964.

374. Shulman, N. R., Marder, V. J., and Weinrach, R. S.: Similarities between known antiplatelet antibodies and the factor responsible for thrombocytopenia in idiopathic purpura: physiologic, serologic, and isotopic studies, Ann. N.Y. Acad. Sci. **124:**499, 1965.

375. Shumway, C. N., Jr., and Miller, G.: An unusual syndrome of hemolytic anemia, thrombocytopenic purpura and renal disease, Blood **12:**1045, 1957.

376. Shumway, C. N., and Terplan, K. L.: Hemolytic anemia, thrombocytopenia, and renal disease in childhood; the hemolytic-uremic syndrome, Pediatr. Clin. North Am. **11:**577, 1964.

377. Shwartzman, G.: Phenomenon of local tissue reactivity and its immunological pathological, and clinical significance, New York, 1937, Paul B. Hoeber, Inc.

378. Siegel, B. M., Friedman, I. A., and Schwartz, S. O.: Hemorrhagic disease in osteogenesis imperfecta, Am. J. Med. **22:**315, 1957.

379. Silverman, F. N.: The roentgen manifestations of unrecognized skeletal trauma in infants, Am. J. Roentgenol. **69:**413, 1953.

380. Simons, S. M., Main, C. A., Yaish, H. M., et al.: Idiopathic thrombocytopenic purpura in children, J. Pediatr. **87:**16, 1975.

381. Singer, D. B.: Postsplenectomy sepsis, Perspect. Pediatr. Pathol. **1:**285, 1973.

382. Sitarz, A. L., Driscoll, J. M., and Wolff, J. A.: Management of isoimmune neonatal thrombocytopenia, Am. J. Obstet. Gynecol. **124:**39, 1976.

383. Skoog, W. A., Lawrence, J. S., and Adams, W. S.: A metabolic study of a patient with idiopathic cyclical thrombocytopenic purpura, Blood **12:**844, 1957.

384. Smith, C. H.: Dermatorrhexis (Ehlers-Danlos syndrome), J. Pediatr. **14:**632, 1939.

385. Smith, J. B., Ingerman, C., Kocsis, J. J., et al.: Formation of an intermediate in prostaglandin biosynthesis and its association with the platelet release reaction, J. Clin. Invest. **53:**1468, 1974.

386. Smith, J. L., and Lineback, M. I.: Hereditary hemorrhagic telangiectasia; nine cases in one Negro family with special reference to hepatic lesions, Am. J. Med. **17:**41, 1954.

387. Smith, T. P., Doss, J. W., and Tartaglia, A. P.: Thrombasthenic thrombopathic thrombocytopenia with giant, "Swiss-cheese" platelets, Ann. Intern. Med. **79:**828, 1973.

388. Solcia, E., Rondini, G., and Capella, C.: Clinical and pathological observations on a case of newborn osteopetrosis, Helv. Paediatr. Acta **23:**650, 1968.

389. Spaet, T. H., and Zucker, M. B.: Mechanisms of platelet plug formation and role of adenosine diphosphate, Am. J. Physiol. **206:**1267, 1964.

390. Spitler, L. E., Levin, A. S., Stites, D. P., et al.: The Wiskott-Aldrich syndrome: results of transfer factor therapy, J. Clin. Invest. **51:**3216, 1972.

391. St. Geme, J. W., Jr., Prince, J. T., Burke, B., et al.: Impaired cellular resistance to herpes-simplex virus in Wiskott-Aldrich syndrome, N. Engl. J. Med. **273:**229, 1965.

392. Steen, E., and Torp, K. H.: Encephalitis and thrombocytopenic purpura after rubella, Arch. Dis. Child. **31:**470, 1956.

393. Stefani, M., Piomelli, S., Mele, R., et al.: Acute vascular purpura following immunization with Asiatic-influenza vaccine, N. Engl. J. Med. **259:**9, 1958.

394. Stein, H., Beck, J., Solomon, A., et al.: Gastroenteritis with necrotizing enterocolitis in premature babies, Br. Med. J. **2:**616, 1972.

395. Stiehm, E. R., Vaerman, J.-P., and Fudenberg, H. H.: Plasma infusions in immunologic deficiency states: metabolic and therapeutic studies, Blood **28:**918, 1966.

396. Stuart, M. J., Murphy, S., and Oski, F. A.: A simple nonradioisotopic technic for the determination of platelet life-span, N. Engl. J. Med. **292:**1310, 1975.

397. Sultan, Y., and Caen, J. P.: Platelet dysfunction in preleukemic states and in various types of leukemia, Ann. N.Y. Acad. Sci. **201:**300, 1972.

398. Sultan, Y., Scrobohaci, M. L., Rendu, F., et al.: Abnormal platelet function, population, and survival time in a boy with congenital absent radii and thrombocytopenia, Lancet **2:**653, 1972.

399. Summer, G. K.: The Ehlers-Danlos syndrome, Am. J. Dis. Child. **91:**419, 1956.

400. Tancer, M. L.: Idiopathic thrombocytopenic purpura and pregnancy: report of 5 new cases and review of the literature, Am. J. Obstet. Gynecol. **79:**148, 1960.

401. Taylor, J. R., and Kellum, R. E.: Anaphylactoid purpura. In Samter, M., ed.: Immunological diseases, Boston, 1971, Little, Brown & Co.

402. ten Bensel, R. W., Stadlan, E. M., and Krivit, W.: The development of malignancy in the course of the Aldrich syndrome, J. Pediatr. **68:**761, 1966.

403. Thomas, D. P., Ream, V. J., and Stuart, R. K.: Platelet aggregation in patients with Laennec's cirrhosis of the liver, N. Engl. J. Med. **276:**1344, 1967.

404. Tidy, H. L.: Haemorrhagic diathesis: angiostaxis, Lancet **2:**365, 1926.

405. Tschopp, R. B., and Weiss, H. J.: Decreased ATP, ADP, and serotonin in young platelets of fawn-hooded rats with storage pool disease, Thromb. Diath. Haemorrh. **32:**670, 1974.

406. Tschopp, T. B., Weiss, H. J., and Baumgartner, H. R.: Interaction of platelets with subendothelium in thrombasthenia: normal adhesion, impaired aggregation, Experentia **31:**113, 1975.

407. Ulutin, O. N.: Qualitative platelet disorders: classification and pathogenesis, Ann. N.Y. Acad. Sci. **201:**174, 1972.

408. Van Loghem, J. J., Dorfmeijer, H., and Van der Hart, M.: Serological and genetical studies on a platelet antigen (Zw), Vox Sang. **4:**161, 1959.

409. van Wieringen, P. M. V., Monnens, L. A. H., and Schretlen, E. D. A. M.: Hemolytic-uremic syndrome: epidemiologic and clinical study, Arch. Dis. Child. **49:** 432, 1974.

410. Vernier, R. L.: Kidney biopsy in the study of renal disease, Pediatr. Clin. North Am. **7:**353, 1960.

411. Vernier, R. L., Farquhar, M. G., Brunson, J. G., et al.: Chronic renal disease in children; correlation of clinical findings with morphologic characteristics seen by light and electron microscopy, Am. J. Dis. Child. **96:**306, 1958.

412. Vernier, R. L., Worthen, H. G., Peterson, R. D., et al.: Anaphylactoid purpura. I. Pathology of the skin and kidney and frequency of streptococcal infection, Pediatrics **27:**181, 1961.

413. Vestermark, B., and Vestermark, S.: Familial sex-linked thrombocytopenia, Acta Paediatr. **53:**365, 1964.

414. Vildosola, J., and Emparanza, E.: Hereditary familial thrombocytopenia. In Proceedings of the tenth international congress of Pediatrics, Lisbon, 1962.

415. Vipan, W. H.: Quinine as a cause of purpura, Lancet **2:**37, 1865.

416. Vitsky, B. H., Suzuky, Y., Strauss, L., et al.: The hemolytic-uremic syndrome: a study of renal pathologic alterations, Am. J. Pathol. **57:**627, 1969.

417. Waldenström, J.: Clinical methods for determination of hyperproteinemia and their practical value for diagnosis, Nord. Med. **20:**2288, 1943.

418. Waldenström, J.: Incipient myelomatosis or "essential" hyperglobulinemia with fibrinogenopenia: a new syndrome? Acta Med. Scand. **117:**216, 1944.

419. Walker, J. H., and Walker, W.: Idiopathic thrombocytopenic purpura in childhood, Arch. Dis. Child. **36:**649, 1961.

420. Wallace, S.: Thrombocytopenic purpura after rubella, Lancet **1:**139, 1963.

421. Walsh, P. N.: Platelet coagulant activities and hemostasis: a hypothesis, Blood **43:**597, 1974.

422. Walsh, P., Mills, D. C. B., Paretti, et al.: Hereditary giant platelet syndrome—absence of collagen-induced coagulant activity and deficiency of factor XI binding to platelets, Br. J. Haematol. **29:**639, 1975.

423. Warshaw, A. L., Laster, L., and Shulman, N. R.: The stimulation by thrombin of glucose oxidation in human platelets, J. Clin. Invest. **45:**1923, 1966.

424. Warshaw, A. L., Laster, L., and Shulman, N. R.: Protein synthesis by human platelets, J. Biol. Chem. **242:**2094, 1967.

425. Weber, F. P.: Multiple hereditary developmental angiomata (telangiectases) of the skin and mucous membranes associated with recurring hemorrhages, Lancet **2:**160, 1907.

426. Wedgewood, R. J. P., and Klaus, M. H.: Anaphylactoid purpura (Schönlein-Henoch syndrome); a long term followup study with special reference to renal involvement, Pediatrics **16:**196, 1955.

427. Weiss, H. J.: Platelet aggregation, adhesion, and adenosine diphosphate release in thrombopathia (platelet factor 3 deficiency): comparison with Glanzmann's thrombasthenia and von Willebrand's disease, Am. J. Med. **43:**570, 1967.

428. Weiss, H. J.: Abnormalities in platelet function due to defects in the release reaction, Ann. N.Y. Acad. Sci. **201:**161, 1972.

429. Weiss, H. J.: The pharmacology of platelet inhibition, Prog. Hemostasis Thromb. **1:**199, 1972.

430. Weiss, H. J.: Platelet physiology and abnormalities of platelet function. Part 1, N. Engl. J. Med. **293:**531, 1975.

430a. Weiss, H. J.: Platelet physiology and abnormalities of platelet function. Part 2, N. Engl. J. Med. **293:**580, 1975.

431. Weiss, H. J., and Aledort, L. M.: Impaired platelet-connective tissue reaction in man after aspirin ingestion, Lancet **2:**495, 1967.

432. Weiss, H. J., and Ames, R. P.: Ultrastructural findings in storage pool disease and aspirin-line defects of platelets, Am. J. Pathol. **71:**447, 1973.

433. Weiss, H. J., Chervenick, P. A., Zalusky, R., et al.: A familial defect in platelet function associated with impaired release of adenosine diphosphate, N. Engl. J. Med. **281:**1264, 1969.

434. Weiss, H. J., and Kochwa, S.: Studies of platelet function and proteins in three patients with Glanzmann thrombasthenia, J. Lab. Clin. Med. **71:**153, 1968.

435. Weiss, H. J., and Rogers, J.: Fibrinogen and platelets in the primary arrest of bleeding: studies on two patients with congenital afibrinogenemia, N. Engl. J. Med. **285:** 369, 1971.

436. Weiss, H. J., and Rogers, J.: Thrombocytopathia due to abnormalities in platelet release function: studies on six unrelated patients, Blood **39:**187, 1972.

437. Weiss, H. J., Tschopp, T. B., Rogers, J., et al.: Studies of platelet 5-hydroxytryptamine (serotonin) in storage pool disease and albinism, J. Clin. Invest. **54:**421, 1974.

438. Weksler, B. B., and Coupal, C. E.: Platelet-dependent generation of chemotactic activity in serum, J. Exp. Med. **137:**1419, 1973.

439. Welch, R. G.: Thrombocytopenic purpura and chickenpox, Arch. Dis. Child. **31:**38, 1956.

440. West, C. D., McAdams, A. J., and Northway, J. D.: Focal glomerulonephritis in children, J. Pediatr. **73:**181, 1968.

441. White, J. G.: Platelet morphology. In Johnson, S. A., ed.: The circulating platelet, New York, 1971, Academic Press, Inc.

442. White, J. G.: Interaction of membrane systems in blood platelets, Am. J. Pathol. **66:**295, 1972.

443. White, J. G., Edson, J. R., Desnick, S. J., et al.: Studies of platelets in a variant of the Hermansky-Pudlak syndrome, Am. J. Pathol. **63:**319, 1971.

444. Wilkinson, T., and Firkin, B.: Idiopathic cyclical acute thrombocytopenic purpura, Med. J. Aust. **1:**217, 1966.

445. Willan, R.: On cutaneous diseases, London, 1808.

446. Willis, A. L., Vane, F. M., Kuhn, D. C., et al.: An endoperoxide aggregator (LASS), formed in platelets in response to thrombotic stimuli: purification, identification, and unique biologic significance, Prostaglandins **8:**453, 1974.

447. Wilson, P., McNicol, G. P., and Douglas, A. S.: Platelet abnormality in human scurvy, Lancet **1:**975, 1967.

448. Wintrobe, M. M.: Clinical hematology, Philadelphia, 1974, Lea & Febiger.

449. Wiskott, A.: Familiarer angeborener Morbus Werlhofii, Monatsschr. Kinderh. **68:**212, 1937.

450. Witebsky, E.: The question of self recognition by the host and problems of autoantibodies and their specificity, Cancer Res. **21:**1216, 1961.

451. Wolfe, S. M., and Shulman, N. R.: Adenyl-cyclase activity in human platelets, Biochem. Biophys. Res. Commun. **35:**265, 1969.

452. Wolff, J. A.: Wiskott-Aldrich syndrome; clinical, immunologic, and pathologic observations, J. Pediatr. **70:**221, 1967.

453. Wright, J. H.: The histogenesis of the blood platelets, J. Morphol. **21:**263, 1910.

454. Wright, J. H., and Minot, G. R.: The viscous metamorphosis of the blood platelets, J. Exp. Med. **26:**395, 1917.

455. Wybran, J., and Fudenberg, H. H.: Cellular immunity to platelets in idiopathic thrombocytopenic purpura, Blood **40:**856, 1972.

456. Yankee, R. A., Graff, K. S., Dowling, R., et al.: Selec-

tion of unrelated platelet donors by lymphocyte HL-A matching, N. Engl. J. Med. **288:**760, 1973.

457. Yankee, R. A., Grumet, F. C., and Rogentine, G. N.: Platelet transfusion therapy: the selection of compatible platelet donors for refractory patients by HL-A typing, N. Engl. J. Med. **281:**1208, 1969.

458. Ylppo, A.: Zum Entschungsmechanismus de Bluttungen bei Fruhgenorenen und Neugeborenen, Z. Kinderheilkd. **38:**32, 1924.

459. Zahavi, J., and Marder, V. J.: Acquired "storage pool disease" of platelets associated with circulating antiplatelet antibodies, Am. J. Med. **56:**883, 1974.

460. Zaidi, Z. H., and Mortimer, P. E.: Congenital thyrotoxicosis with hepatosplenomegaly and thrombocytopenia, associated with aniridia and dislocated lenses, Proc. R. Soc. Med. **58:**390, 1965.

461. Ziegler, Z., Murphy, S., and Gardner, F. H.: Post-transfusion purpura: a heterogeneous syndrome, Blood **45:** 529, 1975.

462. Zinkham, W. H., Medearis, D. N., Jr., and Osborn, J. E.: Blood and bone marrow in congenital rubella, J. Pediatr. **71:**512, 1967.

463. Zucker, M. B., Pert, J., and Hilgartner, M. W.: Platelet function in a patient with thrombasthenia, Blood **28:**524, 1966.

464. Zucker-Franklin, D.: Microfibrils of blood platelets: their relationship to microtubules and the contractile protein, J. Clin. Invest. **48:**165, 1969.

465. Zweiffler, A. J., and Allen, R. J.: Abnormal platelet aggregation in patients with homocystinuria, Circulation **40**(suppl. 3):27, 1969.

25 □ Coagulation disorders

Margaret W. Hilgartner
Campbell W. McMillan

GENERAL CONSIDERATIONS ON THE PLASMA PHASE OF HEMOSTASIS

Clinical disorders of the plasma phase of hemostasis are characterized either by hemorrhage resulting from deficient coagulation or by thrombosis resulting from excessive coagulation. As defined in Chapter 23, the plasma phase of hemostasis includes not only coagulation directly involved in formation of a fibrin clot but also fibrinolysis involved in clot removal and control mechanisms, notably certain natural inhibitors of coagulation and fibrinolysis. However, from a clinical viewpoint abnormalities of any of these three components of the plasma phase are ultimately expressed in a given disorder of coagulation. For example, pathologic fibrinolysis, whether secondary or primary, is clinically expressed in decreased activities of those coagulation factors that are natural substrates of plasmin, i.e., fibrinogen (and fibrin) and factors V, VIII, and XII.

Excessive coagulation expressed in thrombotic disorders may not be as readily measurable; hereditary deficiency of antithrombin III is rarely encountered and in most cases of deep vein or arterial thrombosis no abnormality of coagulation is measurable. In this chapter all clinical disorders of the plasma phase of hemostasis will be presented according to their effects on the coagulation component.

This chapter also includes those thrombocytopenic states, such as purpura fulminans, in which abnormalities of coagulation are fundamental to the clinical disorder. Thrombocytopenic states not characterized by consistent abnormalities of coagulation, notably microangiopathic disease, are discussed in Chapter 24. Disorders such as liver disease and infections that may be associated with coagulation deficiencies and thrombocytopenia through different mechanisms are discussed both in this chapter and in Chapter 24.

Historical perspective

The evolution of concepts about blood coagulation may be arbitrarily divided into three broad phases. The first began with the discovery of Malpighi in 1666 that the solid substance of a blood clot after thorough washing proved to be a meshwork of white strands and not whole blood as previously presumed.[84] A second phase began with a proposal by Morawitz[70] in 1905 of a simple and definitive scheme of coagulation, based on four coagulation factors. The third phase, leading up to the present time, began with the conclusive identification of factor V by Owren[79] in 1947; this factor was the first of a sequence of rapid additions to the coagulation scheme of Morawitz.

Highlights of the first phase, described in detail by Pickering,[84] include the following major discoveries: the confirmation by Ruysch in 1707 and Hewson in 1770 of Malpighi's finding that the solid ingredient of the blood clot is derived from plasma and the naming of this material *fibrin* by Chaptal in 1795; the determination by Denis in 1859 that fibrin is derived from a plasma precursor, which he called plasmine and which was subsequently termed *fibrinogen;* the discovery by Buchanan in 1845 that fibrinogen is converted to fibrin by a substance derived from washings of a fresh blood clot, an observation confirmed and extended by Schmidt,[113] who named the substance *thrombin;* the later suggestion by Schmidt[114] that thrombin is derived from a plasma precursor, *prothrombin,* activated by ill-defined "zymoplastic substances" from tissue and plasma[92]; the discovery by Arthus and Pages[6] in 1890 that *calcium* is required for clotting; and finally, the demonstration by Pekelharing[81] and Hammarsten[31] that calcium is required for the conversion of prothrombin to thrombin but *not* for the action of thrombin on fibrinogen.

In 1905 Morawitz[70] assembled information about coagulation available at that time, including observations of his own, into a comprehensive theory of coagulation that proved to be impregnable through the years. This concept may be summarized in the following two equations[92]:

$$prothrombin + Ca^{++} + thromboplastin = thrombin$$

$$fibrinogen + thrombin = fibrin$$

In this scheme the term "thromboplastin" represents tissue substances required, along with ionic calcium, to convert prothrombin to thrombin. Not included are plasma factors producing fibrinolysis and inhibiting coagulation and fibrinolysis, activities that were dimly recognized at the turn of the century.

In 1947 the first conclusive addition to the coagulation scheme of Morawitz was provided by Owren's[79] discovery of a fifth coagulation factor, termed factor V, through studies of a young woman with a congenital hemorrhagic disorder caused by deficiency of this factor. The four factors recognized prior to that time were, in order, fibrinogen, prothrombin, tissue thromboplastin, and ionic calcium.

The evolution of ideas about coagulation from the time of Morawitz through the discovery of factor V and up to the present has been previously discussed in the introductory section of Chapter 23. However, for the purposes of this chapter certain major highlights should be identified.

The Morawitz concept of coagulation withstood challenges from other theories[11,92] and ultimately was strongly reinforced during the 1930s by the following developments: the introduction by Quick[90] in 1935 of a simple one-stage test of plasma prothrombin activity; the discovery of vitamin K by Dam;[21,22] and the discovery of the direct relationship between mechanisms of lack or inhibition of vitamin K, hypoprothrombinemia, and hemorrhagic disease in human newborns,[129] adults with obstructive jaundice,[90] chicks on purified diets,[91] and Canadian cattle fed spoiled sweet clover.[18,103]

The prothrombin time (PT) test of Quick measures the recalcification time of citrated or oxalated plasma to which is added tissue thromboplastin provided by a saline suspension of dried rabbit brain. The assumption underlying this test during the 1930s was that an abnormal result reflected simply decreased plasma prothrombin activity. The inadequacies of this concept of coagulation became increasingly apparent by the late 1930s, in large part because hemophilia was not explained. Despite the severe bleeding problems and prolonged whole blood clotting time typical of this disorder, the PT was clearly normal.[90] In 1939 Brinkhous made the important observation that the specific prothrombin content of hemophilic plasma is normal but that *conversion* of prothrombin to thrombin is delayed.

The discovery of factor V by Owren[79] in 1947 established the existence of a hitherto unrecognized factor involved in the conversion of prothrombin to thrombin. From then until 1960, six additional clotting factors involved in prothrombin conversion were discovered and ultimately assigned the following Roman numerals, in the order of their discovery: factors VII, VIII, IX, X, XI,

XII.[137] In addition, a factor required for stabilizing fibrin by peptide cross-linkage was discovered by Laki and Lorand[56] and called factor XIII.

These exciting discoveries did not disturb the basic integrity of the Morawitz scheme of coagulation, but they did emphasize the tremendous complexity of prothrombin conversion to thrombin. Furthermore, although the new coagulation factors clearly constituted pieces of the puzzle and knowledge of hemophilia took a giant step forward with the discoveries of factors VIII and IX in 1952,[2,10,116] the manner in which these factors actually fitted together was the subject of lively controversy throughout the 1960s.

However, by the early 1970s a consensus was reached that may be summarized as follows: prothrombin is converted to thrombin by a "prothrombinase" comprised of activated factor X, factor V, ionic calcium, and platelet phospholipids (platelet factor 3); factor X is activated either by a so-called extrinsic pathway involving the interaction of tissue thromboplastin with Ca^{++} and factor VII or an intrinsic pathway involving sequential activation of factors XII, XI, and IX and the interaction of activated factor IX with factor VIII, Ca^{++}, and platelet factor 3.

From a practical viewpoint this concept appears to fit nicely the results of the two major screening tests of coagulation: the PT test of Quick[90] and the test of partial thromboplastin time (PTT) introduced by Langdell et al.[57] The PTT, like the PT, is a modified recalcification time, but, instead of complete tissue thromboplastin, a partial thromboplastin is added in the form of the lipid fraction of thromboplastin or an appropriate equivalent. The PT reflects factor VII in the extrinsic pathway, factors X and V in the prothrombinase or "common pathway," as well as prothrombin itself and fibrinogen. The PTT reflects factors XII, XI, IX, and VIII in the intrinsic pathway as well as factors X and V in the common pathway, prothrombin, and fibrinogen. Strictly speaking, Quick's PT should be renamed the complete thromboplastin time (or its equivalent) since it is now clear that this test measures more than prothrombin activity. Nonetheless, it is an appropriate tribute to Quick to retain the name for this tremendously important test he introduced. Neither the PT nor the PTT reflects factor XIII activity, which requires testing of formed clot solubility in solutions of urea or monochloracetic acid.[3,56]

In the past decade research in the plasma phase of hemostasis has been highly productive through wide-ranging studies of the molecular properties of coagulation factors, fibrinolytic factors, and natural inhibitors of coagulation and fibrinolysis.*

*References 36, 66, 105, 115, 121.

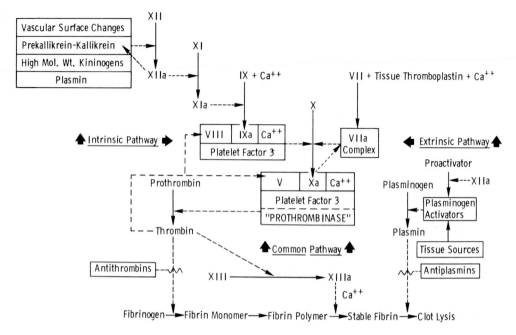

Fig. 25-1. Concept of the plasma phase of hemostasis in 1976. Solid line represents transformation; dashed line, action.

For example, it is now known that thrombin as well as other activated coagulation factors are specialized serine-containing enzymes that are sequentially formed in a "cascade" or "waterfall" fashion, in substantial accord with concepts advanced in 1964 by Macfarlane[63] and Davie and Ratnoff.[23] The tremendous ferment generated during the 1970s by rapid advances in basic knowledge of hemostatic factors in plasma continues to raise questions about how all the pieces fit together. Nonetheless, a consensus does exist and is shown in Fig. 25-1. (See also Figs. 23-1 and 23-2.)

Characteristics of plasma hemostatic factors

Coagulation factors (Table 25-1). Fibrinogen, or factor I, is a macromolecular glycoprotein that is synthesized in the hepatic parenchyma.[29] The molecule consists of two identical parts, each containing three distinct peptide chains designated α, β, and γ; the two halves and their component parts are held together by disulfide bridges.[13] The molecular weight of fibrinogen is 340,000 daltons, and it is specifically altered by thrombin and plasmin, for which it is a natural substrate; thrombin converts the molecule to fibrin monomer by cleaving fibrinopeptides A and B from each of the α- and β- chains, and plasmin progressively degrades fibrinogen to nonclottable fragments D and E with molecular weights of about 90,000 and 50,000 daltons, respectively.[14,66] The average concentra-

tion of fibrinogen in plasma is 300 mg/dl, normally ranging from 150 to 500 mg/dl. The minimum hemostatic level of fibrinogen is unknown but probably lies between 50 and 100 mg/dl. Fibrinogen injected into patients with congenital afibrinogenemia disappears exponentially, with a half-time of 2 to 4 days.[97] Fibrinogen is a nonspecific acute-phase reactant and is increased in most conditions characterized by an increased erythrocyte sedimentation rate.[58]

Prothrombin, or factor II, is a glycoprotein with a molecular weight of about 70,000 daltons; it is synthesized in the hepatic parenchyma.[49,77] Biologically active prothrombin is synthesized in a two-step fashion: intrahepatic ribosomal assembly of the precursor molecule is followed by a vitamin K–dependent step by which carboxyl radicals are added to precisely located glutamic acids, thus enabling the molecule to bind ionic calcium, which is critical to its interaction with prothrombinase and its consequent conversion to thrombin.[64,122] The Ca^{++} binding sites also enable prothrombin and other vitamin K–dependent factors (factors VII, IX, and X) to be adsorbed to barium salts and aluminum hydroxide gel. The plasma concentration of prothrombin, like that of all coagulation factors except fibrinogen, is generally expressed in activity based on functional assays in which the average is arbitrarily taken to be 100%, with a normal range that may extend from about 50% to 200%. Also, although the

Table 25-1. Clinically relevant characteristics of plasma coagulation factors

	Present in fresh whole blood and plasma	Present in aged serum	Concentrated in cryoprecipitate	Adsorbed by BaSO$_4$/Al (OH)$_3$	Dependent on vitamin K
Fibrinogen (I)	+	−	+	−	−
Prothrombin (II)	+	−	−	+	+
Factor V	+	−	−	−	−
Factor VII	+	+	−	+	+
Factor VIII	+	−	+	−	−
Factor IX	+	+	−	+	+
Factor X	+	+	−	+	+
Factor XI	+	+	−	−	−
Factor XII	+	+	−	−	−
Factor XIII	+	−	+	−	−

minimum hemostatic level of prothrombin and other coagulation factors is unknown, such a level probably lies between 25% and 50%. The half-time for exponential disappearance of prothrombin from plasma has been estimated to be 55 to 80 hours.[118]

Thrombin has a molecular weight of about 35,000 daltons and is a serine esterase, i.e., an enzyme that cleaves its substrates by means of an active amino acid serine "tip."[36] The formation of thrombin by stepwise limited proteolysis of prothrombin is illustrated in Fig. 25-2. Free thrombin is cleared so rapidly from the circulation that direct measurement of this enzyme in plasma samples is not possible by current techniques.

Tissue thromboplastin (factor III), ionic calcium (factor IV), and platelet phospholipids (platelet factor 3) play major accessory roles in coagulation. Tissue thromboplastin is a fully recognized but incompletely defined clot-promoting principle of dried tissues, particularly those rich in phospholipid-protein complexes such as brain, lung, and placenta.[135,136] Both lipid and protein components of tissue thromboplastin appear to be necessary for its interaction with factor VII and Ca^{++} to activate factor X via the extrinsic pathway.[65] Platelet factor 3, on the other hand, is a weaker clot-promoting principle than tissue factor III and is a property of lipoproteins in platelet and red cell membranes. More specifically platelet factor 3 activity is ascribed to the phospholipid component of tissue thromboplastin, this component thereby serving as a partial rather than complete thromboplastin.[57] Substantial evidence indicates that phospholipid micelles provide surfaces for optimal concentration and interaction of coagulation factors in the intrinsic and common pathways of thrombin generation.[36] The roles of complete and partial thromboplastins are critical to current concepts of coagulation. These concepts

are unmistakably useful at the present time but there is a somewhat artificial overtone to present distinctions between factors III and 3, which undoubtedly will be relieved in the course of continuing basic research.

Factor IV, ionic calcium, is critical for the biologic activity of the four vitamin K–dependent factors (also known as prothrombin-complex factors): prothrombin and factors VII, IX, and X. Intrahepatic synthesis of all these factors includes a postribosomal vitamin K–dependent step in which glutamic acid residues are carboxylated, enabling these factors to bind Ca^{++}.[30,122,126] These Ca^{++} binding sites are γ-carboxyglutamic acids. Ionic calcium, in turn, anchors each of these factors to phospholipid surfaces at their appropriate positions in the coagulation mechanism: factor IX in the intrinsic pathway, factor VII in the extrinsic pathway, factor X in the common pathway, and prothrombin in its interaction with prothrombinase. However, whereas activities of factors VII, IX, and X are Ca^{++}-dependent in both their procoagulant and activated forms and prothrombin is similarly dependent, thrombin is not. Finally, it should be emphasized that, although Ca^{++} is vital to coagulation, the clinical effects of hypocalcemia do not include a coagulation disorder; life-threatening effects of tetany would occur well in advance of deficient coagulation.

Factor V, previously termed proaccelerin[132] and labile factor,[93] is synthesized in the hepatic parenchyma and has a molecular weight estimated to be 290,000 daltons.[44,77] The exact composition of factor V has not yet been determined, but it is predominantly a protein and appears to contain phospholipid as well.[83] Factor V is consumed during blood coagulation and progressively disappears from oxalated plasma at 37° C but is more stable in citrated plasma. Factor V interacts with activated factor X, Ca^{++}, and platelet factor 3 as prothrombinase in the common pathway to

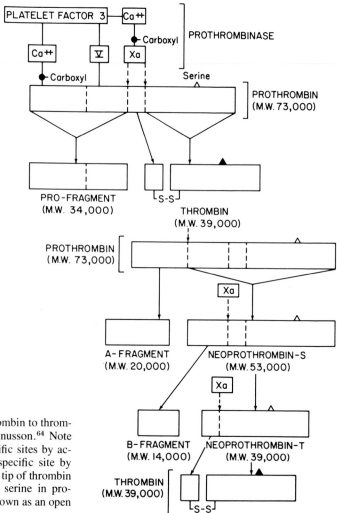

Fig. 25-2. Stepwise conversion of prothrombin to thrombin in accord with the concept of Magnusson.[64] Note that prothrombin is cleaved at two specific sites by activated factor X (Xa) and at a single specific site by formed thrombin itself. The active serine tip of thrombin is shown as a closed triangle; inactive serine in prothrombin and its intermediate forms is shown as an open triangle.

convert prothrombin to thrombin. In this process factor V is not itself converted to an active enzyme, but its action appears to be enhanced by thrombin in a manner that is not yet clear.[36] (See Fig. 25-1.) The half-time for plasma disappearance of transfused factor V activity has been variously reported to be as long as 36 hours[134] and as short as 12 hours.[15]

Factor VI was originally proposed by Owren[79] as the activated form of factor V. The existence of activated factor V is no longer accepted, but it is a fitting tribute to the monumental work of Owren that the factor VI slot has remained undisturbed.

Factor VII, previously termed serum prothrombin conversion accelerator[4] and proconvertin,[80] is a glycoprotein with a molecular weight of 63,000 daltons[89] and is synthesized in the hepatic parenchyma. Factor VII is dependent on vitamin K for postribosomal synthesis of γ-carboxyglutam-

ic acid groups that enable the molecule to bind Ca^{++}. Factor VII becomes activated in the process of forming a complex with tissue thromboplastin and Ca^{++} in the extrinsic pathway and then becomes further activated through its reciprocal interaction with factor X.[73,74,94] Factor VII is stable in plasma and is not consumed in the course of clotting.[43] The half-time of transfused factor VII activity is the shortest of all the known coagulation factors, averaging about 3 hours.[67]

Factor VIII, also termed antihemophilic factor (AHF) or antihemophilic globulin (AHG), is an extremely complex macromolecular glycolipoprotein that in its natural state appears to have a molecular weight of 1 to 2 million daltons.[20,37,69] Despite intensive continuing research and important gains over the past two decades, factor VIII is still a major enigma with respect to its molecular constitution, site(s) of synthesis, genetic control, and relationships of structure to function.[8] One of several interpretations of the factor VIII molecule is that of Wagner and Cooper,[130] who have presented evidence that it is composed of two parts (1) a large carrier protein with a molecular weight of about 2 million daltons that is under autosomal genetic control and possesses the antigenic determinants for heterologous factor VIII antibody, the structural determinant of ristocetin cofactor activity (von Willebrand factor), and the binding site for the functionally active factor VIII fragment, and (2) a smaller protein with a molecular weight of about 100,000 daltons that is under sex-linked genetic control and possesses factor VIII coagulant activity. These workers further suggest that the several functions associated with the large carrier component of factor VIII may be expressed in variable phenotypes. Aside from these unresolved considerations, factor VIII is known to interact with activated factor IX, Ca^{++}, and platelet factor 3 in the intrinsic pathway to activate factor X.[36] In this process factor VIII is not activated, but it is enhanced by trace amounts of thrombin.[82] (See Fig. 25-1.) Like fibrinogen, prothrombin, and factor V, factor VIII is ultimately consumed in the process of clotting. Factor VIII and ristocetin cofactor activities are both concentrated in plasma cryoprecipitate.[71] The disappearance of transfused factor VIII activity from hemophilic plasma is characterized by an initial fall to about 50% of the starting level in 4 to 6 hours, followed by steady exponential decay with a half-time of about 12 hours.[87,88]

Factor IX, also termed Christmas factor[10] and plasma thromboplastin component,[2] is a glycoprotein with a molecular weight of about 90,000 daltons and is synthesized in the hepatic parenchyma under sex-linked genetic control.[5,50] As in the case of prothrombin and factors VII and X, the factor IX molecule is dependent on vitamin K for postribosomal synthesis of γ-carboxyglutamic acids. Factor IX is converted to a serine esterase by activated factor XI in a Ca^{++}-dependent step and then interacts with Ca^{++}, factor VIII, and platelet factor 3 in the intrinsic pathway to activate factor X.[50] Factor IX is stable in plasma and is not consumed in the course of clotting.[42] In patients with Christmas disease the half-time of transfused factor IX, following a rapid initial fall, is about 20 hours.[78]

Factor X, also termed Stuart-Prower factor,[39,127] is a glycoprotein with a molecular weight of 86,000 daltons; it is synthesized in the hepatic parenchyma.[28,41] Like prothrombin and factors VII and IX, factor X is dependent on vitamin K. As noted previously, factor X is situated in the common pathway of thrombin generation and is changed to its active form as a serine esterase both

by factor VII with tissue thromboplastin and Ca^{++} in the extrinsic pathway and by activated factor IX with factor VIII, Ca^{++}, and platelet factor 3 in the intrinsic pathway. In turn, activated factor X interacts with factor V, Ca^{++}, and platelet factor 3 as prothrombinase to convert prothrombin to thrombin. Factor X is stable in plasma and is not consumed in the course of clotting.[39] Following an initial half-time of about 6 hours, factor X transfused into patients with inherited lack of this factor decays steadily with a half-time of about 40 hours.[9,102]

Factor XI, also termed plasma thromboplastin antecedent,[108] is a procoagulant with a molecular weight of about 180,000 daltons; it migrates electrophoretically as a γ_2-globulin.[35,112] The site of its synthesis has not been determined, but decreased plasma factor XI activity has been reported in association with liver disease.[95] Factor XI is converted to an active serine esterase by activated factor XII; activated factor XI, in turn, converts factor IX to its active form in a Ca^{++}-dependent step.[50,112] Factor XI is stable in plasma and is not consumed in the course of clotting.[108] The half-time of factor XI transfused into patients lacking in this factor is about 2.5 days.[109]

Factor XII, also known as Hageman factor,[96] is a protein that migrates electrophoretically with the β-globulins and has a molecular weight of about 80,000 daltons.[100] The site or sites of factor XII synthesis have not been conclusively established. Among the major advances in the past decade has been progress in basic understanding of the central role of factor XII in the initial phase of the intrinsic coagulation pathway and its relation to fibrinolysis. The conversion of factor XII to its active form as a serine esterase is known to be interwoven in a complex manner with the following systems: ill-defined changes of surfaces in contact with factor XII, perhaps electrochemical in nature[76]; the conversion of prekallikrein to kallikrein[138]; the conversion of high molecular weight kininogen to bradykinin[24]; and the fibrinolytic system, including plasmin itself and the conversion of plasma plasminogen proactivator to plasminogen activator.[45,53]

Critical to this body of knowledge was the discovery in 1965 by Hathaway et al.[34] of "Fletcher factor," which was subsequently shown to be prekallikrein.[138] In the mid-1970s there was a burst of reports of patients with another factor XII–related defect, variously termed Fitzgerald factor,[131] Fleaujac trait,[55] Williams trait,[19] and Reid trait[62] — all shown to be functionally identical high molecular weight kininogen.[110] Kaplan et al.[46] have reviewed the current state of the art of factor XII–dependent pathways, and their schematic summary of these pathways is shown in Fig. 25-3.

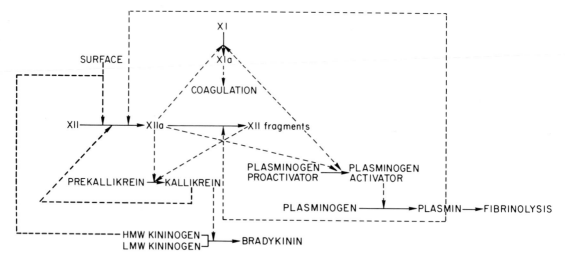

Fig. 25-3. Factor XII–dependent pathways according to Kaplan et al. (From Kaplan, A. P., Meier, H. L., and Mandle, R., Jr.: Semin. Thromb. Hemost. **3**:1, 1976.)

In view of the critical position of factor XII and its related pathways in coagulation and fibrinolysis, it is remarkable that deficiencies of factor XII, prekallikrein, and high molecular weight kininogen are not associated with clinically significant bleeding disorders as a rule. Factor XII is stable in plasma and is not consumed in the course of clotting. The half-time of factor XII transfused into factor XII–deficient patients is about 50 hours.[128]

Factor XIII, also known as fibrin-stabilizing factor or Laki-Lorand factor,[56] is a protein that migrates with the α_2-globulins and has a molecular weight of 320,000 to 350,000 daltons.[25,117] The site or sites of factor XIII synthesis are unknown, but this factor is intimately associated with megakaryocytes and platelets.[68] Factor XIII, activated by thrombin in the presence of Ca^{++},[61] is a transamidase that leads to cross-linkage between adjacent fibrin monomers through the formation of glutamyl-lysine bonds.[85] Factor XIII is stable in plasma but disappears in the course of clotting by adsorption onto fibrin.[60] The half-time of factor XIII transfused into patients with inherited factor XIII deficiency is about 7 days.[16]

Fibrinolytic factors. Fibrinolysis is mediated by the enzyme *plasmin* derived from its inactive plasma precursor *plasminogen* through the action of *plasminogen activators* that in turn are derived both from intrinsic (or plasma) and extrinsic (or tissue) sources.

Plasminogen is a plasma protein with a molecular weight of 92,000 daltons that migrates electrophoretically with the β-globulins.[47] The origin of plasminogen has not been conclusively established, but available evidence suggests that bone

marrow eosinophils and the liver may be sites of plasminogen synthesis.[75,101] Plasmin is formed by loss of one or more small terminal peptides and cleavage of an arginyl-valine bond in the plasminogen molecule, yielding a light chain with a molecular weight of about 30,000 and a heavy chain with a molecular weight of about 50,000 daltons; the two chains are linked by a disulphide bond, and the active serine of the enzyme is located in the light chain.[123,124] Plasmin degrades its substrates by cleaving arginyl-lysine bonds and thus, like trypsin but unlike thrombin, has a wide range of proteolytic specificity.[119] As noted, plasmin participates in the activation of factor XII, and of course its major physiologic substrate is fibrin. The step-wise degradation of fibrinogen by plasmin has been carefully investigated and presented by Marder and Budzynski.[66] (See Fig. 23-3.) Other coagulation factors that may be degraded by plasmin are factors V and VIII.

Naturally occurring plasminogen activators that are extrinsic to plasma are widely distributed among body tissues, fluids, and cells.[54,72,133] The most thoroughly investigated of these is urokinase, a polypeptide with a molecular weight of 54,000 daltons that has been isolated from urine and is probably synthesized in the kidney.[52,59]

The existence of a plasma precursor of plasminogen activator, as distinct from activators derived from tissues, was previously postulated to explain the fibrinolytic effect of streptokinase first identified by Kaplan[48] in 1944; it was suggested that this effect might be the result of a streptokinase-mediated conversion of a plasma "proactivator" to an activator that in turn converts plasminogen to plasmin.[51] More recently it has been

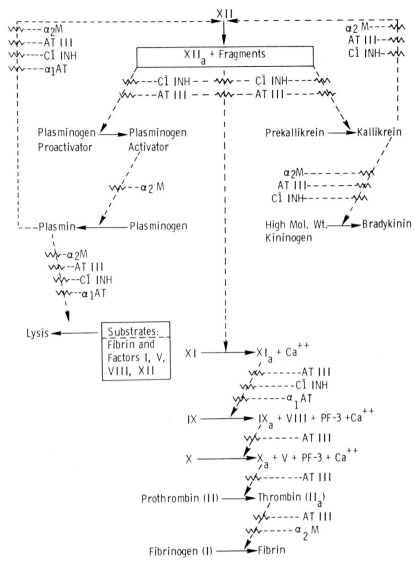

Fig. 25-4. Coagulant and fibrinolytic enzymes inhibited by antithrombin III *(AT III)*, α_2-macroglob-ulin *($\alpha_2 M$)*, C̄Ī inhibitor *(C̄Ī INH)*, and α_1-antitrypsin *($\alpha_1 AT$)*. (Modified from Schreiber, A. D.: Semin. Thromb. Hemost. **3:**43, 1976.)

shown that streptokinase binds to plasminogen itself and exposes an active site on the molecule through a conformational change without actually converting it to plasmin; plasmin is produced by the interaction of reactive streptokinase-plasminogen complexes with unbound plasminogen.[98,99,111]

Other early studies of factor XII suggested a role of this factor in an intrinsic pathway of fibrinolysis.[38,40] In 1972 Kaplan and Austen[45] identified in plasma a proactivator with a molecular weight of 95,000 daltons that is converted to plasminogen activator by activated factor XII. (See Figs. 25-1 and 25-3.) Thus current evidence strongly suggests the existence of intrinsic as well

as extrinsic pathways for the generation of plasminogen activators. Furthermore, it appears that factor XII–dependent activator, like urokinase, enzymatically converts plasminogen to plasmin rather than binding to plasminogen with production of reactive complexes, as in the case of streptokinase.[46]

Natural inhibitors of coagulation and fibrinolysis. The principal natural inhibitors or antiproteases affecting coagulation and fibrinolysis are as follows: antithrombin III, α_2-macroglobulin, α_1-antitrypsin, and the inhibitor of activated C̄Ī. These antiproteases all have overlapping roles in the inhibition of coagulant and fibrinolytic enzymes (see Table 23-4) but antithrombin III and α_2-macroglobulin are the major inhibitors of coagulation and fibrinolysis, respectively.[104,115]

Antithrombin III is an α_2-globulin with a molecular weight of 63,000 daltons, including 15% carbohydrate, and it is probably synthesized in the liver. Among the major accomplishments in coagulation in recent years is the elucidation by Rosenberg et al. of the mechanism of action of this antiprotease and its interaction with heparin.[105-107,120] These workers have shown that the reactive site of antithrombin III is arginine, which interacts with the active serine site of serine-containing esterases, leading to stoichiometric formation of inhibitor-enzyme complexes. Furthermore, heparin changes this interaction from a progressive to an immediate process. Negatively charged heparin binds to positively charged lysine of antithrombin III; this binding presumably produces a conformational change in the antithrombin molecule, which renders its reactive arginine more accessible to interaction with serine in appropriate enzymes. The following serine esterases of the coagulation system are progressively inhibited by antithrombin III and instantly inhibited on the addition of heparin: thrombin and activated forms of factors XII, XI, IX, and X. Plasmin is also a serine protease and is inhibited by antithrombin III with marked enhancement of inhibition by added heparin. However, in mixtures of plasmin, antithrombin III, and α_2-macroglobulin without heparin, approximately twice as much plasmin is bound to α_2-macroglobulin as to antithrombin III.[104]

α_2-Macroglobulin has a molecular weight of 725,000 daltons and, like antithrombin III, may be synthesized in the liver. This antiprotease is capable of binding enzymes of different classes, including serine esterases, but its reactive site or sites have not yet been determined.[7] Available evidence suggests that α_2-macroglobulin is the major inhibitor of plasmin and plasminogen activator and plays a lesser role in the control of coagulant enzymes including thrombin, activated factor XII, and kallikrein.[115] On the other hand, in accord with evidence that plasmin bound to α_2-macroglobulin retains fibrinolytic activity,[32] regulatory protection of certain enzyme activities by this antiprotease may prove to be more significant than its direct inhibitory function.

α_1-Antitrypsin and the inhibitor of the activated CI are both inhibitors of activated factor XII and plasmin. The state of the art in the mid-1970s regarding antiproteases of factor XII–dependent pathways has been comprehensively reviewed by Schreiber[115]; his schematic summary of these pathways is shown in Fig. 25-4.

Table 25-2. Coagulation data for normal subjects in the perinatal period*

Subject	Screening tests†			Coagulation factors†								
	Activated PTT (sec)	PT (sec)	Thrombin time (sec)	I (mg/dl)	II (%)	V (%)	VII + X (%)	VIII (%)	IX (%)	XI (%)	XII (%)	XIII (%)
Normal adult or child	44	13	10	315 ± 60	100	100	100	100	100	100	100	100
Fetus, early (10-15 weeks)	—	—	—	120	—	81	18	—	—	—	—	—
Preterm infant, 27-31 weeks	—	23	—	270 ± 140	30 ± 10	72 ± 25	32 ± 15	70 ± 30	27 ± 10	—	—	100
Preterm infant, 32-36 weeks	70	17 (12-21)	14 (11-17)	226 ± 70	35 ± 12	91 ± 23	39 ± 14	98 ± 40	—	—	30	100
Term infant, average for gestational age	55 ± 10	16 (13-20)	12 (10-16)	246 ± 55	45 ± 15	98 ± 40	56 ± 16	105 ± 35	28 ± 8	30	51	100

*From Hathaway, W. E.: Semin. Hematol. **12:**175, 1975. Used by permission.
†Values represent smoothed means ± standard deviation or ranges from cord blood samples or venous samples in first 24 hours of life.

Plasma phase of hemostasis in the newborn

Neonatal plasma-phase hemostasis has been reviewed by Bleyer et al.[12] and by Hathaway.[33] (See also Chapter 23.) The following comments will be limited to certain highlights of coagulation, fibrinolysis, and control mechanisms in the newborn.

The healthy newborn, whether full-term or premature, is remarkably free of bleeding problems. Nonetheless, numerous studies of neonatal coagulation indicate a rather consistent spectrum of deficits relative to adult values in screening tests (PT, PTT, and TCT) and activities of certain coagulation factors, notably the vitamin K–dependent factors, i.e., prothrombin and factors VII, IX, and X.[1] There is evidence of increased fibrinolytic activity, expressed by increased plasminogen activator activity in plasma and decreased plasminogen levels, but the titer of fibrin and fibrinogen degradation products in serum is usually not significantly increased.[26,27] Natural inhibitors of coagulation and fibrinolysis, notably antithrombin III, are generally decreased in activity and plasma concentration in newborns.[65]

The differences between newborns and adults with regard to the plasma phase of hemostasis, although thoroughly documented, are poorly understood. These differences need to be recognized in interpreting the results of tests of plasma hemostasis in sick newborns, particularly those with bleeding problems. Hathaway[33] has summarized expected values for such tests in newborns of different gestational ages (Table 25-2). The plasma phase of hemostasis in a 1-year-old infant is functionally equivalent to that of an adult.

Classification of coagulation disorders

Coagulation disorders are arbitrarily divided into two major categories: disorders characterized by (1) decreased activity of one or more coagulation factors, i.e., "hypocoagulable," or coagulation deficiency, disorders; and (2) normal or increased activity of one or more coagulation factors, i.e., "hypercoagulable," or thrombotic, disorders. Separate categories for abnormalities of fibrinolysis and natural inhibitors of clotting and fibrinolysis will not be developed since such abnormalities are clinically expressed in coagulation disorders. This classification should be regarded as the final segment of the overall scheme begun in Chapter 24.

A. Coagulation deficiencies (decreased activity of one or more coagulation factors)
  1. Common inherited coagulation deficiencies
    a. Classical hemophilia
    b. von Willebrand's disease
    c. Christmas disease
  2. Uncommon inherited coagulation deficiencies
    a. Congenital fibrinogen deficiencies
      (1) Congenital afibrinogenemia
      (2) Dysfibrinogenemias
    b. Congenital prothrombin deficiency
    c. Congenital factor V deficiency
    d. Congenital factor VII deficiency
    e. Congenital factor X deficiency
    f. Congenital factor XI deficiency
    g. Congenital factor XII deficiency
    h. Congenital factor XIII deficiency
    i. Other inherited coagulation deficiencies
  3. Acquired coagulation deficiencies
    a. Vitamin K deficiency
    b. Disseminated intravascular coagulation
    c. Parenchymal liver disease
    d. Congenital heart disease
    e. Surgical cardiopulmonary bypass
    f. Renal disease
    g. Dysproteinemias
    h. Acquired inhibitors of coagulation (circulating anticoagulants)
    i. Other acquired coagulation deficiencies
  4. Neonatal coagulation deficiencies
    a. Hemorrhagic disease of the newborn
    b. Other neonatal coagulation disorders
      (1) Inherited deficiencies
      (2) Acquired disorders
B. Thrombotic disorders (normal or increased activity of coagulation factors)
  1. Inherited thrombotic disorders
    a. Congenital deficiency of antithrombin III
    b. Other inherited thrombotic disorders
  2. Acquired thrombotic disorders
    a. Drug-induced thrombotic disorders
    b. Other acquired thrombotic disorders
  3. Neonatal thrombotic disorders

Coagulation deficiencies
COMMON INHERITED COAGULATION DEFICIENCIES

The coagulation disorders considered the most common as well as causing the greatest problem in the patient and requiring the greatest proportion of materials to maintain the patient are the sex-linked recessive disorders: classic hemophilia with a deficiency of factor VIII activity and Christmas disease with a deficiency of factor IX activity in the plasma. The less common heritable disorders may be more prevalent than observed since they are of less clinical significance and therefore are identified with less frequency. Von Willebrand's disease, probably the most variable of all the coagulation disorders in its clinical significance and manifestations, is undoubtedly far more prevalent than its recognized incidence suggests.

Classical hemophilia

Classical hemophilia (hemophilia A, factor VIII deficiency, antihemophilic factor deficiency) is an inherited abnormality in the hemostatic mechanism in which the patient has a functional defect of the factor VIII protein resulting in a deficiency of factor VIII clotting activity in the plasma.

Historical perspective. Hemophilia is among the oldest described genetic diseases with records on the Egyptian papyrus and in the Tosefea of the Mishna that Rabbi Judah counseled two families in the second century A.D.[279] In the first family the fourth son of a woman whose first three sons died following circumcision was excused from surgery. The second family involved four sisters, three of whom had sons who bled to death after circumcision. The fourth sister's son was excused. These incidents are frequently quoted in the Talmud.

The "bleeder's" disease was first clearly described by Otto[258] in Philadelphia in 1803 when he described the bleeding into joints and the crippling arthropathy that developed. The description also stated that the disease was sex-linked, found only in the male, and transmitted by the apparently normal female. The name "hemophilia," or love of blood, was given to the disease by Schönlein in 1839, and later Wright[306] showed that the clotting time was prolonged in hemophilia. Addis[142] showed that a globulin fraction prepared by dilution and acidification of normal plasma could correct the clotting defect in hemophilia. Addis assumed that this abnormality was a prothrombin abnormality since the fibrinogen in the globulin fraction of hemophilic plasma had been found normal by Mellanby.[243] The review of the literature and the description of hemophilia by Bulloch and Fildes[167] were the latest developments until the work of Patek and Taylor,[259] who showed that the defect in hemophilia was a result of a deficiency of a globulin fraction referred to as antihemophilic globulin or antihemophilic factor. Later Brinkhous[162] showed that the prothrombin was normal but was converted to thrombin at a slower rate and that this defect could be corrected by blood transfusion. By 1952 hemophilia was defined as a sex-linked recessive disorder caused by a deficiency of the antihemophilic globulin.

The existence of another hemophilioid disorder in males whose plasma corrected that of patients with classical hemophilia was discovered in 1952 by Schulman[275] and Aggeler et al.[143] independently; it was called plasma thromboplastin component deficiency. Neither of these patients had a family history of the disease. However, this hemophilia (hemophilia B) was subsequently named Christmas disease by Biggs et al.[157] after the first patient seen with the disorder in Britain. The disease was inherited in the same manner as classical hemophilia.

The nomenclature of these two disorders as well as the other clotting factors was simplified by the International Committee of the Society of Thrombosis and Haemostasis under Wright[307] when Roman numerals were adopted for clotting factors I to XIII in 1962. The antihemophilic factor is factor VIII, and plasma thromboplastin component is factor IX. Massie has given a description of hemophilia in the celebrated Russian Tsarevich before the advent of modern therapy.[237]

Classification. Patients with classical hemophilia may be classified according to the clinical severity of the disease and the laboratory findings of the deficient factor. Although the clinical severity does not always parallel the laboratory findings and may vary from year to year, the main groupings of patients usually holds steadfast throughout a patient's life, and the group classification is usually constant within a family. Patients may be divided into those with *severe, moderate,* and *mild* disease. Those with severe disease have less than 1% of factor VIII clotting activity in their plasma and have spontaneous bleeding or bleeding without known trauma. The diagnosis is made in infancy, within the first year of life, or following circumcision. Patients with moderate disease have 1% to 5% factor VIII clotting activity and bleed with mild trauma, and those with mild disease have 6% to 50% factor VIII activity and bleed only with severe trauma or surgery. The diagnosis is frequently not made until later in life, often following poor hemostasis with dental extraction.

Incidence. The incidence of hemophilia can not be stated with accuracy at this time because registration of all patients with mild and severe disease is incomplete in most countries. Using prevalent data, however, the figure for classical hemophilia alone has varied from 4.2×10^{-5} in the state of Pennsylvania[282] to 4.5×10^{-5} in Denmark.[149] The figure of 25.8×10^{-5} found by the National Blood Resources Program Pilot Study in 1972 combines moderate and severe factor VIII and factor IX deficiency and is probably somewhat high, but is the figure that is taken as a working estimate until a more precise one can be obtained.[252] It has been reported in all parts of the world and in all races, although rarely in the Chinese.

Etiology. Until recently classical hemophilia has been considered to be simply a plasma coagulation factor deficiency. The low concentrations of the factor VIII protein in normal plasma have hampered biochemical extraction and characterization of the molecule until immunologic methods were applied. Details of the properties are found in extensive reviews by Hershgold et al.,[195] Marchesi et al.,[236] Shapiro et al.,[281] and Legaz et al.[226] They show that the molecular weight is approximately 1.12 million with subunits of 195,000 to 240,000 daltons. The highly purified protein has 5% to 10% carbohydrate with hexose, hexosamine, and sialic acid identified. There is lipid of varying amounts and the amino acids methionine, tyrosine, and tryptophane have been found in small quantities. The specific coagulant activity varies with the investigator and is probably related to inactivation of factor VIII during purification. The factor VIII molecule is in all likelihood a complex of two distinct components, a high molecular weight portion, which contains the antigen and von Willebrand's factor, and the low molecular weight portion, which contains the procoagulant or clotting activity. The two parts can be separated on agarose gel chromatography by varying the salt content in the ionic buffers.[309,311,312] Animals have been immunized with this protein to produce an antiserum to human factor VIII that inactivates factor VIII procoagulant inactivity in a variety of tests that have been used to quantify the factor VIII–related antigen in normal human plasma.[310] Immunoelectrophoresis, Laurel electroimmunoassay, crossed immunoelectrophoresis, tanned red cell hemagglutination, and radioimmunoassay give similar results.[246] Hoyer[206] has shown that there is a correlation between the factor VIII procoagulant factor and the factor VIII–related antigen in normal individuals.

These immunologic studies have been used to distinguish the production of a nonfunctional protein in patients with classical hemophilia and to suggest a heterogeneity of the deficiency state. At least two forms of the disease could be recognized.

In earlier work it was found that 10% of the plasma of hemophilic patients neutralized human naturally occurring anti–factor VIII antibody, whereas the majority did not.* Those plasmas that did not neutralize were "cross-reacting material negative" (CRM− or A−) while those plasmas which did react were "cross-reacting material positive" (CRM+ or A+). The cross-reacting material was consistent within families. However, when Biggs,[156] Gralnick et al.,[189] and Feinstein et al.[182] used rabbit or goat anti–factor VIII antibodies they found all hemophilic plasmas contained the cross-reacting material. The interpretation of these results is that all hemophiliacs synthesize a nonfunctional high molecular weight protein similar to normal factor VIII–related protein, a fact consistent with a normal bleeding time and normal values in the assays for von Wille-

*References 172, 173, 206, 207.

brands's factor, glass bead retention, and ristocetin assay. The difference in antibody response found with the two antibodies, human and animal, however, suggests that a variable type of protein is produced by some hemophiliacs or that there may be conformational differences in the molecules that are recognized differently by the two different antibodies.

Synthesis of the factor VIII complex is discussed in the section on pathogenesis.

Genetics. The mode of inheritance of factor VIII, supported by studies in hemophilic dogs, is characterized by transmission of a sex-linked recessive trait.[163,166,188] Affected males, who are hemizygous, do not transmit the disease to their children but do transmit the abnormal gene to all their daughters, who are heterozygous carriers. All heterozygous women appear clinically normal but transmit the trait and disease to half their sons and the trait to half their daughters, who are heterozygotes. Affected females are produced by the mating of a carrier female and affected male, by lyonization of the defective X chromosome, or by new mutation.[170,187] Male-to-male transmission does not occur.

It has been said that the mutation rate must be very high since 25% of all new patients do not have a positive family history and their mothers therefore are presumed to be noncarriers.[231] However, carrier detection was inaccurate in the past and is still not entirely precise.[155] Merritt[244] suggests that a mutation rate of 2 to 4 × 10⁻⁵ gametes/generation is as accurate an estimation as is possible with present indirect methods, a rate that remains high.

The genetic locus determining classical hemophilia is closely linked to those of a G-6-PD variant and color blindness on the X chromosome but distant from the loci determining Christmas disease, vitamin D–resistant rickets, and the Xgᵃ blood group.[240,276] The closely linked markers are helpful when they occur in the hemophilia carrier.[239]

In 1963 McLester and Graham[241] suggested a "combining subunit" theory of factor VIII synthesis: The molecule is a combination of two gene products—one coded at an autosomal locus (von Willebrand's disease) and the other at the X chromosome locus (hemophilia). Subsequent findings indicate an even greater complexity of factor VIII synthesis, but the concept of combining subunits remains useful.[187,249]

Prenatal diagnosis of hemophilia has not been perfected. Factor VIII antigen and procoagulant activity are not found in amniotic fluid. Therefore determination of the disease state of the newborn infant must await improved techniques of cord sampling. Factor VIII has been found in a 28-

week-old fetus, although in a reduced amount compared to a full-term newborn.[202] Currently only the sex of the fetus may be determined from cells extracted from amniotic fluid and grown in tissue culture for sex chromatin analysis.

Carrier detection was notoriously poor in the past, predictive in only 25% of cases tested and dependent on decreased procoagulant factor VIII activity alone. With the development of immunologic determination of factor VIII–related antigen, a new dimension was introduced into the detection of the obligate carrier. The ratio of factor VIII activity to factor VIII antigen can now be used and is less than 1 in carriers and 1 or more in normal individuals.[312]

Although these techniques do not detect every carrier with certainty, they may be usefully applied to an estimation of probability.[178]

Clinical features. The clinical features of classical hemophilia and Christmas disease are the same; i.e., they are indistinguishable clinically and distinguishable only in the laboratory. The clinical description therefore applies to both disorders. Hemophilia may be present at birth with a prolonged bleeding time from the cord or from the navel after separation, with severe cephalhematoma, or with bleeding from the circumcision site. The diagnosis may be made on cord blood for factor VIII deficiency since the factor VIII molecule is large and does not cross the placenta. Factor IX deficiency may be somewhat more difficult to verify (p. 793). However, it is usually only those infants with severe disease (less than 1% of factor VIII in the plasma) who are identified in the neonatal period. Occasional infants have small submucosal hematomas on erupting teeth, which may ooze when the tooth breaks through the gum. The bleeding stops as the erupting tooth exerts pressure on the receding gum. As the toddler begins to walk, he may develop unusual hematomas on the buttocks, knees, or forehead from falls. Gum or tongue lacerations or a split frenulum is also commonplace. With increased activity of childhood, hemarthrosis and deep muscle hematomas are common. Today 10% to 15% of adolescents have some arthropathy, and 75% of adults have some chronic arthropathy. In the past all patients with severe disease had chronic arthropathy by the age of 10 and those with moderate disease had some degree of chronic arthropathy by adulthood.[215] This statement should not be true today if therapy is instituted at the first sign of bleeding. The philosophy of care has changed radically in the last 10 years, so that the natural history of the disease is different today and changing radically with therapy.

Hemarthrosis. The most common and severe complication is the chronic arthropathy that de-velops following two or more hemarthroses in the same joint. When bleeding occurs within the joint, the joint is opened or put into the position of comfort, usually flexion, to accomodate the blood within the joint. The joint swells and becomes painful, the overlying skin becomes warm, tense, or even shiny, and the joint is tender to palpation. This progression of events takes place within 4 to 6 hours after the onset of bleeding and can be stopped with prompt therapy when the patient first has a stiffness or discomfort within the joint that heralds the onset of bleeding before the objective signs appear. The joints commonly involved are the knees, elbows, ankles, hips, and shoulders, in order of decreasing frequency. Once bleeding has occurred within a joint, deterioration begins and

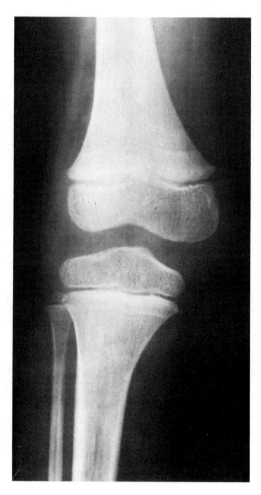

Fig. 25-5. Stage I hemophilic arthropathy. This stage is characterized by soft tissue swelling without bony changes. (From Hilgartner, M. W.: In Schulman, I., et al., eds.: Advances in pediatrics, vol. 21. Copyright © 1974 by Year Book Medical Publishers, Inc., Chicago. Used by permission.)

may progress within several years through subacute and chronic stages to degenerative arthritis.

Arnold and Hilgartner[151] have classified the progression of joint pathology into five stages (Figs. 25-5 to 25-9). The soft tissue swelling of stage I gives way to stage II, in which there is early osteoporosis and overgrowth of the epiphyses. In stage III disorganization of the joint is evident with subchondral cyst formation, squaring of the patella, and widening of the intracondylar notch of the knee and the trochlear notch of the ulna. Thickened boggy synovium is opacified by hemosiderin. This is the final stage at which hemophilic arthropathy may be reversed by medical therapy. In stage IV the cartilage is destroyed and the joint space is narrowed. Stage V is the end stage with fibrous

joint contracture, and complete loss of cartilage and joint space. There is marked painful restriction of motion, and the synovium remains as fibrous unorganized bands. Muscular deformity usually accompanies the bony deformity, making the joint unstable. Bleeding usually follows trauma in early childhood, and when chronic hemarthrosis develops, bleeding may occur without provocation in those with severe and moderate disease. Those with mild disease rarely if ever have hemarthrosis.

Hematuria. Hematuria caused by a bleeding diathesis is usually renal in origin and must be differentiated from nephritis.[285] Bleeding from the kidneys is not unusual in young boys with severe hemophilia over age 4 and has been reported in 7% of the patients 5 to 10 years of age in one series.[225] The incidence progresses to 70% of the adult patients.[264] However, red blood cells are rarely seen on routine urinalysis. Hematuria usually occurs without trauma in the severe disease and is secondary to trauma in moderate and mild hemophilia. In the early stages it is rarely painful, rarely causes a severe blood loss, and may persist for days or weeks. When clotting occurs in the re-

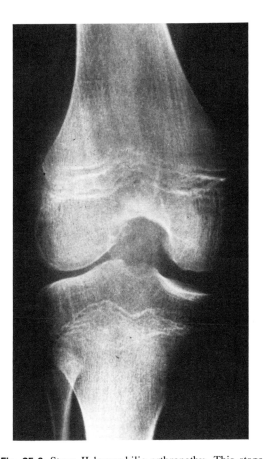

Fig. 25-6. Stage II hemophilic arthropathy. This stage is characterized by early osteoporosis, particularly affecting the epiphyses, and overgrowth of the epiphyses. (From Hilgartner, M. W.: In Schulman, I., et al., eds.: Advances in pediatrics, vol. 21. Copyright © 1974 by Year Book Medical Publishers, Inc., Chicago. Used by permission.)

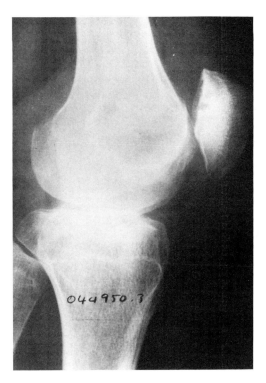

Fig. 25-7. Stage III hemophilic arthropathy. This stage is characterized by disorganization of the joint including patellar squaring, subchondral cysts, and irregularities of the joint surface without significant narrowing of the cartilage space. (From Arnold, W. D., and Hilgartner, M. W.: J. Bone Joint Surg. **59A:**287, 1977.)

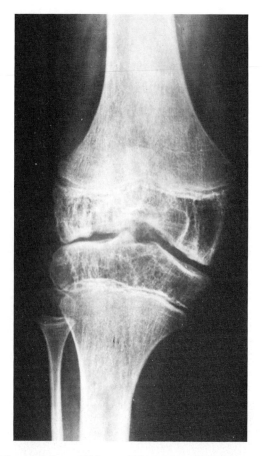

Fig. 25-8. Stage IV hemophilic arthropathy. This stage is characterized by narrowing of the joint space and cartilage destruction. (From Arnold, W. D., and Hilgartner, M. W.: J. Bone Joint Surg. **59A:**287, 1977.)

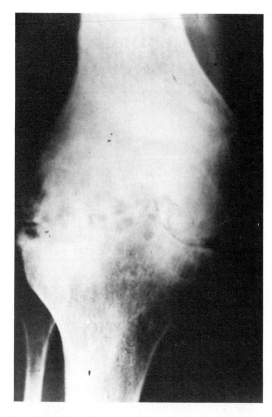

Fig. 25-9. Stage V hemophilic arthropathy. This stage is characterized by fibrous joint contracture, loss of joint space, and marked enlargement of the epiphyses. (From Arnold, W. D., and Hilgartner, M. W.: J. Bone Joint Surg. **59A:**287, 1977.)

nal pelvis and ureter, pain and obstructive uropathy occur. The mechanism for this hematuria is unknown. Lazerson[225] postulates immune complex formation and renal injury as the etiology in patients who have received multiple transfusions. He has collected evidence of lowered serum complement following transfusion for bleeding in a group of hemophiliacs with a history of hematuria. Those patients without a previous history of hematuria had higher baseline levels of serum complement than those with hematuria, which supports his hypothesis of immune injury.

Hematomas. Hemorrhage under the skin and into muscles is not unusual and may have a delayed onset from the time of known trauma. Superficial skin bruises have a characteristic central firm, pale nodule surrounded by the spreading purpuric area. Hematomas are common on the lower extremities, as in all small children.

Hematoma into muscles may be extensive and with serious consequence; e.g., soleus bleeding may produce equinus deformity of the foot in a short time if untreated. Bleeding in the thighs and forearms is also common but easier to control. Bleeding into the forearm can produce Volkman's contracture. Large untreated hematoma may persist and develop into pseudotumors.

Neurologic complications. Bleeding can occur into the central nervous system, into the spinal cord, and into adjacent tissue, which may compress peripheral nerves. In frequency of involvement with significant hemorrhage the nervous system is exceeded only by the musculoskeletal system. Neurologic complications vary in severity, depending on the site of hemorrhage, the rapidity with which the bleeding develops, and the effectiveness of therapy. Hemorrhage may occur following minimal trauma; noted in one recent series the time between the episode of minor trauma and the appearance of bleeding symptoms was 4 days.[181] This lag is not found in the individual with normal hemostatic mechanisms, in whom the severity of bleeding is usually proportional to the severity of trauma. Minor trauma in the hemophiliac may lead to fatal or debilitating complications if not suspected and treated early.[186] Several recent reviews point to the nervous system as a common bleeding site[184] demonstrating an incidence of nervous system bleeding as high as 25.4% in a series of 201 patients over the last 12 years.

CENTRAL NERVOUS SYSTEM. Intracranial bleeding is still considered the major cause of death in hemophiliacs[146,148,218] and may remain the major barrier to the severe hemophiliac reaching a normal life expectancy. The more recent reviews place the incidence for factor VIII deficiency at 12.9%,[181,184,292] a figure that has not changed greatly in 12 years.[218] As expected, those with a greater factor deficiency tend to have more central nervous system bleeding, whereas this site of bleeding is unusual for the patient with mild disease. Furthermore, central nervous system bleeding has been reported to be more prevalent in patients with factor IX deficiency. The mean age of patients with intracranial bleeding was 14.9 years in those with factor VIII deficiency and 15 years in those with factor IX deficiency.[181,218] This occurs in newborns surprisingly rarely, with one case in neonates reported by each of two authors[153,293] and a higher incidence (36%) in infants under 3 years of age in another series.

The relationship of hemorrhage to head trauma is unclear, a history of major head trauma in some instances being unassociated with subsequent intracranial complications. Minor trauma occurred in 55% of the patients in a recent series and was more prevalent in the younger child than the adult.[181]

When there is no history of trauma, the possibility of an underlying congenital lesion or neoplasm must be considered, as in an individual with a normal hemostatic mechanism. Noninvasive procedures should be carried out first, e.g., computerized axial tomography (CAT) of the brain. Appropriate invasive procedures can be done with concentrate coverage. If an inhibitor is present, the diagnostic procedures may still be done with caution and the neurosurgical procedure as necessary.

The common bleeding sites have been reported as subdural or epidural, intracerebral, and subarachnoid.[186] Second episodes of bleeding have been reported within a year of the first episode in 20% of cases. Most authors agree that the mortality has improved remarkably with recent diagnostic suspicion and acumen with both invasive and noninvasive techniques and early and intensive use of replacement material.[220] Once a central ner-vous system lesion is suspected, the hemophiliac should be investigated just as any other patient with a similar set of signs and symptoms under appropriate replacement therapy control. Skull films should be obtained immediately, lumbar puncture and CAT or invasive procedures such as an angiogram when necessary.

Complications have included the minimal brain damage syndrome, seizures, hydrocephalus, and severe problems such as ataxia, hemiparesis, and aphasia. Careful seizure control is important and, although phenytoin (Dilantin) has been the cause of bleeding problems in newborns and older children, these have not been noted in hemophiliacs receiving anticonvulsant drugs.

INTRASPINAL HEMORRHAGE. Intraspinal bleeding is unusual and reported in only 25% of all the cases in two large series.[284,295] Although the three cases at the New York Hospital in the last 25 years have followed trauma, this is not usually present. The symptom complex of back and neck pain with ascending paresis suggesting acute transverse myelitis should alert the physician to the diagnosis.

PERIPHERAL NERVE HEMORRHAGE. Peripheral nerve hemorrhage is probably more common than generally recognized and seems to occur more frequently in older patients. The Oxford group reported that 90% in their series were over 18 years of age and only 10% were children.[145,177] All peripheral nerve lesions are caused by external compression or traction on a nerve.

There have been no proved cases of intraneuronal sheath hemorrhage. Bleeding into the iliacus muscle with subsequent femoral nerve paralysis is the most common peripheral nerve involvement as detailed in several series. This site is followed in frequency by the ulnar, median, sciatic, radial, peroneal, tibial, and dorsal and ventral spinal nerve roots.[186] The neuropathy occurs with external pressure onto a closed compartment as in the arm or leg. The patient has excruciating pain, paresis, and little external sign of swelling, heat, or tenderness. Sensory loss usually precedes the motor loss and may be associated with hip flexion, anorexia, fever, and leukocytosis plus a palpable midinguinal mass that may be confused with appendicitis if it is on the right side. Lesions of the sciatic nerve are frequently associated with buttock hematomas and lesions of the forearm compartment have led to Volkman's contracture.

Most patients with such lesions recover rapidly as soon as replacement therapy is given. However, some neuropathies may require 6 to 12 months for full recovery and necessitate intensive physical therapy in the interim to maintain muscular tone.

Mucous membrane bleeding. Mucous membrane bleeding refers to bleeding in the mouth, the nose, and the stomach; the entire gastrointestinal tract; and the genitourinary tract. The latter has been described in the discussion of hematuria. Gastrointestinal tract bleeding may present within the first year of life as gum bleeding. Small hematomas may form over the crown of the erupting tooth. Mouth bleeding may be common when an unsteady toddler falls and lacerates the frenulum, tongue, or gum. The lacerations rarely heal without replacement therapy. Sutures produce additional puncture sites and tension necrosis and are rarely useful. ε-Aminocaproic acid (EACA, Amicar) has been used for children this young.

Mucous membrane bleeding is frequently associated with loose deciduous teeth. By the time the sharp edges of the exfoliating teeth traumatize the gingival tissue and cause prolonged oozing, the tooth is no longer supported by bone. When the tooth is then tissue borne, it may be easily extracted without replacement therapy. If, however, the tooth is still somewhat in bone, EACA may be useful for a short period of time.[179]

Epistaxis occurs in patients with hemophilia as frequently as in the normal population and is often caused by the wandering fingers of the young. If nosebleeds are extremely frequent and difficult to control, the diagnosis of von Willebrand's disease or a platelet dysfunction should be considered. However, when the nasal mucosa becomes necrotic from multiple bleedings and lacerations of the tissue, replacement therapy may be necessary for healing.

Dental complications. In the past the majority of hemophiliacs had serious problems with periodontal disease and severe dental destruction related to poor dental hygiene and a total lack of prophylactic or restorative care.[302] Dental complications were common when hemophiliacs were afraid to go to the dentist for routine care and the dentist was afraid to treat patients with hemophilia. With the advent of home care, replacement therapy, and the newer high speed dental equipment, good prophylactic and restorative care is now available to all hemophiliacs.[180]

Hazardous bleeding areas. Bleeding in the following areas may be lethal if not treated rapidly: the central nervous system, the retroperitoneal area, and the retropharyngeal space. The central nervous system has been discussed. The retroperitoneal area has been mentioned in the description of peripheral nervous compression from the iliacus muscle bleeding. Bleeding in this area need not be lethal but can be very debilitating from the volume of blood loss, muscle deterioration, and nerve pressure. Bleeding in the retropharyngeal area may accompany pharyngitis or tonsillitis and should be suspected when the throat becomes swollen and swallowing of saliva is a problem. A lateral x-ray film of the neck is often helpful in de-

lineating the magnitude of the problem. When bleeding in this area is suspected, high-dose replacement therapy should be instituted. All three types require rapid and intensive therapy.

Pseudotumors. Hemophilic cysts are peculiar to the patient with hemophilia and have been associated with catastrophic complications in the past.[144] The lesions are enlarging encapsulated hematomas and may occur anywhere in the body. They may develop following subperiosteal hemorrhage; within facial envelopes of muscles; in soft tissue adjacent to bone, producing cortical thinning; or within the bone, expanding the cortex.[199] They may grow over a period of years and are often difficult to treat, requiring intensive medical therapy or radical excision when feasible. The bony defects rarely respond to medical therapy and have frequently required x-ray therapy for healing.[185] They should not be aspirated for diagnosis.[150]

Laboratory evaluation. Historically hemophilia was diagnosed when the whole blood clotting time was prolonged. The currently used tests for abnormalities in the clotting mechanism have been mentioned in Chapter 23. The tests for intrinsic system function—partial thromboplastin time (PTT), prothrombin consumption, and thromboplastin generation time (TGT)—can be used as measures of fibrin clot formation, the clotting ability of a plasma sample. Of these tests, the most widely used is the PTT, because it is fast, reproducible, and inexpensive. There are many commercially available lyophilized platelet lipid substitutes incorporating activators such as kaolin or celite for manual or automated methods. Levels of less than 20% of normal for either factor VIII or factor IX are associated with a prolonged PTT. The PTT may also be used to assay a specific factor by comparing the clotting time of the patient's plasma with that of a known deficient plasma in the test system. Factors VIII, IX, XI, and XII may be assayed in this manner. As stated before, the clinical picture of classical hemophilia and Christmas disease are indistinguishable; they can only be differentiated in the laboratory by specific factor assay. The one-stage assay in the PTT may be used for this differentiation. The TGT has been used in the past but currently is more a research tool than a clinical test for delineating a factor deficiency. If the results of all factor assays are low, an inhibitor against thromboplastin or a specific factor may be present and should be investigated.

These tests, however, only measure clotting activity of plasma. Factor VIII–related protein is determined immunologically by its ability to neutralize an antibody. The level of this inactive clotting protein can be used for carrier detection and for differentiation between von Willebrand's disease and classical hemophilia.[209]

All other commonly used tests for coagulation abnormalities, the PT test, bleeding time, platelet count, and tests for platelet function should be normal. Some confusion with a platelet dysfunction syndrome may arise in patients with classical hemophilia or Christmas disease from the fact that oozing may begin at the site of the bleeding time puncture an hour or more after the test has been done because of a lack of fibrin behind the platelet plug.

Pathogenesis and pathophysiology. Factor VIII–related protein has been found in the plasma of all normal individuals and most patients with classical hemophilia using immunologic techniques. The number of hemophiliacs with the protein varies according to whether the antibody in the test system is human or animal.[172,182,209] Those with the protein are CRM+ and those without the protein are CRM−. The interpretation of these data is that most patients with hemophilia produce a protein that is nonfunctional in the clotting process.[280,311] The production of this molecular variant in classical hemophilia is of practical importance in the separation of affected persons and female carriers from those with von Willebrand's disease; in the latter factor VIII–related antigen and coagulant activity are proportionally decreased.[191,312]

The discovery in recent years of multiple functional properties of factor VIII has led to diversified and frequently confusing terminology for these activities. In 1974 a task force was appointed by the International Committee on Thrombosis and Hemostasis to develop more uniform nomenclature. In 1977 the task force made the following recommendations for designating the three major classes of factor VIII–related activities:

1. *VIII:C*—factor VIII coagulant activity
2. *VIIIR:Ag*—factor VIII–related antigenic activity
3. *VIIIR:WF*—factor VIII–related von Willebrand factor activity generally designating ristocetin cofactor activity or modified appropriately to designate other determinants of platelet function, e.g., bleeding time factor may be designated VIIIR:WF(BT).

For many years an intensive search has been carried out to determine the organ responsible for factor VIII synthesis. The status of the search in 1975 has been reviewed by Webster et al.[300] Certain highlights may be summarized as follows. The liver appears to be the primary site of factor VIII synthesis, and production may be regulated by a negative feedback process[176,261]; the spleen may play a major role in factor VIII storage but not synthesis,[301] and a single spleen transplant in a

hemophilic subject was unsuccessful[193]; the kidneys may be involved in regulation of factor VIII levels but apparently not in its synthesis or storage; factor VIII–like activity associated with lymphocytes[160] is probably a result of tissue factor contamination.[270]

With the development of immunologic techniques, factor VIII–related antigen and von Willebrand's factor have been found in endothelial cells throughout the body.[210] Immunofluorescence studies have demonstrated factor VIII antigen in arteries, arterioles, capillaries and veins, megakaryocytes, and platelets. Both the factor VIII–related antigen and von Willebrand's factor activity have been found in the culture media from cultured human endothelial cells, and evidence has been found of factor VIII antigen synthesis by these cultured cells.[211,212] Factor VIII procoagulant activity could not be found in the media. It is postulated that the procoagulant activity may be made elsewhere or require a specific enzyme interaction for its activity. The answer is not known and Tocantin's theory of factor inaction by an inhibitor may still be valid.[288]

Management. When the hemostatic effect of whole blood was recognized and Brinkhous showed the change in clotting time brought about by fresh frozen plasma, control of most bleeding episodes was available. However, with the discovery by Pool and Shannon[262] of the cryoglobulin precipitate from thawed fresh frozen plasma that was rich in antihemophilic globulin, the era of concentrates of the plasma clotting factors was accelerated. The availability of cryoprecipitate and the concentrates of factors II, VII, VIII, IX, and X has radically changed the treatment of patients with clotting factor deficiencies and brought about a remarkable change in the quality of life and probably the longevity[174] of these individuals. The emphasis is no longer on treatment of the individual bleeding episode but rather on the comprehensive care of the patient. Early outpatient therapy of bleeding episodes is stressed and has produced a decrease in the number of deformities in children born within the last 10 years.[197] Outpatient treatment for bleeding episodes is routine; home treatment or self-infusion is possible for the majority of patients, with hospitalization reserved for rare bleeding episodes and surgical procedures. Aggressive rehabilitation programs and surgical reconstruction have corrected many old deformities. Outreach programs into schools and communities with expert vocational guidance and mental health support have permitted hemophiliacs to become successful, productive members of society. Chronic illness is no longer the burden that it was 10 years ago.

Treatment. Since the current therapeutic management of bleeding episodes in the hemophilias is similar, the treatment of the congenital factor VIII and factor IX deficiencies and Von Willebrand's disease is discussed together.

COMPREHENSIVE CARE. Total comprehensive care requires the support of a large number of individuals, including a primary care physician, pediatrician or internist, hematologist, orthopedist, dental surgeon and general dentist, physical therapist, mental health worker or social worker, and nurse with consultative services of a surgeon, psychiatrist or psychologist, geneticist, and vocational

Table 25-3. Products for replacement therapy of coagulation disorders*

Factor	Therapeutic modality	Storage	Approximate (mg/ml or units/ml)	Reconstitution
Factor I	Fresh frozen plasma	Frozen −20° C	200-400 mg	Thaw at 37° C
	Cryoprecipitate	Frozen −20° C	20-30	With 5-10 ml saline
	Concentrate	4° C	1-22	
Factor II	Fresh frozen plasma	Frozen −20° C	0.75-1 unit	Thaw at 37° C
	Concentrate (prothrombin complex)			
	Konyne (Cutter)	2°-8° C	25	With 20 ml H_2O
	Proplex (Hyland)	2°-8° C	7	With 30 ml H_2O
Factor V	Fresh frozen plasma	Frozen −20° C	0.25-0.50	Thaw at 37° C
Factor VII	Fresh frozen plasma	Frozen −20° C	1	Thaw at 37° C
	Concentrate			
	Konyne (Cutter)	2°-8° C	38	With 20 ml H_2O
	Proplex (Hyland)	2°-8° C	40-110	With 30 ml H_2O
Factor VIII	Fresh frozen plasma	Frozen −20° C	1	Thaw at 37° C
	Cryoprecipitate	Frozen −20° C	5-10	With 5-10 ml saline
	Concentrate			
	Profilate (Abbott)	4° C (28° C for 2 yrs)	20-25	With 10-50 ml saline
	Factorate (Armour)	4°-8° (28° C for 4 wks)	20-25	With 10-50 ml H_2O
	Koate (Cutter)	2°-8° (28° C for 4 wks)	25	With 10-40 ml H_2O
	Hemofil (Hyland)	4°-8° (20°-25° C for 4 wks)	25	With 10-30 ml H_2O
	Humafac (Parke-Davis)	2°-8° C	13-40	With 6-10 ml H_2O
	Lyoc (New York Blood Center)	4° C	6	With 20-30 ml H_2O
	Actif VIII (Merrieux)	2°-3° C	10-15	With 10-50 ml H_2O
von Willebrand's	Fresh frozen plasma	Frozen −20° C	1	Thaw at 37° C
	Cryoprecipitate	Frozen −20° C	2	With 5-10 ml saline
Factor IX	Fresh frozen plasma	Frozen −20° C	1	Thaw at 37° C
	Concentrate (prothrombin complex)			
	Konyne (Cutter)	2°-8° C	25	With 20 ml H_2O
	Proplex (Hyland)	2°-8° C	17-18	With 30 ml H_2O
Factor X	Fresh frozen plasma	Frozen −20° C	1	Thaw at 37° C
	Concentrate (prothrombin complex)			
	Konyne (Cutter)	2°-8° C	31	With 20 ml H_2O
	Proplex (Hyland)	2°-8° C	14-17	With 30 ml H_2O
Factor XI	Fresh frozen plasma	Frozen −20° C	1	Thaw at 37° C
	Cryoprecipitate supernatant	Frozen −20° C	1	Thaw at 37° C
Factor XII	Fresh frozen plasma	Frozen −20° C	1	Thaw at 37° C
Factor XIII	Fresh frozen plasma	Frozen −20° C	1	Thaw at 37° C
Fletcher	Fresh frozen plasma	Frozen −20° C	1	Thaw at 37° C
Fitzgerald	Fresh frozen plasma	Frozen −20° C	1	Thaw at 37° C

*All Concentrates are manufactured from pooled plasma or cryoprecipitate. Each donor unit and final product are screened for HB_sAg by RIA. One international unit of factor is that amount found in 1 ml of fresh normal plasma. Both Konyne and Proplex contain variable amounts of thrombogenic material. Proplex contains 1 unit of heparin/ml of reconstituted material.

guidance counselor. When the patient and his family are first seen and the patient is evaluated hematologically and functionally, comprehensive counseling and treatment plans for the patient can be formulated. This plan may be carried out in a center or at a local hospital if adequate services are available. The patient may then be followed every 3 to 6 months or at yearly intervals, depending on the severity of the disease and the amount of treatment required. Those with the most severe disease should be followed closely and seen at least every 3 months. Counseling, support, and education are ongoing needs and require as close follow-up as the medical needs.[175,198]

FACTOR REPLACEMENT THERAPY. Hemostasis is best achieved by replacement of the missing clotting factor activity. Significant amounts of factor must be given to bring about immediate clot formation and allow regrowth of fibroblasts for adequate healing. The manner in which the clotting factor is delivered depends primarily on the factor deficiency and the magnitude of the bleeding episode. Other parameters, such as age and size of the patient, convenience, acceptability, and cost of product, as well as the method and place of delivery of care to the patient, must also be considered. The available products are listed in Table 25-3.

Fresh frozen plasma contains all of the clotting factors in a concentration of approximately 1 unit of clotting factor activity per milliliter and can be used when only small amounts of clotting factor need to be delivered to the patient. Its use, however, is limited by the volume, since only 10 to 15 ml/kg may be given with safety in one dose, with an expected rise of 15% to 20% of factor activity. Such levels are insufficient for current surgical practices and accepted medical therapy for patients with classical hemophilia and Christmas disease. Fresh frozen plasma, however, may be used in treatment of von Willebrand's disease and factor XIII deficiency and it is the only therapy for deficiencies of factors V, XI, and XII, prekallikrein (Fletcher factor), and high molecular weight kininogen (e.g., Fitzgerald factor).

Fresh frozen plasma is harvested from single donor units and therefore carries less risk of hepatitis than the pooled concentrates. For this reason, it should be considered for those patients with mild deficiency of factor VIII (including von Willebrand's disease) or factor IX and who are therefore treated infrequently.

Cryoprecipitate, the protein that precipitates in fresh frozen plasma when it is thawed at 4° C, is rich in factor VIII and fibrinogen.[262] It is easily prepared in most blood banks capable of component fractionation and is stored at −20° C. Single units can concentrate the factor VIII approxi-

mately tenfold in 10 ml of plasma, and 30% to 60% of the factor VIII can be recovered from the donor plasma. The fibrinogen content may therefore be 3 to 4.5 gm. As a single-donor component, it also carries less hepatitis risk. Great variability exists in the product, however, because of twenty-one steps in its recovery process, which may affect the yield.[261] Pooling of the cryoprecipitate packs may give a more uniform product, but standardization and exact dosage calculation may be difficult. However, administration of this small volume by syringe or drip decreases the possibility of circulatory overload while providing a greater amount of therapeutic material. The cost of this product also varies throughout the country and in some areas may be considerably less than the dried concentrates.

Concentrates of the clotting factor proteins have many advantages and are becoming widely available. Those concentrates available in the United States are listed in Table 25-3, and similar products are available abroad. These lyophilized concentrates are made from pooled plasma obtained by plasmapheresis or a part of a blood bank's program of total donor unit fractionation. The factor VIII concentrates are prepared from cryoprecipitate and purified further by a variety of methods with removal of some fibrinogen.[164,214] They can be stored at 4° C in a refrigerator and reconstituted with sterile water, warmed to body temperature, drawn up into a syringe through a filter needle, and infused slowly by syringe. The more highly purified concentrates with low fibrinogen concentration are extremely desirable at the time of a surgical procedure or for a patient receiving high-dose therapy[213] for an extended period. Because the in vivo half-life of fibrinogen is longer than that of factor VIII, concentrates with a high fibrinogen content are less desirable because of the side effects of hyperfibrinogenemia when patients are maintained at high factor VIII plasma levels for extended periods (Table 25-4). The amount of clotting activity is stated on the bottle label and facilitates dosage calculations. The removal of white cells and platelets in the manufacture of these concentrates virtually eliminates transfusion reactions. The convenience of storage, safety and ease of administration, and standardization of the product have made these concentrates highly acceptable to both physician and patient.

The disadvantages arise from the pooling of the starting plasma. Hepatitis continues to be a problem, although all products and most donors are now tested by third-generation tests, usually radioimmunoassay, for the hepatitis B surface antigen (HB_SAg).[222] Approximately 60% to 80% of plasmas infected with hepatitis B are detected. However, 20% to 40% are not, nor are those in-

Table 25-4. Factor VIII products

	Factor VIII (units/ml)	Dosage (ml)	Fibrinogen (mg/ factor VIII unit)
Cryoprecipitate	5-10	10-15	1.9
Concentrates			
Profilate (Abbott)	12	25-50	0.6.0.8
Factorate (Armour)	10	25-30	0.6-0.9
Koate (Cutter)	22-33	10, 20, 40	0.5-1.0
Hemofil (Hyland)	25	10-30	0.3
Humafac (Parke-Davis)	13-40	6	1.1
Lyoc (New York Blood Center)	4-6	30	4.5
Actif VIII (Merrieux)	10-15	25-50	1.2

fected with the other viral agents that may cause hepatitis, e.g., hepatitis A, E, or "non A–non B." A second disadvantage arises from the fact that significant titers of A and B isoagglutinins may be present and may cause hemolytic anemia in a patient with red cell type A, B, or AB.[255,277,278] Another disadvantage is the cost of the manufacturing procedure since it is closely tied to the cost and availability of plasma. Currently the prices of concentrates are the same as cryoprecipitate in some but not all areas, and cost may be an important consideration in the choice of product for therapy.

The lyophilized concentrates of factors II, VII, IX, and X (prothrombin complex) are marketed primarily for treatment of factor IX deficiency but can be used for bleeding episodes in patients with acquired or congenital deficiencies of factors II, VII, and X.[201,290] The relative amounts of the individual factors found in these concentrates are listed in Table 25-3. Again, the advantages of these concentrates include standardization, storage at 4° C, easy reconstitution with sterile water, and ease of administration with syringe. The disadvantages include a greater concentration of the hepatitis antigen (HbₛAg) than found in factor VIII products with a concomitantly higher incidence of hepatitis associated with their use and increased amounts of thrombogenic material.[244,305] Although the manufacturing procedures are different for the two products available in the United States, these products and those made with the same procedure in other parts of the world contain variable amounts of activated factors IX and X (IXa and Xa).

It has been suggested therefore that these products be administered with great caution in those patients with preexisting liver disease or vascular disease for long-term replacement therapy.[244]

Whole blood is not a product of choice for any hemophilic bleeding episode, and it is unnecessary for anemia. Packed red cells should be used as necessary for anemia.

CALCULATION FOR REPLACEMENT THERAPY. The dosage required to replace a factor deficiency is calculated on the basis of the patient's weight, the assumed plasma volume, and the severity of the bleeding episode. It is convenient to consider the administration of clotting factor in terms of international units per measure of body weight. By definition, 1 international unit of factor VIII or IX is that amount of clotting activity found in 1 ml of fresh normal pooled plasma and 1 international unit is equal to 100% clotting factor activity. For simplified calculations and assuming passage into the extracellular fluid, 1 unit of factor VIII/kg of body weight will raise the patient's plasma level 2%. One unit of factor IX/kg body weight will raise the patient's plasma level 1½%. The difference in plasma level attained is related to the greater amount of factor IX that goes into the extravascular space and may be related to molecular size.[201]

The subsequent dosage is based on the desired plasma level, severity of the bleeding episode, utilization of the infused factor, half-disappearance time and biological half-disappearance time of the infused factor, as well as the length of time desired for replacement therapy. Table 25-5 lists the first half-disappearance time related to diffusion rate or equilibration rate between the intravascular and extravascular spaces and the second half-disappearance time related to the biologic half-life of the clotting factors in nonbleeding patients. For example, the initial half-disappearance time of factor VIII is 4 to 8 hours, while the biologic half-life is 12 to 15 hours.

Previous work has shown that 20% of factors VIII and IX is necessary for hemostasis when therapy is given in a single infusion. For control of acute hemarthrosis a plasma level of 40% to 50% will achieve hemostasis and, allowing for natural decay, still provide some additional replacement coverage for at least 24 hours.[139] This can be given as outpatient therapy and repeated in 48 hours if bleeding is not controlled. Such therapy is ade-

Table 25-5. Half-times of plasma coagulation factors

Factor	First T½ (hr) (diffusion)	Second T½ (hr) (biologic)
Fibrinogen (I)	24-48	80-120
Prothrombin (II)	8	60-100
V	?	12-36
VII	0.5	2-5
VIII (classical hemophilia)	4-8	12-15
VIII (von Willebrand's disease)		
VIII:C	?	29-48*[168]
VIIIR:Ag	?	14-37*[168]
VIIIR:WF (ristocetin cofactor)	?	<8-18*[168]
IX	3-8	18-24
X	2-9	27-31
XI	?	24-48
XIII	?	120-160

*The lower values are results with commercial factor VIII concentrates; the higher values, results with cryoprecipitate.

quate for large bleeding episodes, particularly if the episode has progressed for 6 to 8 hours before therapy is given. Experience suggests that one-half to one-third this amount of therapy may be sufficient for good healing (when therapy is given within 4 hours of onset of a bleeding episode, as on a home care program). Use of adjuvant measures such as ice and an elastic (Ace) bandage continue to be quite useful.[294] Immobilization of a weight-bearing joint for 24 hours is occasionally necessary. When the lyophilized products are used, dosage may be calculated to the nearest vial, using the assayed amount printed on the manufacturer's label. If bags of cryoprecipitate are used, dosage should be calculated using 100 units of factor VIII per bag as the average content.

TREATMENT REGIMENS (TABLE 25-6). The variability of the disease in the patient, the severity of the bleeding episode, and the state of the tissue area in which the bleeding episode occurs determine the treatment regimen. The cost and availability of materials are also determining factors in therapy. The proposed schedule in Table 25-6 is therefore presented as a guide. Dosages are given in amounts that may be administered slowly by syringe or drip unless otherwise stated. Concentrates should be given at a rate of 10 ml/5 minutes. Fresh frozen plasma should be given as quickly as possible.

Hematomas, or hemorrhages under the skin and within muscles, can frequently be controlled by elastic (Ace) bandage pressure and ice. Those that cannot be controlled easily within a few hours and may cause muscle contraction require replacement therapy. Bleeding in certain muscle groups such as

those in the posterior leg, the soleus and gastrocnemius, should be treated early to avoid contraction and scarring that are difficult to rehabilitate. When replacement therapy is necessary, 10 to 20 units/kg given one time should suffice for either classical hemophilia or Christmas disease. Christmas disease can frequently be treated with the lower amount, and fresh frozen plasma may be sufficient to deliver this small amount. Patients with von Willebrand's disease can usually be treated as mild hemophiliacs with the lesser amount of concentrate. Hematomas are considered minor bleeding episodes and are relatively easily controlled.

Hematuria caused by a bleeding diathesis is usually renal in origin and must be differentiated from nephritis. Although disconcerting to the patient, it is rarely the cause of severe difficulty. Pain in the flank area often accompanies clotting in the renal pelvis and signals cessation of gross hematuria. Current treatment includes steroids and factor replacement. Abildgaard et al.[141] reported the effectiveness of steroid administration for 48 hours at the onset of hematuria. However, no benefit from prednisone therapy could be demonstrated in a recent study by Rizza et al.[271] In any event, replacement therapy is occasionally needed. EACA is contraindicated because of protracted renal dysfunction that follows clot formation with EACA on the fibrinogen strands and subsequent lack of clot lysis.[196] Hematuria without trauma is uncommon in other than congenital deficiencies of factor VIII and IX. Hospital admission for replacement therapy may be necessary.

Hemarthrosis occurs only in severe hemophilia and almost never in von Willebrand's disease. Trauma may be followed by hemarthrosis in all grades of the disease, the milder forms as well as the deficiencies of factors X and XI. When synovial changes occur, bleeding may occur without provocation. Table 25-6 details the replacement therapy. Replacement therapy should be given as soon as the patient knows the bleeding has begun, when stiffness or a subjective feeling occurs. Repeat doses may be necessary in 24 to 48 hours if the bleeding is severe or the joint has a chronic arthropathy, but they are not usually required. However, the need for repeat doses should alert the physician to other problems. A nonhealing synovitis requiring short-term prophylaxis, the development of an inhibitor, or an incorrect dosage should be suspected. Bleeding into elbows and wrists may usually be considered minor bleeding episodes and may be treated with smaller amounts of concentrate than when the weight-bearing joints, ankles, knees, and hips, are involved. The latter should always be considered as major episodes and treated with somewhat larger amounts

Table 25-6. Schedules for treatment of bleeding episodes

Type of bleeding	Classical hemophilia	Christmas disease	von Willebrand's disease
Hematoma	Cryoprecipitate, 2 bags/10 kg, or factor VIII concentrate, 20 units/kg Ice, Ace bandage	Fresh frozen plasma, 10 ml/kg Factor IX concentrate, 10 units/kg Ice, Ace bandage	Fresh frozen plasma, 10 ml/kg Cryoprecipitate, 2 bags/ 10 kg Factor VIII concentrate, 10 units/kg Ice, Ace bandage
Hematuria	Steroids, 2 mg/kg, not to exceed 60 mg/day, for 2 days If no visible improvement, start replacement therapy Factor VIII concentrate, 20 units/kg Cryoprecipitate, 4 bags/10 kg for 5 days, or factor VIII concentrate, 40 units/kg for 3-5 days	Factor IX concentrate, 40 units/kg/day for 3 days Steroids, 2 mg/kg, not to exceed 60 mg/day, for 2 days	Steroids, 2 mg/kg for 2 days Fresh frozen plasma, 10 ml/kg q12h for 3 days Cryoprecipitate, 2 bags/10 kg q12h for 3 days Factor VIII concentrate, 10 units/kg q12h for 3 days
Hemarthrosis	Cryoprecipitate, 3-4 bags/10 kg, or factor VIII concentrate, 25-30 units/kg Repeat following day if joint is still painful Prednisone, 2 mg/kg/day for 3 days Consult orthopedist for aspiration if skin is shiny over joint and bleeding extensive or if problem lasts over 1 wk	Factor IX concentrate, 20 units/kg Prednisone, 2 mg/kg/day for 3 days Consult orthopedist for aspiration if skin is shiny over joint and bleeding extensive or if problem lasts over 1 wk	Fresh frozen plasma, 5-10 ml/kg Cryoprecipitate, 2 bags/10 kg Factor VIII concentrate, 10 units/kg
Mucous membrane Mouth	Cryoprecipitate, 6 bags/10 kg once, or factor VIII concentrate, 40 units/kg once EACA, 100 mg/kg q6h for 6 days	Factor IX concentrate, 30 units/kg once EACA, 100 mg/kg q6h for 6 days	Fresh frozen plasma, 20 ml/kg Factor VIII concentrate, 20 units /kg once EACA, 100 mg/kg q6h for 6 days
Deciduous teeth	Should be seen by M.D. If tooth is loose, extract and give replacement therapy Factor VIII concentrate, 40 units/kg once	Should be seen by M.D. If tooth is loose, extract and give replacement therapy Factor IX concentrate, 30 units/kg once	Should be seen by M.D. If tooth is loose, extract and give replacement therapy as for mouth bleeding
Epistaxis	Bilateral pressure on nose for 30 min Pack with epinephrine-soaked Surgicel or Avitene Replacement therapy as for mouth bleeding EACA, 100 mg/kg q6h for 6 days	Same as for classical hemophilia with factor IX instead of factor VIII for replacement therapy	Same as for classical hemophilia except for replacement therapy Replacement therapy as for mouth bleeding
Gastrointestinal	Cryoprecipitate, 6 bags/kg q12h for 3 days, or factor VIII concentrate, 40 units/kg/3 days or for 3 days after bleeding subsides	Factor IX concentrate, 40 units/kg/3 days or for 3 days after bleeding subsides	Fresh frozen plasma, 10 ml/kg q8h for 3 days Cryoprecipitate, 2 bags/10 kg q8h for 3 days Factor VIII concentrate, 10 units/kg q12h for 3 days
Hazardous areas Central nervous system	Cryoprecipitate, 6 bags/10 kg q12h; or factor VIII concentrate, 40 units/kg q12h for first 6 days	Factor IX concentrate, 40 units/kg q12h for 6 days	Fresh frozen plasma, 10 ml/kg q8h for 3 days Cryoprecipitate, 3 bags/10 kg q8h for 3 days

Table 25-6. Schedules for treatment of bleeding episodes — cont'd

Type of bleeding	Classical hemophilia	Christmas disease	von Willebrand's disease
	Cryoprecipitate, 6 bags/10 kg/ day, or factor VIII concentrate, 40 units/kg/day for next 8 days (minimum) Total 14 days of therapy		Factor VIII concentrate, 15 units/kg q8h for 5-8 days
Retropharyngeal	Cryoprecipitate, 6 bags/10 kg, or factor VIII concentrate, 40 units/kg q12h for 4 days	Factor IX concentrate, 40 units/kg q12h for 4 days	Same as for classical hemophilia
Retroperitoneal	Cryoprecipitate, 6 bags/10 kg, or factor VIII concentrate, 40 units/kg q12h for 6 days	Factor IX concentrate, 40 units/kg q12h for 6 days	Same as for classical hemophilia

of concentrate. The use of steroids has been advocated as an anti-inflammatory agent and used with the replacement therapy at the onset of a hemarthrosis.[197,221] Their major effect occurs in those joints in which synovial hypertrophy and synovitis have developed. Shoulder bleeding is rare without provocation and should be treated as a major bleeding episode. Both hip and shoulder hemarthrosis may be deceiving because of the size of the joint into which several deciliters may have bled before symptoms are apparent. Intensive early replacement therapy for bleeding episodes can prevent progression of chronic arthropathy in 80% to 85% of patients in home care programs.[198,229] Brachmann et al.[161] report no arthropathy in his patients on continual prophylaxis three times weekly up to adolescence.

When acute hemarthrosis occurs more than twice in a single joint, initiating the changes of chronic synovitis, short-term prophylaxis with 20 units of factor VIII or IX/kg three times weekly for 4 to 6 weeks and prednisone, 2 mg/kg daily for 1 to 2 weeks, may be necessary. Extensive physical therapy should be carried out with this replacement therapy to prevent further muscular debilitation.[158,175] Occasionally temporary splinting may be necessary to prevent flexion deformities. Long-term bracing is rarely used with current medical therapy. However, it may be required for the chronic arthritis of an adult. Reconstructive surgery with arthroplasty of the hip and knees has been encouraging for adults with painful end-stage arthritis.[151,177]

Ice and Ace bandages are often helpful for hemarthrosis. Additional support to the ankle may be given with firm lace boots. Should a bleeding episode progress sufficiently to cause severe distention of the joint, making the overlying skin tense and shiny, aspiration of the blood may be necessary. Replacement therapy should be given just before the procedure and a firm Ace bandage applied afterwards. Some orthopedists advocate aspiration for all large hemorrhages, but with the institution of replacement therapy within 4 to 8 hours after the onset of bleeding this procedure is usually not necessary.

Peripheral nerve bleeding is not uncommon in severe hemophilia. It is difficult to diagnose and extremely painful. External swelling or tenderness is not seen. Signs of nerve pressure and irritation such as numbness, tingling, and paresis may be the only objective findings. Pain may persist in spite of adequate replacement therapy for a week or more, and paresis for up to 6 months. In the interim, flaccid muscles should be given electrical stimulation and passive exercise to maintain muscle tone. Femoral nerve palsies and ulnar nerve palsies are the most common.

Hazardous bleeding areas include the central nervous system and retropharyngeal and retroperitoneal tissues and are the only bleeding sites requiring mandatory admission for observation and therapy. Bleeding in the first two may be lethal if not treated adequately as may the third, but less rapidly.

Any head injury should be treated as a potential bleeding episode. The extent of therapy depends on the severity of the injury and the objective findings. A severe headache or a headache lasting for more than 12 hours suggests an episode of bleeding in the central nervous system. Clinical evaluation of head trauma in a child is difficult even when the child is observed. For any child with loss of consciousness, vomiting, lethargy, seizures, or weakness even though transient, therapy should be instituted immediately and the physician notified. If a hematoma or laceration occurs, the same procedure should be instituted. In the absence of trauma, any symptoms suggesting intracranial pressure or a headache of more than 12 hours' duration should be treated and followed closely. Any child under the age of 8 to 10 years with mild disease should be treated prophylactically for any injury regardless of how small, because of the unreliability of the history. *The consequence of untreated intracranial bleeding can be so severe that there is no reason to withhold prophylactic treatment today for any patient with a headache or history of trauma.* A documented bleeding episode should be treated for a minimum of 14 days. Children with an uncertain history should be observed and treated prophylactically for 3 days.

Retropharyngeal bleeding frequently accompanies a pharyngitis and should be suspected when a patient complains that he cannot swallow his saliva. With such a complaint, a lateral x-ray film of the neck helps to determine the presence of a retropharyngeal mass and the extent of airway obstruction. With adequate replacement therapy tracheostomy should not be necessary.

Retroperitoneal bleeding presents as lower abdominal pain and iliopsoas muscle irritation and/or contraction. On the right side this may be mistaken for appendicitis. Therefore a dose of replacement material should always be given before a surgeon is called. Replacement therapy for 3 or 4 days usually suffices, but more may be needed. Should any of these bleeding manifestations require operative intervention, the surgeon should be reassured that hemostasis will be as good as in a "normal" patient or one without a known coagulation problem. Normal plasma levels can be maintained as long as necessary and the surgery should be that done for any patient with the same symptom. The surgeon must, however, be meticulous about clamping and ligating as many small vessels as possible. Clamping and cutting between the clamps for delineation of planes is better than blunt dissection, and excessive cauterization is unwise.

Mucous membrane bleeding in the mouth as a result of trauma can be controlled with one dose of replacement therapy and EACA for patients older than 1 year. For younger patients replacement therapy for 4 to 5 days with 25 to 30 units/kg of factor twice daily should suffice.

Exfoliating teeth should be extracted when they become loose and are sitting in the soft tissue. Once they have moved out of the bone, the rough edges may cause oozing that can be controlled with EACA, but bleeding begins again when the drug is withdrawn. One dose of replacement therapy plus EACA usually controls the bleeding with extraction.

Epistaxis is rare in those with normal platelet function and hemophiliacs but common with von Willebrand's disease. Pressure for 30 minutes and packing with Surgicel or Avitene with a pressure pack is usually sufficient. Occasionally a dose of replacement therapy is necessary.

Gastrointestinal bleeding is uncommon but may be an aggravating cause of prolonged bleeding. Therapy should be given for a minimum of 3 days.

Elective surgery is now commonplace for patients with a congenital or acquired clotting factor deficiency and may be undertaken whenever necessary to provide the best medical care to the patient. Certain mandatory prerequisites must be followed to assure a smooth outcome. The laboratory tests listed should be done to confirm the clotting deficiency and to provide for a stockpiling of adequate amounts of clotting factors. An incubated test for inhibitor is necessary to detect a low-titer inhibitor whose anamnestic response might create a postsurgical hazard. The presence of such an antibody is a contraindication to an elective procedure. However, surgical procedures have been done in patients with inhibitors. (See discussion of inhibitors.)

Guidelines for replacement therapy before and after elective surgery

A. Prior to procedure
  1. Complete coagulation work-up.
  2. Conduct incubated test for inhibitors.
  3. Calculate needs and stock-pile therapeutic material in hospital.
  4. Do survival study for recovery of half-life of therapeutic material.
  5. Obtain complete blood count, platelet count, and reticulocyte count.
  6. Determine red cell type.
B. General surgical procedure
  1. Minor
    a. Give dose calculated to bring patient's plasma level to 100% 1 hour prior to procedure (50 units/kg).
    b. Maintain plasma level above 60% for 4 days.
    c. Maintain plasma level above 20% for subsequent 4 days.
    d. Assay daily prior to administration.
  2. Major
    a. Give dose calculated to bring patient's plasma level to 100% 1 hour prior to procedure (50 units/kg).
    b. Maintain plasma level above 60% for 4 days.
    c. Maintain plasma level above 40% for subsequent 4 days or until all drains and sutures are removed.
    d. Assay daily prior to administration.
C. Orthopedic procedure
  1. Give dose calculated to bring patient's plasma level to 100% 1 hour prior to procedure (50 units/kg).
  2. Maintain plasma level above 80% for 4 days (40 units/kg three times daily).
  3. Assay daily prior to administration.
  4. Maintain plasma level above 40% for subsequent 4 days (40 units/kg twice daily).

5. If patient is in cast, discontinue replacement until rehabilitation program.
6. If patient is not in cast, maintain plasma level above 20% for ambulation.
7. For rehabilitation program maintain plasma level above 10% for 3 weeks.

D. Dental procedure
1. Give EACA 100 mg/kg 4 hours before surgery.
2. Give dose calculated to bring patient's plasma level to 100% 1 hour prior to procedure.
3. Continue EACA 100 mg/kg every 6 hours for 7 days.
4. Repeat replacement therapy in 3 days if procedure is extensive.

Although this outline has been divided into major and minor procedures, it is more accurate to say that a surgical procedure is never minor in a hemophiliac and should not be undertaken lightly. The differentiation of the groups lies in the extent of replacement material necessary for fibroblast growth and good scar formation. Orthopedic procedures require more replacement when raw bone surfaces must heal or when a small amount of postoperative bleeding cannot be tolerated. For

example, a small amount of bleeding into or around a prosthetic knee or hip may lead to infection and destruction of the surrounding tissues. On the other hand, when an extremity or operative site is held firm in plaster, or when good surgical apposition of tissues can be achieved with sutures, less extensive replacement therapy is required. Dosages are given broadly and can only be maintained with the assistance of good laboratory support and daily assays of the patient's plasma.

At the University of North Carolina all major surgical procedures in children as well as adults with classical hemophilia are currently being managed with continuous infusion of factor VIII concentrates. It has been observed that this mode of therapy is capable of maintaining a steady level of factor VIII instead of the fluctuating levels characteristic of intermittent therapy.[242] Factor VIII activity is stable in concentrates at room temperature for as long as 24 hours, although infusates are generally renewed every 12 hours. There is a linear relationship between the factor VIII dosage rate and resulting factor VIII activity; 1 factor VIII unit/kg/hour yields a steady level of about 25%. Thus, if it is desired to maintain a steady factor

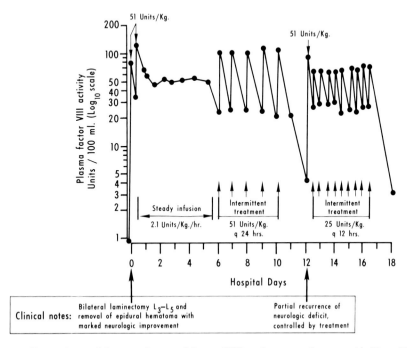

Patient E, Wt. 41 Kg.

Diagnosis: Spinal epidural hematoma

Fig. 25-10. Comparison of three regimens of factor VIII replacement therapy with Hemofil, each totalling 50 to 51 factor VIII units/kg/day, following bilateral laminectomies for removal of epidural hematoma. (From McMillan, C. W., Webster, W. P., Roberts, H. R., et al.: Br. J. Haematol. **18:**659, 1970.)

VIII level of 50% activity, concentrate is continuously infused at 2 units/kg/hour and adjusted as needed. The concentrate is diluted in sterile physiologic saline appropriate for a desired volume and rate of infusion. The length of such treatment for given surgical procedures is the same as that described above for intermittent schedules. A comparison of the effects of continuous and intermittent infusion of factor VIII is shown in Fig. 25-10.

Dental care should formally begin at 3 years of age. For prophylactic care the child with hemophilia should be taught adequate tooth brushing and care of the gums. Fluoride treatments should be given routinely. When restorative work is necessary, hypnosis can be used for relief of fear and anxiety[232] and local analgesia with replacement therapy.[179] Extractions and other surgical procedures can be performed with replacement therapy for 1 day and EACA for 7 days (Table 25-6). The same presurgical screening procedures should be carried out as listed on p. 786. Replacement therapy sufficient to bring the plasma level to near normal should be given once and repeated on the third postoperative day if the procedure has been extensive. The newer hemostatic agents, Ativene and Surgicel, have been useful in packing the sockets. Dental appliances for orthodontics can be used without undue fear of bleeding, with the expected amount of gum or mucous membrane irritation.[251] Hospital admission may be necessary for extensive surgical procedures, but the majority of the care can be given in an outpatient setting.

Adjuvant drug therapy includes analgesics, anti-inflammatory agents, and anti-fibrinolytic agents.

Analgesics have always been an important part of therapy for all hemophiliacs, and although they are not as important now that early replacement transfusions are advocated, it is imperative that the physician know the effect of these drugs on the clotting mechanism. It is not in the patient's best interest to produce a secondary bleeding diathesis.

An ever-increasing list of analgesics contains aspirin and antihistamines, which are known to inhibit platelet aggregation and prolong the bleeding time. Patients should be cautioned against the use of any medication containing aspirin compound and several drugs listed in Table 24-8; propoxyphene (Darvon), acetaminophen (Tylenol), pentazocine (Talwin), codeine, or methadone may be used as alternatives.

The most widely used and best of the anti-inflammatory drugs are the corticosteroids. They have been used in a dose of 1 to 2 mg/kg/day for hematuria and for 48 hours in acute hemarthrosis and chronic synovitis, as already mentioned. Side effects have not been noted for these short courses of therapy. Indomethacin (Indocin) or phenylbutazone (Butazolidine), although excellent drugs for arthritic discomfort, are potentially harmful for the hemophiliac because of inhibition of platelet function caused by these agents; they should be used only with caution. Indomethacin, 25 mg twice daily, is often of great value nonetheless for the patient with severe arthritis. Ibuprofen (Motrin), a known prostaglandin inhibitor with potential in vitro effect, the newest of the drugs used for arthritic pain, may have potential use.

EACA and tranexamic acid (Cyklokapron, AMCA) are antifibrinolytic agents whose action of inhibiting plasminogen activity has been used for a variety of bleeding episodes. They have been used in large-scale trials to prevent spontaneous bleeding and for dental extractions both in Europe and in this country. The results have been singularly unimpressive when EACA was used to prevent joint hemorrhages but quite useful for dental extractions and other mouth bleeding episodes. The study by Walsh et al.[299] showed that multiple teeth could be extracted with one dose of replacement factor and EACA in a dosage of 100 mg/kg every 6 hours for 6 to 7 days. The drug inhibits the plasminogen in the saliva and thereby exerts its activity. A recent study claims a significant reduction in spontaneous bleeding episodes with the use of transexamic acid.[267] The specific prevention of hemarthrosis is not well substantiated.

EACA has not been advocated in the treatment of hemarthrosis since a clot formed with EACA absorbed to the fibrin strands may not dissolve for many months and may contribute to fibrosis and further joint destruction. It has been used with aprotinin (Trasylol), another antifibrinolytic drug, at the time of synovectomy[287] with 24 hours of replacement therapy. Although the results reported a 66% decrease in hemarthrosis, 42% of the patients have no improvement or decreased joint function. Intra-articular fibrosis caused by EACA may contribute to this poor result. However, control studies have not been carried out to either support or discredit this use of EACA.

The methods by which these therapies are given have radically changed with the development of concentrates for therapy. Inpatient therapy is no longer necessary for the majority of bleeding episodes with the exception of bleeding in the central nervous system or retroperitoneal or retropharyngeal areas. All other episodes may be treated in an outpatient facility or, for those patients or family units who qualify for self-transfusion, in a home care program.

Home care programs in which patients or their family members give transfusions of replacement factors away from the hospital were first introduced by Rabiner and Telfer[266] in 1970. Other programs developed in the larger treatment centers with guidelines established by the medical board of the National Hemophilia Foundation.[229,294] Current standards consider home transfusion therapy to be one mode of delivery of replacement therapy within a comprehensive care program. Acceptance of this mode of health care has increased from approximately 10% of the surveyed hemophilic population by the NIH study in 1971 to 36% of all registered hemophiliacs in the recent Pennsylvania report.[282] However, home care programs are not practical for some patients. To qualify for these programs the patient and family members must be free of psychiatric illness, willing to accept some of the responsibility for the patient's medical care, and thoroughly schooled about the disease and its treatment. The patient should be over 4 years of age with a laboratory-proved diagnosis of hemophilia and without an inhibitor. (However, some patients with some types of inhibitors are currently being managed on home care programs.) Mandatory routine follow-up examinations every 3 to 6 months are necessary to maintain good medical care, with the frequency determined by the severity of disease in the patient. Complete patient education concerning the current concept of early treatment, attention to product usage, mechanics of transfusion, complications of therapy, easy access to medical assistance, and in-depth comprehensive follow-up examinations has brought about a remarkable improvement in joint status, school and job attendance, and ultimate functioning of the hemophiliac.[198,229] However, an increased usage of replacement transfusions has come with administration and a greater awareness of its complications. The reader is referred to reports by Rabiner and Telfer,[266] Lazerson,[224] and Levine.[229]

COMPLICATIONS OF THERAPY. The severely affected hemophiliac now uses between 45,000 and 50,000 of concentrate yearly; some use more than 100,000 units of concentrate yearly; some use more than 100,000 units yearly.[229,282] The complications of transfusions of this amount of pooled plasma product are numerous.

Liver function abnormalities may develop. Greater than 50% of patients have persistently elevated levels of SGOT and SGPT, regardless of the product used (either dried concentrate or cryoprecipitate in this country), with somewhat lower enzyme elevations in patients receiving cryoprecipitate in England.* Chronic active disease and acute cirrhosis determined by biopsy are present in 2% to 3%, and splenomegaly in 30%. The incidence of hepatitis B is about 3% per year,

although approximately 80% of the patients have hepatitis B surface antibody.[228] The cause of this high incidence is unclear and the clinical significance remains unknown. Whether the abnormal chemistries are the result of repeated viral infections or to antigen-antibody complex disease is unclear.

Inhibitors were reported in 5% to 20% of patients with hemophilia by Shapiro and Hultin[283] and currently in 14% of 1,200 patients enrolled in a cooperative study of factor VIII inhibitors in classical hemophilia. (See p. 810.)

Significant amounts of *anti-A and anti-B red blood cell isoagglutinins* are concentrated with the factor VIII and cannot be removed in the manufacturing process.[278] This can lead to a Coombs-positive hemolytic anemia in the recipient with type A, B, or AB red cells. The entity resolves when the factor VIII is no longer given but may require steroid therapy while the concentrate is given.

Acute pulmonary problems have been reported with the use of cryoprecipitate because of white blood cell antigens.[268]

Thrombotic episodes have been reported[305] when prothrombin complex concentrates are given to patients with liver dysfunction. The thrombogenic material in the concentrates is thought to be IX_a and X_a. The International Committee on Thrombosis and Hemostasis has recommended the use of an additional 5 units heparin/ml concentrate given when those concentrates are used for high-dose long-term therapy, as for a surgical procedure. It is still recognized that these concentrates are useful and not harmful for the treatment of acute bleeding episodes of the patient with factor IX deficiency.[244]

A *secondary bleeding diathesis* may occur in some patients during intensive replacement therapy with factor VIII concentrates.[192] The disorder is characterized in vitro by defective platelet aggregation and variable prolongation of the TGT, PT, and PTT[152] attributed to effects of either hyperfibrinogenemia or increased circulating levels of fibrinogen degradation products.

Nonspecific febrile and allergic reactions may complicate therapy but are less common with commercial concentrates than with blood bank products.

Two other problems described in persons with hemophilia may or may not be related to effects of replacement therapy.

1. *Hypertension* has been reported by Weisz and Kasper[304] to be significantly increased in persons with hemophilia with onset at 15 years of age. The combined data show that among 159 adult patients, 13.8% had definite and 19.5% had borderline hypertension. The relative contributions of

---

*References 146, 200, 230, 235.

replacement therapy and hemophilia itself to such hypertension are presently unknown.

2. *Renal disease,* appearing as episodic hematuria, begins at 5 years of age and increases with age, with an incidence of approximately 67% in adults.[225,264] Lazerson has found decreased levels of serum complement in patients with a history of hematuria following transfusions of cryoprecipitate and suggests renal injury secondary to immune complex disease. This hypothesis is not established at the present time.

Prognosis. The outlook for the patient with hemophilia is far more hopeful now than in previous years. Although the ultimate impact of improved replacement therapy on longevity has not been established, programs of comprehensive care and home treatment have improved attendance at school and work and should increasingly improve vocational opportunities, psychosocial difficulties, and overall physical capabilities. However, a variety of complications that may attend increased therapy will have to be evaluated closely in the years ahead.[227]

von Willebrand's disease

von Willebrand's disease (VWD, vascular hemophilia, pseudohemophilia) is a highly variable bleeding disorder typically characterized by autosomal dominant expression of platelet dysfunction and factor VIII deficiency. The manifestations of platelet dysfunction consist of a prolonged bleeding time, decreased retention of platelets by glass beads, and decreased ristocetin-induced platelet aggregation. Factor VIII deficiency is typically characterized by corresponding decreases in plasma factor VIII coagulant activity (VIII:C) and factor VIII–related antigen (VIIIR:Ag).

Current evidence indicates that platelet dysfunction in von Willebrand's disease is a result not of an intrinsic platelet defect but rather of a lack of a factor VIII–related principle in plasma known as von Willebrand factor (VIIIR:WF), which is believed to facilitate platelet adhesion in the initial phase of hemostasis. Activity of VIIIR:WF is usually designated by ristocetin cofactor activity, but it is also presumed to be related to the bleeding time and retention of platelets by glass beads.

Historical perspective. The disorder was first described in a young girl and her extended family on the Åland Islands in the Gulf of Bothnia by von Willebrand[296,297] in 1926 and 1931 and reported independently by Minot[248] in 1928 in another family. The original description of the disorder, termed pseudohemophilia by von Willebrand, included autosomal inheritance, mucous membrane bleeding, and a prolonged bleeding time with a normal platelet count, coagulation time, and clot retraction. The disorder was considered to be a thrombocytopathy by von Wille-

brand and Jürgens[298] and continued to be regarded as "a disturbance of platelet function and alteration in the capillary," as originally described by von Willebrand. Macfarlane[234] described bizarre nail bed capillaries in patients with pseudohemophilia.

In 1953 decreased plasma factor VIII activity in this disorder was described independently by Alexander and Goldstein,[147] Larrieu and Soulier,[223] and Quick and Hussey.[265] In 1956 Schulman et al.[274] put together decreased factor VIII levels and capillary abnormalities and termed the disorder vascular hemophilia. The significance of the morphologic abnormality of the capillaries remained obscure, since this was not found in all patients with the disease and was found in patients lacking other characteristic abnormalities. However, Quick continued to believe that the defect was localized in the mechanism that controls the tonus of the microcirculation. In 1957 Jurgens et al.[216] reexamined the original Åland family members and found factor VIII deficiency in those patients as well. Within the past decade the disorder has been increasingly termed von Willebrand's disease, a designation that not only is historically fitting but also implies no assumptions about this complex disease.

In the late 1950s Nilsson et al.[254] found that Blomback fraction I-0 from normal plasma (derived fron Cohn's fraction I) corrected both the factor VIII deficiency and the bleeding time abnormality in von Willebrand's disease and furthermore that this fraction from patients with classical hemophilia was similarly corrective in von Willebrand's disease. The term "von Willebrand factor" was given to the principle in plasma that corrected the bleeding time. These landmark studies and those of others[169] also showed that transfusion of a patient with von Willebrand's disease with either normal plasma or plasma from a patient with classical hemophilia resulted in a prolonged or secondary rise in factor VIII activity between 5 and 24 hours with a subsequent fall that was slower than expected. The half-time of factor VIII activity in these instances was about 40 hours in contrast to the half-time of 12 hours after replacement therapy of patients with classical hemophilia. Infusion of plasma from patients with von Willebrand's disease into patients with classical hemophilia did not result in a rise of factor VIII activity.

Thus the differences between von Willebrand's disease and classic hemophilia became more obvious: the genetic transmission, the bleeding time, and then the response to plasma infusion suggesting stimulation of new synthesis of factor VIII— even by infusions lacking factor VIII coagulant activity.

The next step occurred when Hellem[194] and

Table 25-7. Differentiation of von Willebrand's disease and classical hemophilia

	Bleeding time	Platelet adhesion to glass beads	Platelet aggregation with ristocetin	Factor VIII activity	Factor VIII antigen
Classical hemophilia	Normal	Normal	Normal	Low	High
"Classical" von Wille-brand's disease	Prolonged	Abnormal	Abnormal	Low	Low
Variant I	Prolonged	Abnormal	Normal	Normal	Normal
Variant II	Normal	Normal	Normal	Low	Normal
Variant III	Prolonged	Abnormal	Abnormal	Normal	Low
Variant IV	Prolonged	Abnormal	Abnormal	Low	Normal
Variant V	Normal	Normal	Normal	Low	Low

Borchgrevinck et al.[159] reported poor platelet adhesiveness as well as an abnormal bleeding time in von Willebrand's disease. Then in 1971 another platelet abnormality was described by Howard and Firkin,[204] who reported that the antibiotic ristocetin failed to aggregate platelets normally in platelet-rich plasma from patients with von Willebrand's disease. Abnormal ristocetin-induced platelet aggregation has also been consistently observed in the Bernard-Soulier syndrome, in which the platelet itself is defective, in contrast to the variable deficiency in von Willebrand's disease of a factor VIII–related ristocetin cofactor.[205,303]

Using immunologic techniques Hoyer and Breckenridge[209] and Zimmerman et al.[312] discovered that patients with von Willebrand's disease variably lacked a factor VIII–related antigen that was detected by either a human (homologous) or an animal (heterologous) antibody to factor VIII. Furthermore, deficiencies of factor VIII–related antigen and factor VIII activity were usually proportional in plasma in von Willebrand's disease, whereas factor VIII activity alone was deficient in the plasma of classical hemophilia.

Although this succession of major discoveries about von Willebrand's disease contributed immensely to increased understanding of this disease and of the molecular abnormalities of factor VIII that appear to produce it, at the present time both the molecular and the clinical parts of the puzzle of von Willebrand's disease remain incompletely assembled.

Classification. Because of the marked variability in the clinical expression and laboratory characteristics of von Willebrand's disease, a generally accepted method of classification is not yet available. On the other hand, separation of von Willebrand's disease into "classical" and "variant" forms on the basis of selected laboratory findings may prove to be a useful as well as objective approach to classification (Table 25-7).

Incidence. The true incidence of von Willebrand's disease is unknown. Its observed prevalence is 5 to 10 × 10^{-6} and, in most centers, ranks third in frequency after classical hemophilia and Christmas disease.[238,308] However, some workers think that von Willebrand's disease, including its variants, may be the most common of all heritable deficiencies of coagulation.[233]

Etiology. von Willebrand's disease is the expression of an inherited, poorly understood defect in biosynthesis of the factor VIII molecular complex. Rarely the disorder may be acquired by previously well persons or patients with an underlying disease.[283] The causal relation of an immune inhibitor directed at appropriate functional sites of the factor VIII molecular complex in these instances is suspected but not yet established.

Genetics. It is clear that von Willebrand's disease is transmitted as an autosomal phenotype and is clinically expressed in heterozygotes. However, the heterogeniety of this disorder remains poorly understood and awaits more knowledge about the factor VIII molecule and genetic control of its biosynthesis.

Clinical features. von Willebrand's disease is characterized by a variable mucocutaneous bleeding tendency. Major expressions of the disease include epistaxis, bleeding from the gums, superficial bruises, and prolonged oozing from minor wounds. Menorrhagia is a major manifestation in women. Hematuria is not rare. Hemarthrosis is rare but may occur in patients with very low plasma factor VIII activity, usually below 1%.

Laboratory evaluation. Diagnosis depends on measurement of plasma factor VIII activity, factor VIII–related antigen, and the following platelet studies: bleeding time, platelet retention by glass beads, and ristocetin-induced platelet aggregation. As shown in Table 25-7, classical von Willebrand's disease is characterized by concordant abnormalities of all these measurements; variant forms are characterized by discordant results.

Assay of plasma factor VIII activity can be carried out in systems using the PTT or TGT test. Factor VIII–related antigen can be measured either by immunoelectrophoresis or radioimmunoassay, most commonly using a heterologous antibody. The bleeding time is done most accurately by the Ivy method using a template.[247] The Duke (ear lobe) and Ivy (forearm) methods each have their advocates and for some small children the Duke method may be more practical. There is some incompletely substantiated evidence that the Ivy bleeding time may be the more reliable of the two methods in von Willebrand's disease.[159] Platelet retention by glass beads is tested by comparing platelet counts before and after passage of native or heparinized fresh whole blood through a glass bead–filled column under standard conditions.[194,273] Platelet aggregation studies are done using the antibiotic ristocetin as the aggregating agent with either platelet-rich von Willebrand's disease plasma or a standard suspension of normal platelets in von Willebrand's disease plasma.

Although von Willebrand's disease is typically associated with factor VIII–related defects, comparable platelet dysfunction has been associated with deficiencies of factors IX, X, and XI as well. The connection, if any, between these disorders and factor VIII–related von Willebrand's disease has not yet been clarified.

Differential diagnosis. The principal disorder from which von Willebrand's disease must be differentiated is classical hemophilia, since congenital thrombocytopathies other than von Willebrand's disease are not associated with consistent abnormalities of coagulation. The differential characteristics of classical hemophilia and classic and variant forms of von Willebrand's disease are summarized in Table 25-7. In addition, there are important clinical differences between most cases of von Willebrand's disease and classical hemophilia, but these are not sufficiently objective without laboratory testing.

Pathogenesis and pathophysiology. Major discoveries about von Willebrand's disease up to the present suggest that this disorder is the result of defective biosynthesis and function of the factor VIII molecular complex. Although knowledge of factor VIII is still far from complete, current evidence suggests that this trace glycolipoprotein in plasma is an assembly of at least two structural parts with at least three identifiable functions.[249] The two structural components are presumed to be synthesized separately under sex-linked and autosomal genetic control respectively; the sites and mechanisms of their assembly are unknown. The three functional components of factor VIII are VIII:C, VIIIR:Ag, and VIIIR:WF. Activity of VIIIR:WF is specifically equated with the activity of plasma ristocetin cofactor but is presumably reflected in results of the bleeding time test and glass bead retention of platelets as well.

Variations in the clinical and laboratory expression of von Willebrand's disease are fully recognized.[140,208] All the functional parts of the factor VIII complex may be reduced proportionally as in the classical pattern of von Willebrand's disease, or the parts may be variably deficient (Table 25-7). In accord with studies of structural properties of factor VIII–related protein by Gralnick et al.,[189,190] quantitative deficiency of such protein may account for classical von Willebrand's disease, whereas qualitative defects, including altered molecular weight and carbohydrate content, may underlie variant forms of this disorder.

Nachman et al.[250] have found a glycoprotein I complex on the surface of the human platelet that they believe mediates ristocetin-induced, VIIIR:WF-dependent platelet aggregation. Deficiency of the VIIIR:WF link between platelet glycoprotein and vascular subendothelium may account for platelet dysfunction in von Willebrand's disease in which the platelets themselves appear to be structurally and functionally normal.

Pathology. There are no gross or microscopic pathologic changes that are specifically characteristic of hemorrhage in von Willebrand's disease. Indeed, as suggested, the principal pathology is at the molecular level.

Treatment. In general treatment of von Willebrand's disease has already been discussed in the section on classical hemophilia. Topics that warrent further mention include problems peculiar to the female and the monitoring of hemostatic functions in patients with von Willebrand's disease undergoing major surgery.

Menorrhagia may be severe and in the past has been treated with hysterectomy. If menses are severe enough to require replacement therapy or packed red cells, contraceptive (anovulatory) hormones have been quite useful in controlling hemorrhage.

Childbirth and delivery can be accomplished with no more than normal bleeding if the patient is given cryoprecipitate or fresh frozen plasma the day before delivery, if possible. Treatment should be continued every 6 to 12 hours for at least 2 days to maintain the bleeding time in a normal range.

The general principles for surgical management outlined on p. 786 apply except for the levels of plasma factor VIII activity recommended during the postoperative period. Hemostatic control should not be monitored solely by the factor VIII level because daily replacement therapy that suffices for normal factor VIII activity because of stimulation of de novo factor VIII synthesis in these patients usually does not suffice for normalizing platelet function as well. Furthermore, cryoprecipitate is generally superior to fresh frozen plasma or factor VIII concentrates for postoperative treatment because it combines optimal replacement of ristocetin cofactor activity and correction of the bleeding time as well as stimulation of de novo factor VIII synthesis in the smallest possible infusion volume. On the basis of current evidence,[168] a single dose of 3 bags of cryoprecipitate/10 kg body weight (about 30 units VIII:C/ kg) should produce the following results: a factor VIII coagulant level (VIII:C) above 50% for about 48 hours, ristocetin cofactor activity (VIIIR:WF) above 25% for about 18 hours, and correction of the Ivy bleeding time for about 6 to 12 hours.

Thus the following recommendations are offered for replacement therapy of a child with von Willebrand's disease undergoing a general surgical procedure: 4 bags of cryoprecipitate/10 kg body-weight (40 units VIII:C/kg) preoperatively, followed by 2 bags cryoprecipitate/10 kg every 12 hours for 2 days to promote good platelet function for primary hemostasis, and then 2 bags cryoprecipitate/10 kg once daily for the subsequent 6 days to maintain normal plasma factor VIII activity. Monitoring of hemostatic control should emphasize bedside evaluation of the patient. Ideally measurements of ristocetin cofactor activity, factor VIII activity, and the bleeding time should be carried out once daily to assess hemostatic control more objectively, especially during the first 4 postoperative days. Highly repetitive bleeding time tests may be optimal for monitoring hemostasis in von Willebrand's disease, but such frequency is usually neither necessary nor well tolerated by children. Unfortunately correlation of ristocetin cofactor activity with clinical hemostatic control is not well established at the present time.

Prognosis. On the whole, the prognosis of von Willebrand's disease is quite good. The patient with mild to moderate deficiency of factor VIII will have little or no problem except at surgery. The patient with severe disease may have hemarthroses and be otherwise subject to more clinical problems. However, these difficulties can usually be controlled and minimized with early therapy.

Future perspectives. In their review of von Willebrand's disease in 1964 Barrow and Graham[154] conclude with the statement that its "greatest significance may prove to be the challenge it poses to blood clotting theory." In the late 1970s—more than a decade and many new discoveries later—this statement remains relevant.

Christmas disease

Christmas disease (hemophilia B) is a bleeding disorder that occurs primarily in males; it is characterized by a deficiency of functional factor IX clotting activity and is transmitted as a sex-linked recessive trait. The classification is the same as that of classical hemophilia; i.e., those patients with less than 1% of clotting activity in their plasma have severe disease and may bleed spontane-

ously several times each month. Individuals with moderate disease have 1% to 5% of the clotting factor in their plasma and bleed every 6 to 8 weeks with minor trauma; those patients with 6% to 50% plasma levels have mild disease and bleed only with trauma or surgical procedures.

The determination of severity may be difficult to make in the newborn period because of the physiologic deficiency of factor IX. If the factor IX level is less than 1%, there is no doubt about the diagnosis. However, if the factor IX level is 5% to 10%, the assay should be repeated at 6 months to verify the level.

Historical perspective. The nomenclature has been confusing in the past; hemophilia B, plasma thromboplastin component deficiency, and Christmas disease all refer to the deficiency of factor IX clotting activity in the plasma. The entity was reported in 1947 by Pavlovsky,[260] who found that the blood from one hemophiliac corrected the blood of another hemophiliac. The significance of this report was not recognized until 1952 when Schulman and Smith[275] described a clotting disorder in a hemophilic boy whose defect was similar to classical hemophilia but whose plasma was not corrected by Cohn fraction rich in antihemophilic factor. Later that year Aggeler et al.[143] and Biggs et al.[157] independently described similar cases, and Biggs' group was able to show a sex-linked recessive trait responsible for the disorder in the Christmas family, whose name was then given to the disorder.

Incidence. The incidence appears to be seven to ten times less frequent than that of classical hemophilia with 5,202 approximated in the United States by the NHLI Blood Resource Study of the total 25,400 hemophilic population. Forty percent had severe disease and 55.7% had moderate disease.[252] A mutation rate of 0.5 to 1×10^{-5} gametes/generation has been calculated on this prevalence data of 5.2 by Merritt.[244a]

Genetics. The mode of inheritance of Christmas disease has been well established as an X-linked recessive trait.[163] The carrier female is different from the asymptomatic carrier of classical hemophilia, however, and is more likely to have a low plasma level of factor IX with a bleeding diathesis. The plasma levels may be as low as 25% to 40% and can be used with certainty for carrier detection in one quarter of individuals tested.[217]

Carrier detection is now possible utilizing both the ox brain thromboplastin test (Thrombotest) and the immunologic techniques for factor IX protein, a method similar to that used for factor VIII carrier detection.

Clinical features. Classical hemophilia and Christmas disease cannot be distinguished clinically. It has been stated that the bleeding is less severe in Christmas disease than in classical hemophilia, but this has not been our experience.

Laboratory evaluation. The laboratory diagnosis of both classical hemophilia and Christmas disease and the differential diagnosis are discussed on p. 778. The whole blood clotting time, PTT, and prothrombin consumption, as well as the specific assay for factor IX are all abnormal in the deficiency state. The PT may be prolonged by 1 to 2 seconds and results of the Thrombotest are abnormal in 6% of patients.

Pathogenesis. Christmas disease is the result of a functional deficiency of factor IX, a protein involved in the activation of factor X via the intrinsic pathway. Factor IX molecular substance has been identified both indirectly as cross-reacting material (CRM) through estimation of inhibitor-neutralizing capacity of plasma and directly as antigenic material through radioimmunoassay using heterologous antisera.[272,289] By means of these techniques Christmas disease may be divided into three variant classes according to the presence of antigenic cross-reacting material: CRM−, CRM+, and CRM^R (reduced).[165,253,256] According to different workers the range of CRM is broad, ranging from 0 to 95%[270] with a median of 17% in a recent study by Thompson.[289] In addition, Hougie and Twomey[203] have divided Christmas disease into two classes on the basis of a PT test using ox brain thromboplastin: non-B$_M$, in which this test is normal, and B$_M$, in which the ox brain PT is prolonged. This classification cuts across the CRM categories in that both non-B$_M$ and B$_M$ types of Christmas disease may be CRM+, CRM^R, or CRM−.[173,245,291]

Factor IX is a vitamin K−dependent factor, along with prothrombin and factors VII and X, and is manufactured exclusively in the liver.[171] Available evidence suggests that vitamin K is required for carboxylation of glutamic acid residues in the amino terminal of the vitamin K−dependent molecules, thus enabling them to bind calcium and to participate in coagulation.[286] However, the action of vitamin K has no relevance to the deficiency of factor IX in Christmas disease.

Factor IX normally exists in plasma as a single-chain zymogen and is converted to the active serine protease IXa by factor XIa.[183,257] Animal studies suggest that factor IX is stored in the liver and released when plasma levels are low in accord with a negative feedback process.[300] The exact molecular and physiologic abnormalities of factor IX that produce Christmas disease are not yet established.

Treatment. The general principles of overall management and replacement therapy for Christmas disease have been considered in the discussion of classical hemophilia.

Prognosis. The outlook for this disease is as hopeful as for classical hemophilia. Lyophilized concentrates, early treatment, and home or self-replacement therapy in a total comprehensive care program have greatly improved the life-style and future prospects for these patients. Chronic arthropathy should be minimal and educational and job opportunities should be improved. The complications of therapy may be the only severe problems and will need to be carefully evaluated in the years ahead.

UNCOMMON INHERITED COAGULATION DEFICIENCIES
Congenital fibrinogen deficiencies

An isolated deficiency of fibrinogen is a rare coagulation defect resulting in a variable lack of blood clot formation. In general a complete deficiency is congenital, whereas conditions with reduced amounts of fibrinogen (hypofibrinogenemia) can be either congenital or acquired.

Congenital afibrinogenemia. Congenital afibrinogenemia is a rare inherited hemorrhagic disorder characterized by virtual absence of plasma fibrinogen.[377] This disorder is to be distinguished from hypofibrinogenemia seen in a separate milder entity[390] as well as in some carriers of afibrinogenemia.

The disease has been reported in well over 100 cases, according to Mammen's review in 1974,[371] with none reported since that time. It appears to be transmitted by an autosomal recessive gene with normal fibrinogen or hypofibrinogenemia in the heterozygote and afibrinogenemia in the homozygote. The original patient of Rabe and Solomon[383] was the product of a consanguinous marriage. A similar marital pattern is present in more than half the reported cases.[323,335] A negative family history for bleeding has been described in some cases.

Symptoms of bleeding may occur in the newborn period with hematomas from the trauma of delivery, melena, hematemesis, and bleeding from the umbilicus. Bleeding may occur in the skin or muscles, from mucous membranes with epistaxis and gastrointestinal bleeding, or into joints and the central nervous system. Menstrual bleeding has been reported as both normal and prolonged. Bleeding is frequently spontaneous in origin and, as in the hemophilias, variable in time. Delayed bleeding may occur following surgical procedures.

Since the final substrate for formation of the clot is missing, results of all of the screening tests are abnormal: clotting time, PT, PTT, and thrombin time. Occasionally decreased levels of factors II, V, VII, and VIII have been described. However, in assays using normal plasma or plasma with a normal amount of fibrinogen the deficiency is corrected. Acquired inhibitors of fibrinogen have been described in two persons with congenital afibrinogenemia and also in two previously healthy persons.[396]

Platelet functions have been reported as abnormal, presumably because of the absence of fibrinogen in plasma; bleeding time, adhesion, and aggregation are corrected by the addition of fibrinogen to the test.[404] A small amount of fibrinogen has been found within platelets of patients with the disorder.[375]

Tests for plasma fibrinogen by precipitation and coagulation techniques demonstrate a complete absence of the protein, whereas immunologic procedures may detect trace amounts, 5 mg or less, in patients with homozygous deficiency. Heterozygotes may be detected as partially deficient by the precipitation and coagulation methods.

Bleeding episodes can be controlled by replacement of fibrinogen with fresh frozen plasma, cryoprecipitate, or concentrates of fibrinogen (Cohn fraction I). The dosage should be calculated to raise the fibrinogen level to between 50 and 100 mg/dl. Since the half-life of the protein is approximately 80 hours, the patient may be given infusions every 4 to 5 days when monitored by laboratory control.

Complications have been reported with the concentrates. Hepatitis has been prevalent with the Cohn fraction I concentrates, and antibodies have been formed against the transfused fibrinogen. Thromboembolic complications, particularly pulmonary emboli, have been reported.[356,369] These reports prompted the suggestion of heparinization of the patients prior to fibrinogen infusion. Prolonged and prophylactic therapy therefore must be approached with caution.

Prospects for the future of patients with this chronic disease are greatly improved with the availability of current therapy.

Dysfibrinogenemias. The congenital qualitative abnormalities of the fibrinogen molecule are called dysfibrinogenemias. Patients with the homozygous disease have normal amounts of plasma fibrinogen that fails to form fibrin in the presence of the enzyme thrombin. The first case was described in 1958 in an 8-year-old girl with hypofibrinogenemia and a severe bleeding diathesis.[355] This association with hypofibrinogenemia has not been found in the twenty-six families described since then with dysfibrinogenemia. Each of these twenty-six abnormal fibrinogens was named according to the cities in which it was found, as with the hemoglobinopathies.[320] The abnormalities have been characterized functionally in twenty-four of the twenty-six families and biochemically only in fibrinogen Detroit.[370] The functional defect has been identified according to the phase of fibrin

formation in which it appears, i.e., the first phase, or proteolytic phase, in which thrombin cleaves fibrinopeptide A from the A chain and fibrinopeptide B from the B chain to give the fibrin monomers; the second phase, in which the fibrin monomers aggregate side-to-side and end-to-end to form the fibrin network; and the last, or stabilization phase, in which factor XIII stabilizes the fibrin network. Six of the twenty-four defects were in the proteolytic phase, seventeen in the polymerization phase, and one in the stabilization phase.[371]

The inheritance pattern appears to be autosomal dominant in nature with equal distribution in male and female. Homozygotes have uniformly abnormal fibrinogen molecules. However, most individuals reported have some normal fibrinogen, suggesting that most patients described are heterozygous for the disorder. Only the family with fibrinogen Detroit has been characterized sufficiently well to denote the homozygous state.

The disorder is not uniform in severity, but it is usually mild in presentation. Only members of thirteen of the reported families have had a mild bleeding problem characterized by easy bruising, prolonged bleeding from minor trauma, wound dehiscence, and menorrhagia. Thromboses, however, have occurred in three of the families.[374]

The degree of laboratory abnormality depends on whether the patient is homozygous or heterozygous for the deficiency. In contrast to the patient with afibrinogenemia, a clot forms in dysfibrinogenemia but the appearance of the clot may be abnormal. The whole blood clotting time may therefore be prolonged and the clot will be soft and friable with an increased amount of red cell fallout. The PT and PTT may be normal or abnormal, depending on the degree of deficiency, but the thrombin time and reptilase time are always abnormal. The bleeding time should be normal, as should assays for factors II, V, VII, VIII, IX, X, XI, and XII, and the clot should be insoluble in 5M urea. Fibrinolysis should be normal. Fibrinogen determinations vary with the method used. The precipitation and immunologic methods should give a normal value, whereas the values dependent on clotting in the presence of thrombin are abnormal.

Congenital dysfibrinogenemia must be differentiated from hypofibrinogenemia, and in early infancy from fetal fibrinogen. The three methods for determining fibrinogen—physicochemical, immunochemical, and functional—confirm the presence of dysfibrinogenemia or hypofibrinogenemia. In the former the clotting activity with thrombin is abnormal and in the latter all of the assay methods give the same result. Acquired dysfibrinogenemia has been seen with various diseases such as systemic lupus erythematosus, liver disease, and macroglobulinemia.[381]

The need and efficacy of therapy are not known. However, infused fibrinogen has a normal survival time and may be of value.[317,401]

It is difficult to discuss prognosis with the limited number of cases reported and with the varied symptoms. Affected patients have little or no problem.

Fetal fibrinogen. The observation by Biggs[321] that plasma or fibrinogen from newborn infants, as compared to that from adults, displays a prolonged thrombin clotting time, led to the suggestion that a distinct fetal form of fibrinogen exists. The delay in the thrombin (or reptilase) time of newborn plasma was reported variable in some studies and uniform in others, raising doubts as to the existence of fetal fibrinogen. More recent studies, however, have established that isolated infant fibrinogen from full-term newborn and premature infants of 24 to 35 weeks' gestation displayed prolonged clotting times, particularly under conditions of high ionic strength, and that the clotting times were not attributable to the fetal plasma environment.[340,341] The results were more exaggerated in the plasma of premature infants than of full-term infants, with results of full-term infants falling halfway between those of adults and premature infants. Moreover, the long clotting time has been shown to be a result of the delayed aggregation of fetal fibrin, and it cannot be accounted for by proteolytic alterations or by the relatively high phosphorus content of fetal fibrinogen. Many investigators have examined fetal fibrinogen by immunochemical, physicochemical, electrophoretic, isoelectric focusing, carbohydrate content, and other means but have failed to detect unequivocal structural differences from its adult counterpart.[346,405] It is clear from its functional behavior that a distinct form of fetal fibrinogen exists, but whether it represents posttranslational (nonproteolytic) modifications or a fetal fibrinogen gene remains to be established. This may be an example of "physiologic" dysfibrinogenemia of infancy.

Congenital prothrombin deficiency

Hereditary deficiency of prothrombin is exceedingly rare and is characterized by a mild bleeding disorder with a moderate prolongation of the PT. The disorder was originally described with other deficiencies that have since been found to be deficiencies of other factors in the prothrombin complex, i.e., factors V, VII, and X. The original case of the congenital hypoprothrombinemia was described by Rhoads,[391] and seven other cases have followed in the intervening years.[321,328,359]

Congenital deficiency of prothrombin appears to be inherited as an autosomal recessive defect, ap-

pearing in both males and females. The incidence is too small to calculate prevalence data. The defect appears to be the result of a lack of production of the prothrombin protein. However, the deficiency is not complete, since most homozygous patients can produce approximately 10% of the normal amount of functional prothrombin.

The hemorrhagic manifestations are relatively mild and occur as mucous membrane bleeding, easy bruising, menorrhagia, and bleeding with dental extractions. The laboratory findings are those of a prolonged PT measured by a one- or two-stage assay that is uncorrected by absorbed plasma. The specific assays for factors V, VII, and X and fibrinogen are normal, and a blood thromboplastin inhibitor is not present.

The disorder must be differentiated from dysprothrombinemia. Two nonfunctional prothrombin molecules have been described.[397,398] In prothrombin Barcelona, an inherited autosomal recessive trait, the plasma prothrombin assay using the two-stage method measures a greater amount of prothrombin than the one-stage prothrombin time, a normal amount with the staphylocoagulase method, and normal amounts with the immunologic assay.[358]

The second abnormal prothrombin molecule cannot be completely converted to thrombin. The plasma of these patients contains both normal and abnormal prothrombin molecules.[397]

Therapy for the congenital deficiency is usually unnecessary and vitamin K is of no value. Should replacement therapy be necessary, fresh frozen plasma, 10 to 20 ml/kg body weight, should produce a sufficient rise to approximately 30%. (The hemostatic level is 20%.) Repeat doses should only be necessary every 2 to 3 days. The half-life of the transfused protein is 48 to 120 hours.[322] When gastrointestinal bleeding is present, prothrombin complex concentrate can be used to produce a higher level in the deficient patient without plasma volume overload.

The prognosis for this mild disorder is good.

Congenital factor V deficiency

Factor V deficiency is a mild bleeding disorder affecting both sexes and characterized by bleeding from the mucous membranes and into the skin. The disorder was first described by Owren[379] in 1947 and termed parahemophilia. It has since been described in fifty-two cases with a variable intensity of bleeding and frequency and in association with factor VIII deficiency or a prolonged bleeding time.*

The disease is transmitted as an autosomal recessive trait with intermediate amounts of factor

---

*References 325, 330, 331, 357.

V detected in heterozygous plasma (between 35% and 50%) by specific assay. The nature of the disease appears to be failure of production of this protein, with a complete absence of the protein in the homozygous state. Antisera against human factor V cannot be neutralized by factor V–deficient plasma.[336,338] The protein is unstable in vitro and acts with factor X in the presence of calcium ions and phospholipids to convert prothrombin to thrombin.

Bleeding is usually from the mucous membranes (epistaxis or gastrointestinal bleeding) or into the skin. More severe bleeding may occur with trauma or surgery, and hemarthrosis is unusual. Menorrhagia may be quite severe. Circulating anticoagulants directed against transfused factor V have been reported in both the congenital and acquired states.[336,338]

Both the PT and PTT are prolonged, as is the clotting time. The definitive diagnosis can be made with a specific factor V assay using plasma artificially depleted of factor V or plasma from a patient known to have factor V deficiency.

Bleeding episodes can be treated only with fresh frozen plasma, preferably frozen for less than 1 month. The hemostatic level is approximately 25%, and the half-life of the transfused protein is 36 hours.[402] Transfusion of 1 unit of factor V/kg body weight should give a rise of 1.5% in the plasma level. Treatment therefore may be given once daily for 7 days at the time of an operative procedure and probably not more than once for a minor bleeding episode. All of the clotting factors are present in plasma in a concentration of 1 unit/ml. Therefore transfusion of 10 ml of fresh frozen plasma/kg should raise the plasma level 15%.

In the absence of an inhibitor the prognosis is excellent.

Congenital factor VII deficiency

Factor VII deficiency is a relatively rare clotting disorder that occurs in both males and females and is characterized by mucous membrane bleeding. It is one of the coagulation disorders that is associated with a prolonged PT. The disease was first described by Alexander et al.[315] in 1951, and the missing factor was called serum prothrombin conversion accelerator (SPCA). Owren preferred the term "proconvertin" or "stable factor." All were abandoned and the disease referred to as factor VII deficiency.[365,380] Thirty-six homozygous patients were described in the next 10 years.[344]

The inheritance has been reported as a highly penetrant, incompletely recessive autosomal trait. Heterozygotes have levels of 16% to 42% of normal, and levels of homozygotes are lower.[380] Carriers may have bleeding episodes. Two types of homozygotes have been detected, those without a protein and those with a presumably nonfunctional protein that can neutralize a rabbit antibody prepared by immunization of a rabbit with a crude factor VII preparation.[345]

Although more than fifty-eight cases have been reported, the incidence of this disorder has been difficult to calculate in view of its rarity. It has been estimated as 1/1,000,000 population.

The severity of the bleeding episodes depends on the degree of deficiency. Patients with a 5- to 7-second prolongation of the PT rarely have bleeding problems. Those with a greater prolongation of the PT have more severe bleeding from mucous membranes, epistaxis, and gastrointestinal, skin, muscle, or intracranial bleeding. Fatal intracranial bleeding caused by birth trauma has occurred in newborns.[384] Menstrual bleeding may be severe. Hemarthrosis is rare but has been seen. The acquired deficiency occurs when a patient is given bishydroxycoumarin (Dicumarol) or one of its analogues. The deficiency has been found associated with carotid body tumors. The factor VII level is known to rise in pregnancy and with the use of contraceptive drugs.

The screening tests can be helpful in making the diagnosis of factor VII deficiency. The PTT is completely normal and the PT quite abnormal but corrected by the addition of Russell's viper venom. A specific assay for factor VII confirms the diagnosis. Results of all of the remaining coagulation tests should be normal.

Treatment is not usually necessary but may be required for surgical procedures, severe bleeding, or menstrual bleeding. Serum has been used in the past but is not the best source of factor VII. Fresh frozen plasma is the best source at the present time although the prothrombin complex concentrates do contain appreciable amounts of factor VII and may be of value for small children. The dosage should be calculated to raise the plasma level above 15%, the hemostatic level, and may be difficult to maintain because of the rapid disappearance into the extravascular space. The biologic half-life of the protein is 5 hours. Therapy should be maintained for 4 to 6 days postoperatively, depending on the extent of surgery. Transfusion of 1 unit of factor VII/kg body weight should raise the plasma level 1%.

Congenital factor X deficiency

Factor X deficiency is a rare coagulation abnormality occurring both in males and females and characterized by mucous membrane bleeding, bleeding with trauma, and severe menstrual bleeding. It is similar to factor II and VII deficiencies in its clinical and laboratory abnormalities and its vitamin K dependence.

The disorder was described in 1956 by Telfer

et al.[399] in the Prower family and independently by Hougie et al.[354] in the Stuart family; hence the name Stuart-Prower factor. The factor was subsequently designated factor X by the International Nomenclature Committee.

Three types of factor X molecules have been found with different behavior in vitro, although they produce similar clinical symptoms. The original plasma from Stuart is deficient in a protein that can neutralize an antibody against factor X.[329] The second type neutralized the antibody to factor X and did not have coagulant activity but could be activated by Russell's viper venom.[343] The third type had no coagulant activity and partially neutralized the factor X antibody.[382] Therefore the deficiency in factor X activity may be a complete deficiency of the protein, the presence of a nonfunctional protein, or the presence of a small amount of nonfunctional protein.

Acquired deficiencies of factor X may occur with anticoagulant therapy, with liver disease, in the absence of vitamin K, in newborn infants in the presence of certain drugs that compete for metabolism such as phenytoin (Dilantin), and with amyloidosis.[339] Inactive precursor forms of factor X and all of the vitamin K–dependent factors may be produced in the absence of vitamin K as PIVKA (protein induced by vitamin K absence), PIVKA II, PIVKA VII, PIVKA IX, and PIVKA X.[342]

The incidence of this disorder is extremely low; about twenty cases have been reported in the literature. The deficiency is transmitted as an incompletely recessive trait. Heterozygotes have a decreased level of factor X activity, usually approximately 36% of normal. The disease may occur in infancy with bleeding from the umbilicus. Moderately severe bleeding may occur with epistaxis, hematomas, and occasionally hemarthrosis. Menstrual bleeding may be quite severe. Heterozygotes may have problems with surgical procedures and severe trauma.

The screening PT and PTT are prolonged as are the clotting time, prothrombin consumption, and thromboplastin generation. The special assay using Russell's viper venom may differentiate between factor VII and X, since this agent activates factor X directly.

Fresh frozen plasma can usually deliver sufficient activity for most bleeding episodes. Replacement therapy given as 1 unit of factor X/kg body weight raises the plasma level 1%. Since the hemostatic level is probably about 10%, a plasma level of 15% should be sufficient for surgery and 10% for a usual bleeding episode. The half-life of the protein is 24 to 60 hours, and therapy probably can be given daily for a surgical procedure. For small children any of the prothrombin complex concentrates may be used.

In general the prognosis of factor X deficiency is good.

Congenital factor XI deficiency

Factor XI deficiency is a congenital coagulation disorder occurring in both males and females and characterized by mild bleeding. The disorder was originally described by Rosenthal et al.[393] and given the name "hemophilia C" or "plasma thromboplastin antecedent deficiency." The majority of cases have been reported in Jewish patients, and the inheritance pattern has been demonstrated to be autosomal and incompletely recessive in character.[364,385,396] Heterozygotes may have a factor XI plasma level between 30% and 65% of the normal level and homozygotes less than 20%. Males and females are equally affected. The incidence is about 1×10^{-6} in the population.

The bleeding manifestations are usually mild with epistaxis and menorrhagia the common problems. Bleeding in minor surgical trauma such as tonsillectomy and dental extractions is common, and discovery of the disorder is frequently made at this time. Hemarthrosis is unusual. Bleeding from circumcision or trauma may occur in the newborn, in whom the deficiency is physiologic. Maternal factor XI levels fall during the last trimester of pregnancy. Neonatal levels are below the maternal levels and rise slowly over the first 60 days of life to adult normal levels. Some infants require 9 months to reach the adult normal level.[351]

The factor XI protein is made in the liver, is not dependent on vitamin K for synthesis, and does not cross the placenta. The deficiency in the newborn is presumed to be a result of liver immaturity and does not respond to vitamin K.[351]

The disorder is a true deficiency rather than a dysproteinemia, since coagulant deficiency parallels antigen presence.[387] Acquired deficiencies have been seen in liver disease. Circulating anticoagulants have been reported against factor XI and XII together.[327]

Plasma with this deficiency may or may not show a prolonged clotting time. The prothrombin consumption may be prolonged, and the PTT is abnormal. Specific assay for factor XI using plasma artificially depleted or congenitally deficient of factor XI confirms the diagnosis.[353] In the TGT the defect is seen in both plasma and serum. Results of all other clotting tests should be within the normal range. It is extremely important that the laboratory evaluation be done on a freshly drawn sample, for plasma with this deficiency may be activated if standing or if frozen and may give a falsely normal value for factor XI in the assay. Variant cases have been reported in association with factor VIII deficiency and with a prolonged bleeding time.

Therapy for this disorder may be given with fresh frozen plasma. Only a small amount of the transfused protein goes into the extravascular space. Therefore a rise of 2% should follow transfusion of 1 unit/kg body weight. The hemostatic level is approximately 20%, and the half-life of the transfused protein is 40 to 84 hours, although a 10-hour half-life has been reported in one patient.[352,376] In general the transfusion of 7 to 20 ml of plasma/kg body weight will assure a rise of 25% to 50% in factor XI, an adequate dose for hemostasis of bleeding episodes and surgery. Daily infusions would suffice for the usual patient for postoperative care, but infusions would be necessary every 8 hours for the patient with a 10-hour half life. Laboratory control therefore is a necessity.

Cryoprecipitate supernatant and one of the prothrombin complex concentrates (Konyne) also contain factor XI.[319] These concentrates can be used for those patients requiring prolonged high-dose therapy, as in the postoperative periods.

The prognosis for this mild disorder is good.

Congenital factor XII deficiency

The congenital deficiency of factor XII (Hageman factor or Hageman trait) is a disorder not associated with a hemorrhagic disease.

The disorder was first discovered by Ratnoff[388] in 1955 in a routine preoperative screening of a patient named Hageman. It has since been described in more than 100 cases. The clotting time was grossly abnormal when blood was drawn into plain glass tubes and silicone-coated tubes. Ratnoff termed this factor necessary for the initiation of the clotting process the contact factor.

The genetic transmission is autosomal recessive in character with most heterozygotes having 24% to 60% of normal Hageman factor activity in their plasma. Not all presumptive carriers have been found deficient,[389] and a second family with Hageman trait has been described in which the inheritance appears to be autosomal dominant in character.[318] The incidence of detected cases is quite low, but the numbers are probably inaccurate, since the detection of the disorder is purely happenstance.

Bleeding in this disorder is extremely unusual. Spontaneous bleeding does not occur and there is no bleeding at the time of surgical procedures. Tonsillectomy and adenoidectomy have been performed without bleeding.[313] Rare cases have been reported in which women have had excessive bleeding in childbirth and with dental extraction.

Results of laboratory tests for the first phase of the clotting system are abnormal, while those for the second phase are normal. PTT, prothrombin consumption, whole blood clotting time, and the TGT are abnormal, while the PT is normal. The screening tests are therefore the same as for factor XI deficiency. The differentiation can be made with the specific assay for factor XII using blood that is congenitally deficient in the factor or chicken plasma, which is also deficient in factor XII.

Factor XII protein is absent in the true deficiency and the deficient plasma cannot neutralize an antibody produced against factor XII. The protein is deficient in newborn infants with only 25% of normal adult levels found during the first 6 days of life. Adult levels are reached by 14 days of age.[362] The factor is not deficient in the presence of liver disease, nor is vitamin K necessary for its production. The site of origin is unknown. The function of this factor in the coagulation system remains unclear since deficient patients remain asymptomatic. The activation of the coagulation process in vitro, however, is well recognized, as is the activation of the kinins and the inflammatory process. The later function may be more important than the function in the coagulation process.

Therapy is not usually necessary for this disorder, but should bleeding occur fresh frozen plasma given once should suffice, since the half-life of the protein is 50 to 70 hours.[400]

Congenital factor XIII deficiency

Congenital factor XIII deficiency is an inherited hemorrhagic disorder characterized by poor wound healing and late wound bleeding caused by the formation of a friable clot in the absence of factor XIII. Factor XIII is also called fibrin-stabilizing factor, Laki-Lorand factor, and fibrinase.

In 1944 Robbins[392] discovered a factor that made pure fibrinogen clots insoluble in weak acid and urea. Laki and Lorand[363] confirmed this observation in 1948 and named the factor fibrin-stabilizing factor. The deficiency was described by Duckert et al.[334] in 1960 as the cause of a congenital hemorrhagic disorder, and in 1963 the International Nomenclature Committee recognized the factor and designated it factor XIII.

The disorder is inherited as an autosomal recessive trait with decreased levels of the factor present in the plasma of heterozygotes in some families.[316,368] Consanguinity has been present in several of the reported families. The disorder is quite rare in the general population but has a higher incidence in Pakistanis.[408] It has also been reported in other kindreds in an X-linked inheritance,[390a] although the majority of cases reported are of the autosomal recessive type. A large kindred with factor XII and XIII deficiency has been reported from Newfoundland.[348]

The hemorrhagic defect may be the result of lack of the protein in the patient's plasma or inability of the zymogen to function.[333,347,367]

Infants with the congenital deficiency commonly bleed from the umbilicus and bruise easily, and children may have intracranial bleeding. In adults gastrointestinal hemorrhage is seen and hemarthrosis may occur without residual crippling. Clotting takes place following trauma but bleeding occurs 24 to 36 hours later and may last for several days. Hemorrhage usually does not occur without trauma. Wounds heal slowly, producing large, broad scars. Pregnancy may be interrupted by abortion resulting from severe decidual bleeding.[337]

Levels in newborn infants may be lower than adult normal levels (50% to 76%, compared to 72% to 120%) and reach adult levels by 1 month of age.[324]

Acquired deficiency has been found associated with liver disease, leukemia, lymphomas, and metastatic tumors, anemias, and collagen disorders.[378]

Acquired inhibitors to factor XIII have been reported in several cases, in patients known to have had the factor previously.[373] Results of all of the routine coagulation tests are normal in this disorder. The deficiency should be suspected, however, when the clot appears shaggy and friable. The diagnosis is confirmed by the rapid solubility of the fibrin clot obtained from recalcified plasma when it is placed in 5M urea or a 1% solution of monochloracetic acid. A specific assay may be done using plasma known to be deficient in factor XIII or by testing the transamidation ability of the unknown plasma by quantifying the incorporation of ^{14}C-glycine methyl ester into casein.[366,378]

The delayed bleeding occurs in the absence of factor XIII because of resulting failure in the cross-linkage of fibrin polymer through transamidation, a process in which interfibrin γ-glutamyl–ϵ-lysine isopeptide linkages replace hydrogen bonds between adjacent γ-chains within the polymer. The production of a soft friable clot occurs, and hemorrhage ensues.[360]

Therapy with fresh or fresh frozen plasma given as 1 unit/kg body weight should give a 2% to 3% rise in plasma level of factor XIII. Since the half-life is approximately 6.3 days and the hemostatic level is low (2% to 3%), the replacement therapy need not be repeated more than once weekly.

The prognosis for this disorder is good in the absence of an inhibitor to the factor.

Other inherited coagulation deficiencies

Five other factors have been reported as necessary for the activation of the intrinsic coagulation pathway, fibrinolytic activity, chemotactic activity, and kinin generation. Absence of these factors is not associated with a hemorrhagic disease but may be associated with a prolonged PTT. They are Fletcher factor, Fitzgerald factor, Flaujeac factor, Reid factor, and Williams factor. The last four are probably the same high molecular weight kininogen and will be treated as one entity.[372,407]

Fletcher factor. Deficiency of Fletcher factor does not cause a hemorrhagic diathesis but is associated with a defect in the intrinsic clotting system, in kinin generation, in fibrinolytic activity, and in chemotactic activity caused by the absence of a prekallikrein.

In 1965, Hathaway et al.[349] reported an abnormal whole blood clotting time, and TGT in a Kentucky family named Fletcher. All other clotting factors were normal and the Fletcher plasma was corrected by plasma deficient in factors XII and XI. Hattersley and Hayes[350] reported three more unrelated patients in 1970, and Abildgaard and Harrison[314] noted that the kaolin PTT on the plasma from their patient was corrected by standing 10 minutes, a fact now recognized as diagnostic of this deficiency.

Fletcher factor–deficient plasma is deficient in a prekallikrein that, when activated with kaolin, activates Hageman factor, the coagulation and fibrinolytic systems, and chemotactic activity.[361] Activated prekallikrein or kallikrein releases vasoactive polypeptides (bradykinin) that enhance permeability. Fletcher factor–deficient plasma does not generate bradykinin.[403,406]

Only five families with this deficiency have been reported to date and in these families the inheritance patterns appear to be autosomal recessive. Heterozygotes have Fletcher factor levels of 40% to 72% (normal range 58% to 178%) and homozygotes have a level of 1%. Four of the five families reported are black.

There are no problems associated with the coagulation and fibrinolytic mechanisms or inflammatory response in the patients described. As noted previously, the kaolin PTT is prolonged. The whole blood clotting time, PTT, and TGT are markedly prolonged, and the PTT is shortened by incubation for 10 minutes. All other tests and factor assays are normal.

Treatment is unnecessary for surgical procedures.

Fitzgerald, Flaujeac, Williams, and Reid factors. Fitzgerald, Flaujeac, Williams, and Reid are the eponyms applied to a high molecular weight kininogen associated with fibrinolytic pathways. The deficiency state is not associated with disease in any of the systems mentioned and is discovered in the patient's plasma on routine screening as a prolonged activated PTT.*

The eponyms apply to the same protein, which was found deficient in the patients of those names. Insufficient numbers have been studied to know the inheritance pattern of this deficiency. It appears to have no clinical significance at the present time, but the discovery of these factors, Fletcher factor, and the high molecular weight kininogen have brought about extremely interesting investigations of the interaction of the coagulation and fibrinolytic systems and the inflammatory process.

ACQUIRED COAGULATION DEFICIENCIES
Vitamin K deficiency

Vitamin K deficiency may be acquired as a result of systemic lack or pharmacologic antagonism of vitamin K and is characterized by a variable hemorrhagic tendency because of decreased activities of the vitamin K–dependent coagulation factors, i.e., factors II (prothrombin), VII, IX, and X.

Dietary vitamin K includes a group of naturally occurring, fat-soluble naphthoquinone compounds of which the most important in humans is vitamin K_1: 2-methyl-3-phytyl-1,4-naphthoquinone, or phylloquinone. The daily requirement for vitamin K is small, probably less than 1 μg/kg bodyweight,[452] and is readily obtained from a normal diet, particularly from green leafy vegetables. Dietary vitamin K is largely absorbed from the upper small intestine and transported to the liver, where most of the vitamin is stored.[424,518,530] In older children and adults synthesis of vitamin K by intestinal bacteria does not constitute a significant source since little or no vitamin K is absorbed from the colon; in infants, on the other hand, vitamin K is readily absorbed from the colon, and bacterial synthesis may therefore constitute a major source of the vitamin in this age group.

Vitamin K compounds that have been synthesized for therapeutic use include vitamin K_1 and a variety of water-soluble forms of menadione (2-methyl-1,4-naphtho-quinone).

Historical perspective. The discovery of vitamin K and its relationship to coagulation began with four events widely separated in time and place: (1) increasing recognition during the nine-

teenth century of a bleeding tendency in certain newborns, illustrated by the classical report by Townsend[527] in 1894 in which he introduced the term "hemorrhagic disease of the newborn"; (2) similar recognition of a bleeding tendency in patients with jaundice, illustrated by the recommendation of Osler[496] in 1901 that surgery in such patients should be approached with caution; (3) the recognition by veterinarians in 1921 of a hemorrhagic disease affecting cattle in North Dakota and Ontario[506]; and (4) the observation by Dam[435] in 1929 that chicks fed a purified diet developed a severe hemorrhagic tendency.

In the mid-1930s Dam et al.[436,437,439] suggested that the disease in chicks was caused by lack of a fat-soluble "koagulation vitamin," or simply "vitamin K." In 1939 Dam et al.[438] successfully isolated vitamin K in pure form from alfalfa, and Doisy et al. reported that this vitamin existed in at least two forms: K_1 in alfalfa and K_2 in putrified fishmeal.[418,444] Meanwhile, using his newly developed PT test, Quick[504,505] showed that hypoprothrombinemia was associated with the bleeding disorder in patients with obstructive jaundice and in affected chicks and cattle. In addition, using their two-stage method for measurement of prothrombin, Brinkhous et al.[427] showed in 1937 that "hemorrhagic disease of the newborn" was characterized by hypoprothrombinemia. The correction of decreased prothrombin activity by the administration of vitamin K in the cases of affected newborns, patients with obstructive jaundice, and bleeding chicks firmly established a role for vitamin K in the synthesis of prothrombin.[506] However, the relationship of vitamin K deficiency to hemorrhagic disease in cattle was not established in the course of these developments.

In 1922 Schofield[516] discovered that a toxic ingredient in spoiled sweet clover was responsible for the bleeding disease in cattle, and his observations were extended by Roderick.[511,512] In 1941 Link et al. reported their series of brilliant studies in which they both isolated and synthesized the agent: 3,3-methylene-bis-(4-hydroxycoumarin), or dicumarol.[428,429,521] By the mid-1940s it was established that coumarin somehow interferes with the action of vitamin K in the synthesis of prothrombin.[507]

In the course of discovery of additional coagulation factors during the 1950s it was established that factors VII, IX, and X are also vitamin K dependent.[417] The latest chapter in the story of vitamin K is the discovery that it is involved in the formation of Ca^{++}-binding sites on factors II, VII, IX, and X and not in their overall synthesis as previously presumed.[524,526] In addition, new vitamin K–dependent proteins have been found in cortical bone[503] and bovine plasma[523] and yet others may be identified and characterized in time.

As a final note it should be pointed out that, despite the awesome progress in understanding of this trace substance, the exact mechanisms of its function and pharmacologic inhibition are not yet known.

Classification. An etiologic classification is most appropriate for vitamin K deficiency and this is outlined below. It should be emphasized that deficient activities of factors II, VII, IX, and X associated with parenchymal liver disease and unresponsive to parenteral vitamin K therapy reflect liver dysfunction rather than vitamin K deficiency and are intentionally omitted from this classification.[411]

A. Primary deficiency of vitamin K
 1. Hemorrhagic disease of the newborn
 2. Prolonged unsupplemented parenteral nutrition combined with antibiotic suppression of intestinal flora
B. Decreased absorption of vitamin K
 1. Biliary obstruction, e.g., biliary atresia
 2. Intestinal disorders, e.g., cystic fibrosis
C. Pharmacologic antagonism of vitamin K
 1. Coumarins, e.g., warfarin
 2. Phenytoin (rare)
 3. Salicylates (rare)

Incidence. Vitamin K deficiency caused by simple dietary lack is virtually nonexistent.[531] However, in the context of the several conditions that may interfere with vitamin K utilization by intact liver cells, deficiency of this vitamin is not rare.

Etiology. As in the case of virtually all deficiency states, vitamin K deficiency should be regarded as the expression of an underlying disorder rather than simply a disease within itself. Accordingly its etiology should be considered in terms of the contributing conditions outlined above.

Genetics. In general vitamin K deficiency is acquired. However, in certain instances the mechanisms of deficiency may be caused by a heritable disorder, notably the malabsorption of vitamin K in cystic fibrosis and in cholelithiasis with obstructive jaundice secondary to hereditary hemolytic anemias.

As more is learned about vitamin K, additional principles may be discovered that are involved in the formation of Ca^{++}-binding sites in vitamin K–dependent proteins. Deficiency of such a principle, perhaps genetically determined, is suggested by the "Borgschulte syndrome" of congenital deficiency of factors II, VII, IX, and X, unassociated with malabsorption or liver dysfunction and partially responsive to daily oral administration of pharmacologic doses of vitamin K.[488,510]

Clinical features. The hemorrhagic manifestations of vitamin K deficiency are largely nonspecific and range from a mild bruising tendency or persistent oozing from minor surface wounds to generalized ecchymoses and life-threatening visceral or surface hemorrhage. Of note, however, is that symmetrical purpura, petechiae, and hemarthroses are not characteristic of vitamin K deficiency.

The onset of hemorrhagic signs is usually acute or subacute, typically suggestive of acquired rather than heritable disease. In most cases the history and physical examination should reveal evidence of an underlying disease. If such a disease is not apparent even after vitamin K deficiency is established, additional diagnostic measures should be undertaken. Of particular note in this regard is cystic fibrosis, which may surface in the early months of life with vitamin K deficiency before the disease is otherwise expressed. Hemorrhagic disease of the newborn is discussed on p. 813.

Laboratory evaluation. In general the laboratory diagnosis of vitamin K deficiency is clearcut, reflected in decreased activities of factors II, VII, IX, and X without thrombocytopenia or other abnormalities of coagulation. The PT and PTT are both variably prolonged but the TCT is normal; indeed, vitamin K deficiency is a particularly good example of a coagulation disorder in which the TCT is a helpful adjunct to initial screening with the PT and PTT. Ideally assays of the vitamin K–dependent factors should be carried out as well as assays of other selected factors such as fibrinogen and factors V and VIII. A response to parenteral vitamin K therapy ultimately establishes the diagnosis, even if a full array of assays is not carried out. It should be noted that direct measurements of vitamin K in plasma are not generally available or necessary for the laboratory evaluation of vitamin K deficiency.

Differential diagnosis. The principal hemorrhagic disorders from which vitamin K deficiency must be separated are the thrombocytopenic purpuras, coagulation disorders associated with parenchymal liver dysfunction, and DIC. In most instances laboratory evaluation readily differentiates the effects of vitamin K deficiency from other clinically similar disorders. However, it should be recognized that hepatocellular dysfunction and malabsorption of vitamin K are not mutually exclusive. Thus, if there is evidence for malabsorption, supportive treatment with vitamin K is appropriate even if an optimal response in activities of factors II, VII, IX, and X is not observed.

Pathogenesis and pathophysiology. Beyond the neonatal period the most common cause of vitamin K deficiency is malabsorption of the vitamin from the upper small intestine caused by the underlying diseases listed on p. 802. Suppression of gastrointestinal bacterial flora by antibiotic therapy does not generally produce vitamin K deficiency unless there is a concomitant severe limitation in dietary intake.[452] In those rare instances in which a careful search for causes of vitamin K deficiency is unrewarding, accidental or deliberate ingestion of coumarin agents should be considered.[514,495] Although pharmacologic antagonism of vitamin K may theoretically occur with agents other than coumarin compounds (such as aspirin) significant vitamin K deficiency induced by these agents is rare.

The common denominator of the pathophysiology of vitamin K deficiency is the failure of vitamin K–dependent factors to acquire Ca^{++}-binding sites that are essential for their attachment to phospholipids and consequent interaction with other coagulation factors.

The molecules of factors II, VII, IX, and X are first synthesized in the hepatocyte independent of vitamin K and are complete except for the absence of specific carboxyl radicals; the resulting molecule in each case is functionally inert in terms of Ca^{++} binding or adsorption to barium salts and similar compounds. These PIVKA[461] molecules are now known as descarboxy proteins, e.g., descarboxyprothrombin.[524] In a postribosomal vitamin K–dependent step within the hepatocyte, carboxyl radicals are in some way attached to glutamic acids of the precursor molecule to form γ-carboxyglutamic acids, which then render the molecule functionally competent in terms of Ca^{++}-binding and adsorption to appropriate salts.[447,480,522] Although these generalizations are largely based on studies of prothrombin, available evidence suggests that they are applicable to vitamin K–dependent proteins in general.

Thus vitamin K deficiency caused by a systemic lack of this vitamin or its antagonism by coumarin compounds is characterized not by lack of circulating molecules of factors II, VII, IX, and X but by inability of these molecules to bind Ca^{++} and therefore to participate in coagulation. The mechanism or mechanisms whereby vitamin K performs its vital role and may be blocked by certain pharmacologic agents have not yet been established.

Pathology. There are no specific pathologic findings associated with the functional defects or hemorrhagic manifestations of vitamin K deficiency.

Management. Clinical and laboratory signs of vitamin K deficiency in children are, by definition, corrected in time by the intravenous administration of an arbitrary dose of vitamin K_1, usually about 1 mg. (It should be noted that 1 mg of vitamin K_1 for a 10 kg child is more than 100 times the daily requirement for this vitamin.) The need for additional vitamin K and the route of its administration depend on the nature of the underlying disorder, especially its reversibility. Thus long-term management of vitamin K deficiency, if needed, must be empirically developed on an individual basis.

The intravenous administration of a single dose of vitamin K_1 to a deficient patient is usually followed by clinical cessation of active bleeding within a few hours, substantial improvement in activities of the vitamin K–dependent factors within 1 day, and complete correction of all coagulation functions within about 3 days. In the event of life-threatening hemorrhage complicating vitamin K deficiency, immediate replacement therapy with plasma or a commercially available prothrombin complex concentrate may be considered in addition to vitamin K therapy. However, such replacement therapy is rarely if ever needed. Intravenous vitamin K should be given slowly, about 1 mg/minute, and the remote possibility of an anaphylactic reaction should be kept in mind.

In the event that parenteral vitamin K therapy does not correct hemorrhage and deficiencies of the vitamin K–dependent coagulation factors, simple vitamin K deficiency does not exist and other disorders must be investigated, notably parenchymal liver disease.

Prognosis. Vitamin K deficiency defined in terms of systemic lack or pharmacologic antagonism is a completely curable disorder. Of course, the prognosis hinges on the nature of the underlying disease rather than on the deficiency of vitamin K.

Future perspectives. At the present time the clinical issues of vitamin K deficiency itself do not pose major problems. Diagnosis is well-defined and treatment is both effective and simple. However, the role of vitamin K in coagulation and the mechanisms of its pharmacologic antagonism are not yet completely explained despite the incredible achievements of the past 50 years. Thus the future challenge of vitamin K clearly lies in continuing basic research.

Disseminated intravascular coagulation

Disseminated intravascular coagulation (DIC, consumption coagulopathy, defibrination syndrome) is an acquired hemorrhagic disorder that is associated with an underlying disease and is characterized by multiple deficiencies of hemostasis suggesting uncontrolled activation of coagulation and fibrinolysis. Deficiencies of hemostasis typically include thrombocytopenia; decreased plasma fibrinogen concentration and decreased activities of factors II (prothrombin), V, and VIII; evidence for increased fibrinolytic activity, i.e., an elevated titer of fibrin and fibrinogen degradation products (FDP); and decreased plasma concentration of antithrombin III (AT-III). (DIC is also discussed on pp. 41-42.)

Historical perspective. The clot-promoting property of tissue extracts and its important role in normal hemostasis were firmly established at the turn of the twentieth century.[492] However, for many years thereafter it was not appreciated that pathologic "thromboplastinemia" might occur in humans, resulting in depletion of clotting factors and paradoxically a hemorrhagic state. In 1936 Dieckmann[443] described the occurrence of hemorrhage with unclottable blood in a patient with abruptio placentae. In 1951 Schneider[515] confirmed the finding of defibrination in cases of abruptio placentae and used the term "disseminated intravascular coagulation" to describe the pathophysiology of this disorder. He suggested that the process was initiated by abruption-induced leakage into the circulation of tissue thromboplastin that in turn activated coagulation with consequent disappearance of fibrinogen. He further suggested that treatment of this disorder might consist of anticoagulation during the active process and replacement therapy on its subsidence.

With the explosion of new knowledge about coagulation and fibrinolysis that began in the early 1950s there was a concomitant surge of interest in the pathophysiology and clinical management of DIC, which reached a peak in the late 1960s. The clinical interest in DIC was greatly promoted by encouraging results of heparin therapy for purpura fulminans in children, first described by Little[479] in 1959. During the past decade it has become increasingly clear that heparin is not a panacea for DIC and that, with few exceptions, control of the disease underlying DIC is the key to management rather than therapeutic manipulation of coagulation and fibrinolytic activities.

Since 1950 much literature on DIC has accumulated, including excellent review articles and texts by McKay,[485] Hardaway,[459] and Minna et al.[491]

Classification. Since DIC is a complication of an underlying disease, an etiologic classification is most appropriate:

A. Infections
  1. Parasitic, e.g., malaria
  2. Mycotic
  3. Bacterial, e.g., meningococcemia
  4. Rickettsial, e.g., Rocky Mountain spotted fever
B. Neoplasms, e.g., promyelocytic leukemia
C. Immunologic disorders
  1. Transfusion reactions with intravascular hemolysis
  2. Drug reactions
D. States with extensive tissue damage
  1. Severe trauma
  2. Burns
  3. Heat stroke
  4. Hemorrhagic shock
  5. Postoperative complications
E. Other disorders
  1. Giant hemangioma (Kasabach-Merritt syndrome)
  2. Snakebite
  3. Purpura fulminans
  4. In the newborn, e.g., from obstetrical complications, congenital or perinatal infection, or idiopathic respiratory distress syndrome

Incidence. Although fully expressed and life-threatening DIC is rare in children, its existence should be considered in the evaluation of hemorrhage complicating any underlying disease process.

Etiology. Implicit in the very term "disseminated intravascular coagulation" is an enormous and incompletely verifiable assumption regarding the etiology as well as the pathophysiology of a certain class of hemorrhagic disorders. There is no question that certain diseases may be complicated by hemorrhage associated with progressive depletion of coagulation factors. But there are a number of unresolved problems in applying to deficiencies of coagulation observed in humans a set of ideas largely based on activation of coagulation in test tubes and injection of coagulants into animals.

Genetics. Although genetic determinants may well play a role in DIC, such determinants are not clearly recognized at the present time.

Clinical features. The clinical picture of DIC is as diversified as the diseases with which it may be associated. However, certain salient features may be identified. First and foremost, the clinical hallmarks are impressive purpura, usually ecchymotic, and a pronounced tendency to surface bleeding in a very sick patient. Second, the affected patient typically shows evidence of anemia and variable circulatory failure, manifest by pallor, hypoperfusion of the fingers and toes, tachycardia, and lowered blood pressure if not shock. These features characterize acute DIC, which is the most common form of the disorder in children and adults, e.g., purpura fulminans and DIC complicating meningococcemia. A less fulminating clinical picture is seen in chronic expression of DIC in which the process of intravascular coagulation is apparently sustained in a low-grade fashion with partial compensation by the host, e.g., Kasabach-Merritt syndrome of thrombocytopenia with giant cavernous hemangioma. To identify representative clinical features of acute and chronic DIC in children, further comments about purpura fulminans and the Kasabach-Merritt syndrome may be helpful.

Purpura fulminans is an acute hemorrhagic necrosis of the skin that occurs typically though infrequently after various exanthems in childhood, notably varicella and streptococcal scarlet fever. The major clinical feature of purpura fulminans is highly symmetrical purpura typically involving the buttocks and lower extremities, although the ears, genitalia, and upper extremities may also be involved; the trunk is usually spared. Affected children are very sick and may not survive, although a previous mortality of well above 50% has undoubtedly been lowered since the introduction of heparin therapy by Little[479] in 1959, along with improved measures for supportive care. In surviving children partial amputations of affected extremities may be required for management of gangrene caused by irreversible ischemia.[412]

The Kasabach-Merritt syndrome, as originally described in 1940, is an association of a congenital giant cavernous hemangioma with thrombocytopenic purpura.[469] Since that time it has been shown in several carefully studied cases that thrombocytopenia is associated with abnormalities of coagulation and fibrinolysis, either disseminated or localized within the hemangioma.[462,465,529] The hemangioma is typically a large, solitary, and histologically benign lesion located in the subcutaneous tissue of the trunk, the neck, or an extremity of a young infant. However, Kasabach-Merritt syndrome has also been associated with hemangiomas with other characteristics, i.e., relatively small size, localization in visceral organs or bone, histologic malignancy, and occurrence in older children and adults.[519] The hemorrhagic component of Kasabach-Merritt syndrome is typically low grade and chronic, largely expressed as variable purpura in an otherwise asymptomatic patient. However, afibrinogenemia has been described in this syndrome,[529] and fatal hemorrhage contributes to an overall mortality of approximately 20%.[519] Signs of chronic DIC associated with this syndrome are effectively relieved by any therapeutic measure that successfully eradicates the hemangioma, including surgical excision or radiotherapy.

Laboratory evaluation. The proper laboratory evaluation of DIC constitutes the ultimate challenge to a clinical coagulation laboratory. Ideally such a laboratory should be equipped to perform selected tests covering the entire spectrum of hemostatic function, i.e., platelets, coagulation, fibrinolysis, and natural inhibitors of coagulation and fibrinolysis. Furthermore, such evaluation should be carried out sequentially as well as initially, depending on the clinical course of the patient and the changing expression of DIC.

Initial diagnostic measures should be doubly directed: (1) toward definition of the underlying disease and (2) toward identification of possible DIC in any seriously ill patient, particularly if a bleeding tendency is present. In the latter instance initial tests should consist of a platelet count, examination of all formed elements on a good blood smear with particular attention to shapes of red cells and numbers of platelets, an Ivy bleeding time test (unless prolonged oozing from finger prick or venipuncture sites has already been noted), and the following one-stage plasma screening tests: PT, PTT, and TCT as well if the PT and PTT are significantly prolonged. If these initial times are within normal limits, DIC probably does not exist at that time. But the diagnosis of DIC hinges on sequential clinical and laboratory observations; DIC is *never* ruled out by a single set of findings.

If at any time these initial test results are abnormal, assays for selected coagulation factors and titration of FDPs should be carried out and repeated serially as indicated by clinical events. The following profile is required for a laboratory diagnosis of DIC: a platelet count below 150×10^9/liter or a steadily falling count; significantly prolonged or increasing values of PT, PTT, and TCT; a significantly increased or rising titer of FDPs; and significantly low or falling concentration of fibrinogen and activities of prothrombin and factors V and VIII. Fragmentation of red cells on the blood smear is characteristic of microangiopathic disease and is not of itself indicative of DIC. (See Chapter 24.)

So far there has been relatively little experience in the application of tests of natural inhibitors of coagulation and fibrinolysis to coagulation disorders in general and DIC in particular. It can be confidently anticipated that antithrombin III and α_2-macroglobulin will be especially included in the laboratory evaluation of DIC since these are the principal inhibitors of thrombin and plasmin, respectively. Bick et al.[415] have confirmed evidence that antithrombin III activity is decreased in DIC and reflects the response to heparin therapy in this disorder.

A variety of so-called paracoagulation tests such as the ethanol gelation test[426] may be helpful adjuncts to the laboratory evaluation of DIC, but results of these tests are not sufficiently consistent to be relied on exclusively.

Differential diagnosis. If viewed in the broad context of hemorrhage in a sick patient, the differential diagnosis of DIC would appropriately encompass the entire spectrum of bleeding disorders. Therefore to be objectively separable from many clinically similar disorders DIC must be defined in terms of a rather rigid profile of labora-

Table 25-8. Test results in hemorrhagic states with overlapping characteristics*

| | Platelet tests | | Coagulation screening tests | | | Plasma coagulation factors | | | | | | | Fibrinolysis: FDP |
	Platelet count	Bleeding time	TCT	PT	PTT	I	II	V	VII	VIII	IX	X	
DIC	3	3	3	3	3	3	3	3	2	3	2	2	3
Parenchymal liver disease	2	2	2	3	3	2	3	2	3	1	3	3	2
Primary fibrinogenolysis	1	2	3	3	3	3	1	2	1	2	1	1	3
Cardiopulmonary bypass	2	2	2	2	2	2	1	2	1	2	1	1	2
Vitamin K deficiency	1	2	1	3	3	1	3	1	3	1	3	3	1
Heparin effect	1	2	3	2	3	1	1	2	1	1	3	1	1
Microangiopathic disease	3	3	1	1	1	1	1	1	1	1	1	1	1

*1, Usually normal; 2, variable; 3, usually abnormal.

tory findings in association with an underlying disease. Even so, DIC may be difficult or impossible to differentiate from other conditions that are also characterized by acquired multiple defects of hemostasis, as opposed to isolated platelet disorders and heritable deficiencies of single coagulation factors. Representative disorders with clinical and laboratory effects that may especially overlap with DIC as well as with each other include parenchymal liver disease, vitamin K deficiency, primary fibrinogenolysis, effects of surgical cardiopulmonary bypass, and microangiopathic disease. Differential laboratory characteristics of these disorders are outlined in Table 25-8. It should be emphasized that the members of this group are by no means mutually exclusive, notably DIC and liver failure.[508]

Pathogenesis and pathophysiology. In the face of tremendous advances in knowledge of hemostasis since the early 1950s it is noteworthy that the earliest views of the causes and effects of DIC have been extended but not discarded or replaced by better ideas. For more detailed information the reader should consult other sources previously cited and comprehensive reviews published in 1977.*

DIC is attributed to any underlying pathologic process that activates the coagulation component of hemostasis beyond limits that can be controlled by the host. The coagulation mechanism may be excessively activated by stimuli variously affecting the intrinsic and extrinsic pathways as well as the direct conversion of fibrinogen to fibrin. However, the mechanisms whereby such stimulation is mediated are incompletely understood. For example, the major roles formerly assigned to endothelial damage and activation of factor XII in the pathogenesis of DIC via the intrinsic pathway are increasingly suspect.[494] On the other hand, it is generally accepted that the extrinsic

pathway may be stimulated by circulating thromboplastins such as the products of immune hemolysis, endotoxin-induced lysis of granulocytes, and various neoplasms.

The central pathophysiologic element of DIC is excessive generation of thrombin, combined with secondary generation of plasmin, failure of control mechanisms to harness these and related powerful enzymes, and inability of synthesis to replace losses. As a result, the normally well-ordered cascade system accelerates acutely or chronically, and hemostasis is correspondingly attacked by its own dangerous arsenal of serine protease "arrows" instead of being effectively defended by them. In this process the plasma component of the circulating blood is variably stripped of its coagulation and fibrinolytic factors as well as critical antiproteases and progressively resembles serum. However, intravascular fibrin, unlike the clot in a test tube, tends to be effectively removed by secondary fibrinolysis. Also, activated coagulation factors are rapidly cleared from the circulation by the reticuloendothelial system, particularly the liver.[442]

There is compelling evidence to support this interpretation of DIC, including certain similarities between DIC in humans and the effects of direct injection of coagulants into experimental animals.[431a,500] Also, increased knowledge of the forces involved in the activation and control of hemostasis supports the potentially dire effects of regulatory failure, granting that the clinical application of such knowledge requires assumptions largely derived from studies in vitro.

In any event, confirmation of current concepts of the pathogenesis and pathophysiology of DIC will ultimately depend on proof of the primary role of pathologic generation of thrombin in this disorder. So far all the evidence for intravascular coagulation is based on a constellation of effects that are presumed to be *secondary* to increased thrombin generation, rather than on direct mea-

*References 423, 460, 494, 497.

surements of thrombin itself; this enzyme is cleared from the circulation too rapidly to be detected by current techniques. In the meantime, an impressive case can be made for thrombin as the central enzyme among many in the production of DIC.

Pathology. It should be emphasized that DIC is a pathophysiologic mechanism complicating any primary inflammatory, degenerative, or neoplastic process; it is not itself a pathologic state in an anatomical sense. Therefore DIC is not characterized by specific pathologic findings. Rather, postmortem findings reflect the effects of the underlying disease and the net effect of the interactions between coagulation, fibrinolysis, and control mechanisms in the host at the time of death. Findings relevant to DIC may include widespread fibrin thrombi, particularly in small blood vessels, and variable hemorrhagic necrosis of organ tissues, presumably resulting from sustained ischemia. Such findings may be observed in virtually any organ or tissue, particularly the kidneys, where changes associated with DIC may vary from focal tubular necrosis to bilateral renal cortical necrosis. Autopsy of patients following fully expressed DIC may show no evidence of intravascular fibrin or tissue necrosis necessarily resulting from vascular obstruction.[487] It should be noted that widespread fibrin-containing thrombi in small vessels is characteristic of thrombotic thrombocytopenic purpura,[493] a disease in which DIC is usually not identifiable by customary criteria.[477]

The diversified pathologic findings that may be associated with DIC are described in detail by McKay.[485]

Management. There are three major ingredients of the overall management of DIC: (1) aggressive treatment of the underlying disease, (2) general supportive care of the patient, and (3) specific measures intended to control DIC itself.

The first two principles are unquestionable, particularly treatment of the underlying disease on which the major hope for a successful outcome of the patient largely depends. General supportive measures include whole blood transfusion for hypovolemia and shock, packed red cells for isovolemic anemia, control of significant temperature abnormalities, and careful assessment and management of any organ failure that may be present, notably renal failure. Furthermore, in the case of a patient with active surface bleeding there should be no hesitation to administer initially fresh whole plasma in a dose of 10 to 15 ml/kg body weight (depending on whole blood also given) and 5 bags of platelet concentrates/m² body surface. Such treatment constitutes conservative replacement therapy of depleted platelets and coagulation factors as well as antithrombin III. Rather than ''add-

ing fuel to the fire,'' such treatment has often been associated with objective control of bleeding and in these instances has been continued as indicated by clinical circumstances of the patient.[421] If this initial approach is not helpful, it should be discontinued in favor of measures specifically designed to control intravascular coagulation.

Although there are no generally accepted guidelines for anticoagulant therapy of DIC, there is general agreement that heparin is the single agent of choice and that it should be administered intravenously. Since heparin potentiates the inhibition of thrombin, plasmin, and activated factors XII, XI, IX, and X by antithrombin III, theoretically it is an ideal agent for treatment of DIC, providing there is an adequate level of antithrombin III apart from which heparin has no meaning as an anticoagulant for DIC or any other condition. It is becoming increasingly recognized that previous evaluation of heparin therapy for DIC has not generally included attention to antithrombin III levels; this lack will surely be corrected by future clinical studies and may account for at least some of the failures of heparin therapy in the past. Thus future regimens for DIC will undoubtedly include recommendations not only for heparin but also for replacement of antithrombin III as indicated, perhaps through plasma therapy.

An appropriate daily intravenous dose of heparin for children with DIC is 300 to 600 units/kg given either as intermittent injections of 50 to 100 units/kg every 4 hrs or as a continuous infusion of 10 to 20 units/kg/hr following an initial loading dose of about 50 units/kg. Although there are no definitive studies that have established the relative merits of these two regimens, continuous infusion is increasingly recommended on the grounds that it is more physiologic and possibly safer. There is some evidence that the relatively large doses of heparin that are given intermittently may aggravate existing hemorrhage in certain instances of DIC.[445]

If heparin is effective in the treatment of DIC, depleted plasma factors may be restored rather promptly, e.g., as early as 24 hours after initiation of therapy, while the platelet count tends to rise more slowly.[412] On intermittent schedules all coagulation activities may be measured in preheparin plasma samples, since heparin effects are largely dissipated wthin 4 hours. On continuous infusion the PT may be useful for monitoring coagulation function since it is less responsive to heparin effects than the TCT or PTT;[489] the effects of continuing DIC versus continuous infusion of heparin on prolongation of the TCT and PTT may be difficult to differentiate. On the other hand, a normal or nearly normal PT combined with consistent prolongations of the PTT and TCT within given limits should indicate control of DIC *and* appropriate anticoagulation of patients on continuous infusion of heparin. Other plasma factors and serum FDPs may be measured as desired to monitor progress. The platelet count is a particularly valuable test in children since it is an important indicator of the status of DIC, is generally unaffected by heparin, and does not require venous blood. We think that the whole blood clotting time is not a useful method for monitoring heparin therapy in children.

In heparin-responsive DIC anticoagulation should be maintained until all plasma factors and the platelet count have stabilized at normal levels. Promyelocytic leukemia and purpura fulminans appear to be prime examples of disorders in which associated DIC is frequently responsive to heparin, even without consideration of antithrombin III levels, in these states.*

Heparin is by no means a complete answer to DIC,[432] and failures in its use, including aggravation of bleeding and irreversibility of the underlying disease, are generally more likely than successes. Thus it is appropriate to defer heparinization if the diagnosis is not clear, if the patient's underlying disease is specifically and effectively treatable, and if the patient has evidence of reasonable clinical stability despite DIC.

Given optimal treatment of the primary disease and general supportive care of the patient with DIC, if heparin therapy fails there are no other well-defined options for attempting to control the DIC itself. EACA, a strong inhibitor of plasminogen activator activity and a weak inhibitor of plasmin, has no recognized place in the treatment of DIC; increased fibrinolysis in DIC is usually secondary to activation of coagulation and presumably protects against ischemia by removing intravascular fibrin. On the other hand, EACA is an appropriate agent for treatment of primary fibrinolysis, or more correctly "fibrinogenolysis." Thus in the event of heparin failure in DIC the addition of EACA to heparin therapy may be appropriate if there is evidence for primary fibrinogenolysis, such as rapid lysis of a whole blood clot or a short euglobulin lysis time. However, such findings in DIC are extremely rare. Treatment of DIC with EACA alone is contraindicated since serious thrombotic complications may occur.[486] Dextran has been used with success in the treatment of purpura fulminans,[498] but there has been insufficient experience with this agent in DIC to determine its overall usefulness. This agent is primarily an inhibitor of platelet aggregation with slight heparin-like effects and would not seem as likely to offer benefits for the wide-ranging deficiencies of DIC as heparin itself.

Prognosis. At the present time the prognosis of

*References 410, 412, 454, 456, 463, 479.

DIC must largely be viewed in terms of the prognosis of the underlying disease and the severity of the DIC. A good outcome is associated with those diseases that are susceptible to specific medical or surgical treatment rather than with advances in anticoagulant treatment of DIC, despite the encouraging results of heparin therapy in purpura fulminans.

Future perspectives. It seems unlikely that current concepts of DIC as an expression of uncontrolled thrombin generation and secondary fibrinolysis will be drastically altered. As progress in the understanding of hemostasis continues, the view of DIC will continue to be enlarged, perhaps including better understanding of the manner in which various stimuli drastically disorganize the coagulation cascade and related systems.

Above all, a major future requirement for DIC is improvement in the therapy of DIC itself, apart from treatment of its underlying diseases. An important step has already been taken through Rosenberg's precise definition of antithrombin III as heparin cofactor, along with increasing awareness of the importance of this and other natural inhibitors in the control of coagulation and fibrinolysis. For example, it will be immensely interesting to determine whether closer attention to antithrombin III levels in plasma will improve the results of heparin therapy, at least in some patients.

Parenchymal liver disease

Normal liver function is critical to hemostasis, particularly the coagulation component. This organ is the site of synthesis of fibrinogen, factor V, the vitamin K–dependent factors (prothrombin, VII, IX, and X), and probably other coagulation factors as well as the major natural inhibitors of coagulation and fibrinolysis.[490] The liver is also involved in the clearance from plasma of activated coagulation factors and plasminogen activators.[442,450] Finally, liver disease of virtually any type may be associated with thrombocytopenia from hepatic or splenic platelet sequestration, and qualitative platelet defects have also been described.[481]

Thus it is not surprising that Deutsch[441] found that 85% of patients with liver disease had evidence of one or more abnormalities of hemostasis and 15% of these patients presented clinical bleeding problems. There is no recognized association of a given profile of abnormal coagulation and a given variety of liver disease. However, there is a general correlation between the degree of hepatocellular disease and resulting coagulation abnormalities.[510]

The most characteristic coagulation disorder of parenchymal liver disease is a depression of the vitamin K–dependent factors associated with prolongation of the PT and PTT and unresponsive to parenteral administration of vitamin K. However, the effects of vitamin K deficiency and hepatocellular disease are not necessarily mutually exclusive, as in biliary cirrhosis. The finding of normal or high factor VIII activity in the presence of otherwise defective hemostasis in liver disease may be helpful in differentiating effects of this disease from those of DIC. On the other hand, these two coagulation disorders not only overlap (Table 25-8) but also may coexist.

Major ingredients of treatment for coagulation disorders of liver disease should include parenteral administration of vitamin K to exclude its possible deficiency and conservative replacement therapy with whole plasma and platelets as clinically indicated. Prothrombin complex concentrates should be used with caution if at all in view of possible thrombogenic complications from their use.[419] Likewise heparin and antifibrinolytic agents should be avoided unless clearly indicated by evidence for DIC or fibrinogenolysis, respectively.

Congenital heart disease

A variety of relatively minor abnormalities of hemostasis may be acquired in about 10% of children with congenital heart disease of either cyanotic or noncyanotic types.[484] The most common abnormality appears to be an incompletely defined qualitative platelet defect cited in Chapter 24, but thrombocytopenia and coagulation disorders have also been described. In general the observed defects do not fit well-defined pathophysiologic categories, either within themselves or in relation to the cardiac lesions with which they may be associated. However, in cyanotic congenital heart disease there appears to be a correlation between a variable bleeding tendency, the finding of one or more abnormalities of hemostasis, and the severity of cardiac disease. Indeed, the observation of deficiencies of coagulation combined with thrombocytopenia and activation of fibrinolysis in certain patients with cyanotic congenital heart disease has suggested effects of DIC.[440,473] However, these findings have not been confirmed in other studies of similar patients.[446,468]

From a practical point of view it should be emphasized that apparent deficiency of coagulation in patients with erythrocytosis and cyanotic congenital heart disease can sometimes be instantly "cured" by redrawing a blood sample into a volume of citrate properly adjusted for the high hematocrit. Conventional citration of blood samples with hematocrits ranging above 50% produces proportional overcitration as well as excessive dilution of the plasma sample to be tested.[489]

In any case, careful attention to the clinical history and to selected laboratory tests of hemostasis is clearly warranted in the evaluation of any child with congenital heart disease, especially prior to surgery. However, it is most uncommon for observed abnormalities of hemostasis to contraindicate proceeding with appropriate cardiac surgery. Indeed, such defects are generally relieved in time following successful cardiac repair.

Surgical cardiopulmonary bypass

Cardiopulmonary bypass is now a standard procedure in corrective open-heart surgery in children and adults. However, it is widely recognized that this procedure may be complicated by a variety of hemostatic derangements, occurring in 5% to 25% of cases.[499,528] This subject has been comprehensively reviewed in a series of reports in 1976.*

At the outset it must be emphasized that abnormal bleeding following cardiopulmonary bypass will undoubtedly occur in those patients who have a preexisting bleeding tendency; this discussion assumes that such defects have been ruled out by appropriate preoperative evaluation. There is no satisfactory unitary concept for hemorrhage after cardiopulmonary bypass. For example, although DIC may account for this disorder in certain instances and while the alterations of hemostasis in these two conditions overlap considerably, there is increasing evidence that DIC is not operative in the majority of cases. In his review of this subject Bick[414] suggested that a twofold defect predominates: (1) an incompletely defined thrombocytopathy, occurring in virtually all patients and apparently independent of variable thrombocytopenia that may also be observed, and (2) primary fibrinogenolysis, occurring in the majority of patients and characterized by variably decreased activities of plasmin substrates, i.e., fibrinogen and factors V, VIII, and XII. Aside from such causes and as in the case of any postoperative hemorrhage, incomplete surgical hemostasis must always be considered. In the event of certain specific complications such as hepatic or renal insufficiency from any cause, further variables will be added to the etiology of hemorrhage after cardiopulmonary bypass. Incomplete neutralization of heparin by protamine sulfate may contribute significantly to such hemorrhage.

Since the hemostatic alterations that may follow cardiopulmonary bypass are multifactorial, management must be individualized on the basis of findings in specific cases. However, the following generalizations may be offered in regard to diagnosis and treatment. First, blood for diagnostic studies should never be obtained from venous lines maintained in any fashion with heparin, however dilute. Although tests exist for identifying heparin

---

*References 414, 449, 475, 483.

effects, the separation of local from systemic heparin effects is virtually impossible unless the site of venous sampling is free of extra heparin. Second, while laboratory studies are being carried out to define the bleeding problem treatment should consist of conservative replacement therapy with standard blood products, i.e., administration of appropriate platelet concentrates and, depending on the degree of bleeding and its effects, fresh whole plasma. Empirical trials with specific agents that alter coagulation and fibrinolysis cannot be recommended; their use should be governed by laboratory findings. For example, it has been shown that EACA is clearly useful in the control of hemorrhage associated with objective evidence of excessive fibrinolysis.[472,502] However, as previously noted, the blind use of this agent would be inappropriate and possibly dangerous in a patient subsequently shown to have the findings of DIC.

Renal disease

Inconsistent alterations of coagulation have been described in association with microangiopathic diseases such as the hemolytic-uremic syndrome. However, it is now generally held that thrombocytopenia from accelerated removal of damaged platelets rather than DIC is the central hemostatic defect in these diseases. (See Chapter 24.)

The nephrotic syndrome may be associated with abnormalities of coagulation factor activities.[467] Fibrinogen concentration and factor VIII activity are usually increased, but activities of factors IX[458] and XII[464] may be decreased as a result of their excessive urinary loss. Generally these changes are not clinically significant, but screening tests of hemostasis and an assay of factor IX activity may be appropriate before renal biopsy or major surgical procedures are undertaken.

Dysproteinemias

The dysproteinemias comprise a group of disorders characterized by high circulating levels of abnormal plasma proteins, notably multiple myeloma, Waldenström's macroglobulinemia, and cryoglobulinemia. These disorders are rare in children but may be associated with a bleeding tendency in 15% to 36% of cases along with a wide spectrum of deficiencies of hemostasis affecting coagulation, fibrinolysis, and platelets.[501]

Clinical bleeding appears to be most closely correlated with defective platelet function, perhaps mediated by excessive adsorption onto platelets of abnormal proteins. Defective polymerization of fibrin monomer has also been demonstrated in dysproteinemia and may contribute to the bleeding tendency in some cases.[451] A direct connection between dysproteinemia and defective hemostasis is suggested by an improvement in hemostasis

that usually occurs after the concentration of abnormal proteins is lowered by plasmapheresis.

The dysproteinemias occur almost entirely in adults and therefore rarely warrant consideration in the differential diagnosis of hemostatic disorders in children.

Acquired inhibitors of coagulation (circulating anticoagulants)

For more than two decades it has been recognized that inhibitors of coagulation may be acquired in a variety of clinical circumstances. In recent years the nature of these inhibitors and management of the clinical demands imposed by them have become major subjects of clinical and basic investigation. Acquired inhibitors may be divided into two broad groups: those directed against a single coagulation factor and those directed at interactions among coagulation factors, notably the inhibitor associated with systemic lupus erythematosus, or so-called lupus anticoagulant. Although acquired inhibitors continue to pose major problems in their clinical management, there has been much progress in their immunochemical characterization: they are immunoglobulins, largely of the IgG class, and frequently restricted in subclass composition; usually they do not fix complement.[517] For detailed information about acquired inhibitors the reader should consult the first major review of this subject in 1961 by Margolius et al.[482] as well as more recent articles.*

It should be emphasized that the acquired inhibitors in question are distinct from the following: natural inhibitors of coagulation and fibrinolysis (antithrombin III, α_2-macroglobulin, α_1-antitrypsin, and $C\bar{1}$ inhibitor); therapeutic anticoagulants (heparin and coumarins); and acquired nonimmune inhibitors of hemostasis (FDPs of fibrinolysis and excessive concentration of abnormal proteins in dysproteinemia).

Specific inhibitors. Inhibitors of specific coagulation factors are most commonly acquired by persons with heritable deficiency of a single factor, but they may also arise in association with other disorders as well as in previously healthy persons with no underlying disease. Factor VIII inhibitors occur most frequently, but well-documented inhibitors against the following coagulation factors have also been described: fibrinogen, prothrombin, and factors V, IX, XI, and XIII.[517] Inconclusive evidence exists for inhibitors against factors VII and X. In some instances inhibitors have been doubly directed at factors XI and XII but not XII alone.[434]

Factor VIII inhibitors may be acquired by about 15% of persons with classical hemophilia (usually

*References 416, 420, 448, 517.

in severe cases) as well as by nonhemophilic persons of either sex. The latter group includes postpartum females, persons with underlying diseases or drug reactions, elderly persons, and previously well persons of any age. Certainly in pediatric practice factor VIII inhibitors are largely limited to certain children with severe classical hemophilia.

The reasons for emergence of inhibitors in classical hemophilia as well as in other circumstances are incompletely understood. Undoubtedly this complication develops in relation both to presently unknown intrinsic (genetic?) factors and to the quantity of exposure to factor VIII replacement therapy. Strauss[525] presented evidence that 100 treatment days may represent a critical point at which an inhibitor will have been acquired or else probably will not arise, even with continued treatment. A final answer on this hypothesis is not yet available. In any case, it should be emphasized that the possibility of inhibitor development does not warrant any restrictions on replacement therapy for children with hemophilia. Indeed, the incidence of inhibitor development has not appeared to increase significantly with the advent of factor VIII concentrates and their use in home treatment programs.[470]

In most instances factor VIII inhibitors first appear in childhood. Once established, these inhibitors tend to persist, with rising titers within 2 to 3 weeks after factor VIII exposure, and then gradual fall over months in the absence of such treatment. In nonhemophilic persons factor VIII inhibitors are more likely to disappear in time if the affected person survives the encounter with this complication.

Factor VIII inhibitors are antibodies, largely of the IgG class, with relatively restricted subclass composition; in most cases heavy-chain typing has shown IgG (which does not fix complement), whereas light-chain composition has been more variable.[517] The interaction of factor VIII and its inhibitors is dependent on time and temperature, but the molecular and kinetic properties of this interaction are incompletely understood. However, major progress in more uniform quantitation of factor VIII inhibitors has recently occurred through the introduction of the so-called Bethesda unit, i.e., the activity in 1 ml of inhibitor plasma that reduces the 1 factor VIII unit in 1 ml of normal plasma to 0.5 factor VIII unit after 2 hours of incubation of the mixture under standard conditions.[471] The Bethesda unit is not intended to predict response to factor VIII replacement therapy. However, the definition does suggest an approximate response as follows: if a patient with 10 Bethesda units/ml is given a dose of factor VIII designed to produce a level of 10 units/ml (i.e., 1000%)

the factor VIII activity expected after the infusion would by only 0.5 units/ml (i.e., 50%). It should be readily evident that factor VIII replacement therapy of acquired inhibitors becomes increasingly inappropriate, both financially and logistically, with increasing inhibitor potency.

As to treatment of factor VIII inhibitors, it should be emphasized that the rational principles for replacement therapy of most patients with classical hemophilia simply do not apply. Thus there is not yet a concensus on management of patients with inhibitors although the following two principles are generally held: (1) Treatment is limited to supportive care only unless the bleeding episode is life-threatening or associated with unacceptable pain. (2) Where indicated, treatment is generally designed to provide clinical benefit by effecting a net gain of clot-promoting activity over inhibitor activity. Treatment modalities in the second category include high-dose intermittent or continuous infusion of human factor VIII concentrates, whole blood exchange transfusion and/or plasmapheresis combined with human factor VIII concentrates, animal factor VIII concentrates (porcine or bovine), and infusion of prothrombin complex concentrates. Results of treatment of inhibitors with immunosuppressive agents have been variable and inconclusive.[455]

The use of prothrombin complex concentrates for treatment of factor VIII inhibitors was described by Kurczynski and Penner[474] in 1974. Although the mechanism of action of prothrombin complex concentrate in this setting is unknown, it is presumed that this agent, which contains factor X (along with prothrombin and factors VII and IX), bypasses the block at the factor VIII step of coagulation imposed by the inhibitor. Prothrombin complex concentrates are commercially available in two forms: "regular," containing procoagulants only, and "activated," containing variable coagulant activities of the vitamin K–dependent factors. The relative safety and effectiveness of these two forms in the treatment of acquired factor VIII inhibitors are currently subjects of considerable debate.[422]

This discussion should not be taken to imply that patients with classical hemophilia who develop factor VIII inhibitors are continually in the throes of drastic treatment. Indeed, most children who acquire inhibitors are able to stay at home and go to school since the bleeding tendency is not increased by this complication. The problem is management of those bleeding episodes that do occur, particularly at times when the inhibitor activity may be increased beyond the reach of reasonable factor VIII therapy.

The specific inhibitor of factor VIII that has been described is directed at the coagulation principle of factor VIII. Inhibitors of the von Willebrand factor (ristocetin cofactor) have also been described, both in nonhemophilic persons[457,466] and in a patient with severe von Willebrand's disease.[513]

Specific inhibitors of coagulation factors other than factor VIII are uncommon, especially in children. As in the case of factor VIII inhibitors, the others have appeared in persons with congenital deficiency of a given factor, those without such deficiency but having an underlying disease (notably systemic lupus erythematosus), and normal persons. Of interest among this group is the association of acquired factor XIII inhibitors and chronic isoniazid therapy in four adults whose inhibitors cleared spontaneously on discontinuation of this agent.[517] The cause-and-effect relation in these instances is not conclusive, but the association is probably not entirely coincidental.

It may finally be noted that inhibitors against the following coagulation factors have been described in association with systemic lupus erythematosus: factor VIII,[509] von Willebrand factor,[520] factor IX,[430] factor XI,[430] and factors XI and XII combined.[434] However, these specific factor inhibitors are much less common in systemic lupus erythematosus than the nonspecific inhibitor known as the lupus anticoagulant.

Nonspecific inhibitor: lupus anticoagulant. In 1952 Conley and Hartmann[431] first described a circulating anticoagulant in two adult patients with systemic lupus erythematosus. Since that time the occurrence of a nonspecific anticoagulant in about 6% of patients with systemic lupus erythematosus has been fully established.[448] This inhibitor is primarily expressed in prolongation of the PTT, using both the patient's plasma alone and a mixture of the patient's plasma and normal plasma; the PT may be slightly prolonged, and the TCT is typically normal. Unlike the specific inhibitors described above, the lupus anticoagulant is not directed at a given coagulation factor and therefore does not produce marked factor deficiencies. However, an isolated depression of prothrombin activity may be observed; the reason for this finding is unknown. Likewise, the mechanism of action of the lupus anticoagulant is poorly understood, but available evidence suggests that it inhibits interactions involving formation of prothrombinase (factors V and activated X, platelet factor 3, and Ca^{++}) and/or the conversion of prothrombin to thrombin by prothrombinase.[448,532] The lupus anticoagulant has been associated with IgG antibodies, IgM antibodies, and a mixture of both IgG and IgM antibodies.[476]

The lupus anticoagulant usually is not associated with defective hemostasis, and even major surgery has been uneventfully performed in its presence.[425]

However, at times intensity of the inhibitor may parallel the intensity of the underlying disease.[433] It should be emphasized that the lupus anticoagulant and one or more specific coagulation factor inhibitors are not mutually exclusive findings in systemic lupus erythematosus. Thus individual factor assays should still be performed to identify possible concomitant specific inhibitors; these, unlike the lupus anticoagulant, usually do cause a significant bleeding tendency. Finally, Schleider et al.[514] have shown that twenty-nine of fifty-eight patients with a lupus anticoagulant did not show evidence of concomitant systemic lupus erythematosus.

Other acquired coagulation deficiencies

With the advent of increasingly vigorous chemotherapy for childhood cancer, both oncologists and generalists have become increasingly aware of a spectrum of complications that may result from such therapy. So far, iatrogenic alteration of coagulation as distinct from secondary thrombocytopenia has been largely limited to effects of L-asparaginase.[413] Use of this agent, particularly in the induction of remission in lymphoblastic leukemia, has been associated at times with hypofibrinogenemia. The mechanism of this complication is incompletely understood, but it appears that the cause may be decreased fibrinogen synthesis rather than DIC as initially presumed. Measurement of the plasma fibrinogen concentration is recommended before and during therapy with L-asparaginase, and this agent should be discontinued in the unlikely event of significant hypofibrinogenemia.

Although amyloidosis is virtually nonexistent in children, the reported association of this disorder with isolated factor X deficiency in a few adults[453] deserves brief mention. Following appropriate replacement therapy the selective fall-off of factor X is so rapid in these cases that the plasma level is not raised. Presumably factor X clearance is somehow mediated by the amyloid tissue, since no circulating factor X inhibitor has been demonstrated.[517] Occurrence of this unusual disorder in children has not yet been described.

NEONATAL COAGULATION DEFICIENCIES

The clotting mechanism of all newborn infants is different quantitatively and qualitatively from that of adults. The dysfunction of the platelets has been discussed in Chapter 24. The infant has lower levels of the plasma clotting factors present in the cord blood, which has been called a "physiologic" deficiency. This deficiency is a result of immaturity of the liver enzyme system, which produces all of the clotting proteins and is reflected in lower levels of factors II, VII, IX, X, XI, and XII. These levels decrease further during the first

3 days of life and then rise to the normal adult levels within 2 weeks, with a lag period of as long as 9 months for factors IX and XI in some infants. The levels of prekallikrein Fletcher factor and high molecular weight kininogens (Fitzgerald, Flaujeac, and Williams factors) are also low in newborns and there appears to be a qualitative difference in the type of fibrinogen present, suggesting the presence of a "fetal" fibrinogen. The fall of the levels of factors II, VII, IX, and X within the first 3 days of life is associated with a vitamin K deficiency. Several factors contribute to this physiologic deficiency: the bacteria-free nature of the newborn infant's intestinal tract, which prevents the vitamin K synthesis until intestinal flora are established with food ingestion; a lack of reserve supply of the vitamin; and impaired utilization because of liver immaturity and dysfunction. Although vitamin K crosses the placenta, absolute values in the infant's circulation are dependent on the mother's diet or therapeutic supplements. However, this supply is cut off at delivery and the infant must wait for colonization of his own gut with organisms that produce a vitamin K of questionable value and until intake is sufficient to provide the necessary amount for the synthesis of factors II, VII, IX, and X (<1 $\mu g/kg/day$).

In the premature infant this physiologic deficiency may be even greater than in the full-term infant. Bleyer et al.[533] have shown the physiologic differences from the adult in both full-term and premature infants, as shown in Fig. 25-11. Levels of the vitamin K–dependent factors II, VII, IX, and X are low in both full-term and premature infants. Factor V, also made in the liver, is present in normal adult levels in the healthy full-term infant but levels are low in premature infants. Levels of factor VIII, made in the endothelial cells, are normal in the full-term infant but may be as low as 20% in the 28-week-old premature infant.

Low levels of the clotting factors are reflected in longer normal levels of the screening tests for clotting function. For example, the PT in a normal newborn may be 16 to 18 seconds, with an adult control of 12.5 seconds, and the PTT may be 60 seconds, with an adult control of less than 40 seconds. A bleeding diathesis is not necessarily present unless these screening test examples are exceeded.

Concentrations of 20% to 25% of vitamin K–dependent clotting factors are critical values below which a potential hemorrhagic state exists.

Hemorrhagic disease of the newborn

Hemorrhagic disease of the newborn is a self-limited disease occurring between the first and fifth days of life in full-term infants as a result of a marked deficiency of the vitamin K–dependent clotting factors II, VII, IX, and X. The disease should not occur within the first 24 hours of life or after the fifth day in a well full-term infant. In premature infants the recovery period may be extended and there may be a slower return to normal clotting factor levels — as long as 2 to 3 weeks depending on gestational age. Bleeding may occur spontaneously when values of 5% or lower of one factor are reached or if levels of two or more of the prothrombin complex factors fall below 20%. The incidence was reported as 1/200 to 1/400 births, but it is much less common in full-term infants with improved diets in mothers and the widespread use of vitamin K. The extent to which hemorrhagic disease of the newborn may contribute to more severe bleeding problems in premature than full-term infants is unknown.

Bleeding is rarely massive but consists rather of oozing from the umbilical cord and circumcision site, hematemesis, hematuria, gastrointestinal and vaginal bleeding, ecchymosis, and occasional petechiae. Melena is the most common complaint. Central nervous system bleeding is rare. The diagnosis is made with a PT and PTT elevated above the levels for a normal newborn infant and low values for factors II, VII, IX, and X. The platelet count should be normal and anemia proportional to blood loss. The origin of the blood should be confirmed (whether blood is maternal or fetal in origin), before the clotting tests are done. The characteristics of the hemoglobin in the presence of alkali (Apt test) should help to clarify the origin of the blood, since fetal hemoglobin is alkali resistant and remains pink in solution whereas maternal hemoglobin turns brown.

Treatment consists of 1 mg of vitamin K, preferably in the form of vitamin K_1 (phytonadione) in an aqueous solution administered by intravenous

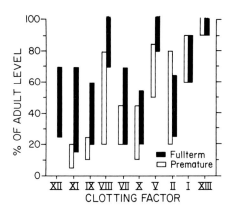

Fig. 25-11. Comparison of full-term and premature newborn coagulation factor activities with those of adults. (From Bleyer, W. A., Hakami, N., and Shepard, T. H.: J. Pediatr. **79:**838, 1971.)

or intramuscular injection. A response should be seen in 4 to 6 hours and additional doses should not be necessary although an additional 1 mg should not be harmful. Only high doses of certain vitamin K analogues (Hykinone) have been found to be complicated by significant hyperbilirubinemia and, in turn, by neurologic complications in the infant. If bleeding has been severe enough to cause the hemoglobin to fall below 12 gm/dl, packed red cells may be indicated, or if bleeding persists in a premature infant, fresh frozen plasma may be indicated to correct the clotting factor deficiency. However, in a full-term infant, if the prothrombin complex factors do not return to normal within 6 hours and bleeding ceases, other causes for the bleeding should be sought.

Today, however, treatment is prophylactic rather than therapeutic. Since vitamin K does cross the placenta, it was suggested by earlier studies that large doses of vitamin K be given to the mother just prior to delivery. But since the time of delivery cannot always be predicted, the final recommendation of the American Academy of Pediatrics[538] has been for the administration of 1 mg of vitamin K to all newborn infants at the time of delivery. This has resulted in the virtual elimination of hemorrhagic disease of the newborn in full-term infants whose mothers have good obstetrical care.

Other neonatal coagulation disorders

Inherited deficiencies. Other coagulation disorders that may cause bleeding in the newborn period have been mentioned as congenital disorders but deserve to be reviewed again. Severe classical hemophilia (factor VIII deficiency), von Willebrand's disease, and Christmas disease (factor IX deficiency) may present with bleeding secondary to trauma of birth. Massive cephalohematoma is not unusual. Bleeding following circumcision or bleeding from the cord may also occur. However, 50% of all severe hemophiliacs do not bleed from circumcision, particularly with the current use of the skin clamp, which by necessity introduces a great deal of tissue thromboplastin into the wound. Prothrombin complex factor deficiencies (factors II, VII, IX, and X) frequently appear as bleeding after the first day that does not respond to vitamin K. Factor XI deficiency is rarely seen in the newborn period but has been misleading. Delayed bleeding from the cord at the time of separation is particularly suggestive of factor XIII deficiency.

Acquired disorders. The infant in utero is in a unique position in that it can acquire a problem only through its mother. A disease that affects the clotting proteins must be present in the mother or in drugs taken by the mother and acquired transplacentally by the infant.

Systemic lupus erythematosus in an exacerbated state in the mother may cause problems in the infant. The lupus antibody against red cells, white cells, and platelets, an IgG antibody, may cross the placenta and cause bleeding at the time of delivery[537] Similarly IgG inhibitors of coagulation, notably the factor VIII inhibitor, may pass from an affected mother into the circulation of the infant.

Drugs prescribed for a specific disease in the mother can be potentially harmful to the infant, whether during gestation, at the time of delivery, or in the neonatal period for a nursing infant.

Anticoagulants given to the mother for thromboembolic disease have been particularly harmful to the infant. Warfarin has been implicated for its teratogenetic effect when taken in the first trimester, an effect reproduced in rats.[540] The deformities are nasal hypoplasia with severe airway obstruction, stippling and poor growth of bones, ophthalmologic abnormalities, mental retardation, and many other developmental abnormalities. The drug crosses the placenta, is excreted slowly with a half-time of 51 hours, and presents an additional cause for poor production of the clotting factors in the newborn infants as well as causing severe hemorrhage at birth. For this reason heparin is suggested for therapy in the last month of pregnancy for any mother with thromboembolic disease, since heparin does not cross the placenta and presents no danger to the infant at delivery. The problems related to heparin therapy appear in the mother and not in the infant.

Warfarin also crosses into the breast milk, and although the data in the literature are conflicting, the drug appears to be present in measurable amounts. There are no good data to show that this amount is harmful to the infant, particularly if he receives other food than mother's milk and is supplemented with 1 mg vitamin K daily.

Drugs directed against platelet function may also cross the placenta. Corby and Schulman[534] have shown that the platelets of the newborn are particularly susceptible to the effects of aspirin and promethazine and have decreased aggregation.

Anticonvulsants, particularly a combination of phenytoin (Dilantin) and phenobarbitol or primidone (Mysoline) given to the mother, were found to be associated with lethal bleeding in infants within the first 24 hours of life in twenty-four cases.[536] The drugs produced a coagulation problem similar to hemorrhagic disease of the newborn with an exaggerated lowering of factors II, VII, IX, and X. Phenytoin and phenobarbitol to a lesser degree compete with vitamin K for glucuronidation and permit the production of PIVKAs, the nonfunctional prothrombin complex proteins.[541] Phenytoin crosses the placenta, it is excreted slowly by the infant, and its effect may be overcome with vitamin K. Additional vitamin K, 1 mg, should be given to the mother daily through the last trimester. The coagulation factor effect is not augmented or decreased when phenytoin is given with phenobarbitol or other anticonvulsant drugs; rather the effect remains the same as phenytoin alone.

Diuretics (in particular the thiazides) given to the mother have been reported to affect the platelets of the infant and in one case to cause bleeding and severe liver disease.[539] These findings have not been confirmed by others.[535]

Thrombotic disorders

INHERITED THROMBOTIC DISORDERS

There are four naturally occurring enzymes that bind thrombin and thereby inhibit its activity. They are α_2-macroglobulin, α_1-antitrypsin, antithrombin III, and $C\bar{1}$ inhibitor. A deficiency of any one of these enzymes may allow the propagation of naturally occurring thrombin in the microcirculation. These antiproteases inhibit other activated coagulants and plasmin as well as thrombin. α_2-macroglobulin inhibits thrombin, plasmin, and kallikrein (activated Fletcher factor)[564] and by its action influences fibrinolytic activity, the early contact phase of intrinsic coagulation, and thrombin activity. Both α_2-macroglobulin and α_1-antitrypsin are known to contribute some plasma antithrombin activity, the latter more than the former. However, their physiologic activity remains unclear. $C\bar{1}$ inactivator, initially identified as an inhibitor of $C\bar{1}$ esterase, is now known to inhibit factors XIIa and XIa, and Fletcher factor. Of these enzymes, antithrombin III is probably the most important inhibitor and the one about which most is known. Human antithrombin III is a single-chain glycoprotein with three disulphide bridges and four prosthetic glucosamine-based oligosaccharide groups.[579]

Congenital deficiency of antithrombin III

Congenital deficiency of antithrombin III is associated with a thrombotic tendency in heterozygous persons. The homozygous state may be incompatible with life.

In 1918 Howell and Holt[569] recognized that a substance in plasma or serum was necessary for the maximum inhibitory effect of heparin against thrombin. Heparin cofactor was necessary for inhibition of the esterase activity of thrombin. Rosenberg[588] described antithrombin III as the heparin cofactor and the enzyme that provided the active site for heparin activity. Its activity was seen as one of slow inhibition of thrombin when acting alone and immediate inactivation of thrombin in the presence of heparin. Antithrombin III also inhibits the activated factors XII, XI, IX, and X in the presence of heparin and thereby inhibits clotting by acting against all of the intermediary clotting enzymes. The enzyme is presumably made in the liver, but little else is known about its metabolism.

The deficiency of antithrombin III was originally described by Egberg[553] and chemically characterized by Abildgaard.[542]

Deficiency of antithrombin III is inherited as an autosomal dominant trait. Only four large kindreds have been reported with the disorder, suggesting that it is uncommon.[546,576] The actual prevalence of antithrombin III deficiency is unknown.

Thrombotic problems usually do not occur until adolescence and may be correlated with a fall in concentrations of antithrombin III and α_2-macroglobulin. Levels of antithrombin III are higher in adult women than men and decrease after 50 years of age in both.

Nonlethal venous thrombosis has occurred in 17% to 70% of three large families with the disorder.[576] Lethal pulmonary embolism has occurred in another family.[546]

Acquired deficiency has been reported in association with liver disease, the nephrotic syndrome, malignancy, sepsis, pulmonary embolism, and DIC; it is not known whether the subnormal levels are due to increased consumption of the factor or decreased production. Patients with the nephrotic syndrome have had antithrombin III levels as low as 30% and are thought to be losing the protein through the kidney.

Results of all of the routine tests for coagulation are normal, as are assays of the clotting factors. Absolute plasma levels of antithrombin III vary with the method of assay, i.e., with whether a one- or two-stage method is used and whether the inhibitor of the enzyme is measured or the residual enzyme is measured with a substrate. Normal values are 80% to 110%. Patients with the disease have levels of 26% to 49%. Newborn levels are half those of normal adults, and normal adult levels are reached by 6 months of age.

Current therapy for any patient with the deficiency is warfarin (Coumadin) in therapeutic doses. Heparin therapy may aggravate deficiency of antithrombin III in affected persons.

Other inherited thrombotic disorders

Homocystinuria, an inborn error of metabolism caused by deficiency of the enzyme cystathionine synthetase, has been associated with ectopia lentis, mental retardation, skeletal deformities, progressive cardiovascular disease, and thromboembolism.[549] Myocardial, cerebral, renal, and pulmonary infarctions are often fatal before the third decade.[377] Platelet destruction is increased with homocystinemia and normalized in some with pyridoxine administration.[550,578,600] Harker et al.[562,563] have found that dipyridamole, 100 mg, and acetylsalicylic acid, 1 gm, daily normalize platelet survival and suggested that these drugs may protect those who are pyridoxine responders from thrombosis. They postulate that the vascular endothelial injury in this disease is chemical in origin because of increased blood levels of homocystine with secondary atherosclerotic lesions, which predispose to platelet thrombosis and decreased platelet survival.

ACQUIRED THROMBOTIC DISORDERS
Drug-induced thrombotic disorders

Thrombosis caused by drugs in children is unusual but must be considered when the following drugs are used.

EACA (Amicar), discussed in the therapy of hemophilia, is an active antifibrinolytic drug that inhibits plasminogen conversion to plasmin, the active enzyme that lyses fibrin. The drug is useful to inhibit the normally occurring urokinase in the urinary tract or in the saliva. However, its use is contraindicated in patients with hemophilia or sickle cell trait who have urinary tract bleeding that is renal in origin in which an unlysed clot might impede renal function for as long as 6 months.[566] EACA should not be used in patients treated with large amounts of prothrombin complex concentrates because activated clotting factors may cause intravascular coagulation.

Oral contraceptives, estrogen, or estrogen-progesterone compounds have been associated with a ''hypercoagulable'' state and with elevated coagulation factors. An extensive body of evidence now exists showing increased peripheral thrombosis and pulmonary emboli in women taking oral contraceptives.*

Other acquired thrombotic disorders

As previously mentioned, acquired deficiency of the naturally occurring inhibitor antithrombin III may contribute to thrombosis.

Thromboembolic disease may also occur during pregnancy and therapy with simple estrogen compounds and contraceptive agents.[552,568] Although these states may be associated with elevated levels of clotting factors and circulating soluble complexes of fibrin monomer, the cause-and-effect relationship of these changes to thrombotic disease has not been established. Foreign surfaces within the vascular tree may be thrombogenic, i.e., indwelling catheters, prosthetic heart valves (in particular the Starr-Edwards valve until it is epitheli-

*References 554, 560, 568

alized), and Dacron vascular splints.[598] The former are becoming more common in children and adolescents, the latter less common.

Diabetes mellitus is associated with a hypercoagulable state with enhanced platelet aggregation in patients with proliferative retinopathy possibly caused by abnormal prostaglandin metabolism and increased levels of factor VIII in the plasma.[552,565] Decreased fibrinolytic activity and lower levels of fibrinogen have also been reported that are reversible with improved control.[585] An increased incidence of arterial thrombosis has been described but not well demonstrated.

A thrombotic disorder has been described with angiographic agents; it is a consumptive disorder similar to DIC with a lowering of the clotting factors and increase in FDPs with subsequent hemorrhage.[573,592]

Thrombosis may complicate the nephrotic syndrome with concomitant elevation of fibrinogen and other procoagulants.[574] The factors are raised to even higher levels with the stimulus of steroid therapy administered for this disease.[570,575,595]

Anticoagulant therapy

Anticoagulant therapy has been proved to be of value for venous thromboembolism but of less value for arterial thrombosis.[556,557,558] In children the use of anticoagulant therapy is limited since deep vein thrombosis is rare. However, the use of a cardiac prosthesis or the diagnosis of microcirculatory thrombosis such as may occur in DIC is becoming more widespread and mandates a discussion of the available modalities of anticoagulation.

Anticoagulation therapy may be divided into two types: that directed against the plasma clotting factors and that directed against the platelets.[559,581] Therapy directed against the plasma clotting factors prevents the action of thrombin on fibrinogen and clot formation, either by inhibiting the transformation of some of the antigenic clotting proteins into the active form and thus interfering with the formation of fibrin or by destroying fibrinogen directly.[545,583] There are three therapeutic modalities available for this purpose. The first involves drugs that affect the utilization of vitamin K in the production of the active clotting factors prothrombin (factor II) and factor VII, IX, and X by the liver through competition of the binding sites on albumin or binding sites in the liver for metabolism. Warfarin (Coumadin), the oldest and best known anticoagulant drug, competes for intrahepatic hydroxylation and glucuronide conjugation by the hepatocytes and thereby decreases the amount of vitamin K available to the liver. PIVKA is therefore produced.[596] PIVKA, according to Stenflo et al.,[593] is antigenetically detected as prothrombin but lacks the modified glutamic acid residues that bind calcium and is therefore non-functioning in blood coagulation. He postulates that the calcium-binding factors VII, IX, and X, whose biosynthesis also requires vitamin K, utilize vitamin K for the same purpose, and therefore the synthesis of all four active clotting factors is inhibited by warfarin.

The second modality involves the use of snake venoms that inhibit fibrin formation and cause defibrination by direct lysis of the fibrinogen molecule. The purified venom in widest use is Ancrod (Arvin) from the Malayan pit viper, *Agkistrodon rhodostoma*.[555,580] This purified venom contains an enzyme that hydrolyzes fibrinogen, removing fibrinopeptide A. The fibrin formed is more susceptible to fibrinolysis than fibrin formed through thrombin activity because factor XIII is not activated and cross-links are not formed. Ancrod produces hypofibrinogenemia by converting fibrinogen to unstable fibrin, which is rapidly cleared. No other clotting factors are affected. There is also some evidence that the FDP produced may act as a platelet antiaggregating agent for additional activity.[591]

The third method of interfering with fibrin formation is with heparin, the mucopolysaccharide from mast cells of bovine tissue and intestinal mucosa of cattle and hogs. It acts with the cofactor antithrombin III to inactivate thrombin and many of the other activated enzymes (IXa and XIa) in the clotting cascade and is degraded in the liver.*

Drugs directed against platelets suppress their adhesion and aggregation by which the normal clotting cascade may be triggered.[559,587] They are particularly valuable if a foreign surface or damaged endothelium susceptible to the formation of a platelet thrombus is exposed. There are three types of drugs whose antiplatelet activity has been recognized in the past 5 years as useful in inhibiting platelet function. They are the nonsteroidal anti-inflammatory drugs and related compounds that inhibit platelet release reactions (aspirin, indomethacin, phenylbutazone, sulfinpyrazone, and fenoprofen), the pyrimido-pyrimidine drugs that inhibit ADP-induced aggregation by increasing cyclic AMP (dipyridamole), and a number of other drugs originally used for quite different purposes (clofibrate and cryoheptadine). Both aspirin and sulfinpyrazone appear to inhibit the release reaction by interfering with the synthesis of prostaglandins. The effect of aspirin exists for 4 to 7 days, or the lifetime of the platelet, but the effect of sulfinpyrazone does not outlast its survival in the circulation. The bleeding times of normal persons can be prolonged by aspirin and indomethacin. The pyrimido-pyrimidine drugs may inhibit primary aggregation in some animals, but their overall usefulness seems much more limited and results of large trials remain controversial. The controlled trials listing the usefulness of aspirin plus sulfinpyrazone or aspirin plus dipyridamole are contradictory but suggest less vascular thrombosis in older patients with atherosclerotic disease. Aspirin seems to be useful in preventing clots in hemodialysis or extracorporeal shunts. The combination of warfarin and one of the antiplatelet drugs seems to be most useful in deep-vein thrombosis, pulmonary embolism, and cardiac prostheses. In DIC heparin is probably not as useful as treatment of the underlying cause, supportive measures, and replacement of clotting factors when the patient is bleeding. The antiplatelet drugs may be of some value for chronic DIC such as seen in the hemolytic uremic syndrome. Controversy persists as to the usefulness of heparin for DIC associated with malignancy and thrombotic thrombocytopenic purpura. The real hazard of its use must be weighed with the benefits in each case.

Schedules of anticoagulant therapy. For anticoagulation with warfarin, the following schedule may be used. The oral dose is absorbed rapidly, reaching maximal concentration in 1 to 9 hours and hypoprothrombinemia in 36 to 72 hours with a duration of action lasting up to 5 days. The clotting factors decrease at a rate consistent with their individual half life: 6 hours for factor VII, 24 hours for factor IX, 40 hours for factor X, and 60 hours for factor II. A loading dose of 10 mg is given to the average adolescent or young adult and 2.5 to 5.0 mg for a child. Therapy should be individualized to maintain a PT (Quick method using rabbit brain-lung thromboplastin with calcium [Simplastin]) of 25 seconds with a control of about 12 seconds. An acceptable range is 20 to 30 seconds. Patients should have periodic PT tests performed, since levels can be affected by diet and other medications. For example, anabolic steroids, chloramphenicol, clofibrate, phenytoin, salicylates, and thyroid hormone can potentiate the anticoagulant effect; allopurinol, barbiturates, diuretics, chronic alcohol usage, and oral contraceptives can antagonize the effects. Worldwide standards continue to be sought for the test thromboplastin to allow travel of all patients receiving anticoagulation with warfarin. However, these standards remain elusive. Periodic determination may be done in laboratories using the same standard throughout the United States.

Heparin may be administered intramuscularly into the abdominal fat pad or intravenously with a constant infusion or intermittent bolus. Each of the methods may be associated with problems. Intra-

---

*References 571, 572, 582, 589.

muscular injections are painful and often associated with local hemorrhage. Bolus administration gives enormous swings of effect on the clotting time from infinity to normal values, while constant infusion requires a constant infusion pump with frequent monitoring to adjust the dosage to the desired amount. Continuous infusion of heparin may provide safer and more effective anticoagulation than intermittent doses.

Commercial heparin is standardized according to its ability to prolong the clotting time of sheep plasma. The number of units per milligram may vary from 130 to 170 units. Orders for the product should therefore be written in units, not milligrams. The dosage should be adjusted to give an activated PTT of 2 to 2½ times the normal, i.e., 80 to 100 seconds using a kaolin-cephalin mixture (Platelin). For children a loading dose of 50 to 75 units/kg may be given as a bolus followed in 2 hours by a constant drip of 10 to 20 units/kg/hour. Since the half-life of heparin is 1½ hours, a PTT taken 1½ hours after the infusion is begun can be used to begin titration. The patient's medical condition, drug therapy, and age effect the amount necessary to maintain anticoagulation. Monitoring twice daily is usually sufficient. In the unlikely event of hemorrhage, stopping therapy may suffice or heparin neutralization can be achieved with protamine sulfate, a basic protein that forms a stable salt with heparin in approximately equal amounts, i.e., 1 mg of protamine sulfate for each 100 units of heparin in circulation, given in a divided dose over a 10- to 15-minute period.

Ancrod is available in limited quantities for investigation in the United States at the present time. In Europe it is given intravenously or subcutaneously to produce hypofibrinogenemia of 50 to 100 mg/dl. One small study by Barrie et al.[544] suggests usefulness in preventing deep vein thrombosis following hip surgery. It has not been used in children.

NEONATAL THROMBOTIC DISORDERS

Thrombotic disorders in the newborn with normal or increased clotting factors are rare and frequently are associated with another disorder.[590] They may be associated with dehydration secondary to adrenal insufficiency or to the hyperviscosity syndrome seen in offspring of diabetic mothers.[561,597] Clotting is presumed to result from a change in the rheology of the vascular system, and with stasis the clotting system may be activated. Hypoxia and a change in pH may also be present in the offspring of diabetic mothers or with adrenal insufficiency. Renal vein thrombosis has been seen in the newborn infant of a diabetic mother[543,548] following birth trauma[586] and aortic thrombosis has been seen with antithrombin III deficiency.[547] Sev-

eral authors have reported hemorrhage following severe birth trauma (shoulder dystocia requiring manipulation for delivery) in which the local thrombosis was sufficient to produce generalized DIC.[551] Intensive care of the small premature infant with indwelling umbilical catheters has also been associated with an increase in embolization and nonbacterial thrombotic endocarditis, presumably because of distorted blood flow around the catheter, or when the catheter is found in the heart.[594]

Thrombosis may also occur following exchange transfusion when the catheter is in the portal vein or its tributaries, leading to infarction and perforation of small and large intestine.[567] The etiology of this progression of events is presumed vessel spasm and back flow of blood during the procedure, with local tissue anoxia. It may be prevented by careful attention to positioning of the umbilical catheter.

In the older child superficial venous thrombosis has been more common with indwelling venous catheters. Spontaneous lower extremity venous thrombosis and pulmonary emboli have been reported following local infections, trauma, and immobilization, as in adults, and the increasing use of oral contraceptives in teenagers has lowered the age at which emboli have been seen.[568,599]

REFERENCES
General considerations on the plasma phase of hemostasis

1. Aballi, A. J.: The action of vitamin K in the neonatal period, South. Med. J. **58:**48, 1965.
2. Aggeler, P. M., White, S. G., Glendening, M. B., et al.: Plasma thromboplastin component (PTC) deficiency: a new disease resembling hemophilia, Proc. Soc. Exp. Biol. Med. **79:**692, 1952.
3. Alami, S. Y., Hampton, J. W., Race, G. J., et al.: Fibrin stabilizing factor (factor XIII), Am. J. Med. **44:**1, 1968.
4. Alexander, B., DeVries, A., Goldstein, R., et al.: A prothrombin conversion accelerator in serum, Science **109:**545, 1949.
5. Aronson, D. L., Preiss, J. W., and Mosesson, M. W.: Molecular weights of factor VIII (AHF) and factor IX (PTC) by electron irradiation, Thromb. Diath. Haemorrh. **8:**270, 1962.
6. Arthus, M., and Pagès, C.: Nouvelle théorie chimique de la coagulation du sang, Arch. Physiol. Norm. Pathol. **2:**739, 1890.
7. Barrett, A. J., and Starkey, P. M.: The interaction of α_2-macroglobulin with proteinases, Biochem. J. **133:**709, 1973.
8. Barrow, E. M., and Graham, J. B.: Blood coagulation factor VIII (antihemophilic factor): with comments on von Willebrand's disease and Christmas disease, Physiol. Rev. **54:**23, 1974.
9. Biggs, R., and Denson, K. W. E.: The fate of prothrombin and factors VIII, IX, and X transfused to patients deficient in these factors, Br. J. Haematol. **9:**532, 1963.
10. Biggs, R., Douglas, A. S., Macfarlane, R. G., et al.: Christmas disease: a condition previously mistaken for haemophilia; Br. Med. J. **2:**1378, 1952.
11. Biggs, R., and Macfarlane, R. G.: Human blood coagu-

lation and its disorders, ed. 3, Oxford, 1963, Blackwell Scientific Publications, Ltd.

12. Bleyer, W. A., Wakami, N., and Shepard, T. H.: The development of hemostasis in the human fetus and the newborn infant, J. Pediatr. **79:**838, 1971.

13. Blombäck, B.: The N-terminal disulphide knot of human fibrinogen, Br. J. Haematol. **17:**145, 1969.

14. Blombäck, B., Blombäck, M., Grondahl, N. J., et al.: Structure of fibrinopeptides: its relation to enzyme specificity and phylogeny and classification of species, Arkiv Kem. **25:**411, 1966.

15. Borchgrevink, C. F., and Owren, P. A.: Surgery in a patient with factor V proaccelerin) deficiency, Acta Med. Scand. **170:**743, 1961.

16. Britten, A. F. H.: Congenital deficiency of factor XIII (fibrin-stabilizing factor), Am. J. Med. **43:**751, 1967.

17. Buchanan, A.: On the coagulation of the blood and other fibriniferous liquids, London Med. Gazette **1:**617, 1845.

18. Campbell, H. A., and Link, P. K.: Studies on the hemorrhagic sweet clover disease. IV. The isolation and crystallization of the hemorrhagic agent, J. Biol. Chem. **138:**21, 1941.

19. Colman, R. W., Bagdasarian, A., Talamo, R. C., et al.: Williams trait: human kininogen deficiency with diminished levels of plasminogen proactivator and prekallikrein associated with abnormalities of the Hageman factor-dependent pathway, J. Clin. Invest. **56:**1650, 1975.

20. Cooper, H. A., Griggs, T. R., and Wagner, R. H.: Factor VIII recombination after dissociation by $CaCl_2$, Proc. Natl. Acad. Sci. **70:**2326, 1973.

21. Dam, H.: Haemorrhages in chicks reared in artificial diets: a new deficiency disease, Nature **133:**909, 1934.

22. Dam, H.: The anti-hemorrhagic vitamin of the chick, Nature **135:**652, 1935.

23. Davie, E. W., and Ratnoff, O. D.: Waterfall sequence for intrinsic blood clotting, Science **145:**1310, 1964.

24. Donaldson, V. H., Glueck, H. I., Miller, M. A., et al.: Kininogen deficiency in Fitzgerald trait: role of high molecular weight kininogen in clotting and fibrinolysis, J. Lab. Clin. Med. **87:**327, 1976.

25. Duckert, F., Jung, E., and Schmerling, D. H.: A hitherto undescribed congenital haemorrhagic diathesis probably due to fibrin stabilizing factor deficiency, Thromb. Diath. Haemorrh. **5:**179, 1960.

26. Ekelund, H.: Fibrinolysis in the first year of life, Acta Paediatr. Scand. **61:**5, 1972.

27. Ekelund, H., Hedner, U., and Nilsson, I. M.: Fibrinolysis in newborns, Acta Paediatr. Scand. **59:**33, 1970.

28. Esnouf, M. P., and Williams, W. J.: The isolation and purification of a bovine-plasma protein which is a substrate for the coagulant fraction of Russell's viper venom, Biochem. J. **84:**62, 1962.

29. Forman, W. B., and Barnhart, M. I.: Cellular site for fibrinogen synthesis, J.A.M.A. **187:**128, 1964.

30. Fugikawa, K., Coan, M. H., Enfield, D. L., et al.: A comparison of bovine prothrombin, factor IX (Christmas factor), and factor X (Stuart factor), Proc. Natl. Acad. Sci. **71:**427, 1974.

31. Hammarsten, O.: Uber die Bedeutung der loslichen Kalksalze fur die Faserstoffgerinnung, Z. Physiol. Chem. **22:**333, 1896.

32. Harpel, P. C., and Mosesson, M. W.: Degradation of human fibrinogen by plasma a_2-macroglobulin-enzyme complexes, J. Clin. Invest. **52:**2175, 1973.

33. Hathaway, W. E.: The bleeding newborn. In Oski, F. A., Jaffe, E. R., and Miescher, P. A., eds.: Current problems in pediatric hematology, New York, 1975, Grune & Stratton, Inc.

34. Hathaway, W. E., Belhausen, H. S., and Hathaway, H. S.: Evidence of a new plasma coagulation factor, I.

Case report, coagulation studies and physiochemical properties, Br. J. Haematol. **26:**521, 1965.

35. Heck, L. W., and Kaplan, A. P.: Substrates of human Hageman factor. I. Isolation and characterization of PTA (factor XI) and its inhibition by α_1 antitrypsin, J. Exp. Med. **140:**1615, 1974.

36. Hemker, H. C.: Interaction of coagulation factors, In Brinkhous, K. M., and Hemker, H. C., eds.: Handbook of hemophilia, Part I, Amsterdam, 1975, Excerpta Medica.

37. Hershgold, E. J.: The subunit structure of human factor VIII (antihemophilic factor), Fed. Proc. **30:**540, 1971.

38. Holemans, R., and Roberts, H. R.: Hageman factor and in vivo activation of fibrinolysis, J. Lab. Clin. Med. **64:**778, 1964.

39. Hougie, C., Barrow, E. M., and Graham, J. B.: Stuart clotting defect. I. Segregation of an hereditary hemorrhagic state from the heterogeneous group heretofore called "stable factor" (SPCA, proconvertin, factor VII) deficiency, J. Clin. Invest. **36:**485, 1957.

40. Iatridis, S. G., and Ferguson, J. H.: Active Hageman factor: a plasma lysokinase of the human fibrinolytic system, J. Clin. Invest. **41:**1277, 1962.

41. Jackson, C. M., and Hanahan, D. J.: Studies on bovine factor X. II. Characterization of purified factor X. Observation on some alterations in zone electrophoretic and chromatographic behavior occurring during purification, Biochemistry **7:**4506, 1968.

42. Johnson, S. A., Rutsky, J., Schneider, C. L., et al.: Activation of purified prothrombin with hemophilic plasma. In Proceedings of the fourth international congress of the International Society of Hematology (1952), New York, 1954, Grune & Stratton, Inc.

43. Johnston, C. L., Jr., Ferguson, J. G., O'Hanlon, F. A., et al.: The fate of factor VII and Stuart factor during the clotting of normal blood, Thromb. Diath. Haemorrh. **3:**367, 1959.

44. Kahn, M. J. P., and Hemker, H. C.: Studies on blood coagulation factor V. A partially purified factor V preparation from human plasma, Coagulation **3:**63, 1970.

45. Kaplan, A. P., and Austen, K. F.: The fibrinolytic pathway of human plasma: isolation and characterization of the plasminogen proactivator, J. Exp. Med. **136:**1378, 1972.

46. Kaplan, A. P., Meier, H. L., and Mandle, R., Jr.: The Hageman factor dependent pathways of coagulation, fibrinolysis, and kinin-generation, Semin. Thromb. Hemost. **3:**1, 1976.

47. Kaplan, A. P., Spragg, J., and Austen, K. F.: The bradykinin forming pathway in human plasma. In Austen, K. F., and Becker, E. L., eds.: Biochemistry of the acute allergic reaction, Oxford, 1971, Blackwell Scientific Publications, Ltd.

48. Kaplan, M. H.: Nature and role of the lytic factor in hemolytic streptococcal fibrinolysis, Proc. Soc. Exp. Biol. Med. **57:**40, 1944.

49. Kisiel, W., and Hanahan, D. J.: Purification and characterization of human factor II, Biochem. Biophys. Acta **304:**103, 1973.

50. Kingdon, H. S., and Lundblad, R. L.: Biochemistry of factor IX. In Brinkhous, K. M., and Hemker, H. C., eds.: Handbook of hemophilia. Part I, Amsterdam, 1975, Excerpta Medica.

51. Kline, D. L., and Fishman, J. B.: Plasmin: the humoral protease, Ann. N.Y. Acad. Sci. **68:**25, 1957.

52. Kucinski, C., Fletcher, A. P., and Sherry, S.: The effect of urokinase antiserum on plasminogen activators: demonstration of immunologic dissimilarity between plasma plasminogen activation and urokinase, J. Clin. Invest. **47:**1238, 1968.

53. Laake, K., and Vennerod, A. M.: Factor XII-in-

duced fibrinolysis: studies on the separation of prekallikrein, plasminogen proactivator, and factor XI in human plasma, Thromb. Res. **4:**285, 1974.

54. Lack, C. H.: Proteolytic activity and connective tissue, Br. Med. Bull. **20:**217, 1964.
55. Lacombe, M. J.: Déficit constitutional en un nouveau facteur de la coagulation intervenant au niveau de contact: le facteur "Fleaujac," C. R. Acad. Sci. **280:**1039, 1975.
56. Laki, K., and Lorand, L.: On the solubility of fibrin clots, Science **108:**280, 1948.
57. Langdell, R. D., Wagner, R. H., and Brinkhous, K. M.: Effect of anti-hemophilic factor in one-stage clotting tests, J. Lab. Clin. Med. **41:**637, 1953.
58. Lascari, A.: The erythrocyte sedimentation rate, Pediatr. Clin. North Am. **19:**1113, 1972.
59. Lesuk, A., Terminiello, L., and Traver, H.: Crystalline human urokinase: some properties, Science **147:**880, 1965.
60. Lorand, L., and Dickenman, R. C.: Assay method for the "fibrin-stabilizing factor," Proc. Soc. Biol. Med. **89:**45, 1955.
61. Lorand, L., and Konishi, K.: Activation of the fibrin stabilizing factor of plasma by thrombin, Arch. Biochem. **105:**58, 1964.
62. Lutcher, C. L.: Reid trait: a new expression of high molecular weight kininogen (HMW kininogen) deficiency, Clin. Res. **34:**47A, 1976.
63. Macfarlane, R. G.: An enzyme cascade in the blood clotting mechanism, and its function as a biological amplifier, Nature **202:**498, 1964.
64. Magnusson, S., Pererson, T. E., Sottrup-Jensen, L., et al.: Complete primary structure of prothrombin: isolation, structure, and reactivity of ten carboxylated glutamic acid residues and regulation of prothrombin activation by thrombin. In Reich, R., Rifkin, D. B., and Shaw, E., eds.: Proteases and biological control, New York, 1975, Cold Spring Harbor.
65. Mahasandana, C., and Hathaway, W. E.: Circulating anticoagulants in the newborn: relation to hypercoagulability and the idiopathic respiratory distress syndrome, Pediatr. Res. **7:**670, 1973.
66. Marder, V. J., and Budzynski, A. Z.: The structure of fibrinogen degradation products, Progr. Hemostasis Thromb. **2:**141, 1974.
67. Marder, V. J., and Shulman, N. R.: Clinical aspects of congenital factor VII deficiency, Am. J. Med. **37:**182, 1964.
68. McDonagh, J., Kiesselbach, T. H., and Wagner, R. H.: Origin of platelet factor XIII (fibrin stabilizing factor), Fed. Proc. **28:**745, 1969.
69. McKee, P. A., Andersen, J. C., and Switzer, M. E.: Molecular structural studies of human factor VIII, Ann. N.Y. Acad. Sci. **240:**8, 1975.
70. Morawitz, P.: Die Chemie der Blutgerinnung. Ergeb. Physiol. **4:**307, 1905.
71. Myhre, B. A., ed.: Blood component therapy, ed. 2, Washington, D.C., 1975, American Association of Blood Banks.
72. Nakahara, M., and Celander, D. R.: Properties of microsomal activator of profibrinolysis found in bovine and porcine heart muscle, Thromb. Diath. Haemorrh. **19:**483, 1968.
73. Nemerson, Y.: The role of lipids in the tissue factor pathway of blood coagulation, Adv. Exp. Med. Biol. **63:**245, 1975.
74. Nemerson, Y.: Biological control of factor VII, Thromb. Haemost. **35:**96, 1976.
75. Niewiarowski, S.: Physiologic implications in fibrinolysis. In Plenary session papers, twelfth congress of the International Society of Hematology, 1968.
76. Nossel, H., Rubin, H., Drillings, M., et al.: Inhibition of Hageman factor activation, J. Clin. Invest. **47:**1172, 1968.
77. Olson, J. P., Miller, L. L., and Troup, S. B.: Synthesis of clotting factors by the isolated perfused rat liver, J. Clin. Invest. **45:**690, 1966.
78. Owen, C. A., Jr., and Bowie, E. J. W.: Infusion therapy in hemophilia A and B. In Brinkhous, K. M., and Hemker, H. C., eds.: Handbook of hemophilia. Part 2, Amsterdam, 1975, Excerpta Medica.
79. Owren, P. A.: The coagulation of blood, investigations on a new clotting factor, Acta Med. Scand. Suppl. 194, 1947.
80. Owren, P. A.: Proconvertin: the new clotting factor, Scand. J. Clin. Lab. Invest. **3:**168, 1951.
81. Pekelharing, G. A.: Über die Bedeutung der Kalksalze für die Gerinnung des Blutes, Int. Beitr. Z. wiss. Med. **1:**433, 1891.
82. Penick, G. D.: Some factors that influence utilization of antihemophilic activity during clotting, Proc. Soc. Exp. Biol. Med. **96:**277, 1957.
83. Philip, G., Moran, J., and Colman, R. W.: Dissociation and association of the oligomeric forms of factor V, Biochem. **9:**2212, 1970.
84. Pickering, J. W.: The blood plasma in health and disease, New York, 1928, The Macmillan Co.
85. Pisano, J. J., Finlayson, J. S., and Peyton, M. P.: Cross-link in fibrin polymerized by factor XIII. ε-(-γ glutamyl) lysine, Science **160:**892, 1968.
86. Pitlick, F. A., and Nemerson, Y.: Binding of the protein complement of tissue factor to phospholipids, Biochem. **9:**5105, 1970.
87. Pool, J. G., and Robinson, J.: Observations on plasma banking and transfusion procedures for haemophilia patients using quantitative assay for antihaemophilic globulin, Br. J. Haematol. **5:**379, 1959.
88. Pool, J. G., and Shannon, A. E.: Production of high-potency concentrates of antihemophilic globulin in a closed-bag system: assay in vitro and in vivo, N. Engl. J. Med. **273:**1443, 1965.
89. Prydz, H.: Some characteristics of purified factor VII preparations, Scand. J. Clin. Lab. Invest. **16:**409, 1964.
90. Quick, A. J.: The prothrombin in hemophilia and obstructive jaundice, J. Biol. Chem. **109:**73, 1935.
91. Quick, A. J.: Coagulation defect in sweet clover disease and in the hemorrhagic chick disease of dietary origin, Am. J. Physiol. **118:**260, 1937.
92. Quick, A. J.: The hemorrhagic diseases and the physiology of hemostasis, Springfield, Ill., 1942, Charles C Thomas, Publisher.
93. Quick, A. J.: On the constitution of prothrombin, Am. J. Physiol. **140:**212, 1943.
94. Radcliffe, R., and Nemerson, Y.: Mechanism of activation of bovine factor VII: products of cleavage by factor Xa, J. Biol. Chem. **251:**4749, 1976.
95. Rapaport, S. I.: Plasma thromboplastin antecedent levels in patients receiving coumarin anticoagulants and in patients with Laennec's cirrhosis, Proc. Soc. Exp. Biol. Med. **108:**115, 1961.
96. Ratnoff, O. D., and Colopy, J. E.: A familial hemorrhagic trait associated with deficiency of a clot-promoting fraction of plasma, J. Clin. Invest. **34:**602, 1955.
97. Rausen, A. R., Cruchaud, A., McMillan, C. W., et al.: A study of fibrinogen turnover in classical hemophilia and congenital afibrinogenemia, Blood **18:**710, 1961.
98. Reddy, K. N. N., and Marcus, G.: Mechanism of activation of human plasminogen by streptokinase: presence of an active center in streptokinase-plasminogen complex, J. Biol. Chem. **247:**1683, 1972.
99. Reddy, K. N. N., and Marcus, G.: Further evidence for an active center in streptokinase-plasminogen com-

plex: interaction with pancreatic trypsin inhibitor, Biochem. Biophys. Res. Commun. **51:**672, 1973.

100. Revak, S. D., Cochrane, C. G., Johnston, A. R., et al.: Structural changes accompanying enzymatic activation of human Hageman factor, J. Clin. Invest. **54:**619, 1974.

101. Riddle, J. M., and Barnhart, M. I.: The eosinophil as a source of profibrinolysin in acute inflammation, Blood **25:**776, 1965.

102. Roberts, H. R., Lechler, E., Webster, W. P., et al.: Survival of transfused factor X in patients with Stuart disease, Thromb. Diath. Haemorrh. **13:**305, 1965.

103. Roderick, L. M.: A problem in the coagulation of the blood "sweet clover disease of cattle," Am. K. Physiol. **96:**413, 1931.

104. Rosenberg, R. D.: Protease inhibitors of blood coagulation. In Human Hemostasis—1975, Washington, D.C., 1975, American Association of Blood Banks.

105. Rosenberg, R. D.: Actions and interactions of antithrombin and heparin, N. Engl. J. Med. **292:**146, 1975.

106. Rosenberg, R. D., and Damus, P. S.: The purification and mechanism of human antithrombin heparin cofactor, J. Biol. Chem. **248:**6490, 1973.

107. Rosenberg, J. S., McKenna, P. W., and Rosenberg, R. D.: Inhibition of human factor IXa by human antithrombin, J. Biol. Chem. **250:**8883, 1975.

108. Rosenthal, R. L., Dreskin, O. H., and Rosenthal, N.: New hemophilia-like disease caused by deficiency of a third plasma thromboplastin factor, Proc. Soc. Exp. Biol. Med. **82:**171, 1953.

109. Rosenthal, R. L., and Sloan, E.: PTA (factor XI) levels and coagulation studies after plasma infusions in PTA-deficient patients, J. Lab. Clin. Med. **66:**709, 1965.

110. Saito, H., Goldsmith, G., and Waldmann, R.: Fitzgerald factor (high molecular weight kininogen) clotting activity in human plasma in health and disease in various animal plasmas, Blood **48:**941, 1976.

111. Schick, L. A., and Castellino, F. J.: Direct evidence of an active site in the plasminogen moiety of the streptokinase: human plasminogen activator complex, Biochem. Biophys. Res. Commun. **57:**47, 1974.

112. Schiffman, S., and Lee, P.: Preparation, characterization, and activation of a highly purified XI: evidence that a hitherto unrecognized plasma activity participates in the interaction of factors XI and XII, Br. J. Haematol. **27:**101, 1974.

113. Schmidt, A.: Ueber den Faserstoff und die Ursachen seiner Gerinnung, Arch. Anat. Physiol. Leipzig, p. 545, 1861.

114. Schmidt, A.: Weitere Beitrage zur Bluthre, Wiesbaden, 1895, Bergmann.

115. Schreiber, A. D.: Plasma inhibitors of the Hageman factor dependent pathways, Semin. Thromb. Hemost. **3:**43, 1976.

116. Schulman, I., and Smith, C. H.: Hemorrhagic disease of an infant due to deficiency of a previously undescribed clotting factor, Blood **7:**794, 1952.

117. Schwartz, M. L., Pizzo, S. V., Hill, R. L., et al.: Human factor XIII from plasma and platelets: molecular weights, subunit structures, proteolytic activation, and cross-linking of fibrinogen and fibrin, J. Biol. Chem. **248:**1395, 1973.

118. Seeler, R. A.: Congenital hypoprothrombinemias, Med. Clin. North Am. **56:**127, 1972.

119. Sherry, S., Alkjaersig, N., and Fletcher, A. P.: Fibrinolysis and fibrinolytic activity in man, Physiol. Rev. **39:**343, 1959.

120. Stead, N., Kaplan, A. P., and Rosenberg, R. D.: Inhibition of activated factor XII by antithrombin-heparin cofactor, J. Biol. Chem. **251:**6481, 1976.

121. Stenflo, J.: Vitamin K, prothrombin, and gammacarboxyglutamic acid, N. Engl. J. Med. **296:**624, 1977.

122. Stenflo, J., Fernlund, P., Egan, W., et al.: Vitamin K dependent modifications of glutamic acid residues in prothrombin, Proc. Natl. Acad, Sci. **71:**2730, 1974.

123. Summaria, L., Hsieh, B., Groskop, R. W. R., et al.: The isolation and characterization of the S-carboxymethyl beta (light) chain derivative of human plasmin, J. Biol. Chem. **242:**5046, 1967.

124. Summaria, L., and Robbins, K. C.: Isolation and characterization of the S-carboxymethyl heavy chain derivative of human plasmin, J. Biol. Chem. **246:**2143, 1972.

125. Summaria, L., and Robbins, K. C.: Isolation and characterization of the S-carboxymethyl heavy chain derivative of human plasmin, J. Biol. Chem. **246:**2143, 1972.

126. Suttie, J. W.: Oral anticoagulant therapy: the biosynthetic basis, Semin. Hematol. **14:**365, 1977.

127. Telfer, T. P., Denson, K. W., and Wright, D. R.: A "new" coagulation defect, Br. J. Haematol. **2:**308, 1956.

128. Veltkamp, J. J., Loeliger, E. A., and Hemker, H. C.: The biological half-time of Hageman factor, Thromb. Diath. Haemorrh. **13:**1, 1965.

129. Waddell, W. W., Guerry, D. P., Bray, W. E., et al.: Possible effects of vitamin K on prothrombin and clotting time in newly-born infants, Proc. Soc. Exp. Biol. Med. **40:**432, 1939.

130. Wagner, R. H., and Cooper, H. A.: Current approaches to the characterization of factor VIII. In Brinkhous, K. M., and Hemker, H. C., eds.: Handbook of hemophilia. Part 1, Amsterdam, 1975, Excerpta Medica.

131. Waldman, R., and Abraham, J. P.: Fitzgerald factor: a hitherto unrecognized coagulation factor, Blood **44:**934, 1974.

132. Ware, A. G., and Seegers, W. H.: Plasma accelerator globulin: partial purification, quantitative determination and properties, J. Biol. Chem. **152:**567, 1948.

133. Warren, B. A.: Fibrinolytic activity of vascular endothelium, Br. Med. Bull. **20:**213, 1964.

134. Webster, W. P., Roberts, H. R., and Penick, G. D.: Hemostasis in factor V deficiency, Am. J. Med. Sci. **248:**195, 1964.

135. Williams, W. J.: The activity of lung microsomes in blood coagulation, J. Biol. Chem. **239:**933, 1964.

136. Williams, W. J.: The activity of human placenta microsomes and brain particles in blood coagulation, J. Biol. Chem. **241:**1840, 1966.

137. Wright, I. S.: The nomenclature of blood clotting factors, Thromb. Diath. Haemorrh. **7:**381, 1962.

138. Wuepper, K. D.: Prekallikrein deficiency in man, J. Exp. Med. **138:**1345, 1973.

Common inherited coagulation deficiencies

139. Abildgaard, C. F.: The management of bleeding in hemophilia, Adv. Pediatr. **16:**365, 1969.

140. Abildgaard, C. F., Simone, J. V., Honig, G. R., et al.: Von Willebrand's disease: a comparative study of diagnostic tests, J. Pediatr. **73:**355, 1968.

141. Abildgaard, C. F., Simone, J. V., and Schulman, I.: Steroid treatment of hemophilic hematuria, J. Pediatr. **66:**117, 1965.

142. Addis, T.: The pathogenesis of hereditary hemophilia, J. Pathol. Bacteriol. **15:**427, 1911.

143. Aggeler, P. M., White, S. G., Glendenning, M. B., et al.: Plasma thromboplastin component (PTC) deficiency: a new disease resembling hemophilia, Proc. Soc. Exp. Biol. Med. **79:**692, 1952.

144. Ahlberg, A. K. M.: On the natural history of hemophilia pseudotumor, J. Bone Joint Surg. **57A:**1133, 1975.

145. Alagille, D., Josso, F., Queneau, P., et al.: Les accidents neurologiques périphériqries chez l'enfant hemophilia, Arch. Fr. Pediatr. **23:**319, 1966.

146. Aledort, L.: Workshop on unsolved therapeutic problems in hemophilia, (March 1-2, 1976, Bethesda, Md.), Pub. No. (NIH)77-1089, U.S. Department of Health, Education, and Welfare.

147. Alexander, B., and Goldstein, B.: Dual hemostatic defect in pseudohemophilia, J. Clin. Invest. **32:**551, 1953.

148. Andonian, A. A., and Whiteman, J. T.: Medical program. In Boone, D. C., ed.: Hemophilia and the regional center concept, Los Angeles, 1971, Los Angeles Orthopaedic hospital.

149. Andreassen, M.: Haemofili i Denmark, Opera Domo Biol. Hered. Hum. (Univ. Hefniensis) **6:**1, 1943.

150. Arnold, W. D.: Pseudotumor of hemophilia, Prog. Pediatr. Hematol. Oncol. **1:**99, 1976.

151. Arnold, W. D., and Hilgartner, M. W.: Hemophilic arthropathy. J. Bone Joint Surg. **59A:**287, 1977.

152. Bark, C. J., and Orloff, M. J.: The partial thromboplastin time and factor VIII therapy, Am. J. Clin. Pathol. **57:**478, 1972.

153. Baehner, R. L., and Strauss, H. S.: Hemophilia in the first year of life, N. Engl. J. Med. **275:**524, 1966.

154. Barrow, E. M., and Graham, J. B.: von Willebrand's disease, Prog. Hematol. **4:**203, 1964.

155. Bennett, B., and Ratnoff, O. D.: Detection of the carrier state for classic hemophilia, N. Engl. J. Med. **288:**342, 1973.

156. Biggs, R.: The absorption of human factor VIII neutralizing antibody by factor VIII, Br. J. Haematol. **26:**259, 1974.

157. Biggs, R., Douglas, A. J., Macfarlane, R. G., et al.: Christmas disease: a condition previously mistaken for haemophilia, Br. Med. J. **2:**1378, 1952.

158. Boone, D. C.: Common musculoskeletal problems and their management, in Boone, D. C., ed.: Comprehensive management of hemophilia, Philadelphia, 1976, F. A. Davis Co.

159. Borchgrevinck, C. F., Egeberg, O., Godal, H. C., et al.: The effect of plasma and Cohn's fraction I on the Duke and Ivy bleeding times in von Willebrand's disease, Acta Med. Scand. **173:**235, 1963.

160. Bouhasin, J. D., Montcleone, P., and Altay, C.: Role of the lymphocyte in antihemophilic globulin production, J. Lab. Clin. Med. **78:**122, 1971.

161. Brachmann, H. H., Hoffman, P., Etzel, F., et al.: Home care in Germany: philosophy of treatment, Thromb. Haematol. **38:**1, 1977.

162. Brinkhous, K. M.: A study of the clotting defect in hemophilia: the delayed formation of thrombin, Am. J. Med. Sci. **198:**509, 1939.

163. Brinkhous, K. M., Dairs, P. D., Graham, J. B., et al.: Expression and linkage of genes for x-linked hemophiliacs A and B in the dog, Blood **41:**577. 1973.

164. Brinkhous, K. M., Shanbrom, E., Roberts, H. R., et al.: A new high potency glycine-precipitated antihemophilic factor (AHF) concentrate, J.A.M.A. **205:**613, 1968.

165. Brown, P. E., Hougie, C., and Roberts, H. R.: The genetic heterogenity of hemophilia B, N. Engl. J. Med. **283:**61, 1970.

166. Buckner, R. G., and Hampton, J. W.: Canine hemophilia, Blood **27:**414, 1966.

167. Bulloch, W., and Fildes, P.: The treasury of human inheritance, London: 1911, Cambridge University.

168. Chediak, J. R., Telfer, M. D., and Green, D.: Platelet function and immunologic parameters in von Willebrand's disease following cryoprecipitate and factor VIII concentrate infusion, Am. J. Med. **62:**369, 1977.

169. Cornu, P., Larrieu, M. J., Caen, J., et al.: Transfusion studies in von Willebrand's disease: effect on bleeding time and factor VIII, Br. J. Haematol. **9:**139, 1963.

170. Czapek, E. E., Hoyer, L. H., and Schwartz, A. D.: Hemophilia in a female, J. Pediatr. **84:**485, 1974.

171. Davie, E. W., and Fugikawa, K.: Basic mechanism in blood coagulation, Ann. Rev. Biochem. **44:**799, 1975.

172. Denson, K. W. E., Biggs, R., Haddon, M. E., et al.: Two types of haemophilia (A+ and A−): a study of 48 cases, Br. J. Haematol. **17:**163, 1969.

173. Denson, K. W. E., Biggs, R., and Manucci, P. M.: An investigation of three patients with Christmas disease due to an abnormal type of factor IX, J. Clin. Pathol. **21:** 160, 1968.

174. Dietrich, S. L.: Comment: Cause of Death in Hemophiliacs, in workshop on unsolved therapeutic problems in hemophilia (March 1-2, 1976, Bethesda, Md.), Pub. No. (NIH)77-1089, U.S. Department of Health, Education and Welfare.

175. Dietrich, S. L.: Comprehensive care for the person with hemophilia, New York, 1977, National Hemophilia Foundation.

176. Dodds, J.: Storage, release, and synthesis of coagulation factors in isolated perfused organs, Am. J. Physiol. **217:**879, 1969.

177. Duthie, R. B., Matthews, J. M., Rizza, C. R., et al.: The management of musculoskeletal problems in the hemophiliac, Oxford, 1972, Blackwell Scientific Publications, Ltd.

178. Elston, R. C., Graham, J. B., Miller, C. H., et al.: Probablistic classification of hemophilia A carriers by discriminate analysis, Thromb. Res. **8:**683, 1976.

179. Evans, B. E.; Dental management. In Progress in Pediatric Hematology/Oncology, vol. 1, Littleton, Mass., 1976, Publishing Sciences Group.

180. Evans, B. E.: Dental treatment for hemophiliacs, Mt. Sinai J. Med. **44:**409, 1977.

181. Eyster, E. M., Hilgartner, M. W., Gill, B., et al.: Central nervous system bleeding in hemophilia, Blood **51:** 1179, 1978.

182. Fernstein, D., Chong, M. N. Y., Kasper, C. K., et al.: Hemophilia A: polymorphism detectable by a factor VIII antibody, Science **163:**1071, 1969.

183. Fugikawa, K., Coan, M. H., Enfield, D. L., et al.: A comparison of bovine prothrombin, factor IX (Christman factor), and factor X (Stuart factor), Proc. Natl. Acad. Sci. **71:**427, 1974.

184. Gendleman, S.: Hemophilia and the nervous system, Mt. Sinai J. Med. **44:**402, 1977.

185. Gilbert, M. S.: Haemophiliac pseudotumors. In Brinkhous, K. M., and Hemker, H. C., eds.: Handbook of hemophilia, Amsterdam, 1975, Excerpta Medica.

186. Gilchrist, G. S., and Piepgras, D. G.: Neurologic complications in hemophilia. In Progress in Pediatric Hematology/Oncology, vol 1, Littleton, Mass., 1976, Publishing Sciences Group.

187. Graham, J. B., Barrow, E. S., Roberts, H. R., et al.: Dominant inheritanct of hemophilia A in three generations of women, Blood **46:**178, 1975.

188. Graham, J. B., Buchwalter, J. A., Hartley, L. J., et al.: Canine hemophilia: observations on its course, the clotting anomaly and the effect of blood transfusion, J. Exp. Med. **90:**97, 1949.

189. Gralnick, H. R., Coller, B. J., and Marchesi, S. L.: Studies of the human factor VIII/von Willebrand's disease factor protein, Thromb. Res. **6:**93, 1975.

190. Gralnick, H. R., Sultan, Y., and Coller, B. S.: von Willebrand's disease: combined qualitative and quantitative abnormalities, N. Engl. J. Med. **296:**1024, 1977.

191. Hathaway, H. S., Lubs, M. L., and Hathaway, W. E.: Carrier detection in classical hemophilia, Pediatrics **57:** 251, 1976.

192. Hathaway, W. E., Mahasandana, C., Clarke, S., et al.: Paradoxical bleeding in intensively transfused hemophilics: alteration of platelet function, Transfusion **13:** 6, 1973.

193. Hathaway, W. E., Mull, M. N., Githens, J. H., et al.: Attempted spleen transplant in classical hemophilia, Transplantation 7:73, 1969.

194. Hellem, A. J.: The adhesiveness of human blood platelets in vitro, Scand. J. Clin. Lab. Invest. 12(suppl. 51): 1, 1960.

195. Herschgold, E. J., Davison, A. M., and Janzen, M. E.: Isolation and some chemical properties of human factor VIII, J. Lab. Clin. Med. 77:185, 1971.

196. Hilgartner, M. W.: Intrarenal obstruction in hemophilia, Lancet 1:486, 1966.

197. Hilgartner, M. W.: Hemophilic arthropathy, Adv. Pediatr. 21:139, 1974.

198. Hilgartner, M. W.: Symposium on home care of patients with hemophilia: current state of the art, Presented at eleventh Congress of World Federation of Hemophilia, Scand. J. Haematol. Suppl. 30:58, 1977.

199. Hilgartner, M. W., and Arnold, W. D.: Hemophilic pseudotumor treated with replacement and radiation therapy, J. Bone Joint Surg. 57A:1145, 1975.

200. Hilgartner, M. W., and Giardina, P.: Liver disease in patients with hemophilia A, B, and von Willebrand's disease, Transfusion 17:495, 1977.

201. Hoag, M. S., Johnson, F. F., Robinson, J. A., et al.: Treatment of hemophilia B with a new clotting factor concentrate, N. Engl. J. Med. 320:581, 1969.

202. Holmberg, L., Henrikson, R., Ekelund, H., et al.: Coagulation in the human fetus: comparison with term newborn infants, J. Pediatr. 85:860, 1974.

203. Hougie, C., and Twomey, J. J.: Hemophilia B$_M$: a new type of factor IX deficiency, Lancet 1:698, 1967.

204. Howard, M. A., and Firkin, B. G.: Ristocetin: a new tool in the investigation of platelet aggregation, Thromb. Diath. Haemorrh. 26:362, 1971.

205. Howard, M. A., Hutton, R. A., and Hardisty, R. M.: Hereditary giant platelet syndrome: a disorder of a new aspect of platelet function, Br. Med. J. 2:586, 1973.

206. Hoyer, L. W.: Immunologic studies of antihemophilic factor (AHF, factor VIII), J. Lab. Clin. Med. 80:822, 1972.

207. Hoyer, L. W.: Immunologic properties of antihemophilic factor, Prog. Hematol. 8:191, 1973.

208. Hoyer, L. W.: von Willebrand's disease, Prog. Hemostasis Thromb. 3:231, 1976.

209. Hoyer, L. W., and Breckenridge, R. T.: Immunologic studies of antihemophilic factor: cross-reacting material in a genetic variant of hemophilia, Blood 32:962, 1968.

210. Hoyer, L. W., de los Santos, R. P., and Hoyer, J. R.: Antihemophilic factor antigen: localization in endothelial cells by immunofluorescent microscopy, J. Clin. Invest. 52:2737, 1973.

211. Jaffe, E. A., Hoyer, L. W., and Nachman, R. L.: Synthesis of antihemophilic factor antigen by cultured human endothilial cells, J. Clin. Invest. 52:2757, 1973.

212. Jaffe, E. A., Hoyer, L. W., and Nachman, R. L.: Synthesis of von Willebrand factor by cultured human endothelial cells, Proc. Natl. Acad. Sci. 71:1906, 1974.

213. Johnson, A. J., Karpatkin, M. H., and Newman, J.: Clinical investigation of intermediate and high purity hemophilia factor (facotr VIII) concentrates, Br. J. Haematol. 21:21, 1971.

214. Johnson, A. J., Newman, J., Howell, M. B., et al.: The preparation and some properties of a chronically useful high purity human antihemophilic factor (AHF), Presented at eleventh congress of the International Society of Blood Transfusion, Sydney, 1965. (Abstract.)

215. Jordan, H. H.: Hemophilic arthropathies, Springfield, Ill., 1958, Charles C Thomas, Publisher.

216. Jürgens, R., Lehmann, W., Wegelius, O., et al.: Mitterlung über den Mangle un antihämophilem globulin (factor VIII) ber der Aolandischen thrombopathie (v. Willebrand-Jürgens), Thromb. Diath. Haemorrh. 1: 257, 1957.

217. Kasper, C. K., Minami, J. Y., and Rapaport, S. J.: Detection of the carrier state in hemophilia B, Clin. Res. 17:116, 1969.

218. Kerr, C. B.: The Management of Hemophilia, Globe, 1963, Australasian Medical Publishing Co., Ltd.

219. Kerr, C. B.: Intracranial hemorrhage in hemophilia, J. Neurol. Neurosurg. Psychiatr. 27:166, 1964.

220. Kinney, T. R., Zimmerman, R. A., Butler, R., et al.: Computerized tomography in the management of intracranial bleeding in hemophilia, J. Pediatr. 91:31, 1977.

221. Kisker, C. T., and Burke, C.: Double-blind studies on the use of steroids in the treatment of acute hemarthrosis in patients with hemophilia, N. Engl. J. Med. 202: 639, 1970.

222. Krugman, S.: Hepatitis: current status of etiology and prevention, Hosp. Prac. 10(1):39, 1975.

223. Larrieu, M. J., and Soulier, J. P.: Déficit en facteur antihémophilique A chex une fille associé à un trouble du saignement, Rev. Hematol. 8:361, 1953.

224. Lazerson, J.: Hemophilia home transfusion program: effect on school attendance, J. Pediatr. 81:330, 1972.

225. Lazerson, J.: Renal disease in hemophilia. In Progress in Pediatric Hematology/Oncology, Littleton, Mass., 1976, Publishing Sciences Group.

226. Legaz, M. E., Schmer, G., Counts, R. B., et al.: Isolation and characterization of human factor VIII (antihemophilic factor), J. Biol. Chem. 248:2946, 1973.

227. Lewis, J. H.: Causes of death in hemophilia, J.A.M.A. 214:1707, 1970. (Letter.)

228. Lewis, J., Maxwell, W. G., and Brandon, J. M.: Jaundice and hepatitis B antigen/antibody in hemophilia, Transfusion 14:203, 1974.

229. Levine, P. H.: Efficacy of self-therapy in hemophilia: a study of 72 patients with hemophilia A and B, N. Engl. J. Med. 291:1381, 1974.

230. Levine, P. H., McVerry, B., Attock, B., et al.: Health of the intensively treated hemophiliac, with special reference to the abnormal liver chemistries and splenomegaly, Blood 50:1, 1977.

231. Li, C. C.: The hemophilia gene in the population. In Brinkhous, K. M., ed.: International conference on hemophilia proceedings, Chapel Hill, 1964, University of North Carolina Press.

232. Lucas, O. N., Carroll, R. T., Finkelmann, A., et al.: Tooth extractions in hemophilia: control of bleeding without use of blood, plasma or plasma fractions, Thromb. Diath. Haemorrh. 8:209, 1962.

233. Lusher, J. M., and Barnhart, M. I.: Congenital disorders affecting platelets. (In press.)

234. Macfarlane, R. G.: The mechanism of hemostasis, Q. J. Med. 10:1, 1941.

235. Manucci, P. M., Capitanis, A., Del Ninno, E., et al.: Asymptomatic liver disease in hemophilia, J. Clin. Pathol. 28:620, 1975.

236. Marchesi, S. L., Schulman, N. R., and Gralnick, H. R.: Studies on the purification and characteristics of human factor VIII, J. Clin. Invest. 51:2151, 1972.

237. Massie, R. K.: Nicholas and Alexandra, New York, 1967, Atheneum Publishers.

238. May, R. B., and McMillan, C. W.: Bleeding disorders in the newborn. In Conn, H. F., and Conn, R. B., eds.: Current diagnosis, Philadelphia, 1977, W. B. Saunders Co.

239. McCurdy, P. R.: Use of genetic linkage for the detection of female carriers of hemophilia, N. Engl. J. Med. 285: 218, 1971.

240. McKusick, V. A.: Mendelian inheritance in man, Baltimore, 1975, Johns Hopkins University Press.

241. McLester, W. D., and Graham, J. B.: Synthesis of plasma antihemophilic factor, Nature **197**:708, 1963.

242. McMillan, C. W., Webster, W. P., Roberts, H. R., et al.: Continuous intravenous infusion of factor VIII in classic hemophilia, Br. J. Haematol. **18**:659, 1970.

243. Mellanby, J.: The coagulation of the blood, J. Physiol. **38**:28, 1909.

244. Menache, D.: Clinical use of factor IX concentrates, Thromb. Diath. Haemaorrh. **33**:597, 1975.

244a. Merritt, A. D.: Population genetics and hemophilia implications of mutation and carrier recognition, Ann. N.Y. Acad. Sci. **240**:121, 1975.

245. Meyer, D., Bidwell, E., and Larrieu, M. J.: Cross reacting material in genetic variants of hemophilia B, J. Clin. Pathol. **25**:433, 1972.

246. Meyer, D., Lavergne, J. M., Larrieu, M. J., et al.: Cross-reacting material in congenital factor VIII deficiencies, Thromb. Res. **6**:93, 1975.

247. Mielke, C. H., Kaneshiro, M. M., Maher, I. A., et al.: The standardized normal Ivy bleeding time and its prolongation by aspirin. Blood **34**:204, 1969.

248. Minot, G. R.: Familial hemorrhagic condition associated with prolongation of bleeding times, Am. J. Med. Sci. **175**:301, 1928.

249. Nachman, R. L.: von Willebrand's disease and the molecular pathology of hemostasis, N. Engl. J. Med. **296**: 1059, 1977.

250. Nachman, R. L., Jaffe, E. A., and Weksler, B. B.: Immunoinhibition of ristocetin-induced platelet aggregation, J. Clin. Invest. **59**:143, 1977.

251. Nakai, T. R., Peterson, J. C., and Law, D. B.: Current concepts in the management of the hemophilic pedontic patient, J. Dent. Child **41**:361, 1974.

252. National Blood Resources Program: Pilot study of hemophilia in the U.S. Bethesda, Md., U.S. Department of Health, Education, and Welfare, National Institutes of Health, 1972.

253. Neal, W. R., Tayloe, D. T., Jr., Cederbaum, A. L., at al.: Detection of genetic variants of haemophilia B with an immunologic technique, Br. J. Haematol. **25**:63, 1973.

254. Nilsson, I. M., Blomback, M., Jorpes, E., et al.: von Willebrand's disease and its correction with human plasma fraction 1-0, Acta Med. Scand. **159**:179, 1957.

255. Orringer, E. P., Koury, M. J., Blatt, P. M., et al.: Hemolysis caused by factor VIII concentrates, Arch. Intern. Med. **136**:1018, 1976.

256. Orstavik, K. H., Osterud, B., Prydz, H., et al.: Electro-immunoassay of factor IX in hemophilia B, Thromb. Res. **7**:373, 1975.

257. Osterud, B., and Flengsrud, R.: Purification and some characteristics of the coagulation factor IX from human plasma, Biochem. **145**:469, 1975.

258. Otto, J. C.: An account of an hemorrhagic disposition existing in certain families, Med. Reposit. **6**:1, 1803.

259. Patek, A. J., Jr., and Taylor, F. A. L.: Hemophilia II. Some properties of a substance obtained from normal plasma effective in accelerating the coagulation depth of hemophilic blood, J. Clin. Invest. **16**:113, 1937.

260. Pavlovsky, A.: Contribution to the pathogenesis in hemophilia, Blood **2**:185, 1947.

261. Pool, J. G.: Cryoprecipitate quality and supply, Transfusion **15**:305, 1975.

262. Pool, J. G., and Shannon, A. E.: Production of high potency concentrates of antihemophilic globulin in a closed bag system; assay in vitro and in vivo, N. Engl. J. Med. **273**:1443, 1965.

263. Pool, J. G., and Spaet, T. H.: Ethionine-induced depression of plasma antihemophilic globulin in the rat, Proc. Soc. Exp. Biol. Med. **87**:54, 1954.

264. Prentice, C. R. M., Lindsay, R. M., Baer, R. D., et al.: Renal complications in hemophilia and Christmas disease, Q. J. Med. **157**:47, 1971.

265. Quick, A. J., and Hussey, C. V.: Hemophilic condition in the female, J. Lab. Clin. Med. **42**:929, 1953.

266. Rabiner, S. T., and Telfer, M. C.: Home transfusion with hemophilia A, N. Engl. J. Med. **283**:1011, 1970.

267. Rainsford, S. G., Jouhar, S. J., and Hall, A.: Tranexamic acid in the control of spontaneous bleeding in severe hemophilia, Thromb. Diath. Haemorrh. **30**:272, 1973.

268. Reese, E. P., Jr., McCullough, J. J., Craddock, P. P.: An adverse pulmonary reaction of cryoprecipitate, in a hemophiliac. Transfusion **15**:583, 1973.

269. Rick, M. E., and Hoyer, L. W.: The molecular structures of factor VIII and factor IX. In Hilgartner, M. W., ed.: Hemophilia in children. In Progress in pediatric hematology/oncology, vol. 1, Littleton, Mass., 1976, Publishing Science Group.

270. Rickles, F. R., Hardin, J. A., Pitlick, F. A., et al.: Tissue factor activity in lymphocyte cultures from normal individuals and patients with hemophilia, J. Clin. Inv. **52**:1427, 1973.

271. Rizza, C. R., Kernoff, P. B., Matthews, J. M., et al.: A comparison of coagulation factor replacement with and without prednisone in the treatment of hematuria in hemophilia and Christmas disease. Thromb. Hemost. **37**:86, 1977.

272. Roberts, H. R., Grizzle, J. E., McLester, W. D., et al.: Genetic variants of hemophilia B: detection by means of a specific PTC inhibitor, J. Clin. Inv. **47**:360, 1968.

273. Salzman, E. W.: Measurement of platelet adhesiveness: a simple *in vitro* technique demonstrating an abnormality in von Willebrand's disease. J. Lab. Clin. Med. **62**:724, 1963.

274. Schulman, I., Smith, C. H., Erlandson, M., et al.: Vascular hemophilia, Pediatrics **18**:347, 1956.

275. Schulman, I., and Smith, C. H.: Hemorrhagic disease in an infant due to deficiency of a previously undescribed clotting factor, Blood **7**:794, 1952.

276. Second international workshop on human gene mapping, Birth Defects **11**:24, 1975.

277. Seeler, R. A.: Hemolysis due to anti-A and anti-B in factor VIII preparations, Arch. Intern. Med. **130**:101, 1972.

278. Seeler, R. A., Telischi, M., Langenhenning, P., et al.: Comparison of anti-A and anti-B titers in factor VIII and IX concentrates, J. Pediatr. **89**:87, 1976.

279. Seligsohn, K.: Hemophilia and other clotting disorders, Isr. J. Med. Sci. **9**:1338, 1973.

280. Shanberge, J. N., and Gore, I.: Studies on the immunologic and physiologic activities of antihemophilic factor (AHF), J. Lab. Clin. Med. **50**:954, 1957.

281. Shapiro, G. A., Anderson, F. C., Pizzo, S. V., et al.: The subunit structure of normal and hemophilic factor VIII, J. Clin. Invest. **52**:2198, 1973.

282. Shapiro, S. S., Eyster, M. E., and Lewis, J.: Collected experience of the Pennsylvania hemophilia program, Thromb. Hemost. **38**:370, 1977. (Abstract.)

283. Shapiro, S. S., and Hultin, M.: Acquired inhibitors to the blood coagulation factors, Semin. Thromb. Hemost. **1**:336, 1975.

284. Silverstein, A.: Intracranial bleeding in hemophilia, Arch. Neurol. **3**:141, 1960.

285. Singher, L. J.: Renal and urologic complications of hemophilia. in Brinkhous, K. M., and Hemker, H. C., Handbook of hemophilia, Amsterdam, 1975, Excerpta Medica.

286. Stenflo, J., Fernlund, P., Egan, W., et al.: Vitamin K dependent modifications of glutamic acid residues in prothrombin, Proc. Natl. Acad. Sci. **71**:2730, 1974.

287. Storti, E., Magrini, U., and Ascari, E.: Synovial fibrino-

lysis and haemophilic haemarthrosis, Br. Med. J. **4:**812, 1971.

288. Tocantins, L. M., Carroll, R. T., and Holburn, R. H.: The clot accelerating effect of dilution on blood and plasma: relation to the mechanism of coagulation of normal and hemophilic blood, Blood **6:**920, 1951.

289. Thompson, A. R.: Factor IX antigen by radioimmunoassay, J. Clin. Invest. **59:**900, 1977.

290. Tullis, J. L., Melin, M., and Jurigan, P.: Clinical use of prothrombin complexes, N. Engl. J. Med. **273:**667, 1965.

291. Twomey, J. J., Corless, J., Thornton, L., et al.: Studies on the inheritance and nature of hemophilia B, Am. J. Med. **46:**372, 1969.

292. Visconti, E. B., and Hilgartner, M. W.: Central nervous system bleeding in hemophilia, an updated view. (In press.)

293. Volpe, J. J., Manica, J. P., Land, V. J., et al.: Neonatal subdural hematoma associated with severe hemophilia A, J. Pediatr. **88:**1023, 1976.

294. Van Eys, J., Hilgartner, M. W., Lazerson, J., et al.: Home care program, physician's manual, New York, 1977, National Hemophilia Foundation.

295. von-Trotsenburg, L.: Neurological complications of hemophilia. In Brinkhous, K. M., and Hemker, H. C., eds.: Handbook of hemophilia, Amsterdam, 1975, Excerpta Medica.

296. von Willebrand, E. A.: Hereditär pseudohemophili, Finska Läk Sällsk Hand. **68:**87, 1926.

297. von Willebrand, E. A.: Über hereditäre pseudohaemophilic, Acta Med. Scand. **76:**521, 1931.

298. von Willebrand, E. A., and Jürgens, R.: Über eine neue Bluterkrankheit, die konstitutionelle Thrombopathie, Klin. Wochenschr. **12:**414, 1933.

299. Walsh, P. N., Rizza, C. R., Matthews, J. M., et al.: Epsilon-aminocaproic acid therapy for dental extractions in haemophilia and Christmas disease: a double blind controlled trial, Br. J. Haematol. **20:**463, 1971.

300. Webster, W. P., Dodds, W. J., Mandel, S. R., et al.: Biosynthesis of factors VIII and IX: organ transplantation and perfusion studies. In Brinkhous, K. M., and Hemker, H. C., eds.: Handbook of hemophilia. Part 1, Amsterdam, 1975, Excerpta Medica.

301. Webster, W. P., Penick, G. D., Peacock, E. E., et al.: Allotransplantation of spleen in hemophilia, N.C. Med. J. **28:**505, 1967.

302. Webster, W. P., Roberts, H. R., and Penick, G. D.: Dental care of patients with hereditary disorders of blood coagulation, Mod. Treat. **5:**93, 1968.

303. Weiss, H. J., Sussman, I. I., and Hoyer, L. W.: Stabilization of factor VIII in plasma by the von Willebrand factor: studies on posttransfusion and dissociated factor VIII in patients with von Willebrand's disease, J. Clin. Invest. **60:**390, 1977.

304. Weisz, J. A., and Kasper, C. K.: Increased prevalence of hypertension in hemophilia. In Fratantoni, J. C., and Aronson, D. L., eds.: Unsolved therapeutic problems in hemophilia, Pub. No. (NIH)77-1089, U.S. Department of Health, Education, and Welfare.

305. White, G. C., Roberts, H. R., Kingdon, H. S., et al.: Prothrombin complex concentrates: potentially thrombogenic materials and clues to the mechanism of thrombosis in vivo, Blood **49:**159, 1977.

306. Wright, A. E.: On a method of determining the condition of blood coagulability for clinical and experimental purposes, and on the effect of the administration of calcium parts in hemophilia and actual or threatened hemorrhage, Br. Med. J. **2:**223, 1893.

307. Wright, I. S.: The nomenclature of blood clotting factors, Thromb. Diath. Haemorrh. **7:**381, 1962.

308. Zieve, P. D., and Levin, J.: Disorders of hemostasis. In Smith, L. H., Jr., ed.: Major Problems in Internal Medicine, Vol. 10, Philadelphia, 1976, W. B. Saunders Co.

309. Zimmerman, T. S., Edgington, T. S.: Factor VIII coagulant activity and factor VIII-like antigen: independent molecular entities, J. Exp. Med. **138:**1015, 1973.

310. Zimmerman, T. S., Hoyer, L. W., Dickson, L., et al.: Determination of the von Willebrand's disease antigen (factor VIII related antigen) in plasma by quantitative immunoelectrophoresis, J. Lab. Clin. Med. **86:**152, 1975.

311. Zimmerman, T. S., Ratnoff, O. D., and Littel, A. S.: Detection of carriers of classic hemophilia using an immunologic assay for antihemophilic factor (factor VIII), J. Clin. Invest. **50:**255, 1971.

312. Zimmerman, T. S., Ratnoff, O. D., and Powell, A. E.: Immunologic differentiation of classic hemophilia (factor VIII deficiency) and von Willebrand's disease with observations on combined deficiencies of anti-hemophilic factor and factor V, J. Clin. Invest. **50:**244, 1971.

Uncommon inherited coagulation deficiencies

313. Abildgaard, C. F., Cornet, J. A., Alcalde, U., et al.: Hageman factor deficiency in a child, Pediatr. **32:**280, 1963.

314. Abildgaard, C. F., and Harrison, J.: Fletcher factor deficiency: family study and detection, Blood **43:**661, 1974.

315. Alexander, B., Goldstein, R., Landwehr, G., et al.: Congenital SPCA deficiency: a hitherto unrecognized coagulation defect with hemorrhage rectified by serum and serum fractions, J. Clin. Invest. **30:**576, 1951.

316. Aziz, M. A., and Siddiqui, A. R.: Congenital deficiency of fibrin-stabilizing factor (factor XIII): a report of four cases (two families) and family members, Blood **40:**11, 1972.

317. Beck, E. A., Charache, P., and Jackson, D. P.: A new inherited coagulation disorder caused by an abnormal fibrinogen (fibrinogen Baltimore), Nature **208:**143, 1964.

318. Bennett, B., Ratnoff, O. D., Holt, J. B., et al.: Hageman trait (factor XII deficiency): a probable second genotype inherited as an autosomal dominant characteristic, Blood **40:**412, 1972.

319. Bennett, E., and Dormandy, K.: Pool's cryoprecipitate and exhausted plasma in the treatment of von Willebrand's disease and factor XI deficiency, Lancet **2:**731, 1966.

320. Bennett, E. H.: Abnormal fibrinogen (fibrinogen "Baltimore") as a cause of familial hemorrhagic disorder, Blood **24:**853, 1964.

321. Biggs, K.: Prothrombin deficiency. Oxford, 1951, Blackwell Scientific Publications, Ltd.

322. Biggs, R., and Denson, K. W. E.: The fate of prothrombin and factors VIII, IX, and X transfused to patients deficient in these factors, Br. J. Haematol. **9:**532, 1963.

323. Bommer, W., Künzer, W., Schröe, H., et al.: Kongenitale afibrinogenämie. Teil I. Ann. Paediatr. **200:**46, 1963.

324. Bouhasin, J., and Altay, C.: Factor XIII deficiency: concentrations in relatives of patients and in normal infants, J. Pediatr. **72:**336, 1968.

325. Breederveld, K., van Royen, E. A., and Ten Cate, J. W.: Severe factor V deficiency with prolonged bleeding time, Thromb. Diath. Haemost. **32:**538, 1974.

326. Coleman, R. W., Bagdasarian, A., Talamo, R. C., et al.: Williams trait: human kininogen deficiency with diminished levels of plasminogen proactivator and pre-kallikrein associated with abnormalities of the Hageman factor-dependent pathways, J. Clin. Invest. **56:**1650, 1975.

327. Cronberg, S., and Nilsson, I. M.: Circulating antico-

agulant against factor XI and XII together with massive spontaneous platelet aggregation, Scand. J. Haematol. **10:**309, 1973.

328. de Bastos, O., Reno, R. A., and Correa, O. T.: A study of three cases of familiar congenital hypoprothrombinemia (factor II deficiency), Thromb. Diath. Haemorrh. **11:**497, 1964.

329. Denson, K. W. E., Lurie, A., DeCataldo, F., et al.: The factor X defect: recognition of abnormal forms of factor X, Br. J. Haematol. **18:**317, 1970.

330. de Vries, A., Mathot, Y., and Shamir, Z.: Familial congenital labile factor deficiency with syndactylism, Acta Haematol. **5:**129, 1951.

331. de Vries, S. I.: Haemorrhagische diathese door tekort aan factor V (proacceleriae), Ned. Tijdschr. Geneesd. **112:**141, 1968.

332. Donaldson, V. H., Glueck, H. I., Movat, H. Z., et al.: Kininogen deficiency in Fitzgerald trait: role of high molecular weight kininogen in clotting and fibrinolysis, J. Lab. Clin. Med. **87:**327, 1976.

333. Duckert, F.: La facteur XIII et al proteine XIII, Nouv. Rev. Fr. Hematol. **10:**685, 1970.

334. Duckert, F., Jung, E., and Shmerling, D. H.: A hitherto undescribed congenital haemorrhagic diathesis probably due to fibrin stabilizing factor deficiency, Thromb. Diath. Haemorrh. **5:**179, 1960.

335. Egbring, R., Andrassy, K., Egle, H., et al.: Diagnotische und therapeutische probleme bei congenitaler afibrinogenämie, Blut **22:**175, 1971.

336. Feinstein, D. I., Rapaport, S. J., McGehee, W. G., et al.: Factor V anticoagulants: clinical biochemical immunological observations, J. Clin. Invest. **49:**1578, 1970.

337. Fisher, S., Rikover, M., and Noar, J.: Factor XIII deficiency with severe hemorrhagic diathesis, Blood **28:**34, 1966.

338. Fratantoni, J. C., Hilgartner, M. W., and Nachman, R. L.: Nature of the defect in congenital factor V deficiency study in a patient with an acquired circulatory anticoagulant, Blood **39:**751, 1972.

339. Furie, B., Greene, E., and Furie, B. C.: Acquired factor X deficiency and systemic amyloidosis: in vivo studies of factor X, N. Engl. J. Med. **297:**81, 1977.

340. Galanakis, D. K., and Mosesson, M. W.: Evaluation of the role of in vivo protcolysis (fibrinogenolysis) in prolonging the thrombin time of human umbilical cord fibrinogen, Blood **48:**109, 1976.

341. Galanakis, D. K., and Mosesson, M. W.: Comparative studies on fetal fibrinogen from full term and premature infants, Thromb. Haemost. **38:**102, 1977.

342. Gaudernack, G., and Prydz, H.: Studies on PIVKA-X, Thromb. Diath. Haemorrh. **34:**455, 1975.

343. Girolami, A., Molano, G., Lazzarin, M., et al.: A new congenital hemorrhagic condition due to the presence of an abnormal factor X (factor X Firiuli): a study of a large kindred, Br. J. Haematol. **19:**179, 1970.

344. Glueck, H. I., and Sutherland, J. M.: Inherited factor VII defect in Negro family, Pediatrics **27:**204, 1961.

345. Goodnight, S. H., Feinstein, D. I., Osterud, B., et al.: Factor VII antibody-neutralizing material in hereditary and acquired factor VII deficiency, Blood **38:**1, 1971.

346. Gullin, M. C., Menache, D.: Fetal fibrinogen and fibrinogen Paris I. Comparative fibrin monomers aggregation studies, Thromb. Res. **3:**117, 1973.

347. Hampton, J. W., Bird, R. M., and Hammarstein, D. M.: Defective fibrinase activity in two brothers, J. Lab. Clin. Med. **65:**469, 1965.

348. Hanna, M.: Congenital deficiency of factor XIII: report of a family from Newfoundland with associated mild deficiency of factor XII, Pediatrics **46:**611, 1970.

349. Hathaway, W. E., Bechasen, L. P., and Hathaway,

H. S.: Evidence for a new plasma thromboplastin factor, Blood **26:**521, 1965.

350. Hattersley, P. G., and Hayse, D.: Fletcher factor deficiency: a report of three unrelated cases, Br. J. Haematol. **18:**411, 1970.

351. Hilgartner, M. W., and Smith, C. H.: Plasma thromboplastin antecedent (factor XI) in the neonate, J. Pediatr. **66:**747, 1965.

352. Horowitz, H., and Fujimoto, M. M.: Survival of factor XI in vitro and in vivo, Transfusion **5:**539, 1965.

353. Horowitz, H., Wilcox, W., and Jujimoto, M. M.: Assay of plasma thromboplastin antecedent (PTA) with artificially depleted plasma, Blood **22:**35, 1963.

354. Hougie, C., Barrow, E. M., and Graham, J. B.: Stuart cltting defect. I. Segregation of an hereditary hemorrhagic state from the heterogeneous group heretofore called "stable factor" (SPCA, proconvertin, factor VII deficiency, J. Clin. Invest. **36:**485, 1957.

355. Imperato, C., and Dettoni, A. G.: Ipofibrinogenemia congenita con fibrinoastenia, Helv. Paediatr. Acta **13:**380, 1958.

356. Ingram, G. I. C., McBrien, D. J., and Spencer, H.: Fatal pulmonary embolism in congenital fibrinogenemia: report of two cases, Acta Haematol. **35:**56, 1966.

357. Jones, J. H., Rizza, C. R., Hardisty, R. M., et al.: Combined deficiency of factor V and factor VIII (antihemophilic globulin): a report of three cases, Br. J. Haematol. **8:**120, 1962.

358. Josso, F., de Sanchez, J. M., Lavergne, J. M., et al.: Congenital abnormality of the prothrombin molecule (factor II) in four siblings: prothrombin Barcelona, Blood **38:**9, 1971.

359. Josso, F., Prou-Wartelle, O., and Soulier, J. P.: Etude d'un cas d'hypoprothrombinémia congénitale, Nov. Rev. Fr. Hématol. **2:**647, 1962.

360. Kanaide, H., and Shainoff, J. R.: Cross-linking of fibrinogen and fibrin by fibrin-stabilizing factor (factor XIII$_a$), J. Lab. Clin. Med. **85:**574, 1975.

361. Kaplan, A. P., and Austen, K. F.: Activation and control mechanism of Hageman factor-dependent pathways of coagulation, fibrinolysis and kinin generation and their contribution to the inflammatory process, J. Allergy Clin. Immunol. **56:**491, 1975.

362. Kurkcouglu, M., and McElfresh, A. E.: The Hageman factor: determination of its concentration during the neonatal period and presentation of a case of Hageman factor deficiency, J. Pediatr. **57:**61, 1960.

363. Laki, K., and Lorand, L.: On the solubility of fibrin clots, Science **108:**280, 1948.

364. Leiba, H., Ramot, B., and Many, A.: Heredity and coagulation studies in ten families with factor XI (plasma thromboplastin antecedent) deficiency, Br. J. Haematol. **11:**654, 1965.

365. Loeliger, A., and Koller, F.: Behavior of factor VII and prothrombin in late pregnancy and in the newborn, Acta Haematol. **7:**157, 1952.

366. Loewy, A. G.: Enzymatic control of insoluble fibrin formation. In Laki, K., ed.: Fibrinogen, New York, 1968, Marcel Dekker, Inc.

367. Lorand, L.: Physiological and clinical significance of disordered cross-linking in fibrin, Thromb. Haemost. **38:**235, 1977.

368. Lorand, L., Urayama, T., Atencio, A., et al.: Inheritance of deficiency of fibrin stabilizing factor (factor XIII), Am. J. Hum. Genet. **22:**89, 1970.

369. MacKinnon, H. H., and Fekete, J. F.: Congenital afibrinogenemia: vascular changes and multiple thrombosis induced by fibrinogen infusions and contraceptive medication, Can. Med. Assoc. J. **140:**547, 1971.

370. Mammen, E. F., Prasad, A. S., Barnhart, M. I. et al.:

Congenital dysfibrinogenemia: Fibrinogen Detroit, J. Clin. Invest. **48:**235, 1969.

371. Mammen, E. F.: Congenital abnormalities of the fibrinogen molecule, Semin. Thromb. Hemost. **1:**184, 1974.

372. Matheson, R. I., Miller, D. R., Lacombe, M. J., et al.: Flaujeac factor deficiency: reconstitution with highly purified bovine high molecular weight-kininogen and delineation of a new permeability-enhancing peptide released by plasma kallikrein from bovine high molecular weight-kininogen, J. Clin. Invest. **58:**1395, 1976.

373. McDevitt, N. B., McDonagh, J., Taylor, H. L., et al.: An acquired inhibitor to factor XIII, Arch. Intern. Med. **130:**772, 1972.

374. Menache, D.: Congenitally abnormal fibrinogen, Thromb. Diath. Haemorrh. **39**(suppl.):307, 1970.

375. Nachman, R. L., and Marcus, A. J.: Immunologic studies of proteins associated with subcellular fractions of thrombasthenic and afibrinogenemic platelets, Br. J. Haematol. **15:**181, 1968.

376. Nossel, H. L., Niemetz, J., Mibashan, R. S., et al.: The management of factor XI (plasma thromboplastin antecedent): diagnosis and therapy of the congenital deficiency state, Br. J. Haematol. **12:**133, 1966.

377. Nuffel, van E., and Verstraete, M.: Un syndrome hémorrhagique rare: l'afibrinogénie presentation clinique d'un cas, Acta Paediatr. Belg. **7:**185, 1953.

378. Nussbaum, M., and Morse, B. B.: Plasma fibrin stabilizing factor activity in various diseases, Blood **23:**669, 1964.

379. Owren, P. A.: Coagulation of the blood: investigations on a new clotting factor, Acta Med. Scand. **194**(suppl.): 1, 1947.

380. Owren, P. A.: Proconvertin, the new clotting factor, Scand. J. Clin. Lab. Invest. **3:**168, 1951.

381. Palascak, J., and Martinez, J.: Dysfibrinogenemia associated with liver disease, J. Clin. Invest. **60:**89, 1977.

382. Prydz, H., and Gladhaug, A.: Factor X immunologic studies, Thromb. Diath. Haemorrh. **25:**157, 1971.

383. Rabe, F., and Salomon, E.: über faserstoffmangel im blut bei einem falle von Haemophilie, Dtsch. Arch. Klin. Med. **132:**240, 1920.

384. Rabiner, S. F., Winick, M., and Smith, C. H.: Congenital deficiency of factor VII associated with hemorrhagic disease of the newborn, Pediatrics **25:**101, 1960.

385. Rappaport, S. I., Proctor, R. R., Patch, M. J., et al.: The mode of inheritance of PTA deficiency: evidence for the existence of major PTA and minor PTA, Blood **18:**149, 1961.

386. Ratnoff, O. D.: Bleeding syndromes, Springfield, Ill., 1968, Charles C Thomas, Publisher.

387. Ratnoff, O. D.: The molecular basis of hereditary clotting disorders, Prog. Hemostasis Thromb. **1:**39, 1972.

388. Ratnoff, O. D., and Colopy, J. E.: A familial hemorrhagic trait associated with a deficiency of a clot-promoting fraction of plasma, J. Clin. Invest. **34:**602, 1955.

389. Ratnoff, O. D., and Steinberg, A. G.: Further studies on the inheritance of Hageman trait, J. Lab. Clin. Med. **59:**980, 1962.

390a. Ratnoff, O. D., and Steinberg, A. G.: Inheritance of fibrin stabilizing factor deficiency, Lancet **1:**25, 1968.

390. Revol, L.: Les grandes hypofibrinémies constitutionelles hemorrhagiques, Hemostase **2:**243, 1962.

391. Rhoads, J. E., and Fitzgerald, T., Jr.: Idiopathic hypoprothrombinemia: an apparently unrecorded condition, Am. J. Med. Sci. **202:**662, 1941.

392. Robbins, K. C.: A study on the conversion of fibrinogen to fibrin, Am. J. Physiol. **152:**581, 1944.

393. Rosenthal, R. L., Dreskin, R. L., and Rosenthal, N.: New hemophilia like disease caused by deficiency of a

third plasma, thromboplastin factor, Proc. Soc. Exp. Biol. Med. **82:**171, 1953.

394. Saito, H., Ratnoff, O. D., Waldmann, R., et al.: Fitzgerald trait: deficiency of a hitherto unrecognized agent, Fitzgerald factor, participating in surface mediated reactions of clotting, fibrinolysis, generation of kinins, and the property of diluted plasma enhancing vascular permeability, J. Clin. Invest. **55:**1082, 1975.

395. Seligsohn, U.: High gene frequency of factor XI deficiency in Ashkenazi Jews, Thromb. Haemost. **38:**187, 1977. (Abstract.)

396. Shapiro, S. S., and Hultin, M.: Acquired inhibitors to the blood coagulation factors, Semin. Thromb. Hemost. **1:**336, 1975.

397. Shapiro, S. S., Martinez, J., et al.: Congenital dysprothrombinemia: an inherited structural disorder of human prothrombin, J. Clin. Invest. **48:**2251, 1969.

398. Soulier, J. P., and Prou-Wartelle, O.: Étude comparative des tours de cofacteur de la staphylocagulase (C.R.T.) et des taux de factor X (prothrombine) dans diverses conditions, Nouv. Rev. Fr. Hematol. **6:**623, 1966.

399. Telfer, T. P., Denson, K. W., and Wright, D. R.: A "new" coagulation defect, Br. J. Haematol. **2:**308, 1956.

400. Veltkamp, J. J., Loeliger, E. A., and Hemker, H. C.: Biological half-time of Hageman factor, Thromb. Diath. Haemost. **13:**1, 1965.

401. von Felten, A., Duckert, F., and Frick, P. G.: Familial disturbances of fibrin monomer aggregation, Br. J. Haematol. **12:**667, 1966.

402. Webster, W. P., Roberts, H. R., and Penick, G. D.: Hemostasis in factor V deficiency, Am. J. Med. Sci. **249:**92, 1964.

403. Weiss, A. S., Gallin, J. J., and Kaplan, A. P.: Fletcher factor deficiency. Diminished rate of Hageman factor activation caused by absence of prekallikrein with abnormalities of coagulation, fibrinolysis, chemotactic activity, and kinin generation, J. Clin. Invest. **53:**622, 1974.

404. Weiss, H. J., and Rogers, J.: Fibrinogen and platelets in the primary arrest of bleeding: studies in 2 patients wtih congenital afibrinogenemia, N. Engl. J. Med. **285:**369, 1971.

405. Witt, I., Muller, H., and Kunzer, W.: Evidence for the existence of fetal fibrinogen, Thromb. Diath. Haemorrh. **22:**101, 1969.

406. Wuepper, K. D.: Prekallikrein-Hageman factor cofactor-Fletcher factor: are they identical? Clin. Res. **21:**484, 1973.

407. Wuepper, K. D., Miller, D. R., and Lacombe, M. J.: Fleaujeac trait: deficiency of human plasma kininogen, J. Clin. Invest. **56:**1663, 1975.

408. Zahir, M.: Congenital deficiency of fibrin-stabilizing factor: report of a case and family study, J.A.M.A. **207:**751, 1969.

Acquired coagulation deficiencies

409. Agle, D. P., Ratnoff, O. D., and Spring, G. K.: The anticoagulant malingerer, Ann. Intern. Med. **73:**67, 1970.

410. Allen, D. M.: Heparin therapy of purpura fulminans, Pediatrics **38:**211, 1966.

411. Ansell, J. E., Kumar, R., and Deykin, D.: The spectrum of vitamin K deficiency, J.A.M.A. **238:**40, 1977.

412. Antley, R. M., and McMillan, C. W.: Sequential coagulation studies in purpura fulminans, N. Engl. J. Med. **276:**1287, 1967.

413. Bettigole, R. E., Himelstein, E. S., Oettgen, H. F., et al.: Hypofibrinogenemia due to L-asparaginase: studies of fibrinogen survival using autologous ^{131}I-fibrinogen, Blood **35:**195, 1970.

414. Bick, R. L.: Alterations of hemostasis associated with cardiopulmonary bypass: pathophysiology, prevention, diagnosis and management, Semin. Thromb. Hemost. **3:**59, 1976.

415. Bick, R. L., Kovacs, I., and Fekete, L. F.: A new two-stage functional assay for antithrombin III (heparin cofactor): clinical and laboratory evaluation, Thromb. Res. **8:**745, 1976.

416. Bidwell, E.: Acquired inhibitors of coagulants, Ann. Rev. Med. **20:**63, 1969.

417. Biggs, R., ed.: Human blood coagulation, hemostasis and thrombosis, Philadelphia, F. A. Davis Co., 1972.

418. Binkley, S. B., MacCorquodale, D. W., Thayer, S. A., et al.: The isolation of vitamin K_1 and K_2 J. Am. Chem. Soc. **61:**1295, 1939.

419. Blatt, P. M., Lundblad, R. L., Kingdon, H. S., et al.: Thrombogenic materials in prothrombin complex concentrates, Ann. Intern. Med. **81:**734, 1974.

420. Blatt, P. M., and Roberts, H. R.: The immunology of inhibitors to clotting factors. In Rose, N. R., and Friedman, H., eds.: Manual of clinical immunology, 1976, American Society of Microbiology, Chapel Hill, N.C.

421. Blatt, P. M., Roberts, H. R., and Saba, H. I.: Consumption coagulopathy, Chapel Hill, 1974, North Carolina Memorial Hospital.

422. Blatt, P. M., White, G. C., II, McMillan, C. W., et al.: Treatment of antifactor VIII antibodies, Thromb. Haemost. **38:**514, 1977.

423. Bleyl, U.: Morphological diagnosis of disseminated intravascular coagulation: histologic, histochemical, and electronmicroscopic studies, Semin. Thromb. Hemost. **3:**247, 1977.

424. Blomstrand, R., and Forsgen, L.: Vitamin K_1-^3H in man: its intestinal absorption and transport in the thoracic duct lymph, Int. Z. Vitaminforsch **38:**45, 1968.

425. Bowie, E. J. W., Thompson, J. H., Jr., and Pascuzzi, C. A.: Thrombosis in systemic lupus erythematosus despite circulating anticoagulants, J. Lab. Clin. Med. **62:**416, 1964.

426. Breen, F. A., and Tullis, J. L.: Ethanol gelation: a rapid screening test for intravascular coagulation, Ann. Intern. Med. **69:**1197, 1968.

427. Brinkhous, K. M., Smith, H. P., and Warner, E. D.: Plasma prothrombin level in normal infancy and in hemorrhagic disease of the newborn, Am. J. Med. Sci. **193:**475, 1937.

428. Campbell, H. A., and Link, K. P.: Studies on the hemorrhagic sweet clover disease. IV. The isolation and crystallization of the hemorrhagic agent, J. Biol. Chem. **138:**21, 1941.

429. Campbell, H. A., Smith, W. K., Roberts, W. L., et al.: Studies on the hemorrhagic sweet clover disease. II. The bioassay of hemorrhagic concentrates by following the prothrombin level in the plasma of rabbit blood, J. Biol. Chem. **138:**1, 1941.

430. Castro, O., Farber, L. R., and Clyne, L. P.: Circulating anticoagulants against factors IX and XI in systemic lupus erythematosus, Ann. Intern. Med. **77:**543, 1972.

431. Conley, C. L., and Hartman, R. C.: A hemorrhagic disorder caused by circulating anticoagulant in patients with disseminated lupus erythematosus, J. Clin. Invest. **31:**621, 1952.

431a. Cooper, H. A., Bowie, E. J. W., and Owen, C. A., Jr.: Chronic induced intravascular coagulation in dogs, Am. J. Physiol. **225:**1355, 1973.

432. Corrigan, J. J.: Heparin should be used cautiously and selectively, in Ingelfinger, F. J., Ebert, R. W., Finland, M., and Relman, A. S., eds.: Controversies in internal medicine, Philadelphia, 1974, W. B. Saunders Co.

433. Corrigan, J. J., Patterson, J. H., and May, N. E.: Inco-agulability of the blood in systemic erythematosus, Am. J. Dis. Child. **119:**365, 1970.

434. Cronberg, S., and Nilsson, I. M.: Circulating anticoagulant against factors XI and XII together with massive spontaneous platelet aggregation, Scand. J. Haematol. **10:**309, 1973.

435. Dam, H.: Cholesterinstaffwechsel in Hühnchen, Biochem. Ztschr. **215:**475, 1929.

436. Dam, H.: Haemorrhages in chicks reared on artificial diets: a new deficiency disease, Nature **133:**909, 1934.

437. Dam, H.: The anti-haemorrhagic vitamin of the chick, Nature **135:**652, 1935.

438. Dam, H., Geiger, A., Glavind, J., et al.: Isolierung des vitamins K in hochgereinigter, Form. Helv. Chim. Acta **22:**310, 1939.

439. Dam, H., Schonheyder, F., and Tage-Hensen, E.: Studies on the mode of action of vitamin K, Biochem. J. **30:**1075, 1936.

440. Dennis, L. H., Stewart, J. L., and Conrad, M. E.: Heparin treatment of hemorrhagic diathesis in cyanotic congenital heart disease, Lancet **1:**1088, 1967.

441. Deutsch, E.: Blood coagulation changes in liver disease, Prog. Liver Dis. **2:**69, 1965.

442. Deykin, D.: The role of the liver in serum-induced hypercoagulability, J. Clin. Invest. **45:**256, 1966.

443. Dieckmann, W. J.: Blood chemistry and renal function in abruptio placenta, Am. J. Obstet. Gynecol. **31:**734, 1936.

444. Doisy, E. A., Binkley, S. B., Thayer, S. A., et al.: Vitamin K, Science **91:**58, 1940.

445. Doughten, R. M., and Pearson, H. A.: Disseminated intravascular coagulation associated with Aspergillus endocarditis: fatal outcome following heparin therapy, J. Pediatr. **73:**576, 1968.

446. Ekert, H., Gilchrist, G. S., Stanton, R., et al.: Hemostasis in cyantoic congenital heart disease, J. Pediatr. **76:**221, 1970.

447. Esmon, C. T., Sadowski, J. A., and Suttie, J. W.: A new carboxylation reaction: the vitamin K dependent incorporation of $H^{14}CO_3$ into prothrombin, J. Biol. Chem. **250:**4744, 1975.

448. Feinstein, D. I., and Rapaport, S. I.: Acquired inhibitors of blood coagulation, Prog. Thromb. Hemost. **1:**75, 1972.

449. Fekete, L. F., and Bick, R. L.: Laboratory modalities for assessing hemostasis during cardiopulmonary bypass, Semin. Thromb. Hemost. **3:**83, 1976.

450. Fletcher, A. P., Biederman, O., Moore, D., et al.: Abnormal plasminogen-plasmin system activity (fibrinolysis) in patients with hepatic cirrhosis: its cause and consequences, J. Clin. Invest. **43:**68, 1964.

451. Frick, P. G.: Inhibition of conversion of fibrinogen to fibrin by abnormal proteins in multiple myeloma, Am. J. Clin. Pathol. **25:**1263, 1955.

452. Frick, P. G., Riedler, G., and Brogli, H.: Response and minimal daily requirement for vitamin K in man, J. Appl. Physiol. **23:**387, 1967.

453. Galbraith, P. A., Sharma, N., Parker, W. L., et al.: Acquired factor X deficiency: altered plasma antithrombin activity and association with amyloidosis, J.A.M.A. **230:**1658, 1974.

454. Gralnick, H. R., Bagley, J., and Abrell, E.: Heparin treatment for the hemorrhagic diathesis of acute promyelocytic leukemia, Am. J. Med. **52:**167, 1972.

455. Green, D.: The use of immunosuppressive agents in patients with factor VIII antibodies. In Brinkhous, K. M., and Hemker, H. C., eds.: handbook of hemophilia. Part 2, Amsterdam, 1975, Excerpta Medica.

456. Hand, J. J., Moloney, W, C., and Sise, H. S.: Coagulation defects in acute promyelocytic leukemia, Arch. Intern. Med. **123:**39, 1969.

457. Handin, R. I., and Moloney, W. C.: Antibody-induced von Willebrand's disease, Blood **44**:933, 1974.
458. Handley, D. A., and Lawrence, J. R.: Factor IX deficiency in the nephrotic syndrome, Lancet **1**:1079, 1967.
459. Hardaway, R. M.: Syndromes of disseminated intravascular coagulation, with special reference to shock and hemorrhage, Springfield, Ill., 1966, Charles C Thomas, Publisher.
460. Heene, D. L.: Disseminated intravascular coagulation: evaluation of therapeutic approaches, Sem. Thromb. Hemost. **3**:291, 1977.
461. Hemker, H. C.: Interaction of coagulation factors. In Brinkhous, K. M., and Hemker, H. C., eds.: Handbook of hemophilia. Part 1, Amsterdam, 1975, Excerpta Medica.
462. Hillman, R. S., and Phillips, L. L.: Clotting and fibrinolysis in a cavernous hemangioma, Am. J. Dis. Child. **113**:649, 1967.
463. Hjort, P. F., Rapaport, S. I., and Jorgensen, L.: Purpura fulminans: report of case successfully treated with heparin and hydrocortisone: review of 50 cases from literature, Scand. J. Haematol. **1**:169, 1964.
464. Honig, G. R., and Lindley, A.: Deficiency of Hageman factor (factor XII) in patients with the nephrotic syndrome, J. Pediatr. **78**:633, 1971.
465. Inceman, S., and Tangman, Y.: Chronic defibrination syndrome due to a giant hemangioma associated with micro-angiopathic hemolytic anemia, Am. J. Med. **46**:997, 1969.
466. Ingram, G. I. C., Prentice, C. R. M., Forbes, C. D., et al.: Low factor-VIII-like antigen in acquired von Willebrand's syndrome and response to treatment, Br. J. Haematol. **25**:137, 1973.
467. Joachim, G. R., Cameron, J. S., Schwartz, M., et al.: Selectivity of protein excretion in patients with the nephrotic syndrome, J. Clin. Invest. **43**:2332, 1964.
468. Johnson, C. A., Abildgaard, C. F., and Schulman, I.: Absence of coagulation abnormalities in children with cyanotic congenital heart disease, Lancet **2**:660, 1968.
469. Kasabach, H. H., and Merritt, K. K.: Hemangioma with extensive purpura, Am. J. Dis. Child. **59**:1063, 1940.
470. Kasper, C. K.: Incidnece and course among patients with classic hemophilia, Thromb. Diath. Haemorrh. **30**:264, 1973.
471. Kasper, C. K., Aledort, L. M., Counts, R. B., et al.: A more uniform measurement of factor VIII inhibitors, Thromb. Diath. Haemorrh. **34**:869, 1975.
472. Kevy, S. V., Glickman, R. M., Bernhard, W. F., et al.: The pathogenesis and control of the hemorrhagic defect in open-heart surgery, Surg. Gynecol. Obstet. **123**:313, 1966.
473. Komp, D. M., and Sparrow, A. W.: Polycythemia in cyanotic heart disease: a study of altered coagulation, J. Pediatr. **76**:231, 1970.
474. Kurczynski, E. M., and Penner, J. M.: Activated prothrombin concentrate for patients with factor VIII inhibitors, N. Engl. J. Med. **291**:164, 1974.
475. Lambert, C. J.: Cardiopulmonary bypass hemorrhage: a surgeon's point of view, Semin. Thromb. Hemost. **3**:90, 1976.
476. Lechner, K.: Acquired inhibitors in auto and isoimmune disease, Thromb. Diath. Haemorrh. **45**:227, 1971.
477. Lerner, R. G., Rapaport, S. I., and Meltzer, J.: Thrombotic thrombocytopenic purpura: serial clotting studies, relation to the generalized Shwartzman reaction, and remission after adrenal steroid and dextran therapy, Ann. Intern. Med. **66**:1181, 1967.
478. Lindhout, M. J., and Kop-Khassen, B. H. M.: Proteins induced by vitamin K antagonists (PIVKA's). In Hemker, H. C., and Veltkamp, J. J., eds.: Prothrombin and

related clotting factors, Leiden, 1975, Leiden University Press.
479. Little, J. R.: Purpura fulminans treated successfully with anticoagulation, **169**:104, 1959.
480. Magnusson, S., Peterson, T. E., Sottrup-Jensen, L., et al.: Complete primary structure of prothrombin: isolation, structure and reactivity of ten carboxylated glutamic acid residues and regulation of prothrombin activation by thrombin. In Reich, R., Rifkin, D. B., and Shaw, E., eds.: Proteases and biological control, New York, 1975, Cold Spring Harbor Laboratory.
481. Mandel, E. E., and Lazerson, J.: Thrombasthenia in liver disease, N. Engl. J. Med. **265**:56, 1961.
482. Margolius, A., Jr., Jackson, D. P., and Ratnoff, O. D.: Circulating anticoagulants: a study of 40 cases and a review of the literature, Medicine **40**:145, 1961.
483. Mason, R. G., Mohammed, S. F., Chuang, H. Y. K., et al.: The adhesion of platelets to subendothelium, collagen, and artificial surfaces, Sem. Thromb. Hemost. **3**:98, 1976.
484. Maurer, H. M.: Hematologic effects of cardiac disease, Pediatr. Clin. North Am. **19**:1083, 1972.
485. McKay, D. G.: Disseminated intravascular coagulation, New York, 1965, Hoeber Medical Div., Harper & Row, Publishers.
486. McKay, D. G., and Muller-Berghaus, G.: Therapeutic implications of disseminated intravascular coagulation, Am. J. Cardiol. **20**:392, 1967.
487. McMillan, C. W., Gaudry, C. L., and Holemans, R.: Coagulation defects and metastatic neuroblastoma, J. Pediatr. **72**:347, 1968.
488. McMillan, C. W., and Roberts, H. R.: Congenital combined deficiency of coagulation factors II, VII, IX, and X: report of a case, N. Engl. J. Med. **274**:1313, 1966.
489. McMillan, C. W., Weiss, A. E., and Johnson, A. M.: Acquired coagulation disorders in children, Pediatr. Clin. North Am. **19**:1029, 1972.
490. Miller, L. L., and Bale, W. F.: Synthesis of all plasma protein fractions except gamma globulins by the liver, J. Exp. Med. **99**:125, 1954.
491. Minna, J. D., Robboy, S. J., and Coleman, R. W.: Disseminated intravascular coagulation in man. Springfield, Ill., 1974, Charles C Thomas, Publisher.
492. Morawitz, P.: Die Chemie der Blutgerinnung, Ergeb. Physiol. **4**:307, 1905.
493. Moschcowitz, E.: An acute febrile pleiochromic anemia with hyaline thrombosis of the terminal aterioles and capillaries, Arch. Intern. Med. **36**:89, 1925.
494. Muller-Berghaus, G.: Pathophysiology of generalized intravascular coagulation, Semin. Thromb. Hemost. **3**:209, 1977.
495. O'Reilly, R. A., and Aggeler, P. M.: Covert anticoagulant ingestion: study of 25 patients and review of world literature, Medicine **55**:389, 1976.
496. Osler, W.: Hemorrhage in chronic jaundice, Am. Med. **1**:152, 1901.
497. Owen, C. A., Jr., and Bowie, E. J. W.: Chronic intravascular coagulation and fibrinolysis (ICF) syndromes (DIC), Semin. Thromb. Hemost. **3**:268, 1977.
498. Patterson, J. H., Pierce, R. B., Anderson, J. R., et al.: Dextran therapy of purpura fulminans, N. Engl. J. Med. **273**:734, 1965.
499. Penick, G. D., Averette, H. E., and Peters, R. M.: The hemorrhagic syndrome complicating extracorporeal shunting of blood: an experimental study of its pathogenesis, Thromb. Diath. Haemorrh. **2**:218, 1958.
500. Penick, G. D., and Roberts, H. R.: Intravascular clotting: focal and systemic, Intern. Rev. Exp. Pathol. **3**:269, 1964.
501. Perkins, H. A., Mackenzie, M. R., and Fudenberg,

H. H.: Hemostatic defect in dysproteinemias, Blood **35:** 695, 1970.

502. Porter, J. M., and Silver, D.: Alterations in fibrinolysis and coagulation associated with cardiopulmonary bypass, J. Thorac. Cardiov. Surg. **56:**869, 1968.

503. Price, P. A., Otsuka, A. S., Poser, J. W., et al.: Characterization of a γcarboxyglutamic acid-containing protein from bone, Proc. Natl. Acad. Sci. **73:**1447, 1976.

504. Quick, A. J.: The prothrombin in hemophilia and obstructive jaundice, J. Biol. Chem. **109:**73, 1935.

505. Quick, A. J.: The coagulation defect in sweet clover disease and in the hemorrhagic chick disease of dietary origin: a consideration of the source of prothrombin, Am. J. Physiol. **118:**260, 1937.

506. Quick, A. J.: The Hemorrhagic diseases and the physiology of hemostasis, Springfield, Ill., 1942, Charles C Thomas, Publisher.

507. Quick, A. J.: The anticoagulants effective in vivo with special reference to heparin and dicumarol, Physiol. Rev. **24:**297, 1944.

508. Rake, M. O., Flute, P. T., Pannell, G., et al.: Intravascular coagulation in acute hepatic necrosis, Lancet **1:**533, 1970.

509. Robboy, S. J., Lewis, E. J., Schur, P. H., et al.: Circulating anticoagulants to factor VIII, Am. J. Med. **49:** 742, 1970.

510. Roberts, H. R., and Cederbaum, A. I.: The liver and blood coagulation: physiology and pathology, Gastroenterology **63:**297, 1972.

511. Roderick, L. M.: The pathology of sweet clover disease in cattle, J. Am. Vet. Med. Assoc. **74:**314, 1929.

512. Roderick, L. M.: A problem in the coagulation of the blood "sweet clover disease of cattle," Am. J. Physiol. **96:**413, 1931.

513. Sarji, K. E., Stratton, R. D., Wagner, R. H., et al.: Nature of von Willebrand factor: a new assay and a specific inhibitor, Proc. Natl. Acad. Sci. **71:**2937, 1974.

514. Schleider, M. A., Nachman, R. L., Jaffee, E. A., et al.: A clinical study of the lupus anticoagulant, Blood **48:** 499, 1976.

515. Schnieder, C. L.: "Fibrin embolism" (disseminated intravascular coagulation) with defibrination as one of the end results of placenta abruption, Surg. Gynecol. Obstet. **92:**27, 1951.

516. Schofield, F. W.: A brief account of a disease in cattle simulating hemorrhagic septicaemia due to feeding sweet clover, Can. Vet. Rec. **3:**74, 1922.

517. Shapiro, S. S., and Hultin, M.: Acquired inhibitors to the blood coagulation factors, Semin. Thromb. Hemost. **1:**336, 1975.

518. Shearer, M. J., Barkhan, P., and Webster, G. R.: Absorption and excretion of an oral dose of tritiated vitamin K in man, Br. J. Haematol. **18:**297, 1970.

519. Shin, W. K. T.: Hemangiomas of infancy complicated by thrombocytopenia, Am. J. Surg. **116:**896, 1968.

520. Simone, J. V., Cornet, J. A., and Abildgaard, C. F.: Acquired von Willebrand's syndrome in systemic lupus erythematosus, Blood **31:**806, 1968.

521. Stahmann, M. A., Huebner, C. F., and Link, K. P.: Studies on the hemorrhagic sweet clover disease. V. Identification and synthesis of the hemorrhagic agent, J. Biol. Chem. **138:**513, 1941.

522. Stenflo, J.: Vitamin K and the biosynthesis of prothrombin. IV. Isolation of peptides containing prosthetic groups from normal prothrombin and the corresponding peptides from dicoumarol-induced prothrombin, J. Biol. Chem. **249:**5527, 1974.

523. Stenflo, J.: A new vitamin K-dependent protein: purification from bovine plasma and preliminary characterization, J. Biol. Chem. **251:**355, 1976.

524. Stenflo, J.: Vitamin K, prothrombin, and gammacarboxyglutamic acid, N. Engl. J. Med. **296:**624, 1977.

525. Strauss, H. S.: Acquired circulating anticoagulants in hemophilia A, N. Engl. J. Med. **281:**866, 1969.

526. Suttie, J. W.: Oral anticoagulant therapy: the biosynthetic basis, Semin. Hematol. **14:**365, 1977.

527. Townsend, C. W.: The hemorrhagic disease of the newborn, Arch. Pediatr. **11:**559, 1894.

528. Verska, J. J., Lonser, E. R., and Brewer, L. A.: Predisposing factors and management of hemorrhage following open-heart surgery, J. Cardiovasc. Surg. **13:**361, 1972.

529. Williams, O. K., Van Buskirk, F. W., Burns, S., et al.: Giant hemangioendothelioma with thrombocytopenia and hypofibrinogenemia, Am. J. Roentgen. **106:**204, 1969.

530. Wiss, O., and Gloor, H.: Absorption, distribution, storage, and metabolites of vitamin K and related quinones, Vitam. Horm. **24:**575, 1966.

531. Woolf, I. L., and Babior, B. M.: Vitamin K and warfarin: metabolism, function, and interaction, Am. J. Med. **53:**261, 1972.

532. Yin, E. T., and Gaston, L. W.: Purification and kinetic studies on a circulating anticoagulant in a suspected case of lupus erythematosus, Thromb. Diath. Haemorrh. **14:** 88, 1965.

Neonatal coagulation deficiencies

533. Bleyer, W. A., Wakami, N., and Shephard, T. H.: The development of hemostasis in the human fetus and the newborn infant, J. Pediatr. **79:**838, 1971.

534. Corby, D. G., and Schulman, I.: The effect of antenatal drug administration on aggregation of platelets of newborn infants, J. Pediatr. **79:**307, 1971.

535. Jerkner, K., Jutti, J., and Victorin, L.: Platelet counts in mothers and their newborn infants with respect to antepartum administration of oral diuretics, Acta Med. Scand. **194:**473, 1973.

536. Mountain, R. R., Hirsh, J., and Gallus, A. S.: Neonatal coagulation defect due to anticonvulsant drug treatment in pregnancy, Lancet **1:**265, 1970.

537. Nathan, D. J., and Snapper, I.: Simultaneous transfer of factors responsible for LE cell formation and thrombocytopenia, Am. J. Med. **25:**647, 1958.

538. Report of Committee on Nutrition: Vitamin K compounds and the water-soluble analogues, Pediatrics **28:**501, 1961.

539. Rodrigues, S. U., Leikin, S. L., and Hiller, M. C.: Neonatal thrombocytopenia associated with antepartum administration of thiazide drugs, N. Engl. J. Med. **270:** 881, 1964.

540. Shaul, W. L., and Hall, J. G.: Multiple congenital anomalies associated with oral anticoagulants, Am. J. Obstet. Gynecol. **127:**191, 1977.

541. Stenflo, J., Fernlund, P., Egan, W., et al.: Vitamin L dependent modifications of glutamic acid residues in prothrombin, Proc. Natl. Acad. Sci. **71:**2730, 1974.

Thrombotic disorders

542. Abildgaard, U.: Purification of two progressive antithrombins of human plasma, Scand. J. Clin. Lab. Invest. **19:**190, 1967.

543. Avery, M., Oppenheimer, E., and Gordon, H.: Renal vein thrombosis in newborn infants of diabetic mothers, N. Engl. J. Med. **256:**1134, 1957.

544. Barrie, W. W., Wood, E. H., Crumlish, P., et al.: Low dosage Ancrod for prevention of thrombotic complications after surgery for fractured neck of femur, Pediatr. Med. J. **41:**130, 1974.

545. Bell, W. R., Pitney, W. R., and Goodwin, J. F.: Thera-

peutic defibrination in the treatment of thrombotic disease, Lancet **1:**490, 1968.

546. Bennett, B., Mackie, M., and Douglas, A. S.: Familial thrombosis due to antithrombin III deficiency: an extensive family study, Thromb. Haemost. **38:**78, 1977.
547. Bjarke, B., Herin, P., and Blomback, M.: Neonatal aortic thrombosis: a possible clinical manifestation of congenital antithrombin III deficiency, Acta Pediatr. Scand. **63:**297, 1974.
548. Blemen, A., Susmano, D., Burden, J., et al.: Non-operative treatment of unilateral renal vein thrombosis in the newborn, J.A.M.A. **211:**1165, 1970.
549. Carson, N. A. J., Aisworth, D. C., Dent, C. E., et al.: Homocystinemia: a new inborn error of metabolism associated with mental deficiency, Arch. Dis. Child. **38:**425, 1963.
550. Carson, N. A. J., and Carri, J. J.: Treatment of homocystinemia with pyridoxine, Arch. Dis. Child. **44:**387, 1969.
551. Edson, J. R., Blaese, R. M., White, J. G., et al.: Defibrination syndrome in an infant born after abruptio placenta, J. Pediatr. **72:**342, 1968.
552. Egeberg, O.: The blood coagulability in diabetic patients, Scand. J. Clin. Invest. **15:**533, 1963.
553. Egeberg, O.: Inherited antithrombin deficiency causing thrombophilia, Thromb. Diath. Haemorrh. **13:**516, 1965.
554. Egeberg, O., and Owren, P. A.: Oral contraception and blood coagulability, Br. Med. J. **1:**220, 1963.
555. Esnuf, M. P., and Tunnah, G. W.: The isolation and properties of the thrombin-like activity from ankistrodon rhodestome venom, Br. J. Haematol. **13:**181, 1967.
556. Gallus, A. S., and Hirsh, J.: Prevention of venous thromboembolism, Semin. Thromb. Hemost. **2:**231, 1976.
557. Gallus, A. S., and Hirsh, J.: Treatment of venous embolic disease, Semin. Thromb. Hemost. **2:**291, 1976.
558. Gallus, A. S., Hirsh, J., Hull, R., et al.: Diagnosis of venous thromboembolism, Semin. Thromb. Hemost. **2:**203, 1976.
559. Genton, E., Ellis, J., and Steele, P.: Comparative effects of platelet suppressant drugs on platelet survival, Thromb. Diath. Haemorrh. **34:**552, 1975.
560. Gordon, J.: Oral contraceptives: risks and benefits, N. Engl. J. Med. **289:**809, 1973.
561. Gross, G. P., Hathaway, W. E., and McGaughey, H. R.: Hyperviscosity in the neonate, J. Pediatr. **82:**1004, 1973.
562. Harker, L. A., Ross, R., Slichter, S. J., et al.: Homocystine induced atherosclerosis, J. Clin. Invest. **58:**731, 1976.
563. Harker, L. A., Slichter, S. J., Scott, C. R., et al.: Homocystinemia, N. Engl. J. Med. **291:**537, 1974.
564. Harpel, P. C.: Studies on human plasma α_2 macroglobulin enzyme interactions, J. Exp. Med. **138:**508, 1973.
565. Hathaway, W. S.: Effect of diabetic plasma in von Willebrand's disease, Pediatr. Res. **1:**213, 1967.
566. Hilgartner, M. W.: Intra renal obstruction in hemophilia, Lancet **1:**486, 1966.
567. Hilgartner, M. W., Lanzkowsky, P., and Lipsitz, P.: Perforation of the small and large intestine following exchange transfusion, Am. J. Dis. Child. **120:**79, 1970.
568. Hougie, C.: Thromboembolism and oral contraceptives, Am. Heart J. **85:**538, 1973.
569. Howell, W. H., and Holt, E.: Two new factors in blood coagulation: heparin and pro-antithrombin, Am. J. Physiol. **47:**528, 1918.
570. Kendall, A. G., Lohmann, R. C., and Dissetor, J. B.: Nephrotic syndrome, a hypercoagulable state, Arch. Intern. Med. **127:**1026, 1971.
571. Kiss, J.: Chemistry of heparin: a short review on recent chemical trends, Thromb. Diath. Haemorrh. **33:**20, 1974.

572. Koller, F.: The physiological function of heparin, Thromb. Diath. Haemorrh. **33:**17, 1974.
573. Krause, W. H., and Lang, A.: Effect of angiography on blood coagulation, Thromb. Haemost. **38:**73, 1977. (Abstract.)
574. Lange, L. G., Carvalho, A., Bagdasanian, A., et al.: Activation of Hageman factor in the nephrotic syndrome, Am. J. Med. **56:**565, 1974.
575. Llach, F., Arieff, A. I., and Massey, S. G.: Renal vein thrombosis and nephrotic syndrome, a prospective study of 36 adult patients, Ann. Intern. Med. **83:**8, 1975.
576. Marciniak, E., Farley, C. H., and DeSimone, P. A.: Familial thrombosis due to antithrombin III deficiency, Blood **43:**219, 1974.
577. McCully, K. S.: Vascular pathology of homocystinemia: implications for the pathogenesis of arteriosclerosis, Am. J. Pathol. **56:**111, 1969.
578. McDonald, L., Bray, C., Field, C., et al.: Homocystinemia thrombosis and the blood platelets, Lancet **1:**745, 1964.
579. Miller-Anderson, M., Borg, H., and Andersson, L. O.: Purification of antithrombin III by affinity chromatography, Thromb. Res. **5:**439, 1974.
580. Muller-Berghaus, G., and Hocke, M. P.: Production of the generalized Schwartzman reaction in rabbits by Ancrod (Arvin) infusion and endotoxin injection, Br. J. Haematol. **25:**111, 1973.
581. Nussbaum, M., Moschos, C. B.: Anticoagulants and anticoagulation: symposium on advances in hematology, Med. Clin. North Am. **60:**855, 1976.
582. Ødegard, O. R., and Teier, A. N.: Antithrombin III, heparin cofactor and antifactor X_a in a clinical material, Thromb. Res. **8:**173, 1976.
583. O'Reilly, R. A.: The pharmacodynamics of the oral anticoagulant drugs, Prog. Hemost. Thromb. **2:**195, 1974.
584. Parkin, T. W., and Kvale, W. F.: Neutralization of the anticoagulant effects of heparin with protamine (sulfate), Am. Heart J. **37:**332, 1949.
585. Peterson, C. M., Jones, R. L., Koenig, R. J., et al.: Reversible hematologic sequelae of diabetes mellitus, Ann. Intern. Med. **86:**425, 1977.
586. Renfield, M. L., and Kraybill, E. N.: Consumptive coagulopathy with renal vein thrombosis, J. Pediatr. **82:**1054, 1973.
587. Robertson, J. J., Douglas, H., Salky, N., et al.; The effect of a platelet inhibiting drug (sulfinpyrazone) in the therapy of patients with transient ischemic attacks (tias) and minor strokes, Thromb. Diath. Haemorrh. **34:**598, 1975.
588. Rosenberg, R. D.: Actions and interactions of antithrombin and heparin, N. Engl. J. Med. **292:**146, 1975.
589. Salzman, E. W., Deykin, D., Shapiro, R. M., et al.: Management of heparin therapy, N. Engl. J. Med. **292:**1046, 1975.
590. Sapire, D. W., Markowitz, R., Valdes-Dapena, M., et al.: Thrombosis of the left coronary artery in a newborn infant, J. Pediatr. **90:**957, 1977.
591. Slade, C. L., Andes, W. A., and Mason, A. D., Jr.: Platelet aggregation following defibrination with Ancrod, Thromb. Haem. **36:**424, 1976.
592. Stein, H. L., and Hilgartner, M. W.: Alteration of coagulation mechanisms of blood by contrast media, Am. J. Roentgen. **104:**458, 1968.
593. Stenflo, J., Fernlund, P., Egan, W., et al.: Vitamin K dependent modifications of glutamic acid residues in prothrombin, Proc. Natl. Acad. Sci. **71:**2730, 1974.
594. Symchych, P. S., Krauss, A. N., and Winchester, P.: Endocarditis following intracardiac placement of umbilical venous catheters in neonates, J. Pediatr. **90:**287, 1977.

595. Thomson, C., Fobes, C. D., Prentice, C. R. M., et al.: Changes in blood coagulation and fibrinolysis in the nephrotic syndrome, Q. J. Med. **43:**399, 1974.

596. Veltkamp, J.: Detection and clinical significance of PIVKA, Mayo Clinic Proc. **49:**923, 1974.

597. Ward, T. F.: Multiple thromboses in an infant of a diabetic mother, J. Pediatr. **90:**982, 1977.

598. Wilner, G. D., Casmella, W. J., Fenoglio, C., et al.: In vivo fibrinopeptide: A generation induced by angiograph-ic catheters, Thromb. Haemost. **38:**73, 1977. (Abstract.)

599. Wise, R. C., and Todd, J. K.: Spontaneous lower extremity venous thrombosis in children, Am. J. Dis. Child. **126:**766, 1973.

600. Zweifler, A. J., and Allen, R. J.: An intrinsic blood platelet abnormality in an homocystinemic boy, corrected by pyridoxine administration, Thromb. Diath. Haemorrh. **26:**15, 1971.

Index

Cyanocobalamin; *see* Vitamins, B$_{12}$
Cyanosis
 congenital heart disease and, 162
 familial, 425-426
 methemoglobinemia and, 363, 364, 365, 366
Cyclic AMP; *see* Adenosine monophosphate, cyclic
Cyclic GMP, 529, 539-542
Cyclophosphamide
 anemias and
   aplastic, 466, 469, 470, 484
   Fanconi's, 487
 Döhle bodies and, 502
 gamma globulin antibody and, 232, 233
 histiocytic diseases and, 670
 Hodgkin's disease and, 630
 idiopathic thrombocytopenic purpura and, 715
 immune hemolysis and, 270
 maintenance therapy with, 613, 614
 marrow transplants and, 471, 476, 479, 481, 482
 neutropenia and, 503, 508
 as non–cell cycle–specific drug, 611
 non-Hodgkin's lymphoma and, 635, 637
 pneumonia and, 483
 remission induction by, 589, 609, 612, 613, 616
Cycloserine, 152
Cyklokapron; *see* Tranexamic acid
Cystadenomas, 220
Cystic fibrosis, 802
Cystine, 112
Cysts
 of bone medullary cavity, 666
 ovarian dermoid, 262
 renal, 220
Cytidine, 346
Cytocentrifuge, 600
Cytochalasin B, 293, 529
Cytochromes, 108-109, 110, 363
 iron deficiency and, 136, 141
 in muscles, 138
Cytomegalovirus
 acquired infection and, 575-576
 Chediak-Higashi syndrome and, 539
 immune disorders and, 569
 leukemias and, 605, 608
 lymphomas and, 631
 marrow transplants and, 483
 thrombocytopenias and, 42
   neonatal, 74, 734, 735
 transfusions and, 77
Cytoplasmic vacuoles, 661, 662
Cytosine arabinoside
 as cell cycle–specific drug, 610
 maintenance therapy with, 613, 614
 megaloblastic anemias and, 174, 204
 myelogenous leukemia and, 616
 neutropenia and, 508, 510
 neutrophils and, 502
 in reinduction therapy, 614
 remission induction by, 589, 609, 615, 616
 viral infections in leukemias and, 608
Cytotoxic drugs, 152, 508; *see also* specific drug

D

D^u gene, 60-61
D-1 trisomy, 384, 599
D-L antibody; *see* Donath-Landsteiner antibody
Dactylitis, 416-417
Dantrolene, 572
Dapsone; *see* Diaminodiphenylsulfone
Daraprim; *see* Pyrimethamine
Darvon; *see* Propoxyphene
Daunomycin, 508, 589, 614, 615

Daunorubicin, 609, 611, 613
DDT; *see* Chlorophenothane
Death
 care of child and, 617-618
 postoperative, sickle cell trait and, 411
Defibrination syndrome; *see* Disseminated intravascular coagulation
Degranulation, 526, 529-530
 defects of, 537-548; *see also* Chediak-Higashi syndrome
 tests for, 540
Dehydration
 neonatal, 818
 sickle cell crises and, 418
Delta-chain variants, 395
Demerol; *see* Meperidine
Dengue-like viruses, 469
Dense bodies, 702, 739
5'-Deoxyadenosylcobalamin, 176
Deoxynucleotidyl transferase, 5
Deoxyribonucleic acid, 22
 anemias and
   dyserythropoietic, 235
   Fanconi's, 487
 erythropoietin and, 219
 Feulgen's stain and, 29
 protein synthesis and, 434
 sensitivity to, 748
 synthesis of
   chloramphenicol and, 468
   iron deficiency and, 141
   megaloblasts and, 173-174
Deoxyribonucleic acid viruses, 592
Dermatitis herpetiformis, 196
Dermatoarthritis, lipid, 665
Dermatofibroma, 664
Dermoid cysts, ovarian, 262
Desferal; *see* Desferrioxamine
Desferrioxamine
 iron stores and, 147, 152
 repeated transfusions and, 231, 232
 thalassemia and, 441-442
Desiccytes, 343
Dexamethasone, 38, 714
Dextran
 disseminated intravascular coagulation and, 808
 erythrocyte membrane and, 293
 erythrocyte removal and, 76
 sickle cell crises and, 418
 thrombocytopathy and, 737
Dextrose, 603
DFP; *see* Diisopropylfluorophosphate
DHAP; *see* Dihydroxyacetone phosphate
2,3-DHB; *see* 2,3-Dihydrobenzoic acid
Diabetes insipidus, 664, 667, 668, 670
Diabetes mellitus
 chemotaxis and, 534
 glucose-6-phosphate dehydrogenase deficiency and, 357, 361
 maternal, 10, 818
 platelets and, 458
 thalassemia and, 438
 thrombotic disorders and, 816
Diagnosis; *see also* Differential diagnosis
 of ABO hemolytic disease of newborn, 280
 anemias and, 93-105
   iron-deficiency, 152-154
 of asplenia, 100
 of disseminated intravascular coagulation, 805
 of fetal-maternal hemorrhage, 127
 of folic acid deficiency, 201-202
 hemophilia and, 777
 of Hodgkin's disease, 628

Erythrocytes—cont'd
  membrane defects of; *see* Membrane defects
  membranes of
    antigen of, alteration in, 227
    binding of immunoglobulin to, 260, 262, 265, 266-268
    biochemistry of, 287-294, 307-308
    failure of, 294; *see also* Membrane defects
    function of, 292-293
    infective agent and, 261-262
    ion transport in, chronic disorders and, 454
    in newborn and premature infants, 12
    sensitivity to, 747-748
  metabolism of, 313-328
    acetylcholinesterase and, 327
    adenine and pyridine nucleotide metabolism and, 325-326
    adenosine triphosphatase and, 326
    capacity and constituents of, 316
    carbonic anhydrase and, 326-327
    defects of; *see* Metabolic defects
    developmental aspects of, 314-316
    galactose pathway and, 326
    glutathione metabolism and, 325
    glycolysis and Embden-Meyerhof pathway in, 316-324; *see also* Embden-Meyerhof pathway
    hexose monophosphate shunt in, 324-325; *see also* Hexose monophosphate shunt
    history and, 313-314
    iron-deficiency anemia and, 140-141
    polyol pathway in, 326
    superoxide dismutase and, 327-328
  in newborn, 11-13, 14, 100
  nucleated, 14, 42, 255, 264, 416, 435
  packed, volume of; *see* Hematocrits
  phase contrast microscopy and, 29-30
  placental transfusion and, 10
  pocked, 100
  polychromatophilic, 99
  primitive, 22
  production of; *see* Erythropoiesis
  protoporphyrin in, 149-150
  size and shape abnormalities of, 96-99
  staining abnormalities and, 99-100
  survival of, 226, 253-254, 330; *see also* Radiochromium; Radioiron
    beta-thalassemia and, 435
    in sensitized individual, 269
    vitamin B$_{12}$ deficiency and, 186
  transfusions of; *see* Transfusions, packed red cell
  utilization patterns and, 224
  vitamin B$_{12}$ deficiency and, 184
  volume of packed; *see* Hematocrit
Erythroid aplasia, 234, 421
Erythroid burst forming unit, 214
Erythroid cells, 14, 157, 314, 315; *see also* Erythroid hyperplasia; Myeloid:erythroid ratio
Erythroid colony forming units, 214
  anemias and
    aplastic, 471, 474
    hypoplastic, 229
  erythropoietin and, 218
  lymphocyte suppressors of, 471, 474
Erythroid-committed precursors, 213
Erythroid hyperplasia, 254-255
  anemias and
    dyserythropoietic, 237
    iron-deficiency, 144
    sickle cell, 416
  hemolytic disease of newborn and, 274
  immune hemolysis and, 265
  in newborn, 5-6, 22
  paroxysmal nocturnal hemoglobinuria and, 304

Erythroid hypoplasia, 234
Erythroid leukemia; *see* Leukemias, erythroid
Erythroid marrow defects, 228-241, 435
Erythroid:myeloid cells; *see* Myeloid:erythroid ratio
Erythroid precursors, 213, 225
Erythrokinetics, 212-214, 222, 227-228; *see also* Ferrokinetics; Kinetics
Erythroleukemia; *see* Leukemias, erythroid
Erythromycin, 607
Erythron, 212-214
Erythrophagocytosis, 265, 274, 665
Erythropoiesis, 23, 212-228; *see also* Anemias, hypoplastic anemias and; *see* Anemias
  beta-thalassemia and, 435
  cellular kinetics of, 212-214
  disorders of, 228-241
    anemias and
      dyserythropoietic, 234-241
      hypoplastic, 228-234
    chronic, 452-453, 454-455
    erythroid marrow defects in, 228-241
  dyserythropoiesis and, 222, 234-241
  ectopic, 226
  erythropoietin and, 216-220; *see also* Erythropoietin
  extramedullary, 226
  fetal, 13, 122, 220-221
  folate and, 191, 196
  hemolytic disease of newborn and, 273
  increase in, 4, 254
  laboratory evaluation of, 222-228
  liver and, 3-4
  microenvironment in, 214-215
  neonatal, 5-6, 221-222
    cessation of, 5-6, 122
  oxygen delivery and, 215-216
  spherocytosis and, 295
  transfusions and, 77, 79-80
  viral infections and, 255
  vitamin B$_{12}$ deficiency and, 186
Erythropoiesis-inhibiting factor, 221
Erythropoietic protoporphyria, 150
Erythropoietin, 216-220
  anemias and
    aplastic, 471
    chronic disorders and, 452, 455
    iron-deficiency, 144
  assays of, 216, 227
  fetus and, 6, 122
  after iron therapy, 157
  kidneys and, 454-455
  in newborn, 122
  nonhematologic conditions with increased, 220
  serum, venous hemoglobin and, 227
Erythropoietin-responsive cells, 213, 218
Erythropoietin-sensitive cells, 213
Erythrose-4-phosphate, 313, 323
Erythrostasis, 649
Escherichia coli
  glucose-6-phosphate dehydrogenase deficiency and, 548
  leukemias and, 605, 608
  marrow transplants and, 483
  myeloperoxidase deficiency and, 548
  neutropenia and, 503, 504
  neutrophilia and, 513
  opsonization disorders and, 535
  protein-calorie malnutrition and, 549
  trapping of, by liver and spleen, 650
ESCs; *see* Erythropoietin-sensitive cells
Esophageal varices, 653-654, 655
Esophageal webs, 134

Hepatitis—cont'd
  glucose-6-phosphate dehydrogenase deficiency and, 357, 360, 361
  hemophilia therapy and, 789
  kernicterus and, 273
  leukemias and, 605, 608
  lymphocytes and, 576
  rubella and, 734
  transfusions and, 77-79
    factor replacement therapy in, 696, 781-782
    platelet, 72
  vitamin B$_{12}$ and, 177
Hepatitis A antigen, 79
Hepatitis B core antigen, 78
Hepatitis B surface antigen, 78-79
Hepatitis C, 79
Hepatocellular disease, 149; *see also* Liver
Hepatomas, 177, 220, 257
Hepatomegaly
  beta-thalassemia and, 437
  granulomatous disease and, 545
  Hodgkin's disease and, 624
  infectious mononucleosis and, 574
  leukemias and, 594, 596, 598, 600
  reticuloendothelial system disorders and; *see* Reticuloendothelial system, diseases of
  sickle cell anemia and, 414-415
  Wiskott-Aldrich syndrome and, 569
Hereditary elliptocytosis; *see* Elliptocytosis
Hereditary persistence of fetal hemoglobin, 408, 410, 424, 447
Hereditary pyropoikilocytosis, 297, 301, 310
Hereditary spherocytosis; *see* Spherocytosis
Hereditary stomatocytosis, 299-301, 310
Hermansky-Pudlak syndrome, 539, 739
Herpesvirus
  leukemias and, 592, 605, 608
  lymphocytes and, 576
  lymphomas and, 631
  marrow transplants and, 483
  neutrophilia and, 513
  thrombocytopenias and, 42
    neonatal, 74, 735
  Wiskott-Aldrich syndrome and, 569
Heterophil agglutination, 574-575, 580
Heterophil antibodies, 572, 574-575
Heterophil-negative mononucleosis syndromes, 575-576
Hexachlorobenzene, 257
Hexadimethrine bromide, 266
Hexokinase
  deficiency of, 330, 331-333
    autohemolysis in, 329
  iron-deficiency anemia and, 140
  leukocyte, 486
Hexokinase-phosphofructokinase system, 319-320
Hexose monophosphate shunt, 324-325
  defects of, 330, 348-362
    gamma-glutamyl-cysteine synthetase deficiency in, 348
    glucose-6-phosphate dehydrogenase deficiency in; *see* Glucose-6-phosphate dehydrogenase, deficiency of
    glutathione peroxidase deficiency in, 349-351
    glutathione reductase deficiency in, 348-349
    glutathione synthetase deficiency in, 348
    6-phosphogluconic dehydrogenase deficiency in, 361-362
  discovery of, 314
  evaluation of, 329
  phagocytosis and, 530, 531
HGPRT; *see* Hypoxanthine-guanine phosphoribosyltransferase
H/h blood group, 58
H/h gene systems, 59
Histamine
  basophils and, 25, 518

Histamine—cont'd
  eosinophils and, 514
  erythropoietin and, 219, 220
  inflammation and, 527
  intrinsic factor and, 176
  stimulation tests and, 187
  in tissue mast cells, 27
Histidine, 112, 200
Histiocytes, 26-27, 101; *see also* Macrophages
  dyserythropoietic anemia and, 237
  foamy, 27
  pigmented lipid, 543, 547
  in sea-blue histiocyte syndrome, 660
  sheets of, 669
Histiocytic medullary reticulosis, 665
Histiocytoma, 664
  giant cell, 665-666
Histiocytosis X and other monocyte-macrophage disorders, 663-671
  eosinophilia and, 517
  leukemias and, 600
  neonatal thrombocytopenia and, 37
  Wiskott-Aldrich syndrome and, 728
Histocompatibility antigens, 64-66, 73, 74, 76, 479-484
  unrelated donors and, 476
Histoplasmosis, 607, 608, 631
HK deficiency; *see* Hexokinase, deficiency of
HK-PFK system; *see* Hexokinase-phosphofructokinase system
HLA antigens; *see* Histocompatibility antigens
Hodgkin's disease, 620-631
  eosinophilia and, 517
  immunology and, 262, 623
  serum ferritin and, 149
  thrombocytopenic purpura and, 718
Holly leaf configuration, 408
Home care programs, 788-789
Homocysteine, 174
Homocystinuria, 815-816
  pyridoxine and, 197-198
  storage pool defects and, 739
  vitamin B$_{12}$ and, 183, 184
Homologous blood syndrome, 81
Hookworm, 130, 515-516
Hormones; *see also* specific hormone
  erythropoietin and, 219-220
  renal failure and, 455
Horned cell, 98-99
Hot-cross bun appearance, 435
Hot spots, 474
Howell-Jolly bodies, 99
  sickle cell anemia and, 415, 416
  spleen and, 649
    congenital absence of, 655
  vitamin B$_{12}$ deficiency and, 184, 185
Howell plasma recalcification time, 685
Hp; *see* Haptoglobin
HSP; *see* Henoch-Schönlein purpura
Humafac; *see* Factor VIII, concentrates of
Human growth hormone, 360
Human placental lactogenic hormone, 219, 220
Humoral inhibitors of hematopoiesis, 471
Humoral mediators of inflammation, 526-528
  deficiencies of, 471
Hunter's syndrome, 663
Hurler's syndrome, 662-663
Hurler variant, 662
HUS; *see* Hemolytic-uremic syndrome
Hyaline thrombi, 724-725
Hybridization, hemoglobin, 389
Hydantoins, 466, 468; *see also* Phenytoin
Hydatid disease, 516

Prednisone
  anemias and
    aplastic, 478
    hypoplastic, 230, 231
    pure red cell, 233
  Chediak-Higashi syndrome and, 543
  2,3-diphosphoglycerate mutase deficiency and, 339
  granulocyte count and, 511
  in hemophilia, 783, 784, 785
  Henoch-Schönlein purpura and, 746
  histiocytic diseases and, 670
  Hodgkin's disease and, 630
  immune hemolysis and, 269
  infectious mononucleosis and, 575
  maintenance therapy with, 613
  myelogenous leukemia and, 617
  as non–cell cycle–specific drug, 611
  non-Hodgkin's lymphoma and, 635
  paroxysmal nocturnal hemoglobinuria and, 306
  potency and dosage of, 714
  purpura and, 732, 733, 748
  with radiation, toxicity of, 615
  remission induction by, 589, 609, 612, 613, 616
  in thrombocytopenias, 38, 714-715, 716, 732, 733
  transfusion reactions and, 81
Pregnancy
  anemias and
    aplastic, 465, 469-470
    sickle cell, 422
  folic acid and, 190, 195-196
  iron supplements in, 120
  teenage, 125
  vitamin B_{12} and, 177
Prekallikrein, 767-768
  deficiency of, 781, 800, 813
Preleukemic syndrome, 335, 592, 737
Prematurity
  anemias and
    blood smears and, 96
    physiologic, 6
  blood and, 10, 13-14, 118
  bone marrow differential counts in, 14
  carbonic anhydrase and, 327
  coagulation in, 8, 688-689, 813
  cord clamping and, 11
  erythrocytes and, 12
    glucose in, 12, 13
    pocked, 100
  erythropoiesis and, 221-222
  exchange transfusion and, 279
  folic acid and, 191, 192, 195
  glutathione peroxidase deficiency and, 350
  granulocytes in, 14
  hemoglobin-oxygen interactions and, 386
  hemorrhage in, 8
  immunoglobulins and, 562
  iron deficit in, 118
  iron supplements and, 155, 160-162
  leukocytes in, 14, 43
  lymphocytes in, 14
  platelets in, 14, 36, 706
  thrombotic disorders and, 818
  vitamin B_{12} and, 178
  vitamin E and, 303
Priapism, 414, 594, 596
Prilocaine, 43, 44
Primaquine
  Heinz bodies and, 100
  sensitivity to, 351, 352, 355-356
Primidone, 198, 814
Primitive cells, 22, 196
Probenecid, 352

Procaine, 20, 291
Procaine amide, 352, 509
Procarbazine, 471, 479, 481, 508, 630
Prochlorperazine, 419, 605
PRO-Ep; *see* Proerythropoietin
Proerythroblast, 23; *see* Pronormoblasts
Proerythropoietin, 217
Profilate; *see* Factor VIII, concentrates of
Progenitor cells, 212, 213
Progesterone, 438, 816
Prolactin, 219, 220
Proliferating differentiated cells, 212, 213-214
Proline, 435
Prolymphocytes, 26
Promazine, 509
Promegakaryocytes, 26
Promethazine
  marrow aspiration and, 20
  to mother, 43, 44, 814
  platelet function and, 605, 706
  thrombocytopathy and, 736
Promonocytes, 25, 500
Promyelocytes, 23-24
  in infancy and childhood, 15
  malignant, 590
  morphology of, 497, 498
  peroxidase staining and, 29
  in premature infants, 14
Pronormoblasts, 23
  erythropoiesis and, 213
  giant, 233
  in infancy and childhood, 15
  in premature infants, 14
  vacuolization of, 467
  vitamin B_{12} deficiency and, 185
Properdin, 529, 650
Propionate, 174-175
Proplex; *see* Prothrombin complex concentrates
Propoxyphene, 788
Propranolol, 220, 438, 500, 509
Propylthiouracil, 466
Prostaglandins
  aspirin thrombocytopathy and, 736
  erythropoietin and, 219, 220
  inflammatory mediators and, 527
  leukemias and, 604
  marrow function and, 471
  platelet aggregation and, 704
Prosthetic heart valves, 816
Protamine sulfate, 70, 687, 818
Protein-calorie malnutrition, 234, 549
Proteinase, 314
Proteins
  cationic, 531
  chloramphenicol and, 467
  dysproteinemias and, 71, 810
  in heme, 108, 251
  hypoproteinemia and, 129, 273
  induced by vitamin K absence, 798, 803
  as inhibitors of respiration, 314
  iron deficiency and, 142
  membrane, 287-288
    elliptocytosis and, 298
    spherocytosis and, 297
  serum, 668, 671
  synthesis of, 433, 434
  transmembrane, 288, 289
  transport, 251
  vitamin B_{12}–binding, 177
  X, 273
  Y and Z, 252, 273, 275
Proteinuria, 181

Thalassemias—cont'd
  silent carrier of beta-thalassemia and, 444
  thalassemia intermedia in, 45, 104, 442
  thalassemia major or beta-thalassemia in, 431-442
    anemias and
      dyserythropoietic, 241
      iron-deficiency, 143, 151, 154
    blood smears and, 97, 143
    cobalt excretion and, 150
    erythroblastopenia and, 234
    erythroid leukemia and, 590
    erythropoiesis and, 222
    ferrokinetics and, 117
    folate deficiency and, 196
    hemoglobin S and, 411, 424-425
    heterozygous, 45
    osseous changes and, 104, 254
    serum ferritin and, 149
    silent carrier of, 444
    thrombocytopenia and, 726
    transfusion-dependent, 45
    transfusions and, 79, 80, 234
  thalassemia minor or thalassemia trait in, 442-443
    blood smears and, 97
    diagnosis of, 444
    glucose-6-phosphate dehydrogenase deficiency and, 353
    iron-deficiency anemia and, 150, 154
    pyropoikilocytosis and, 301
    skeletal changes and, 104
    stomatocytes and, 301
Thiabendazole, 516
Thiamine, 173, 203
Thiamizole; *see* Methimazole
Thiamphenicol, 468
Thiazide diuretics; *see* Diuretics, thiazide
Thiazolsulfone, 352
Thiocyanate, 466, 509
Thioglycolic acid, 509
Thioguanine
  as cell cycle–specific drug, 610
  megaloblastic anemias and, 174, 204
  myelogenous leukemia and, 616
  neutropenia and, 508
  remission induction and, 615, 616
Thio-TEPA, 220
Thiouracil, 43, 508, 509
Thompson-Nelson-Grobelney syndrome, 663
Thorazine; *see* Chlorpromazine
Thorotrast, 509
Thrombasthenia; *see* Glanzmann's disease
Thrombi, hyaline, 724-725; *see also* Thromboses
Thrombin, 765
  discovery of, 679, 762
  excessive generation of, 806
  fibrinogen degradation products and, 687
  inhibition of; *see* Antithrombin III
  platelet aggregation and, 703-705
Thrombin clotting time, 684-685
  disseminated intravascular coagulation and, 805
  dysfibrinogenemias and, 795
  in newborn, 689
Thrombocytopathies
  acquired, 736-737, 809
  Ehlers-Danlos syndrome and, 750
  inherited, 737-740
    with systemic disease, 739
Thrombocytopenias; *see also* Platelets; Thrombocytopenic purpuras
  with absent radii syndrome, 36, 726-727, 734
    aplastic anemia and, 487
    storage pool defects and, 739
  alcoholism and, 198

Thrombocytopenias—cont'd
  anemias and
    aplastic, 472, 475, 477, 485
    iron-deficiency, 144
  Chediak-Higashi syndrome and, 539
  chronic disorders and, 457-459
  congenital heart disease and, 809
  cyclic, 726
  from decreased production and increased destruction, 42
  disseminated intravascular coagulation and, 803
  folic acid deficiency and, 199
  hemangioma and, 41, 750
  hypoplastic, 725-726
  immune, 37-41, 264, 565, 733
  infectious mononucleosis and, 575
  inherited, 37
  leukemias and, 595, 596, 605
  liver disease and, 808
  from maternal autoantibodies, 733
  with maternal drug-induced purpura, 41
  myeloid metaplasia and, 599
  neonatal; *see* Newborn, thrombocytopenias of
  neutropenias with phenotypic abnormalities and, 507
  reticuloendothelioses and, 657, 660, 668
  splenomegaly and, 652
  transfusions and, 71-75, 279
  Wiskott-Aldrich syndrome and, 569, 570
Thrombocytopenic purpuras; *see also* Thrombocytopenias
  acquired, 707-726
    abnormal platelet distribution in, 726
    autoimmune diseases in, 717-718
    cyclic, 726
    decreased or ineffective platelet production in, 725
    hypoplastic, 725-726
    immunologic drug sensitivity in, 718
    infections and, 719
    massive transfusion and, 719
    microangiopathic diseases in, 719-725
    posttransfusion purpura in, 718-719
  giant hemangioma with, 805
  idiopathic, 707-717; *see also* Idiopathic thrombocytopenic purpura
  increased platelet destruction or loss in, 707-719
  inherited, 726-730
  leukemias and, 599, 600
  neonatal; *see* Newborn, thrombocytopenias of
  rubella and, 734-735
  thrombotic, 721, 724-725
  vitamin K deficiency and, 802
Thrombocytosis, 750-751
  chronic disorders and, 458
  iron-deficiency anemia and, 144
  reactive or secondary, 750
  after splenectomy, 439, 649, 716, 750
Thromboplastin
  discovery of, 679, 681
  tissue, 680, 681, 765
Thromboplastin generation test, 681, 683, 684, 778
Thromboplastin time, partial; *see* Partial thromboplastin time
Thrombopoietin deficiency, 727-728
Thromboses; *see also* Thrombotic disorders
  antithrombin III deficiency and, 815
  cardiac, 734
  catheters and, 816, 818
  hemophilia therapy and, 789
  paroxysmal nocturnal hemoglobinuria and, 304, 306
Thrombosthenin, 701, 702, 705
Thrombotest, 793, 794
Thrombotic disorders, 762, 815-818
  neonatal, 734, 818

Thrombotic thrombocytopenic purpura, 724-725
  hemolytic-uremic syndrome and, 721
Thromboxanes, 527
Thrush, 567
Thumb
  absence of, 485
  triphalangeal, 487
Thymectomy, 233, 270
Thymic hypoplasia, congenital, 566-567
Thymidine, ^{3}H-labeled, 601
Thymoma, 232, 262, 456
Thymus transplantation, 567, 572
Thyroid hormone
  anemia and, 456
  anticoagulants and, 817
  2,3-diphosphoglycerate mutase deficiency and, 339
  erythropoietin and, 220
  glucose-6-phosphate dehydrogenase deficiency and, 360
Thyrotoxicosis, 327, 518, 735
Thyrotropic hormone, 518
Thyroxin, 518
TIBC; *see* Total iron-binding capacity
Tiselius' moving boundary method, 388
Tissue basophils, 27
Tissue cell antigens, 64-66
Tissue-derived inflammatory mediators, 527
Tissue eosinophilia, 514
Tissue iron, 115, 118, 145
Tissue macrophages, 500
Tissue mast cells, 27
Tissue thromboplastin, 680, 681, 765
Tocopherol, 161, 173, 303, 441, 537; *see also* Vitamins, E
Tolbutamide, 43, 233, 466, 509, 734
Toluidine blue, 352
Tomography, computerized axial, 627, 633, 777
TORCH syndromes, 42
Total body irradiation, 469, 479, 483
Total hemoglobin mass at birth, 118
Total iron-binding capacity, 114, 146, 452, 453
Total iron-binding transferrin, 546
Total nodal radiotherapy, 630
Toxins
  anemias and
    aplastic, 466-469
    hypoplastic, 233
    pure red cell, 233
  glucose-6-phosphate dehydrogenase deficiency and, 360
  glutathione peroxidase deficiency and, 350
  methemoglobinemia and, 365-366
  neutropenia and, 509
Toxocara canis and *cati,* 515, 516
Toxoplasmosis
  acquired, 576
  Chediak-Higashi syndrome and, 539
  histiocytic diseases and, 667
  leukemia and, 607, 608
  lymphomas and, 631
  thrombocytopenias and, 42, 74, 735
  transfusions and, 77
TPI deficiency; *see* Triose phosphate isomerase deficiency
Tracheal obstruction, 636
Tranexamic acid, 696, 788
Transcobalamin I, 176-177, 182-183, 596
Transcobalamin II, 177, 182, 188
Transcription, 22
Transfer factor, 567, 570, 572, 729
Transfer RNA, 22
Transferrin
  absence of, 162
  biochemistry of, 108, 109, 110
  in fetus, 120
  function of, 113-114, 120

Transferrin—cont'd
  gastroferrin and, 113
  infection and, 139
  in plasma, 114
  saturation of, 144, 145
  serum, 162, 549
  spleen and, 650
  synthesis of, 109, 114
Transfusion-dependent thalassemia major, 45
Transfusion hemosiderosis, 147
Transfusions
  anemias and, 105
    aplastic, 476-477
    hypoplastic, 231-232
    iron-deficiency, 158, 162
    multiple transfusions in, 234
    physiologic, of newborn, 7
    sickle cell, 408, 414, 418, 419, 421, 422
  blood
    calculations of volume for, 68-69
    coagulation inhibitors and, 811
    disseminated intravascular coagulation and, 807
    hemolytic-uremic syndrome and, 724
    iron-deficiency anemia and, 158
    irradiated, 81
    paroxysmal nocturnal hemoglobinuria and, 304
    rubella and, 735
    thrombocytopenias and, 714, 733
  blood components in, 66-81, 83-87, 694, 695
    erythrocytes in; *see* Transfusions, packed red cell
    granulocytes in, 75-77, 85-86
      aplastic anemia and, 477
      Chediak-Higashi syndrome and, 543
      granulomatous disease and, 547
      isoimmune neonatal neutropenia and, 43
    platelets in; *see* Platelets, transfusions of
  coagulation factors and; *see* Factor replacement therapy
  elliptocytosis and, 299
  esophageal bleeding and, 655
  exchange; *see* Exchange transfusions
  fetal-maternal; *see* Fetal-maternal transfusion
  folate level and, 200
  Glanzmann's disease and, 738
  glucose-6-phosphate dehydrogenase deficiency and, 355, 357, 361
  glucose phosphate isomerase deficiency and, 333, 334
  hemochromatosis syndrome and, 230
  hemolytic-uremic syndrome and, 158, 724
  hemophilia and, 780, 781-783
  hexokinase deficiency and, 333
  home, 789
  isoimmune neonatal thrombocytopenic purpura and, 43, 732-733
  leukemias and, 603, 605, 606, 616
  limitations and hazards of, 77-81, 86-87
  marrow transplant rejections and, 482
  maternal-fetal, 11, 35-36, 119; *see also* Maternal-fetal interactions
  maternal hemoglobinopathies and, 44, 45
  multiple
    alloimmunization and, 73
    anemia from 234
    erythropoiesis suppression and, 79-80
    erythropoietin and, 218
    hemophilia and, 776
    reactions to, 80-81
  neutropenia and, 512
  packed red cell, 67-71, 83-84
    adenosine deaminase increase and, 346
    anemias and
      aplastic, 476-477
      iron-deficiency, 158